Danforth's

Obstetrics and Gynecology

Editors

James R. Scott, M.D.

H.A. and Edna Benning Presidential Professor
Department of Obstetrics and Gynecology
University of Utah School of Medicine
Salt Lake City, Utah

Philip J. Di Saia, M.D.

The Dorothy Marsh Chair in Reproductive Biology
Professor, Department of Obstetrics and Gynecology
University of California at Irvine College of Medicine
Orange, California

Charles B. Hammond, M.D.

E.C. Hamblen Professor and Chairman
Department of Obstetrics and Gynecology
Duke University School of Medicine
Durham, North Carolina

William N. Spellacy, M.D.

Professor and Chairman
Department of Obstetrics and Gynecology
University of South Florida College of Medicine
Tampa, Florida

Danforth's
Obstetrics and Gynecology

Eighth Edition

With 61 Contributors
685 Illustrations

Illustrations by
Jennifer Smith, medical illustrator

LIPPINCOTT WILLIAMS & WILKINS
A **Wolters Kluwer** Company
Philadelphia · Baltimore · New York · London
Buenos Aires · Hong Kong · Sydney · Tokyo

Acquisitions Editor: Lisa McAllister
Managing Editor: Susan Rhyner
Manufacturing Manager: Tim Reynolds
Production Manager: Liane Carita
Production Editor: Tony DeGeorge
Cover Designer: Parallelogram
Indexer: Kathy Unger
Compositor: Circle Graphics
Printer: World Color

Printed in the United States of America

9 8 7 6 5 4 3 2 1

Library of Congress Cataloging-in-Publication Data

Danforth's obstetrics and gynecology. — 8th ed. / with 61
   contributors ; Jennifer Smith, illustrator ; [editors, James R.
  Scott . . . [et al.]
      p.   cm.
   Includes bibliographical references and index.
   ISBN 0-7817-1206-8 (alk. paper)
   1. Gynecology—Handbooks, manuals, etc. 2. Obstetrics—Handbooks,
manuals, etc. I. Danforth, David N., 1912– . II. Scott, James
R., 1937– .
   [DNLM: 1. Obstetrics. 2. Genital Diseases, Female. WQ 100D1812
1999]
RG110.D36   1999
618—dc21
DNLM/DLC
for Library of Congress   98-37809
                                            CIP

Contents

——— ◇ ———

Contributors

———— ◇ ————

Marc A. Bernhisel, M.D.
Clinical Assistant Professor
Department of Obstetrics and Gynecology
University of South Florida College of Medicine
Tampa, Florida

Patricia S. Braly, M.D.
Professor and Chief
Section of Gynecologic Oncology
Louisiana State University Medical Center
New Orleans, Louisiana

D. Ware Branch, M.D.
Professor of Maternal-Fetal Medicine
Department of Obstetrics and Gynecology
University of Utah School of Medicine
Salt Lake City, Utah

Robert E. Bristow
Professor
Division of Gynecologic Oncology
Johns Hopkins Medical Institute
Baltimore, Maryland

John R. Brumsted, M.D.
Professor
Department of Obstetrics and Gynecology—
  Reproductive Endocrinology and Infertility
University of Vermont College of Medicine;
Attending Physician
Fletcher Allen Health Care
Burlington, Vermont

Sandra A. Carson, M.D.
Associate Professor and Medical Director
Baylor Assisted Reproductive Technology
Baylor College of Medicine
Houston, Texas

Frank A. Chervenak, M.D.
Professor and Vice Chairman
Department of Obstetrics and Gynecology
The New York Hospital-Cornell Medical Center
New York, New York

Ronald A. Chez, M.D.
Professor of Obstetrics and Gynecology
Professor of Family and Community Health
University of South Florida College of Medicine
Tampa, Florida

Steven L. Clark, M.D.
Professor
Department of Obstetrics and Gynecology
University of Utah School of Medicine
Salt Lake City, Utah

Grace M. Couchman, M.D.
Assistant Professor
Division of Reproductive Endocrinology and
  Infertility
Fertility Clinic
Duke South Hospital
Duke University Medical Center
Durham, North Carolina

Catherine Craven, M.D.
Associate Professor
Department of Obstetrics and Gynecology
University of Utah School of Medicine
Salt Lake City, Utah

Dwight P. Cruikshank, M.D.
Professor and Chairman
Department of Obstetrics and Gynecology
Medical College of Wisconsin
Milwaukee, Wisconsin

Tomas Debrigard, M.D.
Assistant Professor
University of South Florida College of Medicine;
Staff Neonatologist
Tampa General Hospital
Tampa, Florida

John O. L. DeLancey, M.D.
Norman F. Miller Professor
Department of Obstetrics and Gynecology
University of Michigan Health Systems
Ann Arbor, Michigan

Vivian M. Dickerson, M.D.
Associate Clinical Professor
Department of Obstetrics and Gynecology
University of California, Irvine
Orange, California

Philip J. Di Saia, M.D.
The Dorothy J. Marsh Chair in Reproductive
  Biology
Professor of Obstetrics and Gynecology
University of California, Irvine Medical Center
Orange, California

Donald J. Dudley, M.D.
Associate Professor
Department of Obstetrics and Gynecology
University of Utah School of Medicine
Salt Lake City, Utah

David A. Eschenbach, M.D.
Professor
Department of Obstetrics and Gynecology
University of Washington Medical Center
Seattle, Washington

Pamela F. Farrington, M.D.
Assistant Professor
Department of Obstetrics and Gynecology
University of Utah School of Medicine
Salt Lake City, Utah

James V. Fiorica, M.D.
Professor and Chief
Gynecologic Oncology Program
University of South Florida College of Medicine
H. Lee Moffitt Cancer Center
Tampa, Florida

John I. Fishburne, Jr., M.D.
Professor and Chair of Clinical Obstetrics and
  Gynecology
University of Arizona
Maricopa Medical Center
Phoenix, Arizona

Arthur C. Fleischer, M.D.
Professor
Departments of Radiology and Obstetrics and
  Gynecology
Vanderbilt University Medical College
Nashville, Tennessee

Michael A. Gold, M.D.
Clinical Instructor
Department of Obstetrics and Gynecology
University of Oklahoma Health Sciences Center
Oklahoma City, Oklahoma

Charles B. Hammond, M.D.
E. C. Hamblen Professor and Chairman
Department of Obstetrics and Gynecology
Duke University Medical Center
Durham, North Carolina

R. Brian Haynes, M.D., Ph.D.
Professor
Department of Medicine—Clinical Epidemiology
  and Biostatistics
McMaster University Faculty of Health Sciences
Hamilton, Ontario, Canada

Paula J. Adams Hillard, M.D.
Professor
Departments of Obstetrics and Gynecology and
  Pediatrics
University of Cincinnati
Cincinnati, Ohio

Janine K. Jensen, M.D.
Assistant Professor
Department of Obstetrics and Gynecology
University of California, Irvine
Orange, California

Joan G. Jones
Professor and Deputy Director
Department of Anatomical Pathology
Albert Einstein College of Medicine
Bronx, New York

Beth Y. Karlan, M.D.
Director, Gynecologic Oncology
Cedars Sinai Medical Center
Los Angeles, California;
Associate Professor Obstetrics and Gynecology
University of California at Los Angeles School of
  Medicine

William R. Keye, Jr., M.D.
Director
Division of Reproductive Endocrinology and
  Infertility
Beaumont Medical Services
Royal Oak, Michigan

Dennis Yi-Shin Kuo, M.D.
Clinical Assistant Professor
Department of Obstetrics and Gynecology
Cornell Medical College;
New York Hospital Medical Center of Queens
The New York Flushing Hospital Medical Center
Flushing, New York

Maureen P. Malee, M.D., Ph.D.
Assistant Professor
Department of Obstetrics and Gynecology
Brown University School of Medicine
Women and Infants Hospital
Providence, Rhode Island

Byron J. Masterson, M.D.
The J. Wayne Reitz Professor of Gynecologic
  Surgery
University of Florida College of Medicine
Gainesville, Florida

Laurence B. McCullough, Ph.D.
Professor
Center for Medical Ethics and Health Policy
Baylor College of Medicine
Houston, Texas;
Adjunct Professor of Ethics in Obstetrics and
  Gynecology
Cornell University Medical College
New York, New York

Susan F. Meikle, M.D., M.S.P.H.
Division of Reproductive Health
National Center for Chronic Disease Prevention
  and Health Promotion
Centers for Disease Control and Prevention
Atlanta, Georgia

David A. Miller, M.D.
Assistant Professor
Department of Obstetrics and Gynecology
University of Southern California School of Medicine
Women's and Children's Hospital
Los Angeles, California

Howard L. Minkoff, M.D.
Professor
Department of Obstetrics and Gynecology
SUNY Health Science Center at Brooklyn
Brooklyn, New York

Robert M. Nelson, Jr., M.D., M.S.
Professor and Chief
Division of Neonatology
University of South Florida College of Medicine
Tampa General Hospital
Tampa, Florida

Jennifer R. Niebyl, M.D.
Professor and Head
Department of Obstetrics and Gynecology
University of Iowa College of Medicine
University of Iowa Hospitals and Clinics
Iowa City, Iowa

Thomas E. Nolan, M.D.
Professor
Department of Obstetrics and Gynecology
Louisiana State University Medical Center
New Orleans, Louisiana

Donald R. Ostergard, M.D.
Professor of Obstetrics and Gynecology
University of California, Irvine
Director, Division of Urogynecology;
Associate Medical Director for Gynecology
Women's Hospital
Long Beach Memorial Medical Center
Long Beach, California

Michael T. Parsons, M.D., M.B.A.
Professor
Department of Obstetrics and Gynecology
University of South Florida College of Medicine
Tampa, Florida

Richard Paul, M.D.
Chief
Maternal–Fetal Medicine
Department of Obstetrics and Gynecology
University of Southern California School of Medicine
Los Angeles, California

Herbert B. Peterson, M.D.
Chief, Women's Health and Fertility Branch
  Centers for Disease Control and Prevention;
Clinical Professor
Department of Gynecology and Obstetrics
Emory University School of Medicine
Atlanta, Georgia

Margareta D. Pisarska, M.D.
Division of Reproductive Endocrinology and
  Infertility
Department of Obstetrics and Gynecology
Baylor College of Medicine
Houston, Texas

T. Flint Porter, M.D.
Assistant Professor
Department of Obstetrics and Gynecology
University of Utah Medical Center
Salt Lake City, Utah

Daniel H. Riddick, M.D., Ph.D.
Professor
Department of Obstetrics and Gynecology
University of Vermont College of Medicine
Burlington, Vermont

Carolyn D. Runowicz, M.D.
Professor and Director
Division of Gynecologic Oncology
Department of Obstetrics and Gynecology and
*   Women's Health*
Albert Einstein College of Medicine and
*   Montefiore Medical Center*
Bronx, New York

Robert S. Schenken, M.D.
Professor and Frank Harrison Chair in
*   Reproductive Endocrinology*
Department of Obstetrics and Gynecology
The University of Texas Health Sciences Center at
*   San Antonio*
San Antonio, Texas

James R. Scott, M.D.
H.A. and Edna Benning Presidential Professor
Department of Obstetrics and Gynecology
University of Utah School of Medicine
Salt Lake City, Utah

Howard T. Sharp, M.D.
Assistant Professor
Department of Obstetrics and Gynecology
University of Utah School of Medicine
Salt Lake City, Utah

Roya Sohaey, M.D.
Adjunct Assistant Professor of Radiology
University of Utah Medical Center;
Co-Director of Women's Imaging
Grand Valley Radiology
Holland, Michigan

William N. Spellacy, M.D.
Professor and Chairman
Department of Obstetrics and Gynecology
University of South Florida College of Medicine
Tampa, Florida

Robert J. Stillman, M.D.
Clinical Professor
Department of Obstetrics and Gynecology
Georgetown University School of Medicine
Shady Grove Fertility Centers
Washington, D.C.

Irvin Strathman, M.D., F.R.C.S.C.
Assistant Professor
Department of Obstetrics and Gynecology
University of South Florida College of Medicine
Tampa, Florida

Carine I. Stromquist, M.D.
Assistant Professor
Division of Neonatology
University of South Florida College of Medicine
Tampa General Hospital
Tampa, Florida

Suzanne R. Trupin, M.D.
Clinical Professor and Head
Department of Obstetrics and Gynecology
University of Illinois College of Medicine at
*   Urbana—Champaign*
Champaign, Illinois

Joan L. Walker, M.D.
Associate Professor
University of Oklahoma
Oklahoma City, Oklahoma

Kenneth Ward, M.D.
Professor
Department of Obstetrics and Gynecology
University of Utah School of Medicine
Salt Lake City, Utah

Katharine D. Wenstrom, M.D.
Professor and Director
Division of Reproductive Genetics
Department of Obstetrics and Gynecology
University of Alabama at Birmingham School of
*   Medicine*
Birmingham, Alabama

Lance E. Wyble, M.D., M.P.H.
Assistant Professor
Division of Neonatology
University of South Florida College of Medicine
Tampa General Hospital
Tampa, Florida

Preface

⟡

For the past three decades, *Danforth's Obstetrics and Gynecology* has been widely recognized as a standard textbook for medical students, house officers, nurses, and practicing physicians. Previous editions have been translated into several languages and used worldwide. For many, the book has formed the basis of learning and reference in our specialty.

The continued and overwhelming proliferation of subspecialty books, journals, and electronic media has strengthened our view that there is a need (from both a practical and financial standpoint) to preserve this classic text that covers all of obstetrics and gynecology in one volume. It is perhaps now even more important with the current emphasis on primary care for women. However, the practice of obstetrics and gynecology is changing rapidly as we approach the 21st century. Today's physician must be knowledgeable about constantly expanding technology and also adapt to changing economic, social, and political realities.

The purpose of the eighth edition remains much the same as its predecessors. It is designed to cover the modern practice of obstetrics and gynecology as concisely and completely as possible and with maximum authority. We have updated and completely revised the book. Some chapters from the previous edition have been deleted or combined, and new chapters have been added to keep pace with current developments. Increased emphasis has been placed on an evidence-based approach to management, practice guidelines, and cost effectiveness. The co-editors have written or co-authored over one-third of the chapters. The others have been contributed by an elite group of experts chosen because of special expertise in their field. Lists of current references and recommended reading are again provided at the end of each chapter to aid the reader in exploring areas of special interest.

The handbook covering core topics introduced with the last edition has been extremely popular and useful. It is small enough to be carried by students and house staff to enhance the learning process and assist with immediate patient care. The handbook has also been revised and updated.

The editors gratefully acknowledge each of the contributing authors, as well as D. Ware Branch, M.D., for his help with manuscripts and T. Flint Porter, M.D., for his valuable assistance with statistical analysis and odds ratio graphs. We also thank Lisa McAllister and Susan Rhyner at Lippincott Williams & Wilkins and Ladan Hariri at University of California, Irvine for their astute editorial assistance, professionalism, invaluable support, and encouragement given freely during this effort.

James R. Scott, M.D.
Philip J. Di Saia, M.D.
Charles B. Hammond, M.D.
William N. Spellacy, M.D.

Color Plates

———— ◇ ————

Danforth's
Obstetrics
and
Gynecology

CHAPTER 1

Evidence-based Obstetrics and Gynecology

◇

Herbert B. Peterson
Susan F. Meikle
R. Brian Haynes

> The aim of medicine in the broadest sense is to provide for every human being from conception to death, the greatest fullness of health and length of life that is allowed by his genetic constitution and by the accidents of life.
>
> MACFARLANE BURNETT

> Excellent medical practice should be inspired by love and guided by science. Both are essential. If a clinician practices scientific medicine without compassion, he or she becomes an automaton. On the other hand, if a clinician is compassionate but unscientific, he or she may be as dangerous as a well-intended parent feeding chicken noodle soup to a child with meningitis. Evidence-based medicine is not only well-intended, it is well-directed.
>
> DAVID A. GRIMES

◇ RATIONALE FOR EVIDENCE-BASED MEDICINE

Silverman[1,2] chronicled a tragic but instructive story of how the goal of medicine to provide health can be thwarted despite the best of intentions. In 1942 to 1954, more than 10,000 children worldwide were blinded because of a relatively minor change in health care practice. In an effort to improve the survival of premature infants, clinicians exposed newborns to high concentrations of oxygen with the unintended but disastrous consequence of retrolental fibroplasia.

The practice of administering high concentrations of oxygen in the first few days of life was initiated largely on the basis of theoretical considerations and was promulgated in pediatric teaching and research centers. As stated by Silverman,[1] "the retrolental fibroplasia catastrophe would not have been extensive if pediatric leaders had insisted that scientific rules of evidence must be satisfied before any new technique in management of premature infants was used in teaching centers." Silverman[1] also cited cardiologist Eugene Braunwald, who likened the dissemination of medical techniques before proper evaluation "to a genie who has escaped from a bottle—it is virtually impossible to undo the confusion resulting from such unrestrained therapeutic exuberance." Once the use of high-concentration oxygen therapy for premature infants was established, stopping the practice took more than a decade of effort.[1]

The example cited has parallels throughout the history of medicine. The practice of medicine into the 16th century was based largely on the teachings of the Greek physician Galen (*c.* AD 129 to 200), whose pronouncements were embraced without apparent question for centuries.[2] The 17th century saw some questioning of the authority on which medical practice was based. A glimpse of the state of medicine at that time illustrates why such questioning was needed. As King Charles II of England lay dying in 1685, he was cared for by a dozen or more physicians who administered "an enema containing antimony, sacred bitters, rocksalt, mallow leaves, violets, beetroot, camomile flowers, fennel seed, linseed, cinnamon, cardamon seed, saffron, cochineal and aloes." When these measures did not succeed, the king's physicians forced "a mixture of Raleigh's antidote, pearl julep, and ammonia down his throat"[2].

Not until the 19th and 20th centuries, however, did the questioning of traditional medical authorities lead to major advances. A great leap forward occurred in 1865, when Claude Bernard, a French physiologist, described experimental reasoning in his text, *An Introduction to the Study of Experimental Medicine*. This was followed in 1937 with a classic text by A. Bradford Hill[3] describing the use of statistical methods for clinical research.

Randomized, controlled trials conducted in the early to mid-20th century clearly indicated the value of basing medical practice on observation and experiment. Perhaps the most dramatic example of randomized, controlled trials in that period was the United Kingdom Medical Research Council's trial of using streptomycin to treat tuberculosis. Streptomycin became available in 1946, but it was in short supply. The Medical Research Council used a portion of existing supplies to test the drug's effectiveness in treating tuberculosis; those patients receiving streptomycin had a clear survival advantage, compared to those treated with bed rest.

Once the value of scientific inquiry as the basis for clinical practice had been established, Cochrane[4] argued for an ongoing assessment of the effectiveness of available treatments and services, in part as a matter of social justice. He was concerned that the limited resources for health care in the U.K.'s National Health Service be efficiently used for effective treatments, thereby enhancing the likelihood that effective treatments would be more widely available. In his classic text, *Effectiveness and Efficiency: Random Reflections on Health Services,* published in 1971, Cochrane[4] outlined criteria for the evaluation of effectiveness and efficiency in clinical practice. His efforts, along with those of his colleagues at the U.K. Medical Research Council who had conducted early randomized, controlled trials, contributed heavily to what is today termed *evidenced-based medicine.*

The need for evidence-based medicine is as apparent in obstetrics and gynecology as it is in other disciplines. Our history includes bloodletting as standard treatment for eclampsia into the 20th century and the persistence of the practice of routine episiotomy to the present despite the lack of evidence supporting the practice.[5] The rapid incorporation of unproven technologies into widespread use has had a major effect on the practice of obstetrics and gynecology[5]. Conversely, some therapies, such as corticosteroid therapy for women at risk of giving birth prematurely, have been underused despite compelling evidence of their effectiveness.[6]

◊ PRACTICE OF EVIDENCE-BASED MEDICINE

Clinical epidemiologists at McMaster University participating in the Evidence-based Medicine Working Group defined evidence-based medicine as "the conscientious, explicit, and judicious use of current best evidence in making decisions about the care of individual patients."[7] The terms *conscientious* and *judicious* emphasize the need for individualized care. *Conscientious* use requires that evidence be applied consistently when individual circumstances warrant, and *judicious* use requires integration of clinical expertise and evidence to balance risks and benefits of tests and treatments for the individual—based on the individual's circumstance and preferences.[8] By this definition, evidence-based medicine is practiced when clinical expertise is integrated with the best available evidence from a systematic search of the relevant literature. The Working Group[9] further explained that evidence-based medicine "deemphasizes intuition, unsystematic clinical experience, and pathophysiologic rationale as

sufficient grounds for clinical decision-making and stresses the examination of evidence from clinical research."

For these reasons, frequent misinterpretations of evidence-based medicine are that it ignores clinical experience and intuition, does not incorporate an understanding of basic investigation and pathophysiology, and ignores clinical information obtained by history and physical examination. By contrast, as Sackett et al.[7] explained, "Good doctors use both individual clinical expertise and the best available external evidence, and neither alone is enough. Without clinical expertise, practice risks becoming tyrannized by evidence, for even excellent external evidence may be inapplicable to or inappropriate for an individual patient. Without current best evidence, practice risks becoming rapidly out of date to the detriment of patients."[7]

As also noted by Sackett et al.[7], evidence-based medicine is not "cookbook" medicine or "cost-cutting" medicine; nor is it restricted to evaluation of randomized trials and metaanalyses. Evidence-based medicine cannot be cookbook because it integrates clinical expertise, patient choice, and external evidence. Successful integration requires the individualization of therapy; the obstetrician-gynecologist must decide whether or not information obtained from relevant literature pertains to the individual patient, and the obstetrician-gynecologist and patient must determine which evidence-based therapeutic options are preferable.

Evidence-based medicine is not cost-cutting medicine because its focus is not on costs, but on effectiveness and efficiency. The most effective therapy for an individual may also be the most expensive therapy; thus, the practice of evidence-based medicine could lead to increased, not decreased, costs. Finally, evidence-based medicine uses proper randomized, controlled trials and well–conducted metaanalyses when available. However, the best available evidence in medicine, including obstetrics and gynecology, often comes from observational studies.[10]

Grimes[5] identified five barriers to technology assessment that apply to evidence-based medicine in general: (1) the unchallenged acceptance of authority, (2) the acceptance of new technology without critical appraisal, (3) the tendency to let existing dogma prevail, (4) pedantry in medical education, and (5) the practice of medicine by uncontrolled clinical impressions or "the last disaster we encountered or hear about."[5] The practice of evidence-based medicine places a low value on authority[9] and a high value on evidence in decision making about new medical therapies and technologies. New evidence on existing therapies or technologies is also highly valued. Evidence-based medicine discourages reliance on dogma and encourages medical education based not only on understanding of pathophysiology and the clinical insights of faculty but also on acquiring skills necessary to critically appraise evidence and integrate it with clinical expertise and an understanding of the mechanisms of disease. A key assumption of evidence-based medicine is that physicians who base their practice on evidence rather than on uncontrolled impression will provide their patients superior care.[9]

Debate continues about the extent to which new technologies or treatments should be assessed before being incorporated into practice and where the burden of proof for effectiveness should lie. Should promising new interventions be assumed to be effective until there is evidence they are not, or should they be assumed to be ineffective until there is evidence they are effective? Philosophically, the practitioner of evidence-based medicine will in most cases lean toward the latter approach.

◊ A MODEL FOR THE PRACTICE OF EVIDENCE-BASED MEDICINE

Haynes et al.[8] proposed a model for clinical decision making that integrates clinical expertise, research evidence, and patient preferences (Fig. 1). Depending on the circumstances, one component may play a greater role than others in decision making, but ideally all three components are brought into play. The clinical expertise component ensures that the best available evidence is applied to the individual clinical circumstance. It also precludes "the mindless application of rules and guidelines."[8]

The discussion of evidence-based medicine is incomplete without recognizing the existence of substantial gray zones in clinical practice.[11] As with other medical disciplines, the practice of obstetrics and gynecology includes some clinical questions that can be informed by compelling evidence and many others for which adequate evidence is lacking. As noted by Naylor,[11] "Evidence-based medicine offers little help in the many grey zones of practice where the evidence about risk-benefit ratios of competing clinical options is incomplete or contradictory. . . ." Alternatively, "What is black and white in the abstract may rapidly become grey in practice, as clinicians seek to meet their individual patients' needs." The latter circumstance is a gray zone potentially embraced by the model of evidence-based medicine presented here. Clinical expertise is required to ensure that evidence is applied in the best interest of individuals—even though it means practicing in a gray zone. The former circumstance is clearly a constraint on the practice of evidence-based medicine.

Clinicians frequently and readily make decisions in the absence of compelling evidence.[11,12] McDonald[12] argued that such decisions are made by principles, axioms, and *ad hoc* rules or "heuristics" that should be explicit. Formal characterization of the rules of medical decision making in the absence of evidence or in the presence of inconsistent evidence would provide both clinicians and their patients with a better understanding of how medical uncertainty is dealt with.

◊ PUTTING EVIDENCE-BASED MEDICINE INTO PRACTICE

Information to guide medical decision making is proliferating, whereas discretionary time for most clinicians is shrinking. The practice of evidence-based medicine requires the obstetrician-gynecologist to understand and apply principles of clinical epidemiology, to efficiently search the literature, and to critically appraise the literature in solving clinical problems and making the best possible medical decisions.[9] The busy obstetrician-gynecologist has three choices in evaluating available evidence and incorporating that evidence into practice: (1) practicing evidence-based medicine independently, (2) using evidence-based medical summaries developed by others, and (3) using evidence-based practice protocols developed by others.[13] The latter two approaches are briefly addressed here. The former approach is discussed in detail.

Using Evidence-based Medical Summaries

Evidence-based medical summaries go beyond traditional review articles, which have been shown to have little scientific merit. Two sources of summaries are available: One is a journal of secondary publication of structured abstracts and clinical commentaries that have been selected based on explicit criteria intended to select valid and clinically important articles. Such criteria eliminate 98% of the clinical literature.[13] Examples of these journals are *ACP Journal Club*, *Evidence-Based Medicine*, *Evidence-Based Nursing*, and *Evidence-Based Mental Health*. *Evidence-Based Medicine* and *Evidence-Based Nursing* have broad coverage of women's health issues, and all four publications are included in a cumulative database on the Internet and on the CD-ROM, *Best Evidence*.[14]

The second source of summaries is the systematic review of evidence for health care interventions. The most helpful of these currently available are systematic reviews of randomized, controlled trials prepared by Cochrane Review Groups and published in the Cochrane Library.[20] This library is described further in a later section (see "Task 2: Search for Evidence").

Systematic reviews, in contrast to narrative reviews, are intended to answer specific clinical questions in depth.[21] Systematic reviews use specific methods to assemble relevant studies, critically appraise those studies, and synthesize the studies to address a clinical question.[21] Methods for system-

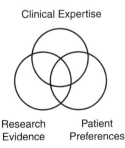

Clinical Expertise

Research Evidence   Patient Preferences

FIG. 1. Transferring evidence from research into practice: the role of clinical care research evidence in clinical decisions. (From ref. 8, with permission.)

atic reviews have been developed to limit systematic error (bias) and random error (chance); the value of a systematic review depends largely on how faithfully these methods have been followed.

When the quantitative results of individual studies in a systematic review are combined using statistical methods, the review is called a *metaanalysis*. Metaanalysis is increasingly used to summarize the obstetric and gynecologic literature.[22,23] A properly done metaanalysis can provide a wealth of information for clinical decision making; a poorly conducted metaanalysis can be misleading. Criteria for evaluating the quality of a metaanalysis have been described (Table 1).

Obstetrician-gynecologists using metaanalyses for decision making should be fully aware that the value of the metaanalysis is constrained by the value of the individual studies being synthesized. The use of metaanalysis may inappropriately confer a cloak of respectability around a collection of poor-quality studies. A collection of studies of poor quality is nothing more than that.

Whether metaanalysis should be restricted to randomized, controlled trials has been debated. Proper randomized trials provide better evidence about health care interventions than do observational studies. A major purpose of metaanalysis is to increase statistical power. Pooling of data from randomized, controlled trials is likely to provide a more precise estimate of a treatment effect than individual trials alone. Pooling observational studies to increase statistical power may introduce bias that is difficult to interpret. Most authorities believe that observational studies should be synthesized separately from randomized, controlled trials, if they are synthesized at all.

Using Evidence-based Practice Protocols

Evidence-based practice protocols have been developed to guide clinical decision making. The stages of development of practice protocols are similar to those to be described for the clinician practicing evidence-based medicine independently: (1) defining the problem, (2) identifying and critically appraising available evidence, and (3) translating the evidence into clinical policy.[24] Rules for developing clinical guidelines have been developed by the Institute of Medicine.[25] The Canadian Task Force on Periodic Health Examination[26] established a process to rate the quality of evidence for guideline development that has been adopted by others, including the United States Preventive Services Task Force[27] and the American College of Obstetricians and Gynecologists (ACOG).[28]

The general intent of practice guidelines is "to inform medical decisions and to decrease variations in care by systematically influencing clinical decisions."[29] However, guidelines may be influenced by the authors' intent—whether it be improving quality of care, saving costs, or reducing liability.[28] Regardless of perspective, the common denominator should be policies firmly based on evidence, where evidence is available. When evidence is not available, the basis on which policy decisions are made should be explicit.

In 1995, ACOG established an evidence-based guidelines process. Guidelines called "Educational Bulletins" are based on evidence that is evaluated and graded. Considerations regarding costs are also addressed.[28]

Evidence suggests that, in general, practice guidelines have the potential to improve patient care.[29] Weingarten[29] argued for careful testing of practice guidelines to determine which improve patient care.

◊ PRACTICING EVIDENCE-BASED MEDICINE INDEPENDENTLY

The obstetrician-gynecologist who practices evidence-based medicine independently needs to be able to accomplish four basic tasks:[13]

◊ Frame the clinical problem into a researchable question.
◊ Design and conduct a thorough search of the literature relevant to the question.
◊ Evaluate the quality of evidence obtained from the literature search, and summarize the best available evidence to address the clinical question.

TABLE 1. *Questions to ask in evaluating a published metaanalysis*

1. Is the purpose of the study (i.e., the hypothesis) clearly identified, and is it an overview of randomized trials of the treatment you are interested in?
2. Does it include a methods section that describes an active, comprehensive effort to include all relevant studies in the analysis?
3. Were explicit inclusion and exclusion criteria used to specify studies eligible for the metaanalysis?
4. Was there an assessment of publication bias (i.e., bias resulting from reporting only those results that are statistically significant, which tends to overestimate the effect under study)?
5. Was a blinded assessment of individual study quality conducted appropriately and systematically?
6. Were the pooled data appropriate for testing the hypothesis?
7. Were multiple raters used to assess coding? If so, were they blinded, and were measures of interrater reliability provided?
8. Were the selection and coding of data based on sound clinical principles or convenience?
9. Was documentation provided that explained how the data were coded and analyzed?
10. Was the comparability of cases and controls assessed?
11. Was heterogeneity testing conducted to assess consistency of results from study to study and reported appropriately?
12. Were results reported in sufficient detail to enable replication of results by the reviewer?
13. Were alternative explanations for observed results considered in the discussion?
14. Were the conclusions generalized appropriately, and did they stay within the domain of the literature review?
15. Were guidelines provided for future research?

(Adapted from refs. 13 and 23.)

◊ Apply the best available evidence to the care of the individual patient, taking into account each patient's circumstances, values, and preferences.

Education in evidence-based medicine works best if clinical questions arise from current dilemmas in patient care. This technique keeps the level of interest high, the applicability pertinent, and the effort current. Convenient access to a computer for on-line searching is preferable, but some searching will take place among journals and textbooks. In this section, we follow one scenario through all four tasks of practicing evidence-based medicine.

Task 1: Ask an Answerable Question

Framing the clinical question is the first and one of the most important steps in practicing evidence-based medicine. The question should be focused and answerable. Sackett et al.[13] have suggested that a well built, answerable question has four parts: (1) a description of the patient or problem, (2) a statement of the intervention being considered, (3) a statement of the alternative to the intervention, and (4) a description of the desired outcome. Many times, the question will be obvious, such as the starting dose of a new medication, and the resource will be handy, such as a formulary book. Other times, the question will not be clear, or there may be several kinds of questions that would apply to a single patient problem. To illustrate how to ask an answerable question, we will present a clinical scenario and follow it through the evidence-based medicine process. The example we have chosen is a question about treatment. Other possible topics for questions include diagnostic tests, prognosis, harm, and the evaluation of guidelines.

Example: A 36-year-old, gravida 2, para 1, presents to labor and delivery at 31 weeks' gestation. She reports leaking fluid for approximately 4 hours. The current pregnancy has been otherwise uncomplicated. Physical examination reveals no signs of infection and confirms membrane rupture. The patient is having a few irregular contractions that she cannot feel; fetal heart tones are 120 beats per minute with good variability.

For this example, we have constructed the following question: In patients who have preterm, premature rupture of the membranes, would steroid therapy to accelerate fetal lung maturity lead to lower mortality or morbidity from respiratory distress syndrome, when compared with observation alone? In our example, the description of the patient is addressed (patients who have preterm, premature rupture of membranes), the intervention being considered is stated (steroid therapy to accelerate fetal lung maturity), as is the alternative (observation alone). The question concludes with a description of the desired outcome (lower mortality or morbidity from respiratory distress syndrome).

There are several different questions that can be framed from this clinical scenario. The first question we framed was designed to select a therapy. A question about determining etiology could be: In patients with a pregnancy resulting in preterm, premature rupture of the membranes, is a culture for group B streptococcus more likely to be positive, compared to patients with rupture of the membranes at term? Similarly, we could have asked about prevention: In patients with a history of preterm, premature rupture of the membranes, does first-trimester screening and treatment for bacterial vaginosis reduce the likelihood of recurrence with subsequent pregnancies, relative to no screening and treatment?

There may be times when it is difficult to identify an answerable question. In other cases, there may be more questions than time to answer them. Prioritization would ensure that the most important issue for the patient or the question most likely to be encountered again in clinical practice will be answered.

Task 2: Search for Evidence

Once the question has been framed, the pertinent evidence must be searched. The first step in this task is determining the resource most likely to be helpful in the search. The best resource may differ depending on the question posed. For treatment effectiveness or safety, the most useful and scientifically sound sources will be randomized, controlled trials and systematic reviews. If one expects that a sufficient number of randomized trials has been conducted to warrant a useful systematic review, a good initial step to assess questions about treatment would be to search the Cochrane Library,[20] hoping to find a review on the subject of interest.

Example: The use of steroids for reducing neonatal morbidity has been a recognized therapy since the 1970s, and enough clinical trials have been reported that systematic reviews have been published. Thus, we chose to search the Cochrane Library, a database with systematic reviews.

After locating the Cochrane Library on the Internet or loading the CD-ROM program from purchased disks, we identify the Cochrane Library introductory page. After clicking on the search icon, we enter the word "steroid" as a key word, and the search is initiated by clicking on the search button. At the top of the page, the index lists the types of information available for our search. Under the heading "systematic reviews" is a subheading "complete reviews." By scrolling down the list under this subheading, we quickly (in less than 1 minute) identify the recent (January 1996) critical review, "Corticosteroids Prior to Preterm Delivery."

The Cochrane Library is one of the specialized databases developed by a group of individuals committed to preparing, maintaining, and disseminating systematic reviews of the effects of health care. These systematic reviews use explicitly defined methods to reduce the effects of bias.[30] The Cochrane Library includes databases of Cochrane and non-Cochrane systematic reviews, as well as a clinical trials database of over 150,000 entries. Although the database of systematic reviews includes unpublished reports and information not available on MEDLINE, it does not yet cover all clinical areas. Nevertheless, perinatal medicine and many topics in women's health are well represented. The Cochrane Library is available through the Internet (after subscribing at http://www.medlib.com) and on disk or CD-ROM from Update Software (Oxford, England), the BMJ Publishing Group (London, England), and the American College of Physicians (Philadelphia, PA).

Sources of Evidence

For some questions and clinical problems, systematic reviews or metaanalyses may not be available. In such cases, the searcher will have to identify individual studies, rate these studies for quality, and then synthesize the best available evidence. The largest available source of medical literature is the National Library of Medicine's MEDLINE, a bibliographic database covering materials from 1966 to the present. Facilitated access to millions of articles from more than 3000 journals has led the way to specialized databases. MEDLINE can be obtained in libraries or purchased through commercial vendors; it is available on-line and on CD-ROM. Members of ACOG can access MEDLINE through ACOGNET. MEDLINE is also free on the Internet (http://igm.nlm.nih.gov and http://www.ncb.nlm.nih.gov/pubmed).

Example: We conduct a separate search on MEDLINE, which takes longer (about 20 minutes) to locate publications under the text words "corticosteroids" and "preterm." Because MEDLINE contains millions of articles and the Cochrane Library contains only systematic reviews, the Cochrane Library provides the best available evidence more efficiently.

ACOG has a World Wide Web site accessible to its members. In addition to MEDLINE, ACOG publications, including evidence-based *Educational Bulletins*, are available on-line. Similarly, the American College of Physicians has a database derived from structured abstracts and clinical commentaries based on a preestablished methodology that screens out poor evidence (http://www.acponline.org).

Consensus guidelines offer another potential source of evidence. However, they often provide summaries of evidence without clearly stating how the evidence was obtained and evaluated. The National Institutes of Health (NIH) has a Web site that makes available its consensus guidelines and workshop proceedings (http://odp.od.nih.gov/consensus).

Example: Through the Internet, we identify an NIH consensus report on the use of corticosteroids to reduce morbidity from prematurity. However, the basis for the NIH report was the Cochrane Library systematic review.

Task 3: Appraise the Evidence

Once we complete our search for the evidence, we assess both the importance and the validity of the evidence for the use of corticosteroids to accelerate fetal lung maturity.

Example: The systematic review, "Corticosteroids Prior to Preterm Delivery," identified in the Cochrane Library, included 18 randomized trials that are of acceptable quality (i.e., meet specified criteria for the elimination of bias, as described in the "Cochrane Collaboration Handbook" included in the Cochrane

Library) and that report clinically relevant outcomes. Thus, we found strong evidence on the general subject of using corticosteroids prior to preterm delivery. Our specific question, however, dealt with the use of corticosteroids in the presence of ruptured membranes. The description of study methods in the review was sufficiently detailed to determine that women with preterm, premature rupture of the membranes were not subjects in two of the 18 studies included in the systematic review. We obtain copies of the other 16 reports and determine that five have data on the risk of neonatal respiratory distress syndrome for women who had preterm, premature rupture of the membranes at 31 weeks' gestation or less and who had corticosteroids administered without other interventions. We use Epi Info, a series of microcomputer programs available online for use by public health professionals (http://www.cdc.gov/epo/epi/epiinfo.htm), to calculate the relative risks. Together, these five reports provide strong support for use of corticosteroids among such women: The summary risk estimate of neonatal respiratory distress syndrome for women who had corticosteroids administered relative to the risk in women who did not have corticosteroids administered is 0.64 (95% confidence interval, 0.48–0.85) (Table 2). Because the 95% confidence interval did not overlap 1.0, the reduction in risk for women who had corticosteroids administered is statistically significant.

While reading the Cochrane Library review, we serendipitously find that randomized trials are available for assessing the use of corticosteroids for reducing perinatal complications other than respiratory distress syndrome, including neonatal mortality and intraventricular hemorrhage. In addition, randomized trials with long-term infant follow-up are available to assess the likelihood of late sequelae of steroid therapy.

Assessing Importance and Validity

The task of appraising the evidence includes assessing both the importance and the validity of the evidence.[13] Some clinicians choose to determine validity before evaluating importance, and others reverse the order. No matter what the order, when the first step is promising, the other must be completed.

An assessment of the importance of a study finding focuses both on the strength of the association between the factor under investigation and the study outcome and on the number of people potentially affected by the finding. Measures commonly used to assess the strength of association in epidemiologic studies are the odds ratio (Fig. 2) and the relative risk (Fig. 3). As discussed below, a properly conducted randomized, controlled trial provides the highest quality of evidence; the relative risk is the measure of association commonly used in such trials.

The obstetrician-gynecologist assessing validity is searching for biases. Sackett et al.[13] provided questions that may aid in an assessment of validity, including those adapted for Table 1 and those included in Table 3. Biases are systematic errors either in design or analysis that could lead to an incorrect conclusion.[31] Biases can result from the way in which study participants were selected (selection bias), from the way in which information was collected from study participants (information bias), and from failure to adjust for factors

TABLE 2. *Selected studies[1] of the effect of corticosteroids after prelabour rupture of the membranes on respiratory distress syndrome*

	Treated		Control		Point estimate (95% Confidence Interval)	Relative risk Graphical				
Study	n	(%)	n	(%)		0	0.5	1	1.5	2.0
Morales et al. (1986)[15]	30/121	(25)	63/124	(51)	0.59 (0.40–0.86)					
Schmidt et al. (1984)[16]	7/24	(29)	6/17	(35)	0.87 (0.34–2.23)					
Collaborative Group on Antenatal Steroid Therapy (1981)[17]	15/153	(10)	17/135	(13)	0.80 (0.41–1.54)					
Taeusch (1979)[18]	7/34	(12)	14/47	(29)	0.74 (0.33–1.68)					
Block (1977)[19]	3/25	(12)	5/26	(19)	0.66 (0.17–2.53)					
Summary relative risk	62/357	(17)	105/349	(30)	0.64 (0.48–0.85)					

[1]Studies were restricted to those in which premature rupture of the membranes could have occurred at 31 weeks gestation. Studies were excluded if interventions other than corticosteroid administration were used. A variety of steroid therapies were used in the included studies.

that influence the study outcome but are extraneous to the study's question (confounders). Biases may distort the measure of study outcomes so greatly that study data may suggest a strong association (a potentially important effect) when in fact no association exists. Conversely, the data may suggest no association when a strong one is present. In other words, biases may lead to a distortion of the truth.

When a recent systematic review of randomized, controlled trials is available, such as those from the Cochrane Library,[20] the obstetrician-gynecologist can (1) accept the conclusions of the reviewer, (2) critically appraise the quality of the review by using criteria such as those in Tables 1 and 2, or (3) conduct an independent search and review of the evidence. When a recent systematic review is not available, the obstetrician-gynecologist must critically appraise the available evidence.

The system for evaluating the quality of evidence proposed by the Canadian Task Force on Periodic Health Examination[26] and adopted by the U.S. Preventive Services Task Force[27] is a useful framework for assessing the relative strengths and weaknesses of different types of epidemiologic studies (Table 4).

Types of Epidemiologic Studies

A basic understanding of epidemiologic methods is necessary for intelligent appraisal of medical evidence. Brief reviews of epidemiologic methods are available,[10,22,23,31] as is a series of articles in the *Journal of the American Medical Association* specifically intended to help clinicians critically appraise the medical literature (Table 5). Standard texts of clinical epidemiology are also helpful.

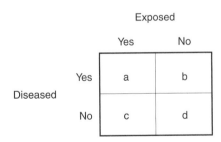

$$\text{Relative risk} \atop \text{odds ratio} = \frac{\text{exposure odds among cases (diseased)}}{\text{exposure odds among controls (not diseased)}}$$

$$= \frac{a/b}{c/d}$$

$$= \frac{ad}{bc}$$

FIG. 2. Calculation of the odds ratio using the 2-×-2 table. The values *a, b, c,* and *d* represent the numbers of people in each of four possible combinations of exposure and disease status.

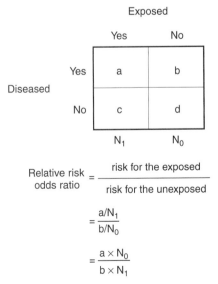

$$\text{Relative risk} \atop \text{odds ratio} = \frac{\text{risk for the exposed}}{\text{risk for the unexposed}}$$

$$= \frac{a/N_1}{b/N_0}$$

$$= \frac{a \times N_0}{b \times N_1}$$

FIG. 3. Calculation of the relative risk using the 2-×-2 table. The values *a, b, c,* and *d* represent the numbers of people in each of four possible combinations of exposure and disease (N_1, total number exposed; N_0, total number unexposed).

TABLE 3. *Are the results of this single study valid?*

The main questions to answer:
1. Was the assignment of patients to treatments random-ized, and was the randomization list concealed?
2. Were all patients who entered the trial accounted for at its conclusion, and were they analyzed in the groups to which they were randomized?

And some finer points to address:
1. Were patients and clinicians kept blind to which treatment was being received?
2. Aside from the experimental treatment, were the groups treated equally?
3. Were the groups similar at the start of the trial?

(From ref. 13, with permission.)

TABLE 5. *Literature available from the Journal of the American Medical Association on using medical articles*

Title	JAMA reference
I. How to get started	1993;270:2093–2095
II. How to use an article about therapy or prevention	
A. Are the results of the study valid?	1993;270:2598–2601
B. What are the results, and will they help me in caring for my patients?	1994;271:59–63
III. How to use an article about a diagnostic test	
A. Are the results of the study valid?	1994;271:389–391
B. What are the results, and will they help me in caring for my patients?	1994;271:703–707
IV. How to use an article about harm	1994;271:1615–1619
V. How to use an article about prognosis	1994;272:234–237
VI. How to use an overview	1994;272:1367–1371
VII. How to use a clinical decision analysis	
A. Are the results of the study valid?	1995;273:1292–1295
B. What are the results, and will they help me in caring for my patients?	1995;273:1610–1613
VIII. How to use clinical practice guidelines	
A. Are the recommen-dations valid?	1995;274:570–574

Most studies in the medical literature relevant to clinical decision making in obstetrics and gynecology are epidemiologic studies. The goal of an epidemiologic study is to accurately measure the relationship between an exposure of interest (e.g., steroid therapy) and an outcome of interest (e.g., neonatal morbidity and mortality from respiratory distress syndrome). The two basic types of epidemiologic studies are experimental and observational.

In experimental studies (e.g., randomized, controlled trials), the exposure is manipulated, and the effect of that manipulation on the outcome is measured directly. When properly conducted, these studies provide the strongest evidence because they are least likely to be affected by bias and thus are most likely to obtain an accurate measure. However, randomized trials are of varying quality. A poorly conducted randomized trial may be of little or no value. The U.S. Preventive Services Task Force requires that randomized trials be "properly conducted" to be considered high-quality evidence (see Table 4). Guidelines for evaluating the quality of randomized trials are available.[32]

TABLE 4. *System for evaluating quality of evidence proposed by the Canadian Task Force on Periodic Health Examination*

I	Evidence obtained from at least one properly randomized controlled trial
II-1	Evidence obtained from well designed controlled trials without randomization
II-2	Evidence obtained from well designed cohort or case–control analytic studies, preferably from more than one center or research group
II-3	Evidence obtained from multiple time series with or without the intervention. Dramatic results in uncontrolled experiments (e.g., the results of the introduction of penicillin treatment in the 1940s) could also be regarded as this type of evidence
III	Opinions of respected authorities, based on clinical experience; descriptive studies and case reports; or reports of expert committees

(From ref. 27, with permission.)

In observational studies (e.g., cohort, case–control, and cross-sectional studies), the exposure is observed rather than manipulated. Observational studies provide a wide range of quality of evidence. The quality of evidence from cohort (follow-up) studies (in which study participants are classified as exposed or unexposed to the factor of interest and then followed over time to see whether or not they develop the outcome of interest) depends on the strength of the study design and analysis. Case–control studies (in which study participants are classified as having or not having the outcome of interest, typically a disease, and are then assessed to determine whether or not they were exposed to a factor of interest in the past) have the same potential range of quality. Although prospective studies (including cohort studies) are often thought to be methodologically superior to retrospective (including case–control) studies, theoretically, a perfectly conducted cohort study will provide the same level of evidence as a perfectly conducted case–control study. In practice, however, retrospective (including case–control) studies are generally more susceptible to bias than are prospective (including cohort) studies.

Cross-sectional studies warrant special mention for the lack of evidence that they typically provide. Cross-sectional studies can be regarded as a snapshot of individuals that provides information about whether or not the individuals have been exposed to the factor of interest and whether they have the outcome of interest at that moment. In these studies, the quality of evidence is typically very low because little information is available about whether the exposure caused the outcome. In fact, in many cross-sectional studies, it is impossible to determine whether the outcome preceded the exposure.

An example concerning the use of condoms for prevention of human immunodeficiency virus (HIV) transmission may be helpful for distinguishing the four types of epidemiologic studies discussed here:

◊ Randomized, controlled trial: Men at risk for acquiring HIV infection are randomized to use or nonuse of latex condoms and then followed over time to determine whether they become infected. Although it would be unethical to assign one study group a known effective strategy for preventing a deadly disease and leaving the other group at risk, a randomized trial of a behavioral intervention to encourage men to use condoms could potentially be conducted without ethical proscriptions.
◊ Cohort (follow-up) study: Men at risk for HIV infection who choose to use latex condoms consistently and men who choose not to do so are followed over time to determine whether or not they become infected. Important differences between men who do and do not use condoms that influence the risk of acquiring HIV infection may bias the estimate of the effect of condom use.
◊ Case–control study: Men with and without HIV infection are selected for study and then asked to provide a detailed record of prior condom use. Men with HIV infection may be more or less likely than uninfected men to recall condom use accurately; differences in recall (a type of information bias) may bias study findings. In the cohort study design, men would be asked to prospectively chart condom use, which would likely lead to a better measure of condom use than reliance on memory alone.
◊ Cross-sectional study: Men with and without HIV infection are asked about current or recent condom use. It is impossible, however, to determine whether the condom use preceded or followed infection with HIV.

Task 4: Apply the Evidence

Once the importance and validity of the evidence have been assessed, the evidence has to be applied to an individual patient. The smaller the number of randomized, controlled trials available to assess the safety and effectiveness of treatment and the narrower the variety of clinical circumstances studied, the more the obstetrician-gynecologist will need to rely on clinical expertise to determine how the available evidence applies to a particular patient. One approach to this task is to ask, "Would my patient satisfy the eligibility criteria for the trial?"[13] or "Is my patient so different from those in the trial that the results don't apply to her?"

Evidence-based medicine also considers the values and preferences of each patient. The values and preferences of the patient may well tip the scale toward or away from treatment, particularly in instances where the balance of risks and benefits of treatment is unclear.

Example: Our review of the evidence indicates that corticosteroids are safe and effective to use for preterm, premature rupture of membranes. The findings applied to a broad range of gestational ages of less than 35 weeks, male and female infants, and across races. No adverse consequences for any subgroups were identified. Thus, there is strong evidence that our patient is an appropriate candidate for corticosteroid therapy. Because the benefits are great and there are no documented risks, the patient will likely agree to steroid therapy.

SUMMARY POINTS

◊ Evidence-based medicine is neither "cookbook" medicine nor "cost-cutting" medicine. Rather, it is the use of the best available evidence in caring for an individual.
◊ Obstetrician-gynecologists can practice evidence-based medicine by using evidence-based medical summaries, systematic reviews, or evidence-based practice protocols.
◊ Obstetrician-gynecologists can also learn to practice evidence-based medicine independently by becoming proficient at four tasks:

1. Framing a researchable question;
2. Conducting a search for evidence to address the question;
3. Critically appraising the evidence;
4. Applying the evidence to the individual patient.

◊ REFERENCES

1. Silverman WA. *Retrolental fibroplasia: a modern parable*. New York: Grune & Stratton, 1980.
2. Silverman WA. *Human experimentation: a guided step into the unknown*. Oxford: Oxford University Press, 1985.
3. Hill AB. *Principles of medical statistics*. New York: Oxford University Press, 1937.
4. Cochrane A. *Effectiveness and efficiency: random reflections on health services*. Cambridge: Cambridge University Press. 1971.
5. Grimes DA. Technology follies: the uncritical acceptance of medical innovation. *JAMA* 1993;269:3030–3033.
6. Grimes DA. Introducing evidence-based medicine into a department of obstetrics and gynecology. *Obstet Gynecol* 1995;86:451–457.
7. Sackett DL, Rosenberg WMC, Gray JAM, Haynes RB, Richardson WS. Evidence-based medicine: what it is and what it isn't. *BMJ* 1996; 312:71–72.
8. Haynes RB, Sackett DL, Gray JAM, Cook DJ, Guyatt GH. Transferring evidence from research into practice: 1. The role of clinical care research evidence in clinical decisions. *ACP J Club* 1996;125:A-14–A-16.
9. Evidence-based Medicine Working Group. Evidence-based medicine: a new approach to teaching the practice of medicine. *JAMA* 1992;268: 2420–2425.

10. Peipert JF, Gifford DS, Boardman LA. Research design and methods of quantitative synthesis of medical evidence. *Obstet Gynecol* 1997;90: 473–478.

11. Naylor CD. Grey zones of clinical practice: some limits to evidence-based medicine. *Lancet* 1995;345:840–842.

12. McDonald CJ. Medical heuristics: the silent adjudicators of clinical practice. *Ann Intern Med* 1996;124:56–62.

13. Sackett DL, Richardson WS, Rosenberg W, Haynes RB. *Evidence-based medicine: how to practice and teach EBM.* New York: Churchill Livingstone, 1997.

14. Haynes RB, Sackett DL, Gray JAM, Cook DJ, Guyatt GH. Transferring evidence from research into practice: 2. Getting the evidence straight. *ACP J Club* 1997;126:A-14–A-16.

15. Morales WJ, Diebel ND, Lazar AJ, Zadrozny D. The effect of antenatal dexamethasone administration on the prevention of respiratory distress syndrome in preterm gestations with premature rupture of membranes. *Am J Obstet Gynecol* 1986;154:591–595.

16. Schmidt PL, Sims ME, Strassner HT, Paul RH, Mueller E, McCart D. Effect of antepartum glucocorticoid administration upon neonatal respiratory distress syndrome and perinatal infection. *Am J Obstet Gynecol* 1984;148:178–186.

17. Collaborative Group on Antenatal Steroid Therapy. Effect of antenatal dexamethasone administration on the prevention of respiratory distress syndrome. *Am J Obstet Gynecol* 1981;141:276–287.

18. Taeusch Jr HW, Frigoletto F, Kitzmillar J, Avery ME, Hehre A, Fromm B, Lawson E, Neff RK. Risk of respiratory distress syndrome after prenatal dexamethasone treatment. *Pediatrics* 1979;63:64–72.

19. Block MF, Kling OR, Crosby WM. Antenatal Glucocorticoid therapy for the prevention of respiratory distress syndrome in the premature infant. *Obstet Gynecol* 1977;50:186–190.

20. *Cochrane database of systematic reviews.* London: BMJ Publishing Group, 1997. (Available from BMJ Publishing Group, PO Box 295, London WC1H9TE, UK. Tel: 44(0)171 383 6185/6245; fax: 44(0)171 383 6662.)

21. Cook DJ, Mylrow CD, Haynes RB. Systematic reviews: synthesis of best evidence for clinical decisions. *Ann Intern Med* 1997;126:376–380.

22. Peipert JF, Bracken MB. Systematic reviews of medical evidence: the use of meta-analysis in obstetrics and gynecology. *Obstet Gynecol* 1997;89:628–633.

23. Thacker SB, Peterson HB, Stroup DF. Meta-analysis for the obstetrician-gynecologist. *Am J Obstet Gynecol* 1996;174:1403–1407.

24. Gray JAM, Haynes RB, Sackett DL, Cook DJ, Guyatt GH. Transferring evidence from research into practice: 3. Developing evidence-based clinical policy. *ACP J Club* 1997;126:A-14–A-16.

25. Institute of Medicine. *Consensus development at the NIH: improving the program.* Washington, DC: National Academy Press, 1990.

26. Canadian Task Force on Periodic Health Examination. *The Canadian guide to clinical preventive health care.* Ottawa: Canada Communication Group, 1994.

27. U.S. Preventive Services Task Force. *Guide to clinical preventive services,* 2nd ed. Baltimore: Williams & Wilkins, 1996.

28. Zinberg S. A guest editorial: evidence-based guidelines: a current perspective. *Obstet Gynecol Surv* 1997;52:65–66.

29. Weingarten S. Practice guidelines and prediction rules should be subject to careful clinical testing. *JAMA* 1997;277:1977–1978.

30. Fullerton-Smith I. How members of the Cochrane Collaboration prepare and maintain systematic reviews of the effects of health care. *Evidence-based Med* 1995;1:7–8.

31. Peterson HB, Kleinbaum DG. Interpreting the literature in obstetrics and gynecology: I. Key concepts in epidemiology and biostatistics. *Obstet Gynecol* 1991;78:710–717.

32. Begg C, Cho M, Eastwood S, et al. Improving the quality of reporting of randomized controlled trials: the CONSORT statement. *JAMA* 1996;276:637–639.

CHAPTER 2

Managed Care in Obstetrics and Gynecology

———— ◇ ————

Byron J. Masterson

◇ ECONOMIC OVERVIEW

The growth of the management of clinical medicine through some form of organized system began late in the 1800s. Prominent among these early efforts were the railroad hospitals and military institutions. The pressures for organizing and managing clinical events, which were handled at random by clinicians paid on a fee-for-service basis, gained momentum in the late 1970s. Initial studies showed the inability of the government or any other institution to pay the projected clinical costs. I began addressing medical audiences in the late 1970s on this very subject, but there was little interest at that time. While the current progress toward global capitation is a driving force in many specialties, obstetrics and gynecology at present is uncommonly capitated. The usual payment to obstetricians is on a discounted fee-for-service basis. The reason for this is essentially that obstetricians themselves have long capitated the obstetric event. In the fee-for-service world, obstetricians rendered an all-inclusive fee for their services, except for a possible surcharge for circumcision and in some instances for a cesarean section. In contrast, the fee for the gynecologist's care usually has been based on the individual service performed (e.g., abdominal hysterectomy, colposcopy, vulvar biopsy, etc.), and therefore gynecologists did not capitate the patient's entire clinical care. In a later section of this chapter, how one derives such capitation fees and how they apply to clinical medicine are discussed.

◇ INDUSTRY PRESSURES FOR COST CONTAINMENT

Fortune 500 companies in the United States usually are heavily involved in world trade. Products made in the United States must therefore be competitive not only in quality but also in price. However, the second largest cost for many major corporations, after salaries, is their health care costs.

The boards of directors of these corporations have had the fiduciary responsibility, as well as simply a good business responsibility, to appropriately manage these costs. A variety of programs designed for cost efficiency have been entertained, but most businesses are now leaning toward "managed care contracting." Leaders in this effort include large companies such as General Telephone and Electronics, which has an extensive program of managing its health care efforts centrally, while in turn using the different health care systems locally that they believe provide the best quality for the funds expended.

The impact of increased managed care shows that health care costs rose only 2.5% last year, but they still cost $3,915 per employee for the average large American company. Even so, this increase in cost compares favorably to the previous years of 1988 through 1990, when health care costs went up more than 15% per year.

◇ FEDERAL PROGRAMS

The pressure for some sort of management of health care costs has been driven from the federal level because of dramatic increases in the Medicare and Medicaid programs over the past 10 years. Medicare programs are currently projected to grow at 8.4% per year, approximately 5% over inflation. Medicare and Medicaid combined produce a figure closer to 7.7%. These percentages represent a definite decrease in their growth rates from those of the 1980s. At these reductions, Medicare will actually cost $60 billion *less* in the years 1998 through 2002 than was forecast just last spring. Medicaid in turn will cost $79 billion less for the same period. These cost containment results are felt to be due almost entirely to the increasing impact of managed care and its growing ability to control the use of more expensive services while decreasing the overall cost of health care spending.

11

◊ SCIENCE AND TECHNOLOGY COSTS

One of the most difficult decisions that caregivers and policy makers have to deal with is determining the impact of new technology on modern health care. While this technology frequently adds greatly to the improved care for the patient (e.g., genetically engineered products that can increase bone marrow production of red and white blood cells), such technology frequently adds greatly to the cost as well (e.g., $1500 to $2000 per course of treatment). However, certain chemotherapy protocols cannot be completed without such bone marrow stimulation or its additional costs and therefore will continue to be used. The widespread use of the high-tech procedures now available in the fields of cardiology and cardiovascular surgery is but another classic example of advanced technology's impact on medical care.

◊ ACADEMIC MEDICAL CENTERS

Control of increasing health care costs has produced a major challenge for academic medical centers because of the high-cost, high-tech care these centers deliver, compared to the care provided at community hospitals. The average cost per case in an academic medical center is approximately $3000 greater than the average cost per case in a nonteaching hospital. Other reasons for the higher costs are varied but frequently center around the more specialized cases, the increasing use of laboratory studies, and poor management systems. Such poor systems are often found in operating rooms and other service areas, where a constant turnover in employees who learn skills but subsequently get promoted or simply leave inevitably produces greater inefficiencies in these areas. As a result, managed care participation is critical to academic medical centers, as they derive one-third or more of their revenue from practice activities, including the majority of their discretionary funds necessary for investment in new projects, equipment, and quality faculty.

Academic Health Centers in a Managed Care Environment

Academic medical centers have several significant advantages in that they have an inherent "aura of quality" with their distinguished faculty and research efforts, large numbers of physicians working within a better coordinated system, tertiary services that would be difficult to maintain in the average small community hospital, and large size that allows them to be very diversified. However, these advantages come with a price, and many payers are increasingly unwilling or unable to pay the higher fees assessed for using academic centers. In addition, faculty members in the academic departments do not always see themselves primarily as caregivers. Often, the high-tech services offered in academic centers cannot sustain themselves when based on the academic practice alone. In addition, it is often quite difficult to communicate and move patients through academic centers that have been organized through the various departments rather than through a group practice that places its focus on the patient.

This structure produces a number of challenges to academic health centers that first must be dealt with by very careful cost analysis. Each activity must add value to the medical center. Every interaction with the patient must be carefully costed, and the price by which such care can be rendered must be determined. The cost of indigent care must be considered and dealt with as well, as academic health centers will no longer be able to provide such care with the current shrinking clinical margins.

Impact of Managed Care on Academic Practice

The ability of academic medical institutions to sustain and support their academic efforts and unfunded research from discretionary funds generated by a practice plan is rapidly disappearing. However, in this era of intense cost analysis, academic health centers must preserve their mission of "teaching, education, and research," or they will lose their very reason for being. These institutions have served our country well and have expanded quite dramatically in the last 45 years. It is now our responsibility to develop the necessary structures to clearly and efficiently demonstrate appropriate costing that will allow these centers to continue to prosper in the future.

◊ PATIENTS' VIEWS OF MANAGED CARE

Most people are familiar with the many anecdotes about the "nurse from hell" who refuses all requests for inpatient care. Likewise, this lack of consideration is also found in the exceptionally poor choice of words by managed care companies in labeling payment for patient services as a *medical loss*," although the only reason for the existence of such organizations is to pay for services that patients need. Indeed, the term should be *medical benefit*. Public perception of managed care companies is surprisingly consistent. As outlined in Table 1, consumers view managed care as giving a restricted choice of providers, doctors, and hospitals and providing less personal care. Many believe that managed care represents a triumph of cost cutting over quality and consequently that the major concern of corporate medicine is greater profit rather than higher quality of care for patients. Many noted the dramatic cost shift from employer to employee. Consumer responses also showed that medical school faculty are not recognized by the general public as true caregivers or researchers, a view that may directly and negatively affect medical schools' ability to bring in new patients for study and treatment.

The public regards the early insertion of inappropriate contract language into managed care contracts in the harshest terms possible. Such language tends to decrease the communication between physicians and patients and has become known as "the gag rule." As a result, many states have now eliminated such contract language by law. Likewise, any sort of reimbursement method designed to reward physicians for

TABLE 1. *Consumer views on managed care*

Less choice of providers, doctors, and hospitals
Less personal care
Triumph of cost cutting over quality
Dramatic cost shift from employer to employee
Concern of corporate medicine is for profit instead of quality of care for patients
Medical school faculty not recognized as caregivers or researchers

(Data from Consumer views on managed care. *Life Science* 1997.)

not providing care is viewed by most people as equally onerous; eventually, language will gradually appear in law that will prevent this type of negative reward system as well.

While there are detractors of managed care companies, it should be remembered that many patients also give hospitals very poor marks (Table 2). Based on a 1997 survey of almost 24,000 patients, the highest percentages of problems reported have involved patient transition, emotional support, and updated information and education. Patients also commented on hospitals' lack of family involvement, poor coordination of medical care, and lack of respect for patients' stated preferences.

A recent American Medical Association survey likewise showed that while 42% of the patients surveyed felt their doctors did explain things well to them, more than half surveyed felt that physicians in general are primarily interested in making money. Over one-third of patients believed that doctors project an attitude that they are "better than others," but almost as many patients agreed that most doctors do spend sufficient time with their patients. With such obviously mixed reviews, it was not surprising to find that 69% of patients surveyed felt that people in general are beginning to lose faith in doctors.

Parenthetically, medical school faculty are often not recognized or credited as being focused on patient care and are often viewed by the public simply as teachers with no active medical practice. The customer (patient) also views the entire health care industry with mixed emotions. Patients may be fondly attached to their personal physician or to their chosen hospital, but the health care industry itself often receives negative reviews.

TABLE 2. *Patients give hospitals poor score card: percentage of patients reporting problems*

Continuity and transition	28.7
Emotional support	26.6
Information and education	23.1
Involvement of family and friends	22.3
Coordination of care	22.9
Respect for patients' preferences	21.8
Physical comfort	10.4

(Data from a survey of 23,768 patients published in Lagnado L. Patients give hospitals poor score card. *Wall Street Journal* Jan, 1997.)

◊ PHYSICIAN AS A SUBSPECIALTY OR PRIMARY CARE PROVIDER

If physicians are to prosper in this market, they must understand it. Each physician must find the position that he or she wishes to take as a practitioner, whether in a partnership or a group, and must clearly differentiate him- or herself from the other physicians in that market. He or she must decide, for instance, whether to be a primary care provider in the field of obstetrics and gynecology or to specialize in subspecialty care. In today's market, this choice will make a great difference both in how many patients a physician may expect to see and for what reason or need that they come. If they are part of a managed care organization, such patients will be coming only with specific tasks or services in mind. However, in choosing to be a subspecialist only, a physician will have obligations for providing care that will be quite different from those expected of the primary care provider.

◊ KEYS TO SUCCESS IN THE MANAGED CARE ENVIRONMENT

As a primary caregiver, a physician must maintain an office located close to patients, with hours that meet the definition of primary care as determined by a managed care company. This may be especially difficult to do if a physician carries a surgical practice and therefore is required to be out of the office a fair amount of the time. There must also be in place in the office an information retrieval system that can support the data requirements of today's managed care companies. The system must be able to provide data indicating how satisfied patients are, how quickly the telephone is answered, or how quickly the office organization is able to respond to requests for information by patients or payers. A managed care company, for example, may request the development of critical paths that require database management, as well as providing such information on a regular basis. The system must also be compatible with the information system used by the managed care company.

Of particular importance to a physician and his or her practice is making certain not to get an adverse case selection. For example, if a primary care obstetrics and gynecology practice capitates a group of patients including one or more cases of acquired immunodeficiency syndrome, one or two patients with a malignant disease, and one very complex obstetric patient, then a physician may find that capitation payments fall woefully short of the amount needed to pay for such complex patient care. Group management systems frequently do not reimburse for this type of loss or may exclude these types of cases from their group of managed care cases on which they currently make payment.

The three potential pitfalls for practitioners in capitation are therefore (1) a challenging case mix, (2) lack of a methodical utilization review, and (3) inadequate information and data tracking systems. The first challenge begins with the adverse case selection, where particular patients having very complex diseases requiring extensive management are capitated at the regular *community rate*—a rate providing only an approximate payment based on people with much simpler problems. Next, a rigorous utilization review system must be put in place, facilitating shorter hospital stays than those of fellow practitioners. Finally, practitioners must be certain that they are not entering into a managed care program with a substandard information system that is inadequate and therefore unable to produce the data required for them to practice effectively in a highly competitive system.

◊ PAYMENT SYSTEMS

Let us now look more closely at the different methods of payment and discuss in some detail the major points of capitation in contrast to the traditional fee-for-service plan. Unlike the fee-for-service system, in which physicians are paid and therefore profit only when they see patients, capitation (literally, per head) guarantees a monthly fee for each plan member regardless of whether or not a service is performed. Capitation plans are designed to emphasize health maintenance and preventive care with an incentive to keep patients healthy and avoid costly procedures. Capitation seeks to provide better outcomes with better utilization of resources: quality care with cost containment. Central to most health care plans being developed today, capitation has become the fastest growing form of provider reimbursement, expected to reach 66% nationwide within the next 5 years.

Revenues created in the fee-for-service world are increased by the performance of more work. In contrast, the clinical practice structured on a capitation basis places its focus on cost. Cost may be defined as follows:

◊ *Fixed costs:* Costs that must be paid regardless of the volume of business performed;

◊ *Variable costs*: Costs that vary with the type and amount of business done.

An example of fixed costs is the payment of office rent or certain employee salaries. In contrast, variable costs are those, for example, for the use of hospital linens and the related costs incurred or added with each new patient seen. In the private practice structure, variable costs may be more significant, and therefore adjustments can be made. In the academic institution, however, more costs are fixed and revolve around payments for salaries. Thus, in this type of managed care model, costs cannot be covered simply by increasing the volume of patients seen because income does not increase. With fixed payment in managed care, costs must be managed within that income. As demonstrated in Figure 1, the fixed income of a managed care system is demonstrated by a straight line that remains "fixed" at the same level regardless of the work performed, unless more patients are added to the practice. In comparison, adjustments can be made in a fee-for-service business system to allow income to continue to rise.

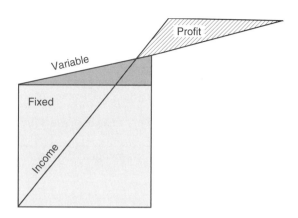

FIG. 1. Relationship between fixed costs, variable costs, and profit.

Fee for Service

In the fee-for-service system, physicians provide a service, and charge and are paid a specific fee for it. This system has the clear market strength of the identification of a unit of work provided with an amount in payment for it. The negative aspect of this system is of course that it records the procedures involved but does not necessarily provide a clear assessment of the patient's health. Physicians have thrived in a fee-for-service system by working very hard, being procedurally oriented, and choosing not to do those things that required a lot of time and yet were not associated with a significant reimbursement source. Procedurally oriented specialists frequently had lifetime incomes two to three times over and above those of office-based physicians such as pediatricians.

Indemnity Insurance Reimbursement System

Indemnity insurance was frequently the primary source of payment in the fee-for-service world. In this system, a patient would pay a chosen insurance company to assume the risk for medical care. If the patient became ill, he or she would see a caregiver, who then rendered a bill that was paid by the insurance company. The insurance company would predict the number of illnesses in a given population and then, through the use of actuaries, would determine their fees prospectively. Patients were able to buy into these pools.

The problem for the insurance companies was that the costs increased faster than they could raise their rates. The health care insurance industry soon became an unattractive business to be involved in, and therefore many companies dropped out of the indemnity insurance business entirely. It is, however, a system that has served the country well for decades, and there most likely will always be some type of indemnity insurance for that portion of the population who can afford the charge.

Closed Panel Health Care System

One additional system that has had some of the qualities of each of the previously described systems is the closed, single-panel health care provision system such as Kaiser-Permanente.

Kaiser owned its own hospitals, had large panels of physicians, provided all of its own services, handled its insurance functions internally, and provided care for a single fee. Many insurance companies sought to copy and develop this model internally for themselves but were often deselected by their patients. This staff-model health maintenance organization (HMO) has been falling steadily from favor, and many of these HMOs have already been disbanded.

Capitation

Capitation is defined as a method of payment that shifts risk and is most commonly used in HMOs with primary care physicians. With capitation, HMOs pay the primary care physician a fixed rate (or capitated fee) per month for all of the patient's primary care needs. Capitation attempts to stimulate preventive care and promote appropriate use of the delivery system by shifting the risk and unifying finance and delivery.

The capitation system can be either a single-specialty capitation, group capitation, group capitation with hospitals, or full capitation including all of the services. Capitation for a single specialty may be calculated by four different methods: fee-for-service, gross income, resource-based, or market-driven.

◊ DISTRIBUTION OF THE HEALTH CARE DOLLAR

The general distribution of health care costs, as well as the general distribution of health care dollars, has undergone drastic change in recent years. Numerous studies report how physicians' portion of health care income has grown, compared to hospitals' share. This change over the years is clearly evident by the continuing decrease in hospitals' portion and the resultant increase in the portion going to physicians in practice. Hospitals have acknowledged this change and in response have begun incorporating and purchasing numerous physician practices.

The following example demonstrates the distribution of health care dollars in managed care (Fig. 2). Let us assume that a managed care company charges $100 per member per month for its premium. The $100 is collected by the HMO, the HMO keeps 10% to 20% for it for administrative fees and profit. This leaves $80 to $90 in monies available to pay all of the various health care expenses. The apportionment of these monies will be divided among the physicians and hospitals, pharmacies and laboratories, ancillary care, home health care, and nontraditional and other kinds of services, with a designated amount going to each groups. Those funds going to physicians will need to be carefully managed as well, which in turn will produce various administrative costs.

Once those costs required to operate the practice have been paid, the remaining sum is the physician's income. However, the physician's ability to see patients is directly limited by the amount of time available. In addition, the agreement is limited by the panel of patients whom the physician is able to take care of, and revenue per month is fixed. Hence, the tremendous importance of managing costs. In the fee-for-service practice, where costs were fixed, income could expand (see Fig. 1), whereas income in the managed care environment is fixed, and costs must therefore be clearly and carefully focused. The provider who manages to have the lowest costs and the best practice location and who can provide the least amount of care consistent with good medical management will be the clear winner in health care of the future.

◊ COSTS OF THE PRACTICE OF MEDICINE

Regardless of the payment system, certain costs will be incurred in managing the care of patients. Today's caregivers must have a good communication system, as it is essential that they or their co-workers be accessible at all times. They must have a practice location that is close to and convenient for patients, an office decor that is acceptable to patients, a

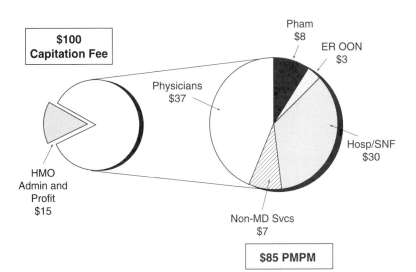

FIG. 2. Capitation rates: average payment per member per month *(PMPM)* with breakdown of payment distribution.

well maintained and clean facility, and adequate supplies and equipment as needed. They must have efficient and reliable employees who are appropriately rewarded and motivated to provide the quality of care that patients will find acceptable. A well organized business office that can effectively meet the needs of physicians, the HMO, and patients is essential to the operation of a successful practice. Lastly, caregivers must be able to be available during those hours when patients wish to be seen. All of these factors produce costs. How the practitioner manages these costs and provides a quality of service that patients find attractive will be the secret to success in the managed care world.

◊ IMPACT OF MANAGED CARE ON MEDICAL STUDENTS

Medical students frequently select the specialty that they wish to practice for their careers based in part on the economic rewards and lifestyle that they believe they ultimately will achieve. If they have to incur significant debt to do this, so be it. The rewards are great, and they can very quickly repay those sums previously borrowed to obtain their specialty certification. However, this scenario becomes a more tenuous thesis when salaries paid for the technical specialties begin to approach those of the cognitive specialties.

An initial effort to make this happen involved the use of relative value systems, which attempted to bridge the gap between procedural and nonprocedural specialties. Second, in a capitated medical practice, a physician who continues to be a very heavy user of higher technology in caring for disease will become an outlier in the group and therefore economically an unacceptable practitioner. Hence, the ability to expand one's efforts in the attempt to pay off heavy loans from student or resident days is greatly diminished. The debt of the average graduating student is quite significant and undoubtedly will affect many students' choice of specialties in the future (Fig. 3).

The number of specialists needed in the managed care environment is estimated to be only about one-half of those currently available. For example, in the tightly managed markets established in California, it is estimated that there are 60% too many cardiologists practicing, and, as a result, many in this particular profession have begun to leave those markets. With the need to achieve the minimum appropriate referrals for each service performed, the number of services will go down.

In addition, the competitive bidding by specialty networks for such services will cause prices to go down. This in turn will greatly affect the income of procedurally oriented specialists, as well as decreasing the opportunity to independently start a practice. All of these decreases negatively affect the ability of fellows and residents to repay the loans used to achieve their subspecialty certification. In response, the marketplace will undoubtedly adjust the numbers of people going into the specialties, as the opportunity for many to find good jobs and practice in their desired specialty will continue to decrease.

Another direct impact on medical students is the decrease in indigent care, which has long provided a source of patients for students and residents to manage and care for over the years. Even though students or residents provide this care at no cost, the supporting costs of approximately 50% of the usual clinical billing must still be provided (i.e., room, nurses, equipment, and supplies). With the falling margins in managed care, teaching institutions will have great difficulty in providing the clinical facilities for indigent care in the absence of a specified future subsidy.

The education and training of medical students and residents will be negatively impacted as well. The very long, repetitive medical record dictations by students and house officers in training, which are time-consuming and hence very expensive to transcribe, will disappear. Patients do not derive any benefit from such lengthy transcription, and the additional costs of this service are needlessly expended in providing such lengthy and often duplicated word processing. This inappropriate use of physicians' time is a significant example of the kind of training that managed care companies no longer wish their physicians to have. Indeed, the teaching

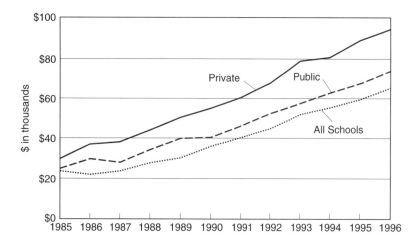

FIG. 3. Educational debt for graduates of public and private medical schools continues to rise.

institution of the future will have to train its students in an entirely different mindset if they are to practice successfully in the managed care environment.

◊ FUTURE OF HEALTH CARE

Physicians should remember that caring for patients is not really determined by the economic system that supports health care. Since the original Medicare bill was passed in 1965, we have seen an economic prospering of the health care enterprise. This system now consumes over 14% of our gross domestic product and indeed has made some other United States' industries no longer cost competitive worldwide. There is great pressure to decrease these expenditures. We spend as much on health care in the United States as the entire gross domestic product of India. And we will continue to be under these pressures. Balanced against control of costs are the increasing age of the population, the growing technology available, and the increased demands of a significant number of the population who do not have the resources to pay for health care. One must constantly remind oneself that this is not the business of medicine. *The true business of medicine is taking care of the sick and promoting wellness. It is not principally to determine the method by which patients are to pay for their health care.*

If physicians realize this and can keep that goal clearly in mind, then these changes will not likely be so devastating emotionally. People will continue to need caregivers, and the role of the physician in this team effort will be one of team leader. Medicine will still be rewarding, exciting, and a wonderful thing to do. Very few people get emotionally attached to their economist or their accountant; however, most patients are greatly appreciative of their physician, as well as the medical care they receive, and physicians will find it their greatest reward. As they go forward in their practice of medicine, they can still look forward to an exciting, rewarding, and important life, regardless of the system that pays for health care.

Some have said that managed care is a system that "neither manages to care nor manages to pay for it." I would suggest that this is neither the issue nor the focus. The primary issue is that the United States needs a health care system that cares for its patients and provides support and skillful service to meet their needs, all in a place where patients can most use it and in a way that they can afford. There is no greater personal satisfaction than being able to provide the wonderful technology, cutting-edge procedures, or specialized care for those patients who cannot afford it and would be economically devastated by such care if they should receive it.

The final chapter has not been written on how we shall provide quality health care in the future. Change will continue to be a part, just as it has been in previous years. Physicians should participate in and lead that change. It will be challenging, but it will surely be exciting.

SUMMARY POINTS

◊ Cost-containment results in Medicaid and Medicare programs have been greatly influenced by the increasing impact of managed care and its ability to control services and the decreasing overall costs of health care spending.

◊ Caregivers and policy makers continue to deal with difficult decisions created by the impact of new technology.

◊ Control of increasing costs is a major challenge for academic medical centers as they compare their high-cost high-tech care to the care provided at community hospitals.

◊ Advantages of the academic health centers include their "aura of quality" in faculty and research, coordination of care through physicians of varied disciplines, availability of tertiary services, and great diversification.

◊ Consumers consistently view managed care as restricting their choice of care providers, being more concerned about profit than quality of care, and decreasing the communication between physician and patient.

◊ In private practice, variable costs can be controlled through adjustments; however, in the academic institution, most costs are fixed and cannot be covered simply with increased volume of patients.

◊ Providers who offer the lowest costs, good practice locations, and the least amount of care consistent with effective medical management will be the most successful in the future health care industry.

◊ Specialty careers for medical students are negatively impacted by heavy debts incurred in obtaining specialty certification, decreasing need for specialist care in the managed care environment, decreased support for indigent care by teaching institutions, and reduction in physicians' available time for specialized training and education.

◊ The future of quality health care will require physicians to embrace, participate in, and be challenged by the changes occurring in the health care system.

◊ GLOSSARY OF TERMS USED IN MANAGED CARE

Capitation   A method of payment that shifts risk and melds finance and delivery to stimulate preventive care and promote appropriate use of the delivery system.

Community rating   Setting premium rates for a region based on the expected utilization and trends of the entire region, not the trends at a specific employer group.

Fee-for-service The traditional health care payment system, under which physicians and other providers receive a payment that does not exceed their billed charge for each unit of service provided.

Health Care Financing Administration (HCFA) Federal agency responsible for the administration of the Medicare and Medicaid programs.

Health maintenance organization (HMO) A system that focuses both on discounted fees and control of utilization. Utilization controls are most advanced in this system and include authorization from primary care physicians to visit specialists, utilization review, and disease management.

Independent practice association (IPA) Loose affiliation of independent private physicians who have created an incorporated business entity for the purpose of contracting with a managed care organization or multiple payors.

Integrated delivery system An organized, closed delivery system of physicians, hospitals, home care, and other providers that acts as a single, contractual delivery system. Patient referrals generally stay within the closed system. The system may be organized by a hospital, or a physician group (e.g., multispecialty group practice), or a carrier (e.g., staff-model HMO).

Per member per month (PMPM) Flat fee paid to each physician under a capitated agreement.

Preferred provider organization (PPO) Network of health care providers offering services on a discounted basis. Contracts are established with providers of medical care, and generally benefits are better if the patient uses the services of a preferred provider.

Primary care physician Physician who cares for the fundamental health needs of a patient population, is focused in internal medicine, family practice, or pediatrics, and acts as the HMO member's primary caregiver. An obstetrician or gynecologist may be considered a primary care physician.

Provider A physician, hospital, group practice, nursing home, pharmacy, or any individual or group of individuals that offers health care services.

Risk-sharing agreements Methods of payment that align economic incentives with goals of appropriate care (e.g., capitation) by sharing the risk of utilization. The provider is compensated based on target appropriateness and outcomes goals.

Staff-model HMO HMO that employs physicians and owns and operates facilities that provide care to its enrollment base. Members typically receive all care in one location.

◊ RECOMMENDED READINGS

Academic health centers in a managed care environment. *American Medical News* July 1994.

Aluise JJ, Konrad TR, Buckner B. Impact of IPAs on fee-for-service medical groups. *Health Care Manage Rev* 1989;14:55–63.

Anderson MV. How to review your own contracts. *J Tenn Med Assoc* 1989; 82:432–433.

Association of American Medical Colleges Task Force. *The financial structure of medical schools: report of the AAMC task force on medical school financing.* Washington, DC: Association of American Medical Colleges, 1996.

Aston G. HHS: managed care applied brakes to '95 health spending. *American Medical News* Feb 17, 1997:5–6.

Boyle K. How to decide which managed health care plans to offer. *Indiana Med* 1988;81:965–966.

Cook JV, Rodnick JE. Evaluating HMO/IPA contracts for family physicians: one group's experiences. *J Fam Pract* 1988;26:325–331.

Copeland EM, Flynn TC, Ross WE. Impact of managed care on one training program. *Arch Surg* 1995;130:930–931.

Desmarais HR, Holmes DE. *Managed care: ethical considerations.* Washington, DC: Association of Academic Health Centers, 1997.

Distribution of health care payment by population. *Managed Care Law Outlook* Sept 1995.

Drucker PF. Marketing 101 for a fast-changing decade. *The Wall Street Journal* November 20, 1990:A20.

Educational debt for graduates of public and private medical schools, 1985–96. AAMC Medical School Graduation Questionnaire, 1996.

Eelkema R. Contract law for physicians: the basics. *Minn Med* 1989; 72:97–101.

Employers rate their most important criteria for selecting an HMO. *Medical Benefits* Sept 15, 1995.

Federal investment in science and technology headed downward. *Life Science* January 21, 1997.

Feldman R, Kralewski J, Shapiro J, Chan H-C. Contracts between hospitals and health maintenance organizations. *Health Care Manage Rev* 1990; 15:47–60.

Fishman LE. *Medicare payments with an education label: fundamentals and the future.* Washington, DC: Association of American Medical Colleges, Division of Health Care Affairs, 1996.

Florida physicians' guide to contracting. Jacksonville, FL: Florida Physicians Association, 1990.

Foster H. *Price vs. quality . . . price wins: factors important to success in the marketplace. Ranking by 102 managed care organizations.* Oak Brook, IL: University Hospital Consortium, 1995.

Hall RT. *Rate setting calculations for capitating specialists.* Atlanta, GA: Towers Perrin IHC, 1996.

Health Care Financing Administration. *Who's in managed care?* HCFA Office of Managed Care, 1996.

Holthaus D. Enter exclusive contracts for right reasons. *Hospitals* 1989; 63(4):40.

Japsen B. Teaching hospitals face hard lessons. *Modern Healthcare* Feb 7, 1994.

Johnsson J. Managed care: CA price competition hot despite fewer contracts. *Hospitals* 1989;63(23):62.

Jones RE. *Academic medicine: institutions, programs and issues,* 7th ed. Washington, DC: Association of American Medical Colleges, Division of Institutions Planning and Development, 1997.

Kalm L, DeMuro PR. Hospital Contracting with PPOs. In: Boland P, ed: *The new healthcare market.* Homewood, IL, Dow Jones-Irwin, 1985.

Lagnado L. Patients give hospitals poor score card. *The Wall Street Journal* January 1997.

Life Science Newsletter Service. Consumer views on managed care. *Life Science* January 22, 1997.

MacStravic S. Market administration in health care delivery. *Health Care Manage Rev* 1989;14:41–48.

Managed care industry overview. Baltimore: Alex Brown & Sons, 1996.

Masterson BJ. Important points in managed care contracts. *Physician Executive J Manage* 1992;18(6):3–11.

McLean RA. Agency costs and complex contracts in health care organizations. *Health Care Manage Rev* 1989;14:65–71.

Medical Leadership Council. *Custom research highlights: winter 1996.* Washington, DC: Advisory Board Company, 1996.

Melnick GA, Zwanziger J, Verity-Guerra A. The growth and effects of hospital selective contracting. *Health Care Manage Rev* 1989;14:57–64.

The role of the tertiary hospital of the future. Washington, DC: Advisory Board Company, September 1996.

Summary of financial support for U.S. medical schools: 1996 AAMC data book. Washington, DC: Association of American Medical Colleges, 1996.

Teaching hospital vs. nonteaching hospital costs. *Hospitals and Health Networks* 1994.

Top ten most frequently capitated specialties. Washington, DC: Advisory Board Company, 1995.

Winslow R. Health-care costs may be heading up again. *The Wall Street Journal* January 21, 1997.

Watson R. *Funding graduate medical education: report to the Florida Medical Association.* February 16, 1996.

CHAPTER 3

Clinical Anatomy of the Female
——— ◊ ———
Philip J. Di Saia

The female reproductive tract is classically divided into external and internal genitalia. This chapter describes the normal anatomy of both as well as the blood, nerve, and lymphatic supplies to the pelvic structures. The pelvic anatomy is described from the abdominal and vaginal routes, because during gynecologic surgery the pelvic anatomy is approached from these perspectives.

◊ BONY PELVIS

The word pelvis is derived from Latin and Greek words meaning a basin or bowl. The bony pelvis is one of several pelvic supportive structures and provides the ultimate attachment of the pelvic soft tissues. The bony pelvis is formed anteriorly and laterally by the innominate bones and posteriorly by the sacrum and coccyx (Fig. 1). These bones are united by several strong ligaments. Unlike the shoulder girdle, which evolved for freedom of motion, the pelvic girdle is adapted for strength, support, and locomotion. In the erect position, the pelvic girdle is inclined forward. The plane of the inlet (Fig. 2) rests at an angle of about 60° with the horizontal, and the axis of the sacrum forms an angle of about 110° with the lumbar spine.

The outline of the plane of the pelvic inlet is regular and connects the promontory of the sacrum with the superior margin of the pubis (see Fig. 3). The circumference of the pelvic outlet is irregular and exhibits median and lateral notches. The median subpubic notch is formed by the union of the pubic rami at the pubic symphysis and is traversed by the urogenital apparatus. Each lateral sciatic notch lies between the lateral margin of the sacrum and coccyx and the ischial tuberosity. The sciatic notch is transformed into greater and lesser sciatic foramina by the sacrospinous and sacrotuberous ligaments. These foramina offer anatomic and pathologic communication between the intrapelvic and gluteal areas.

The bony and ligamentous pelvic mechanism serves to protect the pelvic viscera, support the vertebral column, and facilitate locomotion. The pelvic girdle protects the viscera contained within its cavity from all ordinary trauma, and only through the abdominal wall above or the perineum below are the pelvic contents likely to be injured. In supporting weight transmitted through the spine, the sacrum is forced downward so that the sacral promontory (see Fig. 2) faces forward and downward in the pelvis. In sitting, the weight is transmitted to the ischial tuberosities; in standing, weight is transmitted down the thighs.

The female pelvis differs in form and dimensions from the male pelvis. The female pelvic inlet is oval; the male pelvic inlet is heart-shaped. The female pelvis has a more regular outline than the male pelvis, in which the sacral promontory is more prominent and the sacrum and is longer and more curved. Although the extreme width of the pelvis does not differ materially between the genders, the flares of the ilia are flatter, the pelvic cavity is broader and shallower, the acetabula and ischial tuberosities are set farther apart, the bony walls of the pelvic canal are more vertical, and the subpubic angle is broader in the female than in the male pelvis (see Fig. 1).

The diameters of the pelvic inlet, middle pelvic plane, and the pelvic outlet are of practical importance in obstetrics (see Fig. 2) because the fetus must pass through the narrower opening of the lesser pelvis at birth. The transverse diameter of the pelvic inlet is 13 to 14 cm. The anteroposterior diameter from the sacral promontory to the superior margin of the pubic symphysis is approximately 11.5 cm. The oblique diameter measured from the sacroiliac joint to the opposite pectineal eminence is about 12.5 cm. The greatest anteroposterior diameter of the middle plane of the pelvis, measured from the third sacral vertebra to the middle of the pubic symphysis, is 12 cm. The anteroposterior diameter of the pelvic outlet, which extends from the tip of the coccyx to the inferior margin of the symphysis, is approximately 9 cm, but it may be increased 2 or 3 cm because of the mobility of the coccyx. The transverse diameter of the outlet between the two ischial tuberosities is 10 to 12 cm.

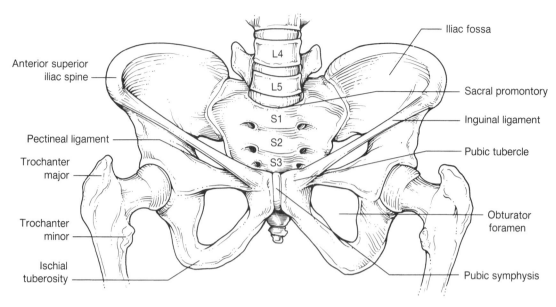

FIG. 1. Anterior view of the pelvic bones.

◊ PELVIC VISCERA

Inside the pelvic cavity rest the pelvic organs most commonly involved in gynecologic surgery: the bladder, uterus, adnexa, and rectum (Fig. 3). In addition to the urogenital organs, the sigmoid colon, cecum, and ileum are components of the pelvic anatomy. As the uterus rises up and forward from the extraperitoneal space during fetal development, it lifts the serosa into a peritoneal covering for the uterine fundus and the contents of the two broad ligaments.

Broad Ligament

The broad ligament is a tent-like reflection of the peritoneum and has an irregularly quadrilateral outline. It contains between its layers the fallopian tube; the ovary and the round ligament; the uterine and ovarian blood vessels, nerves, lymphatics, and fibromuscular and fatty areola tissue; and a portion of the ureter as it passes lateral to the uterosacral ligaments over the lateral angles of the vagina and into the base of the bladder (Fig. 4). The ureter emerges from behind the

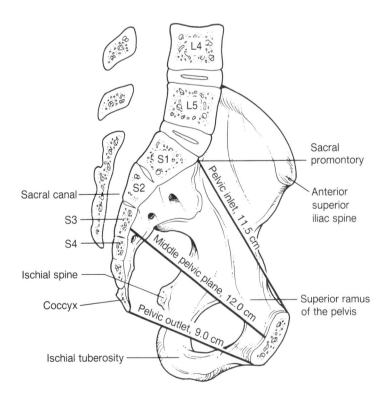

FIG. 2. Lateral view of the pelvic bones.

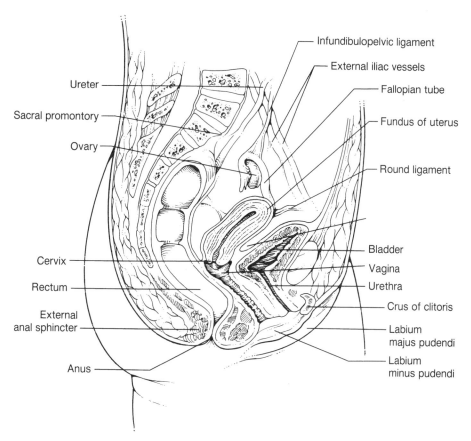

FIG. 3. Lateral view of the pelvic viscera.

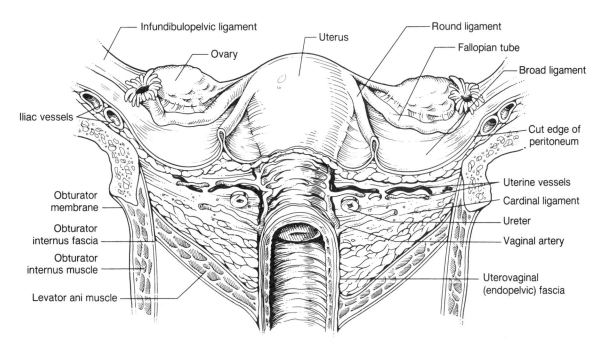

FIG. 4. Ligamentous, fascial, and muscular support of the pelvic viscera.

ovary and under its vessels to pass behind the uterine and superior and middle vesicle arteries (Fig. 5). It then courses near the lateral fornix of the vagina, passing 8 to 12 mm from the cervix and vaginal wall before reaching the bladder. At the bladder, the ureters are about 5 cm apart. They pass through the bladder wall on an oblique 2-cm-long course in an internal, medial, and downward direction. The ureter opens into the bladder by two slit-like apertures, the ureteral orifices, that are about 2.5 cm apart when the bladder is empty.

The 3-mm-thick wall of the ureter has three layers: connective tissue, muscle, and mucous membrane. The muscular coat has an external circular and an internal longitudinal layer throughout its course, and it has an external longitudinal layer in the lower one-third of its course. The mucous membrane is longitudinally plicated and covered by transitional epithelium. The intermittent, peristaltic action of the ureteral musculature propels urine into the bladder. The ureters enter the urinary bladder at the superior lateral angle of its base. Because the ureters pass under the bladder for several centimeters, pressure in the bladder compresses the ureters and prevents the backflow of urine. This oblique passage of the ureter through the bladder wall constitutes a valvular arrangement, although no true valve exists. The circular fibers of the intramural portion of the ureter possess a sphincter-like action.

The pelvic portion of the ureter receives its blood supply from a direct branch of the hypogastric artery, anastomosing superiorly in its adventitia with the branches from the iliolumbar and inferiorly with the branches of the vesical and middle hemorrhoidal arteries. The lymphatic drainage passes along the hypogastric vessels to the hypogastric and external iliac nodes, continuing up the ureters to their middle portion, with drainage directly to the periaortic and precaval nodes.

Bladder

The urinary bladder is located anteriorly in the pelvis, immediately posterior to the pubic symphysis. The upper or posterosuperior surface of the bladder is rounded and is covered by the peritoneum of the anterior wall of the pelvis. Posteriorly, the peritoneum passes on to the uterus at the junction of the cervix and corpus, continuing upward on the anterior surface to form the vesical uterine pouch. When the bladder is empty, the normal uterus rests on its superior surface.

The mucous membrane of the interior of the bladder is rose colored and lies in irregular folds called rugae that become flattened by distention. The three angles of the vesical triangle, called the trigone, are represented by the orifices of the two ureters and the internal urethral orifice. The internal urethral orifice usually is at the lowest point of the bladder, at the junction of the inferolateral and posterior surfaces. The mucosa, the innermost coat of the bladder wall, is a mucous membrane containing transitional epithelium; transitional epithelium is able to stretch. The mucous membrane rests on the submucosa, a layer of areola tissue that connects the mucosa and the two muscular coats of the organ. The blood supply to the bladder comes from branches of the hypogastric artery. The umbilical artery, a terminal branch of the hypogastric artery, gives off the superior vesical artery before its obliterated portion. The middle vesical artery may arise from the superior vessels, or it may come from the umbilical artery itself. The inferior vesical artery usually arises directly from the hypogastric artery. The veins form an extensive plexus on both sides of the bladder and drain to the hypogastric trunk.

Urethra

The female urethra is a small tube that is 2.5 to 5.0 cm long with an average caliber of 2 to 8 mm. The external orifice lies

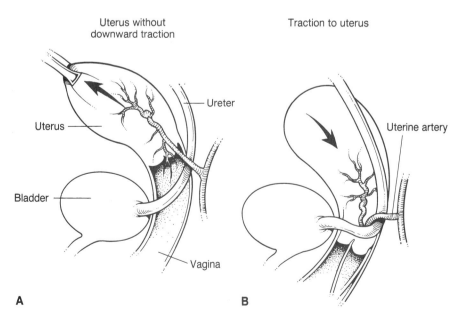

FIG. 5. Ureter placement during **(A)** abdominal hysterectomy and **(B)** vaginal hysterectomy.

between the labia minora immediately anterior to the vaginal opening and posterior to the clitoris. On either side of the midline, close to the posterior margin of the ureteral orifice, lie the minute openings of the paraurethral ducts (i.e., Skene glands). The urethra has pelvic and perineal divisions. The intrapelvic portion, about 2 to 3 cm long, begins at the vesicle orifice 2 to 3 cm behind the pubic synthesis and terminates where the urethra penetrates the urogenital diaphragm. The internal vesical sphincter, which helps to control urination, surrounds the urethra at the vesical neck. The perineal portion is about 1 cm long and traverses the urogenital diaphragm about 1 to 2 cm below the subpubic angle. The urethra opens into the vaginal vestibule about 2 cm posterior to the clitoris.

Vagina

The vagina is a tubular structure extending from the introitus to the cervix uteri. It traverses the urogenital diaphragm and extends through the genital hiatus of the levator ani. It lies in a horizontal position above the levator ani with the uterus angulated above it. The anterior wall of the vagina usually is shorter (9 cm) than the posterior wall (9 to 10 cm).

The vaginal blood supply includes the hypogastric artery, the uterine arteries, the middle rectal artery, and the inferior vaginal artery from the internal pudendal artery.

The sympathetic nervous supply to the vagina is from the hypogastric plexus. Parasympathetic innervation comes from the sacral region (S2–S4) of the cord by way of the pelvic nerve. The inferior pole of the vagina is much more sensitive than the superior vagina because it receives sensory branches from the pudendal nerve.

The vagina is supported by several ligamentous attachments. The lower one-third of the vagina is attached to the pelvic diaphragm, the urogenital diaphragm, and the perineal body. The middle one-third is attached to the pelvic diaphragm and the cardinal ligaments. The upper one-third rests on the levator plate and is attached to the cardinal and uterosacral ligaments.

Perineum

The perineum is divided into the urogenital triangle and the anal triangle (Fig. 6). The urogenital triangle contains the external genitalia or the vulva. The fat pad of the mons is anterior and inferior to the pubic bone. It extends posteriorly as the labia majora. Medial to the labia majora are two folds of skin called the labia minora, and the superior pole of the minora is the clitoris.

The vestibule of the vagina is the opening through which the urethra and vaginal introitus pass to the outside. The vaginal opening is posterior to the urethra. The clitoris is

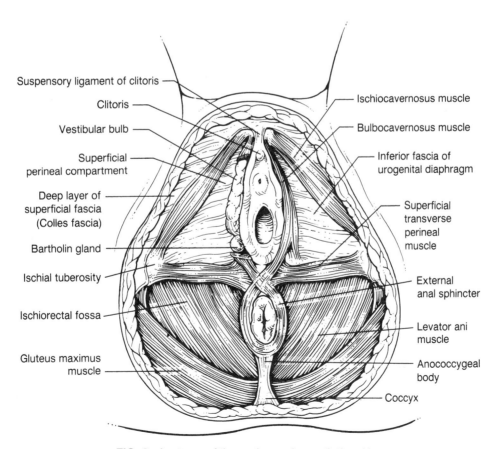

Suspensory ligament of clitoris

Clitoris

Vestibular bulb

Superficial perineal compartment

Deep layer of superficial fascia (Colles fascia)

Bartholin gland

Ischial tuberosity

Ischiorectal fossa

Gluteus maximus muscle

Ischiocavernosus muscle

Bulbocavernosus muscle

Inferior fascia of urogenital diaphragm

Superficial transverse perineal muscle

External anal sphincter

Levator ani muscle

Anococcygeal body

Coccyx

FIG. 6. Anatomy of the perineum beneath the skin.

part of the perineum and part of the vestibule of the vagina, and it makes up the superior aspect of this region. The blood supply to the urogenital diaphragm is the internal pudendal artery, a branch of the hypogastric or internal iliac artery. This area is innervated by the perineal branch of the pudendal nerve, the perineal branch of the posterior femoral cutaneous nerve, and the ilioinguinal and genitofemoral nerves. The posterior femoral cutaneous nerve (S2–S3) supplies the sensory function to the posterior surface of the thigh. The perineal branch may be more important to the area of the urogenital diaphragm. The ilioinguinal and the genitofemoral nerves also supply the mons and the labia majora.

The fascial layers over the urogenital diaphragm are often misunderstood. There are deep fascial layers that cover the muscles, but above them are the superficial fascial layers (i.e., those contiguous with the Scarpa and Camper loose connective tissue planes that are divided by fat and areolar tissue). Infection in these superficial fascial layers and spaces can spread as cellulitis or spread in the form of necrotizing fasciitis onto the abdominal wall.

Vulva

The structures of the vulva are shown in Fig. 7. The mons pubis, an elevation of adipose tissue covered by coarse pubic hair, is anterior and superior to the pubic symphysis. The labia majora extends from the mons to the area of the posterior fourchette and is homologous to the scrotum in men.

The labia minora are two longitudinal folds of skin between the vaginal opening and the labia majora. They form the prepuce and frenulum of the clitoris and are homologous to the penile urethra and skin of the penis. The clitoris is an erectile organ at the anterior junction of the labia minora, at the top of the vaginal vestibule. It is approximately 2 cm long and less than 1 cm wide and consists of two crura attached to the periosteum of the pubic symphysis. A layer of skin called the prepuce is formed at the point where the labia minora unite and cover the body of the clitoris. The exposed portion of the clitoris is the glans. The clitoris is homologous to the glans penis in men.

Anterior to the vaginal orifice and posterior to the clitoris is the urethral orifice. The urethra is a membranous structure

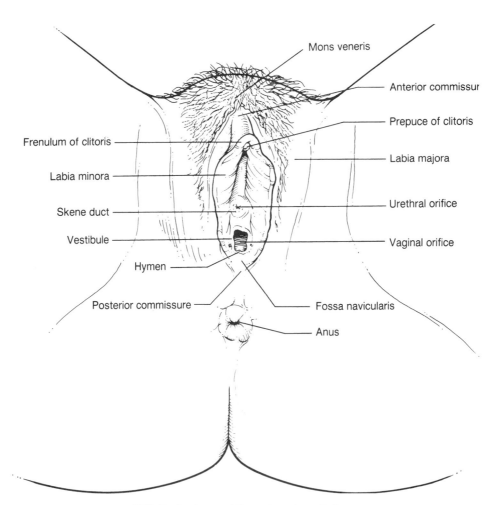

FIG. 7. Anatomy of the external genitalia.

for the passage of urine; in women, it is approximately 3 to 5 cm long. The proximal two-thirds is lined with stratified transitional epithelium, and the distal one-third is stratified squamous epithelium.

On either side of the urethral orifice are the openings of the ducts of the Skene glands, also known as paraurethral glands. The glands secrete mucus, and they empty into the urethra and the vestibule of the vagina. The paraurethral glands are homologous to the prostate.

The Bartholin glands, also called the greater vestibular glands, lie on the posterolateral surface of the vaginal opening. Each gland is covered with cuboidal epithelium, and the duct is lined with transitional epithelium. The glands produce a mucoid secretion. The greater vestibular glands are homologous to the Cowper glands (i.e., bulbourethral glands) in men.

Vasculature

The pelvis contains blood vessels to the lower abdomen, legs, and pelvic organs (Fig. 8). The arteries that supply the pelvic musculature run along the lateral pelvic wall, and the visceral branches to the organ systems travel from their source near the sacroiliac joint.

The main pelvic vasculature is derived from the common or internal iliac artery (i.e., hypogastric artery), which runs retroperitoneally posterior to the ureter and divides into anterior and posterior branches (see Fig. 8). The anterior division is divided into seven branches: umbilical and superior vesical, uterine, vaginal, middle rectal, obturator, internal pudendal, and inferior gluteal arteries. The posterior division divides into the iliolumbar, lateral sacral, and superior gluteal arteries. In 40% of patients, the obturator artery arises from the inferior epigastric artery, a branch of the external iliac artery.

The ovarian arteries are a direct branch of the aorta just inferior to the renal arteries. They traverse retroperitoneally and course bilaterally to enter the infundibulopelvic ligaments. The ovarian veins drain to the vena cava on the right and to the left renal vein on the left. The hypogastric and ovarian arteries can be ligated in a life-threatening bleed without compromise to the pelvic organs because the pelvic collateral circulation is abundant. The course and origin of pelvic blood vessels are highly variable from individual to

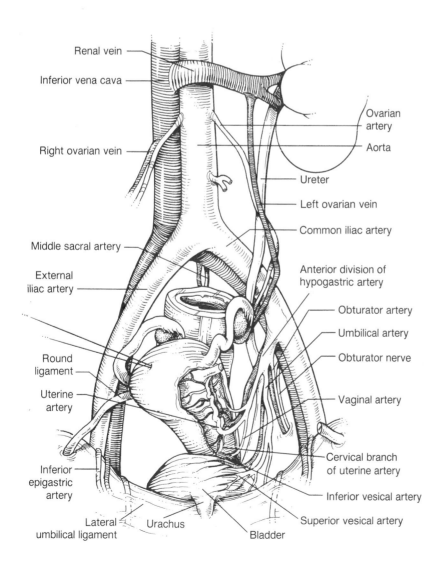

FIG. 8. Blood supply of the pelvis.

individual. Even in the same individual, the blood supply is bilaterally identical only 50% of the time.

Lymphatic System

The lymph nodes follow the arterial system but do not always drain in the same pattern (Fig. 9). The external genitalia, anus, and anal canal drain to the superficial inguinal nodes. The lower one-third of the vagina drains to the sacral nodes and the internal and common iliac nodes but may also connect with the lymphatics of the vulva and drain to the inguinal nodes (Fig. 10). The upper two-thirds of the vagina drains more as the cervix does. The cervix drains to the external or internal iliac and sacral nodes; sampling these nodes is important when a laparotomy is performed for stage I or IIA cancer of the cervix. The lower uterus drains to the external iliac nodes. It is important to perform pelvic node sampling of the external iliac, obturator, and paraaortic areas in patients with endometrial carcinoma because there is an ap-

proximately 10% incidence of lymph node involvement in stage I disease. The upper uterus drains into the ovarian lymphatics to the lumbar nodes. The lymphatics of the ovaries drain out of the pelvis to the lumbar nodes. In vulvar cancer, the primary lesion may be in the midline, where the spread can be to either or both sides, and bilateral dissection of the lymphatics usually is performed. When a vulvar lesion is unilateral, spread to the involved side only is more common.

The vulva contains a multilayered meshwork of lymphatics always limited to an area medial to the genitocrural fold. The lymph nodes of the inguinal area are in two groups. One group is arranged in a pattern parallel and inferior to the inguinal ligament (oblique group of nodes, Fig. 1), and the other group is arranged along the saphenous vein (vertical group). Borgno and his colleagues have clarified the location of the inguinal nodes in relation to the fascia cribrosa, previously described as a partition separating the superficial from the deep inguinal nodes. They demonstrated that the deep inguinal (femoral) nodes are always situated within the open-

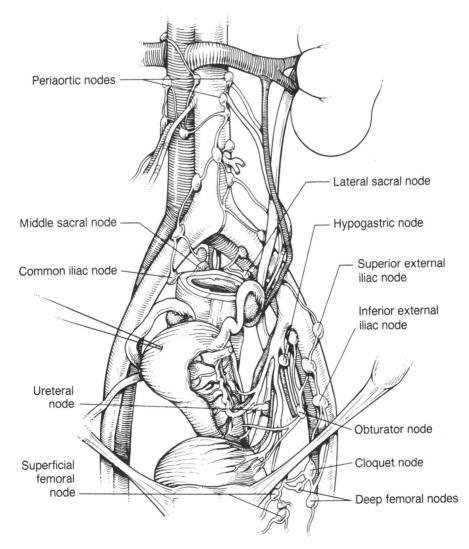

FIG. 9. Lymphatic drainage of the pelvis.

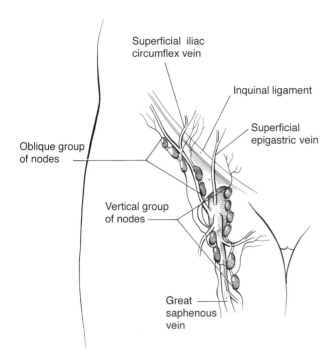

FIG. 10. The superficial inguinal lymph nodes can be divided into the oblique group and the vertical group. (From ref. 5.)

ings in the fascia cribrosa at the fossa ovalis, and there are no lymph nodes distal to the lower margin of the fossa ovalis beneath the cribriform fascia. The implication of this is that an adequate deep inguinal lymphadenectomy does not require removal of the fascia cribrosa because they also report that no lymph nodes were found between the femoral vein and artery or lateral to the artery.

Nerve Supply

The striated muscles of the vaginal outlet and the skin of the perineum receive somatic motor and sensory fibers from the lumbosacral plexus. The pelvic viscera are supplied by the autonomic plexuses, which convey sympathetic and parasympathetic motor and visceral sensory nerves to these organs. The ventral roots of the lumbar and sacral nerves derive from the lumbosacral plexuses. The obturator nerve, the lumbosacral trunk of the lumbosacral plexus, and the entire sacral plexus lie in proximity to the pelvic organs, but only certain branches of the plexuses are directly involved in pelvic innervation.

Sympathetic innervation causes muscular contraction and vasoconstriction, and the parasympathetic supply is responsible for muscle relaxation and vasodilation. Most autonomic fibers enter the pelvis by way of the superior hypogastric plexus. The superior hypogastric plexus runs from the fourth lumbar vertebra to the hollow of the sacrum. It descends into the base of the broad ligament to join the parasympathetic systems from the pelvic plexuses. The motor fibers and accompanying sensory nerves reach the pelvic plexus from S2, S3, and S4 by way of the pelvic nerves called the nervi erigentes. The sensory nerves from the uterus, which accompany the sympathetic nerves and enter the cord at T11 and T12, are responsible for referred pain to the abdomen. The afferents from the cervix (S2 to S4 origin) are referred to the lower back and lumbosacral regions.

The L5, S2, and S3 nerves come from the spinal foramina, merge, and then form the sciatic nerve, which exits between the ischial spine and the inferior border of the piriformis muscle. The internal pudendal nerve arises from the sciatic nerve after it leaves the pelvis (Fig. 11).

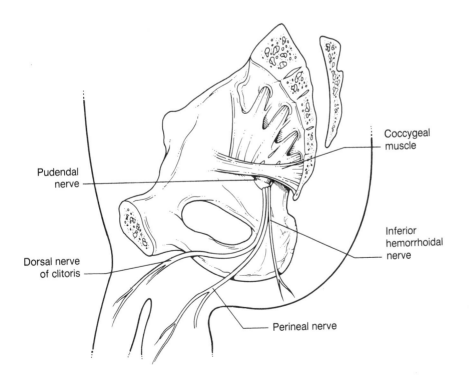

FIG. 11. The pudendal nerve has its origin in the S2 to S4 sacral plexus. As it enters the pudendal canal, it gives off the inferior rectal nerve and then divides into the perineal nerve and the dorsal nerve of the clitoris. The pudendal nerve and its branches innervate the muscles, skin, and erectile tissue of the perineum.

The sacral plexus includes the lumbosacral trunk and the first, second, and third sacral nerves. The S3 and S4 plexuses supply the levator and coccygeus muscles of the pelvic diaphragm, and S4 supplies the perineum. The autonomic innervation to the pelvic organs includes sympathetic, parasympathetic, motor, and visceral sensory fibers. The inferior hypogastric plexus supplies the rectum, uterus, vagina, bladder, and ureter. The visceral afferent pain pathways of the ovary, uterine tube, fundus, body of the uterus, and cervix connect with the spinal cord at the T11 and T12 levels. Pain is referred to the corresponding dermatomes on the skin and is usually from the lower abdomen. Injury to the sacral plexus produces motor and sensory changes that can be disabling.

The genitofemoral nerve (L1 and L2 origin) courses on the belly of the psoas major muscle to the anterior thigh and supplies the labia majora in women and the scrotum in men. Injury produces sensory changes. The obturator nerve (L2 to L4 origin) passes posterior to the iliac vessels and lateral to the hypogastric vessels. It supplies motor branches to the adductor muscles of the leg as well as to the hip, knee joint, and medial thigh. Injury results in loss of thigh adduction, loss of power in internal and external rotation, and sensory losses in the same areas.

◊ RECOMMENDED READINGS

1. Borgno G, Micheletti L, Barbero M. Topographic distribution of groin nodes: a study of 50 female cadavers. *J Reprod Med* 1990;35:1127.
2. Clemente CD. *Gray's anatomy, 30th ed.* Philadelphia: Lea & Febiger, 1985.
3. Crafts RC. *A textbook of human anatomy, 3rd ed.* New York: Wiley & Sons, 1985.
4. DeLancey JOL. Structural aspects of the extrinsic continence mechanism. *Obstet Gynecol* 1988;72:296.
5. Di Saia PJ, Creasman WT. *Clinical gynecologic oncology, 5th ed.* St. Louis: CV Mosby, 1997.
6. Kuhn RJ, Hollyock VE. Observations on the anatomy of the rectovaginal pouch and septum. *Obstet Gynecol* 1982;59:445.
7. Netter FH. *Reproductive system. The Ciba collection of medical illustrations, vol 2.* Summit, NJ: CIBA Pharmaceutical Products, 1984.
8. Nichols DH. *Vaginal surgery, 2nd ed.* Baltimore: Williams & Wilkins, 1983.
9. Wilson DB, Wilson WJ. *Human anatomy, 2nd ed.* Cambridge: Oxford University Press, 1983.
10. Zacharin RF. Functional anatomy of the pelvic floor. *Contemp Ob/Gyn Suppl* 1989;34:111.

CHAPTER 4

Embryo, Fetus, and Placenta: Normal and Abnormal

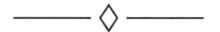

Catherine Craven
Kenneth Ward

Remarkable advances have occurred in our understanding of normal human embryology, placentation, and fetal growth. In an increasing number of pregnancies, an abnormality may be detected early in gestation, and its etiology determined by investigations using sonographic and genetic analysis. A placental examination with gross and microscopic studies will yield additional information about the course of the pregnancy. This chapter reviews reproduction, embryology, fetal development, and placentation in normal human pregnancies. The pathologic findings in pregnancy failure, placental lesions, and some birth defects are discussed.

Specific terms are used to describe events in reproduction and pregnancy. *Pregenesis* defines the time after the formation of the germ cells and before the union of sperm and egg. This period begins with the differentiation of primitive germ cells and their migration from the yolk sac, through the hindgut, to the genital ridge. Pregenesis ends with formation of gametes, or karyogamy. *Aneuploidies,* or abnormal numbers of chromosomes, may occur as a consequence of abnormal meiotic division of chromosomes in gamete formation.

Conception is the fertilization of an ovum by sperm. The time after conception is the *developmental age. Gestational age* is the time calculated from the last menstrual period and by convention exceeds the developmental age by 2 weeks.

The *preembryonic period* is defined as the first 2 weeks after fertilization. The *blastogenetic period* is the first 4 weeks of human development. In days 2 to 4 after fertilization, following a series of cellular divisions, a fertilized oocyte becomes a *blastomere,* or *morula.* At the 8- to 16-cell stage, the blastomere becomes a *blastocyst* as a central cavity is formed. The cells on the outer layer differentiate to become *trophoblasts.* Monozygotic twinning and certain complex fetal anomalies often represents abnormalities of blastogenesis.

The *embryonic disk* is formed from the inner cell mass. With the folding of the disk in week 2 of development, the *embryonic period* begins. *Organogenesis* occurs between 4 and 8 weeks after conception. The conceptus is termed a *fetus* after 8 weeks of life; it has a crown-rump length of 30 mm and a gestational age of 10 weeks. The *fetal period* continues until birth.

◊ PREGENESIS

Human germ cells are first identified in an embryo during week 4 of gestation, developing in the yolk sac near the allantoic stalk (Fig. 1). Germ cells migrate dorsally from the wall of the yolk sac through the hindgut, increasing their numbers by mitosis. The cells accumulate in the genital ridge, near the developing kidneys. By week 7, they condense into cords in the developing gonad. In the presence of a Y chromosome, the gonad becomes a testis. Seminiferous cords[28] are seen in the developing testes beginning in the 10th week. In the female embryo, a few weeks later, primary ovarian follicles form when the oogonia become surrounded by smaller follicular cells.

The formation of the sperm and ovum occurs by a specialized form of cell division called *meiosis.* The process allows the creation of novel gene arrangements through recombination of the DNA and yields a haploid cell. Fertilization returns the germ cells to a diploid state. In the male, the production of sperm does not begin until puberty, but sperm production continues into old age. In the testes, meiosis results in the formation of four haploid sperm. In the female fetus, germ cell meiosis begins *in utero* during the fifth month of development. By the time of birth, most oogonia have become oocytes. Ovarian meiosis yields a single haploid ovum and nonfunctional polar bodies.[28]

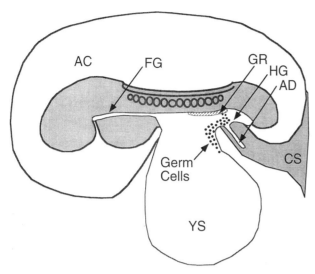

FIG. 1. In developmental week 4, germ cells develop in the yolk sac *(YS)*. These cells increase in number by mitosis and begin to migrate to the genital ridge *(GR)*. The cells traverse the allantoic duct *(AD)* and the hindgut *(HG)* *(AC, amniotic cavity; CS, connecting stalk; FG, foregut)*.

◇ FERTILIZATION AND BLASTOGENESIS

For normal fertilization to occur, *ovulation* is necessary: The ovum must leave the ovary and be carried into the fallopian tube. The unfertilized ovum is surrounded by its zona pellucida. This oocyte has completed its first meiotic division and carries its first polar body. Usually, fertilization occurs within 24 hours after ovulation in the third of the tube adjacent to the ovary. The sperm penetrates the zona pellucida and fuses its plasma membranes with those of the ovum. The sperm nucleus and other cellular contents enter the egg's cytoplasm. Fertilization activates the ovum to complete meiosis II and to discharge an additional polar body.

The next step for a successful pregnancy is *cleavage:* the division of the fertilized egg to form the multicellular blastomere. Normally, 4 days are required to reach the 16-cell stage (Table 1). The blastomere passes from the fallopian tube into the uterine cavity. A central cystic space develops, and the blastomere becomes a blastocyst.[9]

TABLE 1. *Developmental ages*

Postconception day	Formation of tissue or organ
4	Blastula
7–12	Implantation
13	Primitive streak
16	Neural plate
19–21	First somite
23–25	Closure of anterior neuropore
25–27	Arms bud
25–27	Closure of posterior neuropore
28	Legs bud
44	Sexual differentiation

◇ IMPLANTATION

On days 5 to 6 of development, the blastocyst adheres to the endometrium. Specific cellular adhesion molecules are found on the cells of the secretory endometrial surface. These unite with the outer layers of the blastocyst. After attachment, the blastocyst crosses the surface epithelium into the endometrial stroma. There is proliferation of the endometrium in early pregnancy, and the blastocyst becomes embedded in the thickened endometrium.

◇ PLACENTATION

During week 2, cells in the outer cell mass differentiate into trophoblasts. A trophoblastic shell forms the initial boundary between the embryo and the endometrium (Fig. 2). These trophoblasts are the precursor cells for the placenta and membranes. Those trophoblasts nearest the myometrium form the placental disk, while the other trophoblasts form the chorionic membranes.[9]

In early placental development, there is proliferation of the mononuclear cytotrophoblasts in the trophoblastic shell. Multinucleated syncytiotrophoblast cells are seen on the blastocyst surface. Spaces or lacunae appear between the cytotrophoblasts in the trophoblastic shell. Some cytotrophoblasts, termed *X cells,* migrate away from the shell into the decidua and erode into maternal vessels. Maternal red cells may be seen in the trophoblastic lacunae in the second postconception week.[9]

Trophoblastic infiltration of the endometrium and myometrium is associated with alteration of the maternal vessels. The spiral arteries undergo structural alterations that result in the dilation of the vessels. Normal muscular and elastic tissues are replaced by fibrinoid material. Vascular lumina become dilated, and there is infiltration by cytotrophoblasts. The maternal endothelium becomes discontinuous. In this manner, the spiral arteries are transformed into uteroplacental vessels that directly open into the placental intervillous space.[24]

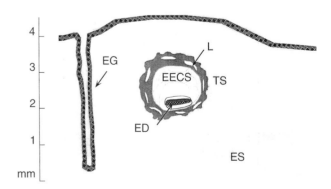

FIG. 2. At 13 days postconception, the blastocyst has implanted into the endometrial stroma *(ES)*. The trophoblast shell *(TS)* isolates the embryonic disk *(ED)* from the surrounding endometrium. Spaces or lacunae *(L)* begin to form in the trophoblast shell *(EECS, extraembryonic coelomic space; EG, endometrial glands)*.

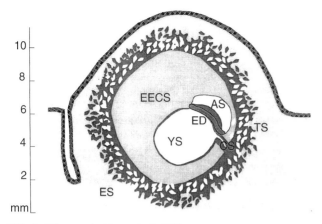

FIG. 3. The trophoblast shell *(TS)* has expanded on day 15, with the formation of primary chorionic villi. The gestational sac seen at ultrasound consists of the extraembryonic coelomic space *(EECS)*, the yolk sac *(YS)* and the amniotic sac *(AS)* *(CS,* connecting stalk; *ES,* endometrial stroma).

Concurrent with the invasion of the trophoblasts into the decidua and the development of uteroplacental vessels, primary placental villi are being formed (Fig. 3). In postconception week 2, cords of trophoblasts grow into the trophoblast shell and expand the lacunae. Some cords of trophoblasts remain attached to the trophoblastic shell and become the anchoring villi. Budding of other cytotrophoblasts into the lacunae form the primary villi.[2]

At about 21 days of life, extraembryonic mesenchymal cells grow into these buds of trophoblasts, transforming the primary villi into secondary villi. A villous core is formed by the ingrowth of fibroblasts. Soon thereafter, embryonic vascular cells grow into the mesenchyme, forming capillaries. The establishment of a vascular network changes the secondary villi to tertiary ones. Umbilical vessels in the connecting stalk join the embryo's blood vessels to the developing placental villi. A closed vascular system is formed, and the human heart begins to beat.[9] The villous tissue proliferates by budding and branching like limbs on a tree (Fig. 4A).[2]

The placenta continues to grow in size as the pregnancy progresses, and it occupies a greater proportion of the endometrial surface. With maturation of the placenta, the trophoblast layer becomes progressively thinner and the villous diameter decreases. To allow nutrient exchange, fetal capillaries enlarge and become apposed to the trophoblastic surface (Fig. 4B). There is a decrease in the distance from the maternal blood to the fetal blood from 50 to 100 μm in the 2nd month of gestation to 4 to 5 μm in the last month of pregnancy.

◊ THE EMBRYO: BLASTOGENESIS AND ORGANOGENESIS

The embryonic disk undergoes a series of developmental steps to become an embryo[23] (Table 1). By developmental day 15, a bilaminar disk has formed. The ectoderm layer is capped by the amniotic cavity (Fig. 3). On the other disk surface, the endoderm layer connects to the yolk sac.

The next step is termed *gastrulation.* Gastrulation encompasses the appearance of midline structures and the formation of the cranial and caudal regions. The embryo develops a left and a right side and a dorsal and a ventral axis. This occurs simultaneously with the development of a mesoderm, resulting in a trilaminar disk.

In developmental days 16 to 24, the mesoderm forms the vascular system and heart (Fig. 5). The placental villi are vascularized. The neural tube is formed by the closure of the neural folds, and there are well defined head and tail regions. Somites appear, and pharyngeal arches begin to form. The endoderm in the foregut fuses to form a tube. Buds from the foregut tube become the pulmonary and hepatic primordia. The urogenital system forms, and germ cells migrate to the developing genital ridges. The hindgut joins to the allantoic duct, which develops in the connecting stalk.

Between days 24 and 28, gastrulation is completed (Fig. 6). The embryo folds to form a curve in the anterior-to-posterior plane. Lateral folding closes the abdominal wall. Limb buds appear. The umbilical cord is formed by the amniotic mem-

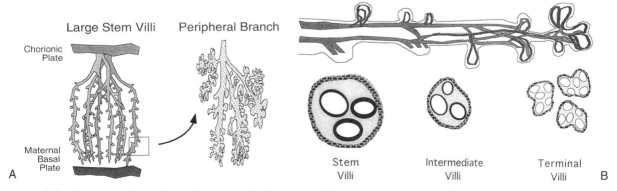

FIG. 4. Arborization of the villous tree. **A:** The stem villi branch as they grow. This process greatly expands the surface area of the placenta, allowing greater exchange of the fetal and maternal circulations. **B:** The stem villi give rise to the intermediate villi, which in turn branch to terminal villi.

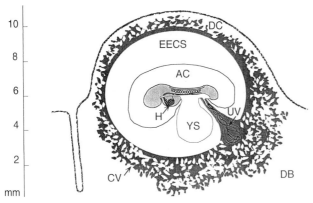

FIG. 5. The embryo at 23 days has developed a beating heart *(H)*. Umbilical vessels *(UV)* in the connecting stalk carry embryonic red cells from the yolk sac *(YS)* to the chorionic villi *(CV)* (*AC*, amniotic cavity; *DB*, decidua basalis; *DC*, decidua capsularis; *EECS*, extraembryonic coelomic space).

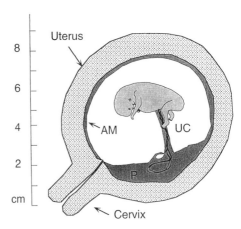

FIG. 7. In weeks 5 and 6, the external structures have formed: head, face, limbs, torso, and body wall. The umbilical cord *(UC)* elongates, giving the lower limbs room to grow. The amniotic membrane *(AM)* fuses with the chorion to form the placental membrane. The uterus has enlarged to accommodate the embryo, amniotic sac, and placenta.

brane encircling the connecting stalk and yolk sac. Placentation is completed by the fusion of the amniotic membrane to the decidua parietalis.

Organogenesis occurs from developmental days 28 to 56. It is characterized by the formation of organs, and histologic differentiation of the tissues (Fig. 7). The face forms by fusion of the frontonasal process and the branchial arches. The heart tube folds, and its chambers and outflow tracts are formed. The intestines undergo elongation and rotation. The urogenital tissues develop into the kidneys, gonads, and associated structures.

The *fetal period* begins after 8 weeks of life and continues until birth. The fetal crown-rump length increases from 1.4 cm to 36 cm. The internal and external structures grow. The fetal weight increases from 5 g to 3400 g. The placenta grows from 5 cm in diameter and 14 g in weight at 8 weeks to 22 cm in diameter and 470 g in weight at 40 weeks. Only the central nervous system continues to undergo significant structural and histologic maturation *in utero*. Myelination of some nerve fibers does not begin until the first year of postnatal life. Maturation of the central nervous system continues for several years in early childhood before maturation is completed.

◊ ABNORMALITIES OF EARLY PREGNANCIES: PREGNANCY FAILURE

The incidence of pregnancy failure depends on the definitions used for pregnancy and pregnancy loss and on the clinical population studied.[6] The probability of the delivery of a live newborn to a healthy, sexually active, fertile woman per menstrual cycle has been estimated at 20% to 30%. This suggests that in 70% to 80% of cycles, an ovum is released, but fertilization, implantation, or continued pregnancy did not occur. In the presence of sperm and egg, a failure of fertilization is estimated to be 10%. This failure of conception contributes to infertility, but not to actual pregnancy failure. Histologic studies of conception and implantation have demonstrated that implantation failure was frequent.[6] Loss of a fertilized ovum due to implantation failure has been estimated at 12% to 15%.

The rates of early spontaneous abortion may be estimated. Currently, the detection of the β chain of human chorionic gonadotropin (β-hCG) is a hallmark of blastomere implantation.[6] This assay is used as presumptive evidence of pregnancy. Before the test was available, pregnancy was diagnosed clinically by cessation of menses and physical changes to the cervix and uterus. Pregnancy failure in women with a positive β-hCG test but without "clinical" pregnancy is about 30%. As many of these pregnancy failures occur at the time of the expected menses, the expelled tissue rarely has been studied to determine an etiology.

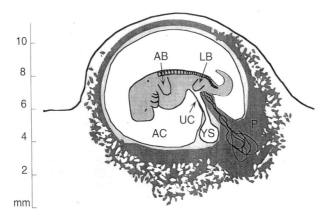

FIG. 6. In postconception week 4, the embryo has undergone later folding to close the abdominal wall. The cranial and caudal regions also curve. The arm buds *(AB)* and leg buds *(LB)* have formed. The amniotic cavity *(AC)* has expanded, nearly obliterating the extraembryonic coelomic space. An umbilical cord *(UC)* is formed when the amnion wraps around the yolk sac *(YS)* duct and the connecting stalk. The discoid placenta *(P)* continues to expand.

Historically, a definitive diagnosis of a viable pregnancy was the detection of fetal heart beats or movement.[6] Transabdominal or endovaginal ultrasound examination of cardiac activity have been used to prove a pregnancy viable. With transabdominal ultrasound, cardiac activity may be visualized after 7 weeks' gestation. The identification of cardiac activity by transabdominal ultrasound has a favorable prognosis for pregnancy: The rate of spontaneous abortions is only 2% to 3% in women who have a viable fetus documented by transabdominal ultrasound.

Endovaginal ultrasound has allowed detection of cardiac activity at an earlier gestational age, 4 to 5 weeks. When these earlier ages were studied, the incidence of spontaneous abortions increased: 9% of embryos with heart activity had subsequent first-trimester pregnancy loss. Two percent of the women in this study presented with blighted ovum, and 6% of the aborted embryos did not demonstrate cardiac function.[6]

◊ THE EMBRYO: ETIOLOGY OF MALFORMATIONS

An aborted embryo is usually malformed.[6] The earlier in gestation that a defect occurs, the more likely it is to cause intrauterine death (Fig. 8). More than 80% of intact embryos examined after delivery have structural malformations. These embryos exhibit major malformations and generalized growth retardation. In more than half of cases studied, the embryonic malformations are associated with a chromosomal abnormality.

Trisomies are the most frequent type of embryonic karyotypic abnormalities, followed by triploidy and monosomy X. These chromosomal abnormalities indicate early failures in meiosis, fertilization, or early zygote division. Nondisjunction of the gamete in meiosis may explain the numerical errors of the chromosomes: triploidy and monosomy X. Fertilization of the ovum by two sperm may yield triploidy. Cases of tetraploidy or mosaicism may occur because of abnormalities of early divisions of the fertilized ovum.[6]

◊ THE FETUS: CLASSIFICATION OF BIRTH DEFECTS

Birth defects have been generally defined as anatomic or functional variation(s) from the normal range in humans.[22] The defects may range from single or multiple anatomic abnormalities; they may represent a minor or severe malformation. *Isolated defects* affect a single body region and often have a multifactorial determination. *Multiple defects* occur in several body regions and are more likely to have a chromosomal or mendelian inheritance.

Isolated birth defects are further characterized. *Anomaly* is defined as a deviation from the expected or average form or function. A *major anomaly* has significant cosmetic or functional consequence, while a *minor anomaly* has little impact on clinical well-being.[22]

A *malformation* is a morphologic defect of a body region or organ resulting from an intrinsically abnormal developmental process, such as chromosomal abnormality, genetic predisposition, or mendelian mutation (Figs. 9 and 10). If a large body region is involved, the defect is one of *blastogenesis*. Single-organ involvement is a defect of *organogenesis*. Because traits in humans have differences in *penetrance* (the presence or absence of a malformation in a gene carrier) and *expressivity* (expression of a trait related to other genes or alleles), no trait in humans is purely genetically determined. Environmental modulation of traits also occurs.[22]

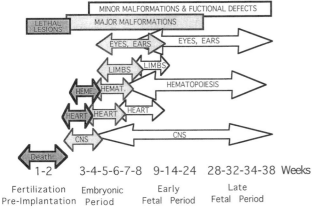

FIG. 8. Embryonic structures develop at different gestational times. The risk of a lethal or major malformation is greater when the defect begins earlier in pregnancy. Failure of adequate cardiac or hematopoietic development prevents a singleton intrauterine life. The risk of birth defects in the nervous system and sense organs may continue throughout the pregnancy. (From Clayton-Smith J, Donnai D. Human Malformations. In: Rimion D, Connor J, Pyeritz R, eds. *Emery and Rimion's Principles and Practice of Medical Genetics.* New York: Churchill Livingstone, 1996:383–394.)

Classification of Errors of Morphogenesis

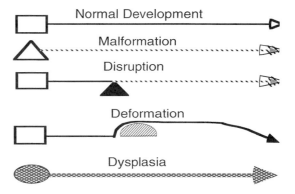

FIG. 9. During development, several mechanisms may result in structural or functional abnormalities. The first line in this figure represents a normal conceptus that continues to develop in time without abnormality. A *malformation* is abnormal from the beginning and continues to be abnormal with maturation. A *disruption* or a *deformation* occurs in a structure that began in a normal fashion. A disruption is a specific event that interferes with normal maturation, yielding an abnormality (e.g., fetal damage secondary to amniotic bands). A deformation is an alteration of normal structures caused by mechanical forces (e.g., the facial and limb features in a fetus with oligohydramnios).

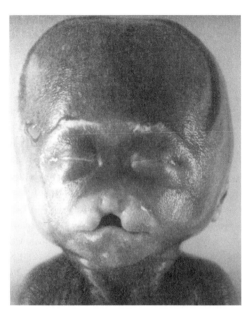

FIG. 10. Malformation. In this fetus with trisomy 18, facial malformations include bilateral cleft lips and midface hypoplasia. These findings are related to the underlying chromosomal defect.

A *disruption* is a morphologic defect of an organ or larger region, resulting in the extrinsic breakdown or interference with an originally normal process (see Fig. 9) For example, an amniotic band may lead to hypoplasia or amputation of a developing limb, as well as interfering with blood flow to adjacent structures. A *deformation* is an abnormal form, shape, or position in a part of the body caused by mechanical forces. These result from a bending of the shape of an otherwise normally developing structure. In oligohydramnios, for example, decreased amniotic fluid leads to deformation of the face and limbs.[23] A tissue *dysplasia* is an abnormal organization of cells into tissues. It may be present in a variety of organs.

A *sequence* is a pattern of multiple anomalies derived from a single anomaly or mechanical factor. The sequence represents a cascade of primary and secondary events that are a result of a single original malformation or disruption.[23] A *syndrome* describes multiple anomalies thought to be pathogenetically related and not representing a sequence. Designation of a condition as a syndrome implies a lower level of understanding of a pattern of pathogenetically related anomalies. With time and additional understanding, a syndrome may be reclassified as a sequence. An *association* is a nonrandom occurrence in one or more individuals of several morphologic defects that are not identified as a sequence or a syndrome.[23]

◊ **TISSUE EXAMINATION IN EARLY
   PREGNANCY FAILURE**

The pathologist has two responsibilities in the examination of the products of conception tissue from a failed pregnancy. The first is to document the failure of intrauterine pregnancy. The second responsibility is determine the possible cause for the abortion. This information is of value for reproductive counseling of couples with recurrent abortion. Even well documented negative pathology findings are valuable. The usefulness of the tissue report for reproductive counseling is dependent on the thoroughness of the pathologist's examination of the abortion tissue. There are excellent texts and monographs about the handling of abortion tissue.[16,21] The following discussion is not intended to replace those, but rather to indicate how a specimen may be handled to increase the information derived from its examination.

For the pathologist to interpret the gross and microscopic findings in an abortus, an adequate maternal clinical history is essential. Information about this pregnancy and the past obstetric and medical history is required for the consultation. In most cases, the reexamination of previous pathology materials and reports will enrich the current interpretation.

The examination of products of conceptions for reproductive counseling should be handled without fixative, as for a frozen section. All tissue expelled spontaneously or obtained at surgery should be submitted. A woman who has had repeated abortions may be counseled to obtain and bring in the gestational tissue in a clean container for examination. The specimen should be kept moist with a small amount of sterile saline and transported cold to the pathology laboratory.

Gross Examination of Tissues in Early Pregnancy Failure

The tissue should be maintained in a sterile manner to allow submission of tissue for cytogenetics. The gross tissue is delicate and will tear or fragment with handling. To prevent this and allow the tissue to expand, the specimen may be floated in a sterile Petri dish with sterile saline. Magnification of the specimen with a hand lens or dissection microscope will demonstrate the fine features. As the gross tissue findings are ephemeral, photographs are usually required.

If a single intact specimen is obtained, it is usually a decidual cast. This should be opened from the narrow end to release the chorionic sac. The size of the sac should be measured and compared to standard tables. The diameter of the sac normally correlates with gestational age, but with the death of the embryo, there is a decreased rate of sac growth. The surface of the normal sac is evenly covered by villi. Abnormal villi have swollen, clubbed, or cystic tips. In some specimens, the villi may be hypoplastic and sparsely distributed.

Within the sac, there may be an embryo, cord, amniotic sac, or yolk sac. The presence or absence of these embryonic structures should be documented with photographs. An embryo should be classified as having normal or abnormal external findings with reference to embryonic development tables. Examination of the internal organs may be possible in some cases, and the heart tube is often preserved when other structures are autolyzed.

Most commonly, an incomplete and fragmented specimen is received. The sac, if present, is ruptured or collapsed. The specimen's contents should be described and photographed.

An occasional specimen consists only of decidua, and the evidence of an intrauterine pregnancy is made by microscopic examination.

Tissues may be submitted for chromosome analysis when the history suggests recurrent spontaneous abortions, a previously morphologically abnormal pregnancy, or an earlier abnormal karyotype of an abortus. Those specimens observed to have abnormal embryonic structures may be submitted for cytogenetic analysis as well. Clinical consultation may determine the additional cases whose pregnancy history suggests the need for cytogenetics: *in vitro* fertilization, chromosomal abnormalities in the parents, previous amniocentesis or chorionic villus sampling for chromosomes, and so on. Tissues from the embryo, amniotic membranes, or villi may be submitted for cytogenetic studies. Villous tissue with hydropic change or other abortion tissues in the appropriate clinical settings may be submitted for flow cytometry for a rapid diagnosis of triploidy.

Histologic Evaluation in Early Pregnancy Failure

There was an initial enthusiasm for the ability of the pathologist to observe villous histology and predict the chromosome findings of the abortus. Subsequent investigators have been unable to make a consistent correlation between histology and karyotype.[10] At present, cytogenetic studies remain the best method for detecting chromosomal abnormalities. *In situ* hybridization techniques have been developed that allow the detection of aneuploidy directly in the abortus tissue. The microscopic findings of villous edema, fibrosis, or fetal hypovascularity should be noted, as they bear on the length of time of intrauterine retention following embryonic death. The tissue should be examined as well for evidence of inflammation, infection, or infarction.

The final pathology report should estimate the gestational age, presence or absence of an embryo, and whether the conceptus is morphologically normal or not. The time of embryonic death may be estimated. Villous histology should be described. Special studies for karyotype, DNA content, or infection should be reported.

◊ PATHOLOGY EXAMINATION IN THE FETUS OR NEONATE

It is often a time of sorrow when a pregnancy ends with the delivery of a stillborn baby or an infant who dies in the neonatal period. Some families will express their grief in an attempt to protect the little one from another procedure: the postmortem examination. Inquiring whether a family has had earlier experiences with an autopsy may introduce the topic in a more general manner. The family may have specific complaints or concerns about the autopsy procedure. These concerns may be specifically addressed, and possibly resolved, before one asks for autopsy permission in *this* perinatal death. It is helpful in the request for an autopsy to reassure the family that the examination will be done in a manner for an open-casket funeral.

In addition, if the family has specific concerns about the invasiveness of a complete autopsy, the care provider may propose that only a limited autopsy be done, directed specifically to the organ system of most concern. An examination limited to the brain or heart, for example, may yield useful information for diagnosis and counseling. The perinatal pathologist may undertake a limited autopsy with visualization of the organs *in situ*, or the examination may be limited only to tissue biopsies. The limited autopsy provides more information than no autopsy at all. The experienced perinatal pathologist understands the family's concern and handles the postmortem examination in an appropriate and dignified manner. Evaluation by a trained perinatal pathologist will generally provide the family with useful information for its grieving. Findings can help the family understand the mechanism of the abnormality or death. The autopsy may suggest an etiology of the birth defect and help relieve the family's guilt or anxiety. It may provide information on the risks of an inherited condition that may recur in other family members.

Consultation between the pathologist and the care providers before, during, and after the postmortem examination is useful to ensure that clinical concerns are addressed. Some essential studies can only be done in a certain time frame after death. Biochemical studies, culture for microorganisms, or tissue isolation for electron microscopy, for example, must be begun at critical times during the autopsy procedure. With these and other studies, a clinicopathologic correlation may be made. These investigations provide valuable information about the diagnosis and treatment choices in this pregnancy and assist in the design of care in future pregnancies.

◊ GUIDELINES FOR PERINATAL AUTOPSY

It is beyond the scope of this chapter to discuss the details of the performance of a perinatal autopsy or the differential diagnosis of the gross and microscopic findings. Excellent descriptions of perinatal pathology are available.[3,11,30] The results of the pathologist's examination of the fetus or neonate will reflect his or her training and interest in perinatal pathology. Often, in community hospitals, the generally trained pathologist will not have enough experience with perinatal pathology to do the best examination. In this setting, the autopsy may be more appropriately referred to a pediatric hospital or medical center with an interest in perinatal pathology.

◊ SPECIAL EMBRYOLOGY: DEVELOPMENT OF THE INTERNAL AND EXTERNAL GENITALIA

The sexual genotype is determined at the time of conception by the sex chromosomes: The presence of a Y chromosome indicates a male conceptus. Anatomic or histologic features of sexual differentiation do not occur for many weeks after fertilization of an egg by sperm. There are different developmental pathways for male and female embryos to form ovaries or testes and internal and external genitalia.[13,28]

As mentioned earlier, the precursor germ cells of sperm and ova are first identified as cells in the caudal portion of the yolk sac near the allantoic stalk (see Fig. 1). In developmental week 5, germ cells begin to migrate toward the genital ridge. The germ cells increase in number by mitosis as they travel.

The mesenchymal cells in the genital ridge signal germ cells to migrate, using chemotactic factors. Germ cell migration causes the accumulation of 10,000 germ cells in the gonad. The germ cells continue to proliferate. Gonadal maturation is induced by the germ cells. A failure of germ cell migration causes the gonad on the genital ridge to remain an undifferentiated streak of mesenchyme. Migration of germ cells requires at least two sex chromosomes: those embryos with 45,XO, a Turner genotype, do not exhibit normal germ cell migration. Their ovaries remain as mesenchymal streaks.

The germ cells arrive at the genital ridge in week 6 and accumulate as sex cords. The genital ridge is composed of mesenchymal and endodermal cells. The primitive gonad is undifferentiated, without features of a testis or ovary (Fig. 11). If a Y chromosome is present, there are signals for the gonad to differentiate into a testis. In the absence of a Y chromosome, an ovary is formed.

Early in developmental week 8, the histologic evidence of sex differentiation is seen. The sex cords in males develop into the seminiferous tubule and rete testis. In females, the sex cords regress, but proliferation of the female germ cells, oogonia, continues into the 15th week. Formation of primordial germ cells begins in the deep cortex.

At 16 weeks, the oogonia enter their first meiotic division. Mesenchymal cells become follicular epithelial cells that surround the germ cell, converting the oogonia to primordial follicles.[20] Even *in utero,* some primordial follicles become atretic and are unable to participate in conception. By developmental week 36, the ovary is filled with primary follicles, although some oogonia are still present. In the ninth month of development, some primordial follicles become graafian follicles with a well defined granulosa cell layer. At the time of birth, the ovary is said to have 400,000 oocytes, although only 400 or so will eventually be released for conception.

The gonadal ridge develops adjacent to the embryonic kidneys: the pronephros, mesonephros, and metanephros (see Fig. 11). The mesonephric urinary collection system, the wolffian duct, becomes the paradidymis, the vas deferens, and the seminal vesicles. These wolffian duct structures regress in the female, persisting as the vestigial structures, the hydatid cyst, epoophoron, paroophoron, and Gartner's duct cyst.

The paramesonephric or müllerian ducts in the female embryo form the fallopian tubes.[13] The uterus is formed by the midline fusion of the two ducts. Incomplete fusion of the two müllerian ducts may lead to a septate or bicornuate uterus (see Fig. 11). Failure of one müllerian tube to form causes aplasia or atresia of one side, resulting in unicornuate uterus.

The external genitalia begin to develop at 4 weeks after conception. The genital tubercle forms adjacent to the cloacal membrane (Fig. 12). In the next few weeks, the cloacal membrane divides to form the urogenital fissure. A phallus and genital swellings can be identified. By the end of week 10, the urethral folds in males fuse to form the penile urethra. Failure of closure leads to hypospadias, occurring in 0.3% of males. The male genital swellings enlarge in anticipation of testicular descent. The testes are found in the scrotal sac in most term infants: 2% to 3% of males have cryptorchid testes at birth. This figure increases to 15% to 30% in premature males. Most cryptorchid testes are found in the inguinal canal.[28]

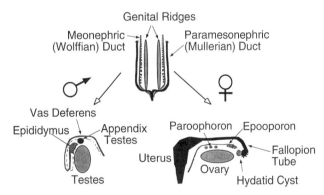

FIG. 11. Development of the internal genitalia. Initially, the genital ridges and mesonephric and paramesonephric ducts are the same in male and female embryos. In the presence of a Y chromosome, the gonad normally becomes a testis. The mesonephric duct becomes the vas deferens and epididymis. The appendix testis is a remnant of the paramesonephric (müllerian) duct. In females, the müllerian ducts form the fallopian tubes and fuse to become the uterus. The mesonephric remnants may cause cyst formation along the course of the original mesonephric (wolffian) duct.

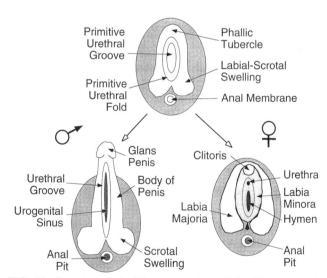

FIG. 12. Development of the external genitalia. The external genitalia develops at different stages in males and females. A phallic tubercle, urethral folds and groove, and labial-scrotal swellings are present. In males, the phallic tubercle enlarges, and the urethral groove closes. The testes descend into the scrotal swelling. In females, the clitoris is formed from the phallic tubercle. The labial swellings and the urethral folds become the labia majora and minora. The urethral groove is modified to become the urethra and vaginal opening.

In females, the labia and clitoris also develop from the genital swelling and phallus (see Fig. 12). Both the müllerian ducts and the urogenital sinus contribute to form the vagina. The vagina is initially a solid structure but becomes a hollow tube by the seventh month. The hymen membranes are a remnant of the solid epithelium.

Various anomalies of the female reproductive tract may occur. A common anomaly is the *arcuate uterus,* in which the fusion of the müllerian tubes is incomplete and there is a notch of the uterus. A septate or duplicated uterus or cervix is a less common finding. Agenesis of one or both müllerian tubes is rare. Agenesis of one tube leads to a unicornuate uterus.

The remnants of the mesonephric (wolffian) ducts are found adjacent to the tubes, uterus, or vagina. These remnants may form cysts, which may become symptomatic. More commonly, the mesonephric remnants are identified as incidental findings. On the fallopian tube fimbria, cysts called the hydatid cyst of Morgagni may occur. Cystic remnants on the broad ligament form parovarian cysts. Adjacent to the vagina, Gartner's duct cyst may be identified.

◊ **COMPARATIVE PLACENTAL ANATOMY**

Review of the anatomy of the articulation of the femur with the pelvis in a series of mammals reveals a similar structure. This ball-in-socket joint is duplicated unmodified in mammals and is seen in birds and reptiles. It is a successful design, and through the forces of natural selection, this joint has been maintained nearly unchanged. On the other hand, if one reviews the comparative anatomy of mammalian placentas, the gross anatomy and microscopic histology vary widely even in related species. The placental shape is discoid in humans, bidiscoid in monkeys, and spread diffusely throughout uterine cavity in horses and pigs. Closely related species such as the European mole and the Pacific mole also vary in gross appearance: In the European mole, the placenta is discoid, while in the Pacific species it is diffuse.

The tissue layers of the maternal fetal barriers vary greatly as well. At one extreme is the epithelial-chorial placenta seen in pigs, sheep, and goats. In these species, oxygen from maternal to fetal red cells crosses six cell layers: the maternal vascular endothelium, maternal connective tissue, maternal endometrial glandular tissue, fetal trophoblastic cells, fetal connective tissue, and fetal endothelium. At the other extreme is the hemomonochorial placenta seen in humans. Maternal red cells directly come in contact with fetal trophoblasts. Oxygen must only cross the trophoblastic cells, connective tissue, and endothelium to reach fetal red cells.

To explain this diversity of structure, Haig[14] observed that there is a genetic conflict in pregnancy. The conceptus has both maternal and paternal genes. These genes may have different survival goals. The mother needs to have good health during this pregnancy and future pregnancies. The mother may need to protect her genetic investment in raising her older children. Careful maternal attention to all her young ensures optimal survival for the maternal genes.

Her overall gene survival is reduced if she is harmed by any one pregnancy.

On the contrary, the paternal genes in the fetus can only be invested in this pregnancy. Causing this fetus to be born large and healthy is more important to the paternal genes than the general health or survival of the mother. Paternal genes affect the trophoblast invasion and support the nutritional needs of the fetus, independently of maternal needs. The most extreme example of a paternal gene expression is the true molar pregnancy. This gestation has no maternal genes but instead two haploids of paternal genes. In such pregnancies, the amount of trophoblastic tissues is increased and placental invasion is greater than that seen when both maternal and paternal genes are present.

The conflict between maternal and paternal genes in this pregnancy may account for the diversity of placental shapes and microanatomy. The paternal genes may attempt to improve the health of *this* fetus by improving the ways in which the fetus gains nutrients from the mother. Paternal genes may attempt to alter the placental structures that interact with maternal tissues. The maternal genes just as effectively must respond to paternal adaptations of the placenta. She must modify her part of the placental design to conserve resources and maintain her health. These dual genetic needs in pregnancy may account for the many placental designs observed in mammals. No one placental design is possible, as the maternal and paternal goals of a single pregnancy are different.

◊ **PLACENTAL FUNCTIONS**

The placenta has numerous functions in pregnancy. It serves the fetus with gas transfer, a task assumed after birth by the lungs. The placenta has excretory functions, water balance, and pH maintenance similar to the postnatal kidneys. It has resorptive functions similar to the gastrointestinal tract. The placenta is hormonally active, secreting β-hCG, human placental lactogen, growth hormones, and others. The placenta serves as a mechanical defensive barrier to protect the fetus from infection or invasion. In addition, the villi contain Hofbauer cells, which are fetal macrophages with scavenger and immunologic functions.

◊ **MATERNAL–PLACENTAL INTERACTIONS**

The endometrium is altered by pregnancy to become decidua. *Decidua basalis* is the endometrium beneath the placenta. *Decidua capsularis* is the decidua lying between the conceptus and the intrauterine cavity. *Decidua parietalis* is found in that endometrium that does not have cellular interaction with trophoblasts.

Maternal red cells are seen in placental lacunae early in pregnancy. However, maternal fetal circulation to the intervillous space is not well established until the second trimester. Then, maternal arterial blood enters the intervillous space through dilated endometrial spiral arteries (Fig. 13). Under pressure greater than the intervillous blood pressure, jets of

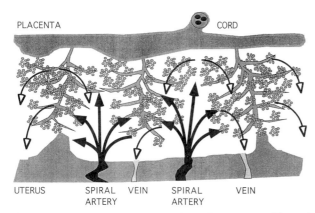

FIG. 13. Maternal perfusion in the intervillous space. The spiral arteries in the uterus are converted to uteroplacental arteries. These are large-bore vessels, capable of carrying large volumes of maternal blood to the placenta. Under pressure, blood spurts into the intervillous space, reaching the chorionic surface of the placenta *(black arrows)*. The blood trickles down, perfusing the spaces between terminal villi. Deoxygenated maternal blood leaves the intervillous space through decidual veins.

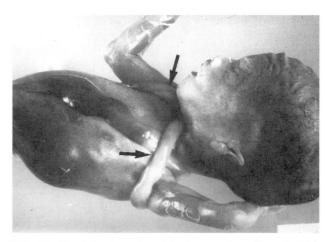

FIG. 14. Fetal demise related to abnormal cord length. This 30-weeks' gestation fetus had a 65 cm long umbilical cord (normal for gestational age: 48 ± 11 cm). The fetus was entangled in the cord, which was wrapped around his neck and upper arms *(arrows)*.

maternal blood shoot up to the chorion beneath the fetal plate. The blood then slowly percolates back to the maternal surface. Nutrient exchange occurs in the terminal villi of the placenta. Deoxygenated maternal blood exits the placenta in the draining decidual veins.[15]

◇ EXAMINATION OF THE PLACENTA IN THE DELIVERY ROOM

A systematic evaluation of the placenta in the delivery room may detect placental abnormalities that warrant additional studies. By routinely examining each part of the placenta with a standard protocol, one is unlikely to miss significant gross features. The placenta presents a tissue history of the pregnancy; an abnormal placenta may explain the unexpectedly poor neonatal outcome.[2] The cord, membranes, fetal surface, and maternal surface are each examined, and the observed features recorded in the delivery report. Abnormalities are carefully noted, as these may correlate with the fetal or neonatal course.

The length of the cord should be estimated.[2] A term delivery with a cord greater than 70 cm is considered a long cord; a cord less than 32 cm is considered short. A long cord predisposes a fetus to entanglement in the cord or cord knots (Fig. 14). Long cords carry a risk of fetal distress or death before or during delivery. Short cords may be seen in the fetus who has reduced motion or who demonstrates abnormal attachment to the amnion.[12] The nature of the coiling umbilical cord vessels is noted: normal, excessive, or reduced. Tightly coiled cords are seen in some cases of intrauterine demise, and cords without normal coiling are associated with perinatal complications.[29] Cords usually twist in a counterclockwise or left-handed manner.

Cord knots, varicosities or *false knots,* cysts, hemorrhages, or areas of narrowing are noted. True knots of the cord are more commonly seen if the cord is long. About 10% of true knots are associated with perinatal mortality (Fig. 15). Cord knots obstruct blood flow and cause fetal ischemia. False knots (Fig. 16) or cysts may be detected, but these are incidental findings and carry no increased risk to the pregnancy. Hemorrhage into the cord is associated with fetal anemia, distress, or death. Attenuated cords may represent a segmental cord constriction or a focal cord obstruction during pregnancy; these have also been associated with fetal loss.

The number of fetal vessels in the cord is counted. A single umbilical artery occurs in about 1% of singleton deliveries and more frequently in twins. Most commonly (70%), the single artery observed is the left umbilical artery. Congenital

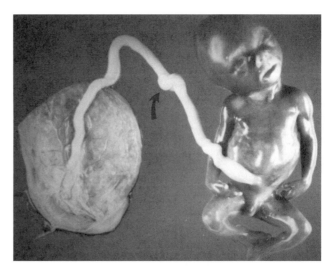

FIG. 15. True cord knots. About 10% of true cord knots *(arrow)* are associated with intrauterine fetal demise.

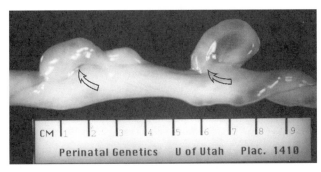

FIG. 16. False cord knots. False knots *(arrows)* are cord varicosities caused by abnormal dilation or positioning of the umbilical vessels. They have no clinical significance.

anomalies and chromosomal defects are increased in infants with a single artery.

The site of the cord insertion is noted. A normal cord inserts into the center of the placenta or eccentrically on the placental disk. The chorionic arteries branch from the cord at the site of the cord insertion. Smaller vessels form and vascularize the complete surface of the placenta (Fig. 17). The placental arteries are more superficial, just beneath the amnion, and cross over the veins.

Umbilical cord insertion at the edge of the placental disk—a *marginal insertion*—occurs in about 7% of deliveries. In about 1% of singleton deliveries, the umbilical cord inserts into the membranes; this is called a *velamentous* insertion. The incidence of velamentous insertion is increased in twins and in placentas with a single umbilical artery. On occasion, major fetal blood vessels are embedded in the placental membranes. When these membranous vessels cross over the uterine os and become the presenting fetal part, the condition is called *vasa previa.* On occasion, the cord may begin its branching to major stem vessels before it inserts into the placenta, called a *furcate* insertion. In these pregnancies, the abnormal insertion of the umbilical or placental vessels predisposes the fetus to distress during delivery. These vessels are

at great risk of tearing during delivery, with fetal hemorrhage. A large hemorrhage during delivery may lead to intrapartum fetal demise. Thrombosis of the these vessels may lead to fetal thrombocytopenia or death.

After the gross features of the cord are noted, the membranes may be examined. In vaginal deliveries, the site of rupture, whether in the sac or at the placental disk, is noted. Torn membranes at the placental edge suggest that the placenta was implanted near the cervical os. Alteratively, if membrane rupture is away from the placental margin, a *placenta previa,* or the placental insertion over the cervical os, is excluded.

The color and texture of the membranes are noted. Green-staining membranes occur when the fetus releases its terminal bowel contents, or meconium, before delivery. This finding is associated with fetal distress before delivery. If the meconium has passed many days before delivery, the green bowel pigment becomes light green or brown. The pigment diffuses into the membranes and is phagocytosed by macrophages. Placental membranes are typically translucent. Membranes may be focally opaque if they sheared away from the uterine wall with the decidua capsularis and parietalis intact. Diffusely opaque membranes may be due to the infiltration of the membranes by neutrophils, termed *acute chorioamnionitis.* Infection should be also suspected when the placenta has a foul odor.

The membranes may be discolored red from acute hemorrhage. Clots adherent to the maternal side of the fetal placental membranes are termed *retromembraneous hemorrhage.* If the hemorrhage occurred days before delivery, the pigment in the membranes may be brown or yellow. The pigment may be distinguished from meconium staining by Perls iron stain on histologic sections of the membranes. Hemoglobin breakdown products contain iron and stain blue, while meconium remains brown-pigmented.

The fetal surface of the membranes and the placental disk are usually shiny without focal lesions. Small white nodules on the membranes, called *amnion nodosum,* are seen in pregnancies with oligohydramnios.[2] The cause of the oligohydramnios may be renal anomalies or amnion leakage. Microscopic examination shows these nodules to be formed of desquamated skin cells. Amnion nodosum is on the fetal surface of the placenta and may be scraped awazy. A similar lesion, squamous metaplasia of the amnion, has white nodules as well, but these are under the amnion, not on its surface.

The insertion of the membranes into the placental disk is examined. In most placentas, the membranes insert into the placental disk at its margin (marginal insertion).[2] A variant of this—*circummarginate insertion*—occurs when the membranes insert away from the placental edge and extend beyond the vascular plate into a white fibrin at the placental edge. The circummarginate insertion may occur completely around the placenta or only focally. These variants of membrane insertion have no clinical significance.

Another form of insertion, termed *circumvallate,* occurs when the membranes insert into the placenta surface in a curved border of folded membranes at the margin[2] (Fig. 18).

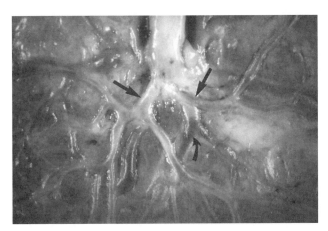

FIG. 17. Normal cord insertion into the fetal surface of the placental disk. The umbilical arteries *(straight arrows)* cross over the umbilical veins *(curved arrow).*

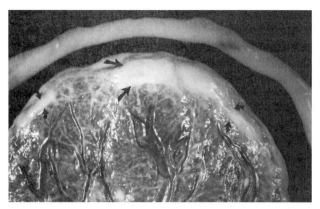

FIG. 18. Circumvallate insertion of the membranes. The *arrows* indicate the raised rim at the placental insertion. Pregnancies with this placental membrane insertion more frequently have hemorrhage or premature rupture of the membranes than those with a marginal or circummarginate insertion.

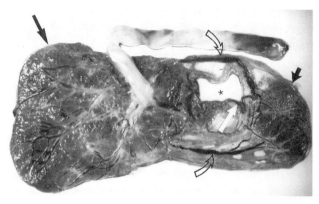

FIG. 19. Placenta with a main *(long arrow)* and accessory (or succenturiate) lobe *(short arrow)*. The membranes ruptured at the site of the *black star,* and delivery ensued through this opening. The *white arrow* identifies a vessel that tore during delivery. The umbilical vessels in the joining membranes are noted by *open arrows.*

This fold elevates the membranes in a white rim above the placental surface. This form of insertion is associated with hemorrhage, premature rupture of the membranes, and prematurity.

Placental membranes are evaluated for the presence of amniotic bands. These may be small strands of amnion torn away from the sac or broad sheets of amnion between the placenta and fetus. Amniotic bands are associated with fetal deformity. The earlier in gestation that these membranes form, the more grave will be the birth defects.

Next, is the fetal surface, with examination of the placental shape. Most placentas are circular or oval in shape. Irregular shapes are associated with abnormal placental implantation. There may have been abnormalities of the maternal uterine surface, such as intrauterine septa, leiomyomata, or scarring from earlier cesarean sections. Pregnancies with irregularly shaped placentas have more frequent perinatal complications, such as hemorrhage, premature separation, or intrauterine retention of placental tissue.

The placenta may not be a single disk. A *bilobed* placenta has two disks of equal size. If the disks are unequal in size, the smaller one is called a *succenturiate* or *accessory lobe* (Fig. 19). The placenta is joined by vessels traveling through the membranes. These vessels carry with them the increased risk of hemorrhage during delivery. An accessory lobe may not be delivered with the larger lobe. A clue to the retained placental disk is the observation that large blood vessels extend to the margin of the placenta but end abruptly. A torn vessel is found at the placental edge.

The fetal surface is examined. Fresh hemorrhages may occur related to the delivery. Shiny white plaques in the chorion under the amnion are frequent and represent deposition of fibrinous material. There may be found a small white oval structure beneath the amnion. This is the remnant of the yolk sac, trapped on the placental surface when the amnion became adherent to the chorion in the first months of pregnancy.

There may be cysts on the fetal surface. Some cysts form from maternal clots in the intervillous space beneath chorion, called *subchorionic thromboses.* The thrombi are believed to form as a consequence of abnormal flow of maternal blood in the intervillous space. The size of the cyst is related to the size of the thrombus. The color of the cyst and its contents are related to when the blood clot formed. A recent cyst may contain red coagulum. A subacute cyst is usually discolored brown or yellow. A cyst formed by a hemorrhage in the distant past contains pale, clear, yellow fluid in its lumen. Hemorrhagic cysts are more common in placentas with abnormalities of maternal circulation.

Another cyst on the placental surface occurs because of the death of a twin early in the pregnancy, termed a *vanishing twin.* This has been documented by sonography in some pregnancies. A twin gestation is initially seen, but later only a single fetus is identified. The cyst on the fetal surface may contain amorphous hemorrhagic debris formed by the degeneration of a fetus and its placenta. In some pregnancies with an early twin demise, the cyst may contain a *fetus papyraceus,* a pale flattened mummified fetus.

Finally, the maternal surface is examined. The basal surface of a normal placenta is lobulated into 10 to 30 lobes, termed *maternal cotyledons.*[2] These lobes correspond to the branching of a chorionic villous vessel in the placenta. The normal basal plate is formed from a mixture of trophoblastic cells, endometrial cells, and matrix. The normal interface between the placenta and endometrium, the *basal plate,* is irregular, with pale and more darkened regions (Fig. 20).

A placenta with a uniformly pale, firm surface is described as having a *maternal floor infarction.* This is a misnomer, as the pallor is due not to infarction, but to a proliferation of trophoblast cells, with senescent placental villi, embedded in a network of proteinaceous matrix. This condition may be associated with intrauterine growth retardation and recurrent fetal loss.[2]

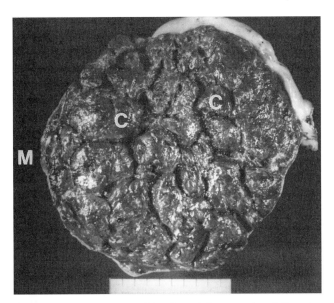

FIG. 20. Normal maternal surface. The margin of the placenta *(M)* has little or no blood clot or fibrin. The cotyledons *(C)* are rounded and full, appearing completely intact. There are no areas of thinning or of adherent blood clots.

Focal areas with pale or dark regions of the cotyledons are seen in placental infarcts (Fig. 21). Infarcts are ischemic necrosis of placental villi. Fresh infarcts are firm and red. Older infarcts are pale or white. Infarcts are more frequently seen in women with pregnancy-induced hypertension. In such pregnancies, the spiral arteries fail to undergo the dilation of physiologic change. Altered blood flow into intervillous space may make villi more susceptible to ischemic necrosis. In a normal term placenta, infarcts may be found at the margins of the placenta or occupy less than 5% of the placental surface. More extensive placental infarction in a term pregnancy or any infarcts in the preterm placenta are abnor-

mal. Placental infarcts are more common in pregnancies complicated by fetal intrauterine growth retardation. Women with a tendency to clot, such as those with factor V Leiden mutation[8] or with autoantibodies to phospholipid or cardiolipin[4] also demonstrate more placental infarctions, as well as a poorer fetal outcome.

Another placental lesion causing irregularities in the surface color or shape is intervillous thrombosis. These represent areas of blood clots that displace the villi, leaving a thin rim of villous tissue. Like infarction, intervillous thrombosis is more common in the placentas of women with pregnancy-induced hypertension; it carries an unfavorable pregnancy outcome.

In some freshly delivered placentas, the basal surface contains fresh blood clots. The clots at the placental edge are called *marginal hemorrhages.* Clots adherent to cotyledons are called *retroplacental hemorrhages* (Fig. 22). As blood will clot on standing, basal plate clots are better assessed in the delivery area rather than later at the pathologist's cutting bench. A formed clot that has compressed adjacent cotyledons and interdigitates into the intervillous space is more likely to be seen following the clinical diagnosis of abruption than the superficially adherent blood clot formed after delivery in the placental container. Fresh hemorrhages are dark red. A marginal hemorrhage that occurred earlier in pregnancy may appear brown or yellow.

The examination of the maternal surface may show irregular areas of the cotyledons, with a torn region depressed from the placental surface. On occasion, the maternal surface does not completely separate from the uterine cavity. A portion of the placenta may detach and remain adherent to the uterus. Placentas having villous tissue that more deeply invades the myometrium, termed *placenta accreta,* will not completely separate. The adherent tissue may cause postpartum bleeding or inflammation. Placentas removed by manual extraction may be incompletely delivered.

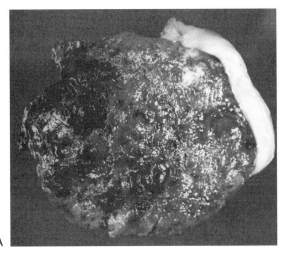
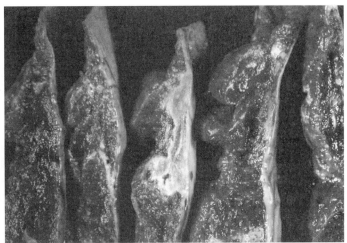

FIG. 21. Maternal plate with areas of pallor and dark discoloration. **A:** There are focal areas of more pale and dark color. This is associated with an irregular thickness of the placental disk. **B:** On cross-section, the placenta is seen to have recent and older infarcts.

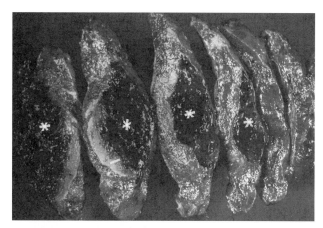

FIG. 22. Retroplacental hemorrhage. Abruption is a clinical diagnosis made when blood hemorrhages between the placenta and the uterus. Large clots may form in the retroplacental space *(white stars)*. Similar clots may form at the placental margin (marginal hemorrhages) or behind the placental membranes (retromembranous hemorrhages).

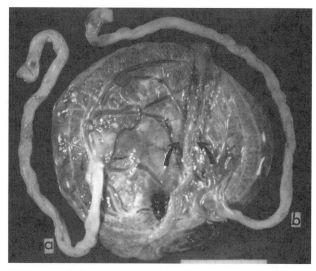

FIG. 23. Twin placenta with a diamniotic, dichorionic dividing membrane *(arrows)*. Such membranes are thicker and more opaque than those that are diamniotic but monochorionic.

◊ PLACENTAL FINDINGS AND BIRTH DEFECTS IN TWIN OR MULTIPLE GESTATION PREGNANCIES

In fraternal twins, placental development of each zygote is the same as that in a singleton pregnancy. The placental disks and membranes of fraternal twins may fuse due to space constraints in the uterus (Fig. 23). The fused placental membranes will be diamniotic and dichorionic, as each embryo has formed its own distinct amnion, chorion, and decidua capsularis.

In monozygotic twins, placentation is more complex.[17] Each twin may form its own placenta and membranes. The dividing membrane will be identical to that of fraternal twins: dichorionic, diamniotic membranes. In other monozygotic twins, the placental chorion layer may be shared, with a single large placenta. Vascular anastomoses may exist in the placenta, joining the two fetal circulations. Injection of the umbilical vessels with milk, other colored liquids, or radiopaque fluids may demonstrate anastomoses on the surface of the twin placenta. In some twin pregnancies, the cords may insert at the same site on the placenta and share surface vessels (Fig. 24). Among monochorionic twins, 2% to 5% are also monoamniotic and share the amniotic sac. These twins are at risk for cord entanglement and death.

In some twin pregnancies, there are differences in the growth of the twins. The umbilical cord of one fetus and its placental distribution may be smaller than the other. Discordant twin fetal growth may occur.

An extreme form of discordant twin development is the acardiac twin pregnancy, in which one twin has acardia or

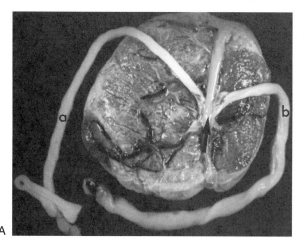

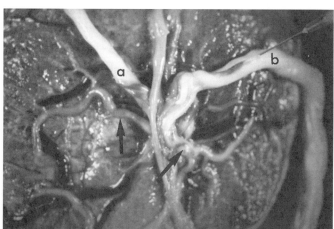

FIG. 24. Common insertion of the umbilical vessels. **A:** The cords from twins *a* and *b* insert together onto the placental surface *(arrow)*. **B:** Injection through the cord *b* demonstrates that the umbilical vessel connects to vessels on both sides of the placental membranes *(arrows)*.

only rudimentary cardiac structures.[19] Placental vascular anastomosis between the twins allows the donor or pump twin to support cardiac function in both. The etiology of acardia iseither a primary heart defect in one twin or reversed arterial perfusion from the "pump" twin to the acardiac twin. The acardiac fetus is usually hydropic, with rudimentary structures. The reversed arterial flow into one twin may cause vascular disruption. Acardiac twin pregnancies are complicated by preterm labor and polyhydramnios. The pump twin may develop intrauterine congestive heart failure and die. About one-third of acardiac fetuses have an abnormal karyotype (monosomy, trisomy, deletions, mosaicism, or polyploidy), while chromosome studies are normal in more than 90% of pump twins. All acardiac twins die, and one-third to one-half of the pump twins die in the perinatal period.

In triplet- or higher-gestation pregnancies, similar placental or fetal anomalies may occur as in twin pregnancies. In multiple-gestation pregnancies, it remains important to examine the placentas carefully. One may investigate the fused membranes and establish the possible zygosities.

◊ BIRTH DEFECTS RELATED TO PLACENTAL MALFORMATIONS

Some birth defects are directly caused by the failure of normal placental development.[7] These are more commonly found in twins, although they may occur in singleton pregnancies.

One such defect is the *body stalk anomaly*. This anomaly should be suspected if prenatal studies detect a fetus with a large abdominal wall defect, fixed to the placenta and the uterine wall. The fetus is joined to the placenta by sheets of amnion. The mechanism for this birth defect is the failure of the amnion to close in a normal manner around the yolk sac duct and connecting stalk. The joining of the embryo by the connecting stalk to the uterine wall may cause deformities of the skeleton, such as kyphosis or scoliosis and lower extremity malposition, contracture, or reduction. The fetus may have intestinal atresia, genitourinary defects such as exstrophy of the cloaca, agenesis of the external genitalia, and neural tube defects such as meningomyelocele. The abdominal viscera are displaced into the extraembryonic coelomic space. Maternal serum alpha-fetoprotein is elevated. This is a fatal birth defect.

A similar lethal abnormality is the *limb–body wall complex with cord agenesis*.[5] The fetus is attached to the placenta by a persistence of the ectodermal–amnion junction with agenesis of the umbilical cord. The shortened umbilical vessels lay in the membranes. There is displacement of the abdominal viscera into the extraembryonic coelomic space. Abnormal fusion of the amnion with the chorion in the first month of life leads to this anomaly. The fetus has limb defects such as amelia, reductions, contractures, talipes, or sirenomelia. Kyphoscoliosis is present. A reduction in thoracic size leads to pulmonary hypoplasia. The genitourinary system has internal and external malformations. Sacral meningomyelocele is common.

◊ PLACENTAL EVALUATION BY A PATHOLOGIST

Most tissues removed at surgery from a patient are routinely submitted for an examination by a pathologist. The tissues usually undergo a gross dissection at the surgical pathologist's cutting bench. Appropriate tissue sections are selected and submitted for histologic analysis. Within 48 hours, as mandated by guidelines of the College of American Pathologists (CAP), a report with appropriate description and diagnoses is returned to the care provider. The portion of the tissue specimen not submitted for histology is held for 2 weeks after the final report is issued. The requisition and accession logs are held for 2 years. Paraffin blocks for histology are kept for 5 years, and glass slides and surgical pathology reports are held for 20 years.

Many hospitals keep paraffin blocks, glass slides, and reports indefinitely. This conservation of surgical tissues and reports permits additional investigations to be done at much later dates. The original diagnoses may be reviewed, and the clinical course correlated with the ultimate patient outcome. Research may be done using the tissue, histologic blocks, or histologic slides to generally improve care for all patients. This stored material also allows reevaluation or reconsideration of the tissue diagnoses, or therapeutic measures undertaken, for those patients whose medical care is eventually evaluated in the courts.

Placentas are handled in a different manner. It is expected that the placenta will be examined in the delivery suite by the obstetrician or midwife. Some placentas are selected to be sent to surgical pathology by the order of the physician or care provider. Other placentas will be discarded after being held in the delivery area for a set period of time.

The guidelines for the selection of placentas that should be referred to a pathologist differ greatly. For example, the American College of Obstetricians and Gynecologists[1] (ACOG) recommended in 1993 that only placentas of stillborn fetuses be routinely examined by a pathologist. This ACOG guideline suggested that all placentas be held for 1 week at 4°C so that they may be sent to surgical pathology for examination if clinical conditions develop or abnormalities are detected.

At the other extreme of recommendations for placental examination, Salafia and Vintzileos[26] suggested that all placentas should be examined by a pathologist. A task force of CAP recommended that placentas be examined in the delivery room by the health care provider performing the delivery. A description of that examination should be recorded in the birth record.[17] Using the results of the gross examination and knowledge of the clinical course, the obstetrician may decide whether or not the placenta needs referral for pathologic examination.

The CAP suggested that some conditions are always an indication for pathologic study (Table 2). Placental examination by a pathologist should be standardized to ensure that complete and relevant information is obtained. Special stud-

TABLE 2. *Recommendations by the College of American Pathologists for examination of a placenta by a pathologist*

Maternal conditions	Fetal conditions
Diabetes mellitus (or glucose intolerance)	Stillbirth or neonatal death
Pregnancy-induced hypertension	Multiple birth
Prematurity (<32 wk)	Congenital anomalies
Postmaturity (>42 wk)	Fetal growth restriction
Maternal history of reproductive failure (≥1 abortion, stillbirth, or neonatal death)	Prematurity (<32 wk)
	Hydrops
	Meconium
	Admission to intensive care
Oligohydramnios	Depression of central nervous system: Apgar ≤3 at 5 min
Maternal fever	Neurologic problems, including seizures
Infection	Suspected infection
Substance abuse	
Repetitive vaginal bleeding	
Abruptio placentae	*Other conditions*
	Suspicion of abnormal pregnancy or delivery of an infant with the potential for litigation
Placenta conditions	
Any gross abnormality of placenta, membranes, or cord	

TABLE 3. *Routine information supplied by pathology report*

Gross report	Microscopic report
Placenta	*Placenta*
Fixed or fresh placenta	Chronic villitis
Trimmed placental weight	Perivillitis or intervillositis
Placenta: complete or incomplete	Basal placental villitis
	Acute intervillous hemorrhage
Placental size	Intervillous fibrin strands
Accessory lobe if present and its size	Acute or chronic ischemia
	Villous infarction
Color of fetal surface	Calcification
Fibrinoid material at fetal surface	Avascular villi
	Chorioangiosis
Amnion nodusum	Hemorrhagic endovasculitis
Infarcts	Dysmaturity
Abruption	Fetal nucleated red cells
Maternal floor abnormalities	Hydrops
	Hemosiderin
	Intervillous fibrin strands
Membranes	Fibrinoid material on villi
Site of placental sac rupture	
Type of membrane insertion	*Membranes*
	Chorioamnionitis (grades 1–3)
Color	
	Umbilical cord
Umbilical cord	Funisitis (Grades 0.5–3)
True and false knots	Vasculitis
Length	
Diameter	
Number of vessels	
Site of cord insertion	

ies that may be coordinated with the pathologist on a case-by-case basis include the following:

◊ Bacterial and viral culture,
◊ Cytogenetic cultures,
◊ Metabolic studies,
◊ Electron microscopy,
◊ DNA studies.

In addition, the CAP recommended that all placentas not referred to pathology be held for several days after delivery to determine whether or not maternal or neonatal complications develop that would indicate the need for examination. The pathology report should address certain specific conditions commonly seen in high-risk pregnancies (Table 3).

Other advocates for pathologic placental examinations are defense lawyers representing obstetricians. These legal experts recommend that a pathology referral be done in any of several clinical conditions[25,27] (Table 4). When a neonate is born less than perfect, the delivering physician may be the target of grief, guilt, and anger. These feelings may lead to malpractice suits. If ligation ensues about a particular delivery, the careful gross and microscopic examination of the placenta at the time of delivery may protect the physician. The placental report may describe preexisting placental or fetal factors that may have caused the untoward neonatal outcome.

A placental examination may not immediately provide the usual information for maternal or neonatal care as that made after delivery. It is often more useful to study the mother and infant directly. However, the placental examination by a qualified pathologist provides a pregnancy record that may benefit the obstetrician, who may later face litigation.

TABLE 4. *Medicolegal indications for placental examination by a pathologist*

Maternal indications	
Diabetes mellitus	Postterm delivery (≥42 wk)
Pregnancy-induced hypertension	Poor previous obstetric history
Premature rupture of membranes	History of drug abuse, including cocaine
Preterm delivery (<36 wk)	Unexplained fever
Fetal or newborn indications	
Neonatal death	Multiple gestation
Prematurity	Intrauterine growth retardation
Congenital Anomalies	Erythroblastosis fetalis
Transfer to neonatal intensive care unit	Meconium
	Apgar <5 at 1 min or <7 at 5 min
Ominous fetal heart tracing	
Placental or cord indications	
Infarcts	Placenta previa
Abruptio placentae	Abnormal appearance

<table>
<tr><td colspan="2">

SUMMARY POINTS

◊ The earlier in gestation that a birth defect develops, the greater will be the risk of fetal death and major structural abnormalities.

◊ The etiology of pregnancy failure or birth defects can often be determined by a careful examination of the intrauterine contents or the placenta and fetus.

◊ A careful and standardized placental examination in the delivery room may detect lesions that relate directly to the perinatal outcome.

◊ Clinical coordination with the perinatal pathologist in the examination of pregnancy-related tissues improves patient care and may play a role in reducing professional liability in the treatment of pregnant women.

</td></tr>
</table>

◊ REFERENCES

1. American College of Obstetrics and Gynecology. Placental pathology. *Int J Gynaecol Obstet* 1993;42:318.
2. Benirschke K, Kaufmann P. *Pathology of the human placenta.* New York: Springler-Verlag, 1995.
3. Bove K. The perinatal and pediatric autopsy. *Arch Pathol Lab Med* 1997;121:368.
4. Branch DW. Thoughts on the mechanism of pregnancy loss associated with the antiphospholipid syndrome. *Lupus* 1994;3:275.
5. Craven CM, Carey JC, Ward K. Umbilical cord agenesis in limb body wall defect. *Am J Med Genet* 1997;71:97.
6. Craven CM, Ward K. Embryology of successful and failed pregnancy. 1997; in press.
7. Craven CM, Ward K. Placental causes of fetal malformations. *Clin Obstet Gynecol* 1996;39:588.
8. Dizon-Townson DS, Nelson LM, Easton K, Ward K. The factor V Leiden mutation may predispose women to severe preeclampsia. *Am J Obstet Gynecol* 1996;175:902.
9. England MA. The human. In: Bard JBL, ed. *Embryos: color atlas of development.* London: Mosby–Year Book Europe, 1994:207.
10. Fox H. Histologic classification of tissue from spontaneous abortions: a valueless exercise? *Histopathology* 1993;22:599.
11. Gilbert-Barness E. *Potter's pathology of the fetus and infant.* St Louis, MO: Mosby–Year Book, 1997.
12. Gilbert-Barness E, Drut RM, Drut R, et al. Developmental anomalies resulting in short umbilical cord. *Birth Defects: Original Articles Series.* White Plains, NY: March of Dimes Birth Defects Foundation, 1993:113.
13. Gray S, Skandalakis J, Broeker B, et al. Female reproductive system. In: Skandalakis JE, Gray SW eds. *Embryology for surgeons: the embryologic basis for the treatment of congenital anomalies,* 2nd ed. Baltimore: Williams and Wilkins, 1994:816.
14. Haig D. Genetic conflicts in human pregnancies. *Q Rev Biol* 1993;68:495.
15. Harris JW, Ramsey EM. The morphology of human uteroplacental vasculature. *Contrib Embryol* 1966;260:43.
16. Kalousek D. Pathology of abortion: the embryo and the previable fetus. In: Gilbert-Barness E. *Potter's pathology of the fetus and infant.* St Louis, MO: Mosby–Year Book, 1997:106.
17. Langston C, Kaplan C. Practice guidelines for examination of the placenta. *Arch Pathol Lab Med* 1997;121:469.
18. Machin G, Still K, Lalani T. Correlations of placental vascular anatomy and clinical outcomes in 96 monochorionic pregnancies. *Am J Med Genet* 1996;61:229.
19. Moore T, Gale S, Benirschke K. Perinatal outcome of forty-nine pregnancies complicated by acardiac twinning. *Am J Obstet Gynecol* 1990;163:907.
20. Nishimura H. *Atlas of human prenatal histology.* Tokyo: Igaku-Shoin, 1983.
21. Novak R, Agamanolis D, Dasu S, et al. Histologic analysis of placental tissue in first trimester abortions. *Pediatr Pathol* 1988;8:477.
22. Opitz J, Wilson G. Causes and pathogenesis of birth defects. In: Gilbert-Barness E. *Potter's pathology of the fetus and infant.* St Louis, MO: Mosby–Year Book, 1997:44.
23. Opitz J, Wilson G, Gilbert-Barness E, et al. Abnormalities of blastogenesis, organogenesis and phenogenesis. In: Gilbert-Barness E. *Potter's pathology of the fetus and infant.* St Louis, MO: Mosby–Year Book, 1997:65.
24. Pijnenborg R. The placental bed. *Hypertens Pregnancy* 1996;15:7.
25. Roberts D. Medical-legal aspects of placental examination. *Obstet Gynecol Surv* 1993;48:777.
26. Salafia C, Vintzileos A. Why all placentas should be examined by a pathologist in 1990. *Am J Obstet Gynecol* 1990;163:1282.
27. Schindler N. The importance of the placenta and cord in the defense of neurologically impaired infant claims. *Arch Pathol Lab Med* 1991;115:685.
28. Skandalakis J, Gray S, et al. Ovary and testes. In: Skandalakis JE, Gray SW, eds. *Embryology for surgeons: the embryologic basis for the treatment of congenital anomalies,* 2nd ed. Baltimore: Williams and Wilkins, 1994:736.
29. Strong TH, Jarles DL, Vegas JS, Feldman DB. The umbilical coiling index. *Am J ObstetGynecol* 1994;170:29.
30. Wigglesworth JS. Causes and classification of fetal and perinatal death. In: Wigglesworth JS, Singer DB, eds. *Textbook of fetal and perinatal pathology.* Boston: Blackwell Science, 1991:77.

CHAPTER 5

Physiology of Reproduction

◇

Grace M. Couchman
Charles B. Hammond

Successful reproduction in women relies on a complex system of communications among the hypothalamus, pituitary, and ovary to achieve pubertal sexual maturity, ovarian follicular development, and ovulation. Pulsatile gonadotropin-releasing hormone (Gn-RH) from the hypothalamus prompts pituitary gonadotropin release and sets into motion the monthly ovarian cycle of follicle development, steroid biosynthesis, and ovulation. Feedback at all levels of communication affects cyclic oocyte development. Pubertal development is under strict neuroendocrine control and relies on appropriate hypothalamic orchestration to achieve the stages of sexual maturation. This chapter examines the fundamental endocrine mechanisms governing reproductive physiology from before puberty to after menopause.

The monthly process of oogenesis and subsequent conception or menstruation depends on the secretion of hypothalamic-releasing and -inhibiting factors: principally, the responsive secretion of anterior pituitary hormones, follicle-stimulating hormone (FSH), and luteinizing hormone (LH) and the consequent ovarian response of follicle development. FSH orchestrates dominant follicle growth, granulosa cell proliferation, and a dramatic increase in estrogen biosynthesis. The rise in estrogen stimulates a midcycle LH surge from the pituitary, triggering ovulation of the dominant follicle and corpus luteum formation. In the absence of conception and human chorionic gonadotropin (hCG) production, withdrawal of LH stimulation results in regression of the corpus luteum, reduction in steroid hormone production, and the initiation of menstruation (Fig. 1). This monthly cycle, which is central to reproduction, depends on the pulsatile release of Gn-RH from the hypothalamus and subsequent episodic pituitary gonadotropin secretion.

◇ HYPOTHALAMUS

The hypothalamus and the pituitary are central to the physiology of reproduction. Structurally, the hypothalamus forms the lateral walls of the ventral aspect of the third ventricle and is part of the junction between the diencephalon and the telencephalon at the base of the brain. The hypothalamus is composed of two groups of nerve fibers: unmyelinated fiber connections within the hypothalamus involved in peptide synthesis and release, such as Gn-RH, and ascending myelinated neuron systems that secrete norepinephrine and serotonin and directly regulate stimulation or inhibition of Gn-RH secretion.

Closely linked to reproductive function is the parvicellular neurosecretory system within the medial hypothalamus, which is composed of two important neuronal bundles: Gn-RH and dopamine fibers. The Gn-RH neurons are located primarily in the preoptic area of the anterior hypothalamus, the arcuate nucleus of the medial basal hypothalamus, and the tuberal hypothalamus, all with projections to the median eminence. The tuberohypophyseal dopamine neurons initiate hormone release. The median eminence is bathed by unique portal capillaries equipped with a fenestrated endothelial lining that permits the passage of large molecules such as Gn-RH, unlike the blood–brain barrier in other parts of the brain (Fig. 2).

Gn-RH secretion is modified by ascending input into the hypothalamus consisting of noradrenergic and serotoninergic projections whose cell bodies lie outside the hypothalamus (Fig. 3). Further insight into reproductive physiology comes with understanding of the physiology of Gn-RH and other hypothalamic hormones.

Hypothalamic Hormones

Pituitary hormone synthesis and secretion are directed by five major hypothalamic peptides: Gn-RH, corticotropin-releasing factor (CRF), growth hormone–releasing factor (GHRF), somatostatin, and thyrotropin-releasing hormone (TRH). Although reproductive physiology is primarily mediated by the pulsatile secretion of Gn-RH, the other metabolic hypothalamic hormones also influence successful reproduction.

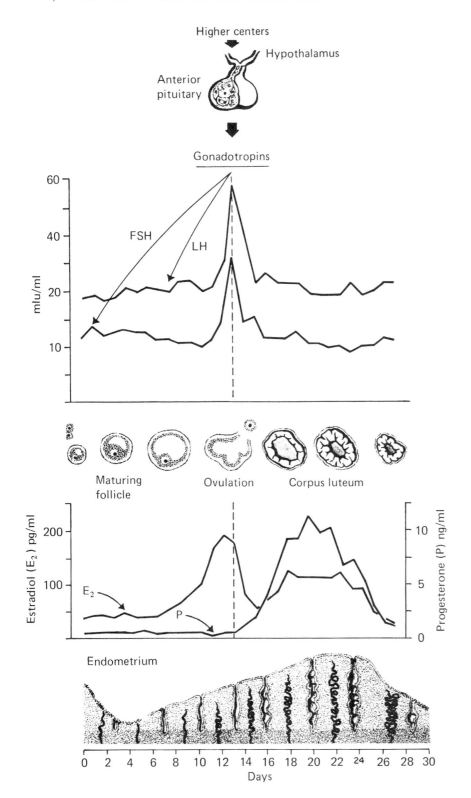

FIG. 1. Coordinated events of the hypothalamus, pituitary, and ovarian and uterine systems. Notice that plasma estradiol peaks around day 12, plasma follicle-stimulating hormone *(FSH)* and luteinizing hormone *(LH)* around day 13, and ovulation around day 14.

Gn-RH is a decapeptide whose episodic release from the hypothalamus occurs every 60 to 90 minutes and stimulates the equally pulsatile anterior pituitary release of FSH and LH. The circulatory half-life of Gn-RH is 2 to 4 minutes, and the amplitude of the Gn-RH pulse is as important as the pulse frequency. Ovariectomized ewes demonstrate pulsatile Gn-RH release that is in synchrony with LH pulses in the peripheral blood and corresponds to Gn-RH pulse amplitude. An increase in the amplitude of pulsatile release of Gn-RH initiates puberty.

Gn-RH axons project primarily from the medial basal hypothalamus to the median eminence, which is bathed in portal blood and contains high levels of all hypothalamic neuro-

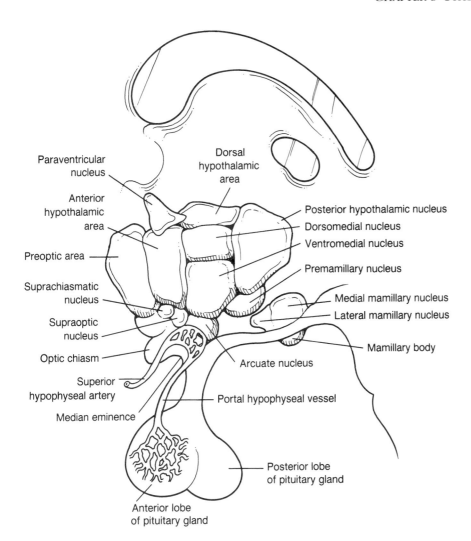

FIG. 2. The hypothalamus and portal hypophyseal vessels. (Adapted from Ganong WF. *Review of medical physiology*, 14th ed. Norwalk, CT: Appleton & Lange, 1989:12.)

peptides. Portal circulation delivers these peptides to the anterior pituitary.

In normal cycling women, the phases of the menstrual cycle demonstrate established pulsatile patterns of gonadotropin release. The follicular phase of the cycle is characterized by high-frequency and low-amplitude pulses; low-frequency, high-amplitude pulses occur in the luteal phase. Infrequent Gn-RH pulsation results in low levels of gonadotropin secretion and concentration and subsequent anovulation and amenorrhea, and higher pulse frequency contributes to a refractory response to FSH and LH and down-regulation of gonadal function.

Gn-RH agonists can increase binding affinity to Gn-RH receptors and resist enzymatic degradation within the hypothalamus and pituitary gland. Administered subcutaneously, intranasally, or in depot form, these compounds down-regulate or restrain the gonadotropin-gonadal axis and mimic a castrated state. They have been used in the treatment of endometriosis, precocious puberty, and fibroids, as potential contraceptives, and in conjunction with assisted reproductive technologies to better control timing of gonadotropin-stimulated cycles. Delivery of pulsatile Gn-RH has been used to induce ovulation in infertile women with ovulatory dysfunction.

CRF, another hypothalamic hormone, controls pituitary secretion of adrenocorticotropic hormone (ACTH). The CRF neuronal system terminates in the median eminence, as does that of Gn-RH. CRF plays a major role in mediating responses to stress and its release is inhibited by circulating cortisol and stimulated by stressful conditions such as hypoglycemia through ascending catecholaminergic pathways. Reproductive dysfunction has been associated with ACTH excess, as in cases of Cushing syndrome, and cortisol excess, as in anorexia nervosa and hypothalamic amenorrhea. An inhibitory effect on Gn-RH may be involved.

GHRF, yet another hypothalamic neuropeptide, triggers episodic growth hormone (GH) synthesis and release from the anterior pituitary. GHRF is localized to the medial basal hypothalamus, and, like Gn-RH and CRF, its axons terminate in the median eminence. GH is involved in many aspects of growth, including regulation of lipolysis and skeletal and muscle development. GH excess results in acromegaly. Pituitary GH is stimulated by the episodic release of GHRF and is under tonic inhibition by somatostatin, a hypothalamic neuropeptide. A decrease in somatostatin results in an increase in GHRF and subsequent GH secretion. GHRF is also

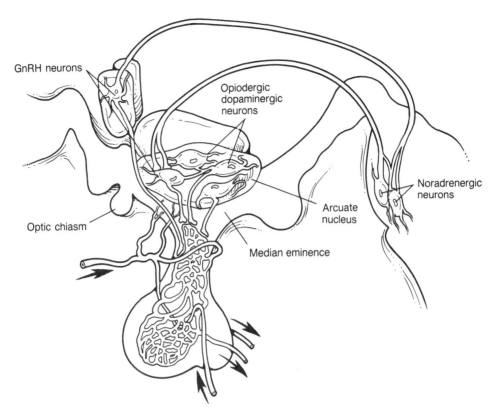

FIG. 3. Neuroanatomic relations of noradrenergic, dopaminergic, opioidergic, and gonadotropin-releasing hormone *(Gn-RH)* neurons within the arcuate-median eminence region and within the preoptic anterior hypothalamic area. (Adapted from Yen SSC, Jaffe RB. *Reproductive endocrinology*, 3rd ed. Philadelphia: WB Saunders, 1991:19.)

inhibited by insulin-like growth factors (IGF) 1 and 2. Somatostatin inhibits GH release, thyroid-stimulating hormone (TSH) release, gastrointestinal hormone secretion, and intestinal blood flow, and it may suppress immune function.

Hypothalamic TRH stimulates pituitary TSH release. TRH neurons are located in the paraventricular nucleus and project to the median eminence. TRH is critical to thyroid hormone regulation. Hypothyroidism and hyperthyroidism are associated with reproductive dysfunction. TRH secretion is stimulated by ascending catecholaminergic axons and is inhibited by feedback from thyroid hormones.

Regulation of Hypothalamic Function

Pulsatile secretion of Gn-RH, which is important to the physiology of reproduction, is regulated by central and peripheral feedback mechanisms: central modulation by norepinephrine, dopamine, and endogenous opioids; pituitary feedback of FSH and LH; ovarian modulation through steroids, activins, and inhibins; and autoregulation of Gn-RH receptors.

The neurotransmitters closely linked to reproduction are norepinephrine, dopamine, and the endogenous opioids. Noradrenergic fibers and their neurotransmitter, norepinephrine, stimulate Gn-RH neurons. Conversely, α-adrenergic blockers in ovariectomized primates suppress Gn-RH pulsation. Further central regulation of Gn-RH secretion is demon-

strated by dopamine, which primarily inhibits Gn-RH release and suppresses prolactin, but some *in vitro* studies of human hypothalami suggest a stimulatory role as well. Neurons within the arcuate nucleus responsible for endogenous opioid secretion inhibit Gn-RH secretion. β-Endorphin administered to normal women results in suppression of Gn-RH and LH pulsation. Neurotransmitters influence reproduction through the regulation of hypothalamic Gn-RH secretion.

Pituitary feedback regulation of the hypothalamus is less well characterized. Pituitary hormones may affect hypothalamic secretion in a short feedback loop by retrograde portal blood flow from the pituitary back to the hypothalamus.

Steroids, primarily estrogen and progesterone, produced by the ovaries feed back to the hypothalamus and pituitary, modulating Gn-RH and consequent gonadotropin pulsation. In ovariectomized and postmenopausal women who lack gonadal feedback, gonadotropin frequency and amplitude remain high. This can be reversed through the administration of estradiol. Circulating estradiol modulates Gn-RH pulse amplitude and subsequent plasma levels of LH and FSH in a biphasic manner, initially inhibiting and then stimulating gonadotropin secretion. The preovulatory surge of gonadotropin is modulated by estradiol. Progesterone decreases LH pulse frequency and increases amplitude, which is consistent with the luteal phase of the menstrual cycle when progesterone levels are high.

Gn-RH can up-regulate or increase the concentration of its own receptors on the pituitary gonadotrophs at physiologic pulsatile frequencies. When pulse frequency is high or tonic, Gn-RH exposure occurs, as in menopause, the number of receptors are down-regulated or decreased, and a refractory gonadotropin response occurs.

◊ PITUITARY

The pituitary rests protected at the base of the brain in the sella turcica and is the second major site of action, after the hypothalamus, within the brain that is central to reproductive physiology. It relies on hypothalamic releasing factors to stimulate secretion of pituitary hormones, which bind primarily to ovarian receptors and regulate gonadal steroidogenesis and gamete production.

Regulation of Pituitary Function

Pituitary hormone secretion is largely under hypothalamic control and is modified by ovarian steroid feedback. The hypothalamic regulatory peptides and neurotransmitters discussed earlier are transported to the pituitary gland through the portal circulation and control the secretion of anterior pituitary hormones. Reproductive physiology centers on the pulsatile release of Gn-RH from the hypothalamus, which binds to high-affinity receptors on the pituitary gonadotrophs and stimulates equally pulsatile release of FSH and LH. The acute release of gonadotropins from storage granules within the gonadotrophs is mediated by calcium-dependent mechanisms. Gonadotropins affect the hypothalamus by way of retrograde portal flow.

Ovarian steroids and inhibin further modify the secretion of FSH and LH (Fig. 4). The pituitary, not the hypothalamus, is the major site of estradiol feedback action. Estradiol has a classic negative feedback effect on gonadotropin secretion. When this loop is abolished by oophorectomy, there is a prompt increase in FSH and LH secretion. Estradiol feedback is biphasic, with inhibitory and stimulatory effects. After the initial inhibitory effect early in the cycle, gonadotropin stimulation increases a few days later. This positive stimulus initiates the preovulatory surge of gonadotropins. Rising progesterone levels enhance the positive feedback of estradiol and amplify the duration of the LH surge, suggesting that the preovulatory follicle itself regulates the timing of ovulation. During the luteal phase, after estrogen priming, progesterone decreases LH pulse frequency and increases the amplitude. Progesterone receptors in β-endorphin neurons in the hypothalamus mediate this effect. β-endorphin decreases Gn-RH pulse frequency.

Other ovarian factors, inhibin and activin, antagonistically interact to affect gonadotropin secretion. A family of inhibin and activin proteins is produced by the granulosa cells of the ovary, composed of α and β subunits. Inhibins are composed of one α and one β subunit and activin is a dimer composed of two inhibin β-subunits. They are members of the trans-

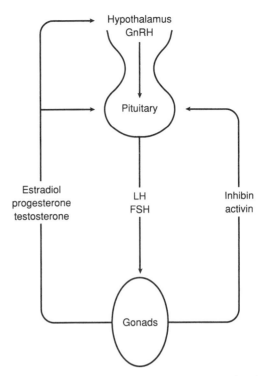

FIG. 4. Feedback control of gonadotropin secretion by gonadal hormones (*FSH*, follicle-stimulating hormone; *Gn-RH*, gonadotropin-releasing hormone; *LH*, luteinizing hormone). (Adapted from Yen SSC, Jaffe RB. *Reproductive endocrinology*, 3rd ed. Philadelphia: WB Saunders, 1991:122.)

forming growth factor β (TGF-β) family. Inhibins, as their name implies, are potent inhibitors of FSH release, and activin is a potent stimulator of FSH release. Follistatin, a binding protein for activin and inhibin, has β-subunit specificity and may be critical in the regulation of important cellular events such as the follicular selection of oocytes and follicular atresia. Other hormone and growth factors, including LH, IGF-1, and vasoactive intestinal peptide, stimulate inhibin production. LH-stimulated androgen production by theca cells is augmented by inhibin. Androgens may selectively stimulate FSH release and inhibit LH release from the pituitary gland.

The control of pituitary prolactin synthesis and secretion differs from that of LH and FSH in that it is under tonic inhibitory control by the hypothalamus, mediated primarily by dopamine release into the portal circulation. The most powerful stimulator of prolactin release is suckling, but how this stimulation is mediated is unknown. It may be decreased dopamine secretion (i.e., decreased inhibition) or a variety of factors such as β-endorphin, vasopressin, TRH, substance P, or angiotensin II that stimulates prolactin release, or a combination of decreased inhibition and increased stimulation may mediate prolactin levels.

Anterior Pituitary Function

The three anterior pituitary hormones most closely linked to reproductive physiology are the gonadotropin, LH, and FSH, together with the polypeptide hormone prolactin. The pituitary cells that synthesize and secrete LH and FSH are called gonadotrophs.

LH and FSH are structurally similar glycoproteins. Both are dimers composed of two α and β subunits (i.e., glycosylated polypeptides) that are tightly bound noncovalently. Human FSH and LH α subunits are essentially identical and share homology with the α subunit of TSH and with hCG. It is the β subunit that has distinctive structure in all of the hormones and is used in plasma assays.

FSH receptors on the ovarian granulosa cells and testicular Sertoli cells promote gamete production in the gonads, specifically the ova-containing follicles within the ovary. FSH acts synergistically with LH, androstenedione, and estradiol to stimulate follicle maturation. It stimulates granulosa cells to aromatize androgens to estradiol. FSH secretion peaks with the midcycle LH surge. The critical sequence of gonadotropin and steroid stimulation for appropriate granulosa cell and follicle maturation seems to be FSH, then FSH and estradiol, followed by FSH, LH, and estradiol.

When LH receptors appear to be under the influence of FSH, LH stimulates theca cells within the ovary to increase the production of androgen, which is aromatized by granulosa cells to increase estradiol biosynthesis. LH stimulates ovum maturation, resumption of the meiotic division that was arrested in fetal life, ovulation, luteinization of granulosa cells, progesterone production, and corpus luteum formation. Disorders of follicle maturation and anovulation, such as polycystic ovarian syndrome, represent a complex disorder of gonadotropin stimulation and follicular response.

During menopause, with the failure of ovarian follicular development and estradiol production, there is a lack of gonadal feedback to the hypothalamus and pituitary, resulting in chronically high levels of FSH and LH. These gonadotropins have been extracted and purified for human use, especially for the treatment of ovulatory dysfunction or for ovulation induction in conjunction with assisted reproductive technologies, such as *in vitro* fertilization and gamete intrafallopian transfer. Serum levels of FSH obtained on day 3 of the menstrual cycle (basal day 3 FSH) reflect ovarian reserve and have been used to predict the chance of achieving a successful pregnancy in assisted reproduction cycles.

Prolactin, a third pituitary hormone, is a single polypeptide of 198 amino acids that is secreted by anterior pituitary cells called lactotrophs. It shares amino acid sequence homology with human GH and human placental lactogen. During pregnancy and lactation, lactotrophs become more abundant. A group of pituitary cells called mammosomatotrophs secrete prolactin and GH. Prolactin affects numerous metabolic processes, but in reproductive physiology it is primarily involved in mammary gland development, initiation of milk secretion, stimulation of established milk secretion, and maintenance of newly formed LH receptor sites during folliculogenesis. Hyperprolactinemia can be a primary cause of infertility and has been associated with decreased gonadotropin secretion, secondary amenorrhea, galactor-

rhea, and menstrual irregularity. The many causes of hyperprolactinemia include pituitary adenomas, hypothyroidism, and medications that affect dopamine action or synthesis. Prolactin is under tonic inhibitory control by dopamine released by the hypothalamus. Therefore, medications that interfere with the metabolism, synthesis, or receptor binding of dopamine can reduce dopamine availability and result in hyperprolactinemia.

Posterior Pituitary Function

The posterior pituitary, or neurohypophysis, and its hormones, oxytocin and vasopressin influence reproductive physiology. The neurohypophysis is an extension of the hypothalamus that retains its neural connections. Oxytocin and vasopressin are synthesized as prohormones (i.e., prooxyphysin and propressophysin) in cell bodies of the supraoptic and paraventricular hypothalamic nuclei. Bound to neurophysin, a large transport peptide, these hormones are packaged and transported in granules to the nerve terminals in the neurohypophysis, where they are stored. Oxytocin and vasopressin can be secreted into the cerebrospinal fluid and directly into the portal circulation. Release of oxytocin and vasopressin is regulated by several factors, including cholinergic and noradrenergic neurotransmitters (Fig. 5).

Posterior Pituitary Hormones

Vasopressin, also referred to as arginine vasopressin or antidiuretic hormone (ADH), is the principal hormone responsible for volume regulation and osmolality in humans. It regulates water diuresis by the kidney and responds to increasing osmotic pressure and decreasing hydrostatic pressure of the blood. Water loading decreases ADH secretion, and plasma osmolarity rapidly increases ADH secretion. ADH regulation probably functions through an anterior hypothalamic osmoreceptor neuron system. A defect in the posterior pituitary system for synthesis and release of ADH can result in excessive water loss (i.e., diabetes insipidus) or excessive retention (i.e., syndrome of inappropriate ADH secretion).

Oxytocin is primarily involved in labor and lactation. It does not appear to initiate labor but is a recognized stimulator of myometrial contractions later in labor. In pregnant women, an increase in the number of myometrial oxytocin receptors is induced by estrogen, and the number of receptors reaches peak levels near term. Oxytocin levels increase in the second stage of labor, when the fetus is expelled, and is important in achieving hemostasis after the placenta is delivered. Oxytocin is used to induce labor and manage obstetric hemorrhage.

Oxytocin plays an important role in milk let-down, which depends on a complex neurogenic reflex arc. The process begins with suckling, which stimulates nerve endings in the nipple. This stimulus travels to the midbrain and hypothalamus through the spinal cord, where it stimulates oxytocin release from the neurohypophysis. Oxytocin causes contractions of the myoepithelial cells of the mammary gland and milk let-down.

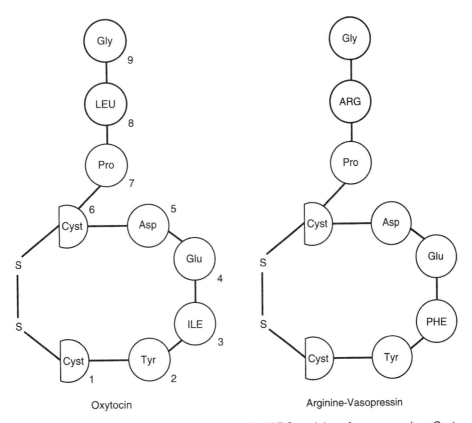

FIG. 5. Structural similarities of oxytocin and vasopressin (*ARG*, arginine; *Asp*, asparagine; *Cyst*, cystine; *Glu*, glutamine; *Gly*, glycine; *ILE*, isoleucine; *LEU*, leucine; *PHE*, phenylalanine; *Pro*; proline; *Tyr*, tyrosine). (Adapted from Speroff L. *Clinical gynecologic endocrinology and infertility*, 4th ed. Baltimore: Williams & Wilkins, 1989:163.)

Pain or fright can block this neurogenic reflex arc and prevent milk let-down. For some women, an infant's crying is enough stimulation to cause oxytocin release and milk expulsion.

Control of Hormonal Secretion

Release of oxytocin and vasopressin from the posterior pituitary is primarily regulated by cholinergic and noradrenergic neurotransmitters and opioid peptides. Acetylcholine stimulation releases the two hormones through nicotinic cholinergic receptors. Tobacco smoking and nicotine use stimulate vasopressin release and subsequent antidiuresis. Noradrenergic fibers also affect oxytocin and vasopressin release. α-Adrenergic neurons stimulate secretion, and β-adrenergic neurons suppress it. Various opioid peptides positively and negatively modulate oxytocin and vasopressin release. Other factors that influence regulation include estrogen, which augments oxytocin receptors, increasing the sensitivity to oxytocin; TRH, which stimulates oxytocin and vasopressin; and angiotensin II, which plays an important role in the regulation of vasopressin secretion.

◊ OVARY

The monthly process of follicle maturation is a complex and orderly task, orchestrated by signals from the hypothalamus and the pituitary, that depends on the ovary to respond with appropriate follicle development and steroid biosynthesis. Primordial germ cells originate from the yolk sac endoderm and migrate to the genital ridge by 5 weeks' gestation. During intrauterine life, persistent mitosis and meiosis increase the total number of germ cells to 6 to 7 million by 20 weeks' gestation. Follicular atresia reduces this peak number to the 1 to 2 million germ cells present at birth. By puberty, approximately 300,000 remain to participate in the reproductive cycle.

The ovarian contributors to follicle development and steroidogenesis include granulosa cells, theca cells, macrophages, and ovarian follicles. FSH-responsive granulosa cells that synthesize estrogen are associated with the oocyte and are separated from the surrounding stroma by the basal lamina. Theca-interstitial cells involved in androgen production reside in the loose stromal connective tissue of the ovary. Leukocytes in the interstitial (i.e., interfollicular) aspect of the ovary probably release regulatory cytokines, including interleukin-1 and tumor necrosis factor, and growth factors, such as basic fibroblast growth factor, TGF-α, and TGF-β, to modulate ovarian function.

Ovarian Hormones

The ovary is involved in the biosynthesis and secretion of three groups of steroid hormones: estrogens, androgens, and progestins. All steroids are lipid-related and share a common carbon ring structure of four fused rings called perhydrocyclopentenophenanthrene (Fig. 6). The family of progestins has 21 carbons, androgens have 19 carbons, and estrogens have 18 carbons.

Cholesterol is the parent compound from which all steroid hormones can be derived (Fig. 7). The cytochrome P-450 is critical in the conversion of cholesterol to steroid hormones because it provides nicotinamide adenine dinucleotide phosphate and activated oxygen necessary for hydroxylation reactions. Cleavage of a six-carbon fragment from cholesterol, a 27-carbon structure, results in pregnenolone, the immediate precursor of progesterone. Oxidation of pregnenolone's hydroxyl group at position 3 and rearrangement of the double bond results in progesterone.

Complete removal of a two-carbon side chain from the 21-carbon compounds, pregnenolone and progesterone, results in the androgenic hormones testosterone and dihydrotestosterone (Fig. 8). The 19-carbon androgens are aromatized to form the estrogenic steroids estrone and estradiol.

Regulation of Ovarian Function

Complex feedback systems, including ovarian steroids, modulate hypothalamic Gn-RH release and pituitary gonadotropin secretion and affect cyclic oocyte development. Oogenesis may be more importantly regulated by local feedback of ovarian hormones, especially estradiol, and other intra-

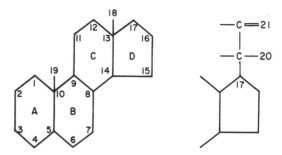

FIG. 6. Cyclopentenophenanthrene ring system. Each ring is identified by a letter from A to D. Carbon atoms are numbered in the sequence shown.

ovarian regulators, including growth factors and neuropeptides that may act locally in a paracrine or autocrine fashion to influence the replication or cytodifferentiation of a developing ovarian cell. The production of ovarian hormones is tied to an orderly process of follicle maturation with follicular, ovulation, and luteal phases.

Follicular Phase

The 10- to 14-day follicular phase consists of a complex, orderly cascade of follicle development and dominant follicle formation, which creates a hormonal microenvironment rich in estradiol and a follicle poised for ovulation.

Despite the growing body of knowledge concerning the physiology of reproduction, it is still unknown what event

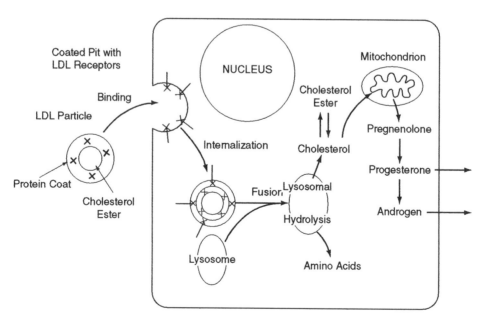

FIG. 7. Circulating low-density lipoprotein (LDL) constitutes the major source of cellular cholesterol substrate for steroidogenesis. Circulating LDL particles, containing a cholesterol ester core surrounded by a protein coat, bind to specific cell membrane receptors. The LDL–receptor complex is internalized and fuses to lysosomes, and the cholesterol esterase is hydrolyzed to cholesterol and the protein coat to amino acids. The free cholesterol is either stored as reesterified cholesterol or transferred to mitochondria, where side-chain cleavage enzymes convert it to pregnenolone. (Modified from Adashi E. Endocrinology of the ovary. *Hum Reprod* 1994;9:817.)

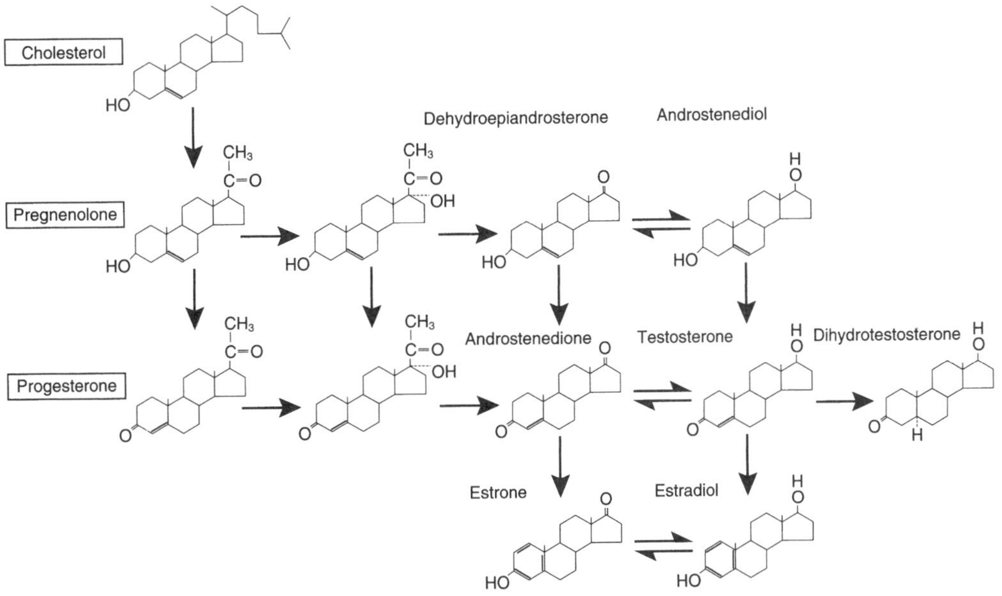

FIG. 8. General scheme for the synthesis of estrogens and androgens. (Adapted from Yen SSC, Jaffe RB. *Reproductive endocrinology*, 3rd ed. Philadelphia: WB Saunders, 1991:159.)

triggers the differentiation of a primordial follicle, an oocyte surrounded by granulosa cell precursors, into a primary follicle, an oocyte surrounded by a single layer of cuboidal granulosa cells. Because FSH receptors do not exist on primordial follicles, this development is considered to be gonadotropin-independent. Granulosa cells of the primary follicle synthesize and secrete mucopolysaccharides, creating the zona pellucida, a halo surrounding the oocyte. Further proliferation of granulosa cells and follicular enlargement result in secondary follicle formation, which is a primary oocyte arrested in the first prophase of the first meiotic division surrounded by several layers of cuboidal granulosa cells. Granulosa cells associated with secondary follicles possess FSH, estrogen, and androgen receptors. Beyond the primordial follicular stage, follicle development depends on gonadotropin stimulation.

As FSH binds to granulosa cell receptors, more receptors are induced, granulosa cells proliferate, and the aromatase enzyme system is stimulated (Fig. 9). The aromatase system is central to ovarian estrogen biosynthesis because it is responsible for the conversion of androgens to estrogen. Patients with congenital enzyme deficiencies, such as 17α-hydroxylase deficiency, do not possess the ability to convert androgens to estradiol. This lack of estrogen and estrogen feedback results in a lack of normal follicle development, sexual immaturity, and primary amenorrhea. In women with normal cycles, the creation of an estrogen-rich follicular microenvironment potentiates follicular growth. Estrogen modifies ovarian function by stimulating granulosa cell proliferation, increasing the number of FSH receptors and their sensitivity to hormone action, and stimulating aromatase activity and further estrogen biosynthesis.

At the same time as granulosa cells proliferate in the secondary follicle, theca cells respond to circulating LH and initiate production of androstenedione, the estrogen precursor, from cholesterol. Androstenedione enters the granulosa cell, where it is aromatized to estradiol. Although estrone is the first estrogen synthesized, it is easily converted to estradiol in the granulosa cell. The granulosa and theca cells are so closely coupled in the process of ovarian estrogen biosynthesis that this interaction is referred to as the two-cell, two-gonadotropin theory of ovarian steroidogenesis (Fig. 10). The system is in delicate balance, as evidenced by the actions of androgen within the granulosa cells. Although androstenedione at low concentrations promotes aromatase action and estrogen biosynthesis, high levels of androgens cause follicular atresia. A microenvironment rich in androgens favors 5α-reductase activity, converting androstenedione to dihydrotestosterone, which cannot later be converted to estrogens. This delicate balance of the hormonal milieu of the follicle contributes to its continued development or atresia.

In the secondary follicle, as granulosa cells proliferate and estrogen is synthesized, follicular fluid accumulates in the intercellular spaces between the granulosa cells and eventually forms a cavity or antrum. Antral fluid reflects the steroidogenesis of surrounding granulosa and thecal cells and contains plasma proteins, proteoglycans, prolactin, and inhibin (Fig. 11). Formation of the antrum transforms the follicle into a small tertiary follicle. The two or three layers of granulosa cells surrounding the oocyte, now located eccentrically, are called the cumulus oophorus. Large preovulatory tertiary follicles are called graafian follicles.

The final stages of follicle development depend on gonadotropin stimulation (Fig. 12). The follicles most likely to

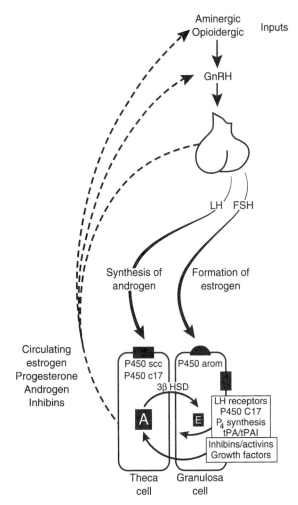

FIG. 9. Representations of the hypothalamic–pituitary–ovarian interaction in the control of the human menstrual cycle. The pulsatile release of luteinizing hormone *(LH)* and follicle-stimulating hormone *(FSH)*, mediated by the hypothalamic gonadotropin-releasing hormone *(Gn-RH)*, induces ovarian theca and granulosa cell steroidogenesis and follicle maturation. The theca cell is endowed with LH receptors, which mediate LH-induced P-450 steroidogenic enzymes and the synthesis of androgens and function as targets of modulators from the paracrine granulosa cells. The multifunctional granulosa cell has the capacity to generate FSH-mediated LH receptors, P-450$_{C17}$ enzyme, and progesterone synthesis *(P₄)*. It has the ability to produce locally a variety of autocrine or paracrine regulators, for example, growth factors and tissue plasminogen activator and inhibitor *(tPA and tPAI)*. (Adapted from Yen SSC, Jaffe RB: *Reproductive endocrinology*, 3rd ed. Philadelphia: WB Saunders, 1991:291.)

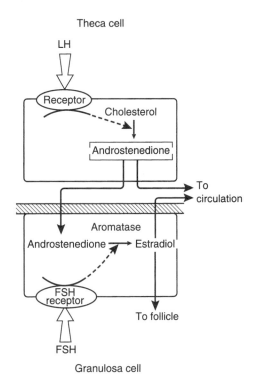

FIG. 10. Coupling of granulosa and theca cells in the two-cell, two-gonadotropin theory of follicular estrogen production *(FSH,* follicle-stimulating hormone; *LH,* luteinizing hormone). (Adapted from Berkowitz R, Barbieri R. The ovary. In: Ryan KJ, Berkowitz R, Barbieri R, eds. *Kistner's gynecology, principles and practice*, 5th ed. Chicago: Year Book Medical Publishers, 1990:259.)

continue to mature, growing in diameter and granulosa cell number, are those with high estrogen levels and low androgen–estrogen ratios. In the luteal phase preceding an ovulatory cycle, follicles that are 1 to 5 mm in diameter constitute the cohort from which the ovulatory follicle will be recruited. Recruitment suggests that a follicle has entered an accelerated development phase and has an opportunity to achieve ovulation. The exponential growth phase, from 5 to 20 mm, largely depends on gonadotropin and occurs during the follicular phase of the ovulatory cycle. It is during this phase that a dominant follicle, the follicle destined to ovulate, is selected. The entire growth phase from small secondary to preovulatory follicle takes approximately 85 days.

By the midfollicular phase, about 1 week before ovulation, one follicle has produced more estrogen than the others and becomes the dominant follicle. This is reflected in the asymmetric measurements of estrogen levels in ovarian venous effluent as early as cycle days 5 through 7. The dominant follicle has the advantage of a higher rate of granulosa cell proliferation, coupled with greater numbers of FSH receptors, greater aromatization ability, and increased estrogen production. The increase in estrogen production is associated with falling circulating levels of FSH. Other developing but nondominant follicles experience decreased estrogen production, have higher androgen–estrogen ratios, and become atretic. The dominant follicle continues with steroid biosynthesis, with peak serum estrogen concentrations occurring approximately 24 to 36 hours before ovulation. Preceding ovulation by 24 to 48 hours, progesterone production accelerates, and a substantial increase occurs 12 to 24 hours before the ovulatory event.

Ovulation

The preovulatory surge of LH and to a lesser extent FSH results from the positive feedback action of estradiol from the

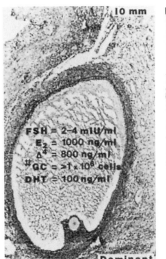
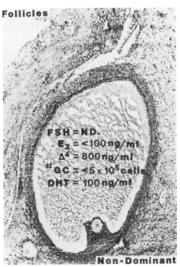

FSH = 2–4 mIU/ml
E₂ = 1000 ng/ml
Δ⁴ = 800 ng/ml
#GC = >1×10⁶ cells
DHT = 100 ng/ml

Dominant

FSH = ND.
E₂ = <100 ng/ml
Δ⁴ = 800 ng/ml
#GC = <5×10⁵ cells
DHT = 100 ng/ml

Non-Dominant

FIG. 11. Differences between the antral fluid microenvironments of a dominant and a nondominant follicle at the midfollicular phase of the menstrual cycle (Δ^4, androstenedione; *DHT*, dihydrotestosterone; E_2, estradiol; *FSH*, follicle-stimulating hormone; *#GC*, number of granulosa cells; *ND*, not detectable). (From Erickson GF, Yen SSC. New data on follicle cells in polycystic ovaries: a proposed mechanism for the genesis of cystic follicles. *Semin Reprod Biol* 1984;2:231; with permission.)

dominant follicle on the pituitary gland. This surge precedes ovulation, the actual rupture of the follicle, by as much as 36 hours and marks the end of the follicular phase. Urinary home LH testing kits are used for diagnostic and therapeutic purposes such as predicting the correct timing for sperm inseminations. Ovulation is preceded by rapid follicular enlargement, but direct measurements of the intrafollicular fluid suggest that it is not under high pressure and that the oocyte–cumulus complex is gently extruded, not explosively expelled, from the follicle. In rats and rabbits, inhibitors of prostaglandin synthesis inhibit ovulation. These and other data suggest that ovulation may be mediated by prostaglandin production. Proteolytic enzymes, such as plasminogen activator, may be involved in digestion of the follicular wall, which is necessary for ovulation to occur.

Luteal Phase

The luteal phase is characterized by reorganization of the granulosa cells of the dominant follicle into the corpus luteum and by increased progesterone production. After ovulation, the dominant follicle, evolving into the corpus luteum, undergoes rapid vascularization. The corpus luteum consists of the surrounding theca-interstitial cells, vascular components, and morphologically changed, or luteinized, granulosa cells. Neovascularization supplies the granulosa-lutein cells with low-density lipoprotein cholesterol, the critical substrate for progesterone production. High levels of progesterone in the presence of estrogen result in powerful negative feedback actions that suppress gonadotropin secretion. The pulse frequency of gonadotropins during the luteal phase of the cycle decreases to every 3 to 4 hours from every 60 to 90 minutes. The corpus luteum is gonadotropin-dependent and relies on continuous tonic support by LH.

Unless pregnancy occurs, demise of the corpus luteum is inevitable 14 ± 2 days after ovulation. The exact mechanisms governing luteolysis are poorly understood, although prostaglandins may play a role. Pregnancy and its associated luteotropic hormone, hCG, maintain luteal function. The hCG, initially secreted by the fetal trophoblast, binds to LH receptors and supports progesterone production in the corpus luteum until placental steroidogenesis is well established. The luteoplacental shift from corpus luteum to placental steroid production occurs at approximately 8 weeks' gestation. With regression of the corpus luteum, progesterone and estrogen production declines, allowing new follicular growth and development with an increase in FSH. The new cycle of follicle development is initiated.

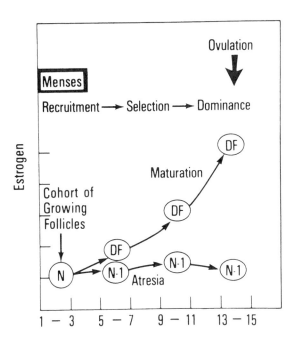

FIG. 12. Recruitment, selection, and ovulation of a dominant ovarian follicle *(DF)*, with atresia of other cohort follicles *(N-1)* in a natural ovarian or menstrual cycle. (From Hodgen, 1982, with permission.)

◊ PUBERTY

The physiology of reproduction depends on the complex and interactive hypothalamic–pituitary–ovarian system. The monthly process of oogenesis, fueled by pituitary gonadotropin secretion of FSH and LH, depends on the pulsatile release of Gn-RH from the hypothalamus (Fig. 13). Puberty, the developmental period during which a person attains sexual maturity and the ability to reproduce, is under strict neuroendocrine control and specifically relies on the hypothalamus to increase the pulsatile secretion of Gn-RH. Puberty is marked by profound neuroendocrine changes, including increases in Gn-RH and gonadotropin pulsatile secretion, changes in ovarian and adrenal steroid production, maturation of the hypothalamic–pituitary–ovarian axis, and subsequent somatic changes, including development of secondary sexual characteristics such as breasts and pubic hair, an acceleration of linear growth, and bone maturation.

Neuroendocrine Development

The prepubertal period is characterized by specific hormonal levels of Gn-RH, gonadotropins, and estradiol. Pulsatile Gn-RH secretion is detectable after 20 weeks' gestation and throughout the first year of life. Thereafter, it gradually declines and reaches a nadir at approximately 6 to 8 years of age. FSH and LH are detectable during the first 25 to 29 weeks' gestation. Gonadotropin levels decrease toward term and fluctuate during the first year or two of life. Thereafter, as with Gn-RH, FSH and LH levels decline and remain low through-

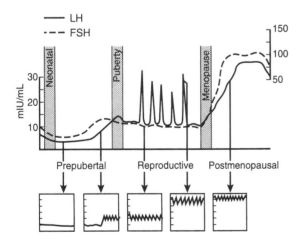

FIG. 13. The changing pattern and ratio of luteinizing hormone *(LH)* to follicle-stimulating hormone *(FSH)* before, during, and after the reproductive phase of a woman's life cycle. The lower boxes illustrate the amplitude of pulsatile LH release through which circulating concentrations are maintained. The *shaded* areas represent periods of nocturnal sleep. Sleep-induced LH rise is uniquely found during pubertal sexual maturation. (Adapted from Yen SSC, Vandenburg G, Tsai CC, Siler T. Causal relationship between the hormonal variables in the menstrual cycle. In: Ferin M, Halberg F, Richart RM, Van de Wiele RL, eds. *Biorhythms and human reproduction.* New York: John Wiley & Sons, 1974:219.)

out childhood until immediately before puberty. Estradiol levels decline dramatically after birth and remain low in the prepubertal years. The hypogonadotropic state associated with prepuberty occurs even in agonadal girls, suggesting that a central mechanism controlling hypothalamic Gn-RH secretion is responsible for the low levels of gonadotropins.

Pulsatile Gn-RH secretion appears to be the limiting factor in the initiation of puberty. Although prepubertal girls demonstrate blunted pituitary responses to exogenous Gn-RH, the administration of pulsatile Gn-RH promotes gonadotropin secretion, follicle maturation, and ovulation, indicating that the pituitary and ovary are not the limiting factors. The initiation of puberty appears to be centrally driven by an increase in hypothalamic pulsatile secretion of Gn-RH. Even in gonadal dysgenesis, in which functional ovaries are absent, puberty is initiated in the same manner. A decline in hypothalamic inhibition or an increase in stimulation may be responsible for the increase in pulsatile Gn-RH secretion by the hypothalamus at the time of puberty, but this mechanism is not well understood. Puberty is heralded by a progressive increase in Gn-RH and LH pulse amplitude without a change in frequency. Nocturnal increase in Gn-RH pulsation is another hallmark of early pubertal development that precedes the ovarian response of folliculogenesis and steroid biosynthesis. Daytime values of FSH and LH may be indistinguishable from prepubertal levels. Maturation of the hypothalamic–pituitary–ovarian axis is required as puberty progresses, and anovulatory cycles indicating dyssynchrony between central and ovarian messages are common in adolescent girls before the complex axis is finally synchronized.

In addition to increased Gn-RH, LH, and FSH pulsation, other hormonal changes occur during the prepubertal and pubertal period (Fig. 14). Before puberty, when the levels of steroids are low, the hypothalamus and pituitary are extremely sensitive to the suppressive effect of small amounts of circulating gonadal steroids. With the start of puberty, the hypothalamic and pituitary gonadostat becomes less sensitive to gonadal steroid feedback, resulting in increased secretion of gonadotropins from the anterior pituitary and consequent increases in ovarian estrogen and progesterone production. LH levels increase 100-fold over prepubertal values, FSH levels increase sixfold, and estradiol levels increase 12-fold.

Prolactin

Prolactin is detectable in the human fetal pituitary as early as 12 weeks' gestation and increases in production and secretion near term. Serum levels fall significantly during the first week of life to reach normal prepubertal levels. During puberty, mean prolactin levels in girls, but not in boys, increase markedly to achieve adult levels.

Growth Hormone

With its acceleration of linear growth, pubertal development is associated with an increase in the episodic release of pitu-

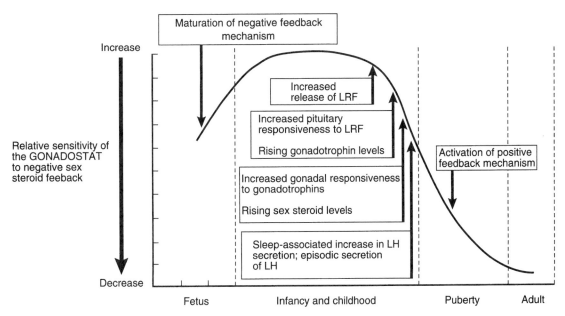

FIG. 14. Schematic illustration of the development of the hypothalamic–pituitary–gonadotropin–gonadal interrelations and the onset of puberty (*LH*, luteinizing hormone; *LRF*, luteinizing release factor). (Adapted from Grumbach et al., 1974.)

itary GH. Once a pubertal pattern of gonadotropin secretion is established, GH appears to enhance the rate of sexual maturation. GH is necessary to stimulate skeletal and muscle growth, regulate lipolysis, and promote cellular uptake of amino acids. IGF-1 and IGF-2 mediate the effects of GH. Episodic release of GH increases during puberty from four to six surges per 24 hours to as many as eight surges per 24 hours, and there is a dramatic increase in the total volume of GH from the prepubertal average daily level of 90 μg to a level of 700 μg in adolescents. Its release is triggered by external stimuli such as sleep and the episodic release of GHRF. GH is probably influenced by tonic inhibition of somatostatin.

Adrenal Androgen

Adrenarche, the increase in adrenal androgen production, is one of the earliest endocrine changes that occurs during puberty. The increase in adrenal steroids occurs as early as 7 to 8 years of age. The activation of adrenal androgen secretion from the zona reticularis results in the secretion of androstenedione, the more potent steroid, and the weaker androgens, dehydroepiandrosterone and its sulfate. The mechanism responsible for the increase in adrenal androgens is not well understood. It is not linked to the pubertal increase in pulsatile Gn-RH and gonadotropin secretion.

Adrenarche and gonadarche, the maturation of gonadal function, are independent events controlled by different mechanisms, and one is not essential for the other. Patients with premature adrenarche associated with high levels of adrenal androgens at very early ages enter puberty within the normal period, demonstrating that precocious puberty does not result from premature acceleration of adrenal androgen production. Children with Addison disease who suffer from adrenal insufficiency and absent or inadequate adrenal androgen secretion typically experience normal pubertal development when supplied with appropriate mineralocorticoid and glucocorticoid replacement therapy, demonstrating that pubertal delay does not occur with inadequate androgen production. Patients with gonadal dysgenesis experience normal adrenarche. Although adrenarche and gonadarche are temporally related, they are independent endocrine events.

Sexual Maturation and Growth during Puberty

Puberty is associated with a host of physical changes, including development of secondary sexual characteristics such as breast, pubic hair, and axillary hair; acceleration of linear growth (i.e., adolescent growth spurt); bone development; and changes in body composition (Fig. 15). In normal girls, external manifestations of puberty are typically seen between 8.5 and 13 years of age, with a mean of 11 years of age and a standard deviation of approximately 1 year for the age at which each pubertal stage is typically reached. By this definition, the appearance of secondary sexual characteristics such as breasts and pubic hair is considered precocious if they occur before 7.5 years of age, and delayed if there are no physical manifestations by 14 years of age. There is great variation in the age at which puberty begins and in the time it takes to achieve mature development. The period from the first sign of puberty to complete maturity can be as short as 1.5 years to more than 6 years. Normal development is most notably characterized by the relations among the pubertal events, and progression through the various stages is more indicative of normal development than the chronologic age at which they appear.

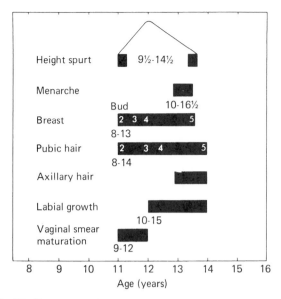

FIG. 15. Sequence of events that occurs in girls at puberty. The numbers under each indicate the normal range of ages within which the event may occur. (From Tanner, 1962, with permission.)

Secondary Sexual Characteristics

Despite wide variations in the timing of pubertal development in normal girls, studies by Tanner on the progression of physical changes during puberty have led to the description of specific stages. These stages include thelarche (breast development), pubarche (pubic hair development), acceleration of linear growth (adolescent growth spurt), and menarche (onset of periodic shedding of the endometrium).

Breast development is typically the first external manifestation of puberty. Thelarche has been described by Tanner in five stages:

Stage 1   Infantile or preadolescent stage that persists from infancy; areola not pigmented, and only papilla is elevated.

Stage 2   Breast bud stage that is the first indication of pubertal breast changes. The areola diameter enlarges; breast and papilla are elevated in a small mound.

Stage 3   Breast and areola enlarge further, with a continuous round contour.

Stage 4   Areola and papilla enlarge and project to form a secondary mound above the remaining breast.

Stage 5   Mature adult breast develops, with resolution of the secondary mound to achieve a smooth, rounded contour with projection of the papilla only.

The duration and stages of breast development vary greatly among girls and are based on genetics and nutritional status. Although the progression from stages 2 through 5 takes an average of 4 years, some women never reach stage 5 until the first pregnancy or later.

Development of the breast as an endocrine organ requires hormonal stimulation, primarily estrogen for ductal growth and progesterone and prolactin for lobuloalveolar development. Prolactin, as discussed earlier, regulates lactation.

Pubic hair development has been described by Tanner as consisting of five stages:

Stage 1   Infantile or preadolescent, with no pubic hair.

Stage 2   Sparse growth of long, slightly pigmented, downy hair, primarily on the labia majora.

Stage 3   Amount of hair increases, with some spread to mons pubis, and hair becomes coarser, darker, and more curly.

Stage 4   Adult-type hair covering a smaller area than in most adults, with no spread to the medial thigh.

Stage 5   Adult distribution of coarse hair with some spread to the medial surface of the thighs, characteristic of normal female escutcheon.

The pubertal increase in adrenal androgen production primarily influences the growth of pubic and axillary hair. Axillary hair appears concomitantly with pubic hair. Although thelarche and adrenarche are temporally related, breast and pubic hair development does not necessarily begin at the same time. Pubic hair may appear before breast enlargement, but typically breast development is the first external sign of puberty and is often quite advanced before pubic hair appears.

Genital development in girls is not defined by standardized data or stages. Attention is given to the mucosal changes indicative of estrogen stimulation that accompanies pubertal development. In the prepubertal period, the epithelium of the vagina and labia are extremely thin and appear bright red on physical examination. As pubertal estrogen levels are attained, the vaginal and vulvar mucosa changes from bright red to pink, and mucoid vaginal secretions appear. Confirmation can be obtained microscopically with vaginal smears. Uterine enlargement is observed during pelvic examination.

Acceleration of Linear Growth

In early childhood, the growth curve is extremely steep and gradually levels off until puberty, at which time growth accelerates, and the curve is again steep. Adolescent girls studied by Marshall and Tanner (1969) in England reached a peak height velocity at 12.1 years of age. The accelerated growth in girls is typically associated with early pubertal changes, such as Tanner breast stage 2 or 3, and most girls experience this growth spurt before menarche. This contrasts markedly with pubertal boys, whose peak height velocity is associated with late puberty, almost 2 years later than girls and usually not until their genitalia are well developed (Fig. 16). Girls and boys have comparable growth spurts (25 and 28 cm, respectively), and the fact that boys experience a longer period of preadolescent growth before acceleration probably accounts for the absolute mean height difference between older boys and girls.

The adolescent growth spurt is governed by GH and gonadal sex steroids, and adrenal androgens appear to play a less critical role in the process. Children with deficient adrenal steroids experience a normal growth spurt, but children with

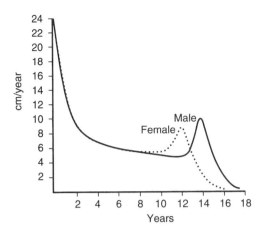

FIG. 16. Velocity curves for length (less than 2 years of age) and height (2 to 18 years of age) for girls and boys show deceleration of growth rate from infancy until the onset of adolescence. (Adapted from Gold JJ, Josimovich JB. *Gynecologic endocrinology*, 4th ed. New York: Plenum Publishing, 1987: 100.)

severe hypogonadism have essentially no growth acceleration. Children deficient in gonadotropins and GH need sex steroids and GH to achieve a growth spurt; GH alone is inadequate. GH apparently augments the rate of sexual maturation after a pubertal pattern of gonadotropin secretion is established. A recent review by Sharara and Guidice (1997) suggests that GH may actually act as a cogonadotropin and augment the actions of FSH and LH on estradiol and progesterone production.

Bone Development

Osseous maturation of the bone (i.e., bone age) more closely correlates with menarche than chronologic age and is a useful index in assessing a child's developmental process. Bone age is assessed from radiographs of a child's hand and wrist, which are compared with standards of normal bone maturation in the general population.

Body Composition

In addition to the development of secondary sexual characteristics and accelerated growth, puberty is associated with significant changes in body composition. In prepubertal children, lean body mass, skeletal mass, and body fat mass are approximately equal. After puberty, women acquire twice as much body fat as men, and men have approximately a 1.5-fold increase in lean body mass, muscle mass, and skeletal mass, compared with women. At approximately the same time as pubic and axillary hair development, axillary and pubic apocrine glands begin to function. Sebaceous glands also become more active in puberty.

◊ MENSTRUAL CYCLE

Menstruation, which is episodic shedding of the endometrium, is the hallmark of the reproductive years, and menarche is one

of the most notable changes of puberty. The mean age for menarche for American girls is 12.3 to 12.8 years, and the mean interval from the first sign of puberty until the menarche is 2.3 ± 1 years. The human menstrual cycle is governed by the complex and orderly functioning of the neuroendocrine system involving the hypothalamic–pituitary–ovarian axis. Pulsatile secretion of hypothalamic Gn-RH stimulates pituitary gonadotropin release and fuels follicle maturation and ovarian theca and granulosa cell steroidogenesis. The physiology of reproduction would not be complete without a discussion of the endometrium or intrauterine environment, the site of preparation for embryo implantation.

Characteristics

Standard menstrual cycle length for women is 28 days. Although there is considerable variation among women, there is relative constancy in the cycles for any one person. A range of 26 to 30 days is considered normal, but the definition remains flexible; an ovulatory woman with a 34-day cycle who is capable of conceiving is not abnormal. The first day of bleeding, which defines the onset of menses, defines the first day of the menstrual cycle, and the day before the next bleeding episode defines the last day of the cycle. The menstrual cycle is divided into the follicular or proliferative phase, which precedes ovulation, and the luteal or secretory phase, which occurs after ovulation and is typically 14 ± 2 days long, the most constant in length of the two cycles.

Menstrual flow typically lasts 4 to 6 days in ovulatory cycles, with an average blood loss of 25 to 60 ml. Normal menstruation occurs after an ovulatory cycle, although anovulatory cycles due to estrogen or progesterone withdrawal can occur because of stress, excessive exercise, travel, or weight loss. Anovulatory cycles are common in the first year after menarche and in the perimenopausal period.

Histologic Phases

The early proliferative phase of the menstrual cycle is characterized by an endometrium less than 2 mm thick. Proliferation of cells of the basal layer and remaining lower uterine segment cells restore the endometrial epithelial surface by day 5 of the cycle. Endometrial glands are tubular, straight, and narrow, with low columnar epithelium. The proliferative phase is marked by increased mitotic activity in stromal and glandular cells. In the late proliferative phase, glandular hyperplasia begins, and the endometrium consequently thickens. There is also an increase in stromal ground substance.

Ovulation marks the change from proliferative to secretory endometrium (Fig. 17). The endometrium has three layers: the basal zone immediately adjacent to the endometrium that undergoes little histologic change, the intermediate spongy zone above the basalis, and the compact zone directly beneath the endometrial surface (Fig. 18). The intermediate and compact zones compose the functional endometrium, which is cyclically shed. Stromal edema occurs,

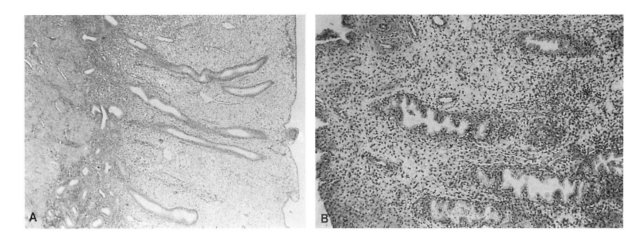

FIG. 17. A: Late proliferative endometrium at or about the time of ovulation. Tortuous, pseudostratified glands with many mitoses are characteristic. Stroma without predecidual reaction may have some degree of edema. **B:** Sixteen-day secretory endometrium. This early postovulatory endometrium is characterized by tortuous-growing glands with irregular vacuolization caused by an accumulation of glycogen in the cytoplasm beneath the nuclei. (Courtesy of Stanley J. Robboy, MD, Duke University Medical Center, Durham, NC.)

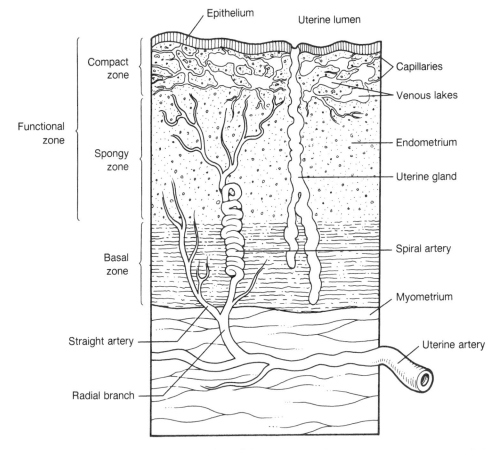

FIG. 18. Diagram of the histologic organization of the secretory-phase human endometrium. (Adapted from Blandau RJ. *Weiss-Greep histology*, 4th ed. New York: McGraw-Hill, 1977:911.)

and glandular epithelial cells accumulate glycogen-rich vacuoles at their bases. The middle- to late-secretory phase is characterized by a 5- to 6-mm-thick endometrium with an edematous stroma, tortuous glands with prominent secretory activity, and developing spiral arteries. The premenstrual endometrium is marked by stromal infiltration by polymorphonuclear and mononuclear leukocytes.

Mechanism of Menstruation

Progesterone withdrawal marks the beginning of menstruation, but whether or not a decline in progesterone is actually the initiator of the menstrual process remains unclear. There may be intermediate regulators. Prostaglandins accumulate in the endometrium during the secretory phase and may contribute to menstrual bleeding by causing vasoconstriction of arterioles. This ischemic process immediately precedes menstruation and causes inadequate perfusion of the upper one-half to two-thirds of the endometrium. As the constricted arteries relax, bleeding begins. Vasoconstriction and the rapid formation of platelet plugs provide hemostasis and limit blood loss with menstruation. Reepithelialization begins almost immediately on day 2 and is completed by day 5.

Progesterone and prostaglandins play major roles in endometrial shedding. After ovulation, there is an increase in lysosomes in the endometrium and an increase in endometrial acid phosphatase activity. Progesterone has a stabilizing effect on lysosomes. If pregnancy does not occur, declining progesterone levels in the late-secretory phase promote disruption of lysosomal membranes and the release of hydrolases, which contribute to cellular disruption, endometrial issue necrosis, and subsequent endometrial sloughing. Local hypoxia associated with prostaglandin secretion is another destabilizing influence on lysosomal membranes. In a cyclic process, lysosomal phospholipases liberate arachidonic acid, which results in increased production of endometrial prostaglandins, particularly prostaglandin $F_{2\alpha}$, a stable prostaglandin that stimulates uterine contraction.

Normal menstrual flow does not form true fibrin clots because it is rich in plasminogen activator, which causes rapid fibrinogenolysis. Small clots that are sometimes described by patients are actually a coagulum containing erythrocytes and vaginal secretions that forms in the vagina. When abnormally brisk uterine bleeding occurs, the blood is clotted because proteolytic enzymes did not have a chance to act. Dark-brown menstrual flow indicates older blood that has been acted on by proteolytic enzymes.

◊ MENOPAUSE

With advancing chronologic age, as menopause approaches, the ovary gradually becomes less responsive to gonadotropins several years before menses cease. Shortly before menopause, circulating levels of FSH increase, and estradiol and progesterone levels fall. FSH levels are higher in perimenopausal women than in younger, reproductive-age women early in the follicular phase, at the time of the midcycle gonadotropin surge, and late in the luteal phase. LH levels appear to be unaffected (Fig. 19). The mechanisms that generate the rise in FSH but not in LH are under investigation. One possible explanation is that inhibin, a glycoprotein produced by the ovarian granulosa cells that is a potent inhibitor of FSH release, is produced in decreasing amounts with aging.

Declining ovarian follicular maturation and its eventual cessation define the menopause, with its associated decrease in estradiol production and absent menstruation. The increase in circulating levels of FSH and LH reflect increased pituitary production, as the metabolic clearance rates of FSH and LH remain essentially unchanged. Gonadotropins have a pulsatile release pattern in postmenopausal women that occurs in 60- to 90-minute intervals.

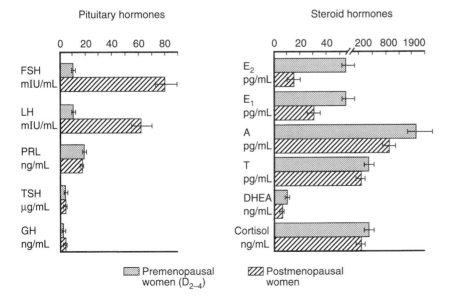

FIG. 19. Circulating levels of pituitary and steroid hormones in postmenopausal women are compared with those in premenopausal women studied during the first week (days 2 to 4 [D_{2-4}]) of the menstrual cycle (A, androstenedione; DHEA, dehydroepiandrosterone; E_1, estrone; E_2, estradiol; FSH, follicle-stimulating hormone; GH, growth hormone; LH, luteinizing hormone; PRL, prolactin; T, testosterone; TSH, thyroid-stimulating hormone). (Adapted from Yen SSC. The biology of menopause. J Reprod Med 1977;18:287.)

Although estrogen production by the postmenopausal ovary is usually minimal, the postmenopausal ovary continues to produce significant amounts of testosterone and androstenedione. These androgens are produced primarily by the ovarian stromal and hilar cells, but the principal source of postmenopausal androstenedione is the adrenal gland. The ovary contributes more significantly to the circulating levels of testosterone than androstenedione. The postmenopausal level of testosterone is approximately equal to that of a premenopausal woman.

In postmenopausal women, circulating levels of estrone are higher than those of estradiol. The low levels of estrogens in postmenopausal women are generated by extragonadal aromatization of adrenal androgens. Androstenedione is aromatized to estrogen in sites outside the ovary and adrenal gland, such as in fat, liver, and kidney. Obese women convert more androgens peripherally than thin women, resulting in greater estrogenic stimulation of the endometrium and a greater risk for endometrial hyperplasia and endometrial cancer.

These two events are independent and controlled by different mechanisms.

◊ Menopause is defined as the eventual cessation of ovarian follicular maturation with its associated decrease in estradiol production and absent menstruation. The increase in circulating levels of FSH and LH reflect increased pituitary production, as the metabolic clearance rates of FSH and LH remain essentially unchanged.

SUMMARY POINTS

◊ Pituitary hormone synthesis and secretion are directed by five major hypothalamic peptides: Gn-RH, CRF, GHRF, somatostatin, and TRH. Although reproductive physiology is primarily mediated by the pulsatile secretion of Gn-RH, the other metabolic hypothalamic hormones also influence successful reproduction.

◊ The three anterior pituitary hormones most closely linked to reproductive physiology are gonadotropin, LH and FSH, together with the polypeptide hormone prolactin. The pituitary cells that synthesize and secrete LH and FSH are called gonadotrophs.

◊ The ovary is involved in the biosynthesis and secretion of three groups of steroid hormones: estrogens, androgens, and progestins. All steroids are lipid-related, are derived from the parent compound cholesterol, and share a common carbon-ring structure of four fused rings called perhydrocyclopentanophenanthrene. The family of progestins has 21 carbons, androgens have 19 carbons, and estrogens have 18 carbons.

◊ Puberty, the developmental period during which a person attains sexual maturity and the ability to reproduce, is under strict neuroendocrine control and specifically relies on the hypothalamus to increase the pulsatile secretion of Gn-RH. Adrenarche, the increase in adrenal androgen production, is one of the earliest endocrine changes that occurs during puberty and is an event that is completely independent of gonadarche, the maturation of gonadal function.

◊ RECOMMENDED READINGS

Adashi EY, Resnick CE, Hernandez ER, et al. Insulin-like growth factor I as an intraovarian regulator: basic and clinical implications. *Ann N Y Acad Sci* 1991;626:161.

Bicsak TA, Tucker EM, Cappel S, et al. Hormonal regulation of granulosa cell inhibin biosynthesis. *Endocrinology* 1986;119:2711.

Dunger DB, Villa AK, Matthews DR, et al. Pattern of bioactive and immunoreactive gonadotrophins in normal prepubertal children. *Clin Endocrinol (Oxf)* 1991;35:267.

Frisch RE, Revelle R. Height and weight at menarche and hypothesis of critical body weights and adolescent events. *Science* 1970;169:397.

Fritz MA, Speroff L. The endocrinology of the menstrual cycle: the interaction of folliculogenesis and neuroendocrine mechanisms. *Fertil Steril* 1982;38:509.

Gainer H, Wray S. Oxytocin and vasopressin. From genes to peptides. *Ann N Y Acad Sci* 1992;652:14.

Grumbach MM, Roth JC, Kaplan SL, et al. Hypothalamic-pituitary regulation of puberty: evidence and concepts derived from clinical research. In: Grumbach MM, Grave GD, Mayer FE, eds. *The control of the onset of puberty.* New York: John Wiley and Sons, 1974:115.

Hodgen GD. The dominant ovarian follicle. *Fertil Steril* 1982;38:281.

Jaffe RB, Plosker S, Marshall L, Martin MC. Neuromodulatory regulation of gonadotropin-releasing hormone pulsatile discharge in women. *Am J Obstet Gynecol* 1990;163:1727.

Katz E, McClamrock HD, Adashi HD, Adashi EY. Ovarian failure including menopause, premature menopause, and resistant ovarian syndrome, and hormonal replacement. *Curr Opin Obstet Gynecol* 1991;2:392.

Kettel L, DePaolo LV, Morales AJ, et al. Circulating levels of follistatin from puberty to menopause. *Fertil Steril* 1996;65:472.

Klein NA, Battaglia DE, Miller PB. *J Clin Endocrinol Metab* 1996;8:1946.

Knight PG. Roles of inhibins, activins, and follistatin in the female reproductive system (review). *Front Neuroendocrinol* 1996;17:476.

Kreiger DT, Liotta AS. Pituitary hormones in brain: where, how and why? *Science* 1979;205:366.

Leong DA, Frawley LS, Neill JD. Neuroendocrine control of prolactin secretion. *Annu Rev Physiol* 1983;45:109.

Marshall WA, Tanner JM. Variations in patterns of pubertal changes in girls. *Arch Dis Child* 1969;44:291.

Pescovitz OH. The endocrinology of the pubertal growth spurt. *Acta Paediatr Scand Suppl* 1990;367:119.

Rasmussen DD, Gambacciani M, Swartz W, et al. Pulsatile gonadotropin-releasing hormone release from the human mediobasal hypothalamus *in vitro:* opiate receptor-mediated suppression. *Neuroendocrinology* 1989; 49:150.

Scott RT, Hofmann GE. Prognostic assessment of ovarian reserve. *Fertil Steril* 1995;63:1.

Sharara FI, Giudice LC. Role of growth hormone in ovarian physiology and onset of puberty. *J Soc Gynecol Investig* 1997;4:2.

Tanner JM. *Growth and adolescence,* 2nd ed. Oxford: Blackwell Science, 1962.

Veldhuis JD, Johnson ML, Seneta E. Analysis of the copulsatility of anterior pituitary hormones. *J Clin Endocrinol Metab* 1991;73:569.

Vermeulen A, Verdonck L. Sex hormone concentrations in postmenopausal women. *Clin Endocrinol (Oxf)* 1978;9:59.

Winter JD, Faiman C. The development of cyclic pituitary-gonadal function in adolescent females. *J Clin Endocrinol Metab* 1973;37:714.

Yen SSC, Tsai CC, Naftolin F, et al. Pulsatile patterns of gonadotropin release in subjects with and without ovarian function. *J Clin Endocrinol Metab* 1972;34:671.

CHAPTER 6

Normal Pregnancy and Prenatal Care

——— ◇ ———

Vivian M. Dickerson
Ronald A. Chez

Concepts about pregnancy and constructs of prenatal care have changed since the early 16th century in Europe when pregnancy and the travails of labor were viewed as punishment for the sins of Eve. The first caretakers of pregnant women were older women in the community who provided advice and attended the actual birth. This evolved into the formalized role of midwife; indeed, the French term for midwife, *sage-femme* (literally, wise woman), reflects these origins.

In the United States, the first organized prenatal care programs began in 1901 with home nurse visits, and the first prenatal clinic was established in 1911. It is not surprising that this focus on maternal and infant health occurred as a direct outgrowth of the women's suffrage movement. The emergence of the physician-obstetrician as the primary caregiver for women of reproductive age has also taken place during this century. This role has become one of partnership with allied health care providers, including nurses, nurse midwives, nurse practitioners, nutritionists, and social workers. This team not only provides medical treatment and advice but also serves as the patient's advocate.

Social and political changes of the last several decades have empowered female patients to take a more active role in their medical care. As women both individually and collectively take increasing responsibility for themselves, they have begun to express their views about and choices for contraception, pregnancy, and child rearing. This has given rise to family- and community-centered care concepts, new venues in which care is received, and a patient–clinician partnership.

Our current emphasis on prenatal care stems from historic pronouncements and retrospective analyses that concluded that women who receive prenatal care have less fetal, infant, and maternal morbidity and mortality.[19,26] However, a firm scientific foundation for the content of prenatal care and its exact relationship to good outcomes is lacking.[9,10] As technology flourishes and resources dwindle, it will become increasingly important to obtain scientifically based evidence demonstrating which of the various components of prenatal care are clinically appropriate, cost-effective, and deserving of preferential funding. At this time, the optimal content and delivery of prenatal care remain the subject of discussion and debate.

◇ PRIMARY AND PRECONCEPTION CARE

Philosophy

Care of the reproductive age woman for both preconception and pregnancy fulfills all of the criteria for primary care as set out by the Institute of Medicine[8] in 1994 and by the American College of Obstetricians and Gynecologists[1] (ACOG) in 1993. Such care is integrated and accessible, focuses on the majority of personal health care needs, represents a sustained partnership between patient and provider, and occurs within the context of family and community. For many women, pregnancy care occurs as one part of the continuum in a long-term primary care relationship.

Content of the Preconception Visit

The preconception visit is a focused interval primary care visit for the woman who is planning to become pregnant in the near future. The content of this interval visit includes a focused history, physical examination, risk assessment and intervention, selected laboratory testing based on the patient's age and the results of the foregoing evaluation, ongoing management of medical conditions, and a plan of care. A purposeful discussion of contraception, sexually transmitted disease prevention, and timing of conception is appropriate. Timely administration of routine immunizations, educational counseling, and advice complete the visit.

Risk Assessment

A goal specific to the preconception interval visit is the systematic identification of potential risks to pregnancy and the implementation of early intervention as necessary. These risks fall into several categories:[13]

Unalterable Factors

These are preexisting factors and cannot at present be altered in any material way by clinical intervention. These include the patient's height, age, reproductive history, ethnicity, educational level, socioeconomic status, and genetic composition.

Factors Benefiting from Early Intervention

Conditions that should or could be modified before pregnancy is attempted include poor nutrition, an underweight or obese body mass index, and poorly controlled medical diseases such as diabetes mellitus, asthma, epilepsy, phenylketonuria, and hypertension.

Some prescription medications that are known teratogens should be discontinued and appropriate substitutions made. These include isotretinoin (Accutane), warfarin sodium (Coumadin), certain anticonvulsants, and some psychotropic agents. Angiotensin-converting enzyme inhibitors should be avoided during the third trimester.

Identification of Unalterable Medical Conditions

Determining the status of a patient's immunity to both rubella, and hepatitis B is appropriate during the preconception visit. In high-risk populations or endemic geographic areas, patients should be assessed for active tuberculosis with skin testing and chest x-ray.

Social Risk Factors

Occupational hazards involving exposure to toxins such as lead and mercury, and hazards in the home such as exposure to toxoplasmosis or toxic chemicals (asbestos, pesticides), are important to identify. Family violence is a particularly important household hazard. Questions such as "Are you in a relationship in which you are being hit, kicked, slapped, or threatened?" should be routinely asked.

Risky Health Habits

The use of illicit drugs or abuse of alcohol represents a significant health hazard to pregnancy. Alcohol is a known teratogen. There is no consensus on the correlation between the quantity of alcohol consumed and the manifestation of adverse fetal effects. Therefore, the best advice to women who wish to become pregnant is to stop drinking.

Smoking cigarettes is associated with adverse pregnancy outcomes including low-birthweight babies, premature birth, and perinatal death. Smoking by both the pregnant woman and members of the household should be avoided during pregnancy and, preferably, not resumed postpartum. Similarly, all illicit drugs have the potential of harming the pregnancy.

Other behaviors that should be avoided are those that promote exposure to sexually transmitted and other infectious diseases. These include unprotected sexual intercourse in a nonmonogamous relationship and the sharing of needles between addicts.

Interventions

The final phase of the preconception visit involves specific interventions derived from the information obtained during the history, physical examination, and risk assessment phases. The specific interventions may include immunization against rubella or hepatitis, changes in prescribed medications, behavior modification, and nutritional and physical activity recommendations.

Folic acid as a supplement can reduce the occurrence or recurrence of neural tube defects. Women who have had previous pregnancies affected by neural tube defects should take 4 mg of folic acid per day, starting 4 weeks prior to conception through the first trimester. For all other women of reproductive age who have the potential to become pregnant, the U.S. Centers for Disease Control and Prevention (CDC) recommends 400 μg (0.4 mg) of folic acid every day.[5]

Smoking has been identified as the leading preventable cause of low birthweight in the United States.[27] The relative risk of intrauterine growth restriction (IUGR) among pregnant smokers has been calculated at 2.2 to 4.2, which clearly indicates a positive association.[12] Because of the morbidity associated with smoking, various methods to assist women to quit smoking should be encouraged prior to pregnancy. Numerous interventions are available, although most are ineffective or only marginally effective (Table 1). Use of the transdermal nicotine patch in pregnancy has been evaluated only on a limited basis[3], and its use is controversial. One benefit of using a nicotine patch is the elimination of exposure to other toxins such as carbon monoxide inhaled in cigarette smoke. Its theoretical risk is that it creates a constant blood level of nicotine, as opposed to the vacillations that occur with smoking.

Approximately 20% of all pregnant women are battered during their pregnancy.[25] About one-half of women who are physically abused prior to pregnancy continue to be battered during pregnancy. For some women, the violence begins with pregnancy. All such patients require information regarding their immediate safety and referrals for counseling and support.

Some patients purposely initiate a preconception visit to determine whether or not their preexisting medical condition is an absolute contraindication to pregnancy. Pulmonary hypertension, for example, although rare, is associated with a 50% maternal mortality and a greater than 40% fetal mortality. It is possible to obtain epidemiologic studies that provide statistics on the morbidity and mortality for mother and fetus for most disease states. These cannot, however, provide specific data for any one patient with her own unique set of medical, demographic, and social variables. Many patients who

TABLE 1. *Smoking cessation in pregnancy*

Study	EXPT n	EXPT %	CTRL n	CTRL %	Odds ratio (95% CI)	Graph of odds ratios and confidence intervals
Effect of anti-smoking advice in pregnancy on continued smoking during pregnancy						
Baric *et al.* (1976)	54/63	85.71	45/47	95.74	0.33 (0.09–1.16)	
Burling (unpub)	62/69	89.86	68/70	97.14	0.30 (0.08–1.16)	
MacArthur *et al.* (1987)	484/493	98.17	483/489	98.77	0.67 (0.24–1.86)	
Lilley and Forster (1986)	73/77	94.81	72/73	98.63	0.31 (0.05–1.82)	
Effect of feedback for smoking cessation in pregnancy on continued smoking during pregnancy						
Bauman *et al.* (1983)	36/36	100.0	43/43	100	1.00 (1.00–1.00)	
Reading *et al.* (1984)	20/39	51.28	20/26	76.92	0.34 (0.13–0.95)	

Graph axis values: 0.01 0.1 0.5 1 2 10 100

CI, confidence interval; CTRL,; EXPT,.
(Adapted from?. In: Chalmers I, Enkin M, Keirse MJNC, eds. *Effective care in pregnancy and childbirth.* New York: Oxford University Press, 1989)

make these inquiries will benefit by reading the relevant medical materials themselves and by obtaining more than one opinion.

How and when to discontinue contraceptive measures are also important to discuss. Patients using medroxyprogesterone acetate (Depo-Provera) injections may experience a several-month delay in the return of regular ovulatory menstrual cycles. An intrauterine device may be removed at any time in the cycle. Likewise, birth control pills may be discontinued at any time prior to attempting conception.

The patient should be advised to seek early prenatal care by making an appointment after missed menses or on confirmation of pregnancy by a home pregnancy test. Unfortunately, in the United States, only 75% of pregnant women receive prenatal care beginning in the first trimester. The goal espoused by the United States Public Health Service for the year 2000 is to have 90% of eligible women enrolled in prenatal care by the end of the first trimester.[21] Ongoing barriers to prenatal care access include lack of money or insurance to pay for care, system undercapacity for appointments, and inadequate transportation (Table 2).[4]

◊ INITIAL PRENATAL VISIT

This visit represents the first detailed assessment of the pregnant patient. The optimal timing of this visit may vary. For women who have been unable to avail themselves of the comprehensive preconception visit (as described above), prenatal visits should begin as soon as pregnancy is recognized. All other women should be seen by about 8 menstrual weeks (6 weeks after conception) of gestation. For all patients, the appropriate content of prenatal care and the first prenatal visit is contained in the antepartum record published by ACOG (see Appendix 1). Identifying data, a menstrual history, and a pregnancy history are obtained. Past medical, surgical, and social history are recorded, along with symptoms of pregnancy. A focused genetic screen, infection history, and risk status evaluation are performed.

Diagnosis of Pregnancy

Evaluation of the signs and symptoms associated with the presumptive diagnosis of pregnancy (Table 3), while a useful ad-

TABLE 2. *Most frequent barriers to prenatal care (PNC) cited by women with insufficient care*

Barrier	Chao et al.	Lake and Nixon	Oxford et al.	Kalmuss et al.	Bowling and Riley	Imershiem et al.	Studies with item in top 4 (%)
Financial	1,2	2	1	1	2	1,2	100
Transportation	—	3	—	—	1	3	50
PNC poorly valued	3	1	1	—	—	—	66
Didn't know was pregnant	—	—	—	3	3	—	33
Limited number of providers	—	—	—	2	4	4	50
Scared	—	—	2	—	—	—	16
Negative institutional practices	—	—	—	4	4	—	33

(Adapted from ref. 4.)

TABLE 3. *Probability of pregnancy based on presumptive signs*

Study	Evidence grade	Characteristic	Pregnant		Likelihood ratio (95% CI)
			Yes	No	
Chadwick (1886)	C	Chadwick sign			
		Present	144	1	28.70 (4.10–200.00)
		Absent	137	55	0.50 (0.44–0.56)
Robinson and Barber (1977)	A	Breast signs			
		Present	549	127	2.71 (2.30–3.20)
		Absent	430	486	0.55 (0.50–0.60)
Robinson and Barber (1977)	A	Vaginal signs			
		Present	172	34	3.17 (2.22–4.51)
		Absent	807	579	0.87 (0.84–0.90)
Robinson and Barber (1977)	A	Palpable fundus			
		Present	84	19	2.77 (1.70–4.51)
		Absent	895	594	0.94 (0.92–0.97)

CI, confidence interval. (Adapted from ref. 2.)

junct, has been largely superseded by the widely available urine pregnancy test.[2] The detection of greater than 35 mIU of human chorionic gonadotropin (hCG) in the first morning void has a very high specificity for pregnancy. Other tests for confirming the presence of pregnancy include a positive serum β-hCG and demonstration of the fetal heart by either auscultation or ultrasound. Using a transvaginal probe, fetal cardiac activity should be seen by postconception week 4. Ultrasound imaging is not routinely indicated to diagnose pregnancy but may be used in the evaluation of a patient who is at increased risk for ectopic pregnancy or missed abortion. In conjunction with early, serial, quantitative serum β-hCG assessments, these conditions can be clearly differentiated from a normal intrauterine pregnancy, and timely therapy initiated (see Chapters 10 and 11).

Gestational Age

Naegele's rule is commonly applied in calculating an estimated date of confinement (EDC). Using the date of the patient's last menstrual period minus 3 months, plus 1 week and 1 year, it is based on the assumptions that a normal gestation is 280 days and that patients all have 28-day menstrual cycles. After adjustment for a patient's actual cycle length, natality statistics indicate that the majority of pregnancies deliver within 2 weeks before or after this estimated date. During prenatal care, the week of gestation can be obtained based on the calculated EDC. When the last menstrual period is unknown or the cycle is irregular, ultrasound measurements between the 14th and 20th week of gestation provide an accurate determination of gestational age (see Chapter 14).

Physical Examination

A targeted physical examination during the first prenatal visit includes special attention to the patient's body mass index (BMI), blood pressure, breasts, and pelvis. On pelvic examination, the cervix is inspected for stigmata associated with diethylstilbestrol exposure and for the presence of condylo-

mata, neoplasia, or infection. A Papanicolaou smear is performed, and cultures for gonorrhea and chlamydia are taken if indicated. A small amount of bright red bleeding may occur after these manipulations, and the patient can be assured that this is normal. On bimanual examination, the cervix is palpated to assess consistency and length and to detect the presence of cervical motion tenderness. Size, position, and contour of the uterus are noted. The adnexae are palpated to assess for masses. The pelvic examination may include evaluation of the bony pelvis, specifically, the diagonal conjugate, the ischial spines, the sacral hollow, and the arch of the symphysis pubis. This evaluation need only be performed once during the pregnancy and may be deferred until the onset of labor (see Chapter 7).

Laboratory Evaluation

Several laboratory tests are routinely done at the first prenatal visit.

Blood Tests

Hematologic testing includes a hemoglobin and hematocrit, a serologic test for syphilis (rapid plasma reagin or VDRL), a rubella titer, a hepatitis B surface antigen, a blood group (ABO), and Rh type and antibody screen. Human immunodeficiency virus (HIV) testing should be offered to all pregnant patients, and refusal documented in the chart. Routine assessment for toxoplasmosis, cytomegalovirus, and varicella immunity is not necessary but may be obtained if indicated.

Urine Tests

Asymptotic bacteriuria occurs in 5% to 8% of pregnant women. Urinary stasis is present during pregnancy secondary to physiologic changes in the urinary system, including decreased ureteral peristalsis and mechanical uterine compression of the ureter at the pelvic brim as pregnancy progresses. Bacteriuria combined with urinary stasis predisposes the patient to pyelonephritis, the most common nonobstetric cause for hospitalization during pregnancy.[23] Asymptomatic bacteriuria is identified using microscopic urine analysis, urine culture (more than 100,000 colonies/ml), or a leukocyte esterase–nitrite dipstick on a clean-catch voided urine.

Cultures

The use of routine genital tract cultures in pregnancy is controversial. While it is clear that chlamydiosis, gonorrhea, group B streptococcal disease, herpes infection, and potentially bacterial vaginosis can be detrimental to the ultimate health of the fetus or newborn, the indications for and timing of cultures for these infections are not clear. The ACOG recommends cultures for chlamydiosis and gonorrhea at the first prenatal visit for high-risk patients. The high-risk patient is defined as less than 25 years of age with a past history or current evidence of any sexually transmitted disease, a new sexual partner within the preceding 3 months, and/or multiple sexual partners.

Miscellaneous Tests

Tuberculosis skin testing in high-risk populations or in certain geographic areas should be done if the patient has not been vaccinated with BCG vaccine. BCG vaccinations are not given in the United States. Appropriate screening for genetic carrier status, if not performed at the preconception visit, includes but is not limited to Tay-Sachs disease, cystic fibrosis, α- and β-thalassemia, and sickle cell disease.

Discussion with the Patient

The first prenatal visit is a time for the caregiver and patient to exchange expectations, to answer questions, and to set the stage for what will occur throughout the rest of normal prenatal care. The timing and content of future visits and the timing and rationale behind further laboratory testing should be explained. The patient should be given authoritative educational resources and materials that are written at the appropriate reading level. She and her partner are encouraged to ask questions about what they will read and to share the concerns they have about the pregnancy. It is important to reinforce that there is no such thing as a meaningless, dumb, or trivial question. Emergency and routine phone numbers should be given to the patient in writing. Social services and community resources, such as Women, Infants, and Children (WIC) programs, may be identified for the patient on an as-needed basis.

Finally, the patient should be made aware of the warning signs and symptoms of infection (fevers, chills, dysuria/hematuria) or threatened pregnancy loss (bleeding, cramping, passage of tissue). Should any of these occur, the patient should seek immediate medical attention. The next prenatal appointment is made at the completion of the first visit.

◊ ROUTINE ANTEPARTUM SURVEILLANCE

Rationale for Routine Prenatal Care

Prenatal care involves the following goals for pregnant women:[19]

◊ To provide continuing, ongoing primary preventive health care;
◊ To maintain or increase maternal health and the capability for self-care and to improve self-image before, during, and after pregnancy;
◊ To reduce the risk of maternal mortality and morbidity, as well as unnecessary pregnancy intervention;
◊ To reduce the risks to health before subsequent pregnancies and beyond the childbearing years;
◊ To promote the development of parenting skills.

The goals of prenatal care for the fetus are as follows:

◊ To reduce the risk of preterm birth, IUGR, retardation, and congenital anomalies;
◊ To enhance fetal health and reduce the need for extended hospitalization after birth;
◊ To promote healthy growth and development, immunization, and health supervision of the infant child;
◊ To reduce the risk of neurologic, developmental, and other morbidities;
◊ To reduce the risk of child abuse and neglect, injuries, and preventable acute and chronic illness.

The goals of prenatal care for the family during pregnancy and the first year of an infant's life are the following:

◊ To promote family development and positive parent–infant interaction;
◊ To reduce the number of unintended pregnancies;
◊ To identify and treat behavioral disorders leading to child neglect and family violence.

Timing and Frequency of Visits

The traditional wisdom for the timing and number of prenatal visits is summarized as follows:

Preconception	Up to 1 year before conception
First prenatal	6 to 8 weeks after missed menses
Monthly	Up to 28 weeks
Bimonthly	Up to 36 weeks
Weekly	Until delivery

The U.S. Public Health Service 1989 report on prenatal care content included a recommendation that the number and timing of individual visits in low-risk patients be modified, based on necessary interventions.[19] The report delineated the interventions and tests deemed minimally necessary in a normal pregnancy and the suggested the timing for each (Table 4). Recent randomized, controlled prospective trials confirm the safety of fewer prenatal visits.[15]

TABLE 4. *Timing in weeks of prenatal care based on specific interventions*

	First visit	6–8[a]	16–18	26–28	32	36	38	39	40
History									
Medical	X								
Psychosocial	X								
Update		X	X	X	X	X	X	X	X
Physical									
General	X								
Blood pressure	X	X	X	X	X	X	X	X	X
Height	X								
Weight	X	X	X	X	X	X	X	X	X
Body mas index	X								
Pelvic exam	X	X							
Breast	X	X							
Fundal height			X	X	X	X	X	X	X
Fetal position				X	X	X	X	X	X
Fetal heart		X	X	X	X	X	X	X	X
Cervical exam	X								
Laboratory									
Hemoglobin/hematocrit	X			X					
Rh Factor	X								
Blood type	X								
Antibody screen	X			X					
Pap smear	X								
GDM screen				X					
Multimarker/MSAFP			X						
Urine									
Dipstick	X								
Protein	X								
Sugar	X								
Culture/urinalysis		X							
Infections									
Rubella	X								
Syphilis	X								
Hepatits B	X								
HIV(offer)	X	X							
Genetic screen	X								

GDM, gestational diabetes mellitus; HIV, human immunodeficiency virus; MSAFP, maternal serum alpha-fetoprotein.

[a]If patient had preconception visit.

(Adapted from ref. 19.)

Content of Subsequent Prenatal Visits

The components of each prenatal visit are the taking of an interval history, assessment of fetal growth and maternal health, risk assessment and identification, intervention as necessary, collection and recording of an ongoing data base (see Appendix I), and education, advice, and support of the patient and her family.

Interval History

Each prenatal visit begins with information gathering. Patients should be asked questions about their general health (see "Concerns and Questions Particular to Pregnancy" below), their diet, sleeping patterns, and fetal movement. Questions regarding warning signs such as bleeding, contractions, leaking of fluid, headache, or visual disturbances are also appropriate. Patients should be given the opportunity to raise their own questions and concerns at each visit.

Physical Examination

The patient is weighed, and total weight gain and trends are evaluated (see "Nutrition" below). The blood pressure is taken, and trends are assessed for possible pregnancy-induced hypertension or preeclampsia. As blood pressure tends to decrease during the second trimester, increases of 30 mm Hg systolic or 15 mm Hg diastolic over first trimester pressures are considered abnormal.

The fundal height is measured with a tape from the top of the symphysis pubis, over the uterine curve, to the top of the fundus (Figs. 1 and 2). This technique places an emphasis on change in growth patterns rather than the absolute measurement in centimeters, which can vary between patients. Ges-

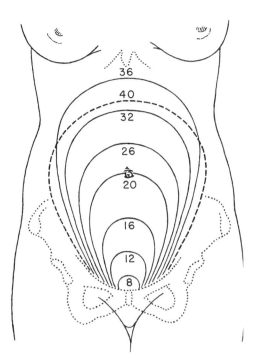

FIG. 1. The height of the fundus at comparable gestational dates varies among patients. Those shown are the most common. A convenient rule of thumb is that at 20 weeks' gestation, the fundus is at or slightly above the umbilicus.

tational age is approximately equal to fundal height in centimeters from 16 to 36 weeks' gestation. Measurements that are several centimeters smaller than expected for week of gestation are suspicious for oligohydramnios, IUGR, fetal anomaly, abnormal fetal lie, or premature fetal descent into the pelvis. Conversely, larger than expected measurements may indicate multiple gestation, polyhydramnios, fetal macrosomia, or leiomyomata. These concerns can be resolved with ultrasound examination.

Fetal heart rate is auscultated, with care taken to differentiate fetal from maternal rates. The normal fetal heart rate throughout pregnancy is between 120 and 160 beats per minute.

Fetal position has been traditionally evaluated with the use of Leopold maneuvers. These are initiated at midpregnancy when fetal body parts are more clearly identified. The maneuvers consist of four parts; the first three are performed with the examiner standing to one side of the patient and facing her head, and the last with the examiner facing the patient's feet.

◇ The *first maneuver* answers the question, "What fetal part occupies the fundus?" (Fig. 3). The examiner palpates the fundal area and differentiates between the irregular, firm breech and the round, hard head.

◇ The *second maneuver* answers the question, "On which side is the fetal back?" (Fig. 4). The palms of the hands are placed on either side of the abdomen. On the one side, the linear continuous ridge of the back is felt, while the other side contains compressible areas and nodular parts.

◇ The *third maneuver* answers the question, "What fetal part lies over the pelvic inlet?" (Fig. 5). A single examining hand is placed just above the symphysis to grasp between the thumb and third finger the fetal part that overrides the symphysis. If the head is unengaged, it is readily recognized as a round, hard object that frequently can be displaced upward. After engagement, the back of the head or a shoulder is felt as a relatively fixed, knob-like part. In breech presentations, the irregular, nodular breech is felt in direct continuity with the fetal back.

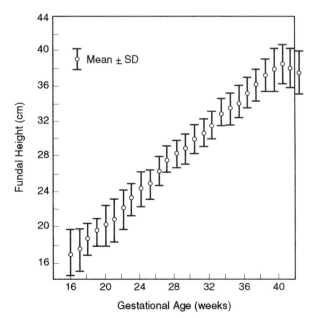

FIG. 2. Fundal heights versus gestational age.

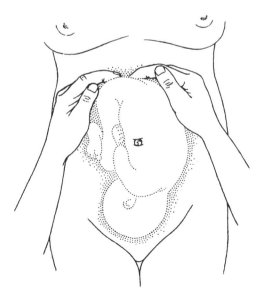

FIG. 3. The first Leopold maneuver reveals what fetal part occupies the fundus.

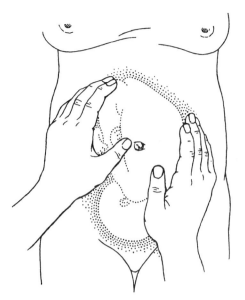

FIG. 4. The second Leopold maneuver reveals the position of the fetal back.

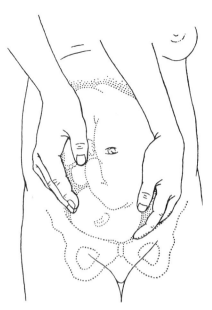

FIG. 6. The fourth Leopold maneuver reveals the position of the cephalic prominence. In a flexion attitude, the cephalic prominence is on the same side as the small parts.

◊ The *fourth maneuver* answers the question, "On which side is the cephalic prominence?" (Figs. 6 and 7). This maneuver can be performed only when the head is engaged; if the head is floating, the maneuver is inapplicable. The examiner faces the patient's feet and places a hand on either side of the uterus, just above the pelvic inlet. When pressure is exerted in the direction of the inlet, one hand can descend farther than the other. The part of the fetus that prevents the deep descent of one hand is called the cephalic prominence.

The routine examination is completed by evaluating the patient for edema. A finding of new-onset edema of the face and hands in association with proteinuria and elevated blood pressure is consistent with preeclampsia. Dependent pitting edema of the ankles and legs in the absence of other findings is normal in late pregnancy. It responds well to resting with the legs elevated and therefore is usually absent on rising in the morning.

Routine examination of the cervix is not necessary unless the patient is at risk for cervical incompetence or is being evaluated for preterm labor.

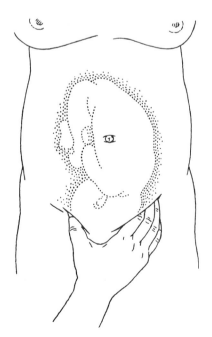

FIG. 5. The third Leopold maneuver reveals what fetal part lies over the pelvic inlet.

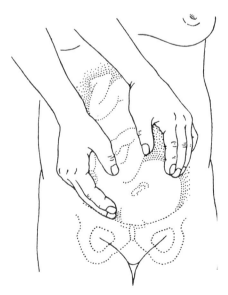

FIG. 7. In the fourth Leopold maneuver, in an extension attitude, the cephalic prominence is on the same side as the back.

Laboratory Evaluation

Five laboratory tests are offered to all patients. These include screening for serum alpha-fetoprotein, gestational diabetes, Rh antibodies, bacterial vaginosis, and group B streptococci.

Maternal Serum Screening Test

Screening for maternal serum alpha-fetoprotein (MSAFP) is performed to detect fetal neural tube defects. During pregnancy, AFP is produced in sequence by the fetal yolk sac, the fetal gastrointestinal tract, and finally the fetal liver. Its peak concentration in fetal serum occurs at the end of the first trimester of pregnancy. Excretion of AFP in fetal urine results in high levels of AFP in the amniotic fluid. Transfer of AFP to the maternal serum occurs via the placenta and transamniotically. MSAFP levels continue to rise until approximately 30 weeks' gestation (Fig. 8). The interpretation of the MSAFP screening test is gestational age dependent and should be performed at the 15th to 20th menstrual weeks of pregnancy.

MSAFP levels are reported as multiples of the median from the database of the individual laboratory. Elevated maternal serum and amniotic fluid levels of AFP detect 85% of open neural tube defects (open spina bifida and anencephaly). Other causes for elevated MSAFP levels include omphalocele and gastroschisis, multiple gestation, fetal demise, and incorrect dates. Patients with abnormal MSAFP levels require evaluation with targeted fetal ultrasonography (Fig. 9) (see Chapter 12).

The risk of fetal trisomy 21 is related to gestational age–normalized concentrations of MSAFP, total β-hCG, and unconjugated estriol. Thus, these three biochemical markers may be used in conjunction with the maternal age–related risk of fetal trisomy 21 to derive a more precise risk of fetal trisomy 21 in a given pregnancy. Called the triple screen because three biochemical markers are used, this scheme assumes that computed risks for fetal trisomy 21 greater than 1 in 270 (in the first trimester, the midtrimester risk of fetal trisomy 21 in a 35-year-old woman) should prompt consideration of genetic amniocentesis. Using such a scheme, prospective studies show that approximately 60% of fetal trisomy 21 will be detected, with a false-positive rate of 5%. Maternal serum screening is not recommended in women aged 35 years and older because current recommendations hold that women in this age group should be offered chorionic villus sampling or amniocentesis. It is important to counsel a patient about the differences between a screening test and a diagnostic test. The possibility of false-positive and false-negative test results should also be explained.

Screening for Gestational Diabetes

The 1-hour, 50-g oral glucose screen is used to detect glucose intolerance in pregnancy. Following an abnormal screen, a 3-hour glucose tolerance test, commencing with a fasting blood sugar, followed by a 100-g glucola, is currently recommended. Two or more abnormal values on this test are considered diagnostic of gestational diabetes mellitus (GDM).

Universal screening is controversial. Risk factors for GDM include (1) maternal age greater than 30 years; (2) previous macrosomic, malformed. or stillborn infant; (3) GDM in a previous pregnancy; (4) family history or diabetes; (5) maternal obesity; (6) persistent glucosuria; or (7) chronic use of certain drugs such as β-sympathomimetics or corticosteriods. Proponents of universal screening argue that screening only those patients with risk factors will detect no more than half of patients with glucose intolerance. Opponents argue that the inconvenience and expense of testing are not necessary in patients without these risk factors, because the incidence of frank GDM in this population is so low.

Routine screening, if used, is performed on all patients between 24 and 28 weeks' gestation. Selective screening based on risks may be performed earlier and repeated as needed. A patient may be tested in the fasting or nonfasting state. One hour after administration of a 50-g glucose load, the patient's blood is drawn. A patient with a glucose value greater than 140 mg/dl of serum is a candidate for a 3-hour, 100-g glucose tolerance test.

The significance of GDM lies not in an increased risk of fetal loss but in the risk of excessive fetal growth with its attendant birth-related morbidities. In addition, women with GDM have a 60% likelihood of developing overt diabetes mellitus within 16 years.

Rescreening for Rh Antibodies

All Rh-negative women who are unsensitized at the beginning of pregnancy should be retested at approximately 26 to 28 weeks' gestation. If the antibody screen remains negative, the mother should receive $Rh_0(D)$ immune globulin, 300 mg, at 28 weeks to prevent isoimmunization in the third trimester.

Screening for Bacterial Vaginosis

Bacterial vaginosis (BV) is a condition in which the normal flora of the vagina (specifically lactobacilli) are reduced in

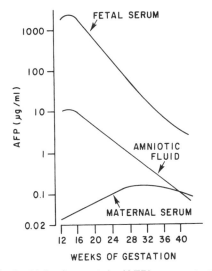

FIG. 8. Alpha-fetoprotein (AFP) concentrations in fetal serum, amniotic fluid, and maternal serum throughout gestation. (From Seppala M, ed. *Amniotic fluid*, 2nd ed. New York: Excerpta Medica, 1978; with permission.)

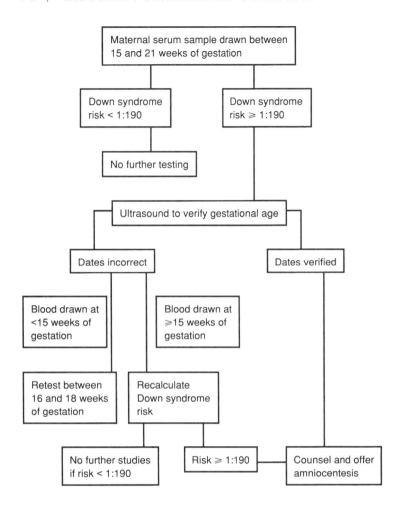

FIG. 9. Screening for Down syndrome during pregnancy by measuring markers in maternal serum. (Adapted from Haddow JE, Palomaki GE, Knight, GJ, et al. Prenatal screening for fetal Down Syndrome with the use of measurement of maternal serum markers. *N Engl J Med* 1992;327:588.)

number and replaced by an overgrowth of anaerobic organisms. Some studies have linked BV with an increased incidence of preterm labor, endometritis, and premature rupture of the membranes.[11,16] A simple and effective screen, performed late in the second trimester, consists of a pelvic examination and wet mount to detect BV. A Gram stain may provide even greater accuracy.

The treatment for women who are positive for BV includes either metronidazole (intravaginal or oral) or intravaginal clindamycin cream (Cleocin). Because BV is often asymptomatic, a test of cure may be appropriate.

Testing for Group B Streptococci

Group B streptococci (GBS) are part of the normal vaginal, genitourinary, and gastrointestinal tract flora in up to 20% of healthy women. GBS have been implicated in preterm labor, as well as in amnionitis, endometritis, and wound infection in the mother. Vertical transmission during labor or delivery may result in generalized sepsis in the newborn and related long-term morbidity or neonatal death.

Prevention strategies have focused on detection of the bacteria in the mother and early onset of GBS disease in the newborn. A decision analysis, comparing 19 different strategies for GBS screening, was published by Rouse et al.[24] Effectiveness, cost, and possible adverse consequences were taken into account. There are no randomized, prospective, controlled trials that have shown any one strategy to be preferable; and no such trials are likely to be forthcoming because of the large numbers of subjects required to show a significant difference, if one exists. A choice of one of two strategies therefore has been recommended by the ACOG, the American Academy of Pediatrics, and the CDC.

One strategy involves routine anogenital cultures of all pregnant women at 35 to 37 weeks' gestation. Cultures are obtained from the lower third of the vagina and perianal area; cervical cultures are not reliable, and a speculum is not necessary to obtain an adequate culture sample. Culture-positive women are treated during labor with antibiotic prophylaxis to prevent fetal-neonatal GBS infection. The second, equally acceptable strategy is antibiotic prophylaxis during labor, treating only women with risk factors for fetal-neonatal GBS infection. In this strategy, routine culture for GBS is not required. Risk factors include preterm labor (less than 37 weeks' gestation), rupture of the membranes more than 18 hours prior to delivery, birth of a previous infant with GBS infection, or maternal fever during labor (greater than 38°C or 100.4°F).

Testing Based on Symptoms or Clinical Risk Assessment

A part of prenatal care of the normal patient consists of ongoing risk assessment and intervention, or referral if a risk is identified. Several clinical signs or symptoms warrant further evaluation. Symptoms suggestive of urinary tract infections should prompt immediate microscopic examination of a clean-catch urine specimen and cultures when appropriate. High-risk behaviors, identified during the course of a pregnancy, should prompt a test (or retest) for HIV infection and other sexually transmitted diseases (STDs), or performance of a urinary drug screen. Repeated testing of hemoglobin should be done if the patient is symptomatic or at nutritional risk for anemia.

Other testing, performed on an as-needed basis, includes ultrasound to detect abnormal fetal growth, antepartum fetal monitoring to assess fetal oxygenation status, or comprehensive targeted ultrasound examinations. A more thorough discussion of antepartum fetal monitoring can be found in Chapters 14 and 15.

Discussion with Patients and Families: Answering Questions

Patients need the opportunity to engage in dialogue with their *health care provider* and to feel confident that their concerns are heard. It is a time to emphasize the involvement of the entire family in the pregnancy process, including the role of the father and the impact of the pregnancy on any siblings. Therefore, an important part of the prenatal visit is discussion with the patient, her partner, and/or her family both to exchange questions and answers and to provide reassurance and education. The exact content of these discussions will vary from visit to visit. Reaffirming the importance of appropriate social behaviors, such as smoking cessation, is beneficial, as are periodic evaluations of the social support systems and help in the home both now and after the birth of the infant.

Ongoing risk assessment requires that the patient be educated about the signs and symptoms of preterm labor and preeclampsia. The list of warning signs for which an emergent telephone call is warranted includes the following:

◊ Vaginal bleeding,
◊ Leaking of fluid from the vagina,
◊ Rhythmic cramping pains of more than 6 per hour,
◊ Abdominal pain of a prolonged or increasing nature,
◊ Fever or chills,
◊ Burning with urination,
◊ Prolonged vomiting with inability to hold down liquids or solids for more than 24 hours,
◊ Severe continuous headache, visual changes, or generalized edema,
◊ A pronounced decrease in the frequency or intensity of fetal movements.

◊ CONCERNS AND QUESTIONS PARTICULAR TO PREGNANCY

Pregnancy is a time of change, expectation, and anticipation; it may also be a time of heightened anxiety, emotionality, concern, and uncertainty. Many symptoms that the nonpregnant patient might view as minor may indicate a cause for alarm during pregnancy. Daily life events and practices may take on a new meaning when being shared with the unborn fetus. The provision of direct, concise, and accurate information in a compassionate and reassuring manner will assuage many of these worries and provide direction for day-to-day activities.

Nutrition

The objectives of nutritional assessment and counseling are to develop, in concert with the patient, an analysis of maternal nutritional risk, a goal for total weight gain, and a diet plan that will fit the patient's life style and is ethnically sensitive.

The overriding principle of good nutrition is that there is a positive linear relationship between maternal weight gain and newborn weight *and* that prepregnant maternal body mass index (BMI) can affect fetal weight independently of the amount gained by the mother during pregnancy. Together, initial weight and weight gain have an impact on IUGR and low birthweight.

The BMI is a calculation that relates the patient's weight to her height, thereby providing a more accurate indirect estimate of the patient's body fat distribution than can be obtained by weight alone. The BMI is calculated by dividing weight in kilograms by height in meters squared. If pounds and inches are used, the quotient is multiplied by 700. The BMI of a patient is categorized as underweight, normal weight, overweight, or obese (see Appendix II).

Maternal Weight Gain

The ideal weight gain for an individual patient during pregnancy depends on several factors. The most important of these are the prepregnant BMI and the type of gestation (single versus multiple). It is important to note that weight gain for a normal BMI is 25 to 35 lb (11 to 16 kg), but the optimal weight gain for an underweight teenager carrying a singleton pregnancy approaches 40 lb (18.2 kg), or 5 lb every 4 weeks in the second half of pregnancy (Fig. 10). An obese woman, on the other hand, may need to gain no more than 15 lb (6.8 kg). Figure 11 illustrates the components of weight gain in a normal pregnancy. During the first and second trimesters, most of the weight gained reflects maternal growth, while fetal growth is most rapid in the last trimester, with the fetus more than tripling its weight. According to Pederson et al.,[20] a patient carrying twins regardless of her BMI should be counseled to gain more that 40 lb to decrease the risk of both preterm labor and low birthweight.

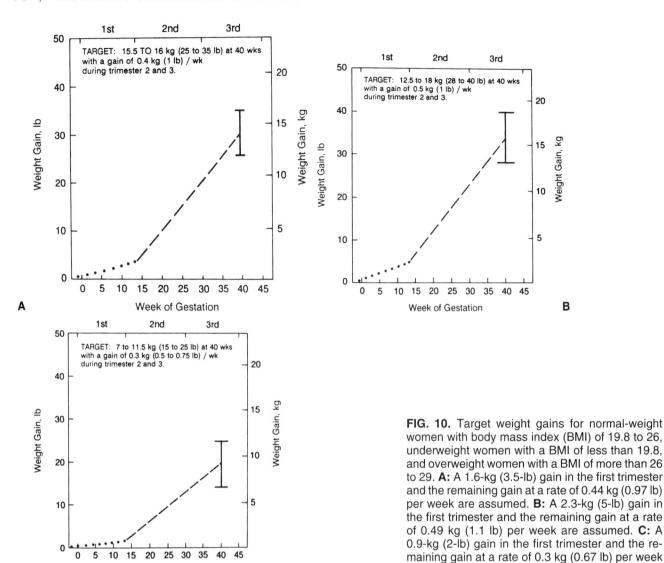

FIG. 10. Target weight gains for normal-weight women with body mass index (BMI) of 19.8 to 26, underweight women with a BMI of less than 19.8, and overweight women with a BMI of more than 26 to 29. **A:** A 1.6-kg (3.5-lb) gain in the first trimester and the remaining gain at a rate of 0.44 kg (0.97 lb) per week are assumed. **B:** A 2.3-kg (5-lb) gain in the first trimester and the remaining gain at a rate of 0.49 kg (1.1 lb) per week are assumed. **C:** A 0.9-kg (2-lb) gain in the first trimester and the remaining gain at a rate of 0.3 kg (0.67 lb) per week are assumed.

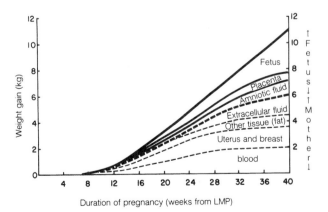

FIG. 11. Pattern and components of weight gain during pregnancy (*LMP*, last menstrual period). (From Pitkin RM. Nutritional support in obstetrics and gynecology. *Clin Obstet Gynecol* 1976;19:489; with permission.)

Maternal Diet

The diet is a means of achieving the optimal goal for total weight gain and should be evaluated periodically. While weight gain is an important gauge of caloric intake, the quality of the diet and the frequency of meals may also affect patient and fetal well-being. A diet should be balanced by containing foods from all of the basic food groups, as outlined in the Food Guide Pyramid published by the U.S. Department of Agriculture in 1992. Specifics of a diet will vary considerably according to patient preference, family eating patterns, and cultural and ethnic background.

Increased nutritional requirements during pregnancy reflect the needs of the fetus for growth, as well as maternal physiologic needs. To meet the overall increasing energy needs, the average woman must consume an additional 300 kcal per day beyond her baseline needs. The appropriate daily caloric content of a diet required to supply energy needs and achieve appropriate weight gain can be estimated by multiplying the patient's optimal body weight in kilograms by 35 kcal and adding 300 kcal to the total (Table 5).

Vitamin and Mineral Supplementation

Multivitamin supplements are not routinely necessary in a woman eating a well balanced diet. However, 400 μg of supplemental folic acid daily is necessary because the requirement cannot be met with food alone. Additional folate may be necessary for women with a hemoglobinopathy or twin gestation, or for women on antiseizure medications. Vitamin D supplementation is not generally required, unless there is inadequate exposure to sunlight.

Mineral supplementation is also not needed in healthy women. The exception is iron. The iron requirements of pregnancy total about 1 g. Due to the monthly menses, most women have less than optimal iron stores during their reproductive years. Therefore, supplementation with 30 mg of elemental iron is recommended in the second and third trimesters to prevent anemia and to meet this requirement. One tablet of iron salts per day, ingested between meals or at bedtime, is sufficient to meet this requirement. Women with iron deficiency anemia require 60 to 120 mg of ele-

mental ferrous iron per day. Additional zinc (15 mg) and copper (2 mg) are then needed, as iron inhibits the absorption of these ions.

Calcium supplementation is not necessary in women with a diet that includes adequate dairy foods. Absent this, calcium supplementation may be used on an as-needed basis to meet the recommended dietary allowance (RDA) of 1200 mg per day during pregnancy. Zinc is a trace mineral. A zinc deficiency may be teratogenic in humans, although this has not yet been conclusively demonstrated. Zinc levels in amniotic fluid correlate with antimicrobial activity, suggesting that zinc plays a role in protecting against intrauterine infection. Low dietary intake of zinc has been associated with IUGR, although it does not cause IUGR. The RDA for zinc during pregnancy is increased from 15 to 20 mg per day.[18]

Other Dietary Considerations

Vegetarianism

Lactoovovegetarians should have no particular nutritional deficiency, with the possible exceptions of iron and zinc, which may be supplemented. The strict vegan, however, must design a diet of sufficient vegetable proteins to provide all of

TABLE 5. *Recommended dietary allowances for women of reproductive age and for pregnant and lactating women*

Nutrient	Nonpregnant women	Pregnant women	Increase (%)	Lactating women	Sources
Energy	2200 kcal	2500 kcal	+14	640 kcal	Protein, fat, carbohydrate
Protein	50 mg	60 mg	+20	65 g	Meats, fish, poultry, dairy
Fat-soluble vitamins					
Vitamin A	800 μg	800 μg	No change	1300 μg	Dark green, yellow, or orange fruits, vegetables, liver
Vitamin D	5 μg	10 μg	+100	10 μg	Fortified dairy products
Vitamin E	8 μg	10 μg	+25	12 μg	Vegetable oils, nuts, leafy vegetables
Vitamin K	—	65 μg	—	65 μg	Green vegetables, dairy products
Water-soluble vitamins					
Vitamin C	60 mg	70 mg	+17	95 mg	Citrus fruits, tomatoes
Thiamine	1.1 mg	1.5 mg	+36	1.6 mg	Enriched grains, pork
Riboflavin	1.3 mg	1.6 mg	+23	1.8 mg	Meats, liver, grains
Niacin	15 mg	17 mg	+13	20 mg	Meats, nuts, legumes
Vitamin B_6	1.6 mg	2.2 mg	+37	2.1 mg	Poultry, fish, liver, eggs
Folate	180 μg	400 μg	+120	280 μg	Leafy vegetables, liver
Vitamin B_{12}	2 μg	2 μg	+10	2.6 μg	Animal proteins
Minerals					
Calcium	800 mg	1200 mg	+50	1200 mg	Dairy products
Phosphorus	800 mg	1200 mg	+50	1200 mg	Meats
Magnesium	280 mg	320 mg	+14	355 mg	Seafood, legumes, grains
Iron	15 mg	30 mg	+100	15 mg	Meats, eggs, grains
Zinc	12 mg	15 mg	+25	19 mg	Meats, seafood, eggs
Iodine	105 μg	175 μg	+17	200 μg	Iodized salt, seafood
Selenium	55 μg	65 μg	+18	75 μg	Seafood, liver, meats

(Adapted from ref. 18.)

the essential amino acids normally found in animal protein. Due to the decreased protein density of most vegetables, this may cause an unusually high weight gain. Supplementation of zinc, vitamin B_{12}, and iron is necessary.

Food Restriction

Dieting and fasting on a chronic basis in an otherwise healthy woman can result in suboptimal fetal growth. Eating disorders such as bulimia and anorexia nervosa reflect extreme forms of food restriction and malnutrition. There are limited data about these disorders in pregnancy, but anoretics in particular place their fetus at risk. Bulimic women may suffer from electrolyte imbalance and a deficit of trace minerals.

Many pregnant women in the United States are not eating an optimal diet due to poverty and inadequate resources to purchase food. It is appropriate to inquire about resources in impoverished women and to refer these patients to groups such as WIC and for food stamps.

Pica

Pica is the compulsive ingestion of nonfood substances with little or no nutrient value. The practice most commonly involves ice, clay (geophagia), or starch (amylophagia). Although pica is most commonly recognized during pregnancy, it is not specific to the gravid state. Neither the cause nor the medical implications of pica are well understood. It is unusual for pica to cause significant harm if the diet is otherwise nutritionally adequate.

Phenylketonuria

Women with phenylketonuria who are not on a phenylalanine-controlled diet are at increased risk of bearing fetuses with microcephaly, growth retardation, and mental retardation. The goal of dietary management is to minimize these adverse fetal outcomes by reducing the maternal serum phenylalanine levels to less than 20 mg/dl before and during the pregnancy.

Megadose Vitamins

The misuse of megadose nutrients can be categorized as a fad type of dietary manipulation. Water-soluble vitamins such as vitamin C cannot be consumed in harmful quantities because they are readily excreted in the urine. However, a problem occurs with fat-soluble vitamin A. There is an association between high doses of supplemental vitamin A and birth defects similar to those seen with isotretinoin. Although the minimum teratogenic dose in humans has not been identified, it may be a little as 10,000 IU per day. Beta-carotene is a provitamin of vitamin A, but it does not produce similar toxicity. Most prenatal vitamins contain less than 5,000 IU of vitamin A, and until further data are available, this should be considered the maximum safe supplemental dose.[22]

Caffeine

Caffeine is contained in numerous foodstuffs such as coffee, tea, chocolate, and cola beverages. A naturally occurring substance, it is the most widely used psychoactive drug in the United States. It is a central nervous system stimulant and is physically and psychologically addictive. Withdrawal symptoms include nausea, lethargy, malaise, and headache. The only evidence for teratogenic effects of caffeine comes from animal studies using doses not compatible with human consumption. Several large human studies have failed to show that caffeine has deleterious effects on the fetus, when ingested in customary amounts. Thus, moderate caffeine intake is probably safe in pregnancy. Adverse maternal effects of caffeine include insomnia, acid indigestion, reflux, and urinary frequency. As these problems are already exaggerated in pregnancy, moderation in the consumption of caffeine is advisable.

Exercise

Over the past two decades, an increasing number of women of reproductive age have made exercise a routine part of their daily activities. For the normal healthy woman, a low-impact exercise regimen may be continued throughout pregnancy.

While there are no data to indicate that pregnant women must decrease the intensity of their exercise or lower their target heart rates, physiologic changes of pregnancy may alter the effect of various exercises on the body or may limit the body's ability to perform certain types of exercise. Body position as a modulator of cardiac output is particularly important in the third trimester, when either motionless standing or the supine position can result in decreased venous return and cardiac output. In some instances, this will result in hypotension or syncope.

Both oxygen uptake and baseline oxygen consumption are increased during pregnancy. Deep breathing is more difficult, particularly in later pregnancy, due to uterine size and decreased diaphragmatic excursion. These changes combine to make less oxygen available for aerobic activity, thereby decreasing maximum exercise performance.

Data regarding the fetal response to maternal exercise are conflicting. While most are very reassuring, problems include faulty research design and sample size inadequate to achieve statistical significance. Moderate (submaximal) exercise may cause a significant increase in maternal core body temperature and thereby the fetal temperature, which remains a constant 1°F above that of the mother. There is no evidence, however, that the slight increase in core body temperature associated with moderate exercise poses a risk to the fetus. Studies of the fetus following submaximal maternal exercise (65% to 70% aerobic capacity) have not shown any associated changes in the fetal heart rate. Adverse exercise-induced effects on the fetus, including malformations, retardation, growth restriction, or lowered birthweights, have not been demonstrated in humans.

Recommendations

Women who exercise regularly before pregnancy should be encouraged to continue. They may be counseled that performance capacity tends to fall, but this is not a sign that they should forgo regular moderate exercise. Indeed, exercise may relieve stress, diminish anxiety, and increase self-esteem. It has also been shown that women who exercise regularly have significantly shorter labor.[6]

Specific exercise regimens should be individualized, and patients who have not been physically active prior to pregnancy are advised to proceed slowly. General recommendations include the following:

◊ Exercise should be regular rather than sporadic and intermittent;
◊ Exercise should be stopped if signs and symptoms of oxygen deprivation, such as extreme fatigue, dizziness, or extreme shortness of breath occur;
◊ To avoid becoming overheated, pregnant women should exercise in a cool area, and stay well hydrated and wear appropriate clothing;
◊ Exercise that requires prolonged time in the supine position should be avoided during the second and third trimesters;
◊ The form of exercise chosen should not be one with significant risk of trauma (especially to the abdomen) or falls;
◊ Caloric intake should be increased in direct proportion to the additional energy requirements of exercise.

Contraindications

Relative contraindications to exercise during pregnancy include the following:

◊ Evidence of IUGR,
◊ Persistent vaginal bleeding,
◊ Incompetent cervix or cervical cerclage placement,
◊ Risk factors for preterm labor,
◊ Rupture of membranes,
◊ Pregnancy-induced hypertension,
◊ Chronic medical conditions that might be adversely impacted by vigorous exercise.

Nausea and Vomiting

Recurrent nausea and vomiting during the first trimester occurs in about one-half of pregnancies. While the term *morning sickness* is well known, it is a misnomer, as these symptoms can occur at any time throughout the day or night. The etiology of this problem is not clear. Hormonal, as well as emotional, factors have been investigated without consistent results. Symptoms can be mild or so severe that the patient becomes dehydrated and risks electrolyte imbalance and caloric malnutrition. Nonpharmacologic measures often suffice to alleviate, if not completely relieve, the symptoms. These include avoidance of fatty or spicy foods, eating small, more frequent meals, drinking ginger teas, inhaling peppermint oil vapors, wearing motion sickness bands on the wrists, and increasing rest periods each day. In severe cases of emesis, various pharmacologic agents have been used with varying success. These include pyridoxine, a variety of antihistamines, promethazine, metoclopramide, and trimethobenzamide. More recently, intravenous droperidol and diphenhydramine show promise in treating the most severe manifestation of nausea and vomiting, hyperemesis gravidarum.[17] Because supplemental vitamin and mineral preparations may exacerbate symptoms of nausea, they should be stopped until the symptoms have resolved.

Ptyalism

Ptyalism is the increased production of saliva, probably induced by the consumption of starch. There is no cure, although reducing carbohydrate intake may be helpful. The problem is often self-limiting.

Heartburn

Heartburn is a reflux esophagitis caused by both mechanical factors (enlarging uterus displacing the stomach above the esophageal sphincter) and hormonal factors (progesterone causing a relative relaxation of the esophageal sphincter). Treatment consists of eliminating acidic and spicy foods, decreasing the amount of food and liquid at each meal, limiting food and liquid intake before bedtime, sleeping in a semi-Fowler's position or propped up on pillows, and use of antacids. Liquid forms of antacids and H_2-receptor inhibitors provide the most consistent relief of symptoms. Patients should be cautioned that antacids containing aluminum may cause constipation, while diarrhea may be associated with use of those containing magnesium.

Constipation

Progesterone-induced relaxation of the intestinal smooth muscle slows peristalsis and increases bowel transit time. Dietary management of this common condition includes increased fluids and liberal intake of high-fiber foods. Iron salts may exacerbate the problem. Over-the-counter (OTC) products containing psyllium draw fluid into the intestine and promote a more rapid transit time. Enemas, laxatives, and strong cathartics should be avoided.

Varicosities and Hemorrhoids

Varicosities most often occur in the lower extremities but may be seen in the vulva as well. Contributing factors include genetic predisposition, advanced maternal age, increased parity, and prolonged standing. Manifestations can range from mild cosmetic effects to chronic pain and superficial thrombophlebitis. Treatment includes avoidance of garments that constrict at the knee and upper leg, support stockings, and increased periods of rest with the legs elevated.

Hemorrhoids, varicosities of the rectal veins, are due to mechanical compression by the enlarging uterus, as well as from constipation and straining at stool. Treatment includes OTC topical preparations, cool sitz baths, and stool softeners. If thrombosis of a hemorrhoid occurs, the clot can be excised to relieve pain and swelling.

Leg Cramps

Almost half of all pregnant women suffer from recurrent painful spasms of the muscles of the lower extremities, especially the calves. Leg cramps are more frequent at night and usually occur during the third trimester. Various prophylactic and therapeutic options have been suggested, most notably, calcium lactate, but there are no data from controlled trials to show benefit over placebo for any of these. Massage and placing the affected muscle(s) on stretch relieves the cramps when they occur.

Backache

Most pregnant women experience lower backaches as pregnancy progresses. These are usually alleviated by minimizing the amount of time spent standing, by increasing rest, by wearing a specially designed support belt over the lower abdomen, and by taking an analgesic such as acetaminophen. Exercises to increase muscular strength of the back and abdomen are sometimes helpful. Shoes with good support and avoidance of high heels that exaggerate the lordotic posture are essential. Increasingly severe or abrupt-onset back pain requires orthopedic consultation. Rhythmic cramping pains originating in the back may be a sign of preterm labor and necessitate appropriate evaluation.

Round Ligament Pain

This pain most frequently occurs during the second trimester when women report sharp, bilateral or unilateral groin pain. The pain may be increased with sudden movement or change in position. Resolution of unremitting ligament pain is sometimes achieved by having the patient assume a position on the hands and knees and lower the head to the floor, while keeping the buttocks in the air.

Headache

Generalized headaches are not uncommon during the first trimester of pregnancy. Muscle tension headaches may occur intermittently. The frequency and intensity of migraine headaches may increase or decrease during pregnancy. Headaches during the second and third trimesters are not an expected symptom of pregnancy. Pathologic headaches that occur with preeclampsia are discussed in Chapter 22.

Sexual Relations

There are no data to support restriction of coital activity during a normal pregnancy. The couple can be counseled regarding positions of comfort and possible changes in sexual desire. Nipple stimulation, vaginal penetration, and orgasm can cause uterine contractions secondary to the release of prostaglandins and oxytocin. However, there are no proven adverse effects on the fetus or the onset of labor. The question of the effect of coitus in women at risk for preterm labor or early spontaneous pregnancy loss remains unanswered. Couples at risk may prefer to avoid sexual relations to minimize any feelings of guilt or responsibility if a problem occurs subsequently.

There are two concrete interdictions to coitus during pregnancy. The first is that intercourse should not occur after membranes rupture or in the presence of known placenta previa. The second is that forceful introduction of air into the vagina should be avoided because of the risk of fatal air embolism.

Employment

Most patients are able to continue to work throughout their pregnancy. In general, work activities that increase the risk of falls or trauma, especially to the abdomen, should be avoided. Hazardous toxic or chemical exposures should be identified early and avoided. Strenuous physical activity to the point of exhaustion and prolonged standing may be associated with poor pregnancy outcomes, and the work routine should be modified accordingly.[14]

Urinary Frequency

Patients often experience urinary frequency during the first 3 months of pregnancy, as the enlarging uterus compresses the bladder, and again during the last weeks, as the fetal head descends into the pelvis. If frequency occurs in conjunction with dysuria, hematuria, or urgency/hesitancy, the patient should be evaluated for a urinary tract infection.

Leukorrhea

An increase in the amount of vaginal discharge is physiologic and expected during pregnancy. Discharge accompanied by itching or burning or a malodorous discharge should be evaluated and treated accordingly. Douching has no place in the treatment or management of leukorrhea in pregnancy.

Syncope

Venous pooling in the lower extremities increases as the pregnancy progresses. This can lead to dizziness or light-headedness, especially after standing upright abruptly or for long periods of time. Other causes of syncope include dehydration, hypoglycemia, and the shunting of blood flow to the stomach after eating a large meal. Syncope during exercise is a sign of overexertion. In general, syncopal episodes resolve rapidly and should be managed acutely, just as in a nonpregnant patient. Syncope in the supine position is avoidable by resting in either the left or right lateral recumbent position, thereby relieving uterine compression of the vena cava.

X-rays/Ionizing Radiation

The adverse effects on the fetus of ionizing radiation are dose-dependent. While there is no single diagnostic procedure that results in a dose of radiation high enough to threaten the fetus or embryo, cumulative exposures or multiple procedures should be avoided, especially during the first trimester when the fetus is at highest risk for possible anomalies. Patients may undergo dental x-rays as needed, provided that the abdomen is fully covered by a lead apron. Studies using radioactive isotopes are best avoided. As in all diagnostic procedures, the risks and the potential benefits must be evaluated and individualized for each patient.

Travel

Most issues concerning travel involve the comfort of the mother. When prolonged sitting is involved, the patient should try to stretch her legs and walk for 10 minutes every 2 hours to decrease the risk of thrombosis that can occur secondary to the hypercoaguable pregnancy state and mechanical compression of venous blood flow from the extremities. Dependent edema may also be more pronounced after prolonged sitting. If the patient will be away from home for a significant period of time, she should take a copy of her medical record with her. Pregnant women can and should always wear seatbelts when riding in a car. Travel in a pressurized airplane presents no additional risk to pregnant women. In traveling abroad, especially to underdeveloped countries, the usual precautions should be taken regarding ingestion of unpurified drinking water and uncooked fruits and vegetables.

Immunizations

Four immunizations using vaccines containing live viruses should be avoided during pregnancy. These are measles, mumps, rubella, and yellow fever. The risks for the fetus from the administration of rabies vaccine are unknown, and each case must be considered individually, since the indications for prophylaxis are not altered by pregnancy.

◊ PREPARING FOR CHILDBIRTH

Prenatal Education Classes

Few empiric studies have examined the impact of prepared childbirth education on perinatal outcomes, but such education is generally believed to be helpful and valuable. The landmark volume *Birth of a Child* by Grantley Dick-Read, published in 1958, changed the face of childbirth education forever. Formal childbirth classes evolved rapidly in a multi-

plicity of settings. The goals of these classes are to educate and to answer questions in a conducive environment, so that both the patient and her partner have the opportunity to decrease their anxiety level and increase their knowledge. Classes are designed to be an empowering experience, helping the parent(s) become a part of the process rather than objects of the actions of others. The content of childbirth classes varies but usually includes topics such as normal labor and delivery, anesthesia, breathing and concentration techniques, obstetric complications and interventions, and obstetric operations. Many instructors encourage patients to formulate a "birth plan," to put it in writing, and to share it with their clinician. This can facilitate communication between the parents themselves and between patient and caregiver.

There are also decisions that are best considered and made prior to the delivery. These include issues such as breastfeeding, postpartum contraception, return to work, and circumcision of a male infant. It is helpful if parents are given information in a nonjudgmental, nonthreatening environment so that they may make appropriate, well considered, and informed decisions.

Signs of Labor

The final element in preparing for childbirth is knowledge of when labor is occurring and when it is appropriate to notify the health care provider. Patients should be given a 24-hour phone number to call for assistance. A course of action should be made clear to the patient and her partner (see Chapter 7). As has been reinforced throughout pregnancy, any warning signs of potential adverse outcomes mandate an immediate telephone call.

◊ CONCLUSION

The future of effective and efficient prenatal care in this country depends largely on access, our ability to demonstrate clear benefit, and the incorporation of evidence-based data and practices that have well defined outcomes and utilize cost-effective methods.

Of equal importance to the content of prenatal care is the manner in which it is delivered. A crucial determinant of effective prenatal care is the clinician–patient relationship. Virtues of trust and honesty and ethical treatment are integral to achieving the goal of prenatal care to ". . . allow the patients to flourish, not to alienate them from themselves. The skill of a caregiver can prevent the alienating experience of a bad outcome; but caregivers who look for a solution to their own powerlessness in the domination of patients or the domination of natural processes can make good outcomes alienating experiences for their patients. Effective caregivers recognize their own powerlessness and work with patients. Effective caregivers are aware of cultural diversity and assess the care they give, not in terms of their own needs or the needs of a profession or a medical organization, but in terms of those who have entrusted them with care."[7]

SUMMARY POINTS

◊ Pregnancy is a normal physiologic event in a woman's life, and most pregnancies are normal.

◊ The preconception visit is a focused interval primary care visit that allows systematic identification of potential risks and the implementation of early interventions.

◊ The appropriate content of the first prenatal visit and subsequent prenatal care is contained in formalized published forms.

◊ A firm scientific foundation for the content and timing of prenatal care visits and the relationship of such care to maternal and newborn outcomes is lacking.

◊ Pregnancy is a time of change, expectation, anticipation, concern, and uncertainty for many women and their families; the provision of direct, concise, and accurate information in a compassionate and reassuring manner by the clinician is therapeutic.

◊ The future of effective and efficient prenatal care depends on access to care, an informed and motivated patient, an ability to demonstrate benefit from the tests and procedures used, and the incorporation of evidence-based practices.

◊ REFERENCES

1. American College of Obstetricians and Gynecologists. *The obstetrician-gynecologist and primary preventive health care.* Washington, DC: American College of Obstetricians and Gynecologists, 1993.
2. Bastian LA, Piscitelli JT. Is this patient pregnant? Can you really rule out early pregnancy by clinical examination? *JAMA* 1997;278:586.
3. Benowitz NL. Nicotine replacement during pregnancy. *JAMA* 1991; 266:3174.
4. Brown SS, ed. *Prenatal care: reaching mothers, reaching babies.* Washington, DC: National Academy Press, 1988.
5. Centers for Disease Control and Prevention. Recommendations for the use of folic acid to reduce the number of cases of spina bifida and other neural tube defects. *MMWR* 1992;41(RR-14):1.
6. Clapp JF III, Little KD. The interaction between regular exercise and selected aspects of women's health. *Am J Obstet Gynecol* 1995;173:2.
7. DeVries RJ. Care givers in pregnancy and childbirth. In: Chalmers I, Enkin M, Keirse MJNC, eds. *Effective care in pregnancy and childbirth.* New York: Oxford University Press, 1989:143.
8. Donaldson M, Yordy K, Vanselow N, eds. *Defining primary care: an interim report.* Washington, DC: National Academy Press, 1994.
9. Enkin MW. Randomized controlled trials in the evaluation of antenatal care. *Int J Techol Assess Health Care* 1992;8:40.
10. Fiscella K. Does prenatal care improve birth outcomes? A critical review. *Obstet Gynecol* 1995;85:468.
11. Hiller SL, Nugent RP, Eschenbach DA, et al. Association between bacterial vaginosis and preterm delivery of low birth weight infants. *N Engl J Med* 1995;333:1737.
12. Institute of Medicine: Committee to Study the Prevention of Low Birthweight. *Preventing low birthweight.* Washington, DC: National Academy Press, 1985.
13. Jack B, Culpepper L. Preconception care. In: Merkatz I, Thompson J, eds. *New perspectives on prenatal care.* New York: Elsevier Science, 1990;69.
14. Luke B, Mamelle N, Keith L, et al. The association between occupational factors and preterm birth: a U.S. nurses study. *Am J Obstet Gynecol* 1995;173:849.
15. McDuffie RS Jr, Beck A, Bischoff K, Cross J, Orleans M. Effect of frequency of prenatal visits on perinatal outcome among low-risk women: a randomized controlled trial. *JAMA* 1996;275:847.
16. McGregor JA, French JI, Seo K. Premature rupture of membranes and bacterial vaginosis. *Am J Obstet Gynecol* 1993;169:463.
17. Nageotte MP, Briggs GC, Towers CV, Asrat T. Droperidol and diphenhydramine in the management of hyperemesis gravidarum. *Am J Obstet Gynecol* 1996;174:1801.
18. National Academy of Sciences. *Recommended dietary allowances.* Washington, DC: National Academy Press, 1989.
19. National Institutes of Health. *Caring for our future: a report of the Public Health Service expert panel on the content of prenatal care.* Washington, DC: NIH, 1989. NIH publication 90-3182.
20. Pederson AL, Worthington-Robets B, Hicko DE. Weight gain patterns during twin gestation. *J Am Diet Assoc* 1989;89:642.
21. Public Health Services. *Healthy People 2000: national health promotion and disease prevention objectives.* Washington, DC: US Department of Health and Human Services, 1991.
22. Rothman KJ, Moore LL, Singer MR, Nguyen US, Mannino S, Milunsky A. Teratogenicity of high vitamin A intake. *N Engl J Med* 1995; 333:1369.
23. Rouse DJ, Andrews WW, Goldenberg RL, Owen J. Screening and treatment of asymptomatic bacteriuria of pregnancy to prevent pyelonephritis a cost-effectiveness and cost-benefit analysis. *Obstet Gynecol* 1995; 86:119.
24. Rouse DJ, Goldenberg RLL, Cliver SP, Cutter GR, Mennemeyer ST, Fargason CA Jr. Strategies for the prevention of early-onset neonatal group B streptococcal sepsis: a decision analysis. *Obstet Gynecol* 1994;83:483.
25. Stewart DE, Cecutti A. Physical abuse in pregnancy. *Can Med Assoc J* 1993;149:1257.
26. US Congress, Office of Technology Assessment. *Healthy children: investing in the future.* Washington, DC: Government Printing Office, 1988. Publication OTA-H-345.
27. US Department of Health and Human Services. *The health consequences of smoking for women: a report of the Surgeon General.* Washington, DC: Government Printing Office, 1980. Publication HHS-396.

Appendix I

DATE _____

NAME _____
      LAST   FIRST   MIDDLE

ID # _____ HOSPITAL OF DELIVERY _____

NEWBORN'S PHYSICIAN _____ REFERRED BY_____

FINAL EDD_____ PRIMARY PROVIDER/GROUP _____

BIRTH DATE	AGE	RACE	MARITAL STATUS	ADDRESS:

MONTH DAY YEAR   S M W D SEP

OCCUPATION   EDUCATION   ZIP: PHONE: (H)   (O)
- ☐ HOMEMAKER   (LAST GRADE COMPLETED)   INSURANCE CARRIER / MEDICAID #
- ☐ OUTSIDE WORK
- ☐ STUDENT   Type of Work

HUSBAND/FATHER OF BABY: PHONE: EMERGENCY CONTACT: PHONE:

TOTAL PREG	FULL TERM	PREMATURE	AB, INDUCED	AB, SPONTANEOUS	ECTOPICS	MULTIPLE BIRTHS	LIVING

MENSTRUAL HISTORY

LMP ☐ DEFINITE ☐ APPROXIMATE (MONTH KNOWN)   MENSES MONTHLY ☐ YES ☐ NO   FREQUENCY: Q _____ DAYS   MENARCHE _____ (AGE ONSET)
    ☐ UNKNOWN ☐ NORMAL AMOUNT/DURATION   PRIOR MENSES _____ DATE   ON BCP AT CONCEPT. ☐ YES ☐ NO   hCG + ____ / ____ / ____
    ☐ FINAL _____

PAST PREGNANCIES (LAST SIX)

DATE MONTH / YEAR	GA WEEKS	LENGTH OF LABOR	BIRTH WEIGHT	SEX M/F	TYPE DELIVERY	ANES.	PLACE OF DELIVERY	PRETERM LABOR YES / NO	COMMENTS / COMPLICATIONS

PAST MEDICAL HISTORY

	O Neg + Pos.	DETAIL POSITIVE REMARKS INCLUDE DATE & TREATMENT		O Neg + Pos.	DETAIL POSITIVE REMARKS INCLUDE DATE & TREATMENT
1. DIABETES			16. D (Rh) SENSITIZED		
2. HYPERTENSION			17. PULMONARY (TB, ASTHMA)		
3. HEART DISEASE			18. ALLERGIES (DRUGS)		
4. AUTOIMMUNE DISORDER			19. BREAST		
5. KIDNEY DISEASE / UTI			20. GYN SURGERY		
6. NEUROLOGIC/EPILEPSY					
7. PSYCHIATRIC			21. OPERATIONS / HOSPITALIZATIONS (YEAR & REASON)		
8. HEPATITIS / LIVER DISEASE					
9. VARICOSITIES / PHLEBITIS					
10. THYROID DYSFUNCTION			22. ANESTHETIC COMPLICATIONS		
11. TRAUMA/DOMESTIC VIOLENCE			23. HISTORY OF ABNORMAL PAP		
12. HISTORY OF BLOOD TRANSFUS.			24. UTERINE ANOMALY/DES		

	AMT/DAY PREPREG	AMT/DAY PREG	#YEARS USE			
				25. INFERTILITY		
				26. RELEVANT FAMILY HISTORY		
13. TOBACCO						
14. ALCOHOL				27. OTHER		
15. STREET DRUGS						

COMMENTS: _____

ACOG ANTEPARTUM RECORD (FORM A)

The American College of Obstetricians and Gynecologists, 409 12th Street, SW, PO Box 96920, Washington, DC 20090-6920

SYMPTOMS SINCE LMP

GENETIC SCREENING/TERATOLOGY COUNSELING
INCLUDES PATIENT, BABY'S FATHER, OR ANYONE IN EITHER FAMILY WITH:

	YES	NO		YES	NO
1. PATIENT'S AGE ≥ 35 YEARS			12. MENTAL RETARDATION/AUTISM		
2. THALASSEMIA (ITALIAN, GREEK, MEDITERRANEAN, OR ASIAN BACKGROUND): MCV < 80			IF YES, WAS PERSON TESTED FOR FRAGILE X?		
3. NEURAL TUBE DEFECT (MENINGOMYELOCELE, SPINA BIFIDA, OR ANENCEPHALY)			13. OTHER INHERITED GENETIC OR CHROMOSOMAL DISORDER		
4. CONGENITAL HEART DEFECT			14. MATERNAL METABOLIC DISORDER (EG. INSULIN-DEPENDENT DIABETES, PKU)		
5. DOWN SYNDROME			15. PATIENT OR BABY'S FATHER HAD A CHILD WITH BIRTH DEFECTS NOT LISTED ABOVE		
6. TAY–SACHS (EG, JEWISH, CAJUN, FRENCH CANADIAN)					
7. SICKLE CELL DISEASE OR TRAIT (AFRICAN)			16. RECURRENT PREGNANCY LOSS, OR A STILLBIRTH		
8. HEMOPHILIA			17. MEDICATIONS/STREET DRUGS/ALCOHOL SINCE LAST MENSTRUAL PERIOD		
9. MUSCULAR DYSTROPHY					
10. CYSTIC FIBROSIS			IF YES, AGENT(S):		
11. HUNTINGTON CHOREA			18. ANY OTHER		

COMMENTS/COUNSELING: _____

_____

_____

INFECTION HISTORY	YES	NO		YES	NO
1. HIGH RISK HEPATITIS B/IMMUNIZED?			4. RASH OR VIRAL ILLNESS SINCE LAST MENSTRUAL PERIOD		
2. LIVE WITH SOMEONE WITH TB OR EXPOSED TO TB			5. HISTORY OF STD, GC, CHLAMYDIA, HPV, SYPHILIS		
3. PATIENT OR PARTNER HAS HISTORY OF GENITAL HERPES			6. OTHER (SEE COMMENTS)		

COMMENTS: _____

_____

_____ **INTERVIEWER'S SIGNATURE** _____

INITIAL PHYSICAL EXAMINATION

DATE _____ / _____ / _____   PREPREGNANCY WEIGHT _____   HEIGHT _____   BP_____

	NORMAL	ABNORMAL				
1. HEENT	☐ NORMAL	☐ ABNORMAL	12. VULVA	☐ NORMAL	☐ CONDYLOMA	☐ LESIONS
2. FUNDI	☐ NORMAL	☐ ABNORMAL	13. VAGINA	☐ NORMAL	☐ INFLAMMATION	☐ DISCHARGE
3. TEETH	☐ NORMAL	☐ ABNORMAL	14. CERVIX	☐ NORMAL	☐ INFLAMMATION	☐ LESIONS
4. THYROID	☐ NORMAL	☐ ABNORMAL	15. UTERUS SIZE	_____ WEEKS		☐ FIBROIDS
5. BREASTS	☐ NORMAL	☐ ABNORMAL	16. ADNEXA	☐ NORMAL	☐ MASS	
6. LUNGS	☐ NORMAL	☐ ABNORMAL	17. RECTUM	☐ NORMAL	☐ ABNORMAL	
7. HEART	☐ NORMAL	☐ ABNORMAL	18. DIAGONAL CONJUGATE	☐ REACHED	☐ NO	_____ CM
8. ABDOMEN	☐ NORMAL	☐ ABNORMAL	19. SPINES	☐ AVERAGE	☐ PROMINENT	☐ BLUNT
9. EXTREMITIES	☐ NORMAL	☐ ABNORMAL	20. SACRUM	☐ CONCAVE	☐ STRAIGHT	☐ ANTERIOR
10. SKIN	☐ NORMAL	☐ ABNORMAL	21. SUBPUBIC ARCH	☐ NORMAL	☐ WIDE	☐ NARROW
11. LYMPH NODES	☐ NORMAL	☐ ABNORMAL	22. GYNECOID PELVIC TYPE	☐ YES	☐ NO	

COMMENTS (Number and explain abnormals): _____

_____

_____ **EXAM BY** _____

ACOG ANTEPARTUM RECORD (FORM B)

NAME _____

LAST   FIRST   MIDDLE

DRUG ALLERGY:

RELIGIOUS/CULTURAL CONSIDERATIONS _____	ANESTHESIA CONSULT PLANNED ☐ YES ☐ NO

PROBLEMS/PLANS	MEDICATION LIST:	Start date	Stop date
1.	1.		
2.	2.		
3.	3.		
4.	4.		
5.	5.		
6.	6.		

EDD CONFIRMATION

INITIAL EDD:

LMP ____ / ____ / ____ = EDD ____ / ____ / ____

INITIAL EXAM ____ / ____ / ____ = ____ WKS = EDD ____ / ____ / ____

ULTRASOUND ____ / ____ / ____ = ____ WKS = EDD ____ / ____ / ____

INITIAL EDD ____ / ____ / ____ INITIALED BY _____

18–20-WEEK EDD UPDATE:

QUICKENING ____ / ____ / ____ +22 WKS = ____ / ____ / ____

FUNDAL HT. AT UMBIL. ____ / ____ / ____ +20 WKS = ____ / ____ / ____

FHT W/ FETOSCOPE ____ / ____ / ____ +20 WKS = ____ / ____ / ____

ULTRASOUND ____ / ____ / ____ = ____ WKS = ____ / ____ / ____

FINAL EDD ____ / ____ / ____ INITIALED BY _____

VISIT DATE _____ (YEAR)

Column headers (diagonal): WEEKS GEST. (BEST EST.) | FUNDAL HEIGHT (CM) | PRESENTATION | FHR | FETAL MOVEMENT | PRETERM LABOR SIGNS/SYMPTOMS; +=PRESENT O=ABSENT | CERVIX EXAM (DIL./EFF./STA.) | BLOOD PRESSURE | EDEMA | WEIGHT | URINE (GLUCOSE/ALBUMIN) | NEXT APPOINTMENT | PROVIDER (INITIALS)

COMMENTS:

PROBLEMS: _____

COMMENTS: _____

ACOG ANTEPARTUM RECORD (FORM C)

LABORATORY AND EDUCATION

INITIAL LABS	DATE	RESULT	REVIEWED
BLOOD TYPE	/ /	A B AB O	
D (Rh) TYPE	/ /		
ANTIBODY SCREEN	/ /		
HCT/HGB	/ /	_____ % _____ g/dL	
PAP TEST	/ /	NORMAL / ABNORMAL / _____	
RUBELLA	/ /		
VDRL	/ /		
URINE CULTURE/SCREEN	/ /		
HBsAg	/ /		
HIV COUNSELING/TESTING	/ /	☐ POS. ☐ NEG. ☐ DECLINED	

OPTIONAL LABS	DATE	RESULT	
HGB ELECTROPHORESIS	/ /	AA AS SS AC SC AF $\uparrow A_2$	
PPD	/ /		
CHLAMYDIA	/ /		
GC	/ /		
TAY–SACHS	/ /		
OTHER			

8–18-WEEK LABS (WHEN INDICATED/ELECTED)	DATE	RESULT	
ULTRASOUND	/ /		
MSAFP/MULTIPLE MARKERS	/ /		
AMNIO/CVS	/ /		
KARYOTYPE	/ /	46, XX OR 46, XY / OTHER ____	
AMNIOTIC FLUID (AFP)	/ /	NORMAL ____ ABNORMAL ____	

24–28-WEEK LABS (WHEN INDICATED)	DATE	RESULT	
HCT/HGB	/ /	_____ % _____ g/dL	
DIABETES SCREEN	/ /	1 HOUR _____	
GTT (IF SCREEN ABNORMAL)	/ /	____ FBS ____ 1 HOUR ____ 2 HOUR ____ 3 HOUR	
D (Rh) ANTIBODY SCREEN	/ /		
D IMMUNE GLOBULIN (RhIG) GIVEN (28 WKS)	/ /	SIGNATURE _____	

32–36-WEEK LABS (WHEN INDICATED)	DATE	RESULT	
HCT/HGB (RECOMMENDED)	/ /	_____ % _____ g/dL	
ULTRASOUND	/ /		
VDRL	/ /		
GC	/ /		
CHLAMYDIA	/ /		
GROUP B STREP (35–37 WKS)	/ /		

COMMENTS/ADDITIONAL LABS

PLANS/EDUCATION   (COUNSELED ☐)

☐ ANESTHESIA PLANS _____
☐ TOXOPLASMOSIS PRECAUTIONS (CATS/RAW MEAT) _____
☐ CHILDBIRTH CLASSES _____
☐ PHYSICAL/SEXUAL ACTIVITY _____
☐ LABOR SIGNS _____
☐ NUTRITION COUNSELING _____
☐ BREAST OR BOTTLE FEEDING _____
☐ NEWBORN CAR SEAT _____
☐ POSTPARTUM BIRTH CONTROL _____
☐ ENVIRONMENTAL/WORK HAZARDS _____

☐ TUBAL STERILIZATION _____
☐ VBAC COUNSELING _____
☐ CIRCUMCISION _____
☐ TRAVEL _____
☐ LIFESTYLE, TOBACCO, ALCOHOL _____

REQUESTS _____

TUBAL STERILIZATION	DATE	INITIALS
CONSENT SIGNED	____ / ____ / ____	_____

AA128   12345/10987

PROVIDER SIGNATURE (AS REQUIRED) _____

NAME _____
LAST   FIRST   MIDDLE

ID # _____

Supplemental Visits

VISIT DATE (YEAR)	WEEKS GEST. (BEST EST.)	FUNDAL HEIGHT (CM)	PRESENTATION	FHR	FETAL MOVEMENT	PRETERM LABOR SIGNS/SYMPTOMS: + =PRESENT O=ABSENT	CERVIX EXAM (DIL/EFF./STA.)	BLOOD PRESSURE	EDEMA	WEIGHT	URINE (GLUCOSE/ALBUMIN)	NEXT APPOINTMENT	PROVIDER (INITIALS)	COMMENTS:
														_____
														_____
														_____
														_____
														_____
														_____
														_____
														_____
														_____
														_____
														_____
														_____
														_____
														_____
														_____

Progress Notes

_____

_____

_____

_____

_____

_____

_____

_____

_____

PROVIDER SIGNATURE (AS REQUIRED) _____

ACOG ANTEPARTUM RECORD (FORM E)

NAME _____
LAST   FIRST   MIDDLE

ID # _____

Progress Notes

_____
_____
_____
_____
_____
_____
_____
_____
_____
_____
_____
_____
_____
_____
_____
_____
_____
_____
_____
_____
_____
_____
_____
_____
_____
_____
_____
_____

PROVIDER SIGNATURE (AS REQUIRED) _____

The American College of Obstetricians and Gynecologists, 409 12th Street, SW, PO Box 96920, Washington, DC 20090-6920

ACOG ANTEPARTUM RECORD (FORM F)

Appendix II

The following table shows the body mass index (BMI) for weight and height. From the bottom line: Every number below the first dark line is "underweight." Every number between the first and second dark line is "normal weight." Every number between the second and third dark line is "overweight." The rest of the chart above the third dark line represents "obese."

BMI for weight and height

Weight — Height [in (cm)]

lb	kg	55.9 (142)	56.7 (144)	57.5 (146)	58.3 (148)	59.1 (150)	59.8 (152)	60.6 (154)	61.4 (156)	62.2 (158)	63.0 (160)	63.8 (162)	64.6 (164)	65.4 (166)	66.1 (168)	66.9 (170)	67.7 (172)	68.5 (174)	69.3 (176)	70.1 (178)	70.9 (180)	71.7 (182)	72.4 (184)	73.2 (186)	74.0 (188)
226	100	49.6	48.2	46.9	45.7	44.4	43.3	42.2	41.1	40.1	39.1	38.1	37.2	36.3	35.4	34.6	33.8	33.0	32.3	31.6	30.9	30.2	29.5	28.9	28.3
218	99	49.1	47.7	46.4	45.2	44.0	42.8	41.7	40.7	39.7	38.7	37.7	36.8	35.9	35.1	34.3	33.5	32.7	32.0	31.2	30.6	29.9	29.2	28.6	28.0
216	98	48.6	47.3	46.0	44.7	43.6	42.4	41.3	40.3	39.3	38.3	37.3	36.4	35.6	34.7	33.9	33.1	32.4	31.6	30.9	30.2	29.6	28.9	28.3	27.7
213	97	48.1	46.8	45.5	44.3	43.1	42.0	40.9	39.9	38.9	37.9	37.0	36.1	35.2	34.4	33.6	32.8	32.0	31.3	30.6	29.9	29.3	28.7	28.0	27.4
211	96	47.6	46.3	45.0	43.8	42.7	41.6	40.5	39.4	38.5	37.5	36.6	35.7	34.8	34.0	33.2	32.4	31.7	31.0	30.3	29.6	29.0	28.4	27.7	27.2
209	95	47.1	45.8	44.6	43.4	42.2	41.1	40.1	39.0	38.1	37.1	36.2	35.3	34.5	33.7	32.9	32.1	31.4	30.7	30.0	29.3	28.7	28.1	27.5	26.9
207	94	46.6	45.3	44.1	42.9	41.8	40.7	39.6	38.6	37.7	36.7	35.8	34.9	34.1	33.3	32.5	31.8	31.0	30.3	29.7	29.0	28.4	27.8	27.2	26.6
205	93	46.1	44.8	43.6	42.5	41.3	40.3	39.2	38.2	37.3	36.3	35.4	34.6	33.7	33.0	32.2	31.4	30.7	30.0	29.4	28.7	28.1	27.5	26.9	26.3
202	92	45.6	44.4	43.2	42.0	40.9	39.8	38.8	37.8	36.9	35.9	35.1	34.2	33.4	32.6	31.8	31.1	30.4	29.7	29.0	28.4	27.8	27.2	26.6	26.0
200	91	45.1	43.9	42.7	41.5	40.4	39.4	38.4	37.4	36.5	35.5	34.7	33.8	33.0	32.2	31.5	30.8	30.1	29.4	28.7	28.1	27.5	26.9	26.3	25.7
198	90	44.6	43.4	42.2	41.1	40.0	39.0	37.9	37.0	36.1	35.2	34.3	33.5	32.7	31.9	31.1	30.4	29.7	29.1	28.4	27.8	27.2	26.6	26.0	25.5
196	89	44.1	42.9	41.8	40.6	39.6	38.5	37.5	36.6	35.7	34.8	33.9	33.1	32.3	31.5	30.8	30.1	29.4	28.7	28.1	27.5	26.9	26.3	25.7	25.2
194	88	43.6	42.4	41.3	40.2	39.1	38.1	37.1	36.2	35.3	34.4	33.5	32.7	31.9	31.2	30.4	29.7	29.1	28.4	27.8	27.2	26.6	26.0	25.4	24.9
191	87	43.1	42.0	40.8	39.7	38.7	37.7	36.7	35.7	34.9	34.0	33.2	32.3	31.6	30.8	30.1	29.4	28.7	28.1	27.5	26.9	26.3	25.7	25.1	24.6
189	86	42.7	41.5	40.3	39.3	38.2	37.2	36.3	35.3	34.4	33.6	32.8	32.0	31.2	30.5	29.8	29.1	28.4	27.8	27.1	26.5	26.0	25.4	24.9	24.3
187	85	42.2	41.0	39.9	38.8	37.8	36.8	35.8	34.9	34.0	33.2	32.4	31.6	30.8	30.1	29.4	28.7	28.1	27.4	26.8	26.2	25.7	25.1	24.6	24.0
185	84	41.7	40.5	39.4	38.3	37.3	36.4	35.4	34.5	33.6	32.8	32.0	31.2	30.5	29.8	29.1	28.4	27.7	27.1	26.5	25.9	25.4	24.8	24.3	23.8
183	83	41.2	40.0	38.9	37.9	36.9	35.9	35.0	34.1	33.2	32.4	31.6	30.9	30.1	29.4	28.7	28.1	27.4	26.8	26.2	25.6	25.1	24.5	24.0	23.5
180	82	40.7	39.5	38.5	37.4	36.4	35.5	34.6	33.7	32.8	32.0	31.2	30.5	29.8	29.1	28.4	27.7	27.1	26.5	25.9	25.3	24.8	24.2	23.7	23.2
178	81	40.2	39.1	38.0	37.0	36.0	35.1	34.2	33.3	32.4	31.6	30.9	30.1	29.4	28.7	28.0	27.4	26.8	26.1	25.6	25.0	24.5	23.9	23.4	22.9
176	80	39.7	38.6	37.5	36.5	35.6	34.6	33.7	32.9	32.0	31.3	30.5	29.7	29.0	28.3	27.7	27.0	26.4	25.8	25.2	24.7	24.2	23.6	23.1	22.6
174	79	39.2	38.1	37.1	36.1	35.1	34.2	33.3	32.5	31.6	30.9	30.1	29.4	28.7	28.0	27.3	26.7	26.1	25.5	24.9	24.4	23.8	23.3	22.8	22.4
172	78	38.7	37.6	36.6	35.6	34.7	33.8	32.9	32.1	31.2	30.5	29.7	29.0	28.3	27.6	27.0	26.4	25.8	25.2	24.6	24.1	23.5	23.0	22.5	22.1
169	77	38.2	37.1	36.1	35.2	34.2	33.3	32.5	31.6	30.8	30.1	29.3	28.6	27.9	27.3	26.6	26.0	25.4	24.9	24.3	23.8	23.2	22.7	22.3	21.8
167	76	37.7	36.7	35.7	34.7	33.8	32.9	32.0	31.2	30.4	29.7	29.0	28.3	27.6	26.9	26.3	25.7	25.1	24.5	24.0	23.5	22.9	22.4	22.0	21.5
165	75	37.2	36.2	35.2	34.2	33.3	32.5	31.6	30.8	30.0	29.3	28.6	27.9	27.2	26.6	26.0	25.4	24.8	24.2	23.7	23.1	22.6	22.2	21.7	21.2
163	74	36.7	35.7	34.7	33.8	32.9	32.0	31.2	30.4	29.6	28.9	28.2	27.5	26.9	26.2	25.6	25.0	24.4	23.9	23.4	22.8	22.3	21.9	21.4	20.9
161	73	36.2	35.2	34.2	33.3	32.4	31.6	30.8	30.0	29.2	28.5	27.8	27.1	26.5	25.9	25.3	24.7	24.1	23.6	23.0	22.5	22.0	21.6	21.1	20.7
158	72	35.7	34.7	33.8	32.9	32.0	31.2	30.4	29.6	28.8	28.1	27.4	26.8	26.1	25.5	24.9	24.3	23.8	23.2	22.7	22.2	21.7	21.3	20.8	20.4
156	71	35.2	34.2	33.3	32.4	31.6	30.7	29.9	29.2	28.4	27.7	27.1	26.4	25.8	25.2	24.6	24.0	23.5	22.9	22.4	21.9	21.4	21.0	20.5	20.1
154	70	34.7	33.8	32.8	32.0	31.1	30.3	29.5	28.8	28.0	27.3	26.7	26.0	25.4	24.8	24.2	23.7	23.1	22.6	22.1	21.6	21.1	20.7	20.2	19.8
152	69	34.2	33.3	32.4	31.5	30.7	29.9	29.1	28.4	27.6	27.0	26.3	25.7	25.0	24.4	23.9	23.3	22.8	22.3	21.8	21.3	20.8	20.4	19.9	19.5
150	68	33.7	32.8	31.9	31.0	30.2	29.4	28.7	27.9	27.2	26.6	25.9	25.3	24.7	24.1	23.5	23.0	22.5	22.0	21.5	21.0	20.5	20.1	19.7	19.2
147	67	33.2	32.3	31.4	30.6	29.8	29.0	28.3	27.5	26.8	26.2	25.5	24.9	24.3	23.7	23.2	22.6	22.1	21.6	21.1	20.7	20.2	19.8	19.4	19.0
145	66	32.7	31.8	31.0	30.1	29.3	28.6	27.8	27.1	26.4	25.8	25.1	24.5	24.0	23.4	22.8	22.3	21.8	21.3	20.8	20.4	19.9	19.5	19.1	18.7
143	65	32.2	31.3	30.5	29.7	28.9	28.1	27.4	26.7	26.0	25.4	24.8	24.2	23.6	23.0	22.5	22.0	21.5	21.0	20.5	20.1	19.6	19.2	18.8	18.4
141	64	31.7	30.9	30.0	29.2	28.4	27.7	27.0	26.3	25.6	25.0	24.4	23.8	23.2	22.7	22.1	21.6	21.1	20.7	20.2	19.8	19.3	18.9	18.5	18.1
139	63	31.2	30.4	29.6	28.8	28.0	27.3	26.6	25.9	25.2	24.6	24.0	23.4	22.9	22.3	21.8	21.3	20.8	20.3	19.9	19.4	19.0	18.6	18.2	17.8
136	62	30.7	29.9	29.1	28.3	27.6	26.8	26.1	25.5	24.8	24.2	23.6	23.1	22.5	22.0	21.5	21.0	20.5	20.0	19.6	19.1	18.7	18.3	17.9	17.5
134	61	30.3	29.4	28.6	27.8	27.1	26.4	25.7	25.1	24.4	23.8	23.2	22.7	22.1	21.6	21.1	20.6	20.1	19.7	19.3	18.8	18.4	18.0	17.6	17.3
132	60	29.8	28.9	28.1	27.4	26.7	26.0	25.3	24.7	24.0	23.4	22.9	22.3	21.8	21.3	20.8	20.3	19.8	19.4	18.9	18.5	18.1	17.7	17.3	17.0
130	59	29.3	28.5	27.7	26.9	26.2	25.5	24.9	24.2	23.6	23.0	22.5	21.9	21.4	20.9	20.4	19.9	19.5	19.0	18.6	18.2	17.8	17.4	17.1	1.67
128	58	28.8	28.0	27.2	26.5	25.8	25.1	24.5	23.8	23.2	22.7	22.1	21.6	21.1	20.5	20.1	19.6	19.2	18.7	18.3	17.9	17.5	17.1	16.8	16.4
125	57	28.3	27.5	26.7	26.0	25.3	24.7	24.0	23.4	22.8	22.3	21.7	21.2	20.7	20.2	19.7	19.3	18.8	18.4	18.0	17.6	17.2	16.8	16.5	16.1
123	56	27.8	27.0	26.3	25.6	24.9	24.2	23.6	23.0	22.4	21.9	21.3	20.8	20.3	19.8	19.4	18.9	18.5	18.1	17.7	17.3	16.9	16.5	16.2	15.8
121	55	27.3	26.5	25.8	25.1	24.4	23.8	23.2	22.6	22.0	21.5	21.0	20.4	20.0	19.5	19.0	18.6	18.2	17.8	17.4	17.0	16.6	16.2	15.9	15.6
119	54	26.8	26.0	25.3	24.7	24.0	23.4	22.8	22.2	21.6	21.1	20.6	20.1	19.6	19.1	18.7	18.3	17.8	17.4	17.0	16.7	16.3	15.9	15.6	15.3
117	53	26.3	25.6	24.9	24.2	23.6	22.9	22.3	21.8	21.2	20.7	20.2	19.7	19.2	18.8	18.3	17.9	17.5	17.1	16.7	16.4	16.0	15.7	15.3	15.0
114	52	25.8	25.1	24.4	23.7	23.1	22.5	21.9	21.4	20.8	20.3	19.8	19.3	18.9	18.4	18.0	17.6	17.2	16.8	16.4	16.0	15.7	15.4	15.0	14.7
112	51	25.3	24.6	23.9	23.3	22.7	22.1	21.5	21.0	20.4	19.9	19.4	19.0	18.5	18.1	17.6	17.2	16.8	16.5	16.1	15.7	15.4	15.1	14.7	14.4
110	50	24.8	24.1	23.5	22.8	22.2	21.6	21.1	20.5	20.0	19.5	19.1	18.6	18.1	17.7	17.3	16.9	16.5	16.1	15.8	15.4	15.1	14.8	14.5	14.1
108	49	24.3	23.6	23.0	22.4	21.8	21.2	20.7	20.1	19.6	19.1	18.7	18.2	17.8	17.4	17.0	16.6	16.2	15.8	15.5	15.1	14.8	14.5	14.2	13.9
106	48	23.8	23.1	22.5	21.9	21.3	20.8	20.2	19.7	19.2	18.8	18.3	17.8	17.4	17.0	16.6	16.2	15.9	15.5	15.1	14.8	14.5	14.2	13.9	13.6
103	47	23.3	22.7	22.0	21.5	20.9	20.3	19.8	19.3	18.8	18.4	17.9	17.5	17.1	16.7	16.3	15.9	15.5	15.2	14.8	14.5	14.2	13.9	13.6	13.3
101	46	22.8	22.2	21.6	21.0	20.4	19.9	19.4	18.9	18.4	18.0	17.5	17.1	16.7	16.3	15.9	15.5	15.2	14.9	14.5	14.2	13.9	13.6	13.3	13.0
99	45	22.3	21.7	21.1	20.5	20.0	19.5	19.0	18.5	18.0	17.6	17.1	16.7	16.3	15.9	15.6	15.2	14.9	14.5	14.2	13.9	13.6	13.3	13.0	12.7
97	44	21.8	21.2	20.6	20.1	19.6	19.0	18.6	18.1	17.6	17.2	16.8	16.4	16.0	15.6	15.2	14.9	14.5	14.2	13.9	13.6	13.3	13.0	12.7	12.4
95	43	21.3	20.7	20.2	19.6	19.1	18.6	18.1	17.7	17.2	16.8	16.4	16.0	15.6	15.2	14.9	14.5	14.2	13.9	13.6	13.3	13.0	12.7	12.4	12.2
92	42	20.8	20.3	19.7	19.2	18.7	18.2	17.7	17.3	16.8	16.4	16.0	15.6	15.2	14.9	14.5	14.2	13.9	13.6	13.2	13.0	12.7	12.4	12.1	11.9
90	41	20.3	19.8	19.2	18.7	18.2	17.7	17.3	16.8	16.4	16.0	15.6	15.2	14.9	14.5	14.2	13.8	13.5	13.2	12.9	12.6	12.4	12.1	11.9	11.6
88	40	19.8	19.3	18.8	18.3	17.8	17.3	16.9	16.4	16.0	15.6	15.2	14.9	14.5	14.2	13.8	13.5	13.2	12.9	12.6	12.3	12.1	11.8	11.6	11.3

Appendix III

Maternal and child health care currently accounts for a large proportion of health care dollars spent annually in the United States. This is due to the large numbers of patients and the numerous procedures performed during pregnancy and the first months of life.

The effectivenesss of prenatal care is still often measured in terms of finite outcomes such as maternal and infant mortality. While these end points do not take into account such parameters as patient satisfaction, emergency interventions, length of hospitalization, and degree of access, they are used as a crude measure of quality of care of mothers and infants and are often cited in comparisons between states and countries, even when the actual data and methodologies for obtaining them are diverse and incomparable. The definitions currently used by the National Center for Health Statistics when collecting data on maternal and infant mortality and morbidity are included below for reference:

◊ *Live birth:* the complete expulsion or extraction from the mother of a product of human conception, regardless of the duration of the pregnancy, that then breathes or shows any other evidence of life, whether or not the umbilical cord has been cut or the placenta is attached.
◊ *Fetal death (stillbirth):* death before the complete expulsion or extraction from the mother of a product of human conception, regardless of the duration of the pregnancy. This definition excludes terminations of pregnancy.
◊ *Early neonatal death:* death of a liveborn infant during the first 7 days of life.
◊ *Late neonatal death:* death of an infant after 7 days but before 29 days of life.

◊ *Fetal death rate:* the number of stillborn infants per 1000 infants born.
◊ *Neonatal mortality rate:* the number of infant deaths before 29 days of life per 1000 live births.
◊ *Perinatal death rate:* a combination of fetal and neonatal deaths per 1000 total births.
◊ *Birth rate:* the number of births per 1000 members of the population.
◊ *Fertility rate:* the number of live births per 1000 female members of the population between the ages of 15 and 44 years.
◊ *Maternal mortality:* the death of a woman from any cause related to or aggravated by pregnancy or its management, regardless of duration or site of pregnancy (but not from accidental or incidental causes), occurring during the pregnancy or up to 42 days after the pregnancy. It includes direct and indirect obstetric deaths.
◊ *Direct obstetric death:* the death of a woman from obstetric complications of pregnancy, labor, or the puerperium, resulting from interventions, omissions, or treatment, or from a chain of events resulting from any of these.
◊ *Indirect obstetric death:* the death of a woman resulting from a previously existing disease or a disease that developed during pregnancy, labor, or the puerperium that was not related to direct obstetric causes, although the physiologic effects of pregnancy were partially responsible for the death.
◊ *Maternal mortality rate:* maternal deaths per 100,000 live births.

CHAPTER 7

Normal Labor, Delivery, and Puerperium

———— ◊ ————

Pamela F. Farrington
Kenneth Ward

◊ NORMAL LABOR

Labor is defined as regular, rhythmic, progressive uterine contractions that produce effacement and dilation of the cervix. If the estimated gestational age is accurate, labor usually begins within 2 weeks of the estimated date of confinement (EDC). The EDC is 266 days or 38 weeks after conception (280 days or 40 weeks after first day of the last menstrual period). Only 3% to 5% of patients actually deliver on their EDC.

An understanding of normal labor and delivery is essential for obstetric practice, yet many practitioners do not adapt their management of labor to the latest evidence. Many obstetricians continue to use a style that they were taught as residents. Some women criticize their physicians for using a "programmed" approach to labor, and some react by choosing delivery alternatives that may not be as safe. Midwives claim that the obstetrician's approach is not individualized or supportive enough. Consumer groups have reported that nurse-midwives have a cesarean section rate that is half the national average and their rate of vaginal birth following cesarean section is 2.8 times the national average. At the same time, some of our colleagues are advocating an even more programmed "active management" approach to labor. Clearly, the management of normal labor remains a controversial subject that affects almost every obstetric patient; there is still a need for further thought and study.

The normal stimulus for the biochemical cascade that results in labor is unknown. Prior to the onset of true labor, there is a general softening and stretching of pelvic ligaments and the soft tissues of the vagina. There is also shortening and dilatation (ripening) of the cervix. Braxton Hicks contractions (weak, irregular, regional, rhythmic contractions) usually occur for weeks before the onset of actual labor. It is hypothesized that a "placental clock" gene is active from the earliest stages of pregnancy and that this gene determines the length of gestation and the timing of parturition. One signal controlled by this clock is the placental hormone corticotropin-releasing factor (CRF). CRF is released into the maternal circulation early in the second trimester, and its concentration rises exponentially as pregnancy advances. CRF regulates the secretion of adrenal cortisol, which can increase the strength of uterine contractions. CRF also stimulates production of oxytocin by the fetus and prostaglandins by the placenta.

Other factors probably play a role. For instance, progesterone inhibits and estrogen stimulates uterine contractility. Like CRF, estrogen also stimulates the production of oxytocin receptors in the uterus. Thus, as progesterone levels decline near term, estrogen may stimulate myometrial contractility. Mechanical stretch can also increase uterine contractility, as occurs with twin gestations and pregnancies complicated by polyhydramnios. Once labor is initiated, the process is thought to involve multiple positive feedback loops. For instance, contractions stimulate the cervix to stretch. Stretching of the cervix elicits a reflex contraction by the uterus, pushing the fetal head against the cervix to stretch it more, and so on. A clearer understanding of the mechanisms of spontaneous labor will help in the management of women in whom labor must be induced, and aid in our attempts to stop the progress of preterm labor.

Phases of Labor

Three stages of labor have been defined to help follow progress in labor and identify those women who are experiencing labor abnormalities that would be helped by intervention. Emanuel Friedman carefully studied thousands of normal and abnormal labors with serial cervical examinations to define the expected rate of progress and detect patterns that may indicate a labor disorder. A graphic labor curve (partogram) such as that in Figure 1 can be very helpful in caring for a woman in labor. These graphs are typically referred to as a Friedman curve.

The first stage of labor begins with the onset of regular uterine contractions and ends with complete cervical dilation. The first stage is itself divided into three phases: the latent phase, the active phase, and the deceleration phase. During the latent phase, contractions become progressively stronger, longer, more frequent, and better coordinated. The cervix effaces but shows minimal dilation. The mother's discomfort can be minimal to severe, depending on the ripeness of the cervix. The latent phase may be intermittent over several days, or it may last only a few hours, averaging 8 hours in nulliparas and 5 hours in multiparas. During the active phase, the contractions are usually strong and very regular, occurring every 2 to 3 minutes. The cervix dilates from 3 to 4 cm to full dilation, and the presenting part descends well into the pelvis. This phase of labor is predictably associated with increased discomfort for the mother. The length of the active phase is more predictable, lasting about 5 hours in nulliparas and 2 hours in multiparas. The deceleration phase goes unnoticed in many labors, occurring at the end of the active phase, and simply represents the observed relative slowing of dilation when the cervix is close to being completely dilated.

The second stage is defined as the period from complete cervical dilation to delivery of the baby. During the second stage, contractions are strong and regular, with a frequency of every 1 to 3 minutes. The baby's head descends more deeply into the pelvis, with each contraction stimulating a strong urge to push in patients who do not have regional anesthesia. The uterine contractions and the maternal pushing efforts work together to achieve delivery of the baby. The second stage typically lasts about 60 minutes in nulliparas and 15 minutes in multiparas. Epidural or caudal anesthesia tend to lengthen the second stage.

The third stage of labor is defined as the period from delivery of the baby to delivery of the placenta. Delivery of the placenta may occur immediately after the birth of the baby, or it can take up to 30 minutes. The progress of labor depends on three critical components:

◊ *Powers*—uterine contractions and maternal pushing;
◊ *Pelvis*—the bony pelvis and the overlying soft tissues;
◊ *Passenger*—the baby's size and positioning.

The power of labor can be clinically assessed by palpation of the uterus during contractions or with the use of an

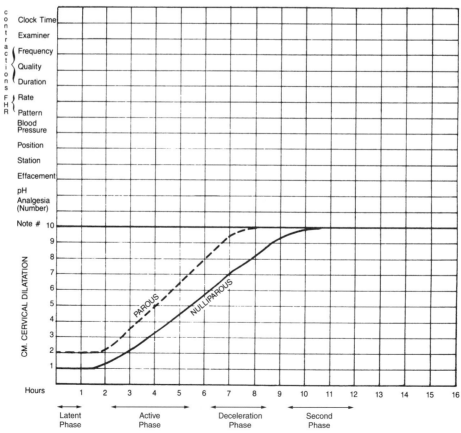

FIG. 1. Flow sheet for following labor progress.

intrauterine pressure catheter if the adequacy of the contractions is in question. While some consider evaluation of the bony pelvis a lost art with the decreased utilization of forceps to achieve vaginal delivery, thoughtful assessment of clinical pelvimetry continues to be valuable in the evaluation of progress in labor and especially dysfunctional labor. Clinical pelvimetry should be performed at the first prenatal visit and repeated upon presentation in labor. This evaluation involves consideration of the pelvic inlet, midpelvis, and outlet:

◊ *Pelvic inlet:* The transverse diameter of the pelvic inlet averages 13 cm. It cannot be measured clinically, but a narrow inlet is a very rare cause of dystocia. The anteroposterior (AP) diameter of the inlet is most important. It is estimated clinically by determining the distance between the lower margin of the symphysis pubis and the sacral promontory (Fig. 2). This value is known as the diagonal conjugate. The obstetric conjugate—or true AP diameter—is 1.5 to 2.0 cm shorter. If the diagonal conjugate is 12 cm or greater, the pelvic inlet is an adequate size for a normal fetus.

◊ *Midpelvis:* The specific diameters of the midpelvis cannot be measured clinically. Contraction of the midpelvis is suspected if the ischial spines are quite prominent, the pubic arch is narrow, the pelvic side walls converge, or the sacral concavity is quite shallow (Fig. 3).

◊ *Pelvic outlet:* The transverse diameter of the pelvic outlet should be greater than 8 cm. This diameter can be estimated by placing a fist on the perineum to measure the distance between the ischial tuberosities. The AP diameter is estimated by noting the angle made by the pubic rami. A contracted outlet is rarely the sole cause of dystocia; however, it is often associated with midpelvis contraction.

Consideration of the above measurements allows assignment to one of the various pelvic types, and thus an appreciation of how and where labor may be stalled if the pelvis is not favorable for childbirth (Fig. 4). Careful evaluation of the midpelvis is most important, as those women found to have a contracted midpelvis (prominent ischial spines, flat sacrum, sacrosciatic notch less than two fingerbreadths wide) are poor candidates for forceps-assisted vaginal delivery. However,

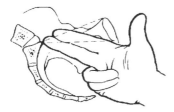

FIG. 2. The pelvic inlet anteroposterior diameter is estimated from the diagonal conjugate.

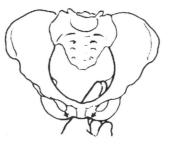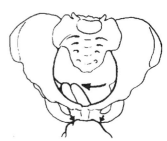

FIG. 3. The transverse diameter of the midpelvis is estimated by evaluating the distance between the ischial spines.

because the fetal skull has the ability to mold, borderline pelvimetry is not a contraindication to a trial of labor.

From the perspective of the baby, labor involves movement progressively downward through the pelvis in the following *cardinal movements* (Fig. 5).

◊ *Engagement* occurs days to weeks prior to labor for primigravidas and at the onset of labor for multigravidas.

◊ *Flexion* of the neck allows the occiput to lead, and the smallest possible diameter of the fetal head travels downward through the pelvis.

◊ *Descent* is progressive as the cervix thins, and the lower uterine segment lengthens.

◊ *Internal rotation* occurs during descent. The vertex rotates from transverse to either a posterior or anterior position to pass the ischial spines.

◊ *Extension* occurs as the fetal head distends the perineum and the occiput passes beneath the symphysis.

◊ *External rotation* of the head after delivery to a transverse position allows the shoulders to rotate internally to an AP position.

Management of Labor and Delivery

Antepartum Instructions

All women should be advised of the circumstances that should prompt them to seek evaluation. These include (1) possible rupture of the membranes, (2) regular uterine contractions, (3) heavy bleeding per vagina, (4) back, pelvic, or abdominal pain greater than they are anticipating, (5) and a change in their baby's activity. Especially with a woman's first pregnancy, false labor or Braxton Hicks contractions are likely to be confused with true labor. The contractions of false labor tend to be irregular both in intensity and in interval, and the associated discomfort, if any, is typically limited to the lower abdomen and groin. The contractions of false labor usually abate with time, analgesia, or sedation. With true labor, the contractions progressively increase in intensity. They occur every 2 to 4 minutes and cause discomfort in the abdomen and back with the associated sensation of increasing pelvic pressure. For many women, labor will be preceded by the passage of bloody show (a small amount of blood with mucous discharge from the cervix). In 10% of pregnancies, the amniotic and chorionic sac (the membranes) rupture before labor be-

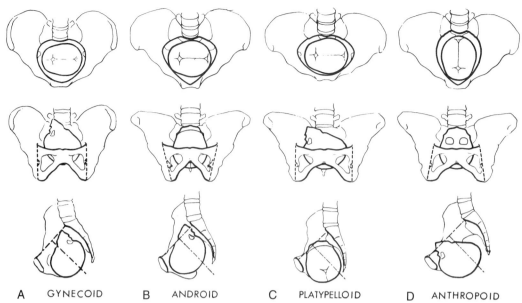

A   GYNECOID   B   ANDROID   C   PLATYPELLOID   D   ANTHROPOID

FIG. 4. Pelvic types. **A:** Gynecoid pelvis—most common, round to oval inlet, ischial spines not prominent, curved sacrum, wide pubic arch; best suited for childbearing. **B:** Android pelvis—heart-shaped inlet,
narrow midpelvis with anterior sacrum, prominent ischial spines, convergent side walls, narrow pubic
arch. **C:** Platypelloid pelvis—least common, decreased anteroposterior dimensions at all levels with wide
transverse dimensions. **D:** Anthropoid pelvis—narrow inlet, midpelvis, and pubic arch.

gins, and amniotic fluid leaks through the cervix and out of the
vagina. Of women with rupture of the membranes prior to
labor at term, 80% to 90% will go into labor spontaneously
within 24 hours. Often, the only way to confirm the diagnosis
of true labor is observation over several hours and examination of the cervix for change.

Admission

The most important step in management of normal labor is
the correct diagnosis upon admission. If the patient is having contractions, their time of onset and frequency should
be recorded. Questions should focus on spontaneous rupture
of the membranes, presence or absence of bleeding, fetal activity, any allergies, use of any medications, and most recent oral intake. A review of her prenatal record should take
specific note of her expected date of confinement and its reliability, as well as her past medical history and details of
previous pregnancies: number, gestation, fetal size, duration of labor, and any complications. The patient's total
weight gain during the pregnancy should be calculated, and
any recent rapid weight gains noted. Prenatal laboratory
data should be reviewed, including blood type, hematocrit,
$Rh_0(D)$ immune globulin requirements, VDRL test, rubella
immunity, and hepatitis and human immunodeficiency
virus (HIV) status.

The admission physical examination should include vital
signs (temperature, pulse, blood pressure), thyroid palpation,
examination of the chest and extremities, and a brief neurologic examination. Leopold maneuvers should be performed
to assess fetal position (Fig. 6), and the uterus should be pal-

pated to determine the frequency, intensity, and duration of
uterine contractions. Fundal height should be evaluated and
a clinical assessment of fetal weight should be performed.
Fetal heart tones should be auscultated with specific evaluation of the response of the fetal heart rate (FHR) to the uterine contractions.

On pelvic examination, the vulva should be examined for
herpetic lesions, condylomata, and lacerations. For women
with possible rupture of the membranes, it is appropriate
to confirm the leaking of amniotic fluid. This is most commonly done with a sterile speculum examination for pooling
of fluid at the top of the vagina. The pH of the pooled fluid can
be checked with nitrazine paper, which turns blue in the presence of amniotic fluid, and an air-dried sample of the fluid can
be examined under a microscope for the characteristic "fern"
pattern that confirms the presence of amniotic fluid. Since cervical mucus and maternal serum can demonstrate a fern pattern, care must be taken in collection of this sample. Palpation
of the cervix includes attention to the following:

◊ Assessment of the softness or firmness of the cervix,
◊ Degree of effacement (Fig. 7),
◊ Dilation of the cervical os,
◊ Location of the cervical os with respect to the axis of the
  birth canal (vagina), noted as anterior or posterior,
◊ Development of the lower uterine segment.

The presenting part should be palpated to confirm whether
it is the head, foot, buttock, or shoulder. Station is determined
by noting the position of the fetal presenting (bony) part relative to the ischial spines (Fig. 8). The fetal position is determined by noting the orientation of occiput relative to the ma-

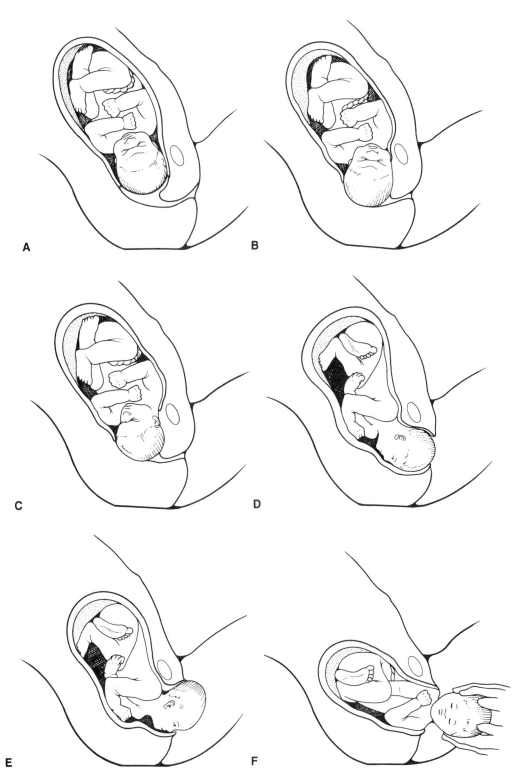

FIG. 5. Cardinal movements of labor. **A:** Engagement. **B:** Flexion. **C:** Descent and internal rotation. **D, E:** Extension. **F:** External rotation.

ternal pelvis (Fig. 9). The attitude of the fetal head is the position of the fetal head relative to the fetal chest and any lateral flexion of the head (Figs. 10 to 12). Clinical pelvimetry should be repeated (as above). Pelvimetry using computed tomography is indicated in women who have suffered a prior

injury to the bony pelvis and in those with a breech presentation in whom other criteria for vaginal breech delivery have been met (see Chapter 27).

In women at term with rupture of the membranes prior to the onset of labor, it is appropriate to defer digital examina-

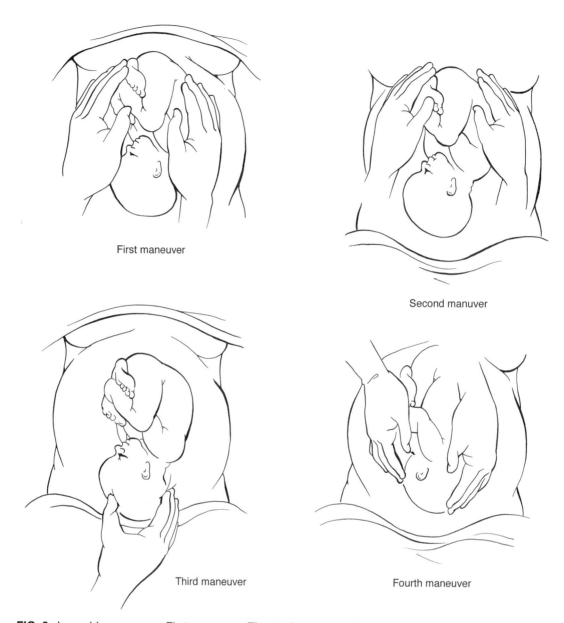

First maneuver

Second manuver

Third maneuver

Fourth maneuver

FIG. 6. Leopold maneuvers. First maneuver: The uterine contour is outlined; the fundus is palpated, allowing identification of the fetal parts. Second maneuver: By palpation of the sides of the maternal abdomen, the location of the fetal back is determined. Third maneuver: The presenting part is grasped, identified, and evaluated for engagement. Fourth maneuver: With palpation toward the pelvis, the identity of the presenting part is confirmed, and flexion or extension of the fetal head is evaluated.

tion of the cervix until they are in active labor, to decrease the risk of chorioamnionitis. It is important, however, to confirm the baby's presentation, and an ultrasound examination should be performed if the presentation is not clear by Leopold examination.

Management of the First Stage of Labor

Critical for management of the first stage of labor is an appreciation of the tremendous range of normal. The primary goals are to monitor the baby's well-being, support the woman through what can be a very long and uncomfortable

time, and offer intervention as it may become appropriate. This may be viewed as maximizing the joy of this miraculous event and helping allay the fears associated with labor. Support of the woman through labor includes allowing her to assume whatever position is most comfortable (or least uncomfortable) for her. All forms of monitoring, be it intermittent auscultation, external fetal monitoring, or internal monitoring, can be accomplished in a sitting or upright position. The only time a healthy woman's free movements must be limited is when she has received analgesia and would not be steady on her feet. Much study has been done on the effect of maternal position in labor on uterine blood flow, and certainly

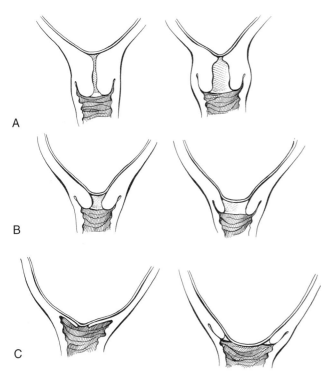

FIG. 7. Degree of cervical effacement. **A:** No effacement. **B:** 75% effacement. **C:** 100% effacement.

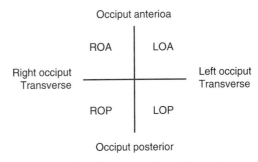

FIG. 9. Fetal position. The orientation of the vertex presentation within the maternal pelvis.

Vital signs should be monitored at least every 4 hours, or more frequently as clinically indicated. If a woman develops an intrapartum fever, defined as greater than 38°C (100.4°F), evaluation and treatment for chorioamnionitis may be indicated. When a woman's membranes are ruptured for longer

the left lateral recumbent position has been demonstrated to be optimal and should be utilized whenever there is concern about the baby's tolerance of labor. No particular position other than avoidance of the supine position has been shown to affect outcome for the healthy baby.

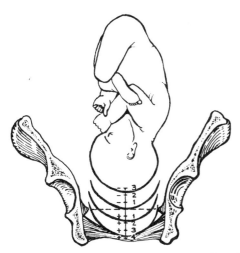

FIG. 8. Stations of the fetal head. At the 0 station, the fetal head is at the ischial spines and fills the maternal sacrum. Positions above the ischial spines are referred to as −1, −2, and −3, referring to the number of centimeters that the head is positioned above the spines. As the head descends past the ischial spines, the stations are referred to as +1, +2, +3, and +4.

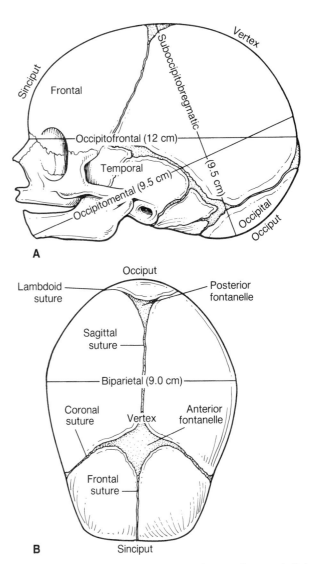

FIG. 10 A and **B.** The bones, sutures, fontanelles, and clinically important diameters of the fetal head.

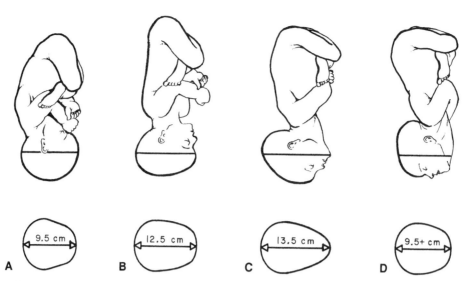

FIG. 11. Fetal attitude and dimensions of a term-size fetus. **A:** Full flexion presents the smallest circumference of the fetal head to the narrower planes of the pelvis. **B:** Military attitude usually changes to full flexion with descent into the pelvis. **C:** Brow presentation usually converts to full flexion or a face presentation, as the occipitomental diameter is too large for all except the largest pelves to accommodate. **D:** Face presentation presents dimensions that allow descent through the pelvis, unless the chin is posterior. Persistent mentum posterior must be delivered by cesarean section.

than 18 hours, prophylactic antibiotics are recommended, specifically intravenous penicillin G, 5 million U, followed by 2.5 million U every 4 hours in an attempt to decrease the risk of early-onset group B streptococcal sepsis in the neonate.

Placement of an intravenous line is not necessary for all women in labor. However, women who are dehydrated from the efforts of a long latent phase or have experienced significant vomiting in labor will benefit from intravenous hydration. All women in whom conduction anesthesia is used require preloading with intravenous fluid to avoid hypotension and the consequent decrease in uterine blood flow with the development of a sympathetic block. Women at increased risk of postpartum hemorrhage (i.e., those with prior postpartum hemorrhage, prolonged labor, or overdistended uterus)

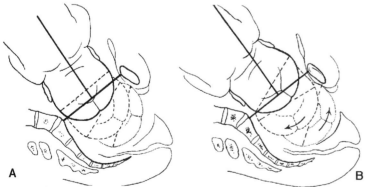

FIG. 12. Fetal attitude and lateral flexion of the fetal head. **A:** Synclitism: The plane of the biparietal diameter is parallel to the plane of the inlet. **B:** Asynclitism: Lateral flexion of the fetal head leads to anterior parietal or posterior parietal presentation.

should be advised to have an intravenous access established for administration of fluids and medication, should these be necessary.

Laboratory evaluation upon presentation in labor is quite minimal for women who have received prenatal care and have had a recent evaluation of their hemoglobin or hematocrit. Certainly, if a woman has hypertension on admission, she should be thoroughly evaluated for possible preeclampsia. In women who have not had any prenatal care, it is appropriate to order a complete blood cell count, blood type, and Rh status, an antibody screen, a rubella titer, and syphilis, hepatitis, and HIV screens. These women should also be offered gonococcal and chlamydial screening.

There are no strict criteria for how often the cervix should be examined during the first stage of labor. In general, frequent examinations in the latent phase of labor serve little purpose. Frequent cervical checks increase a woman's expectation for progress in labor that may not be realistic; in addition, such examinations are uncomfortable and increase risk for infectious morbidity. At the same time, if the membranes have ruptured and the presenting part was not engaged on the prior examination, then a cervical check should be performed, and the FHR auscultated. When women enter the active phase of labor, monitoring the progress of labor with cervical examinations every 2 hours allows identification of those women who are not making normal progress and who should therefore be evaluated for oxytocin augmentation.

A full discussion of anesthesia and analgesia is presented in Chapter 8. It is very helpful for women to be advised of the potential options for labor anesthesia and analgesia during their prenatal education so that they can best participate in the choice of medication, should that be necessary. Many patients prefer a natural childbirth that avoids anesthesia and allows both partners to play an active role in the delivery. The Lamaze method (after Dr. Fernand Lamaze, a French obstetrician) is a natural childbirth approach that emphasizes a conditioned learning technique in which the mother tries to control her fear and pain with muscle control and relaxation. The Leboyer method (after French obstetrician Frederick Leboyer) stresses the importance of a gentle delivery and minimal trauma for the newborn. This method suggests that the baby should be born into a dimly lit room that is kept relatively silent. Immediately after birth, the child is placed on the mother's abdomen to be gently massaged, in the belief that tactile stimulation and early contact can soothe the baby and promote bonding. For more adventurous individuals, the water birth technique is proposed to further ease a child's entry into this world by delivery under water. None of these various options has been subjected to rigorous scientific evaluation to determine effectiveness, although none has been demonstrated to be harmful to mother or baby. Unfortunately, routine obstetric techniques have been slow to evolve in response to scientific data as well. Couples can have a profound sense of disappointment when labor does not allow adherence to a "birth plan." Some are so committed to one plan and so afraid that various providers will interfere with their plan that they take additional risk and plan a home birth to ensure that their wishes are not disregarded. Every effort should be made to accommodate individual needs and desires to provide to all women and their families the increased safety of a birthing center or hospital birth.

To monitor the baby's well-being and tolerance of labor, assessment of the FHR is utilized. Electronic fetal monitoring is currently used in an increasing percentage of labors without clear evidence that this technology has improved outcome for the low-risk baby or mother, compared to intermittent auscultation. During the active phase of the first stage of labor, the FHR should be evaluated at least every 30 minutes, preferably following a uterine contraction when intermittent auscultation is used. If continuous electronic fetal monitoring is used, the tracing should be evaluated at least every 30 minutes. During the second stage of labor, the FHR should be evaluated and recorded at least every 15 minutes when auscultation is used and should be evaluated at least every 15 minutes when electronic fetal monitoring is utilized.

Amniotomy, more correctly referred to as artificial rupture of the membranes (AROM), has become such a common practice that it is difficult to make a recommendation regarding its appropriateness in normal labor. Most studies show that amniotomy shortens the total length of labor but that it may increase maternal discomfort and the incidence of variable decelerations. Indications for amniotomy have included allowing placement of internal fetal monitoring for those with concerning tracings, assessment of the amniotic fluid for meconium, and most commonly accelerating labor. As with all interventions, AROM should be performed for an indication, as this procedure carries with it some, albeit a small, risk for cord prolapse and development of an abnormal FHR. To prevent these complications, elective AROM in the setting of normal labor should be performed only when the presenting part is well applied to the cervix, and preferably during a contraction to minimize the chance for dislodging the baby's head.

Management of Second Stage of Labor

The onset of the second stage of labor with complete dilation of the cervix is usually noted by the woman as the presenting part descends into the vagina and she experiences the urge to push with contractions. Even with regional anesthesia, most women will become aware of increased pelvic pressure and specifically a sense of rectal pressure, giving them the urge to push. The cervix should be examined at this time to confirm complete dilation. The position and station of the presenting part should be checked, and descent of the presenting part with maternal pushing should be assessed. During the second stage of labor, the FHR should be auscultated at least every 15 minutes through a contraction and the recovery phase. Support of a woman in the second stage involves allowing her to find the most comfortable and effective position for pushing, as well as encouraging her efforts. Preparations for delivery should be made when the presenting part begins to distend the perineum and possibly sooner for multigravidas. Local or pudendal anesthesia, if necessary, should be administered at this time.

An episiotomy is an incision in the perineum used to facilitate vaginal delivery. It is useful for patients in whom the perineum does not readily stretch and when delivery must be rushed. Episiotomy has been routinely recommended in the past, since the procedure substitutes a surgical incision for excessive stretching and possible tearing of the perineal tissues. It was argued that a surgical incision is easier to repair than a tear and that episiotomy decreases painful anterior tears, as well as future problems with pelvic relaxation. While this procedure has a long history, there is little evidence to support most of its purported benefits. What is known is that episiotomy will prevent a perineal laceration in many women; however, a midline episiotomy increases the risk of extension through the anal sphincter and into the rectum, and thus the risk for rectovaginal fistula formation and sphincter dysfunction.

There are two basic types of episiotomy: midline and mediolateral. The benefits of a midline episiotomy include anatomic end results, easy repair, and lower incidence of postpartum pain or dyspareunia. Episiotomy should not be performed until delivery is imminent. A midline incision is made with scissors from the midpoint of the posterior fourchette directly backward toward the rectum (Fig. 13). The midline episiotomy is subdivided into first degree—through the mucosa only; second degree—through the mucosa and subcutaneous tissues, including the muscles of the perineal body; third degree—through the anal sphincter; and fourth degree—through the rectal mucosa. A mediolateral episiotomy is less likely to ex-

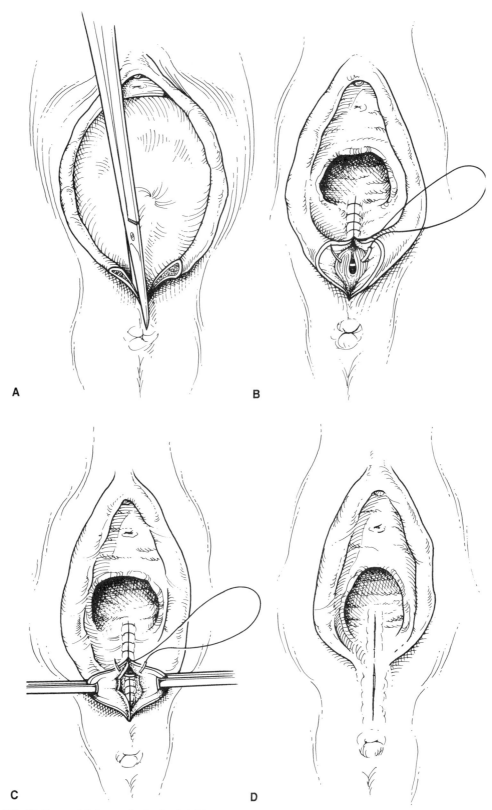

FIG. 13. Midline episiotomy. **A:** As the fetal head distends, with the perineum under adequate anesthesia, the episiotomy is cut through the perineal body and the tissues of the vagina and the rectovaginal septum. **B:** The episiotomy is repaired by reapproximating the vaginal mucosa in a running fashion with a delayed absorbable suture. **C:** The submucosal tissue of the vagina and the subcutaneous tissue and fascia of the perineal body are then closed. **D:** The skin is then reapproximated with a running subcuticular suture.

tend through the sphincter but more likely to cause pain during healing, dyspareunia, or excessive blood loss. A mediolateral incision is made with scissors from the midpoint of the posterior fourchette at a 45-degree angle laterally on either side. Although a mediolateral episiotomy does not usually extend into the sphincter or rectum, postoperative pain and healing time are increased. Care must be taken during the repair to achieve a good anatomic result.

Regardless of use of an episiotomy, tears and extensions into the rectum are best prevented by keeping the baby's head well flexed until the occiput passes beyond the subpubic arch. As the vertex appears beneath the symphysis, the perineum is supported by direct pressure from a draped hand over the coccygeal region. As the head delivers, it will rotate to a transverse position, the mother should be encouraged to continue to push to achieve delivery of the anterior shoulder. A quick check should be done for the presence of wrapping of the umbilical cord around the baby's neck (nuchal cord). The cord can usually be slipped around the baby's head or double-clamped and cut if it is too tight to reduce. The maternal pushing efforts can be assisted by placing gentle downward traction on the baby's head. With delivery of the anterior shoulder, a moment can be taken to suction the baby's nose and mouth with a bulb or DeLee trap. Gentle upward traction assisting renewed pushing by the mother will achieve delivery of the posterior shoulder. The baby's body generally delivers easily following the shoulders. Care must be taken only to support the baby's head and ensure that the baby does not slip from one's grip. After confirmation of good respiration and normal heart rate (easily checked at the cord insertion at the umbilicus), the baby should be given to the mother to cradle. The cord is then double-clamped and cut, and cord blood collected. The baby should be dried and wrapped soon following delivery to maintain its body temperature.

Management of the Third Stage of Labor

The third stage of labor begins following the delivery of the baby and ends with the delivery of the placenta. Following the birth, one should watch for signs of placental separation, including lengthening of the umbilical cord, a gush of blood coming from the uterus, and the uterus becoming more globular and rising in the maternal abdomen. Once these signs are observed, with palpation of the fundus and pressure of the thumb just above the symphysis pubis, gentle traction may be placed on the umbilical cord, resulting in delivery of the placenta (Fig. 14). Whenever traction is placed on the cord, attention must be made to the potential and serious obstetric complication of uterine inversion. It is far preferable to perform a manual extraction of the placenta than to deal with the consequences of an iatrogenically inverted uterus. If at any time heavy bleeding occurs during the third stage of labor or if the placenta is not delivered within 30 minutes of the birth, the placenta should be manually removed. The anesthesiologist should be alerted at this time, as general anesthesia may

be required for patients who have no regional anesthesia and dilation and curettage may be necessary if the placenta does not readily separate from the uterine wall. The placenta should then be carefully inspected for cord insertion, confirmation of a three-vessel cord, and completeness of the placenta and membranes. If any portion of the placenta or the membranes is missing, the uterine cavity should be manually explored. Some advocate routine exploration of the uterine cavity to reduce the risk of infection and bleeding from retained placental fragments. The benefit of this examination in women without regional anesthesia must be weighed against the discomfort it causes, as well as disrupting the interaction of the mother with her newborn. The uterus should be frequently palpated following delivery of the placenta to ensure that it remains well contracted. Oxytocin, 10 to 20 U intramuscularly or diluted in a liter of intravenous fluid, has been demonstrated to decrease the incidence of postpartum hemorrhage secondary to uterine atony. The birth canal, including the cervix, vagina, and perineum should be inspected for lacerations requiring repair. During this time, the baby should be kept with the family and placed to the breast to nurse within the first 10 to 20 minutes after birth. This first suckling not only stimulates endogenous oxytocin release but also begins the process of milk production and successful breast-feeding.

Management of the "Fourth Stage" of Labor

Because many complications of birth occur or become evident during the first hour after delivery, this time has been referred to as the "fourth stage" of labor, though not officially defined as a stage of labor. The new mother should be seen at least every 15 minutes by a trained labor and delivery nurse checking vital signs and looking for any evidence of uterine atony or postpartum hemorrhage. The perineum should be inspected for any signs of hematoma formation. The newborn should undergo its initial assessment at this time and be observed closely for any signs of compromise.

Postpartum Care

After the first 24 hours, postpartum recovery is rapid. A regular diet should be offered as soon as the patient requests food, sometimes shortly after delivery. Full ambulation is encouraged as soon as possible. Exercises to improve tone and strengthen abdominal muscles may be started after 1 day. The perineum should be cleansed with warm water two or three times daily after voiding or bowel movements. Shower baths can be encouraged, but vaginal douching is prohibited during the early puerperium to avoid the risk of introducing infection into the uterus. Pain from an uncomfortable perineal laceration or episiotomy can be relieved with warm sitz baths and an analgesic (e.g., acetaminophen, 650 mg, with or without codeine or ibuprofen, 600 to 800 mg) (Table 1).

Especially when regional anesthesia is used, care must be taken to avoid problems with urinary retention and bladder overdistention. Women should be encouraged to void every

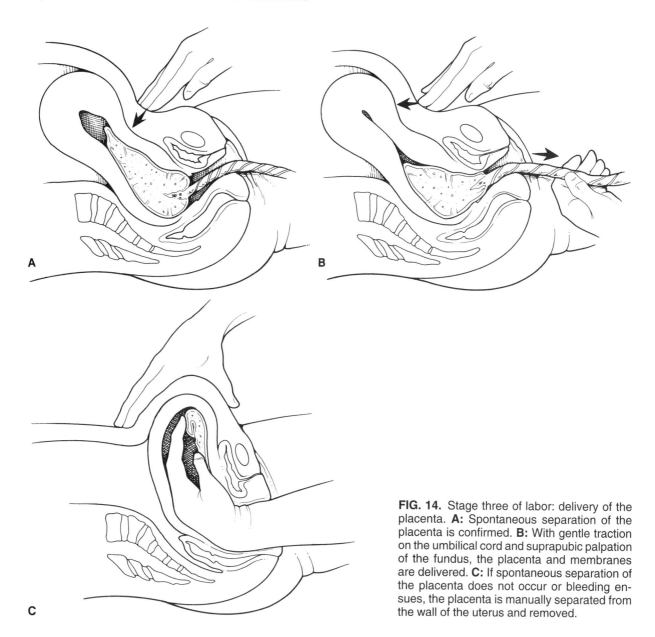

FIG. 14. Stage three of labor: delivery of the placenta. **A:** Spontaneous separation of the placenta is confirmed. **B:** With gentle traction on the umbilical cord and suprapubic palpation of the fundus, the placenta and membranes are delivered. **C:** If spontaneous separation of the placenta does not occur or bleeding ensues, the placenta is manually separated from the wall of the uterus and removed.

2 to 3 hours, even if they are not aware of any sensation of bladder fullness, as rapid diuresis may occur following delivery, especially when oxytocin is discontinued.

Prior to discharge, a complete blood cell count should be checked if there is any concern that a woman has experienced heavier than normal postpartum bleeding. In addition, seronegative women should be immunized against rubella on the day of discharge. If the mother is Rh-negative, is not sensitized, and has an Rh-positive infant, she should be given $Rh_0(D)$ immune globulin to prevent sensitization from occurring. As discharge from the hospital now occurs anywhere from 12 to 48 hours following an uncomplicated birth, most women have not begun milk production prior to their discharge. To support breast-feeding, it is critical to advise women of the availability of assistance, should they experience any difficulty with nursing. If

the mother does not plan to breast-feed, she should be advised to bind and avoid any stimulation of the breasts. She should also take aspirin, acetaminophen, or ibuprofen if engorgement becomes uncomfortable.

The length of inpatient hospitalization has changed remarkably over the past two decades, reflecting the decreasing risk of postpartum complications and changing medical and societal attitudes toward birth, as well as pressures from third-party payers. Numerous reports, including three randomized, controlled trials have shown early discharge, 12 to 24 hours postdelivery, *with* appropriate follow-up in the home results in a low and acceptable rate of readmission of mothers and babies. Several studies showed that longer hospital stays improve maternal postpartum adjustment and breast-feeding success. Stays of 12 to 24 hour are only acceptable when patients have adequate help in the home and the community has

TABLE 1. *Examples of orders after routine vaginal delivery: immediately postpartum*

Oxytocin, 10 U IM
Bed rest and vital signs every 15 min for 1 h postpartum
    then every 4 h
Regular diet
Ambulation as tolerated when stable
Ice pack to the perineum
Tucks to the perineum as required
Sitz baths three times daily and at bedtime, as needed
IV line (if present): discontinue when vital signs are stable
    and uterine bleeding is normal
Urethral catheterization if unable to void in 6–8 h
Breast binder if not nursing
Complete blood cell count on postpartum day 1
Type and crossmatch for Rh$_0$(D) immunoglobulin if indicated
Medications
    Vitamins: continue prenatal vitamins; additional ferrous
        sulfate if anemic
    Pain: ibuprofen, 400–600 mg PO of 4–6h, f
        or cramping/pain
    Bowels: docusate sodium, 100 mg PO BIO,
        Milk of Magnesia, 30 ml/d PO, as needed; bisacodyl,
        10 mg PO or per rectum, as needed

a home care nursing program with 24-hour coverage, 7 days a week. Home care services, while not always necessary, can be very helpful and appear to increase the safety of early discharge. All women and their babies discharged within 24 hours of birth should be offered a minimum of one home visit or an appointment for outpatient follow-up in the first few days following discharge.

◊ PUERPERIUM

The puerperium is the 6 to 8 weeks following delivery of the placenta, in which the uterus returns to its normal state. Following delivery of the placenta, the uterus contracts to less than half its size prior to the birth. The involution that then occurs over the next several weeks is most rapid in women who breast-feed their newborns. The postpartum discharge, or lochia, changes as the uterus involutes. Initially, the discharge is grossly bloody (lochia rubra), persisting for 3 to 4 days. It then decreases in volume and changes to pale brown and becomes thinner (lochia serosa), persisting for 10 to 12 days. Finally, the discharge becomes yellowish white, occasionally tinged with blood (lochia alba), and may persist for several weeks. The total volume of lochia is about 250 ml, and women are usually encouraged to use external pads to absorb it, rather than intravaginal tampons, to minimize the risk of infection. When followed closely, a woman's hematocrit may actually rise due to diuresis following delivery and autotransfusion occurring as the uterus involutes. After 1 week, the uterus is firm and nontender and extends to about midway between the symphysis and the umbilicus. By 2 weeks postpartum, the uterus should no longer be palpable abdominally. The contractions of the involuting uterus may be painful, especially during the first few days following delivery. This discomfort usually is readily relieved with acetaminophen or ibuprofen.

Prior to discharge, women should receive instructions regarding what they can expect during the puerperium and recommendations for activity. In general, women should be encouraged to rest and gradually increase their activity following delivery. They do not need to be restricted in terms of ambulation but potentially should be cautioned against driving in the early postpartum period due to distraction by discomfort and delay in reaction in case of an emergency. Women can resume a regular diet, with encouragement to push fluids due to increased requirements while nursing. As the perineum heals and any swelling decreases, women should note decreasing perineal discomfort. Any exacerbation in pain should prompt seeking evaluation for possible infection or hematoma formation. A return of normal bladder function should be noted, but women should be cautioned that they may experience some difficulty with stress and urge incontinence, which can be expected to gradually improve in the months following delivery.

Parents should receive information regarding lochia, expected volume, changes, and duration; activities; care of the breasts, perineum, and bladder; and dietary and, specifically, fluid requirements. The specific signs of complications should be stressed, including fever, chills, leg pain or swelling, episiotomy pain or drainage, and abnormal duration or volume of bleeding.

Couples should be advised that they can safely resume coitus when desired and comfortable, usually abstaining for at least 2 weeks following the birth. They should be forewarned of potential discomfort of the perineum and problems with vaginal dryness due to atrophic vaginitis, as well as changes in libido related to pregnancy and delivery.

Couples' options regarding contraception should be reviewed. While barrier methods of contraception are often utilized during nursing, hormonal methods can safely be used by the breast- or bottle-feeding mother. The progesterone-only pill, or minipill, is appropriate and effective for breast-feeding mothers and can be started about 2 weeks postpartum. Women who are not nursing and desire a combination oral contraceptive can safely be started on one 1 to 2 weeks following delivery. Long-acting progestin contraception such as medroxyprogesterone acetate (Depo-Provera) injections or levonorgestrel implants (Norplant System) can be started or placed anytime following delivery. Many wait until 6 to 8 weeks following delivery to begin these methods of contraception to avoid confusion of normal lochia following birth with abnormal bleeding while using these methods of contraception. A diaphragm should be fitted only after complete involution of the uterus at 6 to 8 weeks postpartum. In the meantime, condoms and spermicidal foam or jelly should be used. Intrauterine devices can be placed immediately following delivery of the placenta; however, due to increased rates of expulsion and increased risk for uterine perforation, waiting until 8 weeks postpartum for placement is most often recommend.

In nonlactating women, ovulation usually occurs about 6 weeks postpartum. The first menses following delivery is often an anovulatory cycle; however, conception has been reported as early as 2 weeks postpartum, so contraception must be advised even in the early postpartum period. While women who exclusively breast-feed their babies usually do not ovulate for at least 3 months following delivery, an occasional nursing mother will ovulate early, and thus use contraception should be advised. Women who receive rubella immunization, which is a live vaccine, are advised to delay pregnancy for at least 3 months. Women should be cautioned about postpartum depression. Instructions from the pediatrician regarding care of the neonate should be reinforced, as well as encouraging follow-up should any problems occur.

At the visit 4 to 6 weeks postpartum, inquiries should be made regarding breast-feeding, continued bleeding, resumption of sexual intercourse, use of appropriate contraception, and any difficulty with regard to voiding or bowel movements. Physical examination should include weight, blood pressure, breast examination, and abdominal examination, as well as a thorough pelvic examination. The perineum should be inspected for adequate healing of any episiotomy or laceration. The uterus should be completely involuted, and a Papanicolaou smear obtained as appropriate. Women should be counseled regarding emotional lability in the postpartum period and and reassured that intervention is available should she experience clinically significant depression.

◊ COMPLICATIONS OF THE PUERPERIUM

Puerperal Infection

Fever is the most commonly observed sign of puerperal infection. Whenever a woman's temperature rises above 38°C (100.4°F) in the first 24 hours postpartum, she must be evaluated for endometritis. The differential diagnosis includes infections of the perineum, vagina, uterus, parametrium, bladder, kidneys, or breast. Noninfectious causes of fever, such as dehydration, femoral thrombophlebitis, or thyroid storm, must also be considered. Women suffering with puerperal infection frequently complain of chills, headache, malaise, and anorexia. Physical examination reveals pallor and tachycardia, and the uterus is soft, large, and tender. Lochia may be diminished if the cervix is blocked, or it may be profuse and malodorous. Parametrial involvement, peritonitis, and pelvic thrombophlebitis may complicate the illness. Endotoxic shock or a virulent puerperal sepsis may develop in a relatively short time and can be fatal. Prompt and aggressive management with broad-spectrum antibiotics—and potentially surgery—is mandatory.

Endometritis commonly follows chorioamnionitis during labor. Various maternal conditions increase the risk, including anemia, preeclampsia, prolonged rupture of the membranes, prolonged labor, traumatic delivery, repeated examination, retention of placental fragments within the uterus, and postpartum hemorrhage. Puerperal infections can be caused by normal vaginal flora or bowel contaminants, typically *Escherichia coli*, β-hemolytic streptococci, *Streptococcus faecalis,* and anaerobic organisms such as *Clostridium perfrin-*

gens. Most infections involve mixed flora, but progression to an anaerobic infection is a particular risk following cesarean delivery. Prevention of puerperal infections should be an ongoing goal of all labor and delivery units, and working to decrease the number of digital examinations in labor, preventing postpartum hemorrhage, and preventing retained placental fragments or membranes by careful placental examination contribute to that goal.

Postpartum Hemorrhage

Postpartum hemorrhage has been defined as a blood loss of greater than 500 ml during or after the third stage of labor. This definition is somewhat burdensome, as careful measures of blood loss following delivery reveals that the average approximates 500 ml. After infection, postpartum hemorrhage is the major cause of maternal mortality. The causes include uterine atony (resulting from overdistention, prolonged labor, grand multiparity, or uterine relaxants), unrecognized lacerations, retained products of conception, or hypofibrinogenemia. Most serious hemorrhages occur within the first 24 hours but can occur weeks after delivery.

Once again, treatment begins with prevention. Antepartum correction of anemia, recognition and anticipation of uterine atony, and knowledge of a history of puerperal hemorrhage are helpful. In these particularly high-risk women, active management of the third stage of labor is appropriate. After placental separation, oxytocin, 10 U intramuscularly, or dilute oxytocin drip, 10 U per 1 liter, generally ensures uterine contraction and reduces the inevitable blood loss. The placenta must be examined thoroughly for completeness. If it is incomplete, the uterus must be explored manually, and missing fragments recovered. If the placenta does not separate spontaneously within 30 minutes after delivery, manual removal is advised. Rarely, curettage is required to remove placental fragments and decidua.

If hemorrhage occurs, bimanual uterine massage and intravenous oxytocin drip are required. If bleeding persists, the uterus, cervix, and vagina should be explored for lacerations or retained secundines. The cervix and the vagina are also examined. Intramuscular injection of methylergonovine maleate or prostaglandin $F_{2\alpha}$ can aid in stimulating contraction of the atonic uterus. Preparation should be made to replace blood and blood products as necessary to prevent the development of a consumptive coagulopathy. If contractions cannot be stimulated in a refractory atonic uterus, hypogastric artery ligation or hysterectomy may be required. If bleeding from a vaginal wall laceration is persistent, packing, angiography, and selective embolization may be helpful.

Depression

Many mothers feel an emotional letdown during the first few days after delivery. In its mild form, the "baby blues" is characterized by bouts of sadness or crying. Mild degrees of depression are quite common and usually short-lived. More extreme postpartum depression can last for weeks to months and is characterized by insomnia, pessimism, lethargy, feelings of inadequacy, inability to cope, and fatigue. In patients with these symptoms, it is important to rule out postpartum hypothyroidism. If this depression is profound and lasts longer than 72 hours or is associated with lack of interest in the infant, suicidal or homicidal thoughts, hallucinations, or psychotic behavior, it is pathologic and requires consultation with a psychiatrist. True puerperal psychosis is usually the emergence of preexisting mental illness in response to the physical and psychic stress of pregnancy and delivery, and psychotherapy is required.

While a number of situational factors contribute to this emotional letdown (e.g., lack of sleep, emotional stress, parental anxiety), it is clear that hormonal factors also contribute. The endorphins produced during labor quickly decrease after delivery. Similarly, the extraordinarily high levels of estrogens and progesterone abruptly decline following delivery of the placenta. The majority of women who suffer with postpartum depression do not require a psychiatric consultation but rather can be managed by their obstetrician utilizing monotherapy or a combination of a short course of an antidepressant, psychologic support and help, and parenting education.

Breast-feeding

While numerous problems and frustrations can occur during nursing, the greatest challenge to those caring for women and their newborns is to provide the support and assistance necessary to allow women to begin and maintain successful breast-feeding. Beginning with prenatal education regarding the benefits of nursing, including optimal nutrition, decreased neonatal infections, and decreased food allergies, support for breast-feeding must continue in the labor and delivery room, in the recovery room following cesarean section, and on the postpartum floor and nursery. Since most women are discharged before their milk comes in, most questions and problems with breast-feeding must be handled as an outpatient. Therefore, to achieve successful, sustained breast-feeding among their patients, physicians' office staff must have the ability to field questions and promptly correct problems with nursing.

In response to the hormonal stimulation early in pregnancy, the breast undergoes growth and development of the terminal portion of the duct system, with an increase in the number of alveoli and infiltration of the interstitial tissue with lymphocytes, plasma cells, and eosinophils. During this time, there is a significant decrease in the supporting stroma, adipose, and connective tissue. The breasts are ectodermal glands that develop from the milk lines, and residual mammary tissue may be present anywhere along these lines. This mammary tissue may become engorged with milk when lactation begins, and it is necessary to reassure women that the mass on their abdomen or mons is not pathologic and will

resorb. The glands are merocrine glands, similar to other protein-secreting glands in the body. The fatty component of milk arises as lipid droplets that project into the lumen of the gland and are dropped off, covered by a thin layer of cytoplasm and cell membrane.

The hormonal control of milk production is rather involved. Declining progesterone levels appear to be the initial stimulus for milk production. However, interestingly, progesterone does not have a significant inhibitory effect on established lactation. Prolactin is necessary for normal milk production. However, mammary development and milk secretion have been reported in women with low levels of prolactin. Historically, bromocriptine given for 2 to 3 weeks postpartum would inhibit prolactin secretion and effectively inhibit lactation. Due to concerns regarding central nervous system side effects and the incidence of rebound lactation upon discontinuing bromocriptine, it is no longer approved for this use. Estrogen enhances the effect of prolactin on breast development but antagonizes prolactin by inhibiting secretion of milk. Thus, even low-dose estrogen-containing birth control pills given in the early postpartum period have been shown to decrease milk supply, whereas no effect on volume or composition has been associated with progestin-only pills. Suckling triggers secretion of oxytocin and prolactin. There is a dramatic increased sensitivity of the breast to stimulation within 24 hours postpartum, which continues for several days. In women who must inhibit lactation, decrease in stimulation by binding the breast is the key to success. No increase in prolactin secretion occurs until sucking actually begins. Once lactation is established, oxytocin levels can increase in response to hearing a baby cry or seeing a picture of one's newborn, which can cause let-down to occur at unexpected times. Oxytocin stimulates contraction of the myoepithelial cells providing milk for the current meal. Prolactin stimulates the synthesis and secretion of milk into the alveolar spaces, preparing for the next meal. Prolactin levels do not correlate well with milk volume, and late in lactation prolactin levels are low despite plenty of milk.

Breast-fed babies drink more than 500 ml of milk per day. Mothers who exclusively breast-feed twins or triplets can produce 2 to 3 liters per day. While lactation is being established, the frequency of nursing is related to milk volume, but once lactation is established, there is little, if any, relationship between nursing frequency and infant milk intake. Thus, two babies may be very different in terms of how often they nurse, but they take in similar total amounts of milk. Maternal age, parity, exercise, and nutrition (except in the extreme) have little, if any, influence on milk volume. Infants respond to solid food by reducing breast milk intake, and many mothers report that their babies drop feedings when they start on solid food. Smoking and high levels of alcohol intake have an adverse effect on milk volume. The concentration of the individual constituents of mature human milk have been shown to vary considerably. The greatest variations have been observed from woman to woman; however, composition changes from the beginning of a feeding to the end, from day to day, and with the onset and progression of lactation.

Colostrum is the fluid secreted by the breast immediately following childbirth. The intense yellow color of colostrum is indicative of the high concentration of carotenoids, about 10-fold higher than that of mature milk. Over the 4- to 7-day period of colostrum production, the concentrations of fat and lactose increase, while those of protein and minerals decrease.

There are substantial differences between the milk of mothers who deliver preterm and those who deliver at term. Preterm milk has higher protein, sodium, and chloride concentrations and lower lactose concentrations than milk secreted by mothers of full-term infants. Mineral concentrations also vary. There is some evidence that extremely premature infants have demands for calcium and phosphorus that exceed those available in preterm breast milk, and it appears that a combination of breast milk and low-birthweight formulas may be optimal for growth and development in these babies.

Maternal nutrition is primarily important for the mother's health. As in pregnancy, the baby will get what it needs in the breast milk at the expense of the mother. Women are able to produce milk with adequate content of protein, fat, carbohydrate, and most minerals, even when their supply of nutrients is limited. The nutrients in human milk most likely to be present in lower than normal concentrations in response to chronically low maternal intake are the vitamins, especially vitamins B_6, B_{12}, A, and D. Nutrients maintained at the expense of maternal stores or tissues include the macronutrients, most minerals, and folate. The kinds of fatty acids present in human milk are strongly influenced by maternal diet. However, maternal total fat and cholesterol intake have no apparent influence on the total fat and cholesterol contents of human milk. Fluid requirements obviously increase during nursing, but forced increased fluids will not increase milk supply. Other than encouraging breast-feeding women to follow a well balanced, varied diet, there are no specific dietary restrictions. Women who are strict vegetarians and those who do not eat dairy products may benefit from dietary supplements. Some babies appear to dislike certain foods in their mother's diets, and it appears that rarely food allergens, especially from cow's milk, may account for some cases of colic and gastrointestinal problems in breast-fed infants.

Human milk is ordinarily a complete source of nutrients for the exclusively breast-fed infant for the first 6 months of life. Breast- and bottle-fed babies grow similarly for the first 2 to 3 months; however, the rate of weight gain of breast-fed infants is less rapid over the subsequent 9 months. This appears related to differences in caloric intake. The only supplementation that may be indicated for the breast-fed baby is vitamin D, if exposure to sunlight is limited or if the mother's intake is low, and B_{12}, if the mother is a complete vegetarian and her B_{12} intake is low. Low-income women, black women, and adolescents characteristically have diets low in iron, calcium, magnesium, and vitamin A. It is reasonable to recommend a multivitamin with iron supplementation to all nursing women. Exclusively breast-fed infants ordinarily maintain a normal

iron status for their first 6 months of life, regardless of maternal iron intake, and providing solid foods may reduce the percentage of iron absorbed by the partially breast-fed infant, making it important in such cases to ensure that adequate iron is provided in the diet. In areas of the country where the water supply is not fluoridated, supplemental fluoride is recommended to strengthen developing teeth.

Surprisingly, few infections are transmitted through human milk. Cytomegalovirus is common in milk produced by seropositive women, and as many as 70% of seropositive lactating women have the virus in their milk at some time. Although infants become infected by ingesting the virus, the colonization does not progress to disease, possibly because of specific IgG antibodies transferred via the placenta during pregnancy and immune substances provided in the mother's milk. Both the wild and vaccine strains of rubella virus have been recovered from human milk. As a consequence of this transmission, mild clinical rubella has been reported, but severe disease has not. Women who live in regions endemic for hepatitis B virus (HBV) commonly have the surface antigens in their milk, but there is no evidence that breast-feeding is a route of HBV transmission and infection. As newborns can now be actively and passively immunized against HBV, it is not a contraindication for breast-feeding. However, until a vaccine for hepatitis C virus is developed, hepatitis C infection is a contraindication to nursing. Because of the documentation of transmission of HIV through breast milk, the Centers for Disease Control and Prevention recommends that mothers seropositive for HIV-1 not breast-feed. Caffeine, alcohol, drugs, and environmental contaminants can be passed through the breast milk. Maternal consumption of two to three caffeinated beverages per day is not associated with unacceptable levels of caffeine. Concerns about cigarette smoking are primarily related to the long-term health of women; however, smoking has been related to decreased milk volume. Exposure of infants to nicotine is much more significant through the respiratory tract than through breast milk. Women should be encouraged to stop smoking and those who cannot should be encouraged to avoid smoking around their baby, but they should not be discouraged from nursing. Women with known heavy exposures to the pesticide DDT, polychlorinated biphenyls, and heavy metals can be offered testing to determine their blood levels and make recommendations regarding nursing. Interestingly, concentrations of heavy metals are higher in certain water supplies, cow's milk, and reconstituted formula than in human milk. Exposure of infants to radionuclides has been shown to be significantly higher among formula-fed babies.

While breast-feeding is not completely protective, food allergies appear to be less frequent in infants who are exclusively breast-fed. In infants with a family history of atopic disease, breast-feeding delays the onset of disease, and that delay may be enough to reduce disease severity. We do not know how breast milk and breast-feeding provide protection to babies. It is known that secretory antibody and other immunologic factors are important. It also appears that the infant's respiratory defenses are stimulated by the soluble immune factors. In addition,there may be behavioral and physiologic effects that have a significant impact.

Breast-feeding has several significant effects on the mother. Nursing suppresses the pulsatile release of gonadotropin-releasing hormone from the hypothalamus and stimulates the release of prolactin, which affects the release of luteinizing hormone from the pituitary, causing suppression of ovulation. The frequency of the suckling rather than the total duration of suckling appears to be related to the suppression of ovulation. Mothers whose baby early on sleeps through the night can expect to have an earlier return of ovulation and thus menstruation. Nursing women have a greater delay in resumption of intercourse, compared to those who bottle-feed. In some women, this is clearly attributable to discomfort due to relative vaginal atrophy and decreased lubrication from low estrogen levels. It is reasonable to encourage the use of lubrication during intercourse. If that does not provide relief for women with a well established milk supply, a vagina estrogen cream is very effective. Decreased sexual interest may also be related to low androgen levels. Maternal stress and fatigue can certainly play a part in decreased libido at any time.

Producing breast milk requires approximately 1000 kcal of energy per day. Virtually all women have stored extra fat during pregnancy in anticipation of lactation. Lactating women eating self-selected diets typically lose 1 to 2 lb (0.45 to 0.91 kg) of weight per month in the first 4 to 6 months of nursing. However, roughly 20% of lactating women maintain or gain weight.

Studies that have followed women from before conception until 4 months after they stop nursing have found a loss of bone mineralization with pregnancy and lactation and a recovery of losses in the postlactation period. Perhaps more important, no relationship has been found between reproductive history and the occurrence of hip and forearm fractures in postmenopausal women. In fact, bone mass studies in menopausal women have found higher bone mass associated with a history of pregnancy and breast-feeding.

Not working or working part-time is associated with longer breast-feeding. However, working is rarely the reason given by women for not breast-feeding. The barriers to breast-feeding while working include lack of flex-time or part-time work, inadequate maternity leave and job security, lack of on-site day care, and lack of an appropriate place to pump or breast-feed. Often, the biggest problem facing a mother trying to work and breast-feed is the people around her who do not understand why she bothers.

In the hospital, the goal should be let the mother and baby find the positions most comfortable for them. The key is establishing a sense of confidence in the mother and supporting her with simple answers to questions when they arise. The important part of early breast-feeding is to put the baby to the breast frequently for short periods of time to stimulate milk production.

Nursing Problems

Evaluating problems with nursing requires observing the mother and baby nursing, which the office setting is not always conducive to—and thus the advantage of lay assistance and lactation specialists. Adequate rest is important, and encouragement to rest should accompany almost all calls about problems with nursing.

Concerns about Insufficient Milk Supply

Encouragement to rest applies especially to concerns about insufficient milk supply, the most common reason women give for weaning. In the mother who wants to nurse, this is when encouragement is most important. She needs to have confidence that a decrease in her milk supply is temporary and can be quickly built back up. She will simply need to rest and keep herself hydrated and well nourished.

Sometimes, problems with milk supply relate to problems with let-down. Normally, within 1 minute of suckling, the first myoepithelial contraction occurs, associated with a pins-and-needles sensation within the breast as let-down occurs. Let-down can be inhibited by cold, pain, and emotional stress and can be elicited by auditory and visual stimuli. The let-down reflex can be difficult to achieve using a breast pump. A quiet, private setting and pictures of the baby to look at may help. Therapy for those having trouble with let-down should first be directed to the above factors. Oxytocin in nasal-spray form has also been used for therapy. The spray contains 40 USP units (IU) per milliliter, and one uses one spray into one or both nostrils 2 to 3 minutes prior to nursing or pumping.

Often, concerns about milk supply are actually frustrations about frequency of feeding. Babies empty their stomachs about every 90 minutes. When the composition of human milk was compared to that of other animals, it most closely resembled the milk of animals that nurse their young almost constantly. In those societies where newborns are held or carried continuously, the babies nurse for short bursts several times an hour. For the mother having trouble with frequent feedings, asking her to keep a record of feeding times can be extremely helpful: Often a schedule emerges, or she finds that her infant is sleeping longer than she thought.

Engorgement

Engorgement is a common problem, especially for the woman who is breast-feeding for the first time. It involves congestion and increased vascularity, as well as accumulation of milk. Some engorgement is normal. When the woman finds areolar engorgement and flattening the nipple, it is best to express some of the milk manually, so that the areola and nipple soften enough for the baby to grasp. For engorgement of the body of the breast, it is helpful to support the breast with a nursing bra, massage the breast, use cold packs to decrease vascularity, and express some milk while showering. It is common for women with engorgement to feel achy and run a low-grade fever, for which acetaminophen will help. The cornerstone of therapy is frequent nursing.

Painful Nipples

Painful nipples are usually caused by problems with positioning and latching on. For some women, comfort will be gained by leaving their nipples exposed and using either a lamp or hair dryer to dry their nipples after feedings. In general, nipple shields should be avoided, as they decrease the volume of milk that the baby receives; however, for short periods, they may help healing of a painful nipple and allow some women who were ready to give up on nursing to get through a rough time.

Mastitis

Mastitis usually occurs after breast-feeding is fully established in the weeks to months after delivery. Women report fever, flu-like symptoms, and unilateral pain and erythema usually limited to one quadrant of the breast. An antibiotic that covers staphylococcal infections usually is curative. Neglected or recurrent infections and infections with resistant organisms can lead to a breast abscess. Treatment of an abscess usually involves intravenous antibiotics and surgical drainage.

Jaundice

Jaundice is more common in breast-fed babies. Bilirubin levels are related to passage of stool, and bottle-fed babies excrete more stool and more bilirubin in the first 3 days than breast-fed infants. Supplementation with water or dextrose solution does not help. When early jaundice, which peaks on about day 3, is diagnosed, more frequent nursing may be helpful, with supplementation only as necessary. The syndrome of breast milk jaundice becomes apparent, and the bilirubin continues to rise past day 3, peaking at around the 7th day. There is no correlation with weight loss or gain, and stools are normal.

This syndrome has been attributed to a substance in the milk of some mothers that inhibits the hepatic enzyme glucuronyltransferase, preventing the conjugation of bilirubin. Seventy percent of previous children of a given mother whose infant has breast milk jaundice have had jaundice. For the diagnosis of breast milk jaundice, a bilirubin reading is obtained 2 hours after a breast-feeding, and then breast-feeding is discontinued for at least 12 hours, when formula is used. The bilirubin level is then measured again; a drop of more than 2 mg/100 ml is diagnostic.

Treatment of breast milk jaundice involves discontinuing breast-feeding for a time until the bilirubin level drops below 15 mg/100 ml. Usually, breast-feeding can be resumed, with periodic follow-up for 10 to 14 days to be sure the fall continues. Rarely, breast milk jaundice persists, requiring one or two feedings per day of formula to dilute the effect of the breast milk and very rarely requiring discontinuation of breast-feeding.

Special Problems and Concerns

Some mothers and infants have special problems and concerns. Feeding infants with oral defects is obviously a challenge but can be done if the mother has the desire and the patience. Mothers of babies with physical and/or neurologic problems often want to provide breast milk, even when the prognosis is guarded. Likewise, women in such situations may need permission to wean a baby if the task of care and pumping is overwhelming. Breast augmentation does not cause an interruption of ducts or nerve or blood supply, and breast-feeding is both possible and successful. Concerns about changes in contour of the breast are real, but the changes in the breasts related to the pregnancy will be more significant than those caused by nursing. Women who have had reduction mammoplasty may have difficulty, as sometimes the procedure used interrupts the ducts and/or the nerve supply, especially when repositioning of the nipple is necessary. Often, contacting the plastic surgeon can provide guidance, and binding the breasts is appropriate for those advised against breast-feeding.

SUMMARY POINTS

◊ Labor is the effacement and dilation of the cervix produced by uterine contractions.

◊ Critical to the management of labor is the correct diagnosis upon admission of where a woman is in the course of labor.

◊ Understanding the normal variation in labor will allow one to offer appropriate intervention to those women needing assistance.

◊ Decreasing the complications of puerperal infection and postpartum hemorrhage are the ongoing goals of a low-risk labor and delivery unit.

◊ Encouraging and providing support for breast-feeding has significant benefits for both infants and mothers.

◊ RECOMMENDED READINGS

Allman AC, Genevier ES, Johnson MR, Steer PJ. Head-to-cervix force: an important physiological variable in labour. 1. The temporal relation between head-to-cervix force and intrauterine pressure during labour. *Br J Obstet Gynaecol* 1996;103:763–768.

Brisson CG, Fraser W, Breart G, Krauss I, Thornton J. The effect of routine early amniotomy on spontaneous labor: a meta-analysis. *Obstet Gynecol* 1996;87:891–896.

Carbonne B, Benachi A, Leveque ML, Cabrol D, Papiernik E. Maternal position during labor: effects on fetal oxygen saturation measured by pulse oximetry. *Obstet Gynecol* 1996;88:797–800.

Ely JW, Howser DM, Dawson JD, Bowdler NC, Rijhsinghani A. Practice patterns during the third stage of labor: the effect of physician age and specialty. *J Fam Pract* 1996;43:545–549.

Fleissig A. Are women given enough information by staff during labour and delivery? *Midwifery* 1993;9:70–75.

Fraser WD, Marcoux S, Moutquin JM, Christen A. Effect of early amniotomy on the risk of dystocia in nulliparous women. The Canadian Early Amniotomy Study Group. *N Engl J Med* 1993;328:1145–1149.

Frigoletto FJ, Lieberman E, Lang JM, et al. A clinical trial of active management of labor. *N Engl J Med* 1995;333:745–750.

Fuentes A, Williams M. Cervical assessment. *Clin Obstet Gynecol* 1995;38:224–231.

Garite TJ, Porto M, Carlson NJ, Rumney PJ, Reimbold PA. The influence of elective amniotomy on fetal heart rate patterns and the course of labor in term patients: a randomized study. *Am J Obstet Gynecol* 1993;168: 1827–1831.

Goffinet F, Fraser W, Marcoux S, Breart G, Moutquin JM, Daris M. Early amniotomy increases the frequency of fetal heart rate abnormalities: Amniotomy Study Group. *Br J Obstet Gynaecol* 1997;104:548–553.

Halldorsdottir S, Karlsdottir SI. Empowerment or discouragement: women's experience of caring and uncaring encounters during childbirth. *Health Care Women Int* 1996;17:361–379.

Husslein P, Leitich H. Some aspects on the mechanism of human labor and delivery. *Eur J Obstet Gynecol Reprod Biol* 1995;59:S3–S7.

Juntunen K, Kirkinen P. Partogram of a grand multipara: different descent slope compared with an ordinary parturient. *J Perinat Med* 1994; 22:213–218.

Kruse J. The physiology of labor and management of prolonged labor. *Prim Care* 1993;20:685–704.

Lawrence R. *Breastfeeding: a guide for the medical profession.* St. Louis, MO: Mosby–Year Book, 1994.

Leppert PC. Anatomy and physiology of cervical ripening. *Clin Obstet Gynecol* 1995;38:267–279.

Maggi M, Baldi E, Susini T. Hormonal and local regulation of uterine activity during parturition: part I—the oxytocin system. *J Endocrinol Invest* 1994;17:739–756.

Maggi M, Baldi E, Susini T. Hormonal and local regulation of uterine activity during parturition: part II—the prostaglandin and adrenergic systems. *J Endocrinol Invest* 1994;17:757–770.

Malone FD, Geary M, Chelmow D, Stronge J, Boylan P, D'Alton ME. Prolonged labor in nulliparas: lessons from the active management of labor. *Obstet Gynecol* 1996;88:211–215.

Myers DA, Nathanielsz PW. Biologic basis of term and preterm labor. *Clin Perinatol* 1993;20:9–28.

O'Driscoll K. Active management of labour: true purpose has been misunderstood. *BMJ* 1994;309:1015.

Peaceman AM, Socol ML. Active management of labor. *Am J Obstet Gynecol* 1996;175:363–368.

Romero R, Baumann P, Gomez R, et al. The relationship between spontaneous rupture of membranes, labor, and microbial invasion of the amniotic cavity and amniotic fluid concentrations of prostaglandins and thromboxane B_2 in term pregnancy. *Am J Obstet Gynecol* 1993;168: 1654–1664.

Slade P, MacPherson SA, Hume A, Maresh M. Expectations, experiences and satisfaction with labour. *Br J Clin Psychol* 1993;32:469–483.

Steinborn A, Gunes H, Halberstadt E. Signal for term parturition is of trophoblast and therefore of fetal origin. *Prostaglandins* 1995;50: 237–252.

CHAPTER 8

Obstetric Analgesia and Anesthesia

◇

John I. Fishburne, Jr.

The purpose of this chapter is to acquaint the obstetrician with the various techniques of obstetric analgesia and anesthesia and to describe their indications, advantages, disadvantages, and complications. The technical aspects, including the methods of administration, will not be described in detail, as these are usually beyond the purview of the obstetrician-gynecologist. Readers seeking specific information on how to perform the various obstetric anesthetic techniques are referred to the recommended readings list at the end of this chapter (see Hawkins, 1998).

Obstetric analgesia or anesthesia refers to the multiple techniques useful for the alleviation of the pain associated with labor or delivery. The anesthetic chosen must be appropriate for the mother and her fetus because the drugs used to provide maternal analgesia or anesthesia usually cross the placenta and may adversely affect the fetus. The choice of an appropriate analgesic technique must be made by the patient, the obstetrician, and the anesthesiologist and should take into consideration her anatomy and physiology, the status of her fetus, and the pharmacology of the drugs to be employed.

◇ PAIN OF PARTURITION

Studies of animals and humans have documented that the pain that occurs during labor and delivery is caused by increasing dilation of the cervix, contraction and distention of the uterus, and distention or rupture of the vagina, vulva, and perineum. Pain may be generated through stretching or application of pressure to adjacent pelvic organs.

The pain that occurs in the first stage of labor increases in severity as the cervix becomes more dilated. The onset of pain lags approximately 15 to 30 seconds behind the onset of the uterine contraction and is first perceived when the intraamniotic pressure reaches 15 mm Hg above that of resting tonus. In the second stage of labor, sharp pain occurs as the tissues of the vagina and perineum are stretched. Stretching stimulates the second, third, and fourth sacral nerve roots, which carry nociceptive information to the spinal cord through the sensory fibers of the pudendal nerve.

Adnexal pressure and traction on the bladder, urethra, rectum, and peritoneum also contribute to the pain of parturition. Compression of the lumbosacral plexus by the fetal head, particularly in the occiput posterior position, may cause pain even before the onset of labor.

The pain of uterine contractions is conducted through small sensory nerve fibers of the paracervical and inferior hypogastric plexuses to join the sympathetic nerve chain at L2-3. The ascending fibers enter the spinal cord through the nerve roots of T-10 to T-12, with a variable contribution from L-1 (Fig. 1). Because the cutaneous branches of the lower thoracic and upper lumbar nerves migrate caudally for a considerable distance before they innervate the skin, the pain of uterine contractions is often referred to the area over the upper sacrum and the lower lumbar spine.

Pain from the uterus and cervix is transmitted through the small-diameter myelinated delta A fibers and unmyelinated C fibers. These fibers enter the spinal cord by the dorsal nerve roots and converge in Lissauer's tract, ascending or descending for several segments before turning medially to innervate laminae I, II, or V of the dorsal horn (Fig. 2). Because there are relatively fewer nociceptive afferent nerves from visceral structures than from somatic structures, visceral pain is perceived as being diffuse and difficult to localize. These visceral afferents also synapse on and excite the same dorsal horn neurons as afferents from somatic structures. This arrangement is responsible for the phenomenon of referred pain.

Several ascending pathways transmit painful stimuli from the dorsal horn neurons to the higher centers of the brain, including the lateral spinothalamic tract, the spinomesencephalic tract, and the spinoreticular tract. Neurons in the central regions project to other supraspinal structures, such as the somatosensory cortex, to complete the sequence needed for the interpretation of pain.

The afferent transmission of nociceptive information from the periphery and the spinal cord to supraspinal structures is modulated by inputs originating from a variety of nuclei, including those in the periaqueductal gray matter and rostral

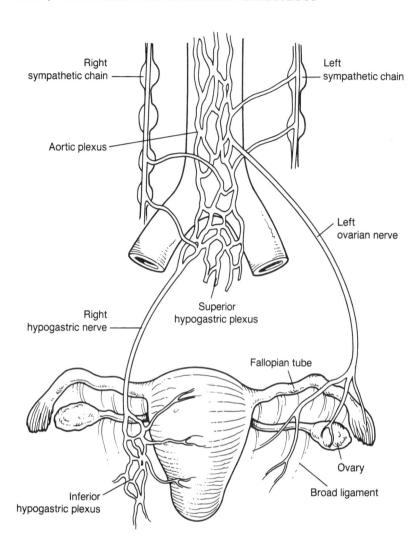

FIG. 1. Sympathetic nerve supply of the uterus from the pelvic and abdominal distribution. The uterine nerves arise from the upper part of the uterus (i.e., upper uterine segment), the contraction of which contributes to pain; from the lower part of the uterus (i.e., lower uterine segment), the distention of which contributes to pain; and from the cervix, the dilatation of which contributes to pain. The ovarian nerve supplies the ovary, fallopian tube, broad ligament, round ligament, and the side of the uterus, and it communicates with the uterine plexus. The sympathetic efferent and afferent fibers are shown together. (Adapted from Abouleish E. *Pain control in obstetrics.* Philadelphia: JB Lippincott Co, 1977.)

medulla. Stimulation of these nuclei inhibits afferent transmission of pain impulses in the spinal cord.

The gate theory of Melzack and Wall holds that stimulation of the large cutaneous beta A nerve fibers closes a gate in the substantia gelatinosa of the spinal cord, preventing pain impulses from being carried rostrally by the delta A and C nerve fibers. This theory forms the basis for the use of acupuncture, transcutaneous electrical nerve stimulation, and intracutaneous nerve stimulation with sterile water papules for the relief of pain associated with parturition.

Pregnancy appears to reduce anesthetic requirements. It has been postulated that high progesterone levels lead to increased quantities of endogenous endorphins, which may increase the maternal threshold to pain. One study correlated pain intensity during labor and plasma levels of β-endorphin. The lowest endorphin levels were found after abolition of labor pain by epidural analgesia. The highest concentrations were observed in the first few minutes after delivery, immediately after cessation of the severe pain of expulsive labor.

The obstetrician must understand the mechanisms of pain activation and transmission, so that appropriate analgesia may be selected. The nature of the pain of labor varies in intensity with the stages of labor. The intensity of pain is related to physical factors such as the strength and duration of uterine contractions, the rapidity of cervical dilation, the degree of distention of the vaginal and perineal tissues, the requirement for operative delivery, and the size, presentation, and position of the infant. Augmentation of labor with oxytocin increases the strength of uterine contractions and increases the pain. The primiparous woman may perceive greater pain than the multipara who enters labor with more advanced cervical dilation. Exhaustion, psychologic factors, and protracted nausea and vomiting may also increase the parturient's perception of labor pain.

The obstetrician should appreciate the importance of providing pain relief during early labor through the use of systemic analgesics or regional block analgesia. As labor progresses, additional analgesia must be provided through perineal extension of a segmental epidural or through the use of paracervical, pudendal, or spinal blocks.

◊ SYSTEMIC ANALGESIA AND SEDATION

In the management of labor pain, systemic narcotics are usually considered to be the first step beyond the less invasive or

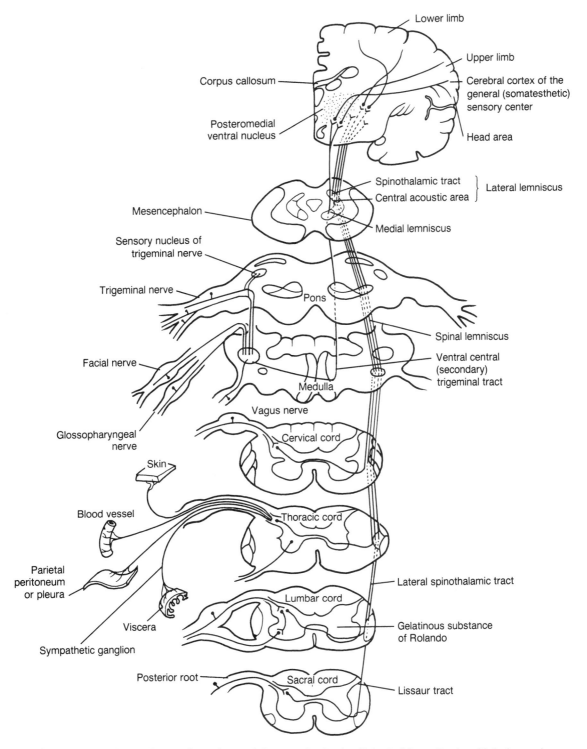

FIG. 2. Nociceptive pathways from the periphery to the brain. (Adapted from Bonica JJ. Labor pain: mechanisms and pathways. In: Marx GF, Bassel GM, eds: *Obstetric analgesia and anesthesia.* New York: Elsevier, 1980:173.)

"natural" methods. Although narcotics may be highly effective in relieving the pain of labor, their side effects prohibit the use of large doses. The physician must walk a tightrope between oversedation, with its attendant maternal and neonatal respiratory depression, and effective relief of the pain of labor. The most feared newborn side effect is respiratory depression. The maternal side effects, in addition to respiratory depression, include nausea, vomiting, hypotension, obtundation of protective reflexes, and decreased gastrointestinal motility.

Systemic Narcotics

Meperidine

Meperidine (Demerol) has achieved the widest popularity for systemic analgesia during labor. It is preferred over morphine because it produces less emesis and does not penetrate the immature fetal blood–brain barrier as easily as morphine. It can be administered intravenously or intramuscularly during labor. Current usage most often consists of small, incremental intravenous doses of 25 to 50 mg. Placental transfer of meperidine occurs rapidly, and typical cord–maternal concentration ratios of 0.75 to 1.63 are reported. Meperidine has been recovered from the fetus within 2 minutes of administration to the mother. The degree of newborn depression is related to the quantity of drug transferred to the fetus. Maximal depression of the infant occurs when delivery takes place 2 to 4 hours after maternal intravenous or intramuscular administration. Delivery of the infant within 1 hour of administration produces little evidence of newborn depression.

Meperidine has as its principal metabolite the compound normeperidine, which is slowly metabolized but is equipotent with meperidine in its ability to produce respiratory depression. Repeated intravenous administration of small doses of meperidine leads to increasing maternal and fetal levels of normeperidine. Meperidine has an elimination half-life in neonatal blood of 22.7 hours, and that of normeperidine is measured in days.

Morphine

Morphine is pharmacologically more potent than meperidine by a factor of approximately 10. Morphine is alleged to cross the immature fetal blood–brain barrier, producing newborn respiratory depression. Because of this reputation, morphine has virtually disappeared from the armamentarium of analgesic drugs used by the obstetrician for the management of labor.

Fentanyl

Fentanyl (Sublimaze) is a potent synthetic narcotic with analgesic activity approximately 100 times that of morphine. Its onset of action is rapid, and its duration of activity is short (i.e., 20 to 30 minutes) because of its rapid distribution from plasma. Only 5% of the injected dose remains in the plasma 5 minutes after intravenous injection. The terminal drug elimination half-life after a single small dose is 1 to 2 hours. Fentanyl is highly bound to protein, which may limit its placental transfer. It has no active metabolites. Fetal–maternal blood concentration ratios average 0.31 over the first 10 minutes after intravenous administration. Fentanyl produces moderate analgesia and mild sedation. The onset of analgesia is rapid, lasting for approximately 45 minutes. There is a brief period of decreased fetal heart rate (FHR) variability, which may persist for as long as 30 minutes, but no other disturbing FHR patterns have been reported. Compared with neonates exposed to no narcotics or to other analgesics, no differences have been found in the frequencies of low Apgar scores, depressed respirations, or abnormal neurologic and adaptive capabilities. Comparative studies with meperidine indicate that the need for newborn naloxone (Narcan) administration is greater after use of meperidine than after administration of fentanyl. Evidence suggests that the latter drug seems to be underused in the management of labor in the United States.

Nalbuphine

Nalbuphine (Nubain) is a potent narcotic agonist-antagonist agent that at equianalgesic doses produces respiratory depression equivalent to that of morphine. The advantage of nalbuphine is that a ceiling effect is seen for analgesia and respiratory depression as the dosage is increased. Maximal respiratory depression occurs with a dose of 30 mg in a 70-kg adult. Apnea is unlikely after administration of an excessively large dose. However, in the absence of overdosage, respiratory depression is equivalent to that of morphine. Nalbuphine has been compared with meperidine for use in active labor. Maternal cardiovascular parameters, pain intensity, progress of labor, and FHR recordings during labor have been related to side effects and neonatal outcome, but neither drug has shown a significant advantage over the other. However, a possible transient depressive effect of nalbuphine on the fetal central nervous system (CNS) has been identified.

Butorphanol

Butorphanol (Stadol) is another synthetic narcotic with agonist-antagonist properties. It is five times more potent than morphine and 40 times more potent than meperidine. It has achieved moderate popularity in the United States in the management of the pain of the first stage of labor. It is usually administered intravenously in doses of 1 to 2 mg. Butorphanol exhibits the same ceiling effect for analgesia and respiratory depression as nalbuphine. Studies comparing butorphanol to meperidine indicate significantly greater butorphanol-induced analgesia (i.e., 30 to 60 minutes after intravenous injection), with few drug-related maternal side effects other than sedation.

Newer Opioids

The newer synthetic opioids, sufentanil and alfentanil, have been used to augment epidural and spinal anesthesia and analgesia, but they have not been studied extensively for systemic analgesia during labor.

Patient-controlled Systemic Analgesia

Patient-controlled analgesia (PCA) is widely available and provides pain relief through self-administration of intravenous opioids. Morphine and meperidine are the analgesics most commonly employed with this technique. Unfortunately, the episodic and increasing nature of labor pain undermines the effectiveness of systemic PCA. In a study comparing patient-controlled with nurse-administered meperidine, Rayburn et al. (1989a) found pain relief to be equivalent. Maternal side effects occurred with equal frequency in both groups, but neonatal naloxone therapy was required more often when meperidine was administered by the patient than by the nurse. PCA with systemic opioids was not found to be advantageous over nursing administration of these drugs.

In a study by Rosenblatt et al. (1991), metoclopramide (Reglan) was used as an analgesic adjunct to PCA for patients undergoing prostaglandin induction of labor for second-trimester termination of pregnancy. Patients were given intravenous metoclopramide, 10 mg, or saline placebo followed by PCA-administered morphine. Those receiving metoclopramide used 54% less morphine and had lower pain scores.

Narcotic Antagonists

Naloxone

Because all narcotics cross the placenta and can produce respiratory depression in the neonate, availability of an effective antagonist is essential. Naloxone reverses opioid-induced respiratory depression without producing side effects of its own. Because it also reverses analgesia, its prophylactic use is not advised. Naloxone may be administered to the parturient as an intravenous bolus of 0.4 mg to treat maternal respiratory depression. Care must be taken to titrate naloxone to the desired effect, since large doses have been implicated in the causation of myocardial infarction and other cardiovascular problems. Naloxone, 0.01 mg/kg, may also be administered intravenously or intramuscularly to the newborn to reverse the respiratory depressant effects of placentally transferred narcotics. The effect is usually apparent within a few minutes and persists for as long as 2 hours. The neonate must be carefully observed for evidence of renarcotization, which may occur because the half-life of naloxone is less than that of most narcotics.

Naltrexone

Naltrexone (ReVia) is an oral opioid antagonist that is useful in treating pruritus, which can occur when epidural opioid is used for control of pain after cesarean section. Its use during labor has not been recommended.

Nonnarcotic Drugs

Benzodiazepines

The principal benzodiazepine drugs are diazepam (Valium) and midazolam (Versed). Diazepam has been used extensively in other parts of the world for seizure prophylaxis in patients with severe preeclampsia. However, because of its side effects on the newborn, it has found little favor in the United States. Newborns exposed to diazepam characteristi-

cally exhibit hypotonicity, hypoactivity, and impaired temperature regulation and metabolic response to cold stress.

Midazolam is a newer benzodiazepine anxiolytic, a sedative drug with significant amnestic properties. It is two to five times more potent than diazepam and is soluble in water, a property that reduces pain associated with intravenous administration. Midazolam crosses the sheep placenta, achieving a fetal–maternal concentration ratio of 0.15. Its metabolites are inactive, and the drug is excreted more rapidly than diazepam. Midazolam has been used as an induction agent for cesarean section, but because of its ability to cross the placenta, it has produced neonatal respiratory depression and decreased body tone and temperature. Midazolam has not been recommended for use as a tranquilizer-sedative in labor, although its amnestic properties may prove beneficial, if given in small doses.

Barbiturates

Barbiturates were once popular for sedation in the latent phase of labor. Although they cause maternal sedation and decreased anxiety, barbiturates lack analgesic properties and may increase the perception of pain when given without concomitant administration of a narcotic. Most barbiturates have long elimination half-lives and readily cross the placenta. Prolonged neonatal effects have been the cause of the virtual elimination of these drugs from the obstetrician's armamentarium.

Other Sedatives

Phenothiazine derivatives, such as promethazine (Phenergan), have been used in obstetrics to relieve anxiety and reduce the requirements for narcotics. Some drugs of this family, such as chlorpromazine (Thorazine), have weak α-adrenergic blocking activity and should be avoided if epidural or spinal analgesia is contemplated because they may potentiate hypotension.

Hydroxyzine, although not a phenothiazine, has similar properties when used in combination with narcotics. Maternal sedation is achieved without significant maternal or newborn side effects. Hydroxyzine is considered an effective tranquilizer that may potentiate the effects of narcotics.

Ketamine (Ketalar), when administered intermittently at low doses (10 to 15 mg), can produce analgesia in parturients without causing maternal loss of consciousness or neonatal respiratory depression. An improvement on this technique using low-dose ketamine infusion has been described by Maroof et al. (1998). In this study, patients were given an intravenous bolus of ketamine, 0.5 mg/kg, upon achieving 4 cm of cervical dilation. This was followed by an infusion of ketamine at 0.25 mg/kg per hour. The mean duration of labor was 3.2 ± 1.1 hours, and the mean dose of ketamine required was 87.2 ± 9.7 mg. Patients served as their own controls, evaluating labor with and without the benefit of ketamine. Pain scores were significantly better with ketamine. The authors concluded that ketamine infusion produced acceptable analgesia throughout labor and was not associated with delirium or loss of consciousness in any patient. In addition, neonatal respiratory depression was not noted.

Use of Systemic Medications

Because the use of systemic narcotics and tranquilizers does not require special training or the availability of anesthesia personnel, they are used extensively in this country to provide labor analgesia. These compounds do not induce FHR abnormalities other than changes in variability and rarely sinusoidal heart rate pattern, nor do they cause fetal acidosis. The drug-related adverse maternal effects of narcotics can include nausea, vomiting, sedation, decreased gastric motility, and respiratory depression. The neonatal effects of these agents include CNS depression, respiratory depression, impaired early breast-feeding, altered neuroadaptive behavior, and decreased ability to regulate body temperature. To minimize these side effects, the lowest effective dosage should be employed, and the timing with respect to delivery must be carefully considered.

Resuscitation equipment should be kept at hand, and naloxone, used to antagonize opioids, should be readily available. Benzodiazepine toxicity may be reversed with flumazenil (Romazicon), an antagonist drug recently made available for this purpose.

Before 1970, inhalational analgesia was commonly used for management of the first and second stages of labor. Agents employed for this purpose included trichloroethylene, methoxyflurane, and nitrous oxide. Trichloroethylene was administered by hand-held inhalers and provided adequate analgesia. Unfortunately, its toxic metabolites caused it to be abandoned. Methoxyflurane is highly lipid soluble and very slowly eliminated from fat reservoirs in the mother and newborn. High-output renal failure associated with overdosage contributed to the decline in its use.

Nitrous oxide can be inhaled periodically with contractions in a 50% mixture with oxygen. During a painful contraction, the mother breathes from a mask connected to the regulator valve of a breathing circuit. A scavenging system eliminates exhaled waste anesthetic gases. Unfortunately, nitrous oxide does not fully control the pain of uterine contractions, largely because of the latent period that follows its inhalation. When it is breathed at the onset of a contraction, maximal analgesia is achieved only after the contraction has ended. Proper timing of inhalation is essential to the provision of adequate pain relief using this technique. When nitrous oxide is used in conjunction with meperidine, maternal oxygen saturation may decrease. Use of a pulse oximeter to ensure adequate maternal oxygenation is recommended.

◊ REGIONAL ANALGESIA

Local Anesthetic Agents

Most local anesthetic agents share a common structure consisting of a hydrophilic amino group connected by an intermediate chain to a lipophilic aromatic residue. Their presumed mechanism of action is to block exchange of sodium and potassium ions across the cell membrane, probably through mechanical interruption of ion flow through cell wall channels.

Local anesthetic drugs are manufactured as chloride salts. In solution, they dissociate into cation amines and chloride anions. The amine moiety further dissociates into a nonionized base and a hydrogen ion. The hydrogen ion is taken up by tissue buffers, and the base diffuses to the nerve membranes, in which recombination with tissue hydrogen ions results in the reformation of the active cationic form that produces the nerve block.

Studies of sensory nerve action potentials after injection of lidocaine (Xylocaine) demonstrated that the sensory nerve action potential decreases more sharply in pregnant women than in nonpregnant women. This implies that pregnant women have an increased susceptibility to the effects of local anesthetic agents.

Local anesthetics belong principally to two groups, those of ester and amide configurations. Ester drugs are generally characterized by their rapid onset of action, short duration, and low toxicity. Chloroprocaine (Nesacaine) is a representative of this group and is commonly used for lumbar epidural analgesia. It is rapidly metabolized by serum pseudocholinesterase, forming paraaminobenzoic acid. Lidocaine, bupivacaine, and ropivacaine are representatives of the amide group. These drugs are more highly bound to protein and have a slower onset and a longer duration of action. They are metabolized in the liver. Toxicity is usually greater than for drugs of the ester group (Table 1).

Local anesthetic drugs distribute throughout the maternal tissues and into the fetus. Distribution to the fetus depends on maternal tissue uptake, maternal blood concentration, uterine blood flow, and maternal and fetal metabolism and excretion. Fetal-tissue drug distribution is also affected by asphyxia. Fetal asphyxia leads to increased P_aCO_2, which results in cerebral and coronary vessel dilation and increased brain and myocardial blood flow. The increased perfusion of these organs with anesthetic drug leads to greater toxicity. The decrease in pH seen with fetal asphyxia results in diminished protein binding and increased free drug concentrations in the fetal circulation and tissues, a phenomenon referred to as ion trapping.

Side Effects of Local Anesthetic Drugs

Systemic Toxicity

Major complications involving the use of local anesthetics include toxic blood levels of the drug and epinephrine, psychomotor, and allergic reactions, as well as reactions due to epinephrine that is often added to local anesthetic solutions to retard systemic absorption and prolong duration of action.

Maximal safe doses for healthy young adults are 7 mg/kg (300 mg) of lidocaine, 2 to 3 mg/kg (175 mg) of bupivacaine, and 20 mg/kg (800 to 1000 mg) of chloroprocaine (see Table 1). Absorption is accelerated with topical use on mucosal surfaces, and the maximal safe dose should be reduced to 40% of that used for local infiltration.

TABLE 1. *Characteristics, concentrations, and properties of local anesthetics*

	Chloroprocaine (Nesacaine)	Tetracaine (Pontocaine)	Lidocaine (Xylocaine)	Bupivacaine (Marcaine)
Characteristics				
Type	Ester	Ester	Amide	Amide
Potency	Moderate	High	Moderate	High
Duration	Short	Long	Intermediate	Long
Physiochemical properties				
Molecular weight	302	300	234	325
Plasma protein binding (%)	—	75	64	95
Concentrations				
Infiltration (%)	1–2	—	0.5–1	0.125
Field block (%)	1	—	0.50–1	0.125–0.25
Pudendal, paracervical (%)	1.5	—	1	0.25–0.50
Spinal (mg)	—	4–12	20–100	5–15
Epidural block	—	—	—	—
Labor (%)	1.5–2	—	1–1.5	0.25–0.5
Surgery (%)	3	—	2	0.50
Maximal initial dose (mg/kg)	20	1.5	7	2–3

(From Akamatsu TA, Bonica JJ. Spinal and extradural analgesia: anesthesia for parturition. *Clin Obstet Gynecol* 1974;17:183; with permission.)

Another common reason for high blood levels of local anesthetic drugs is accidental intravascular injection. This most commonly occurs when a paracervical block is used or when an epidural catheter erodes into a vein. To minimize accidental intravenous injection, gentle aspiration should be undertaken before each injection. Injection should be done slowly and incrementally with 2 to 5 ml of local anesthetic drug to reduce the chance of a sudden increase in plasma levels.

The infiltration of a local anesthetic agent into an area rich in vessels, such as the region of the uterine artery (e.g., paracervical block) or the epidural space, may be associated with absorption of the drug through blood vessel walls. The serum levels tend to rise slowly, and toxic manifestations usually occur only after multiple injections.

Repeated injections of slowly metabolized local anesthetic drugs, such as the amides, may lead to accumulation in the serum such that toxic levels are achieved. This phenomenon does not occur readily with esters such as chloroprocaine, which are rapidly metabolized (maternal serum half-life of 21 seconds and fetal serum half-life of 43 seconds for chloroprocaine). To minimize the likelihood of producing high serum levels, care should be taken to record the amount and concentration of local anesthetic solution and to limit use to approximately 25% less than the maximal safe dose.

Signs and symptoms of local anesthetic drug toxicity include, in order of their appearance, a relaxed feeling, drowsiness, lightheadedness, tinnitus, circumoral paresthesias, metallic taste, slurred speech, blurred vision, unconsciousness, convulsions, and cardiac dysrhythmias and arrest. In 1983, the U.S. Food and Drug Administration issued an advisory, warning that 0.75% bupivacaine should no longer be used in obstetrics because of reports of bupivacaine-induced cardiac arrest occurring at blood levels of only 3 to 5 μg/ml. The advisory stated that the resuscitation in these cases had been "difficult or impossible despite apparently adequate prepara-

tion and appropriate management." Inadvertent intravascular injection causes high serum levels, which produce cardiac arrest through blockade of the cellular sodium channels, inhibiting repolarization of the nerve cell membranes of the conduction system of the heart. Bupivacaine has been found to bind avidly to nonspecific cardiac protein–binding sites, slowing the conduction of impulses arising in pacemaker cells and causing a dose-dependent reduction in the strength of systolic myocardial contractions, leading to cardiac arrest.

During the course of a toxic reaction, CNS stimulation is usually followed by generalized depression. CNS excitation symptoms and signs, including twitching, apprehension, and convulsion, occur first. These are followed by cardiovascular excitation signs of hypertension, tachycardia, arrhythmia, and convulsion. Respiratory effects are variable and include apnea, hypoxia, obstruction, and increased risk of pulmonary aspiration of gastric contents.

When blood levels rise slowly to toxic levels, depression usually occurs alone, without prior stimulation. CNS features include stupor, unconsciousness, coma, and a postictal state. Cardiovascular effects are those of vasodilation, hypotension, shock, bradycardia, ventricular fibrillation, and cardiovascular collapse. Respiratory changes include respiratory depression, apnea, hypoxia, and pulmonary arrest.

Management is best accomplished through prevention, as described previously. The only therapy is symptomatic. Only signs and symptoms that are present are treated. Treatment includes the use of mask oxygen, a reliable intravenous line, and measures to ensure and protect the airway. These include use of the head-down and lateral positions, cricoid pressure to occlude the esophagus, the availability of adequate suction, and the capability to perform endotracheal intubation, if needed.

Adequacy of respirations must be ensured by means of positive pressure ventilation with a high fraction of inspired oxygen. CNS hyperreactivity and convulsions are treated with thiopental (Pentothal) in small, incremental doses of 25 to 50 mg given intravenously or with 2.5 to 5 mg of diazepam given intravenously. In the event of cardiovascular depression, the head-down position should be used, with elevation of the lower extremities and left uterine displacement. Vasoactive drugs such as ephedrine, phenylephrine, epinephrine, and calcium may be employed to support the circulation. If cardiopulmonary resuscitation is indicated, the fetus should be delivered promptly to relieve maternal central venous compression.

Convulsions should not be treated primarily with muscle relaxants, because these control only the motor manifestations of the seizure and do not affect CNS hyperactivity with its attendant increased oxygen use. Cricoid pressure should be applied until the trachea can be intubated to reduce the likelihood of the acid pulmonary aspiration syndrome. Convulsions caused by accidental intravascular injection of local anesthetic drugs are usually short-lived.

Effects on the Fetus and Uterus

Use of bupivacaine for epidural analgesia has been associated with FHR decelerations. In a study of 150 patients receiving lidocaine, bupivacaine, or chloroprocaine for labor analgesia, 8 of 50 fetuses had late deceleration patterns after maternal epidural administration of bupivacaine 0.5%. Only 3 of 50 exposed to lidocaine 1.5% and none of 50 exposed to chloroprocaine 2% experienced late deceleration patterns. These patterns were not associated with maternal hypotension.

Steiger and Nageotte (1990) studied the intrauterine pressure associated with FHR decelerations after epidural bupivacaine. They observed an increased incidence of FHR decelerations when baseline tonus was elevated, but neonatal outcomes were unaffected by these minor FHR changes.

Chloroprocaine 3% with sodium bisulfite as a preservative has been associated with neurologic deficits when accidentally injected into the subarachnoid space. Chloroprocaine solution without preservative is now available for regional block analgesia and should be used in 1% and 2% concentrations.

Use of Local Anesthetics

Local Infiltration of the Perineum

Local infiltration of the perineum is commonly performed when an episiotomy is needed and time or fetal head position does not allow a pudendal block to be administered. An average of 10 to 20 ml of local anesthetic solution is employed. The preferred drugs are lidocaine 1% or chloroprocaine 2%.

Pudendal Block

The pudendal block provides analgesia of the vaginal introitus and perineum. There are several advantages of this analgesic technique. Because the elapsed time between administration and delivery is short, there is relatively little systemic absorption and therefore little opportunity for the drug to di-

rectly affect the fetus. The block is easy to accomplish and provides analgesia of the perineum only. The disadvantages include the need for large drug doses (i.e., 10 ml on each side) and the possibility of infection leading to retropsoas or subgluteal abscess.

With the transvaginal approach, the ischial spine must first be identified. Through a guide, a needle is inserted into the vagina and directed laterally and posteriorly to the ischial spine. A submucosal wheal is made, and the needle is advanced into the sacrospinous ligament, where resistance is felt. As the needle passes the ligament, a loss of resistance is felt. The needle has now entered the pudendal canal, which contains the pudendal nerve and associated vessels (Fig. 3). After aspirating the needle for blood, 3 to 5 ml of local anesthetic solution (usually lidocaine 1%) is injected, and the needle is advanced another 0.5 to 1 cm. If aspiration is again negative, 5 to 7 ml of solution is injected. A total of 10 ml is injected on each side. Approximately 10 minutes are required for anesthesia to occur. Chloroprocaine 1% to 2% or bupivacaine 0.5% may also be used for this block. Analgesia with chloroprocaine lasts less than 1 hour, but bupivacaine analgesia is much more prolonged.

Paracervical Block

Paracervical block (PCB) anesthesia may be used when the active phase of labor begins, and it can be employed until approximately 8 cm of dilation has been achieved. Although formerly popular, this block has fallen into relative disuse since the description of bradycardia after PCB and its proven association with fetal acidosis. The PCB is useful when anesthesia personnel are unavailable and the obstetrician is not skilled in other methods such as epidural or caudal block.

The PCB relieves the pain associated with uterine contractions, but it is not effective for pain associated with distention of the pelvic floor. The two drugs of choice are chloroprocaine and lidocaine in 1% concentrations. Typically, 6 ml of drug is administered superficially, just under the vaginal mucosa, at the 4- and 8-o'clock positions (Fig. 4). In this way, bradycardia, which occurs in 10% to 30% of cases, is less likely to appear. The landmark study by Baxi et al. (1979), using a transcutaneous oxygen electrode attached to the fetal scalp, demonstrated that bradycardia is related to decreasing fetal oxygenation, which becomes marginal approximately 10 minutes after injection. This research has been corroborated by the study of isolated human uterine artery segments and by work in animals, indicating that direct uterine artery vasoconstriction and uterine hypertonus in response to the injection of a local anesthetic drug diminish uterine blood flow and fetal oxygenation.

Lumbar Epidural Analgesia

Standard Technique

Lumbar epidural analgesia was first performed in 1884 by Corning, who recognized that analgesia could still occur

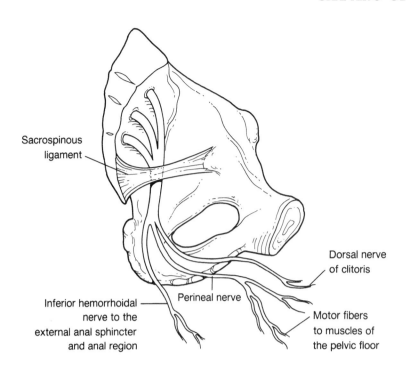

FIG. 3. The pudendal nerve and its branches. The inferior hemorrhoidal nerve can arise higher up from the pudendal nerve or separately from the sacral plexus. (Adapted from Abouleish E. *Pain control in obstetrics.* Philadelphia: JB Lippincott Co, 1977.)

when attempted spinal analgesia failed. In 1921, Pages applied the technique to surgery. Obstetric applications were made by Graffagnino and Seyler in 1935.

The most commonly used anesthetic agents for lumbar epidural analgesia are chloroprocaine 1% to 2%, lidocaine

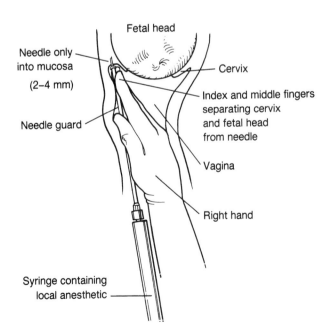

FIG. 4. Technique of paracervical block. Notice the position of the hand and fingers in relation to the cervix and fetal head and the shallow depth of the needle insertion. No undue pressure is applied at the vaginal fornix by the fingers or needle guide. (Adapted from Abouleish E. *Pain control in obstetrics.* Philadelphia: JB Lippincott Co, 1977.)

1% to 2%, bupivacaine 0.0625% to 0.5%, and ropivacaine 0.25% to 0.5%.

The technique of lumbar epidural analgesia involves the insertion of a 17- or 18-gauge Tuohy needle through the ligamentum flavum into the epidural space at the L4-5, L3-4, or L2-3 interspace. Although the hanging-drop technique for identification of the epidural space is generally effective, most physicians prefer the lack-of-resistance technique as the one that affords the least risk of penetration of the dura. Use of air to identify the dural space produces a higher incidence of failed segmental blocks, although a repeat injection usually corrects this problem. A fine catheter is passed through the epidural needle in a cephalad direction for a distance of 2 to 3 cm within the epidural space. This catheter is securely taped in place and serves as an avenue for intermittent or continuous injection of local anesthetic agents or opioids.

Epidural Opioids in Labor

Epidural injection of opioids alone has been shown to be of limited value for the relief of labor pain. High doses of morphine (7.5 mg) have provided satisfactory analgesia, but only during the first stage of labor. Because of its slow onset of action (often 1 hour or more), morphine is not a satisfactory agent for this use. Fentanyl used alone has yielded much the same result. Epidural narcotics, when given as the sole analgesic, have fallen far short of their early promise. Fortunately, the addition of opioids to dilute concentrations of epidural local anesthetics has been proven to be quite effective in the relief of labor pain. The combination is a rational one because local anesthetic solutions relieve somatic pain preferentially, whereas opioids are more effective in relieving visceral pain.

Fentanyl and Bupivacaine. It has become fashionable to employ ever smaller doses of opioids and local anesthetic drugs for epidural analgesia. Chestnut, McGrath, et al. (1994) investigated the continuous epidural infusion of bupivacaine 0.0625% with fentanyl 0.0002% during the second stage of labor. They concluded that this mixture provides better second-stage analgesia than a saline placebo but does not significantly increase the incidence of instrumental delivery. The addition of fentanyl approximately doubles the analgesic efficacy of any concentration of bupivacaine, while shortening the time to complete analgesia.

Sufentanil and Bupivacaine. When sufentanil (20 to 30 μg) combined with 10 ml of bupivacaine 0.25% is administered extradurally, analgesia begins more quickly than when sufentanil is excluded from the mixture. Labor analgesia seems to be improved, and top-up requirements are reduced. Large doses of sufentanil are unnecessary because 0.2 to 0.3 μg/ml of the mixture give results similar to those with tenfold higher concentrations. It is also possible to potentiate the action of very low concentrations of bupivacaine while minimizing motor block, enabling ambulation during the first stage of labor.

Alfentanil and Bupivacaine. Alfentanil is a synthetic opioid with a short duration of action and a low potential for systemic toxicity. When used alone, epidural alfentanil produces early, excellent analgesia that becomes inadequate in the latter part of the first stage and for the second stage of labor. With doses as high as 30 μg/kg per hour, neonatal hypotonia has been recognized. Alfentanil elimination is delayed in the neonate.

Opioid and Chloroprocaine Mixtures. Mixtures of opioids with chloroprocaine have not been shown to be useful, as chloroprocaine appears to antagonize the analgesic effects of the opioid, while increasing its side effects, particularly nausea and pruritus. The mechanism of this unfavorable interaction is unknown. Chloroprocaine may also prolong the onset of morphine analgesia and decrease the effectiveness of bupivacaine if used before these agents. The most satisfactory analgesia appears to be produced when opioids are combined with bupivacaine rather than with other local anesthetics.

The beneficial effects of epidural opioids in labor appear to be the following:

◊ Reduction in motor block, allowing improved mobility of the patient;
◊ Reduction in shivering;
◊ Decreased incidence of hypotension;
◊ Use of lower doses of local anesthetic agents;
◊ Greater maternal satisfaction with the analgesia that they provide.

Effects of Epidural Analgesia on Labor

Epidural analgesia from local anesthetic drugs has had variable effects on the progress of labor. The first stage of labor is unaffected, but the second stage may be prolonged, depending on the technique used. If the block is initiated before the active phase of labor (i.e., 5 to 6 cm of cervical dilation) and in the absence of oxytocin stimulation, diminished uterine contractility and slowed progress in labor have been reported. When administered in the active phase of labor, lumbar epidural analgesia causes only a transient reduction in the frequency and intensity of uterine contractions. This effect may be potentiated by epinephrine-containing solutions. The slowing of labor seldom persists beyond 20 to 30 minutes and then is followed by restoration of the preinjection pattern. Guidozzi et al. (1992) reported on their work with 56 patients given continuous epidural infusions with bupivacaine 0.125% during the first stage of labor. They measured uterine work, which they expressed in Alexandria units and as the area under the pressure curve. Their study showed that continuous low-dose epidural analgesia had no significant effect on uterine work during the active phase of the first stage of labor when cervical dilation was 5 cm or more.

It is commonly thought that lumbar epidural analgesia prolongs the second stage of labor because of diminished reflex-induced voluntary pushing. Several studies have demonstrated that a well coached patient usually accomplishes a spontaneous vaginal delivery, if she is encouraged to delay pushing with her contractions until the fetal head passes the ischial spines or is visible at the introitus. Data from St. Mary's Hospital in London suggest that operative intervention should be based on the rate of progress rather than the elapsed time in the second stage of labor. Second-stage labors lasting as long as 3 hours do not seem to carry undue risk for the fetus if the prolongation is caused by epidural analgesia.

Hawkins et al. (1995) evaluated the association between instrumental delivery and epidural analgesia. In their two-component study, they first conducted a retrospective analysis of the medical records of 14,804 parturients having a vaginal delivery before and after the implementation of an active epidural analgesia service. Despite a tenfold increase in the use of epidural analgesia, there was similar usage of instrumental delivery in both the epidural and nonepidural groups. In addition, the epidural-forceps association was noted to be twice as strong for parous patients as for nulliparous patients (odds ratios: 9.74 and 4.52, respectively). The second component was a case control study designed to determine which other factors, in addition to epidural analgesia, might be associated with an increase in instrumental delivery. While epidural analgesia was one factor, the others identified were gestational age greater than 41 weeks, second stage of labor greater than 2 hours, occiput posterior or transverse fetal position, and previous cesarean section. Each of these factors was individually and independently associated with an increase in the incidence of instrumental delivery, independent of epidural use.

The effect of epidural analgesia on duration and outcome of induced labor was evaluated by Rojansky et al. (1997). They prospectively studied 210 women admitted for induction of labor. Of these, 112 were given an epidural block, while 98 served as controls. Using multiple regression analysis, they showed that epidural analgesia significantly prolonged labor and was associated with an increase in instrumental delivery rates. Also observed was a significant reduction in intrapartum complication rates, such as FHR changes and meconium passage. The cesarean section rate and Apgar scores were found not to be influenced by epidural analgesia.

It has been suggested that epidural analgesia increases the primary cesarean section rate and numerous studies support both sides of this debate. A study by Thorp et al. (1990) compared nulliparous women at term who received epidural analgesia in labor with a control group consisting of those who received narcotics or no analgesia. The frequency of cesarean section for dystocia was significantly greater in the epidural group than in the control group. They concluded that "epidural analgesia in labor may increase the incidence of cesarean section for dystocia in nulliparous women." In another study, Lieberman et al. (1996) retrospectively examined 1733 low-risk term nulliparous patients in whom labor began spontaneously. The cesarean delivery rate among women receiving epidural analgesia was 17%, compared with 4% among those who did not receive epidural analgesia. They determined that the risk of cesarean section was 3.7, with a confidence interval of 2.4 to 5.7. The cesarean risk was highest when epidural analgesia was administered early in labor. Turcot et al. (1997) prospectively studied 925 nulliparous women in spontaneous labor at term. They found the adjusted odds ratio of operative delivery in the presence of epidural analgesia to be 3.4 (95% confidence interval, 2.0 to 5.8). The association persisted independently of dystocia. In

yet another study, Ramin et al. (1995) randomly offered epidural bipivacaine-fentanyl or intravenous meperidine analgesia to 1300 women with uncomplicated term pregnancies and in spontaneous labor. They noted that epidural analgesia provided superior pain relief, but its use was associated with prolonged labor and a two- to fourfold increased risk of cesarean delivery. A metaanalysis published in 1994 comprised six studies for primary analysis and two others for secondary analysis. It was determined that the cesarean delivery rate for women undergoing epidural analgesia was 10% greater than for women who labored without epidural analgesia. The authors concluded that their metaanalysis strongly supported an increase in cesarean delivery associated with epidural analgesia during labor. In a recent 1998 metaanalysis, the Cochrane Pregnancy and Childbirth Group reviewed randomized clinical trials comparing epidural to nonepidural analgesia in labor. Figure 5 graphically illustrates the outcome of this review. The authors stated that there is an increase in the cesarean delivery rate overall (data from four studies) and the major reason for this seems to be dystocia. This analysis concluded that epidural block is likely to provide more effective pain relief than alternative methods, but at the cost of increased rates of operative delivery. Further research is needed to define the adverse effects more accurately, as well as to evaluate the effects of different regional analgesia techniques.

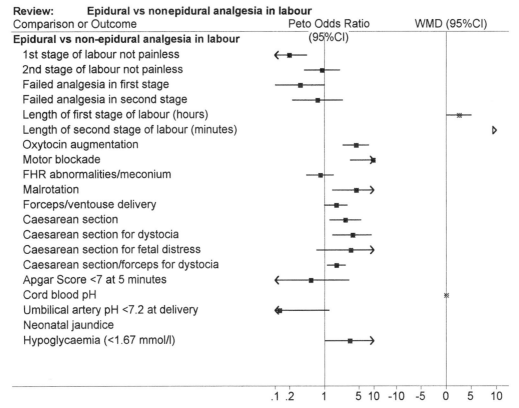

FIG. 5. Epidural versus nonepidural analgesia in labor. (From *The Cochrane Library* 1998; Issue 1, P1, from the Cochrane Pregnancy and Childbirth Group.)

There is also evidence supporting the other side of the debate. Gribble and Meier (1991) evaluated labor outcomes at a time when epidural analgesia could be obtained on demand and compared them to a time when no epidural service was available. The primary cesarean section rate was 9% without the epidural service and 8.2% after the epidural service began. The investigators found that the availability of on-demand epidural analgesia did not increase the primary cesarean section rate. Similarly, following the introduction of a full epidural analgesia service, Bailey and Howard (1983) reported a slight increase in the rate of forceps deliveries, but no change in the cesarean section rate. Naulty et al. (1998) reported a decline in the overall incidence of cesarean delivery despite an increase in the percentage of parturients who received epidural analgesia when the epidural technique was changed from intermittent boluses of lidocaine or bupivacaine to infusions of bupivacaine plus fentanyl. Ploeckinger et al. (1995) investigated the influence of epidural analgesia on surgical delivery rates, intrapartum fever, and blood loss. Although intrapartum fever and greater blood loss were associated with epidural analgesia, there was no difference in the cesarean delivery rate when epidural analgesia was employed. In two studies, Chestnut et al. (1994) evaluated the effect of early administration of epidural analgesia on obstetric outcome in nulliparous women in spontaneous labor and in women receiving intravenous oxytocin. They concluded that early administration of epidural analgesia did not prolong labor or increase the incidence of operative delivery, when compared with intravenous nalbuphine analgesia followed by late administration of epidural analgesia. These findings were independent of whether patients were in spontaneous labor or were receiving intravenous oxytocin. Finally, Nageotte et al. (1997) compared epidural analgesia with combined spinal–epidural (CSE) analgesia in nulliparous women during labor. They postulated that because CSE analgesia permits ambulation during labor, it would be associated with a lower incidence of dystocia than continuous lumbar epidural analgesia. However, they found no significant difference in the overall rate of cesarean delivery, the incidence of dystocia, or the degree of overall satisfaction between the two techniques. They noted, however, that dystocia necessitating cesarean delivery was significantly more likely when analgesia was administered with the fetal vertex at a negative station (odds ratio: 2.5; $p<0.001$) or the cervix had reached less than 4 cm of dilation (odds ratio: 2.2; $p<0.001$).

Thus, it would appear that there are many variables with the potential to affect the risk of cesarean delivery. These would include patient-related factors such as parity, labor pattern, and oxytocin use, as well as obstetrician-related factors such as active or passive management. Epidural-related factors would include the timing of the epidural block with respect to cervical dilation, the level of block achieved, the pattern of drug injection (intermittent, continuous, or patient-controlled epidural analgesia), and the variety, volume, concentration, and mixture of drugs employed. It should be clear from the foregoing that there is no pat an-

swer to the question of whether or not epidural analgesia affects the cesarean section rate.

Effects of Epidural Analgesia on Uterine Blood Flow

Studies investigating changes in intervillous blood flow and mean arterial pressure with lumbar epidural analgesia in adequately preloaded patients have demonstrated only a negligible reduction in these parameters with the onset of effective analgesia. Well hydrated patients with preeclampsia have experienced improvement in intervillous blood flow along with a slight decrease in blood pressure.

Advantages and Disadvantages of Lumbar Epidural Analgesia

There are three principal advantages of lumbar epidural analgesia: (1) The parturient remains awake and cooperative. (2) The incidence of complications is very low when the technique is used correctly. (3) Epidural technique can be used to provide analgesia or anesthesia for a vaginal delivery or a cesarean section delivery. The disadvantages of lumbar epidural analgesia include (1) the possibility of poor perineal analgesia, (2) the presence of "hot spots," where analgesia is insufficient, (3) delayed onset of action, (4) technical difficulty, (5) intravascular injection, (6) accidental dural puncture, and (7) hypotension. Technical failure occurs in approximately 4% of cases.

Hypotension is common, occurring in as many as 50% of patients undergoing epidural anesthesia for cesarean section. It often occurs despite left uterine displacement and use of an adequate vascular preload. Treatment should consist of the following steps:

1. Ensure or verify left uterine displacement.
2. Increase intravenous fluid infusion to the maximal available rate.
3. Administer oxygen by facemask.
4. If hypotension does not immediately resolve, administer ephedrine intravenously in 5- to 10-mg increments until hypotension resolves.

The use of phenylephrine has been advocated, but it should be used only after failure of all other methods, and then only in very small doses of 20 to 40 µg per bolus, because its pure α-adrenergic effects may further compromise uteroplacental blood flow.

Indications and Contraindications for Lumbar Epidural Analgesia

Indications for lumbar epidural analgesia include pain in labor, management of the patient with preeclampsia who does not have a coagulation abnormality, management of labor in patients with certain cardiac lesions, and management of breech delivery.

Van Zundert et al. (1991) demonstrated that expulsion times in patients with breech delivery under lumbar epidural analgesia can be short despite the presence of adequate perineal analgesia during the expulsion phase. They believed that correctly managed epidural analgesia enhances delivery of the breech presentation.

There are absolute and relative contraindications to the induction of lumbar epidural analgesia. Absolute contraindications include the following: patient refusal, infection at the anticipated site of puncture, and absence of resuscitation equipment. Relative contraindications are include fever, preexisting CNS disease, severe anemia, hypovolemia, severe hypertension, hypotension, extreme obesity, lack of experience by the anesthetist, precipitate labor, and blood coagulation defects.

Although an arbitrary platelet count of 100,000/mm³ has been advocated as the lower limit for safe lumbar epidural analgesia, successful blocks without epidural bleeding complications have been obtained with platelet counts as low as 50,000/mm³. In a recent report, Beilin et al. (1997) described a study of 80 women who presented for labor and delivery and had platelet counts less than 100/mm³ during the peripartum period. Of these 80, 30 were given an epidural anesthetic. The range of platelet counts was 69,000 to 98,000/mm³. No patient had any documented neurologic complication. These authors concluded that regional anesthesia should not necessarily be withheld when the platelet count is less than 100,000/mm³.

The threshold for bleeding time should be 10 minutes or less. However, the bleeding time is difficult to measure accurately, and significant discrepancies exist, depending on the technique used. The best indicator of potential bleeding is a patient history of bruises, contusions, petechiae, bleeding from the gums, and so on.

Patient-controlled Epidural Analgesia

Patient controlled epidural analgesia (PCEA) is a technique by which the patient self-administers on-demand doses of an analgesic mixture via an epidural catheter, whenever she perceives discomfort. To avoid overdosage, a lockout period follows each self-administration. This technique has been reported to be associated with a decreased need for anesthetic drugs and less demand on staff time, compared to continuous epidural infusion (CEI). A recent prospective randomized trial compared PCEA with CEI. All patients received a continuous infusion of bupivacaine 0.125% with fentanyl 2 μg/ml, with the CEI group receiving 10 ml per hour and the PCEA group receiving a basal infusion of 6 ml per hour and a demand dose of 3 ml with a 10-minute lockout. Groups were compared for duration of infusion, length of first-stage analgesia, length of second stage of labor, total administered analgesic mixture, and time spent by the anesthesia care provider. No statistical differences between the CEI and the PCEA groups were found. Another recent prospective, double-blinded, randomized study compared CSE analgesia with standard epidural analgesia in spontaneously laboring nulli-

parous parturients. There was no difference in the rate of progress of labor, the amount of epidural local anesthetic required and the incidence of instrumental deliveries between the CSE and the standard epidural analgesia groups. However, analgesia was more complete and there was higher patient satisfaction in the CSE group than in the epidural analgesia group.

Caudal Analgesia

Caudal analgesia was first introduced by Hingson and Edwards in 1942 and was used as a single method for relief of labor discomfort and the pain associated with vaginal delivery. Because it necessitated large doses of local anesthetic drugs, toxicity was not uncommon. This technique has been virtually supplanted by the lumbar approach to the epidural space. However, caudal analgesia has enjoyed a resurgence for the relief of pain in laboring women in whom lumbar epidural analgesia has failed to provide relief of rectal or low sacral pain, for forceps delivery in women who do not have perineal analgesia, for manual removal of the placenta in association with a segmental lumbar epidural block, and for analgesia in patients undergoing cervical cerclage.

Complications have been rare. The literature records four cases of fetal local anesthetic intoxication secondary to accidental injection of the fetal scalp or skull, with two deaths. There was one documented case of maternal intravascular injection in 795 caudal blocks and no case of sacral epidural infection.

Subarachnoid Analgesia

Subarachnoid or spinal analgesia has become less popular for vaginal delivery since epidural analgesia has increased in use. The primary reason is the concern that hypotension will occur and that dural penetration will lead to postpartum dural puncture headache (PDPH). Spinal analgesia has continued to enjoy popularity for cesarean section delivery because use of longer-acting agents such as tetracaine (Pontocaine) and bupivacaine enables a single injection to suffice for the duration of the surgery. Hypotension is commonplace and is frequently seen with the high block needed for cesarean section, even with an adequate fluid preload and careful lateral displacement of the uterus.

The major advantages of spinal analgesia include (1) use of a very low dosage of local anesthetic or narcotic analgesic drug and (2) the excellent analgesia provided. Onset of action is rapid, and satisfactory muscle relaxation occurs. Uterine activity is not affected. The disadvantages include (1) poor motor function with resultant inability of the mother to assist vaginal delivery through pushing, (2) hypotension, (3) technical difficulty, and (4) the possibility of PDPH.

Morphine and fentanyl have provided analgesia during labor and after cesarean section when administered intrathecally in small doses. Labor analgesia may persist as long as 24 hours and is not accompanied by muscle relaxation. The major disadvantages include pruritus, which affects as many as 40% of patients, and PDPH. Pruritus can be antagonized with small doses of intravenous naloxone or oral naltrexone. PDPH can be minimized through the use of 26- to 29-gauge Quincke, Whitacre, or Sprotte needles. New evidence suggests that the pencil-point Sprotte needle is the least likely (1% incidence) to produce PDPH.

A 30- to 32-gauge microcatheter can be passed through 26-gauge spinal needles, permitting the use of continuous spinal analgesia in labor and surgery. Unfortunately, there is evidence suggesting that neural injury may result from the use of these fine catheters, perhaps because of the high concentrations of the solutions that directly bathe the spinal cord and filum terminale.

Combined Spinal–Epidural Analgesia

Spinal analgesia has been combined with placement of an extradural catheter using the needle-through-needle technique. With this technique, a 26-gauge long spinal needle is passed into the subarachnoid space through a 16-gauge Tuohy needle that has been placed epidurally. After injection of the spinal anesthetic solution, an epidural catheter is threaded and taped in place for later use. Typically, this block is started with injection of morphine sulfate, 100 to 250 µg, or fentanyl, 50 µg, with or without 1 to 2 mg of bupivacaine, into the subarachnoid space. Injection of saline or bupivacaine into the epidural space will extend the subarachnoid block, presumably due to compression of the dural sac by the extradural injection. Analgesia with minimal motor block allows ambulation during labor. When the subarachnoid analgesia begins to wear off, injections may be made through the epidural catheter.

A recent study by Felsby et al. (1995) compared the efficacy of CSE analgesia with epidural for labor analgesia. Critics of CSE have argued that, compared to epidural analgesia, CSE takes longer to perform and requires a greater number of patient interventions, such as treatment of pruritus, fetal bradycardia, hypotension, and nausea. The investigators in this study therefore devised it to compare CSE with epidural analgesia with respect to these parameters. The study included 51 parturients randomized in double-blind fashion to one technique or the other. There was no difference in the time required to perform CSE, as compared to epidural analgesia, but there were significantly more interventions in multiparous patients. The rapid onset of action of both techniques resulted in similar degrees of patient satisfaction.

Complications of Regional Block Analgesia

Postpartum Dural Puncture Headache

When a large-bore epidural needle (e.g., 18-gauge Tuohy) penetrates the dura and arachnoid membranes, the incidence of PDPH approximates 50%. A possible cause is the decrease in cerebrospinal fluid (CSF) volume secondary to blood loss during delivery or straining during the second stage of labor. Furthermore, normal postpartum diuresis decreases CSF for-

mation. Other factors governing the frequency of PDPH include the number of times the dura has been punctured, the direction of the bevel, and the type of needle used.

PDPH occurs because a decrease in CSF volume causes compensatory vasodilation and traction on the pain-sensitive vessels and supporting structures of the brain. Assumption of the erect position increases traction on these structures and aggravates the pain. Therefore, the main diagnostic criterion of PDPH is that it is postural. Ocular and auditory symptoms, such as vertigo, ataxia, and sixth cranial nerve palsy, and nausea and loss of appetite may be associated with PDPH.

Many different treatment regimens have been employed for this condition, including prompt administration of 3 liters of intravenous or oral fluid, administration of saline through the epidural catheter, the use of abdominal binders, the administration of intravenous or oral caffeine, bed rest, analgesics, and epidural blood or Gelfoam patches. The most effective of these is the epidural blood patch.

Evidence suggests that prophylactic epidural blood patch can substantially reduce the incidence and severity of PDPH. In a recent study by Lowinwirt et al (1998), patients with accidental dural puncture with 16- or 17-gauge needles were randomized and allocated to two treatment groups. In one group, patients received 15 to 20 ml of autologous blood through the indwelling epidural catheter at least 5 hours following the last dose of local anesthetic and just before catheter removal. Patients in the control group were managed conservatively with intravenous hydration, bed rest, theophylline, or caffeine. Eighty-three percent of patients receiving the prophylactic epidural blood patch avoided PDPH. Only 4% of patients treated conservatively avoided PDPH. Use of prophylactic epidural blood patch was not associated with any complications, and the patients receiving it experienced considerably less suffering.

Chronic Low-back Pain

Low-back pain is a common complaint in the postpartum period. A controversy exists as to the role that epidural analgesia for labor and delivery might play in the subsequent development of low-back pain. Whereas several retrospective studies have demonstrated an association, other prospective studies have shown no increased risk of acute low-back pain after epidural use. A recent study by Macarthur et al. (1997) examined the risk of low-back pain 1 year after delivery in patients who received epidural analgesia, as compared with those who did not. This prospective follow-up study showed no difference in the prevalence of low-back pain at 1 year after delivery. Therefore, it seems unlikely that epidural analgesia makes any significant contribution to the 19% to 33% prevalence of low-back pain among women.

Neurologic Complications

Neurologic complications of epidural and spinal analgesia are rare. Most postblock neurologic sequelae are related to intraoperative positioning problems. An example is foot drop associated with pressure on the lateral popliteal nerve and caused by an improperly placed stirrup. In the lithotomy position, pressure applied on the femoral cutaneous nerve by the inguinal ligament may cause pain and numbness in the lateral thigh. Pain and numbness in the distribution of the sciatic nerve may result from forceps delivery or passage of the baby's head through the pelvis.

Spinal nerve root neuropathy may be caused by traumatic insertion of a spinal needle or an epidural needle or catheter. In this case, pain and paresthesias along the distribution of the nerve are perceived immediately, but they tend to disappear when the needle or catheter is removed. Rarely, symptoms may appear as long as 2 days after the procedure. Recovery usually occurs in 1 to 2 weeks, but injury can be permanent.

Accidental injection of an irritant solution (e.g., thiopental) or a prep solution into the CSF may produce adhesive arachnoiditis, which can cause permanent loss of spinal cord function. Epidural abscess usually is caused by hematogenous spread and not by injection of contaminated anesthetic solutions.

Epidural hematoma is a serious complication that, although rare, may occur in conjunction with coagulopathy. A hematoma should be suspected if recovery from the block is slow or absent or if neurologic function worsens after a period of initial recovery. The primary symptoms are pain and weakness, which may progress rapidly to paralysis. Early surgical drainage provides the only chance for recovery of neurologic function.

Neurologic complications after spinal or epidural analgesia are rare, occurring with an incidence of approximately 19 in 10,000 deliveries.

◊ OTHER METHODS OF PAIN RELIEF

Prepared Childbirth

Prepared childbirth techniques are based on the belief that pain can be eliminated or reduced by conditioned reflexes of controlled relaxation and that education about the birth process can diminish the pain resulting from fear of the unknown. Parturients and significant others are offered a series of five to ten weekly lectures and are educated about pregnancy, labor, and the delivery process. The parturient is taught how to relax and engages in exercises to strengthen her back and abdominal muscles. She also learns specific breathing patterns to be used while she experiences the discomfort of uterine contractions. Effective courses also teach her that additional methods of pain relief are available and that these do not cause harm to her fetus. Parturients should be advised that to ask for these other methods does not imply that she is a failure.

Hypnosis

Hypnosis is a state of altered consciousness that requires deep concentration. The patient is not asleep, but she initiates a trance as labor begins and continues it until delivery is completed. The patient must undergo a time-consuming series of training sessions with a hypnotist, and this technique is not always successful.

Acupuncture

Acupuncture has been used to help control labor pain in China and the Far East for many years. Since the early 1970s, mixed reports of its efficacy have been published in the West. Some studies indicate that acupuncture can significantly lower pain scores and may decrease the duration of the first stage of labor. Although enthusiasm for the technique is mixed in western countries, the Chinese continue to report 99% rates of excellent and good success. When acupuncture is used for cesarean section in conjunction with intravenous meperidine and local anesthetic infiltration, blood pressure, pulse rate, and respirations are stable, and the degree of patient acceptance is reported to be high.

Biofeedback

Biofeedback is a method of pain relief that involves no risk to the mother or her fetus. Biofeedback is provided by a portable electromyographic device through an audible sound and visual monitor. Electrodes placed over the maternal abdomen monitor tension of the abdominal musculature. This technique may be helpful during the first stage of labor and may reduce its duration and the use of systemic medications.

Transcutaneous Electrical Nerve Stimulation

Transcutaneous electrical nerve stimulation (TENS) analgesia is based on the observation that application of a mild electric current to the skin can result in reduction of pain. Activation based on the gate theory and release of enkephalins are possible modes of action. Three studies evaluating the effectiveness of TENS suggested that, although the method does no harm, it probably does little good and should not be advocated for widespread use for labor analgesia (see Kaplan, 1997; Kaplan, 1998; Carroll, 1997).

Intracutaneous Nerve Stimulation

Expanding on earlier work regarding the relief of pain through counterirritation, Bengtsson and associates in 1981 successfully treated the pain of urolithiasis with intracutaneous injections of sterile water. Trolle et al. (1991) evaluated the analgesic effect of intradermal sterile water blocks in women complaining of severe low-back pain during labor. Saline solution was used as a control. Sterile water or saline (0.1 ml) was injected at four different spots in the low-back area, approximately corresponding to the borders of the sacrum. Eighty-nine percent of women in the sterile water group reported an analgesic effect, compared with 45% in the saline group. Although initial pain scoring did not show any significant differences between the groups, there were highly significant differences by 2 hours after the block. Meperidine use in the two groups was similar, as were the rates for oxytocin use and dystocia. The cesarean section rate in the sterile water group was significantly lower. This technique is free of adverse effects and enjoys a high degree of patient acceptance. Additional work is necessary before it can be routinely advocated.

◊ ANESTHESIA FOR CESAREAN SECTION DELIVERY

There are three anesthetic choices for cesarean delivery. Selection of one over the others depends on the patient's desires, medical status, and the urgency of the operation.

Epidural Analgesia

Epidural analgesia accounts for approximately one-third of anesthetics used for cesarean section. It offers the advantages of minimizing the risk of aspiration pneumonitis and sparing of airway-protecting reflexes.

To carry out a cesarean section operation, a sensory dermatome level of at least T-6 is required. Anesthesia to this level eliminates proprioception from the respiratory muscles of the chest wall, and the parturient may experience a subjective sensation of suffocation. Reassurance and sedation usually allay this fear. The patient should be placed on the operating table with the uterus displaced laterally through elevation of the right hip or by tilting of the operating table, so that the heavy gravid uterus does not compress the inferior vena cava and impede venous return to the heart.

A vascular preload of 1000 to 1500 ml of a non–glucose-containing crystalloid solution should be administered before dosing of the epidural needle or catheter with the anesthetizing solution. Bupivacaine 0.5% with or without added opioid is administered through the catheter in 3- to 5-ml increments. An alternate technique involves administration of the anesthetizing solution directly through the needle, with placement of the catheter after the 10- to 15-ml dose has been incrementally administered. The patient should be given oxygen by nasal prongs or by mask. One study failed to reveal any differences in the clinical condition of neonates, as assessed by Apgar scores and blood gas analyses, when oxygen administration by these two modalities was compared.

A recent study by Arsiradam et al (1998) compared ropivacaine 0.75% with bupivacaine 0.5% for epidural analgesia in elective cesarean delivery. The two groups were analyzed for level of block, median time to block, pain at delivery, quality of analgesia, blood pressure changes, Apgar scores, and neurologic and adaptive capacity scores. There were no significant differences in any of these parameters. The authors concluded that ropivacaine 0.75% can be safely administered epidurally in doses up to 187.5 mg and provides excellent analgesia for elective cesarean section.

Epidural opioids have been useful for relieving pain of visceral origin, which affects as many as one-third of the women who have cesarean sections under epidural anesthesia. Visceral pain occurs primarily during bladder retraction, exteriorization of the uterus, and suturing of the peritoneum. The

addition of fentanyl to bupivacaine reduces the time of onset of analgesia to the level of T-6 and increases the quality of analgesia. Sufentanil has also been added to bupivacaine for epidural analgesia for cesarean section. Sufentanil significantly improves the quality of anesthesia, without depressing the neurobehavioral status of the newborn.

Studies of fentanyl concentrations in neonates demonstrate that fentanyl crosses the placenta and is in the serum of the newborn. Even high maternal doses (e.g., 100 μg) of fentanyl yield safe levels in the newborn, but the drug should not be administered in cases of suspected fetal compromise.

Morphine is associated with the greatest degree of postoperative analgesia, but sufentanil and fentanyl cause less pruritus and vomiting.

There are several advantages to using epidural analgesia for cesarean section delivery: (1) If an epidural catheter is already in place, it can be used expeditiously for the cesarean section delivery. (2) Maternal hypotension is less pronounced with epidural than with spinal anesthesia. (3) Headache is usually avoided, unless the patient sustains an accidental dural puncture. (4) The length of anesthesia is controllable in case surgery is prolonged. (5) The technique is adaptable for postoperative pain relief by using continuous or intermittent injections of local anesthetics, opioids, or both. The disadvantages include (1) the slower onset of analgesia, (2) the requirement for a larger amount of anesthetic solution with its attendant increased risk of systemic toxicity, and (3) the lower success rate than that experienced with subarachnoid block.

Subarachnoid Block Anesthesia

A subarachnoid block provides excellent analgesia for cesarean section delivery. Approximately one-third of cesarean sections are performed using this technique. It is generally reserved for patients having elective or urgent cesarean sections; those with more emergent need are subjected to general anesthesia. Prehydration is administered with 1500 to 2000 ml of a non–dextrose-containing crystalloid solution. A 26-gauge or smaller spinal needle is inserted into the subarachnoid space, which is identified by observing the egress of spinal fluid through the needle and the characteristic feel of the needle penetrating the dura. If longer-duration analgesia is desired, tetracaine, 10 to 12 mg, in dextrose or bupivacaine 0.75%, 10 to 12 mg, with dextrose is administered. Analgesia of shorter duration is obtained with the use of lidocaine 5% in 7.5% dextrose.

Opioids may also be administered intrathecally to improve cardiovascular stability. Spinal narcotics are associated with a high incidence of nausea, vomiting, pruritus, and somnolence, as well as with the potential for delayed respiratory depression. Morphine and fentanyl, however, may be administered with hyperbaric bupivacaine and have improved intraoperative analgesia while providing postoperative analgesia that may last for 18 to 24 hours. Because of its high lipid solubility, fentanyl has a shorter duration of action than morphine.

Contraindications to spinal anesthesia include patient refusal, septicemia, infection of the puncture site, acute or chronic hypovolemia, and abnormal clotting parameters. Spinal anesthesia is usually avoided in obstetric patients with acute CNS disease. Use of intrathecal morphine increases the likelihood of recurrent herpetic infections.

The most common complication of spinal anesthesia is hypotension. This should be treated promptly with fluid administration and intravenous ephedrine (5- to 10-mg bolus). Oxygen should be given, and the parturient's oxygen saturation should be monitored with a pulse oximeter. In the event of a total spinal block, cricoid pressure should be applied and endotracheal intubation performed to prevent aspiration of gastric contents.

An unexpectedly high level of anesthetic block may be achieved with epidural and spinal analgesia because of inadvertent injection of a large volume of local anesthetic solution into the subarachnoid space instead of the epidural space, accidental subdural injection, or faulty positioning of the patient after appropriate spinal injection.

Subdural (supraarachnoid) block is a rare complication that characteristically demonstrates a delayed onset of 20 to 30 minutes, with cephalad extension, minimal hypotension, unilateral block, and minimal motor block. The diagnosis of a subdural block is made retrospectively by the injection of a radiopaque solution through the catheter.

A total spinal block generally occurs within 90 seconds after injection, but it may be delayed for as long as 20 minutes. Dyspnea, hypotension, unconsciousness, and apnea are signs and symptoms of total spinal block. Treatment includes ventilation through an endotracheal tube and, if needed, cardiocirculatory support. The likelihood of inadvertent spinal analgesia while attempting epidural block can be minimized through gentle aspiration of the catheter combined with using a test dose of sufficiently small volume that it is unlikely to produce a high block.

With the increasing use of spinal narcotics, pruritus is becoming a commonplace adverse effect. It is also seen with epidural use, and its incidence approaches 60% when epidural morphine is employed. The cause seems to be related to stimulation of opioid receptors rather than to release of histamine. Naloxone can be used to control pruritus, but the dose must be titrated carefully to avoid antagonism of analgesia. Nalbuphine may also be used and is less likely to antagonize analgesia. Pruritus occurs less commonly with more highly lipid-soluble narcotics such as fentanyl.

Approximately 23% of women experience shivering during normal labor and delivery, and the rate increases to approximately 68% with epidural analgesia. Shivering can be diminished or abolished through epidural injection of opioids (e.g., sufentanil, 100 µg).

General Anesthesia

General anesthesia is used for cesarean section when the patient refuses regional analgesia or has a contraindication to regional analgesia or when a need exists for rapid delivery because of fetal distress, cord prolapse, shoulder dystocia, or maternal hemorrhage.

The American College of Obstetricians and Gynecologists in *Committee Opinion No. 104* (March 1992) cited the risk factors for failed intubation and urged obstetricians to be alert to the presence of the factors that place parturients at increased risk for complications from emergency general anesthesia. Among these are marked obesity, severe facial and neck edema, extremely short stature, short neck, difficulty opening the mouth, a small mandible, protuberant teeth, arthritis of the neck, anatomic abnormalities of the face or mouth, a large thyroid gland, asthma, serious medical or obstetric complications, and a history of problems with anesthetics. If any of these factors is identified, a member of the anesthesia team should be consulted to prepare for the unexpected need to induce general anesthesia.

Pneumonitis resulting from aspiration of gastric contents has long been feared as a complication of general anesthesia for obstetrics. A recent report by Warner et al., in which the incidence and consequences of pulmonary aspiration of gastric contents during 215,488 anesthetic procedures was reviewed, revealed that aspiration of gastric contents occurred in only one of every 3216 procedures, with a mortality of only one in 71,829 procedures. Sixty-four percent of patients who experienced aspiration of gastric contents had no adverse sequelae. Only three patients in this series died, and all three had severe predisposing conditions, such as gastrointestinal obstruction. Nonetheless, the prudent anesthetist administers a nonparticulate oral antacid, such as sodium citrate, given prophylactically to increase the gastric pH. If time allows, an H_2-blocker (e.g., ranitidine, 50 mg intravenously) should be administered. Intravenous metoclopramide, 10 mg, hastens gastric emptying and increases gastroesophageal sphincter tone.

Before induction of anesthesia, the patient should be preoxygenated with 100% oxygen by mask for at least 3 minutes. Induction is commonly carried out using thiopental (4 mg/kg intravenously). Propofol (Diprivan) also has been advocated. Propofol is associated with a blunted hypertensive response to endotracheal intubation and has yielded similar and satisfactory Apgar scores. Neurologic and adaptive capacity scores and umbilical cord blood gas analyses are also satisfactory. If propofol infusion is prolonged before delivery, neonatal blood levels are high, and neurologic and adaptive capacity scores may be impaired.

Intubation is facilitated by use of succinylcholine. Cricoid pressure is maintained during induction of anesthesia until the endotracheal tube is in place, the cuff has been inflated, and respirations have been auscultated. These actions minimize the risk of pulmonary aspiration of gastric contents, but care must be taken not to occlude the airway completely with excessive manual pressure. After successful intubation, a mixture of equal parts of nitrous oxide and oxygen is administered, and a low dose of an inhalational agent, such as halothane 0.5%, enflurane 1%, or isoflurane 0.75%, is administered to optimize maternal analgesia and amnesia. These low concentrations have minimal effects on uterine contractility and are not associated with postpartum hemorrhage. After delivery of the infant, the nitrous oxide concentration may be increased to 70%, and narcotics may be given intravenously to supplement the anesthesia. Midazolam may be used to decrease the risk of maternal recall.

The advantages of general anesthesia include (1) reliability of the technique, (2) rapidity of induction of anesthesia, and (3) avoidance of sympathetic blockade and hypotension. The disadvantages include (1) the risks of maternal aspiration of gastric contents, (2) failed intubation, (3) maternal awareness, and (4) hypertension during manipulation of the larynx.

If the cords are poorly visualized during laryngoscopy, no more than three attempts at endotracheal intubation should be made before beginning a failed intubation drill. The initial maneuver in the failed intubation drill depends on the obstetric indication for cesarean section. If the operation is not emergent, the patient should be awakened and an epidural or spinal block performed. If a regional anesthetic cannot be accomplished, an awake blind oral or nasal intubation should be considered. In an obstetric emergency, the patient must be ventilated with bag and mask, and anesthesia must be maintained with nitrous oxide, oxygen, and an inhalational agent throughout the remainder of the cesarean section. The continuation of cricoid pressure with adequate patient paralysis is important to reduce the maternal risk of aspiration. If it should prove impossible to ventilate the patient with bag and mask, an emergency maneuver such as cricothyroidotomy must be performed. Transglottic jet ventilation or use of an esophageal gastric tube airway or laryngeal mask may enable adequate ventilation.

Failure to perform endotracheal intubation after multiple attempts (an eightfold increase in obstetrics) was deemed responsible for 16 maternal deaths in the United Kingdom in 1982 and continues to contribute significantly to anesthetic causes of maternal mortality.

Anticipation of a difficult intubation allows the anesthesia team to be prepared to use preanesthetic direct laryngoscopy or make available a flexible fiberoptic laryngoscope.

Analgesia after Cesarean Section

In recent years, considerable advances have been made in the management of pain after cesarean section. The availability of epidural narcotics has enabled the anesthesia team to provide the postsurgical patient with effective, long-term analgesia. Morphine is probably the most commonly used epidural opioid, but because of its delayed onset of action, high incidence of pruritus, concern about delayed respiratory depression, and increased incidence of recurrent herpes simplex, many other opioids have been studied. Epidural fentanyl, sufentanil, and alfentanil have all been found to be efficacious in providing postoperative analgesia. Sufentanil, 30 μg, appears to give analgesia similar in efficacy and duration to fentanyl, 100 μg.

The most feared complication is respiratory depression. The rate of analgesia-related respiratory depression is approximately 0.09%. Because this complication is rare, patients receiving postoperative epidural opioid analgesia may be safely nursed on the general ward, if the nurses are appropriately educated in monitoring the degree of somnolence and the respiratory rates of their patients. Naloxone should be readily available to antagonize respiratory depression.

◇ RECOMMENDED READINGS

Abboud TK, Lee K, Zhu J, et al. Prophylactic oral naltroxone with intrathecal morphine for cesarean section: effects on adverse reactions and analgesia. *Anesth Analg* 1990;71:367.

Arsiradam NM, Maliti Z, Rocke DA. Ropivacaine 7.5 mg/ml for epidural anesthesia in elective cesarean section: a comparison with 5 mg/ml bupivacaine. *Anesth Analg* 1998;86:S361(abst).

Bacigalupo G, Riese S, Rosendahl H. Quantitative relationships between pain intensities during labor and beta-endorphin and cortisol concentrations in plasma: decline of the hormone concentrations in the early postpartum period. *J Perinat Med* 1990;18:289.

Bailey PW, Howard FA. Epidural analgesia and forceps delivery: laying a bogey. *Anaesthesia* 1983;38:282.

Baxi LV, Petrie RH, James LS. Human fetal oxygenation following paracervical block. *Am J Obstet Gynecol* 1979;135:1109.

Beilin Y, Zahn J, Comerford M. Safe epidural analgesia in thirty parturients with platelet counts between 69,000 and 98,000 mm⁻³. Anesth Analg 1997;85:385.

Birnback DJ. What's new in obstetric anesthesiology? *Int J Obstet Anesth* 1997;6:32.

Carroll D, Tramer M, McQuay H, Nye B, Moore A. Transcutaneous electrical nerve stimulation in labour pain: a systematic review. *Br J Obstet Gynaecol* 1997;104:169–175.

Chestnut DH, Vincent RD, McGrath JM, et al. Does early administration of epidural analgesia affect obstetric outcome in nulliparous women who are receiving intravenous oxytocin? *Anesthesiology* 1994;80:1193.

Chestnut DH, McGrath JM, Vincent RD, et al. Does early administration of epidural analgesia affect obstetric outcome in nulliparous women who are in spontaneous labor? *Anesthesiology* 1994;80:1201.

Chestnut DH, Laszewski LJ, Pollack KL, et al. Continuous epidural infusion of 0.0625% bupivacaine–0.0002% fentanyl during the second stage of labor. *Anesthesiology* 1990;72:613.

Coalson DW, Glosten B. Alternatives to epidural analgesia. *Semin Perinatol* 1991;15:375.

Dan U, Rabinovici Y, Barkai G, et al. Intravenous pethidine and nalbuphine during labor: a prospective double-blind comparative study. *Gynecol Obstet Invest* 1991;32:39.

Douglas MJ. Potential complications of spinal and epidural anesthesia for obstetrics. *Semin Perinatol* 1991;15:368.

Faure EA. The pain of parturition. *Semin Perinatol* 1991;15:342.

Felsby S, Juelsgaard P. Combined spinal and epidural anesthesia. *Anesth Analg* 1995;80:821.

Gribble RK, Meier PR. Effect of epidural analgesia on the primary cesarean rate. *Obstet Gynecol* 1991;78:231.

Guidozzi F, Graham KM, Buchmann EJ, Christophers GJ. The effect of continuous low-dose epidural analgesia on uterine work during the active phase of the first stage of labour. *S Afr Med J* 1992;81:361.

Harke S, Mandell G, Ramanathan S. Patient-controlled epidural analgesia versus continuous infusion for labor pain relief. *Anesth Analg* 1998; 86:S371(abst).

Hawkins JL. New techniques for labor analgesia: IARS 1998 review course lectures. *Anesth Analg* 1998;(suppl):57–60.

Hawkins JL, Hess KR, Joyce T, et al. A reevaluation of the association between instrument delivery and epidural analgesia. *Reg Anesth* 1995;20:50.

Hepner DL, Gaiser RR, Cheek TG, Gutsche BB. Efficacy analysis between the combined spinal-epidural and epidural for labor analgesia. *Anesth Analg* 1998;86:S373(abst).

Hughes SC. Analgesia methods during labour and delivery. *Can J Anaesth* 1992;39:R18.

Hunt CO. Spinal anesthesia for obstetrics. *Int Anesthesiol Clin* 1989;27:26.

Kaplan B, Rabinerson D, Pardo J, Krieser RU, Neri A. Transcutaneous electrical nerve stimulation (TENS) as a pain-relief device in obstetrics and gynecology. *Clin Exp Obstet Gynecol* 1997;24:123–126.

Kaplan B, Rabinerson D, Lurie S, Bar J, Krieser UR, Neri A. Transcutaneous electrical nerve stimulation (TENS) for adjuvant pain-relief during labor and delivery. *Int J Gynaecol Obstet* 1998;60:251–255.

Lieberman E, Lang JM, Cohen BA, et al. Association of epidural analgesia with cesarean delivery in nulliparas. *Obstet Gynecol* 1996;88:993.

Lowenwirt I, Cohen S, Zephyr J, et al. Can prophylactic epidural blood patch reduce the incidence and severity of postpartum dural puncture headache in obstetrics? *Anesth Analg* 1998;86:S378(abst).

Macarthur AJ, Macarthur C, Weeks SK. Is epidural anesthesia in labor associated with chronic low back pain? A prospective cohort study. *Anesth Analg* 1997;85:1066.

Maroof M, Hakin S, Khan RM, Ahmed S. Low-dose ketamine infusion is effective in relieving labor pain. *Anesth Analg* 1998;86:S380(abst).

McIntosh DG, Rayburn WF. Patient-controlled analgesia in obstetrics and gynecology. *Obstet Gynecol* 1991;78:1129.

Miller AC. The effects of epidural analgesia on uterine activity and labor. *Int J Obstet Anesth* 1997;6:2.

Morton SC, Williams MS, Keeler EB, Kahn KL. Effect of epidural analgesia for labor on the cesarean delivery rate. *Obstet Gynecol* 1994;83:1045.

Nageotte MP, Larson D, Rumney P, et al. Epidural analgesia compared with combined spinal-epidural analgesia during labor in nulliparous women. *N Engl J Med* 1997;337:1715.

Naulty JS. Continuous infusions of local anesthetics and narcotics for epidural analgesia in the management of labor. *Int Anesthesiol Clin* 1990;28:17.

Naulty JS, Smith R, Ross R. Effect of changes in labor analgesic practice on labor outcome. *Anesthesiology* 1998;69:A660(abst).

Pan PH, Moore C, Fragneto R, et al. Do obstetric outcomes differ between early combined spinal-epidural and epidural anesthesia in spontaneously laboring nulliparous parturients? *Anesth Analg* 1998;86:S382(abst).

Paterson CM, Saunders NS, Wadsworth J. The characteristics of the second stage of labour in 25,069 singleton deliveries in the North West Thames Health Region, 1988. *Br J Obstet Gynaecol* 1992;99:377.

Pilkington S, Carli F, Dakin MJ, et al. Increase in Mallampati score during pregnancy. *Br J Anaesth* 1995;74:638.

Ploeckinger B, Ulm MR, Chalubinski K, Gruber W. Epidural anaesthesia in labour: influence on surgical delivery rates, intrapartum fever and blood loss. *Gynecol Obstet Invest* 1995;39:24.

Ramin SM, Gambling DR, Lucas MJ, et al. Randomized trial of epidural versus intravenous analgesia during labor. *Obstet Gynecol* 1995;86:783.

Rayburn WF, Leuschen MP, Earl R, et al. Intravenous meperidine during labor: a randomized comparison between nursing- and patient-controlled administration. *Obstet Gynecol* 1989;74:702.

Rayburn WF, Rathke A, Leuschen MP, et al. Fentanyl citrate analgesia during labor. *Am J Obstet Gynecol* 1989;161:202.

Rojansky N, Tanos V, Reubinoff B, et al. Effect of epidural analgesia on duration of outcome of induced labor. *Int J Gynaecol Obstet* 1997;56:237.

Rosenblatt WH, Cioffi AM, Sinatra R, et al. Metoclopramide: an analgesic adjunct to patient-controlled analgesia. *Anesth Analg* 1991;73:553.

Saunders NS, Paterson CM, Wadsworth J. Neonatal and maternal morbidity in relation to the length of the second stage of labour. *Br J Obstet Gynaecol* 1992;99:381.

Steiger RM, Nageotte MP. Effect of uterine contractility and maternal hypotension on prolonged decelerations after bupivacaine epidural anesthesia. *Am J Obstet Gynecol* 1990;163:808.

Thorp JA, McNitt JD, Leppert PC. Effects of epidural analgesia: some questions and answers. *Birth* 1990;17:157.

Trolle B, Moller M, Kronborg H, Thomsen S. The effect of sterile water blocks on low back labor pain. *Am J Obstet Gynecol* 1991;164:1277.

Turcot L, Marcoux S, Fraser WD, et al. Multivariate analysis of risk factors for operative delivery in nulliparous women. *Am J Obstet Gynecol* 1997;176:395–402.

Van Zundert A, Vaes L, Soetens M, et al. Are breech deliveries an indication for lumbar epidural analgesia? *Anesth Analg* 1991;72:399.

Warner MA, Warner ME, Weber JG. Clinical significance of pulmonary aspiration during the perioperative period. *Anesthesiology* 1993;78:56–62.

Westmore MD. Epidural opioids in obstetrics—a review. *Anaesth Intensive Care* 1990;18:292.

Wiklund RA, Rosenbaum SH. Anesthesiology. *Med Prog* 1997;337:1215.

Yau G, Gin T, Ewart MC, et al. Propofol for induction and maintenance of anaesthesia at caesarean section: a comparison with thiopentone/enflurane. *Anaesthesia* 1991;46:20.

CHAPTER 9

Newborn Assessment and Care

◊

Robert M. Nelson
Carine I. Stromquist
Lance E. Wyble

This chapter reviews important issues related to the transition from fetus to newborn and assessment and care issues of the newborn in the first minutes to days of life. Emphasis is placed on a review of neonatal resuscitation, the initial physical examination of the newborn, and the problems of meconium aspiration and sepsis. We have attempted to use recent review articles, which means that original articles and primary research are not directly referenced. The Cochrane Library was also used, as data in it come from a wide range of bibliographic databases, including unpublished evidence. Neonatal clinical problems are being addressed by combining these sources and developing expert opinions (http://hiru.hirunet.mcmaster.ca/cochrane/). Because of the relative ease of updating such sources, they may increasingly play an essential part in evaluating new therapies.

◊ FETUS-TO-NEONATE TRANSITION

The transition from life as a fetus to life as a newborn is among the most perilous and complicated trips that any human will make. At birth, an infant must make the change from dependence on mother and placenta to independence.[22] The lung must establish itself as an organ of gas exchange by clearing lung liquid, as well as secreting surfactant so that it does not collapse with each expiration. Blood must now perfuse the lung. Changes in vascular pressures as a result of this increased pulmonary blood flow and clamping of the umbilical cord, close shunts (foramen ovale and ductus arteriosus) that were present *in utero*.[10] An infant must establish a consistent and persistent respiratory pattern to ensure adequate ventilation. Finally, temperature regulation, likewise previously dependent on the mother, now must activate systems not utilized *in utero* (nonshivering thermogenesis).[23] All of these and many other quantitatively less immediate important changes may be affected by the normal changes of labor. The

process of active labor results in an intermittent decrease in uterine blood flow, leading to increased levels of carbon dioxide, decreased levels of oxygen, and acidemia. For example, the interplay of hypercarbia, hypoxia, and acidosis may have an adverse effect on the dilation of the pulmonary vascular bed, thereby shunting blood away from the lung and increasing hypoxia, hypercarbia, and acidosis. Inadequate response to environmental temperature may similarly affect an infant's ability to make this transition.[13] The catecholamine surge, especially norepinephrine release, plays a major role in this transition. Norepinephrine causes cessation of fetal lung liquid secretion but is also important in producing the newborn's ability to establish nonshivering thermogenesis.

◊ RESUSCITATION

Resuscitation of the newborn should begin before complete asphyxia, defined as progressive hypoxemia, hypercarbia, and acidosis that ultimately results in multiorgan system disease. Two clinical situations that most closely resemble the total asphyxia seen in animal models are complete compression of fetal vessels (prolapsed cord) and total premature separation of the placenta (abruption). Undoubtedly, the more common situation is partial asphyxia. The infant's response to this challenge is dependent on its history and the level of asphyxia.

Data from animal models of total asphyxia demonstrate specific changes in respiratory pattern, heart rate, and blood pressure. There is an initial period of rapid breathing followed by a period of primary apnea. A period of secondary apnea follows and, if prolonged, results in the inability to resuscitate the individual. Infants seen in primary apnea can easily be resuscitated. However, one is not able to prospectively determine primary from secondary apnea, and therefore in infants one must always assume that secondary apnea is occurring.

131

After the initial period of heart rate acceleration, corresponding to the onset of primary apnea, bradycardia will develop and persist when resuscitation occurs. Blood pressure will increase until the time of irregular gasping occurs between primary and secondary apnea and then will begin to fall. Once the blood pressure has decreased beyond 50% of the premorbid state, resuscitation becomes progressively more difficult. Events such as cold or material in the mouth and trachea will prolong resuscitation.[3]

◊ MATERNAL–FETAL HISTORY

It should be noted that the need for resuscitation might have nothing to do with the birth process itself; various conditions will result in a depressed newborn. The individual responsible for the resuscitation of that newborn should be conversant with these possibilities. They can be divided into two categories: those primarily related to the mother and those primarily related to the infant.

Mother-related issues often involve a maternal drug history of both recreational drug use (e.g., cocaine or heroin) and therapeutic drugs taken during the pregnancy or labor (e.g., meperidine). More women with chronic diseases that would not previously have allowed successful pregnancy are now able to conceive and carry a pregnancy. It is important that physicians caring for newborns be aware of the effects of maternally used medications on infants. Maternal analgesia history during labor and delivery is of obvious importance. Any history suggestive of viral infections or acute bacterial infection (chorioamnionitis) during labor is also important. Sepsis in the neonatal period has all of the signs and symptoms that one associates with asphyxia; however, it requires additional therapies.

Infant-related conditions include prematurity, congenital anomalies involving the airway, congenital diaphragmatic hernias, or central nervous system lesions. The presence of meconium in the amniotic fluid represents a special case that is considered more thoroughly later.

◊ EQUIPMENT, DRUGS, AND PEOPLE

An understanding of and familiarity with the appropriate equipment and drugs are essential in resuscitation. The major piece of equipment is a radiant heater for warming an infant. Today, these generally come equipped for providing oxygen and suctioning and have drawers for additional equipment such as laryngoscopes and endotracheal tubes. Each brand is slightly different, and practitioners should familiarize themselves with important parts before needing to use it. Laryngoscopes and their blades should be checked regularly. Batteries and bulbs can malfunction with aging. The most commonly used Miller type is 0 or 1 in size.

Resuscitation bags can be either the anesthesia type, in which the practitioner controls a valve that determines the pressure delivered and inflation of the bag, or the self-inflating type. The latter is preferred, since it's less likely that too high a pressure will inadvertently be used during the resuscitation. Regardless of the type of bag, it should be checked before it is needed to ensure proper functioning. Oxygen delivery and suction capabilities similarly need to be present and functioning.

According to the American Academy of Pediatrics and American Heart Association Neonatal Resuscitation Program (NRP), only a few drugs are needed in the delivery room.[3] Epinephrine, sodium bicarbonate, naloxone, and volume expanders are the essentials. Naloxone needs to be available to reverse maternal narcotic analgesics. Pressor agents such as dopamine are less commonly used in the delivery room, although they may be needed to support blood pressure after the initial phase of the resuscitation. As with the equipment, it is essential for practitioners involved in resuscitation to know the dosages and delivery routes of each of these agents.

◊ PROCEDURES

Successful resuscitation is dependent on having trained and efficient personnel whose focus is on the infant. The particular disciplines available will vary among institutions. However, physicians, nurses, and respiratory therapists may each have essential roles. The pediatric physician as head of the team, if present, should assign specific duties to each of the other disciplines to ensure that all parts of the resuscitation are being efficiently accomplished. It is the goal of the NRP to assure that at least one individual trained in resuscitation of the newborn is present at each delivery. Pursuant to that, each hospital that delivers infants should ensure that NRP-qualified individuals are available for every birth. Resuscitation of the newborn is most effective when it is individualized to the response of the patient. The NRP, as with other formalized resuscitation skill-building certifications, emphasizes that all activities done should be viewed as a decision/action evaluation cycle. Therefore, if the appropriate action is decided on and performed and the expected response does not occur for any given patient, then further evaluation and actions are indicated.

The initial steps in resuscitation of the newborn are outlined in Figure 1. As with resuscitation of older patients, the hallmark of effective neonatal resuscitation is establishment of an airway, consistent respirations or breathing, and maintenance of the circulation. Important signs of the infant's status are its respirations, heart rate, and color. Figure 1 outlines the steps to be taken for infants who respond to measures prior to the use of drugs. The infant is first placed under a radiant warmer and thoroughly dried. Suctioning of the mouth and nose should occur. Presence of meconium in the amniotic fluid represents a specific issue that will be discussed separately.

If there are spontaneous respirations and the heart rate is above 100 beats per minute, the skin color is then evaluated and oxygen is given if necessary. If no respirations are present or those present appear to be ineffective, a bag and mask should be used to provide respiratory support. In general, a positive pressure of 15 to 20 cm of water is needed to ex-

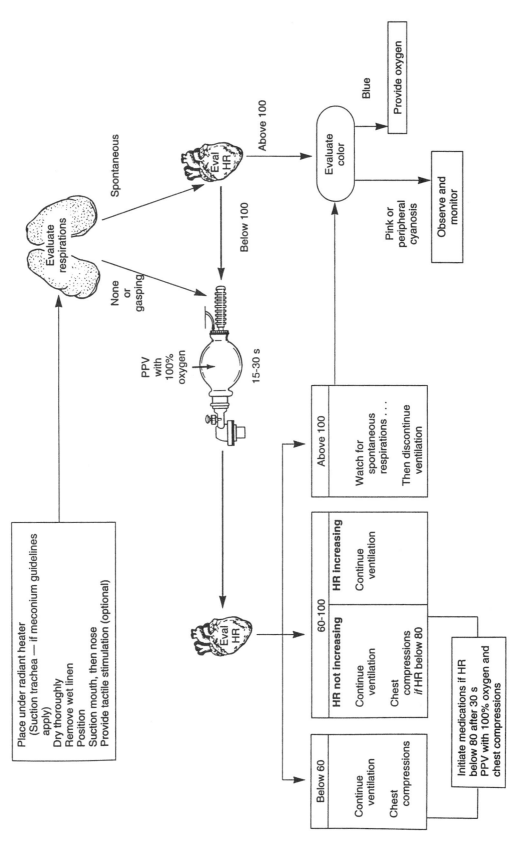

FIG. 1. Initial decision points and actions of resuscitation. (Adapted from ref. 3.)

pand the lung. In some situations, especially in the infant with lung disease, a greater pressure may be required. Once this is begun, the heart rate is determined. If it is now above 100 beats/minute, one can delay further actions and watch for spontaneous respirations. If bag-and-mask positive pressure ventilation has occurred for some time, the carbon dioxide level may have been lowered to such an extent that a few moments need to pass for the infant to develop respiratory stimulation to breathe.

If the heart rate is below 60 beats/minute, positive pressure ventilation is continued, and chest compressions should begin. The indications for bag-and-mask ventilation versus direct endotracheal intubation depend on the need for prolonged ventilatory support and other factors, including the available skills. All individuals who may be placed in the position of resuscitating newborns should have demonstrated proficiency in bag-and-mask ventilation. It should be remembered that the NRP does not by itself certify an individual in the ability to place an endotracheal tube.

The use of medications for resuscitation is shown in Figure 2. When the heart rate is very low or not present, epinephrine via the endotracheal tube or into an umbilical vein is then indicated. For prolonged resuscitation, there should be some consideration of giving sodium bicarbonate. If there is any evidence or suspicion of acute blood loss or signs of hypovolemia, volume expanders can be given. This can be as albumin, normal saline, or perhaps other agents. Recent data suggest that normal saline may have advantages over albumin, including cost. Administration of a volume expander may need to be repeated if evidence of hypovolemia persists. With severe asphyxia, some signs may suggest hypovolemia. If used in this setting, volume expansion should be done slowly, since the issue may be cardiac contractility rather than inadequate intravascular volume. When low blood pressure persists, one should consider starting dopamine. At that point, one should also consider other entities that may be affecting the ability to resuscitate, including pneumothorax. If the mother has received narcotics for analgesia within 4 hours before delivery, naloxone may reverse the effects of the drugs.

◊ APGAR SCORES

The Apgar score has been used for almost 50 years as a way of assessing the status of newborns. Almost all newborns in the United States have 1- and 5-minute Apgar scores assigned to them. However, the Apgar score has taken on meanings over its 40-year history beyond that either intended or appropriate.[8] Although the Apgar score is not determined until 1 minute of age, resuscitation of an infant should not wait until then. The individual practitioner should immediately examine the baby after birth to determine the appropriate response. The NRP recommends that Apgar scores be assigned every 5 minutes up until 20 minutes or until two scores are 8 or greater. While this undoubtedly suggests something about the status of the infant at those times, it gives additional infor-

mation on prognosis. Apgar scores are of limited use alone to predicate long-term central nervous system outcome.[16] Cerebral palsy can occur in infants with normal Apgar scores.

◊ MECONIUM

Meconium is the first fecal material that a fetus or newborn eliminates. In 8% to 20% of deliveries, meconium is passed *in utero.* Aspiration of meconium into the fetal or neonatal airway can result in severe pulmonary disease with a risk of death. In the mid-1970s, several studies suggested that early intervention by the obstetrician and pediatrician resulted in a markedly decreased incidence of meconium aspiration syndrome (MAS).[6] Interventions consisted of suctioning of the oropharynx by the obstetrician with the head at the perineum and then tracheal suctioning by the neonatal physician by direct laryngoscopy. The majority of published studies were either nonrandomized nor controlled. The weight of evidence for a decrease in MAS incidence resulted in a change in practice pattern, so that standard of care became suctioning by the obstetrician and pediatrician. Later studies, however, reported that MAS was not totally eliminated.[24] In 1988, Linder et al.[15] reported on a randomized trial of selective tracheal suction. Infants who had a normal 1-minute Apgar score, a normal vaginal delivery, and spontaneous breathing before being handed to the pediatrician, and were suctioned demonstrated a higher incidence of respiratory complications than those who were not suctioned. Yoder[25] also suggested that a selective approach was indicated. An expert panel suggested that for the infant who was vigorous at birth with thin meconium and whose oropharynx had been suctioned, tracheal intubation is not indicated.[9] Only the Linder et al.[15] study was randomized, controlled, and prospective.

At present, the recommendations are as follows:

◊ Careful suctioning of the oropharynx with the head at the perineum is indicated.
◊ For infants who are depressed, suctioning via an endotracheal tube is indicated prior to positive pressure ventilation. (While data suggest that such infants may have shorter courses, changes in incidence of MAS are not noted.)
◊ Tracheal suctioning is indicated if meconium is thick and contains particulate material.
◊ Endotracheal suctioning is not indicated if meconium is thin in an active infant who has had oropharyngeal suctioning.

It is clear that while the policies of the last 20 years and more have resulted in decreased morbidity, a number of issues are still unresolved and/or controversial. Readers are referred to the work of Wiswell and Bent[24] and Katz and Bowes[14] for an understanding of the two most disparate views. The former authors are convinced that the more aggressive approach to suctioning is probably indicated. The latter authors are equally convinced that MAS is a complex entity that occurs *in utero* and tracheal suctioning should not

Medications
Epinephrine
Volume Expander
Sodium Bicarbonate

Dopamine

Naloxone
Hydrochloride

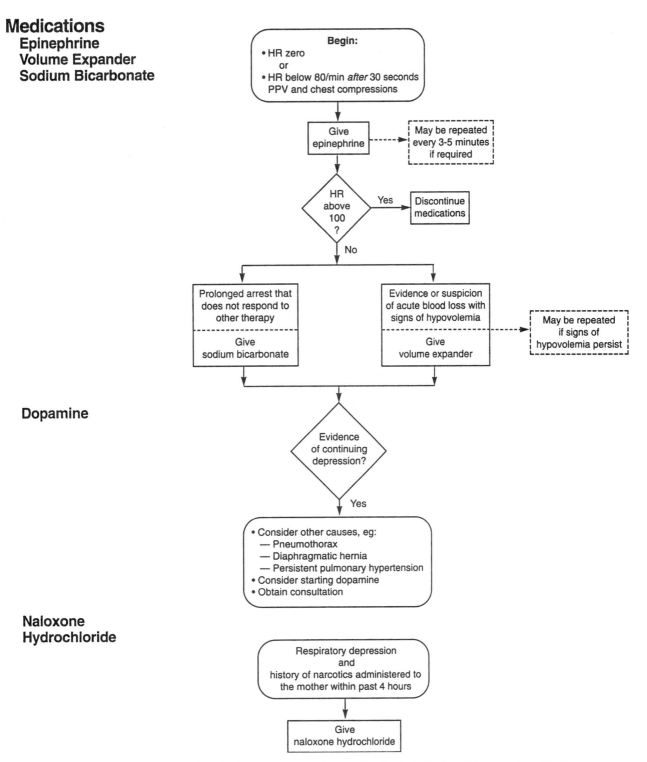

FIG. 2. Decision points and action items of the most severely affected infant and the use of medications. (Adapted from ref. 3.)

be performed in the vigorous term infant. Both utilize, however, either retrospective studies or inferential data to make their points.

Amnioinfusion has been suggested as a way of improving the outcome in such patients. However, a recent review by

Glantz and Letteney[12] came to the conclusion that it has not proven effective in reducing MAS.

One of the decision points for the management of meconium-stained amniotic fluid is its consistency. The consistency of the amniotic fluid with meconium in it is dependent on its volume and the volume of meconium evacuated into the amniotic space. The majority of studies on prevention of MAS do not quantify this consistency; they only describe it as thin and watery at one extreme and like thick pea soup with particles at the other. We are not aware of any studies that either demonstrate interobserver reliability in describing its consistency or quantify its consistency by other means. There are other unresolved issues. Recent studies suggest that meconium-stained amniotic fluid is associated with increased maternal infectious morbidity and the use of antibiotic prophylaxis may decrease these problems.[1] The authors support the recommendations noted earlier in this chapter but would suggest that additional studies are warranted to resolve the issues.

◊ NEWBORN ASSESSMENT AND INITIAL CARE

After the initial evaluation and therapy required for resuscitation, a more thorough examination of the patient should occur. This can be done within a few minutes of birth to be followed by a complete examination at 12 to 24 hours of age.

A review of maternal history will point to portions of the examination that require increased attention. The offspring of the mother with juvenile-onset diabetes mellitus should be thoroughly examined for evidence of congenital malformations, hypoglycemia, and respiratory distress. Mothers with exposures to viruses such as cytomegalovirus or to therapeutic and/or recreational drugs may have infants with particular physical features. Finally, any abnormal prenatal ultrasound findings emphasize specific areas of the examination.

General Appearance

Gestational age assessment is an essential component of the examination. A standard examination is used to assess gestational age.[2] Infants who are either premature or postmature are at risk for conditions requiring specific follow-up. Plotting the weight, length, and head circumference versus gestational age identifies small- and large-for-age infants.

The importance of assessing the infant's general appearance must be emphasized. Infants go through phases of activity in the first hours of life. A baby who is active and crying, whose color is pink, and who is in no cardiorespiratory distress is most likely making a good transition to postnatal life. An infant whose body is cyanotic or pale needs further investigation. An organized look at the baby lying on the warmer will allow the practitioner to recognize when a more extensive examination is needed. For example, an infant who is moving only one arm might suggest the need to consider Erb's palsy of the affected arm.

The nurse attending the infant normally takes vital signs. Respiration rate should normally be 40 to 60 and heart rate between 120 and 160 beats/minute. The temperature will reflect maternal core temperature but may fall rapidly by 2° to 3°C if appropriate drying and wrapping did not occur. Changes in these vital signs from the abnormal toward the

normal over brief periods of time are more important than initial abnormal findings.

Cardiovascular Assessment

Examination of the heart and lungs prior to disturbing the infant may be most productive. Evidence of poor perfusion—a pale appearance or prolonged capillary refill time beyond 3 seconds—suggests the need for further evaluation. The presence of a hyperactive precordium may suggest cardiac anomalies. The heart is best heard at the left lower sternal border. The practitioner should remember that it is easier to hear normal flow turbulence in an infant; hence, murmurs are frequently heard. Closing of the patent ductus arteriosus can also result in the presence of a murmur. Examination of the pulses for equality on both sides and presence in the lower extremities may suggest problems such as coarctation of the aorta. Blood pressure readings are not routinely done in the first hours after birth but deferred till later, unless signs such as poor perfusion are present.

Assessment of Chest and Lungs

Observation of the chest for asymmetries may point toward conditions such as pneumothorax or malformations of the chest wall. In the first 1 to 2 hours after birth, it is common to see infants with respiratory rates slightly higher than normal. If this value is improving and the infant's color is normal, watchful waiting is indicated. Today, the availability of pulse oximetry allows the infant's oxygen levels to be determined easily. An infant who is having periods of apnea or is showing increased work of breathing by retractions requires more extensive investigation. The presence of equal breath sounds is important while listening to the chest. However, especially with small infants, the presence of equal breath sound does not eliminate the possibility of pneumothorax, since the chest is small enough to transmit sounds. It is uncommon to hear many rales or rhonchi after the first few breaths. Persistence of these findings suggests the need for further investigation. Stridor, an extra sound during inspiration or expiration audible by the unaided ear, should be investigated. Grunting, nature's way of providing positive end-expiratory pressure, that lasts beyond a few minutes suggests pulmonary disease.

Head Assessment

Visual inspection of the head may identify hemangiomas or wounds at the site of scalp electrodes. With vaginal births, molding of the head occurs and is associated with edema of the scalp (caput succedaneum). If a vacuum device was used to deliver the infant, discoloration of the scalp may be noted at the site. Cephalohematoma, a subperiosteal hemorrhage confined to a single bone, occurs during the birth but becomes more obvious on days 2 and 3 of life. Cranial sutures should be examined to determine whether they are fused, narrow, or wide. There is a broad range of normal. The presence of craniotabes, softening of bone especially in the area close to the suture line, is neither uncommon nor pathologic. A similar feeling throughout the skull is a greater concern.

Assessment of Eyes, Ears Nose and Throat

Examination of the face may provide important information. Abnormal positioning of the eyes—either too wide or too narrow—and gross malformations of the eye can be noted immediately. Asymmetry of the face may suggest specific malformation syndromes. The oral cavity examination in an otherwise normal infant can be confined to its gross appearance. A practitioner may use a small finger to feel the palate for posterior clefts. Frequently, retention cysts, called Epstein's pearls, are observed on the alveolar ridge. Choanal atresia should be susepcted when a baby cannot breathe unless its mouth is open. Attempts to pass catheters through the nares can suggest the need for further workup. Examination of the neck for webbing or dermal fistula is important. Abnormally low-placed ears or abnormally formed ear lobes may be indicative of a syndrome.

Abdomen Assessment

Immediate observation should demonstrate any wall defects or the appearance of a concave or convex abdomen, which may suggest the presence of a diaphragmatic hernia or abdominal masses. The umbilical cord is examined for the presence of two arteries and a vein. If only two vessels are found, anomalies should be suspected. The abdominal examination by palpation is perhaps best done in the immediate postbirth period because the wall is most relaxed at that point. The liver edge is palpable to 1 to 2 cm, and both kidneys and the spleen may be normally palpable.

Genital–Perineal Assessment

Male and female external genitalia show gestational age differences. Female infants may have small vaginal tags. An imperforate hymen may be associated with obstruction of the urinary system. Male infants with the presence of scrotal masses such as hydrocele are common. The presence of a painful mass with bluish discoloration should lead to investigation for testicular torsion by ultrasound. The presence of ambiguous-appearing genitalia should result in further evaluation. Some advocate obtaining a rectal temperature to ensure patency of the rectum.

Back and Extremities Assessment

The back should be examined for any midline lesions. Assessment of the extremities should include their movement. The Moro reflex may demonstrate asymmetry of movements of the upper extremities. The hips should be examined for evidence of dislocation. Syndactyly or polydactyly may in some cases suggest specific syndromes. Extra digits connected only by a narrow neurovascular pedicle may be familial.

Skin Examination

A preterm infant's skin is thin and translucent, whereas a term infant's skin is thicker. During the first 6 to 24 hours especially, peripheral vascular lability results in a variety of skin findings. Classic acrocyanosis or blue appearance of the peripheral extremities is normal. A less common finding is the harlequin sign, a difference in body color from the right to the left side, which, while dramatic, is not physiologically important. The presence of petechiae throughout much of the body's surface may imply thrombocytopenia or other clotting abnormalities. Petechiae confined only to the presenting part or the head and neck in the presence of a nuchal cord imply only a pressure phenomenon. A baby who has a ruddy complexion may have an elevated hematocrit and blood hyperviscosity, while a pale infant may have a low hematocrit. The presence of nevi, hemangioma, and scalp defects should be noted.

Milia in neonates are most commonly seen on the nose. A dramatic-appearing rash is neonatal pustular melanosis, which appears as white pustular lesions that later become hyperpigmented. It should not be confused with vesicular lesions, such as those from herpes simplex virus. Though not clinically important, mongolian spots are deeply pigmented areas, noted most commonly on the buttocks and in dark-skinned infants. Jaundice in the first 24 hours always requires further investigation.

Neurobehavioral Examination

The neurobehavioral examination changes over the first minutes and hours of life. Maternal conditions and gestational age also affect these findings. The initial examination and findings are best interpreted by these evaluations over time.

The term infant normally stays in a flexed position. The preterm infant, in contrast, has extremities that are extended. Any asymmetry of position or movement should be noted. A lethargic infant or one who is very jittery requires immediate further evaluation. The presence of extra movements—of a random nature—should be noted for duration, effect on any cardiorespiratory signs, and whether or not they cease or start when an infant is stimulated to assist in the diagnosis of seizures.

The behavior of infants in these first minutes and hours of birth has been well studied. The first period of activity lasts between 15 and 30 minutes; infants are quite vigorous and responsive. From 1 to 2 hours, infants are usually in a quiet, alert state. This is an excellent time for parents to spend time with an infant, undisturbed by the medical team. The rapid initial physical examination can be accomplished before this, so that parents and infant can be undisturbed. Infants will then go through a sleep period between 2 and 6 hours of age followed by a second period of reactivity. During this time, they may be somewhat more tachypneic and pass meconium.

◊ ROUTINE CARE ISSUES

Most nurseries have specific protocols as to which laboratory tests are routinely performed. Protocols are based on the likelihood of either finding an abnormality or not missing one. The most common test is blood glucose screening. Most infants screened have risk factors, such as largeness or smallness for gestational age, maternal diabetes, or maternal drug therapy (e.g., β-mimetics). Routine screening of hematocrit depends on specific clinical findings in an infant: A plethoric-appearing infant is at risk for an elevated hematocrit, whereas a pale infant may have a low hematocrit. The normal hematocrit in neonates is between 45 and 60 ml/dl. Hematocrits above 70 ml/dl and below 40 ml/dl need further investigation. Most states have mandated screening for some inborn errors of metabolism, such as phenylketonuria and hypothyroidism. This usually occurs at 48 hours after birth but may be mandated at other specific times and/or on discharge. It should be noted that certain maternal diseases, such as human immunodeficiency virus infection, require specific testing in the infant.

Vitamin K for prevention of hemorrhagic disease should be given to all infants. This should be done by injection, since oral dosing does not totally prevent the disease. Eye prophylaxis against *Neisseria gonorrhoeae* conjunctivitis should also be performed. Hepatitis B vaccine is recommended for all newborns. If the mother's hepatitis B status is not known in the first 12 hours, then not only a vaccine but also hepatitis B immune globulin should be administered.[21] If the mother is positive for hepatitis B surface antigen, the infant should receive the immune globulin within 7 days.

◊ PARENT CARE

It would be inappropriate not to mention the care of the family, as the parents will be the ongoing caregivers of the infant. Providing the family–infant group appropriate care and information at this time is important. The infant's first period of quiet, alert state 30 minutes to 2 hours after birth can be used to establish breast-feeding. Physicians who deliver infants and have an understanding of the initial examination and assessment of newborns may allay the the mother or father's concerns.

◊ NEONATAL SEPSIS

The early diagnosis of neonatal bacterial sepsis remains a difficult task. Delayed treatment may result in preventable morbidity or mortality. Outcome evaluations consistently demonstrate advantages to careful patient selection, whether the clinician is considering intrapartum antibiotic prophylaxis for the mother or empiric antibiotic therapy for the neonate. A significant problem of neonatal sepsis is that it may start with nonspecific symptoms. Since treatment of neonatal sepsis is low risk, while the disease is high risk, clinical practice has dictated that more babies than are actually later documented to have infection are evaluated and treated in intensive care nurseries. Improvement in diagnostic accuracy is a necessary requirement in a world pressured by shrinking revenue and family expectations of earlier discharge following delivery. Risk of empiric antibiotic therapy includes alteration of normal flora, intravenous infiltrates, and risk of invasive disease due to resistant flora. Clinicians must pay careful attention to the prenatal history to assess the risk of sepsis in newborns. Asymptomatic infants at high risk should receive empiric antibiotic therapy pending culture results, whereas those at low risk may be evaluated and observed. Medium-risk infants are either treated or observed, depending on the relative risk of suspected sepsis by the clinician. While clinician behavior has continued to be inconsistent, it is hoped that clinicians will understand the single and additive risk for various historical factors and implement a rational approach to patient management. Each physician should determine a risk level, based on specific evidence, at which he or she will treat empirically with antibiotics. Gerdes[11] has summarized the increased risk for sepsis seen with specific clinical factors. In general, these factors increase the risk from 0.8% to as high as 10%. The data also suggest that different factors may result in similar risks. For example, a term infant with prolonged rupture of membranes and chorioamnionitis should be managed in the same way as a preterm infant with prolonged rupture of membranes but no amnionitis, based on equivalent risk (3% to 8%). Other clinical settings that should prompt great suspicion of neonatal sepsis are hemodynamic instability, transient abdominal distension, 5-minute Apgar score less than 6, and unexplained elevated bilirubin levels.

Adjunctive Testing for Sepsis of the Newborn

The difficulties in accurately identifying the septic neonate have prompted evaluation of many adjunctive tests to indicate infection. Because of the severity of the disease, high sensitivity and high negative predictive accuracy are optimal. To achieve these goals, however, one must be willing to treat some infants who are not truly infected and thereby accept a lower specificity and a lower positive predictive accuracy. The most frequently used adjunctive test is the white blood cell (WBC) and the differential cell counts. The past decade has witnessed an increased use of these values through the establishment of normal reference ranges for total neutrophil count and indices of immature neutrophils.[16] The stated lower limits for normal total neutrophil count in newborns begins at 1800 cells/mm^3, rises to 7200/mm^3 at 12 hours of age, and then declines and persists at 1800/mm^3 beyond 72 hours of age. A similar time curve has been demonstrated for the total immature neutrophil count, which peaks at 1400/mm^3 at 12 hours of age, and the ratio of immature to total neutrophils (I/T ratio), which is 0.16 or less at birth and declines to a peak value of 0.12 beyond 72 hours of age. Neutropenia is believed to be the best predictor of sepsis, whereas neutrophilia does not correlate well. Manroe et al.[16] observed a 100% negative predictive value if the total neutrophil count, immature neutrophil count, and I/T ratio were all normal. Subsequent studies have failed to identify such a reliable predictive value in sepsis. Rodwell et al.[20] developed a seven-point hematologic scoring system based on the WBC count, total and immature neutrophil counts and I/T ratio, degenerative changes in neutrophils, and thrombocytopenia. This approach was useful in that a 96% sensitivity and 99% negative predicted value were obtained. However, the pitfalls noted above continued to result in failure to identify all septic infants and left this score as a useful but not definitive test. Additional adjunctive and nonspecific diagnostic tests include C-reactive protein, erythrocyte sedimentation rate, and other acute-phase reactants, as well as direct visualization of bacteria in neutrophils stained by acridine orange after a cytospin or Gram stain and culture of a gastric aspirate. Most of these tests have even lower sensitivity than the WBC parameters.[11] The U.S. Food and Drug Administration has warned against the use of latex agglutination for group B streptococcus identification in neonatal urine. Evaluation has failed to find accuracy using this body fluid. This technique is still useful when used with spinal fluid and blood.

Group B Streptococcus Disease in the Newborn

In May 1996, the Centers for Disease Control and Prevention[7] published recommendations aimed at the prevention of group B streptococcus (GBS) disease in newborns. Two approaches—universal maternal GBS screening at 35 to 37 weeks or identification of risk factors for neonatal sepsis—were adopted for the evaluation and treatment of mothers with or at risk of having GBS disease. Intrapartum antimicrobial prophylaxis (IAP) was recommended for mothers with GBS disease or risk factors associated with a higher risk of maternal GBS disease. A great deal of discussion has been generated as to which mothers should receive IAP. The final recommendations provided an algorithm for empiric management of neonates born to a mother who had received IAP. It is identified as "one possible algorithm," with the suggestion that "other management approaches" developed by physicians may represent appropriate alternatives, such as that shown in Figure 3.

Neonate with Signs Compatible with Sepsis

The most important feature to identify is whether or not the neonate has signs compatible with sepsis. In this situation, clinical judgment is required in deciding the degree of evaluation and whether or not to start therapy. In general, if sepsis cannot be ruled out, a full workup, including blood cultures and a lumbar puncture (if the neonate is stable), is recommended, and therapy is initiated. Neonates with clinical signs compatible with sepsis have died when antibiotic therapy was not started because of reliance on a normal WBC count.[21] Thus, *in the presence of signs compatible with sepsis, especially if evident soon after birth, the decision to start therapy should not be guided by WBC counts.* If the physician decides on clinical grounds that the patient is not septic

and the signs do not warrant further investigation, this is documented in the medical record.

Asymptomatic Neonate at Risk of Sepsis

Key epidemiologic work and randomized, controlled clinical trials in the 1980s demonstrated that prevention of neonatal GBS disease, if possible, depends on a prenatal strategy.[4] This strategy consists of identifying whether a mother (1) is a GBS carrier or (2) has risk factors associated with an increased incidence of neonatal GBS disease. If either of these pertains, then the mother is given IAP, and the risks of colonization and sepsis of the neonate are significantly reduced, but not eliminated. It should be noted that the only controlled trial to show a significant reduction in neonatal sepsis involved not only maternal IAP but also neonatal therapy every 12 hours until cultures proved negative.[4, 18] After birth, the approach to the evaluation and therapy of the asymptomatic neonate varies according to degree of risk and consists of observation alone, limited laboratory evaluation and then observation, or more extensive laboratory evaluation and therapy. The decision also involves considerations of staff availability to care for the babies in the nursery and the experience of staff in recognizing and treating neonatal sepsis. The purpose is to emphasize that clinical judgment should always play a major role in decision making.

Asymptomatic neonates at risk for sepsis can be divided into three groups:

Group 1   Neonates at high risk for sepsis—those less than 34 weeks of age or the sibling of a neonate who had GBS sepsis in this pregnancy (i.e., a twin or other multiple sibling with current GBS sepsis): Immediate evaluation and therapy are recommended.[19]

Group 2   Neonates whose mothers have identified risk factors or have received IAP: Evaluation and therapy will be determined by the specific risk of sepsis according to the number and type of risk factors and the adequacy of maternal IAP (defined as therapy more than 4 hours before delivery).

Group 3   Neonates with no identified risk factors: Observation is appropriate. This group may include neonates whose maternal GBS status was not evaluated.

A normal complete blood cell count with differential at 6 to 12 hours is highly specific for health in the asymptomatic baby.[11] Discharge of asymptomatic at-risk neonates is not advised for at least 48 hours. The family is informed of the plans, and the management strategy is documented in the medical record.

Therapy and Discharge of the Asymptomatic At-risk Neonate

Opinion about the extent of investigation and the time to start therapy varies among physicians, and there are no controlled clinical trials to provide an unbiased answer. With or without

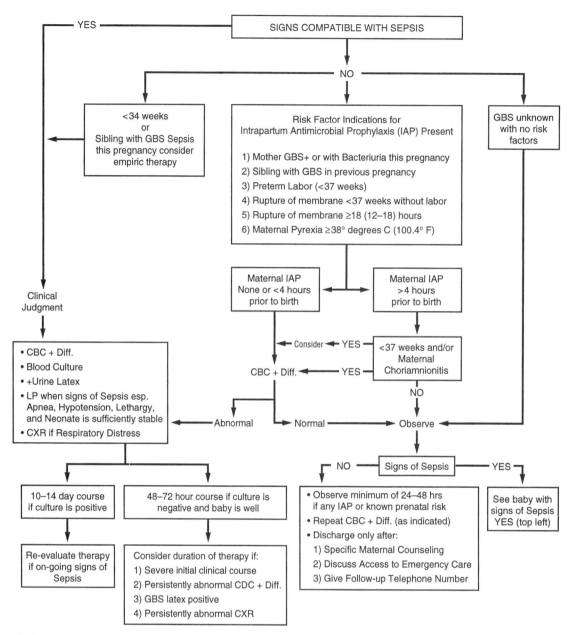

FIG. 3. Algorithm developed by the agency for Health Care Administration, Florida Society of Neonatologists, on the management of the infant with potential neonatal sepsis.

maternal IAP, if asymptomatic at-risk babies remain clinically well and after 2 to 3 days their blood culture report is negative and blood cell counts and differentials are normal, then it is appropriate to stop antibiotics and discharge the babies on the same day. For the treated asymptomatic neonate with a positive blood culture, the duration of antibiotic therapy generally recommended is 10 to 14 days. No clinical controlled trial exists to guide the practitioner.

◊ CONCLUSIONS

Today, medical care teams face pressures to discharge mothers and neonates rapidly. However, when we are uncertain,

medical wisdom dictates that we err on the safe side. Nowhere is this truer than in the case of the asymptomatic newborn baby at risk for sepsis. It is recommended that these babies should not be discharged before 48 hours postnatally. The medical care team must educate both the patient caregivers and medical managers that the current prenatal management strategies aimed at prevention are not foolproof in early neonatal sepsis. The evidence to support current postnatal management approaches is largely of the opinion variety. The development of practice guidelines will assist in defining and refining the basis of therapy. To be useful tools in medical care, practice guidelines should be flexible, updated rapidly as new information surfaces, widely disseminated, and above all based, if possible, on solid research data.[5] In this era of evidence-based medicine and computerized communication, practice guidelines can have a practical impact and stimulate questions and research to improve medical care while minimizing costs.

SUMMARY POINTS

◊ Steps in the transition from fetal to neonatal life include lung liquid clearance and replacement of liquid by gas. Changes in blood flow to the lung, including elimination of vascular shunts, a consistent respiratory pattern, and the ability to control temperature are also necessary. Maternal status may affect this transition.

◊ Effective resuscitation of the newborn depends on the availability of trained practitioners who are efficient and knowledgeable in the resuscitation procedure.

◊ Meconium-stained amniotic fluid should be suctioned from the oral pharynx after delivery of the head. Infants who are depressed at birth, have not had oropharyngeal suctioniong, or are born in thick meconium need tracheal suctioning. Amnioinfusion has not eliminated the risk of MAS.

◊ Knowledge of the normal neonate examination can assist the practitioner in identifying at-risk infants, while providing initial information to the parents.

◊ Reduction in early-onset sepsis in the neonate requires the joint efforts of the obstetric practitioner and the pediatric practitioner to treat at-risk mother–infant dyads. A management algorithm is presented.

◊ REFERENCES

1. Adair C, Ernest J, Sanchez-Ramos L, et al. Meconium-stained fluid-associated infectious morbidity: A randomized, double-blind trial of ampicillin-sulbactam prophylaxis. *Obstet Gynecol* 1996;88:216–220.
2. Ballard J, Khoury J, Wedig K, et al. New Ballard score: expanded to include extremely premature infants. *J Pediatr* 1991;119:417–423.
3. Bloom R, Cropley C, the AHA/AAP Neonatal Resuscitation Program Steering Committee. *Textbook of neonatal resuscitation.* Philadelphia: American Heart Association, 1995.
4. Boyer K, Gotoff S. Prevention of early-onset neonatal group B streptococcal disease with selective intrapartum chemoprophylaxis. *N Engl J Med* 1986:314:1665–1669.
5. Campazzi E, Lee D. How to assess clinical guidelines In: Casanova J, ed. *Tools for the task: role of clinical guidelines.* Tampa, FL: American College of Physician Executives, 1997:77–92.
6. Carson B, Losey R, Bowes W, et al. Combined obstetric and pediatric approach to prevent meconium aspiration syndrome. *Am J Obstet Gynecol* 1976;126:712–715.
7. Centers for Disease Control and Prevention. Perinatal group B streptococcal disease: a public health perspective. *MMWR* 1996:45(no. RR-7): 1–24.
8. Committee on Fetus and Newborn, American Academy of Pediatrics, and Committee on Obstetrics Practice, American College of Obstetricians and Gynecologists. Use and abuse of the Apgar score. *Pediatrics* 1996:98:141–142.
9. Committee on Neonatal Ventilation/Meconium/Chest Compressions. Guidelines proposed at the 1992 National Conference on Cardiopulmonary Resuscitation and Emergency Cardiac Care, Dallas. *JAMA* 1992:268:2276–2281.
10. Friedman A, Fahey J. The transition from fetal to neonatal circulation. *Semin Perinatol* 1993;17:106–121.
11. Gerdes J. Clinicopathologic approach to the diagnosis of neonatal sepsis. *Clin Perinatol* 1991;18:361–380.
12. Glantz JC, Letteney DL. Pumps and warmers during amniofusion: is either necessary? *Obstet Gynecol* 1996;87:150–155.
13. Hopper S. Fetal metabolic response to hypoxia. *Reprod Fertil Dev* 1995;7:527–538.
14. Katz V, Bowes W. Meconium aspiration syndrome: reflections on a murky subject. *Am J Obstet Gynecol* 1992;166:171–183.
15. Linder N, Aranda J, Tsur M, et al. Need for endotracheal intubation and suction in meconium-stained neonates. *J Pediatr* 1988;112:613–615.
16. Manroe B, Weinberg A, Rosenfeld C, et al. The neonatal blood count in health and disease: I. Reference values for neutrophilic cells. *J Pediatr* 1979;95:89–98.
17. Nelson K, Emery E. Birth asphyxia and the neonatal brain: what do we know and when do we know it? *Clin Perinatol* 1993;20:327–344.
18. Ohlsson A, Myhr T. Intrapartum chemoprophylaxis of prenatal group B streptococcal infections: a critical review of randomized controlled trials. *Am J Obstet Gynecol* 1994;170:910–917.
19. *1997 Red book: report on the committee on infectious diseases.* Elk Grove, IL: American Academy of Pediatrics, 1997.
20. Rodwell R, Leslie A, Tudehope D. Early diagnosis of neonatal sepsis using an hematologic scoring system. *J Pediatr* 1988;12:761–767.
21. Rozycki H, Stahl G, Baumgart S. Impaired sensitivity of a single early leukocyte count in screening for neonatal sepsis. *Pediatr Infect Dis J* 1987;6:440–442.
22. Sansoucie D, Cavaliere T. Transition from fetal to extrauterine circulation. *Neonatal Network* 1997;16:5–11.
23. Symonds M, Bird J, Clarke L, et al. Nutrition, temperature and homeostasis during perinatal development. *Exp Physiol* 1995;80:907–940.
24. Wiswell T, Bent R. Meconium staining and the meconium aspirations syndrome. *Pediatr Clin North Am* 1993;40:955–981.
25. Yoder B. Meconium-stained amniotic fluid and respiratory complications: impact of selective tracheal suction. *Obstet Gynecol* 1994; 83:77–84.

CHAPTER 10

Early Pregnancy Loss
◊

James R. Scott

The term *abortion,* which has a negative connotation to many patients, is gradually being replaced by the word *miscarriage.* Both terms originally defined pregnancy losses prior to 20 weeks' gestation, but they were more commonly used by physicians to describe first-trimester losses. These arbitrary time limits have become less useful with advances in developmental biology and diagnostic sonography. The preembryonic period is defined as conception through the first 5 weeks of pregnancy from the first day of the last menstrual period. The embryonic period begins at 6 to 9 weeks' gestation, and the fetal period is from 10 weeks until delivery.

◊ EPIDEMIOLOGY

Human reproduction is relatively inefficient, and miscarriage is the most common complication of pregnancy, with an incidence of approximately 15% among pregnancies that are clinically recognized. However, histologically defective ova found in hysterectomy specimens (Fig. 1) and data on early pregnancies detected only with sensitive β-human chorionic gonadotropin (β-hCG) assays indicate that the very early and often unrecognized pregnancy loss rate is two to three times higher.[1,2] The prevalence of miscarriage also increases with maternal age from 12% in women younger than 20 years of age to over 50% in women older than 45 years of age (Fig. 2).

◊ ETIOLOGY

In view of the complicated genetic, hormonal, immunologic, and cellular events that require precise integration for fertilization and nidation, it is remarkable that successful pregnancy occurs so often. When early pregnancy loss occurs, it can be due to a number of embryonic and parental factors.

Embryonic Factors

Most single sporadic losses are caused by nonrepetitive intrinsic defects in the developing conceptus, such as abnormal germ cells, defective implantation, defects in the developing placenta or embryo, accidental injuries to the fetus, and probably other causes as yet unrecognized. Fifty percent of women presenting with spotting or cramping already have a nonviable conceptus by sonogram, and many of these embryos are morphologically abnormal.[3] About one-third of abortus specimens from losses occurring before 9 weeks' gestation are anembryonic. Some cases of empty gestational sacs or "blighted ova" actually represent pregnancy failures with subsequent embryonic resorption.[4] The high proportion of abnormal aborted conceptuses is apparently the result of a selective process that eliminates about 95% of morphologic and cytogenetic errors.

The frequency of chromosomally abnormal spontaneously aborted products of conception in the first trimester is approximately 60% and decreases to 7% by the end of week 24 (Fig. 3). The rate of genetic abnormalities is even higher in anembryonic miscarriages.[3] Autosomal trisomies are the most common (51.9%), but the relative frequency of each type of trisomy differs considerably.[4,5] Trisomy 16, which accounts for about one-third of all trisomic abortions, has not been reported in liveborn infants and is therefore highly lethal; trisomy 22 and 21 follow in frequency. The next most common chromosomal abnormalities, in decreasing order, are monosomy 45,X (the most common single karyotypic abnormality), triploidy, tetraploidy, translocations, and mosaicism.

Parental Factors

In most instances, the couple is chromosomally normal and an abnormal conceptus occurs in a random, sporadic fashion. In a small percentage of cases, one member of the couple is the carrier of a balanced translocation, and the offspring of these parents may be repeatedly aborted.[5] Media publicity tends to give the impression that a variety of agents such as infections, video display terminals, cigarette smoking, coffee, ethanol, chemical agents, and drugs (see Chapter 13) markedly increase the risk of miscarriage. In reality, extrinsic factors account for very few cases of early pregnancy loss.[5,6]

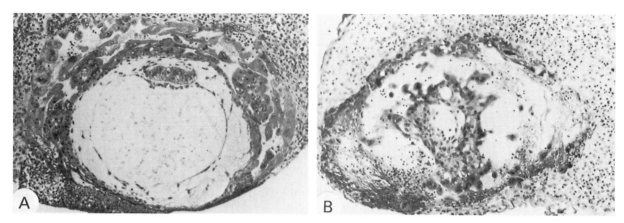

FIG. 1. Histologic comparison of **(A)** a morphologically normally implanted human ovum estimated to be about 11 to 12 days of age with **(B)** an abnormal conceptus, showing a defective trophoblast with pathologically large lacunae and an empty chorionic sac that is destined to abort. (From Hertig AT, Rock J, Adams EC. *Am J Anat* 1956;98:435; with permission.)

◊ PATHOLOGY

Most miscarriages occur within a few weeks after the death of the embryo or rudimentary analog. Initially, there is hemorrhage into the decidua basalis, with necrosis and inflammation in the region of implantation. The conceptus is partially or entirely detached and becomes a foreign body in the uterus. Uterine contractions and dilation of the cervix usually result in expulsion of most or all of the products of conception. When the sac is opened, fluid is often found surrounding a small macerated embryo, or there may be no visible embryo in the sac. Histologically, hydropic degeneration of the placental villi caused by retention of tissue fluid is common.

◊ CLINICAL FEATURES AND TREATMENT

An unrecognized pregnancy episode should always be considered a possibility in any woman of reproductive age with abnormal bleeding or pain. Each new pregnant patient should also be instructed to notify her physician promptly about vaginal bleeding or uterine cramps. Since management depends on a number of factors, it is convenient to consider the clinical aspects of miscarriage under the following subgroups.

Threatened Miscarriage

Any bloody vaginal discharge or uterine bleeding that occurs during the first half of pregnancy has traditionally been assumed to be a threatened miscarriage. Because as many as 25% of pregnant women have some degree of spotting or bleeding during the early months of gestation, it is a common diagnosis.

Bleeding associated with threatened miscarriage is typically scanty, varies from a brownish discharge to bright red bleeding, and may occur repeatedly over the course of many days. It usually precedes uterine cramping or low backache. On pelvic examination, the cervix is closed and uneffaced, and no tissue has passed. The differential diagnosis includes ectopic

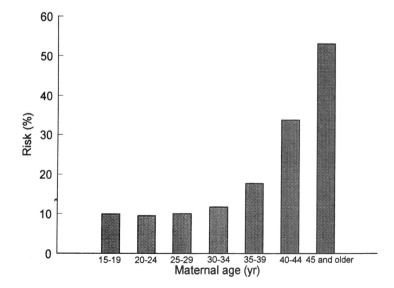

FIG. 2. Relation of maternal age to the risk of spontaneous abortion. (Data from Warburtin D, Kline J, Stein Z, et al. Cytogenetic abnormalities in spontaneous abortions of recognized conceptions. In: Porter IH, ed. *Perinatal genetics: diagnosis and treatment.* New York: Academic Press, 1986:133.)

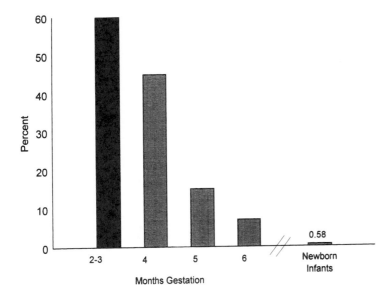

FIG. 3. The frequencies of chromosomal anomalies among 3040 spontaneously aborted fetuses related to the duration of pregnancy. For comparison, the frequency of chromosomal anomalies among 54,749 newborn infants is shown. (Data from Shiota K, Uwabe C, Nishimaura H. High prevalence of defective human embryos at the early implantation period. *Teratology* 1987;35:309; Boue J, Boue A, Lazar P. Retrospective and prospective epidemiological studies of 1500 karyotyped spontaneous human abortions. *Teratology* 1975;12:11; Lauritsen JG. Aetiology of spontaneous abortion: a cytogenetic and epidemiological study of 288 abortuses and their parents. *Acta Obstet Gynecol Scand Suppl* 1976;52:1; and Creasy MR, Crolla JA, Alberman ED. A cytogenetic study of human spontaneous abortions using banding techniques. *Hum Genet* 1976;31:177.)

pregnancy, molar pregnancy, vaginal ulcerations, cervicitis with bleeding, cervical erosions, polyps, and carcinoma.

A viable conceptus can be detected with modern ultrasound as early as 5.5 weeks of gestation.[7,8] The ability to visualize the embryo and embryonic heart motion has made evaluation and management of threatened miscarriage more precise. However, accurate knowledge of gestational age is necessary for proper interpretation. Ultrasound findings are unreliable at 3 to 4 weeks' gestation, and what appears to be an empty uterus can be misinterpreted as an abnormal intrauterine or ectopic pregnancy when it is actually a very early normal gestation. If there is any doubt of normalcy, it is best to perform follow-up β-hCG measurements and sonograms. From 5 to 6 weeks, the yolk sac and gestational sac are visible by vaginal ultrasound, and the embryo with cardiac activity is seen soon after that. Abnormal gestational sac and yolk sac size, an embryo small for dates, and slow embryonic heart rates are signs indicative of impending pregnancy loss.[7–9] More than 95% of pregnancies continue if a live embryo is demonstrated ultrasonically at 8 week's gestation.[9] These embryos have a very low mortality rate during the next few weeks,[7] and the subsequent pregnancy loss rate is only 1% if a live fetus is seen at 14 to 16 weeks' gestation.

Although there is no convincing evidence that any treatment regimen favorably influences the course of threatened miscarriage, a sympathetic attitude by the physician along with continuing support and follow-up are important to patients. This includes a tactful explanation about the pathologic process and favorable prognosis when the pregnancy is viable. An optimistic but cautious approach is prudent, since a few of these women will have a later embryonic or fetal death. It is reasonable to advise patients to remain at home or near a telephone until it can be determined whether the symptoms will persist or cease. Continued observation is indicated as long as bleeding and cramping are mild, the cervix remains closed, quantitative β-hCG levels are increasing normally,

and a normal embryo or fetus is evident on follow-up sonogram. If the bleeding and cramping progressively increase, the prognosis becomes worse. An unfavorable outcome is also associated with negative or falling β-hCG values, sonographic evidence of an embryo or fetus decreasing in size (Fig. 4), a slow heart rate, and a uterus that is not increasing in size on pelvic examination.[7,8] If careful clinical evaluation indicates that the conceptus is no longer viable, the treatment options are expectant management or evacuation of the uterus. In women with minimal intrauterine tissue by ultrasound, waiting for spontaneous passage of the products of conception is possible.[10] The complication rate may be decreased by elective uterine curettage in patients with significant amounts of tissue[11] (see "Missed Miscarriage").

Inevitable and Incomplete Miscarriage

Early pregnancy loss is a process rather than a single event. Previously classified as different entities, inevitable and incomplete miscarriages present a similar clinical picture and are treated in the same way. A miscarriage is inevitable when bleeding or gross rupture of the membranes is accompanied by pain and dilation of the cervix. The miscarriage is incomplete when the products of conception have partially passed from the uterine cavity, are protruding from the external os, or are in the vagina with persistent bleeding and cramping. Placental tissue is more likely to be retained when this occurs in the second trimester. Bleeding can be profuse and occasionally produces hypovolemia. A careful vaginal examination usually establishes the diagnosis. Rarely, one conceptus is aborted, and a normal retained twin proceeds to delivery at term. This unusual situation can be diagnosed by ultrasound at the time of first-trimester bleeding. There is otherwise no fetal survival in inevitable or incomplete miscarriages. Evacuation of the uterus is advisable to prevent maternal complications from further hemorrhage or infection.

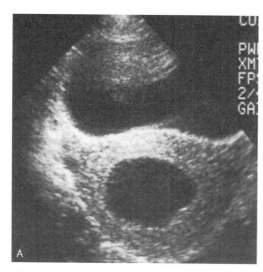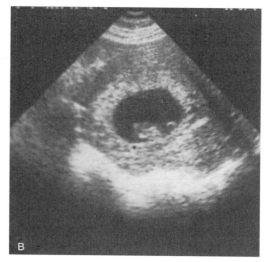

FIG. 4. Ultrasonic comparison of **(A)** an anembryonic pregnancy with no fetal tissue that is destined to abort with **(B)** a normal gestational sac with a transonic area, echogenic rim, and fetal pole.

In most cases, a vacuum or suction curettage can be performed promptly and safely in an outpatient setting using analgesia, a paracervical block, and an intravenous infusion of normal saline containing 10 to 20 U of oxytocin. Often, the cervix is dilated, and the products of conception can be removed from the cervical canal and lower uterine segment with ring forceps to facilitate uterine contractions and hemostasis. Suction curettage is performed using a plastic curette and vacuum pressure. As the curettage proceeds, tissue can be seen as it flows through the curette and suction tubing. The curette is rotated 360 degrees clockwise as it is withdrawn, and the procedure is repeated in a counterclockwise direction. When a grating sensation is noted and no more tissue is obtained, the endometrial cavity has been emptied.

Preparation is necessary to anticipate any problems such as allergic reactions to medication, uterine atony, uterine perforation, seizure, or cardiac arrest. A hemoglobin level should be obtained, and blood replacement may be necessary if hemorrhage occurs. If measures taken in the emergency room fail to promptly control bleeding, the patient should be transferred to the operating room for an examination under anesthesia and evacuation of the uterus. After curettage, the patient is observed for several hours. When stable, she is discharged and followed as an outpatient. Rh-negative women should receive 50 µg or the standard 300-µg dose of Rh immune globulin to prevent Rh immunization. The tissue obtained should be examined to confirm the presence of products of conception and rule out the possibility of ectopic pregnancy.

Complete Miscarriage

Patients followed for a threatened miscarriage are instructed to save all tissue passed, so it can be inspected. When the entire products of conception have passed, pain and bleeding soon cease. If the diagnosis is certain, no further therapy is necessary. In questionable cases, ultrasound is useful to de-termine that the uterus is empty. In some circumstances, curettage may be necessary to be sure that the uterus is completely evacuated. Removal of remaining necrotic decidua decreases the incidence of bleeding and shortens the recovery time.

Missed Miscarriage

In this situation, expulsion of the conceptus does not occur despite a prolonged period after embryonic death. The reason that some dead embryos do not abort spontaneously is not clear. Typically, the patient's symptoms of pregnancy regress, the pregnancy test becomes negative, and no fetal heart motion is detected by ultrasound. Most patients do eventually abort spontaneously, and coagulation defects due to retention of a dead fetus are rare in the first half of pregnancy. However, expectant management is emotionally trying, and many women prefer to have the uterus evacuated. During the first trimester, this is done by suction curettage preceded by insertion of laminaria if the cervix is closed. The procedure is often performed in a hospital setting with intravenous fluids and blood available in case significant bleeding occurs.

In the second trimester, the uterus can be emptied by dilation and evacuation (D&E) or induction of labor with intravaginal prostaglandin E_2 (PGE$_2$) or misoprostol (Cytotec). D&E is an extension of the traditional dilation and curettage (D&C) and vacuum curettage. It is especially appropriate at 13 to 16 weeks' gestation, although many proponents use this procedure through 20 weeks. The cervix is usually first dilated with laminaria to avoid trauma, and the fetus and placenta are mechanically removed with suction and instruments. If vaginal PGE$_2$ is used, one 20-mg suppository is placed high in the posterior vaginal vault every 4 hours until the fetus and placenta are expelled. Between 2.5 and 5 mg of diphenoxylate given orally and 10 mg of prochlorperazine (Compazine) given intramuscularly can control diarrhea and nausea, and narcotics or epidural anesthesia can be used to control pain. In this situation, a retained placenta is relatively common and may require manual removal and uterine curettage. Misoprostol in 200-μg tablets applied to the external os of the cervix at 12-hour intervals is equally effective.[12]

Septic Miscarriage

Septic abortion, once a leading cause of maternal mortality, has become a less frequent occurrence because changes in abortion laws have made pregnancy terminations by physicians available to women with unwanted pregnancies. However, any type of spontaneous miscarriage can also be complicated by infection. The infection is most commonly endometritis but can progress to parametritis and peritonitis. These patients present with fever, abdominal tenderness, and uterine pain. In severe cases, local infection progresses to septicemia and septic shock. The polymicrobial infection mirrors the endogenous vaginal flora and includes *Escherichia coli* and other aerobic, enteric, gram-negative rods, group B β-hemolytic streptococci, anaerobic streptococci, *Bacteroides* species, staphylococci, and microaerophilic bacteria.

The initial evaluation and management of septic abortion should include several steps:

◊ Physical and pelvic examination;
◊ Complete blood cell count and determination of electrolyte, blood urea nitrogen, and creatinine levels;
◊ Type and screen or crossmatch of blood;
◊ Smears from cervix for Gram stain;
◊ Aerobic and anaerobic cultures of endocervix, blood, and available products of conception;
◊ Indwelling Foley catheter;
◊ Intravenous fluids (e.g., saline, Ringer's lactate) through a large-bore angiocatheter;
◊ Administration of 0.5 ml of tetanus toxoid, given subcutaneously for immunized patients, or 250 U of tetanus immune globulin, administered deep within the muscle;
◊ Supine and upright radiographs of the abdomen to detect free air or foreign bodies.

Optimal therapy consists of evacuation of the uterus and aggressive use of parenteral antibiotics before, during, and after removal of necrotic tissue by curettage (Table 1). Prompt removal of the infected tissue is important and should be performed within a few hours after beginning intravenous antibiotics. Numerous antibiotic regimens have been recommended, but high-dose, broad-spectrum coverage as outlined in Table 1 is essential. Although most patients with septic abortions respond favorably to treatment, the septic shock syndrome is a serious complication that requires aggressive management in an intensive care setting (see Chapter 30).

Recurrent Miscarriage

Recurrent miscarriage, traditionally defined as three or more consecutive first-trimester spontaneous losses, affects about

TABLE 1. *Antibiotic regimens for septic abortion*

Gram-positive anaerobe and aerobic organism coverage:
1. Aqueous penicillin G, 4–5 million U IV q4–6h (20–30 million U each 24 h); or
2. Ampicillin, 2 g IV q4–6h; or
3. Clindamycin (Cleocin), 600 mg IV q6h or 900 mg IV q8h; or
4. Cephalothin (Keflin) (or other cephalosporin), 2 g IV q4–6h (for penicillin-allergic patients, there is a 10% cross allergy); or
5. Imipenem-cilastatin (Primax), 250–500 mg q6h (must decrease dose for patients weighing < 70 kg or with renal compromise)

Resistant gram-negative aerobic organism coverage:
1. Gentamicin, 1–1.5 mg/kg IV q8h (adjust dose according to peak and through levels, monitor for nephrotoxicity and ototoxicity, decrease dose in patients with renal compromise); or
2. Aztreonam (Azactam), 1–2 g IV q8–12h or q6h in cases of serious infection (alternate antibiotic for patients who develop gentamicin toxicity; decrease dose in patients with renal compromise); or
3. Imipenem-cilastatin (see previous dose schedule)

Gram-negative anaerobic organism coverage:
1. Clindamycin, 600 mg IV q6h or 900 mg q8h; or
2. Metronidazole, 1 g IV loading dose, followed by 500 mg q6h; or
3. Imipenem-cilastatin (see previous dose schedule)

The usual approach is to start one drug from each group. Recommended regimens are based on clinical effectiveness and may change as new antibiotics become available.

1% of couples. Primary aborters are sometimes defined as women who have never had a successful pregnancy, and secondary aborters are those whose repetitive losses follow a live birth. There is no specific classification for women who have multiple miscarriages interspersed with normal pregnancies. It is generally agreed that a workup for possible causes of recurrent pregnancy loss (RPL) is indicated in most patients after three consecutive miscarriages and is reasonable in some women over age 30 to 35 years with two miscarriages.

The management of couples with RPL is controversial. This clinical entity has received much attention in the lay and medical literature during the past decade. Despite publicity to the contrary, there is little evidence that poor nutrition, infections, unrecognized diabetes, toxic agents, or psychologic trauma are significant etiologic factors.[5,6] Moreover, various new diagnostic tests for RPL are continually being proposed to replace those that have been disproved and discarded over the years. Those most recently proposed include antithyroid antibodies,[13] elevated follicular-phase luteinizing hormone levels,[14] circulating maternal embryotoxic factor,[15] and abnormal lymphocyte subset ratios (elevated CD56+ levels).[16] It is beyond the scope of this chapter to critically analyze each assay, but the mechanism of pregnancy loss and potential relationship to each of these remains largely theoretical. Until effective treatments are identified and proven by properly designed studies, these screening tests have little utility in the routine evaluation of patients with RPL.

Classically, investigation of anatomic, hormonal, genetic, and autoimmune factors has been recommended (Fig. 5).[5,17,18] Even these are coming under closer scrutiny because treatments advocated are empirical, have not been submitted to controlled trials, and are not totally successful.

Structural Uterine Defects

Hysterosalpingography, magnetic resonance imaging, hysteroscopy, and laparoscopy can be used to diagnose septate uterus, other müllerian anomalies, uterine defects associated with diethylstilbestrol exposure, submucous myomas, and intrauterine synechiae.[19] The prognosis for successful pregnancies in patients with müllerian anomalies is related to the type of malformation, with asymmetric fusion defects carrying the worst prognosis and septate, bicornuate, and didelphic uteri carrying increasingly better prognoses. In patients with RPL, the prevalence of these anatomic defects is approximately 10% to 15%.[18,19] The cause of pregnancy loss in women with uterine anomalies is uncertain, but a diminished blood supply interfering with normal implantation and placentation and the reduced size of the uterine cavity are often cited.

Abdominal metroplasty has been replaced in most cases by the hysteroscopic removal of uterine septa. This procedure can be accomplished in an outpatient setting and eliminates the need for cesarean delivery. The subsequent live-birth rate is greater than 80%.[5,18,19] Removal of synechiae and submucous myomas can also be performed hysteroscopically (see Chapter 45).

Endocrine Problems

Luteal-phase deficiency (LPD) is a controversial entity attributed to abnormal ovarian function with insufficient progesterone production or an inadequate progesterone effect on the endometrium.[20] Patients with LPD characteristically have short cycles, postovulatory intervals less than 14 days, and secondary infertility with recurrent early losses. The exact pathogenesis of pregnancy loss in patients with LPD is unclear, but progesterone secreted by the corpus luteum is necessary to support the endometrium until placental production begins at about 6 to 8 weeks' gestation. Potential underlying causes of LPD include decreased gonadotropin-releasing hormone, decreased follicle-stimulating hormone, inade-

quate luteinizing hormone, inadequate ovarian steroidogenesis, and endometrial receptor defects.

The true incidence is unknown because there is little agreement on the criteria necessary to make the diagnosis. Endometrial biopsy or luteal-phase serum progesterone levels are the most widely accepted diagnostic tests. Both are timed for the late luteal phase of the cycle. The endometrial biopsy is histologically dated, and a lag greater than 2 to 3 days is considered suspect. However, this should be confirmed by repeat biopsy, because delayed endometrial histology can occur sporadically in women with no reproductive problems.

The rationale for progesterone replacement therapy for LPD was derived from observations in which spontaneous abortion occurred when the corpus luteum was surgically removed before 6 to 8 weeks' gestation. The most commonly advocated treatment is a 25-mg progesterone suppository inserted into the vagina morning and night beginning after ovulation and continued until menses begin or through the first 8 to 10 weeks of pregnancy. Comparable doses of oral micronized progesterone have also been used. Successful pregnancy rates up to 90% have been reported, but there have been no controlled studies, and a missed miscarriage can be the result. Clomiphene and other ovulatory agents have been tried to improve follicular development and corpus luteum function, but the results have been variable.

Chromosomal Abnormalities

Parental chromosomal anomalies are found in approximately 5% of couples with RPL.[4,5,21] Cytogenetic examination of both partners is helpful to predict recurrence and forms the basis for genetic counseling. Most abnormalities are balanced translocations, with two-thirds being reciprocal translocations and one-third Robertsonian translocations.[4,5] Couples with balanced translocations have spontaneous loss rates ranging from 50% for reciprocal translocations to 25% for Robertsonian translocations. All couples with a parental chromosomal abnormality deserve counseling about genetic amniocentesis or chorionic villus sampling in any future pregnancy to exclude a serious fetal chromosomal abnormality. Parental chromosomal abnormalities do not usually preclude further attempts at pregnancy, because most couples eventually have normal offspring. For the rare homologous Robertsonian translocation

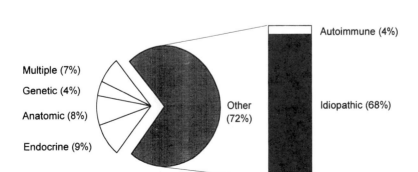

FIG. 5. Factors considered responsible for recurrent pregnancy loss in more than 400 patients evaluated at the University of Utah.

that prevents successful pregnancy, therapeutic possibilities include artificial donor insemination, *in vitro* fertilization with donor oocytes, and adoption.

Chromosomal analysis of the products of conception is also clinically useful, particularly in the evaluation of the reason for failure of a treatment regimen.[4,5]

Molecular mutations that may be shown in the future to cause recurrent miscarriages include lethal, single-point mutations, possibly linked to *MHC* genes; mutations in genes that code for products critical for normal development; mutations in homeobox genes that control transcriptional regulation; mutations that lead to severe metabolic errors and embryonic death; and disorders of protooncogenes and oncogenes.

Autoimmunity

Antiphospholipid syndrome (APS) has been recognized as a proven cause of pregnancy loss for over a decade (see Chapter 24). Approximately 5% of women with RPL have lupus anticoagulant (LA), medium-to-high levels of anticardiolipin (aCL), or both.[21] These acquired antiphospholipid autoantibodies are induced by as yet unknown stimuli in the setting of aberrant immunoregulation. Low levels of IgG or IgM aCL are of questionable significance,[22,23] and there is little evidence that other antiphospholipid antibodies contribute to the management of RPL patients.

The most important finding in these patients is the high rate of late first- or second-trimester death of a fetus determined to have cardiac activity. Patients with high levels of aCL or a history of prior fetal death are at greatest risk of another fetal loss. The cause of fetal death appears to be a decidual vasculopathy that results in decidual infarction and insufficient blood flow to the placenta. Intervillous thrombosis has also been described. However, these lesions are nonspecific, and the degree of pathology is not always sufficient to explain the fetal death. The mechanisms by which aCL may cause decidual vasculopathy and fetal death are unknown. An imbalance of local prostacyclin and thromboxane production leading to vasoconstriction, platelet aggregation, intravascular thromboses, decreased activation of protein C, and decreased trophoblast annexin V has been proposed.

The presence of a positive LA or aCL does not invariably indicate a poor prognosis, and some patients have achieved successful pregnancies without specific medical therapy. However, many reports suggest that women with APS and previous pregnancy loss can be treated during subsequent pregnancies to improve the chance of delivering a live infant. At present, heparin with low-dose aspirin appears to be the most effective and safest treatment (Table 2).[24–28] One treatment regimen includes one low-dose aspirin taken daily throughout pregnancy. Subcutaneous heparin (7500 U every 12 hours) is begun with first-trimester documentation of a live fetus, and the dose is adjusted upward in the second trimester to achieve anticoagulation. Concomitant use of a corticosteroids and heparin should be avoided, because this combination has not been shown to be better than either alone

TABLE 2. *Live-birth rate with heparin treatment for patients with antiphospholipid syndrome*

Investigation[a]	Reference	Pregnancies (n)	Live births (%)
Rosove (1990)	24	15	14 (93)
Cowchock et al. (1992)	25	8	6 (75)
Branch et al. (1992)	26	19	16 (84)
Kutteh (1996)	27	25	20 (80)
Rai et al. (1997)	28	45	32 (71)
Total		112	88 (79)

[a]It is not possible to compare series because of different selection factors, criteria used for diagnosis, and treatment regimens.

in achieving a live birth. Moreover, several cases of severe osteoporosis with fractures have occurred. The use of high-dose intravenous immunoglobulin also has generated interest due to anecdotal reports of successful pregnancies with lowered aCL levels, but no controlled trials have been performed. Even with treatment, patients with APS require careful antepartum management (see Chapter 24).[26,27]

Thrombophilic Disorders

RPL has recently been linked to hypercoagulable states, hyperhomocystinemia, and deficiencies in activated factor XII (Hageman factor). Deficiencies of antithrombin III, protein C, or protein S are associated with a higher percentage of both first-trimester miscarriages and fetal deaths, while factor V Leiden mutation increases the risk of second-trimester pregnancy loss. Abnormal factor V resistance to anticoagulant effects of activated protein C is numerically the most important cause of a familial thromboembolic disease.[30] It is usually associated with the factor V Leiden mutation in the factor V gene, present in approximately 2% to 5% of the general population. It is not yet clear which RPL patients would benefit from screening for thrombophilias, and properly designed trials are needed to determine whether aspirin or anticoagulant therapy can decrease the risk of pregnancy in these women.[30]

Idiopathic Causes

Because most cases of RPL have no discernible cause, alloimmune factors have long been suspected. These have yet to be proven, largely because little is known about the mechanisms that prevent immunologic rejection of the conceptus in successful pregnancies (see Chapter 24). Early reports proposed that HLA compatibility between couples, the absence of maternal leukocytotoxic antibodies, or the absence of maternal blocking antibodies were related to RPL. The importance of these factors has not been substantiated, and these expensive tests are no longer clinically indicated.[32] Contemporary research is focused on local decidual or trophoblast immunosuppressive factors such as cytokines, growth factors, hormones, enzymes, and endometrial proteins. Some of these immunoactive factors appear to be necessary for implantation and growth and development of the early placenta and embryo, and others may cause abortion, when expressed. There are no practical clinical tests available for these factors, and the diagnosis of alloimmune-mediated RPL is one of exclusion.

Although no alloimmune mechanism has been unequivocally shown to cause RPL in humans, several types of immunotherapy have been advocated. Originally, the attempt to improve maternal immunotolerance in recurrent aborters was based on evidence that pretransplant blood transfusions decreased rejection of organ allografts and that the rate of resorptions or abortions in animal models was reduced by prior immunization with spleen cells from a paternally related strain. The most popular regimen involves injections of the husband's leukocytes, but there is no consensus about the dose, route, or indications for this treatment. Immunization using viable leukocytes carries the risks of any blood transfusion, such as hepatitis, human immunodeficiency virus, and cytomegalovirus infections. Reactions have been uncommon but include soreness and redness at the injection site, cutaneous graft-versus-host–like reaction, fever, maternal platelet and leukocyte alloimmunization, and blood group sensitization.[32]

The efficacy of this treatment has often been questioned because of the reasonable chance of a successful pregnancy even without treatment.[5,18,32] When data from prospective randomized trials were combined in a recent metaanalysis, there appeared to be a slight benefit to leukocyte immunization (Fig. 6). The live-birth rates were 68% for immunized versus 61% for control patients.[33] Several other metaanalyses have also been completed, and the conclusions are highly dependent on the methods used for the analysis (Fig. 7).[34–36] It is still unclear whether paternal leukocyte alloimmunization is an efficacious treatment for patients with unexplained RPL, and a more definitive answer may be forthcoming from a recently completed multicenter randomized trial. Intravenous immune globulin has been proposed as an alternative therapy in patients with unexplained RPL. Three controlled trials have been reported, and the results are conflicting.[32,36] Nevertheless, this treatment seems to be no more successful than paternal cell immunization.

Cautious interpretation of the results of immunotherapy is warranted until the effectiveness and long-term safety are clearly established. One scheme for a reasonable and cost-effective management of patients with recurrent miscarriage is summarized in Table 3. Treatment of maternal nonimmunologic factors is effective and rewarding in well selected cases. If the initial workup is negative, further attempts at pregnancy without treatment may be justified, depending on age, situation, and wishes of the couple. However, an earlier and more aggressive approach is reasonable if the patient has few reproductive years left, has had an infertility problem, or has had multiple miscarriages. If further immunologic evaluation and experimental immunotherapy are considered, it is perhaps best to refer these patients to legitimate research centers with an interest in this problem.

A sympathetic attitude by the physician is important. Establishment of trust and rapport and a sincere appreciation of the distress and grief experienced by these couples permit tactful and thorough discussions with patient and husband.

Cervical Incompetence

Incompetent cervix, more appropriately called premature cervical dilatation, is an important cause of second-trimester

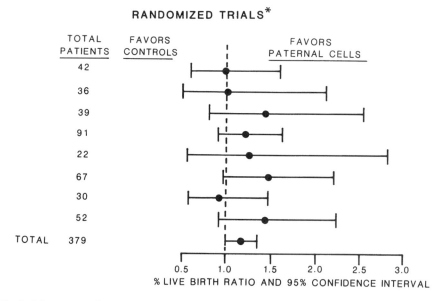

FIG. 6. Odds ratios and 95% confidence intervals of successful pregnancy outcome with paternal leukocyte immunization. (Data from ref. 33.)

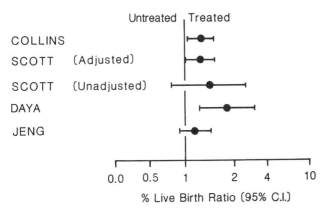

FIG. 7. Odds ratios for placebo/no treatment versus paternal leukocyte immunization calculated from pooled data from prospective randomized trials. Although live-birth rates favor paternal white cell immunization, the results are statistically significant in only three of the five analyses.

loss. It is an obstetric entity characterized by gradual, painless dilatation of the cervix with bulging and rupture of the membranes and subsequent expulsion of a fetus too immature to survive. Pregnancy loss from this cervical abnormality usually occurs in the second trimester and is thought to be an entirely different and distinct entity from a first-trimester miscarriage or premature labor in the third trimester. It results from different factors, presents a distinctive clinical picture, and requires different management. Moreover, miscarriage and premature labor are common, but midtrimester premature cervical dilatation is relatively rare.

The cervix is fundamentally a connective tissue structure, unlike the rest of the uterus, which is basically muscular. The

TABLE 3. *Suggested routine evaluation for recurrent miscarriage*

History
Determine pattern and trimester of pregnancy losses and whether a live fetus was present; clues suggestive of autoimmune disease; unusual exposure to environmental toxins, drugs, infections; previous gynecologic disorders or surgery, including dilatation and curettage; and previous diagnostic tests and treatments[a]

Physical
Abnormalities on pelvic examination, including findings suggesting abnormal cervix, diethylstilbestrol exposure, or uterine anomalies

Tests
Hysterosalpingogram
Luteal-phase endometrial biopsy
Parental chromosome analysis
Screening test for lupus anticoagulant and anticardiolipin
Other laboratory tests if suggested by history and physical examination

[a]Ultrasound examination at 6 weeks of gestation in the next pregnancy and chromosome analysis of the products of conception from any subsequent spontaneous abortion.

cause of cervical incompetence is obscure, and various etiologic factors have been proposed.[37,38] Previous surgery or trauma to the cervix such as D&C, amputation, conization, cauterization, loop electrosurgical excision procedure (LEEP), or traumatic delivery seem to be factors in some cases. In other instances, congenital cervical structural defects, uterine anomalies, or abnormal cervical development associated with *in utero* diethylstilbestrol exposure appear to play a role.

There is little agreement regarding the diagnosis of cervical incompetence, except that it is one of exclusion that requires careful evaluation to rule out other potential causes of midtrimester pregnancy loss. Other causes include abruptio placentae, chorioamnionitis, and uterine anomalies, but they usually present different clinical pictures. Whether or not the condition can be diagnosed during the nonpregnant state by methods designed to calibrate the diameter of the endocervical canal or during early pregnancy by sonographic findings is questionable. The absolute diagnosis of cervical incompetence can be made only by seeing the fetal membranes bulging through the partially dilated cervix of a patient in the middle trimester of pregnancy who is not in labor. A presumptive diagnosis is most reliably made from the characteristic history of repeated silent dilatation of the cervix followed by rupture of the membranes and a relatively painless, rapid labor with delivery of an immature infant. On inspection in the nonpregnant state, the cervix may be shortened with a patulous os or may be deformed with lacerations that sometimes extend to the vaginal fornix.

Although bed rest, various intravaginal devices, and pharmacologic agents have been used with some success, the generally accepted treatment for incompetent cervix is surgical. Various methods have been described, but the McDonald or Shirodkar procedures (Fig. 8) are most commonly employed prophylactically.[37,38] These are techniques performed vaginally, usually under regional anesthesia, that are designed to reinforce the cervix at the level of the internal os. If there is insufficient cervical tissue to allow placement of a cerclage vaginally, an abdominal approach is sometimes used.[39,40] The reinforcement suture is usually placed toward the end of the first trimester after ultrasound documentation of a live fetus, after the risk of miscarriage has passed, and before the cervix starts to dilate.

Often, the history is not classical, and it is difficult to determine whether or not premature cervical dilatation will occur in a subsequent pregnancy. These patients are usually followed with frequent vaginal examinations and serial sonograms to diagnose potential cervical changes. Ultrasound can be used to accurately assess cervical length, but it not clear whether there is a difference in the ultimate outcome for pregnancies with and without abnormal results of ultrasound examinations.[38] Preliminary studies suggest that the technique may be a useful adjunct to follow patients thought to be at risk for cervical incompetence.

Placement of the cerclage in the second trimester after cervical change has occurred is sometimes necessary but is less effective.[41] The procedure should not be used if the diagno-

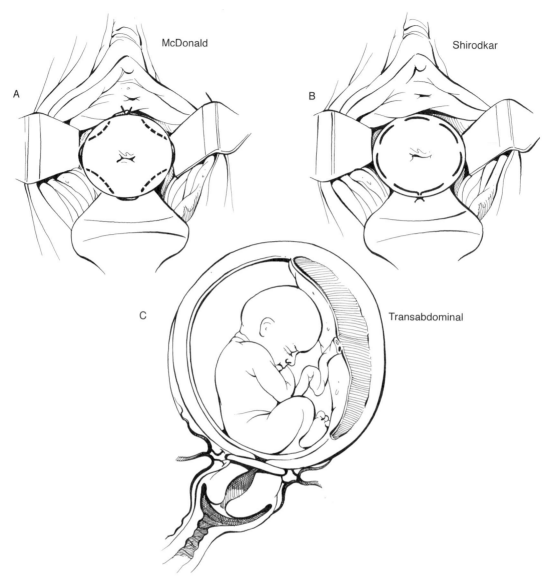

FIG. 8. Incompetent cervix can be treated by three procedures. **(A)** In the McDonald cerclage procedure, a multiple-bite suture using large, monofilament nylon is placed around the cervix and tied securely to reduce the diameter of the cervical canal to a few millimeters. **(B)** In the Shirodkar procedure, Mersaline tape encircling the cervix is passed under the mucosa and anchored to the cervix anteriorly and posteriorly with interrupted sutures. **(C)** With transabdominal cervicoisthmic cerclage, a Mersaline band is placed in an avascular space medial to the uterine vessels at the level of the cervicouterine junction.

sis is in doubt, if membranes are ruptured, or if vaginal bleeding and cramping are part of the clinical picture. There is no evidence that postoperative antibiotics, progesterone, or tocolytic agents are useful adjuvants. If membranes rupture or labor ensues at any time, the cerclage should be removed to prevent chorioamnionitis, sepsis, cervical laceration, and rupture of the uterus. Otherwise, the suture is removed when fetal maturity is achieved, usually after 37 weeks' gestation, which is often followed by the onset of labor and a relatively rapid delivery. If the patient desires further pregnancies, some physicians leave the cerclage in place and deliver by cesarean section.

The effectiveness of cerclage has often been questioned, even in women with a classic clinical picture. Nevertheless, when patients are carefully selected, this type of management is 80% to 90% successful in preventing delivery of an immature fetus. There is little difference in the fetal survival rates between the McDonald and Shirodkar techniques. The procedure has also been used prophylactically for patients with previous preterm deliveries with less convincing evidence for cervical incompetence. However, prospective randomized studies show there is no difference in perinatal outcome between treated and untreated groups when the procedure is used in this manner.[38,42]

SUMMARY POINTS

⬦ Miscarriage is the most common complication of pregnancy, and the most frequent etiology is a chromosomal abnormality of the conceptus.

⬦ Ultrasound is helpful in determining whether or not the embryo is viable, and appropriate modern management may be either observation or evacuation of the uterus.

⬦ Recurrent early pregnancy loss is sometimes associated with underlying maternal abnormalities that can be detected with standard tests. However, immunologic tests and immunotherapy proposed to prevent further miscarriages remain controversial.

⬦ REFERENCES

1. Wilcox AJ, Weinberg CR, O'Connor JF, et al. Incidence of early pregnancy loss. *N Engl J Med* 1988;319:189.
2. Fantel AG, Shepard TH. Morphological analysis of spontaneous abortuses. In: Bennett MJ, Edmunds DK, eds. *Spontaneous and recurrent abortion.* Oxford: Blackwell Scientific Publications, 1987:8.
3. Goldstein SR. Sonography in early pregnancy. *Clin Obstet Gynecol* 1994;37:681.
4. Byrne JLB, Ward K. Genetic factors in recurrent abortion. *Clin Obstet Gynecol* 1994;37:693.
5. Scott JR, Branch DW. Evaluation and treatment of recurrent abortion. In: Keye WR, Chang RJ, Rebar RW, Soules MR, eds. *Infertility: evaluation and treatment.* Philadelphia: WB Saunders, 1994:230.
6. Brent RL, Beckman DA. The contribution of environmental teratogens to embryonic and fetal loss. *Clin Obstet Gynecol* 1994;37:646.
7. Goldstein SR. Embryonic death in early pregnancy: a new look at the first trimester. *Obstet Gynecol* 1994;84:294.
8. Achiron R, Tadmor O, Mashiach S. Heart rate as a predictor of first-trimester spontaneous abortion after ultrasound-proven viability. *Obstet Gynecol* 1991;78:330.
9. Simpson JL, Mills JL, Holmes LB, et al. Low fetal loss rates after ultrasound-proved viability in early pregnancy. *JAMA* 1987;258:2555.
10. Hemminki E. Treatment of miscarriage: current practice and rationale. *Obstet Gynecol* 1998;91:247.
11. Hurd WW, Whitfield RR, Randolph JF, Kercher ML. Expectant management versus elective curettage for the treatment of spontaneous abortion. *Fertil Steril* 1997;68:601.
12. Nuutila M, Toivonen J, Ylikorkala O, et al. A comparison between two doses of intravaginal misoprostol and gemeprost for induction of second-trimester abortion. *Obstet Gynecol* 1997;90:896.
13. Pratt DE, Kaberlein G, Dudkiewicz A, et al. The association of antithyroid antibodies in euthyroid nonpregnant women with recurrent first trimester abortions in the next pregnancy. *Fertil Steril* 1993;60:1001.
14. Clifford K, Rai R, Watson H, et al. Hypersecretion of luteinizing hormone, infertility and miscarriage. *Lancet* 1996;ii:1141.
15. Ecker JL, Laufer MR, Hill JA. Measurement of embryotoxic factors is predictive of pregnancy outcome in women with a history of recurrent abortion. *Obstet Gynecol* 1993;81:84.
16. Coulam CB, Goodman C, Roussev RG, et al. Systemic CD56+ cells can predict pregnancy outcome. *Am J Reprod Immunol* 1995;33:40.
17. Plouffe L, White EW, Tho SP, et al. Etiologic factors of recurrent abortion and subsequent reproductive performance of couples: have we made any progress in the past 10 years? *Am J Obstet Gynecol* 1992;167:313.
18. Scott JR. Habitual abortion: recommendations for a reasonable approach to an enigmatic problem. In: Soules MR, ed. *Controversies in reproductive endocrinology and infertility.* New York: Elsevier Science, 1989:95.
19. Patton PE. Anatomic uterine defects. *Clin Obstet Gynecol* 1994;37:705.
20. Coulam CB, Stern JJ. Endocrine factors associated with recurrent spontaneous abortion. *Clin Obstet Gynecol* 1994;37:730.
21. Portnoi MF, Joye N, Van Den Akker J. Karyotypes of 1142 couples with recurrent abortion. *Obstet Gynecol* 1988;72:31.
22. Branch DW, Silver RM, Pierangelli SS, et al. Antiphospholipid antibodies other than lupus anticoagulant and anticardiolipin antibodies in women with recurrent pregnancy loss, fertile controls, and antiphospholipid syndrome. *Obstet Gynecol* 1997;89:549.
23. Silver RM, Porter TF, van Leeuwen I, et al. Anticardiolipin antibodies: clinical consequences of "low titers." *Obstet Gynecol* 1996;87:494.
24. Rosove MH, Tabsh K, Wasserstrum N, Howard P, Hahn BH, Kalunian KC. Heparin therapy for pregnant women with lupus anticoagulant or anticardiolipin antibodies. *Obstet Gynecol* 1990;75:630–634.
25. Cowchock FS, Reece EA, Balaban D, et al. Repeated fetal losses associated with antiphospholipid antibodies: a collaborative randomized trial comparing prednisone to low-dose heparin treatment. *Am J Obstet Gynecol* 1992;166:1318.
26. Branch DW, Silver RM, Blackwell JL, et al. Outcome of treated pregnancies in women with antiphospholipid syndrome: an update of the Utah experience. *Obstet Gynecol* 1992;81:614.
27. Antiphospholipid syndrome. *ACOG Educ Bull* 1998;244:1.
28. Rai R, Cohen H, Dave M, Regan L. Randomized controlled trial of aspirin and aspirin plus heparin in pregnancy in women with recurrent miscarriage associated with phospholipid antibodies. *BMJ* 1997;314:253.
29. Kutteh WH. Antiphospholipid antibody-associated recurrent pregnancy loss: treatment with heparin and low-dose aspirin is superior to low-dose aspirin alone. *Am J Obstet Gynecol* 1996;35:1584.
30. Preston FE, Rosendaal FR, Walker ID, et al. Increased fetal loss in women with heritable thrombophilia. *Lancet* 1996;348:913.
31. Rouse DJ, Goldenberg RL, Wenstrom KD. Antenatal screening for factor V Leiden mutation: a critical appraisal. *Obstet Gynecol* 1977;90:848.
32. Kutteh WH, Stovall DW, Scott JR. The immunologic diagnosis and treatment of recurrent pregnancy loss. *Infertil Reprod Med Clin North Am* 1997;8:267.
33. Coulam CB, Clark DA, Collins J, Scott JR. Worldwide collaborative observational study and meta-analysis on allogeneic leukocyte immunotherapy for recurrent spontaneous abortion. *Am J Reprod Immunol* 1994;32:55.
34. Daya S, Gunby J. The recurrent miscarriage immunotherapy trialist group. The effectiveness of allogeneic leukocyte immunization in unexplained primary recurrent spontaneous abortion. *Am J Reprod Immunol* 1994;32:294.
35. Jeng GT, Scott JR, Burmeister LF. A comparison of meta-analytic results using literature vs. individual data. *JAMA* 1995;274:830.
36. Scott JR. Immunotherapy for recurrent miscarriage. *Cochrane Library* 1997;3:1.
37. Gomez-Lobo V. Cervical cerclage. *Postgrad Obstet Gynecol* 1993;13:1.
38. Barth WH. Cervical incompetence and cerclage: unresolved controversies. *Clin Obstet Gynecol* 1994;37:831.
39. Novy MJ. Transabdominal cervicoisthmic cerclage: a reappraisal 25 years after its introduction. *Am J Obstet Gynecol* 1991;164:1635.
40. Scibetta JJ, Sanko SR, Phipps WR. Laparoscopic transabdominal cervicoisthmic cerclage. *Fertil Steril* 1998;69:161.
41. Aarts JM, Brons JTJ, Bruinse HW. Emergency cerclage: a review. *Obstet Gynecol Surv* 1995:459.
42. MacNaughton MC, Chalmers IG, Dubowitz V, et al. Final report of the Medical Research Council/Royal College of Obstetricians and Gynaecologists multicentered randomized trial of cervical cerclage. *Br J Obstet Gynaecol* 1993;100:516.

CHAPTER 11

Ectopic Pregnancy

———— ◊ ————

Margareta D. Pisarska
Sandra A. Carson

The uterus evolved to interface between the developing gestation and the maternal organism, facilitating the nourishment and protection of the fetus while limiting the physiologic drain on the mother. When pregnancy occurs outside the specially adapted uterus, it becomes a life-threatening event and precludes successful gestation. The obstetrician-gynecologist is frequently called on to accurately diagnose and promptly treat this relatively common phenomenon, ectopic pregnancy. Choosing the optimal therapeutic approach is crucial not only to prevent mortality but also to optimize subsequent fertility while minimizing medical costs. This chapter utilizes an evidence-based approach in considering the incidence, risk factors, diagnosis, treatment modalities, and cost analysis of ectopic gestation.

◊ INCIDENCE

Ectopic pregnancies have steadily increased over the past three decades in the United States from 4.5 per 1000 pregnancies in 1970 to 16.8 per 1000 pregnancies in 1989, based on hospitalizations.[75] In 1992, the Centers for Disease Control and Prevention estimated 108,800 ectopic pregnancies (19.7 per 1000 pregnancies), reflecting both hospitalizations (reported by the National Hospital Discharge Survey) and outpatient management (reported by the National Hospital Ambulatory Medical Care Survey). This 2% incidence includes outpatient hospital records, but it may still underestimate the total number of ectopic pregnancies because patients managed in private physician offices were not included.[55]

There are at least two reasons for the apparent increased incidence of ectopic pregnancies. First, this increase parallels the increase in the prevalence of risk factors for ectopic pregnancy.[55] Second, the advent of sensitive pregnancy tests and transvaginal ultrasound facilitates earlier diagnosis, detecting some ectopic pregnancies that in the past may have resolved spontaneously prior to diagnosis.[44]

Improved diagnosis and prompt therapy have also contributed to the concomitant decline in deaths due to ectopic pregnancies. Between 1979 and 1986, 13% of maternal deaths were secondary to ectopic pregnancy;[79] by 1992, this dropped to 9%.[152] Yet ectopic pregnancies continue to be the leading cause of maternal death in the first trimester, 90% as a result of hemorrhage.[79]

Incidence by Location

Ectopic pregnancy is the implantation of a fertilized ovum outside the uterine corpus.[44] The most common site of ectopic pregnancy is the fallopian tubes, accounting for 98.3% of all ectopic gestations. Implantation in the ampulla accounts for 79.6% of tubal ectopic pregnancies; 12.3% are in the isthmus, 6.2% in the fimbrial end, and the remaining 1.9% in the interstitial region. Ectopic nidation outside the fallopian tubes is rare; only 1.4% of ectopic pregnancies are abdominal pregnancies, 0.15% ovarian, and 0.15% cervical (Fig. 1).[24]

◊ PATHOGENESIS AND RISK FACTORS

Ectopic pregnancy is most often associated with risk factors leading to tubal damage and altered embryo transport.[179] A metaanalysis of risk factors, excluding contraception, identified the factors listed in Figure 2 as the most influential in causing ectopic pregnancy.[8]

Tubal Damage/Infection

Documented tubal pathology carries a 3.5-fold common adjusted odds ratio for ectopic pregnancy.[8] Patients with a previous ectopic pregnancy were six to eight times more likely to experience another ectopic pregnancy. Additional clinical series revealed that 8% to 14% of patients experienced more than one ectopic pregnancy.[85,88,105,184,186,193] It follows that

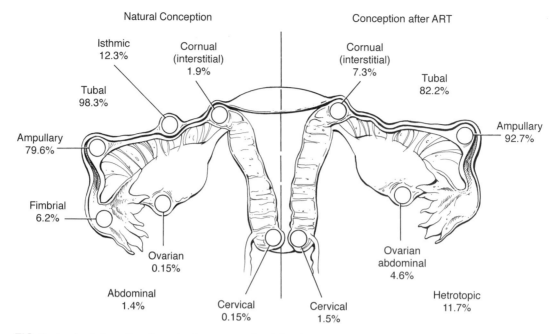

FIG. 1. Implantation sites for ectopic pregnancies following natural cycles **(left)** and assisted reproductive technology **(right)**.

patients with a history of tubal surgery have a 21-fold common adjusted odds ratio of ectopic pregnancy.[8]

Tubal pathology is frequently the result of an infectious process. Patients with a history of pelvic infections, including gonorrhea, serologically confirmed chlamydiosis, and pelvic inflammatory disease have a two- to fourfold common adjusted odds ratio for developing an ectopic pregnancy.[8,30,44,210] In a cohort study by Westrom,[232] the ectopic pregnancy rate was 4% in women with laparoscopy-proven salpingitis, compared to 0.7% in women with normal tubes. In a study evaluating histologic specimens of 121 cases of ectopic pregnancy, microscopic evidence of inflammatory disease was present in 38% of cases.[21] Recurrent episodes of pelvic infections increase the likelihood of tubal occlusions: 12.8% after one infection, 35.5% after two infections, and 75% in patients with three or more infections.[232]

Salpingitis Isthmica Nodosa

Salpingitis isthmica nodosa is an anatomic thickening of the proximal portion of the fallopian tubes with multiple lumen diverticula. This tubal pathology increases the incidence of ectopic pregnancy by 52% in age- and race-matched controls.[133]

Diethylstilbestrol

In utero exposure to diethylstilbestrol (DES) alters fallopian tube morphology, resulting in absent or minimal fimbrial tissue, a small os, and decreased length and caliber of the tube.[179] Abnormal tube anatomy accounts for the fivefold common odds ratio for ectopic pregnancy.[8]

Cigarette Smoking

Patients who smoke cigarettes are at a slightly increased risk of ectopic pregnancy. It is difficult to imagine the link between ectopic pregnancy and cigarettes. Theories include impaired immunity in smokers predisposing them to pelvic infections,[44] alterations in tubal motility[8] or a representation of certain lifestyles associated with increased risk.[8]

Douching

Vaginal douching has been associated with a slightly increased risk of ectopic pregnancy. Patients who douche may be exposed to more pelvic infections and subsequent tubal damage than those who do not.[8]

Contraception

Intrauterine devices (IUDs) have been associated with ectopic pregnancy. A multicenter case–control study conducted by the World Health Organization[234] in 10 countries found an odds ratio of 6.4 for ectopic pregnancy in current IUD users compared to pregnant controls, whereas the odds ratio was only 0.5 when the comparison was made to nonpregnant controls. Similarly, in the Oxford Study of 17,032 contraceptive users, the proportion of unplanned pregnancies that were ectopic was higher in women using an IUD compared to women taking an oral contraceptive.[229] Thus, IUDs effectively prevent pregnancy, but if pregnancy occurs in a woman using an IUD, there is an increased likelihood that the pregnancy will be ectopic.[148,229] Interestingly, in one multicenter study, a higher

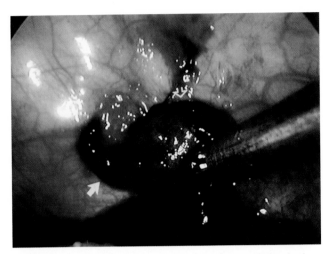

PLATE 1. Characteristic features of a primary abdominal pregnancy are complete abortion of the gestational sac *(open arrow)*, leaving a discrete crater *(closed arrow)* and massive hemoperitoneum. (From ref. 86, with permission.) (This plate is printed in black and white as Figure 11-3.)

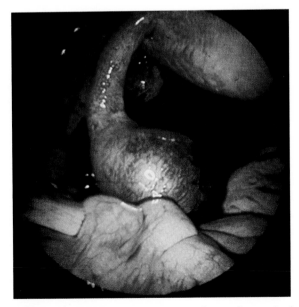

PLATE 2. Laparoscopic visualization of ampullary ectopic pregnancy. (This plate is printed in black and white as Figure 11-4.)

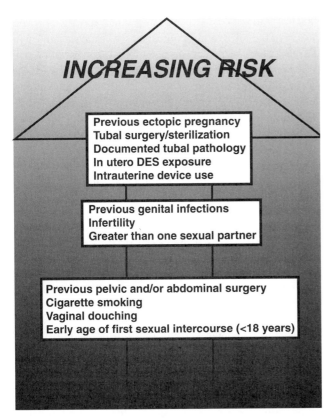

FIG. 2. Risk factors associated with ectopic pregnancy.

proportion of ovarian ectopic pregnancies occurred in IUD users (5.5%), compared to 0% in nonusers.[234]

Ectopic pregnancy after tubal ligation follows a similar pattern to that observed with current IUD use. A metaanalysis using case–control studies found the common odds ratio for tubal sterilization to be 9.3 when compared to pregnant controls and 0.52 when compared to nonpregnant controls,[148] a finding confirmed by two additional multicenter case–control trials.[158,234] As with the IUD, tubal ligations effectively prevent pregnancy, but if pregnancy does occur, the suspicion for an ectopic pregnancy should be high.

The risk of ectopic pregnancy may be higher after electrocoagulation procedures than other forms of tubal sterilization,[142] possibly resulting from tubal recanalization[25,39,44,93,192] or uteroperitoneal fistula formation. McCausland[141] found uteroperitoneal fistulas in 75% of 42 hysterectomy specimens from women with previous tubal ligations in which the tubes were cauterized flush with the uterus.

In direct contrast, women taking oral contraceptives are at reduced risk of ectopic pregnancies when compared to nonpregnant controls, but at an elevated risk when compared to pregnant controls.[148] This protection is due to the overall efficacy of oral contraception in preventing all pregnancy. Similarly, barrier contraception (condoms, spermicides, and diaphragms) also reduces the odds ratio of ectopic pregnancy, as demonstrated by two multicenter studies.[158,234] An additional advantage may be attributed to the decreased risk of sexually transmitted diseases in women using these methods.

Evidence-based Recommendation

Women with a previous ectopic pregnancy, tubal surgery or pathology, or *in utero* DES exposure are at high risk for ectopic pregnancy. Women who experienced genital infections, infertility, or more than one sexual partner have a moderate risk of ectopic pregnancy. Previous pelvic or abdominal surgery, smoking, vaginal douching, or early age of first sexual intercourse only slightly increases the risk of ectopic pregnancy.

Contraception, if used properly, is an effective way of reducing pregnancy, both intrauterine and extrauterine. If pregnancy does occur in patients with an IUD or tubal ligation, the suspicion for ectopic pregnancy should be high. (Strength of recommendation: A.)

◊ SIGNS AND SYMPTOMS

Ectopic pregnancies today can be diagnosed prior to the development of symptoms. The classic triad of amenorrhea, irregular vaginal bleeding, and lower abdominal pain continues to be the most common symptoms of ectopic pregnancy.[231] Sudden, severe, unilateral abdominal pain[103] is the most common complaint in 90% to 100% of women with ectopic pregnancy.[231] Pain radiating to the shoulder,[103] syncope,[103] and shock[43] as a result of hemoperitoneum occur in up to 20% of patients.

The most common signs are related to the abdominal examination. Abdominal tenderness is present in 90% of patients and rebound tenderness in 70%.[43] The pelvic examination is usually nonspecific; cervical motion tenderness is present in up to two-thirds of patients,[43] and a palpable adnexal mass is present in 50%.[231]

◊ ABDOMINAL PREGNANCY

The incidence of abdominal pregnancy is estimated at 1 in 8000 births, and abdominal pregnancy represents 1.4% of ectopic pregnancies.[177] The prognosis is poor, with an estimated maternal mortality rate of 5.1 per 1000 cases.[11] The risk of dying from an abdominal pregnancy is 7.7 times higher than from other forms of ectopic pregnancy.[11]

Abdominal pregnancies can be categorized as primary or secondary. Primary abdominal pregnancies are rare and occur as a result of primary peritoneal implantation. They usually abort early in the first trimester due to hemorrhagic disruption of the implantation site and hemoperitoneum (Fig. 3). Secondary abdominal pregnancies occur with reimplantation after a partial tubal abortion or intraligamentary extension.[86] Historical criteria to distinguish between primary and secondary abdominal pregnancies are moot, because treatment is directed by clinical presentation.

Risk factors associated with abdominal pregnancies are pelvic infections,[12] ectopic gestation,[12] endometriosis,[12] history of infertility,[86] prior tubal surgery,[86] and threatened abortion.[86] Amenorrhea, lower abdominal pain, and vaginal bleeding were the commonly reported symptoms in a series of abdom-

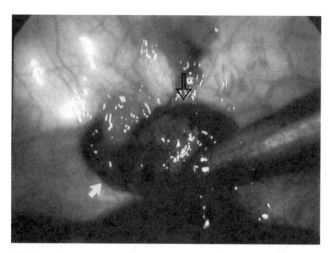

FIG. 3. Characteristic features of a primary abdominal pregnancy are complete abortion of the gestational sac *(open arrow)*, leaving a discrete crater *(closed arrow)* and massive hemoperitoneum. (From ref. 164a, with permission.) (This figure is printed in color as Plate 1.)

inal pregnancies, and the most common sign was abdominal tenderness.[86] Advanced abdominal pregnancies should be suspect in cases of hemoperitoneum, abnormal presentations, painful fetal movements, fetal death, and spurious labor.[86] Ultrasound[128] is the diagnostic tool of choice.

If the fetus is near viability, hospitalization is recommended.[12] If time permits, bowel preparation, administration of prophylactic antibiotics, and adequate blood replacement should be made available prior to delivery.[86] Unless the placenta is implanted on major vessels or vital structures, it should be removed.[86] If the placenta is left in place, many complications can occur, including sepsis, abscess formation, secondary hemorrhage, intestinal obstruction, wound dehiscence, amniotic fluid cyst formation, hypofibrinogenemia, and preeclampsia.[12] Methotrexate is unlikely to accelerate retained placental absorption, because the trophoblasts are no longer actively dividing.

The survival rate of livebirths more than 30 weeks' gestation is 63%, but malformations occur in 21.4% of fetuses.[196] Compression deformities of the skull and extremities from oligohydramnios[38] occur in 20% to 40% of living infants[12]. In addition, intrauterine growth retardation from placental insufficiency can contribute to infant morbidity.[195]

◊ OVARIAN PREGNANCY

Ovarian pregnancy, the most common form of abdominal pregnancy,[84] is rare, accounting for less than 3% of all ectopic gestations.[80] Clinical findings are similar to tubal ectopic gestations: abdominal pain, amenorrhea, and abnormal vaginal bleeding.[84,174] In addition, hemodynamic instability as a result of rupture occurred in 30% of patients in one series.[174]

Women with ovarian pregnancies are usually young and multiparous,[84,174] but the causes of ovarian pregnancies are not clear. Hallat[84] found that 20% of ovarian pregnancies were as-

sociated with IUD use, whereas in a series reported by Raziel et al.,[174] 90% of ovarian pregnancies were associated with IUD use. However, others have not found an association with IUD use.[123] As in tubal pregnancy, inflammatory disease was present in 45.8% of ovarian pregnancies;[80] unlike tubal pregnancies, there are no reports of recurrent ovarian pregnancies.

Diagnosis is usually made by the pathologist because many ovarian pregnancies are mistaken for a ruptured corpus luteum. Only 28% of cases were diagnosed correctly at time of laparotomy.[84] The recommended treatment is cystectomy, wedge resection, or oophorectomy at laparotomy,[174] although two cases of laparoscopic removal have been successful.[47,180]

◊ CORNUAL (INTERSTITIAL) PREGNANCY

Interstitial pregnancy accounts for 4.7% of ectopic gestations and carries a 2.2% maternal mortality.[60] Almost all cases are diagnosed after the patient is symptomatic. The most frequent symptoms are abdominal pain, amenorrhea, abnormal vaginal bleeding, and shock, resulting from the hemorrhage of uterine rupture.[60] Due to myometrial distensibility, rupture is usually delayed, occurring at 9 to 12 weeks.[177]

A unique risk factor for interstitial pregnancy is previous salpingectomy, present in about 25% of patients.[13,78]

Only high suspicion and repeated ultrasound examination with Doppler flow studies enable early diagnosis. With early diagnosis, alternatives to the traditional cornual resection at laparotomy have been performed successfully. Togas et al.[218] successfully treated four patients with laparoscopic cornual resection. Other treatments include systemic methotrexate,[19,64,74,108,212] local injection of methotrexate,[74,157,217] potassium chloride,[217] and removal by hysteroscopy.[217] Regardless of initial treatment used, if uncontrolled hemorrhage occurs, hysterectomy is warranted.[60]

◊ CERVICAL PREGNANCY

The incidence of cervical pregnancy ranges from 1 in 2500 to 1 in 12,422.[223] The most common predisposing factor is a prior dilation and curettage, present in 68.6% of patients; 31% were performed for termination of pregnancy. Other predisposing factors implicated in cervical pregnancies are previous cesarean delivery and *in vitro* fertilization. Asherman syndrome, IUD use, infertility, or prior ectopic pregnancy does not appear to play an important role.[223]

The most common presenting symptom of cervical pregnancy is painless vaginal bleeding. In reported cases, 91% of patients presented with vaginal bleeding, and 29.2% had massive bleeding.[223] Abdominal pain occurred with vaginal bleeding in only 25.8% of cases.[223] The cervix is usually enlarged, globular or distended. On occasion, it appears cyanotic, hyperemic, and soft in consistency.[223] Sonography and magnetic resonance imaging have improved diagnosis of cervical pregnancy: Up to 81.8% of patients were correctly diagnosed with ultrasound identification of the intracervical gestational sac below a closed internal cervical os, and trophoblastic invasion into the endocervical tissue.[223]

Conservative therapy is commonly employed. Dilation and evacuation with cervical tamponade successfully treated 62.3% of patients with cervical pregnancy.[223] A 26-French Foley catheter with a 30-ml balloon successfully tamponaded 92.3% of cervical bleeding.[223] Preoperative preparation for cervical bleeding, such as ligation of cervical branches of the uterine arteries, Shirodkar cerclage placement, or uterine artery embolization, results in a higher success rate for conservative therapy. Similar to tubal ectopic pregnancy, medical management for cervical pregnancy has recently been employed. Systemic and local treatment with various agents carries an overall success rate of 81.3%.[223] Short series of cases document successful methotrexate treatment of cervical pregnancy in the first trimester: Hsu et al.[96] successfully treated three cervical pregnancies with methotrexate, and Timor-Tritsch et al.[216] directly injected five cervical pregnancies under ultrasound guidance with 100% success and cited four other case reports. Unfortunately, massive hemorrhage may occur despite conservative measures, and hysterectomy is warranted.

◊ HETEROTOPIC PREGNANCY

Heterotopic pregnancy is the coexistence of an intrauterine and ectopic gestation.[177] In 1948, the spontaneous heterotopic pregnancy rate was calculated as 1 in 30,000 pregnancies, based on an ectopic pregnancy incidence of 0.37% and dizygous twinning rate of 0.8%.[53] In the 1980s, the calculation rose to 1 in 10,000 due to an increased ectopic pregnancy rate.[175] Today, heterotopic pregnancies actually occur in 1 in 3889[18] to 1 in 6778[87] pregnancies. In a review of 66 heterotopic pregnancies by Reece et al.,[175] 93.9% were tubal, and 6.1% ovarian.

Simultaneous existence of intra- and extrauterine pregnancies poses several diagnostic pitfalls. Heterotopic pregnancies are diagnosed in most cases after clinical signs and symptoms develop, and 50% of patients are admitted for emergency surgery following rupture.[177]

Similar to tubal ectopic pregnancies, the most common complaint is lower abdominal pain, occurring in 81.8% of patients. Peritoneal irritation occurs in 43.9% and vaginal spotting in 31.8%.[175] Routine ultrasound detects only about 50% of tubal heterotopic pregnancies, and the remainder are diagnosed at laparoscopy or laparotomy when patients become symptomatic.[177] Serial levels of the β subunit of human chorionic gonadotropin (β-hCG) are not helpful due to the concomitant intrauterine pregnancy.

If patients are hemodynamically unstable, an exploratory laparotomy is warranted. If the diagnosis is suspected or the patient is symptomatic but hemodynamically stable, laparoscopy can be performed. Expectant management is not recommended, since β-hCG levels cannot be monitored adequately. Systemic methotrexate is contraindicated if a viable intrauterine pregnancy is present. Local injection of methotrexate with potassium chloride was not successful in a small case series.[82]

◊ ECTOPIC PREGNANCY AND ASSISTED REPRODUCTIVE TECHNOLOGY

Incidence

The risk of ectopic pregnancy is increased in patients undergoing an assisted reproductive technology (ART) procedure, compared to the 2% rate in the general population. This increased risk of ectopic pregnancy has been attributed to the cause of infertility for which most patients seek treatment, that is, tubal factor infertility. Information on ectopic pregnancies resulting from ART comes from data obtained from all institutions in the United States and Canada reporting to the Society for Assisted Reproductive Technology. From 1988 to 1992, 5% to 5.7% of all clinical pregnancies resulting from ART were ectopic.[5] These rates were calculated from all forms of ART, including *in vitro* fertilization (IVF), gamete intrafallopian transfer (GIFT), and zygote intrafallopian transfer (ZIFT). From 1992 to 1994 ectopic pregnancy rates were calculated for individual procedures: 4.4% to 4.9% after IVF, 3.2% to 4% after GIFT, and 2.8% to 3.9% after ZIFT.[6,9,10]

Location

As in naturally occurring ectopic pregnancies, the fallopian tube is the most common site for ectopic pregnancies following IVF. Data obtained from three case–control studies revealed that 82.2% of ectopic pregnancies were tubal. When tubal location was specified, 92.7% were ampullary, and 7.3% interstitial. Extratubal ectopic nidations were as follows: 4.6% ovarian/abdominal, 1.5% cervical, and 11.7% heterotopic pregnancies (see Fig. 1).[54,107,135,171]

Tubal Pathology

The most important predisposing factor for ectopic pregnancy in patients undergoing IVF is tubal pathology. Ectopic pregnancies are four times higher in patients with tubal-factor infertility compared to patients with normal tubes.[54,91,242] In two case–control studies, hydrosalpinx was more commonly associated with ectopic pregnancy than other causes of tubal pathology.[54,171] Prior tubal reconstructive surgery (salpingostomy) increases the risk of ectopic pregnancy by 10% above that in patients with tubal-factor infertility without prior surgery.[242]

Thus, it is not surprising that patients with previous pelvic inflammatory disease have a sixfold increase in ectopic pregnancy after IVF.[135] However, a history of prior ectopic pregnancy does not seem as important a risk factor in IVF cycles as in natural cycles. In one small case–control study, a twofold increase in ectopic pregnancy was found in patients with a history of ectopic pregnancy,[107] whereas another case–control study did not confirm this increase.[135]

Ovulation Induction

Hormone alterations during ovulation induction theoretically alter tubal function. Estrogen administration results in functional tubal blockage and embryo arrest in the fallopian tube in animal studies.[170,226] In humans, steroid hormones alter tubal function and contractility, thus affecting tubal peristalsis.[107,127] Multiple small studies found that ovulation-inducing agents, including clomiphene citrate, increase ectopic pregnancy rates;[63,140,226] yet other studies have not found this to be so.[135,137] One case–control study found peak estradiol levels were significantly higher in patients with ectopic pregnancies, but in the same study a number of ectopic pregnancies occurred in frozen embryo transfers with normal estradiol levels, thus refuting the association of ectopic pregnancies with elevated estradiol levels.[107]

Embryo Transfer

Knutzen et al.[112] injected 50 µl of radiopaque fluid in mock embryo transfers and found that the material entered the tubes either partially or totally in 44% of subjects, suggesting misplacement of embryos into the fallopian tubes. Embryo catheter placement was also implicated in the increased risk of ectopic pregnancies, which occurred more frequently in patients who underwent deep fundal transfer versus midcavity placement.[153,240] Although transfer techniques may increase the chances of embryos reaching the fallopian tubes, ectopic pregnancies may result from tubal pathology preventing the embryos from moving back into the uterus.[91]

Heterotopic Pregnancy

Heterotopic pregnancies occur in 1% to 3% of pregnancies following an ART procedure. This increased prevalence of heterotopic pregnancies following ART may be related to ovarian hyperstimulation and multiple ovum development. Of 111 heterotopic pregnancies following ART, 88.3% were tubal, 6.3% cornual, 2.7% abdominal, 1.8% cervical, and 0.9% ovarian.[177]

Evidence-based Recommendation

Patients with tubal factor infertility are at higher risk of ectopic gestation after ART than patients with other causes of infertility and should be monitored accordingly. Heterotopic and extratubal ectopic pregnancies are increased following ART compared to natural cycles. (Strength of recommendation: B.)

◊ DIAGNOSIS

Today, ectopic pregnancy can be diagnosed before 6 weeks of amenorrhea, often as early as 4.5 weeks' gestation, prior to the onset of symptoms.[36] The traditional laparoscopic visualization of ectopic pregnancy (Fig. 4) is now rarely necessary and frequently impossible at the early gestational age that other methods can make the diagnosis. Diagnostic tests routinely used today are serial measurements of β-hCG, ultrasonography, serum progesterone, and uterine curettage.[204,205,208] The diagnostic algorithm in Figure 5 proved 100% efficacious in diagnosing ectopic pregnancy when it was tested randomly against confirmatory laparoscopy.[205]

β-hCG

β-hCG determinations used today are based on the enzyme-linked immunosorbent assay (ELISA), detecting low β-hCG concentrations in urine and serum, 20 mIU/ml and 10 mIU/ml, respectively.[45] The β-hCG, produced by trophoblastic cells in normal pregnancy doubles about every 2 days.[124,126] Abnormal pregnancies, whether intrauterine or ectopic, have impaired β-hCG production with prolonged doubling time. Failure of the β-hCG concentration to rise after 48 hours diagnoses a nonviable pregnancy and allows uterine curettage. If a viable intrauterine gestation is not visible by transvaginal ultrasound when the β-hCG is above 2000 mIU/ml (First International Reference Preparation),[16,17,34,68,77,155,215] uterine curettage can be performed for treatment of a nonviable intrauterine pregnancy or as a diagnostic measure for an ectopic gestation.[16] This β-hCG concentration is not universal, and each institution must identify its own values to avoid terminating healthy intrauterine pregnancies.

β-hCG determinations are further employed for the diagnosis of ectopic gestations: After uterine curettage, if the β-hCG fails to decline by 15%,[36] the pregnancy is ectopic and treatment is indicated.

Serum Progesterone

The serum progesterone level reflects the production of progesterone by the corpus luteum that is stimulated by a viable pregnancy. During the first 8 to 10 weeks of gestation, serum progesterone concentrations change little; as pregnancy fails, the levels decrease.[204] Thus, progesterone measurements are used to distinguish between a normal intrauterine pregnancy and an abnormal gestation (nonviable

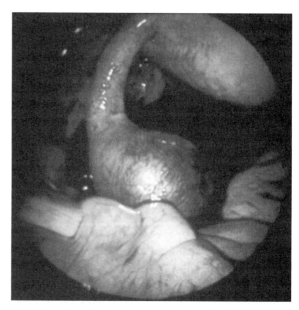

FIG. 4. Laparoscopic visualization of ampullary ectopic pregnancy. (This figure is printed in color as Plate 2.)

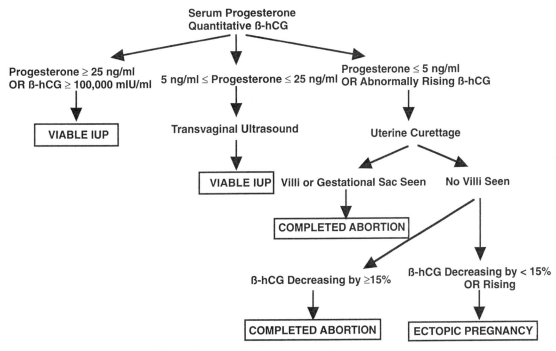

FIG. 5. Diagnostic algorithm for ectopic pregnancy.

intrauterine pregnancy or ectopic pregnancy). The measurement of progesterone contributes to the diagnosis of an ectopic pregnancy in three ways:

◊ It is an inexpensive screening test that can identify patients who need to undergo further testing. Further diagnostic testing in patients with low serum progesterone reduced the prevalence of ruptured ectopic pregnancy in an emergency room setting by 50%.[206]

◊ It excludes ectopic pregnancy with a 97.5% sensitivity when concentrations are greater than 25 ng/ml (greater than 79.5 nmol/l).

◊ It identifies nonviable pregnancies with 100% sensitivity when concentrations are less than 5 ng/ml (less than 15.9 nmol/l). Thus, a single progesterone value of less than 5 ng/ml allows diagnostic uterine evacuation when ectopic pregnancy cannot be distinguished from spontaneous intrauterine abortion.[204,205,208]

Transvaginal Ultrasound

The high resolution of transvaginal ultrasound reliably detects intrauterine gestation when β-hCG levels are between 1000 and 2000 mIU/ml (First IRP),[16,17,34,68,77,155,215] as early as 1 week after missed menses.[106,111,155]

Diagnosis of an ectopic pregnancy can be made with 100% specificity but with low sensitivity (15% to 20%) if an extrauterine gestational sac containing a yolk sac or embryo is identified (Fig. 6).[27,156] A complex adnexal mass without an intrauterine pregnancy improves sensitivity to 21% to 84% at the expense of lower specificity (93% to 99.5%).[27,156] In a review of 10 studies, Brown and Doubilet[27]

concluded that the presence of any noncystic, extraovarian adnexal mass in the absence of an intrauterine gestation was diagnostic of an ectopic pregnancy with 98.9% specificity, 96.3% positive predictive value, 84.4% sensitivity, and a 94.8% negative predictive value. Despite the high resolution of transvaginal ultrasound, an adnexal mass will not be found in 15% to 35% of patients with an ectopic pregnancy.[69,156,178,181]

Serum β-hCG concentrations and transvaginal ultrasound predict ectopic pregnancy with a positive predictive value of 95%[7]. Diagnosis is routinely made by the absence of an intrauterine pregnancy at a designated β-hCG concentration. Barnhart et al.[16] were able to identify all viable intrauterine pregnancies by ultrasound when the β-hCG was greater than 1500 mIU/ml (First IRP). However, Braffman et al.[23] found

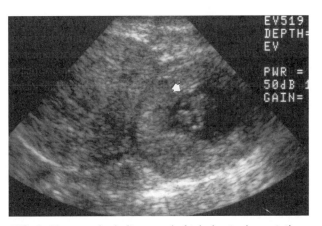

FIG. 6. Transvaginal ultrasound of tubal ectopic gestation.

the diagnostic accuracy of ultrasound to be 81% when the β-hCG was greater than or equal to 1500 mIU/ml (First IRP), and in those patients with an "indeterminate" ultrasound, 24% had an ectopic pregnancy. Thus, ultrasound alone cannot diagnose all ectopic pregnancies, and further diagnostic modalities are warranted.

The availability of color Doppler was initially believed to improve the diagnostic capabilities of transvaginal ultrasound, increasing sensitivity to 87% and specificity to 99%,[57] but later studies have not confirmed a marked improvement over two-dimensional imaging alone[1] and B-mode sonography.[42]

Uterine Curettage

Uterine curettage, which may be performed in the office, is necessary when ultrasound is not sufficient for diagnosis. Curettage should be performed after a nonviable pregnancy has been documented on the basis of a progesterone level less than or equal to 5 ng/ml or a plateauing β-hCG level.[204,205,208] Visualization of villi in the tissue obtained at curettage (by flotation in saline) indicates the occurrence of a spontaneous intrauterine abortion. In the absence of villi, a decrease in the β-hCG level of 15% or more 8 to 12 hours after curettage is diagnostic of a complete abortion.[204] If the β-hCG titer plateaus or rises, the trophoblast was not removed by curettage, and ectopic pregnancy is diagnosed.[204]

Evidence-based Recommendation

A screening serum progesterone maximizes the diagnostic yield of subsequent testing in patients at risk for ectopic pregnancy. Serial β-hCG, transvaginal ultrasound, and uterine curettage allow laparoscopy to be avoided in the early diagnosis of ectopic pregnancy. (Strength of recommendation: A.)

◊ SURGICAL TREATMENT

Since the first successful salpingectomy was performed by Tait[211] in 1884, ectopic pregnancies have traditionally been treated by salpingectomy at laparotomy. Historically, ectopic pregnancies were diagnosed at the time of emergency surgery, when concern for the patient's life superseded any concerns for her future fertility. It was not until 1953, when Stromme[209] performed the first conservative procedure (salpingotomy) for an ectopic pregnancy, that subsequent successful pregnancy outcomes were reported, confirming fertility preservation after salpingotomy.[224] Subsequently, other conservative surgical procedures, such as fimbrial expression and segmental resection with later reanastomosis, have been performed to preserve fertility; all have been modified for the laparoscope. Today, medical therapy has become an alternative treatment to surgery for the patient with an unruptured ectopic pregnancy.

Ruptured Ectopic Pregnancy

Early diagnosis and treatment of ectopic pregnancy account for the decrease in hemodynamically unstable patients presenting for emergency surgery today. In the 1970s, 13.5% to 17.8% of patients with ectopic pregnancies presented in hypovolemic shock,[118,213] whereas in the early 1980s only 4.4% of patients were in hypovolemic shock.[118] Today, the estimate for patients presenting in shock is at most 10%,[138] and laparotomy with salpingectomy is the treatment of choice.

Once contraindicated due to the decreased venous return from intraperitoneal insufflation,[102,136] laparoscopic salpingectomy was successful in 30 of 33 patients presenting in hypovolemic shock. Three patients required a laparotomy, and 88% of patients required blood transfusions. Unfortunately, a comparison to laparotomy was not performed to evaluate whether or not morbidity was similar.[198] In the hands of a skilled laparoscopist, with advanced cardiac monitoring and anesthesia, laparoscopic salpingectomy may be an alternative to laparotomy in this subgroup of patients, but further evidence is required before any recommendations can be made.

Stable Ectopic Pregnancy

Salpingectomy, considered radical surgical therapy for an unruptured ectopic pregnancy, is rarely performed today because of the efficacy of conservative surgical therapy. Salpingectomy can be performed either at laparotomy or laparoscopy using cautery or sutures (laparoscopic or endoloops). Yao and Tulandi[235] compared reproductive outcome from one case–control study,[51] one cohort study[197] and 7 case series.[14,119,159,165,194,214,222] Of the 2635 patients treated, 528 patients treated with conservative surgery and 1246 patients treated with radical surgery desired fertility. Subsequent to conservative surgery, 53% of patients had an intrauterine pregnancy, compared to 49.3% after radical surgery. Recurrent ectopic pregnancy rates were slightly higher after conservative surgery: 14.8% compared to 9.9%. Laparoscopic salpingectomy is preferred over salpingotomy in cases of uncontrollable bleeding not resolved with conservative measures, extensive tubal damage, and recurrent ectopic pregnancy in the same tube, as well as for sterilization.[26]

The recommended conservative surgical procedure for an ampullary ectopic pregnancy is the linear salpingotomy, because the ectopic nidation is located between the endosalpinx and serosa, not in the tubal lumen.[31] A linear salpingotomy is made through a longitudinal incision by electrocautery, scissors, or laser over the bulging antimesenteric border of the fallopian tube. Products of conception are removed with forceps or suction. After maintaining hemostasis, the incision is left to heal by secondary intention.

Isthmic pregnancies are routinely treated with segmental excision followed by intraoperative or delayed microsurgical anastomosis.[15] The tubal lumen is narrower and the muscularis is thicker in the isthmus than in the ampulla, predisposing the isthmus to greater damage after salpingostomy and greater rates of proximal obstruction.[122]

Fimbrial expression, also known as "milking," should only be used when the trophoblastic tissue is aborting through the fimbriae.[15]

Laparoscopy has several advantages over laparotomy, including less blood loss,[151] less analgesia,[151] and improved postoperative recovery, as measured by shorter hospitalizations[131,228] and length of time to resume normal activity.[131] In addition, cost analysis resulted in significant savings in three randomized trials.[131,151,228]

Conservative laparoscopic surgery, salpingotomy, or fimbrial expression was evaluated in 32 studies: seven randomized controlled studies (I), two well designed controlled trials (II-1), two cohort studies (II-2), and 21 case series (II-3) (Table 1). Of the 1614 patients treated between 1980 and 1997, treatment was successful in 93.4% (required no additional therapy). Of the 207 patients evaluated for tubal patency using either hysterosalpingogram or laparoscopy, 77.8% had patent tubes. Of the 647 women desiring subsequent fertility, 56.6% had an intrauterine pregnancy and 13.4% developed another ectopic pregnancy.

TABLE 1. *Overview of outcomes of studies on the treatment of stable ectopic pregnancy*

Method	Studies[a] (n)	Patients (n)	Success[b]	Tubal Patency[b]	Subsequent Fertility[b]	
					IUP	EP
Conservative laparoscopic surgery	32 **I:** 66, 67, 83, 150, 160, 228, 241 **II-1:** 109, 166 **II-2:** 29, 188 **II-3:** 3, 22, 28, 40, 41, 48, 50, 89, 97, 104, 110, 121, 143, 146, 161, 167, 189, 196, 197, 225, 237	1614	1508 (93.4)	161/207 (77.8)	366/647 (56.6)	87/647 (13.4)
Variable-dose methotrexate	12 **I:** 83 **II-2:** 101 **II-3:** 33, 76, 99, 114, 129, 147, 168, 169, 183, 208	325	305 (93.8)	127/161 (78.9)	55/95 (57.9)	7/95 (7.4)
Single-dose methotrexate	6 **II-2:** 201 **II-3:** 73, 81, 90, 173, 200	304	265/304 (87.2)	61/75 (81.3)	39/64 (61.0)	5/64 (7.8)
Direct injection methotrexate	21 **I:** 61, 66, 67, 150, 160, 241 **II-1:** 166 **II-3:** 49, 58, 62, 113, 116, 144, 145, 162–164, 185, 189, 221, 233	668	502 (75.1)	130/162 (80.2)	87/152 (57.2)	9/152 (5.9)
Expectant management	13 **II-3:** 35, 37, 52, 65, 71, 117, 130, 134, 183, 190, 219, 239 **III:** 39	598	402 (67.2)	60/79 (75.9)	12/14 (85.7)	1/14 (7.1)

I, randomized, controlled studies; **II-1**, controlled trials; **II-2**, cohort studies; **III-3**, case series; **III**, case reports.
[a] Study references are listed according to quality of evidence.
[b] Percentages are in parentheses.

Yao and Tulandi[235] evaluated subsequent fertility, combining three randomized trials, and found that intrauterine pregnancy rates were similar: 61% for laparoscopy and 53% for laparotomy. Recurrent ectopic pregnancy rates were 7% after laparoscopy and 14% after laparotomy—numbers too small for firm conclusions.[132,151,227,235]

The increased rate of persistent ectopic pregnancies has been a criticism of conservative laparoscopic therapy. Compared to laparotomy, two studies found an increased rate of persistent ectopic pregnancies after laparoscopy.[131,151] Another study failed to confirm these findings, with a 3.3% rate for both treatment groups.[228]

Evidence-based Recommendation

Due to lower morbidity and equal efficacy, laparoscopic surgery is preferable to laparotomy in the treatment of ectopic pregnancy. Salpingectomy by laparotomy is best reserved for the hemodynamically unstable patient. (Strength of recommendation: A.)

◊ MEDICAL MANAGEMENT

Methotrexate therapy of ectopic pregnancy, first introduced by Tanaka et al.,[212] was used successfully in many trials. A folic acid antagonist, methotrexate inhibits *de novo* synthesis of purines and pyrimidines, interfering with DNA synthesis and cell multiplication.[46] Actively proliferating trophoblasts are particularly vulnerable to methotrexate.[122,182] Hemodynamically stable patients with an unruptured ectopic pregnancy measuring less than or equal to 4 cm by ultrasound are eligible for methotrexate therapy.[205,208] Patients with larger masses or evidence of acute intraabdominal bleeding are ineligible for methotrexate therapy.[201,205,208] Two commonly employed treatment regimens are shown in Table 2.

Variable-dose Methotrexate

Multiple-dose methotrexate therapy is tailored to the patient and ectopic pregnancy aggressiveness. Outcomes of 12 studies—one randomized control trial (I), one cohort study (II-2), and 10 case series (II-3) comparing variable-dose systemic methotrexate with laparoscopic salpingostomy—are presented in Table 1. Between 1982 and 1997, 325 cases of ectopic pregnancy treated with variable-dose methotrexate were reported. Of these cases, 93.8% were treated successfully with variable-dose systemic methotrexate (no subsequent therapy was required), and 78.9% of the 161 women tested had patent oviducts; in addition, of the 95 women desiring pregnancy, 57.9% had a subsequent intrauterine pregnancy and 7.4% developed a recurrent ectopic pregnancy. These rates all compare favorably with conservative surgical management.

There is only one randomized clinical trial comparing laparoscopic salpingostomy with systemic methotrexate.[83] In it, 75 patients with laparoscopy-confirmed ectopic pregnancy were randomly treated with systemic methotrexate or

TABLE 2. *Two commonly employed methotrexate regimens*

Regimen	Monitor
Variable dose	
Methotrexate, 1 mg/kg IM, alternate days (days 1, 3, 5, 7)	β-hCG weekly until undetectable
Leucovorin calcium, 0.1 mg/kg IM, alternate days (days 2, 4, 6, 8)	Initial blood count, platelets, and liver enzymes
Continue until β-hCG drops ≥ 15% in 48 h **OR** 4 doses methotrexate given	
Single dose	
Methotrexate, 50 mg/m² IM	β-hCG days 4 and 7, then weekly until undetectable
Repeat dose if	Initial blood count, platelets, and liver enzymes
Day 7 β-hCG ≥ day 4 β-hCG	

β-hCG, human β-chorionic gonadotropin.
(Modified from ref. 36.)

laparoscopic salpingostomy. In the 38 patients treated with methotrexate, three (8%) required surgical intervention for active bleeding and/or tubal rupture. An additional course of methotrexate was required in two patients (5%) for persistent trophoblast. Of the 37 patients in the salpingostomy group, two patients (5%) failed and required salpingectomies, and eight patients (22%) were treated with methotrexate for persistent trophoblast. Tubal patency was present in 14 of 21 patients (67%) in the methotrexate group, and 14 of 23 (61%) in the salpingostomy group. This study confirms the effectiveness of methotrexate therapy as a more definitive treatment modality than salpingostomy.

Single-dose Methotrexate

Single-dose methotrexate, although more convenient, is not as efficacious as multidose methotrexate. The high success rates in the initial study utilizing single-dose methotrexate was most likely due to the inclusion of spontaneously aborting intrauterine pregnancies.[207] Six studies of single-dose methotrexate therapy were evaluated: one cohort (II-2) and five case–control studies (II-3) involving 304 patients (see Table 1). Although overall success of treatment, measured as no surgical intervention, is 87.2%, 11.5% of patients required more than one dose. Of the patients considered to be treated successfully (either with one or more doses), tubal patency was found in 81.3% of the 75 women evaluated. The subsequent intrauterine pregnancy rate was 61%, and for ectopic pregnancies 7.8%, in the 64 patients desiring future fertility in the same group (those treated with either one or more doses of methotrexate).

Safeguards

During methotrexate therapy, a patient should be examined by only one examiner only once.[205,208] The physician and the patient must recognize that transient pain is common. Transient pelvic pain frequently occurs 3 to 7 days after the start of therapy, lasts 4 to 12 hours, and is presumably due to tubal abortion.[205,208] Perhaps the most difficult aspect of methotrexate therapy is learning to distinguish the transient abdominal pain of successful therapy from that of a rupturing ectopic pregnancy. Objective criteria help; surgical intervention is necessary only when pain is accompanied by orthostatic hypotension or a falling hematocrit. Physicians may prefer to hospitalize the patient with pain for observation (usually about 24 hours). In addition, colicky abdominal pain is common during the first 2 or 3 days of methotrexate therapy, and the patient should avoid gas-producing foods, such as leeks and cabbage. Finally, the patient should avoid exposure to the sun because photosensitivity can be a complication.[154]

Methotrexate by Direct Injection

In 1987, Feichtinger and Kemeter[59] instilled 1 ml (10 mg) of methotrexate into an ectopic gestational sac under transvaginal ultrasound, and resolution occurred within 2 weeks. Direct injection delivers concentrations of methotrexate to the site of implantation at higher concentrations than those achieved with systemic administration. Thus, less systemic distribution of the drug decreases toxicity. However, this approach has the substantial disadvantage of requiring laparoscopic or ultrasonographic needle guidance.

Outcomes in 21 studies involving direct injection of methotrexate are presented in Table 1; these studies include six randomized, controlled trials (I), one controlled trial without randomization (II-1), and 14 case series (II-3), evaluating methotrexate by direct injection into the gestational sac either laparoscopically or by transvaginal ultrasound guidance. Between 1989 and 1997, only 75.1% of 668 cases of ectopic pregnancy were treated successfully with methotrexate by direct injection, and some patients required more than one injection. Tubal patency and subsequent pregnancy rates were comparable to conservative laparoscopic surgery and systemic methotrexate: 80.2% of the 162 women tested had patent oviducts, and of the 152 women desiring pregnancy, 57.2% had a subsequent intrauterine pregnancy and 5.9% developed a recurrent ectopic pregnancy.

The randomized, controlled trials (I) resulted in successful treatment with methotrexate by direct injection in 86.2% of the 138 patients. Again, successful therapy included some patients who received more than one injection. Tubal patency was present in 85.1% of the 47 women evaluated, and intrauterine pregnancy occurred in 73.1% of the 26 women desiring subsequent fertility. One of the earlier randomized, controlled trials was discontinued because three of seven patients assigned to laparoscopic injection of methotrexate required additional laparoscopic surgery.[150] Even with the higher success rate in the randomized trials, these rates are still unacceptably low for direct injection of methotrexate to be considered as a therapeutic alternative for ectopic pregnancy.

Methotrexate by Tubal Cannulation

Instillation of methotrexate by hysteroscopically directed tubal cannulation has also been described. Risquez et al.[176] reported resolution of 27 of 31 cases by this method, with the remaining four ultimately requiring surgery. Although these results are encouraging, this approach seems to have no major advantage over other methods, except that methotrexate can be instilled into very small ectopic gestational sacs without the gestational sac actually being visualized.

Side Effects

High doses of methotrexate can cause bone marrow suppression, acute and chronic hepatotoxicity, stomatitis, pulmonary fibrosis, alopecia, and photosensitivity.[114] These side effects are infrequent in shorter treatment schedules used in ectopic pregnancy and can be attenuated by the administration of leucovorin (citrovorum factor).[183,208] A literature review of the side effects with methotrexate was performed by Kooi and Kock.[115] Of the 23 studies evaluated, 16 studies reported side effects, all of which resolved within 3 to 4 days after methotrexate therapy was discontinued. Impaired liver function was the most common side effect, reported in 17 of 141 patients receiving systemic methotrexate. Of 141 patients, stomatitis developed in nine, gastritis/enteritis in three, and bone marrow suppression in one. Local therapy, direct injection into the ectopic gestation, resulted in fewer side effects as a result of less systemic absorption. One of 91 patients developed impaired liver function tests, one developed gastritis/enteritis, and one bone marrow suppression.[115] Additional case reports exist in the literature. Two cases of life-threatening neutropenia and febrile morbidity were reported after a single dose and after three doses of intramuscular methotrexate, requiring hospitalization for 1 month and 13 days, respectively.[100] Two cases of transient pneumonitis from methotrexate therapy for ectopic pregnancy have been reported.[95,187] One patient was reported to develop reversible alopecia (a loss of 33% to 50% of her scalp hair) on two separate occasions following single-dose therapy for an ectopic pregnancy.[220] One hematosalpinx and two pelvic hematoceles were reported as late sequelae of methotrexate following the normalization of β-hCG levels. All three patients presented with pelvic pain, abnormal bleeding, and a pelvic mass, requiring surgical intervention, 3 to 5 months after initial therapy.[243] Although there are reports of complications as a result of methotrexate therapy, these cases are rare, and methotrexate for the treatment of ectopic pregnancy remains a safe alternative to surgical therapy.

Direct Injection of Cyotoxic Agents

Prostaglandins,[58,98,125] hyperosmolar glucose,[76,120,237] potassium chloride, and saline by direct injection have been tried as therapeutic alternatives to methotrexate.

Prostaglandins cause strong tubal muscular contractions and are local vasocontrictors. Attempts using prostaglandin (PG) E_2 injections directly into the ectopic gestation were abandoned because of untoward side effects, including severe discomfort, vomiting, and cramps.[58] Subsequently, direct injection of $PGF_{2\alpha}$ into the affected tube and the ovary containing the corpus luteum was successful in 24 of 26 (92%) women treated,[125] and Husslein[98] reported an 84% success rate in 152 patients from eight centers in Austria. In addition to the limited criteria for prostaglandin use, namely, a β-hCG level less than 2500 mIU/ml and ectopic gestation less than 2 cm, serious cardiopulmonary side effects have been reported, including pulmonary edema,[56] making this therapeutic alternative unfavorable.

Similarly, hyperosmolar glucose has been injected either laparoscopically[76,120,237] or by transvaginal ultrasound guidance.[76] In two small series, glucose therapy was successful in 100% of 16 patients and 94% of 16 patients, respectively.[120,237] A larger randomized trial comparing hypertonic glucose injection with laparoscopy versus transvaginal ultrasound guidance had poorer success rates: 51.2% after a single injection in the laparoscopic group and 74.4% in the transvaginal group.[76]

The limited experience with prostaglandins and hypertonic glucose, poor success rates, and the need for laparoscopic or transvaginal aspiration makes these treatment alternatives unacceptable at present.

Evidence-based Recommendation

Variable-dose methotrexate is the medical treatment of choice for ectopic pregnancy. (Strength of recommendation: A.)

◊ EXPECTANT MANAGEMENT

Ectopic pregnancies do resolve spontaneously. In a cavalier experiment in 1955, Lund[130] hospitalized 119 women with ectopic pregnancy for observation; all were at least 6 weeks' gestation. Some required multiple large transfusions, and many were hemodynamically unstable. However, 68 resolved without surgery. Twelve additional studies reported in the literature since Lund's found similar results: 11 case series (II-3) and one study reporting on five cases (III) (see Table 1). Of these 13 studies, 67.2% of the 598 ectopic pregnancies resolved without surgery. Thus, both conservative medical and surgical therapy overtreats at least 50% of these patients. We are left to accept this overtreatment rate until a marker is uncovered that identifies this subgroup of patients who can be treated with expectant management.

Recent attempts at uncovering such markers have failed. Carson et al.[37] discontinued a prospective trial that separated

observed from treated patients based on their levels of human chorionic somatomammotropin (human placental lactogen) because three of nine patients designated as safe to observe required treatment. Creatinine kinase also failed to detect the ectopic pregnancies destined for absorption.[172] β-hCG level and size of the ectopic pregnancy also have little bearing on whether it will spontaneously resorb, unless the β-hCG level is less than 1000 mIU/ml. Even in such cases, only 88% resolve spontaneously.[219] Furthermore, declining β-hCG concentrations in laparoscopy-confirmed ectopic pregnancy failed to predict spontaneous absorption in 32 of 60 women (53.3%).[190]

Evidence-based Recommendation

Until a marker for ectopic pregnancies destined for spontaneous resolution is identified, expectant management must be abandoned in lieu of safe, conservative therapy. (Strength of recommendation: A.)

◊ PERSISTENT ECTOPIC PREGNANCY

Persistent ectopic pregnancy occurs when there is incomplete removal of trophoblastic tissue following conservative surgical therapy; it is diagnosed by a plateauing or rising β-hCG concentration following surgical therapy.[94] Due to the limited number of reported cases and small series of cases, there is no single optimal treatment. In the largest series, all 19 patients with persistent ectopic pregnancies were successfully treated using single-dose systemic methotrexate.[94] Successful treatment has also been reported with salpingectomy, repeat salpingostomy, RU 486 (mifepristone), and expectant management.[94]

Evidence-based Recommendation

The low morbidity and optimal outcome obtained with methotrexate suggest that it is the safest and most effective treatment modality for persistent ectopic pregnancy. (Strength of recommendation: B.)

◊ Rh FACTOR

All unsuccessful first-trimester pregnancies, including ectopic pregnancies, in women at risk for Rh sensitization require $Rh_0(D)$ immune globulin, 50 μg.

◊ COST ANALYSIS

In 1990, total costs for ectopic pregnancies were estimated to be $1.1 billion. Direct costs, expenditures for health care, accounted for 77% of the total costs, and the remainder were incurred as a result of lost wages and/or household responsibilities not performed due to illness (indirect costs). Direct costs from hospital charges were estimated at $6079 per case, with hospital accommodations (mean length of stay, 3.47 days) and operating room charges accounting for the majority of the hospital expense, 36% and 40%, respectively. An additional $3254 for professional fees increased inpatient charges to $9333, and $149 for postoperative follow-up visits increased the total direct cost to $9482 per case. Indirect costs for a 28-day disability were estimated at $250.5 million, 67% as a result of lost wages and the remainder from lost household duties.[230]

Today, with the continuing rise in ectopic pregnancies, treatment strategies must consider cost effectiveness after patient safety. Traditionally, ectopic pregnancies have been treated by laparotomy. More recently, surgical management has been directed toward laparoscopy. In a retrospective cohort, direct costs per patient for laparoscopic surgery was lower than the same procedure performed by laparotomy. The cost of laparoscopic conservative surgery or salpingectomy was $2125 and $1872, respectively. Costs for conservative treatment or salpingectomy via laparotomy were higher, $3420 and $3490, respectively. Length of hospital stay accounted for the higher cost for open surgery.[149] In addition, three randomized, controlled trials (I) found direct cost savings of laparoscopy over laparotomy equaling $1200,[151] $1500,[227,228] and 4641 Swedish krones.[131,132] Although one study did not find a difference in average direct costs between laparoscopy and laparotomy, recovery was significantly shorter in the laparoscopy-treated group, 2.4 versus 4.6 weeks,[92] similar to the decreased recovery period found in two randomized trials.[131,132,151] This shorter recovery period can be extrapolated to lower indirect costs.

Although laparoscopy is a more cost-effective treatment alternative to laparotomy, it is nonetheless associated with the high costs of operating rooms, anesthesia, and surgeon's fees. Medical therapy is not only less invasive but more cost-efficient. At a university-based teaching facility, direct costs for medical and surgical therapy of 60 consecutive patients treated for ectopic pregnancy were retrospectively analyzed. All ectopic pregnancies in this group resolved with medical therapy alone. Charges for 21 patients treated with methotrexate averaged $1563 (range, $1169 to $2300). Of the 15 patients treated with laparoscopy, the average charge was $6626 (range, $4625 to $10,429), with an average hospital stay of 2.5 days. Patients requiring laparotomy, due to hemodynamic instability, incurred an average charge of $8001 (range, $3171 to $22,082). Average length of stay following laparotomy was 5.2 days.[202] Similar results were found in another retrospective direct cost analysis from Canada. The direct costs for the methotrexate group were based on success rates of 72.5% with treatment failures included, and 95% success rates for the laparoscopic surgery group. The total cost of methotrexate therapy was Canadian $35,180, with a mean cost per patient of $880 ± 160. The total cost for the laparoscopic group was Canadian $73,440, with a mean cost per patient of $1840 ± 150. Although the mean cost per patient after methotrexate failures was $2330 ± 220, the low cost of successful treatment with methotrexate (mean $330 ± 67) accounted for the overall lower cost of methotrexate therapy than laparoscopic surgery.[236]

Direct costs from third-party payers have been calculated for single-dose methotrexate therapy and laparoscopic treatment, including cost of treatment failures. Calculated costs for single-dose systemic methotrexate are based on treatment cost, medication administration, weekly laboratory tests, and repeat follow-up visits for a total of 6 weeks. Based on successful therapy after a single injection, the estimated cost is $439. If a second dose is required, an additional cost of $148 is incurred. A worst case scenario for methotrexate therapy was assessed, with an initial failure rate of 42%. Even with surgical intervention for this percentage of failures, the cost of methotrexate therapy would still only be $1390 per case due to the low cost of treatment successes. Direct costs from third-party payers for laparoscopic surgery were calculated from cost of operation, anesthesia, surgery and pathology fees, associated laboratory tests, and one follow-up visit with a β-hCG assay. Total cost amounted to $2506 for successful initial therapy. Based of the worst treatment success of 83%, with 17% requiring further therapy, the cost rose to $2536 per case in patients treated with laparoscopy. With the cost of methotrexate therapy ranging from $439 to $1390 and the cost of laparoscopic therapy ranging from $2506 to $2974, methotrexate therapy resulted in savings ranging from $1124 to $2536 per patient treated over laparoscopic therapy, depending on worst/best case scenarios.[4]

More recently, a randomized clinical trial of 58 patients compared systemic multidose methotrexate with laparoscopic salpingostomy. Direct costs were calculated by multiplying medical resources used by resource unit prices. Indirect costs were obtained from questionnaires, which included transportation, additional costs, and costs incurred from lost productivity. Treatment failures with alternative therapeutic modalities were included in the analysis. When confirmative laparoscopy was included, the cost of methotrexate therapy was $4058 per patient. Without confirmatory laparoscopy, the cost decreased to $3191 per patient. Since laparoscopy is no longer required for diagnosis, the lower cost for medical therapy is more realistic. Compared to the cost of $3902 for laparoscopic salpingostomy, methotrexate still resulted in a 20% decrease in the cost of treatment.[20]

Evidence-based Recommendation

On consideration of cost effectiveness, systemic methotrexate is the treatment of choice for unruptured ectopic pregnancy. Direct costs are substantially decreased with methotrexate therapy. Although there are not enough data on indirect cost savings, the calculated $250.5 million in indirect costs lost for ectopic pregnancy, based on a 28-day disability, will also be substantially decreased as a result of shorter disability from outpatient medical treatment. In addition to its cost effectiveness, systemic methotrexate does not subject patients to surgical intervention and the complications associated with it. (Strength of recommendation: B.)

SUMMARY POINTS

◊ The life-threatening ectopic pregnancy is found most commonly in patients with tubal pathology after both natural conception and ART.

◊ Technologic advances in serum screening, sensitive β-hCG testing, and transvaginal ultrasound allow avoiding expensive laparoscopy for diagnosis and enable medical therapy.

◊ Conservative surgical therapy and medical therapy for ectopic pregnancy have similar success rates and subsequent fertility rates. However, cost analysis alone suggests medical therapy is the ideal choice.

◊ Variable-dose methotrexate is preferable to single-dose methotrexate, direct injection, or tubal cannulation.

◊ REFERENCES*

1. Achiron R, Goldenberg M, Lipitz S, Mashiach S, Celsner G. Transvaginal Doppler sonography for detecting ectopic pregnancy: is it really necessary? *Isr J Med Sci* 1994;30:820–825.

2. Agarwal SK, Wisot AL, Garzo G, Meldrum DR. Cornual pregnancies in patients with prior salpingectomy undergoing *in vitro* fertilization and embryo transfer. *Fertil Steril* 1996;65:659–660.

3. Aharoni A, Guyot B, Salat-Baroux J. Operative laparoscopy for ectopic pregnancy: how experienced should the surgeon be? *Hum Reprod* 1993;8:2227–2230.

4. Alexander JM, Rouse DJ, Varner E, Austin JM Jr. Treatment of the small unruptured ectopic pregnancy: a cost analysis of methotrexate versus laparoscopy. *Obstet Gynecol* 1996;88:123–127.

5. American Fertility Society, Medical Research Institute, Society for Assisted Reproductive Technology. *In vitro* fertilizaton embryo transfer (IVF-ET) in the United States: 1990 results from the IVF-ET Registry. *Fertil Steril* 1992;57:15–23.

6. American Fertility Society, Society for Assisted Reproductive Technology. Assisted reproductive technology in the United States and Canada: 1992 results generated from the American Fertility Society Society for Assisted Reproductive Technology Registry. *Fertil Steril* 1994;62:1121–1128.

7. Ankum WM, Hajenius PJ, Schrevel LS, Van der Veen F. Management of suspected ectopic pregnancy. *J Reprod Med* 1996;41:724–728.

8. Ankum WM, Mol BWJ, Van der Veen F, Bossuyt PMM. Risk factors for ectopic pregnancy: a meta-analysis. *JAMA* 1996;65:1093–1099.

9. Assisted reproductive technology in the United States and Canada: 1994 results generated from the American Society for Reproductive Medicine/Society for Assisted Reproductive Technology Registry. *Fertil Steril* 1996;66:697–705.

10. Assisted reproductive technology in the United States and Canada: 1993 results generated from the American Society for Reproductive Medicine/Society for Assisted Reproductive Technology Registry. *Fertil Steril* 1995;64:13–21.

11. Atrash HK, Friede A, Hogue CJR. Abdominal pregnancy in the United States: frequency and maternal mortality. *Obstet Gynecol* 1987;69:333–337.

12. Attapattu JAF, Menon S. Abdominal pregnancy. *Int J Gynaecol Obstet* 1993;43:51–55.

13. Auslender R, Arodi J, Pascal B, Abramovici H. Interstitial pregnancy: early diagnosis by ultrasonography. *Am J Obstet Gynecol* 1983;146:717–718.

14. Badawy SZA, Taymour E, Shaykh ME, et al. Conservative surgical treatment of tubal pregnancy: factors affecting future fertility. *Int J Fertil* 1986;31:187–192.

15. Balasch J, Barri PN. Treatment of ectopic pregnancy: the new gynaecological dilemma. *Hum Reprod* 1994;9:547–558.

16. Barnhart K, Mennuti M, Benjamin I, Jacobson S, Goodman D, Coutifaris C. Prompt diagnosis of ectopic pregnancy in an emergency department setting. *Obstet Gynecol* 1994;84:1010–1015.

17. Bateman BG, Nunley WC Jr, Kolp LA, Kitchin JD III, Felder R. Vaginal sonography findings and hCG dynamics of early intrauterine and tubal pregnancies. *Obstet Gynecol* 1990;75:421–427.

18. Bello GV, Schonholz D, Moshirpur J, Jeng D-Y, Berkowitz RL. Combined pregnancy: the Mount Sinai experience. *Obstet Gynecol Surv* 1986;41:603–613.

19. Benifla JL, Sebban E, Pennehouat G, et al. Treatment with methotrexate of 4 interstitial, unruptured pregnancies. *Contracept Fertil Sex* 1993;21:845–847.

20. Bianchi S, Fedele L, Portuese A, Borruto F, Dorto M. Transrectal ultrasonography in the assessment of rectovaginal endometriosis. Presented at the 52nd annual meeting of the American Society for Reproductive Medicine, Boston, MA, November, 1996. ASRM supplement: abstract P-089.

21. Bone NL, Greene RR. Histological study of uterine tube with tubal pregnancy: a search for evidence of previous injection. *Am J Obstet Gynecol* 1961;82:1166.

22. Bornstein S, Kahn J, Fausone V. Treatment of ectopic pregnancy with laparoscopic resection in a community hospital. *J Reprod Med* 1987;32:590–591.

23. Braffman BH, Coleman BG, Ramchandani P, et al. Emergency department screening for ectopic pregnancy in an emergency department setting. *Radiology* 1994;190:797–802.

24. Breen JL. A 21-year survey of 654 ectopic pregnancies. *Am J Obstet Gynecol* 1970;106:1004–1019.

25. Brenner PF, Benedetti T, Mishell DR. Ectopic pregnancy following tubal sterilization surgery. *Obstet Gynecol* 1977;49:323–324.

26. Brezinski A, Schenker JG. Current status of endoscopic surgical management of tubal pregnancy. *Eur J Obstet Gynecol Reprod Biol* 1994;54:43–53.

27. Brown DL, Doubilet PM. Transvaginal sonography for diagnosing ectopic pregnancy: positivity criteria and performance characteristics. *J Ultrasound Med* 1994;13:259–266.

28. Bruhat MA, Manhes H, Mage G, Pouly JL. Treatment of ectopic pregnancy by means of laparoscopy. *Fertil Steril* 1980;33:411–414.

29. Brumsted J, Kessler C, Gibson C, Nakajima S, Riddick DH, Gibson M. A comparison of laparoscopy and laparotomy for the treatment of ectopic pregnancy. *Obstet Gynecol* 1988;71:889–892.

30. Brunham RC, Binns B, McDowell J, et al. *Chlamydia trachomatis* infection in women with ectopic pregnancy. *Obstet Gynecol* 1986;67:722–726.

31. Budowick M, Johnson TRB, Genadry R, Parmley TH, Woodruff JD. The histopathology of the developing tubal ectopic pregnancy. *Fertil Steril* 1980;34:169–171.

32. Buster JE, Carson SA. Ectopic pregnancy: new advances in diagnosis and treatment. *Curr Opin Obstet Gynecol* 1995;7:168–176.

33. Byrjalsen C, Toft B. Medical treatment of ectopic pregnancy. *Ann Chir Gynaecol* 1991;80:381–383.

34. Cacciatore B, Stenman U, Ylostalo P. Diagnosis of ectopic pregnancy by vaginal ultrasound in combination with a discriminatory serum hCG level of 1000 IU/1(IRP). *Br J Obstet Gynaecol* 1990;97:904–908.

35. Carp HJ, Oelsner G, Serr DM, Mashiach S. Fertility after nonsurgical treatment of ectopic pregnancy. *J Reprod Med* 1986;31:119–122.

36. Carson SA, Buster JE. Ectopic pregnancy. *N Engl J Med* 1993;329:1174–1181.

37. Carson SA, Stovall TG, Ling FW, Buster JE. Low human chorionic somatomammotropin fails to predict spontaneous resolution of unruptured ectopic pregnancies. *Fertil Steril* 1991;55:629–630.

38. Cartwright PS, Brown JE, Davis RJ, Thieme GA, Boehm FH. Advanced abdominal pregnancy associated with fetal pulmonary hypoplasia: report of a case. *Am J Obstet Gynecol* 1986;155:396–397.

39. Chakravarti S, Shardlow J. Tubal pregnancy after sterilization. *Br J Obstet Gynaecol* 1975;82:58–60.

40. Chapron C, Querleu D, Crepin G. Laparoscopic treatment of ectopic pregnancies: a one hundred case study. *Eur J Obstet Gynecol Reprod Biol* 1991;41:187–190.

*The 25 most important references are printed in boldface.

41. Chapron C, Fouly JL, Wattiez A, et al. Results of conservative laparoscopic treatment of isthmic ectopic pregnancies: a 26 case study. *Hum Reprod* 1992;7:422–424.

42. Chew S, Anandakumar C, Vanaja K, Wong YC, Chia D, Ratnam SS. The role of transvaginal ultrasonography and colour Doppler imaging in the detection of ectopic pregnancy. *J Obstet Gynaecol Res* 1996;22:455–460.

43. Chez RA, Moore JG. Diagnostic errors in the management of ectopic pregnancy. *Surg Gynecol Obstet* 1963;117:589–596.

44. Chow W, Daling JR, Cates W, Greenberg RS. Epidemiology of ectopic pregnancy. *Epidemiol Rev* 1987;9:70–94.

45. Christensen H, Thyssen H, Schebye O, et al. Three highly sensitive "bedside" serum and urine tests for pregnancy compared. *Clin Chem* 1990;36:1686–1688.

46. Chu E, Drake JC, Boarman D, Baram J, Allegra CJ. Mechanism of thymidylate synthase inhibition by methotrexate. *J Biol Chem* 1990; 265:8470–8478.

47. Coevering RJV, Fisher JE. Laparoscopic management of ovarian pregnancy: a case report. *J Reprod Med* 1988;33:774–776.

48. Daniell JF, Herbert CM. Laparoscopic salpingostomy utilizing the CO_2 laser. *Fertil Steril* 1984;41:558–563.

49. Darai E, Benifla JL, Naouri M, et al. Transvaginal intratubal methotrexate treatment of ectopic pregnancy: report of 100 cases. *Hum Reprod* 1995;11:420–424.

50. DeCherney AH, Diamond MP. Laparoscopic salpingostomy for ectopic pregnancy. *Obstet Gynecol* 1987;70:948–950.

51. DeCherney AH, Kase N. The conservative surgical management of unruptured ectopic pregnancy. *Obstet Gynecol* 1979;54:451–455.

52. Dericks-Tan JS, Scholz C, Taubert HD. Spontaneous recovery of ectopic pregnancy: a prelimary report. *Eur J Obstet Gynecol Reprod Biol* 1987;25:181–185.

53. DeVoe RW, Pratt JH. Simultaneous intrauterine and extrauterine pregnancy. *Am J Obstet Gynecol* 1948;56:1119–1126.

54. Dubuisson JB, Aubriot FX, Mathieu L, Foulot H, Mandelbrot L, de Joliniere JB. Risk factors for ectopic pregnancy in 556 pregnancies after *in vitro* fertilization: implications for preventive management. *Fertil Steril* 1991;56:686–690.

55. Ectopic pregnancy—United States, 1990–1992. *JAMA* 1995;273:533.

56. Egarter C, Husslein P. Prostaglandins in the treatment of tubal pregnancy. *Geburtshilfe Frauenheilkd* 1988;48:361–363.

57. Emerson DS, Cartier MS, Altieri LA, et al. Diagnostic efficacy of endovaginal color Doppler flow imaging in an ectopic pregnancy screening program. *Radiology* 1992;183;413–420.

58. Feichtinger W, Kemeter P. Treatment of unruptured ectopic pregnancy by needling of sac and injection of methotrexate or PGE_2 under transvaginal sonography control. *Arch Gynecol Obstet* 1989;246: 85–89.

59. Feichtinger W, Kemeter P. Conservative treatment of ectopic pregnancy by transvaginal aspiration under sonographic control and methotrexate injection. *Lancet* 1987;1:381–382.

60. Felmus LB, Pedowitz P. Interstitial pregnancy: a survey of 45 cases. *Am J Obstet Gynecol* 1953;66:1271–1279.

61. Fernandez H, Baton C, Lelaidier C, Frydman R. Conservative management of ectopic pregnancy: prospective randomized clinical trial of methotrexate versus prostaglandin sulprostone by combined transvaginal and systemic administration. *Fertil Steril* 1991;55:746–750.

62. Fernandez H, Benifla JL, Lelaidier C, Baton C, Frydman R. Methotrexate treatment of ectopic pregnancy: 100 cases treated by primary transvaginal injection under sonographic control. *Fertil Steril* 1993;59:773–777.

63. Fernandez H, Coste J, Job-Spira N. Controlled ovarian hyperstimulation as a risk factor for ectopic pregnancy. *Obstet Gynecol* 1991;78: 656–659.

64. Fernandez H, De Ziegler D, Bourget P, Feltain P, Frydman R. The place of methotrexate in the management of interstitial pregnancy. *Hum Reprod* 1991;6:302–306.

65. Fernandez H, Lelaidier C, Baton C, Bourget P, Frydman R. Return of reproductive performance after expectant management and local treatment for ectopic pregnancy. *Hum Reprod* 1991;6:1474–1477.

66. Fernandez H, Pautheir S, Doumerc S, et al. Ultrasound-guided injection of methotrexate versus laparoscopic salpingotomy in ectopic pregnancy *Fertil Steril* 1995;63:25–29.

67. Fernandez H, Pauthier S, Sitbon D, Vincent Y, Doumerc S. Role of conservative therapy and medical treatment in ectopic pregnancy: literature review and clinical trial comparing medical treatment and conservative laparoscopic treatment. *Contracep Fertil Sex* 1996;24: 297–302.

68. Fossum GT, Davajan V, Kletzky OA. Early detection of pregnancy with transvaginal ultrasound. *Fertil Steril* 1988;49:788–791.

69. Frates MC, Laing FC. Sonographic evaluation of ectopic pregnancy: an update. *AJR* 1995;165:251–259.

70. Frates MC, Brown DL, Doubilet PM, Hornstein MD. Tubal rupture in patients with ectopic pregnancy: diagnosis with transvaginal US. *Radiology* 1994;191:769–772.

71. Garcia AJ, Aubert JM, Sama J, Josimovich JB. Expectant management of presumed ectopic pregnancies. *Fertil Steril* 1987;48:395–400.

72. Gjelland K, Hordnes K, Tjugum J, Augensen K, Bergsjo P. Treatment of ectopic pregnancy by local injection of hypertonic glucose: a randomized trial comparing administration guided by transvaginal ultrasound or laparoscopy. *Acta Obstet Gynecol Scand* 1995;74:629–634.

73. Glock JL, Johnson JV, Brumsted JR. Efficacy and safety of single-dose systemic methotrexate in the treatment of ectopic pregnancy. *Fertil Steril* 1994;62:716–721.

74. Goldenberg M, Bider D, Oelsner G, Admon D, Mashiach S. Treatment of interstitial pregnancy with methotrexate via hysteroscopy. *Fertil Steril* 1992;58:1234–1236.

75. Goldner TE, Lawson HW, Xia Z, Atrash HK. Surveillance for ectopic pregnancy—United States, 1970–1989. *MMWR* 1993;42(no. SS-6): 73–85.

76. Goldstein DP. Treatment of unruptured ectopic pregnancy with methotrexate with folic acid rescue. Presented at the 34th annual meeting of the American College of Obstetricians and Gynecologists, New Orleans, LA, May 3–8, 1986. Washington, DC: American College of Obstetricians and Gynecologists, 1986:40(abst).

77. Goldstein SR, Snyder JR, Watson C, Danvon M. Vaginal sonography versus serum human chorionic gonadotropin in early detection of pregnancy. *Am J Obstet Gynecol* 1988;158:608–612.

78. Graham M, Cooperberg PL. Ultrasound diagnosis of interstitial pregnancy: findings and pitfalls. *J Clin Ultrasound* 1979;7:433–437.

79. Grimes DA. The morbidity and mortality of pregnancy: still risky business. *Am J Obstet Gynecol* 1993;170:1489–1494.

80. Grimes HG, Nosal RA, Gallagher JC. Ovarian pregnancy: a series of 24 cases. *Obstet Gynecol* 1983;61:174–180.

81. Gross Z, Rodriguez JJ, Stalnaker BL. Ectopic pregnancy: nonsurgical, outpatient evaluation and single-dose methotrexate treatment. *J Reprod Med* 1995;40:371–374.

82. Guirgis RR. Simultaneous intrauterine and ectopic pregnancies following *in vitro* fertilization and gamete intra-Fallopian transfer: a review of nine cases. *Hum Reprod* 1990;5:484–486.

83. Hajenius PJ, Engelsbel S, Mol BW, et al. Systemic methotrexate versus laparoscopic salpingostomy in tubal pregnancy: a randomized clinical trial. Presented at the 52nd annual meeting of the American Society for Reproductive Medicine, Boston, MA, November, 1996. ASRM supplement: S132(abst).

84. Hallatt JG. Primary ovarian pregnancy: a report of twenty-five cases. *Am J Obstet Gynecol* 1982;143:55–60.

85. Hallatt JG. Repeat ectopic pregnancy: a study of 123 consecutive cases. *Am J Obstet Gynecol* 1976;122:520–524.

86. Hallatt JG, Grove JA. Abdominal pregnancy: a study of twenty-one consecutive cases. *Am J Obstet Gynecol* 1985;152:444–449.

87. Hann LE, Bachmann DM, McArdle C. Coexistent intrauterine and ectopic pregnancy: a reevaluation. *Radiology* 1984;152:151–154.

88. Helvacioglu A, Long EM, Yang SL. Ectopic pregnancy: an eight-year review. *J Reprod Med* 1979;22:87–92.

89. Henderson SR. Ectopic tubal pregnancy treated by operative laparoscopy. *Obstet Gynecol* 1989;160:1462–1469.

90. Henry MA, Gentry WL. Single injection of methotrexate for treatment of ectopic pregnancies. *Am J Obstet Gynecol* 1994;171:1584–1587.

91. Herman A, Raphael R, Golan A. The role of tubal pathology and other parameters in ectopic pregnancies occurring in *in vitro* fertilization and embryo transfer. *Fertil Steril* 1990;54:864–868.

92. Hidlebaugh D, O'Mara P. Clinical and financial analyses of ectopic pregnancy management at a large health plan. *J Am Assoc Gynecol Laparosc* 1997;4:207–213.

93. Honore LH, O'Hara KE. Failed tubal sterilization as an etiologic factor in ectopic tubal pregnancy. *Fertil Steril* 1978;29:509–511.

94. Hoppe DE, Bekkar BE, Nager CW. Single-dose systemic methotrexate for the treatment of persistent ectopic pregnancy after conservative surgery. *Obstet Gynecol* 1994;83:51–54.

95. Horrigan TJ, Fanning J, Marcotte MP. Methotrexate pneumonitis after systemic treatment for ectopic pregnancy. *Am J Obstet Gynecol* 1997; 176:714–715.

96. Hsu JJ, Chiu TH, Lai IM, Soong Yk. Methotrexate treatment of cervical pregnancies with different clinical parameters: a report of three cases. *J Reprod Med* 1995;40:246–250.

97. Huber J, Hosmann J, Vytiska-Binstorfer E. Laparoscopic surgery for tubal pregnancies utilizing laser. *Int J Gynaecol Obstet* 1989;29: 153–157.

98. Husslein P. Conservative treatment for ectopic pregnancy by local application of prostaglandins. *Eur J Obstet Gynecol Reprod Biol* 1993; 49:72.

99. Ichinoe K, Wake N, Shinkai N, Shiina Y, Miyazaki Y, Tanaks T. Nonsurgical therapy to preserve oviduct function in patients with tubal pregnancies. *Obstet Gynecol* 1987;156:484–487.

100. Isaacs JD, McGehee RP, Cowan BD. Life-threatening neutropenia following methotrexate treatment of ectopic pregnancy: a report of two cases. *Obstet Gynecol* 1996;88:694–696.

101. Isaacs J, Meeks RG, Hampton HL, et al. Treatment of unruptured ectopic pregnancy with methotrexate. *J Miss Med Assoc* 1992;33:81–85.

102. Ivankovich AD, Miletich DJ, Albrecht RF, et al. Cardiovascular effects of intraperitoneal insufflation with carbon dioxide in dogs. *Anesthesiology* 1975;42:281–287.

103. Jehle D, Krause R, Braen GR. Ectopic pregnancy. *Emerg Med Clin North Am* 1994;12:55–71.

104. Johns DA, Hardie RP. Management of unruptured ectopic pregnancy with laparoscopic carbon dioxide laser. *Fertil Steril* 1986;46:703–705.

105. Jones DH. Ectopic pregnancy: an analysis of one hundred consecutive cases. *Br J Clin Pract* 1966;20:377–383.

106. Kadar N, Devore G, Romero R. Discriminatory zone: its use in the sonographic evaluation for ectopic pregnancy. *Obstet Gynecol* 1981; 58:156–160.

107. Karande VC, Flood JT, Heard N, Veeck L, Muasher SJ. Analysis of ectopic pregnancies resulting from *in vitro* fertilization and embryo transfer. *Hum Reprod* 1991;6:446–449.

108. Karsdorp VH, Van der Venn F, Schats R, Boer-Miesel ME, Kenemans P. Successful treatment with methotrexate of five vital interstitial pregnancies. *Hum Reprod* 1992;7:1164–1169.

109. Karsten U, Seifert B. Introduction and results in the endoscopic treatment of extrauterine pregnancy. *Zentralbl Gynakol* 1990;112:467–473.

110. Keckstein J, Hepp S, Schneider V, Sasse V, Steiner R. The contact Nd:YAG laser: a new technique for conservation of the fallopian tube in unruptured ectopic pregnancy. *Br J Obstet Gynaecol* 1990;97:352–356.

111. Kim DS, Chung SR, Park MI, Kim YP. Comparative review of diagnostic accuracy in tubal pregnancy: a 14-year survey of 1040 cases. *Obstet Gynecol* 1987;70:547–554.

112. Knutzen V, Scoto-Albers CE, Fuller D, Sher G, Shynock K, Behr B. Mock embryo transfer in early luteal phase, the cycle prior to *in-vitro* fertilization and embryo transfer. Presented at the 45th annual meeting of the American Fertility Society, San Francisco, CA, November 13–16, 1989. AFS program supplement: S152(abst).

113. Kojima E, Abe Y, Morita M, Ito M, Hirakawa S, Momose K. The treatment of unruptured tubal pregnancy within intratubal methotrexate injection under laparoscopic control. *Obstet Gynecol* 1990;75:723–725.

114. Kooi GS. Methotrexate: a nonsurgical treatment of ectopic pregnancy. Tilburg, the Netherlands: St. Elizabeth Hospital, 1991. Doctoral thesis.

115. Kooi S, Kock HC. A review of the literature on nonsurgical treatment in tubal pregnancies. *Obstet Gynecol Surv* 1992;47:739–749.

116. Kooi GS, Kock HCLV. Treatment of tubal pregnancy by local injection of methotrexate after adrenaline injection into the mesosalpinx: a report of 25 patients. *Fertil Steril* 1990;54:580–584.

117. Korhonen J, Stenman UH, Ylostalo P. Serum human chorionic gonadotropin dynamics during spontaneous resolution of ectopic pregnancy. *Fertil Steril* 1994;61:632–636.

118. Kranz SG, Gray RH, Damewood MD, Wallach EE. Time trends in risk factors and clinical outcome of ectopic pregnancy. *Fertil Steril* 1990; 54:42–46.

119. Kucera E, Mack F, Novak J, Andrasova V. Fertility after operations or extrauterine pregnancy. *Int J Fertil* 1969;14:127–129.

120. Lang PF, Weiss PAM, Mayer HO, Haas JG, Hönigl W. Conservative treatment of ectopic pregnancy with local injection of hyperosmolar glucose solution or prostaglandin F_2. *Lancet* 1990;336:78–81.

121. Largtebrekke A, Sornes T, Urnes A. Fertility outcome after treatment of tubal pregnancy by laparoscopic laser surgery. *Acta Obstet Gynecol Scand* 1993;72:547–549.

122. Leach RE, Ory SJ. Modern management of ectopic pregnancy. *J Reprod Med* 1989;34:324–338.

123. Lehfeldt H, Tietz C, Gorstein F. Ovarian pregnancy and the intrauterine device. *Am J Obstet Gynecol* 1970;108:1005–1009.

124. Lenton EA, Neal L, Sulaiman R. Plasma concentrations of human chorionic gonadotropin from the time of implantation until the second week of pregnancy. *Fertil Steril* 1982;37:773–778.

125. Lindblom B, Hahlin M, Lundorff P, Thorburn J. Treatment of tubal pregnancy by laparoscope-guided injection of prostaglandin F_2. *Fertil Steril* 1990;54:404–408.

126. Lindblom B, Hahlin M, Sjoblom P. Serial human chorionic gonadotropin determinations by fluoroimmunoassay for differentiation between intrauterine and ectopic gestation. *Am J Obstet Gynecol* 1989;161:397–400.

127. Lindblom B, Hamburger L, Ljung B. Contractile patterns of isolated oviductal smooth muscles under different hormonal conditions. *Fertil Steril* 1980;33:283–288.

128. Little KJ, Green MM. Abdominal gestation. *J Emerg Med* 1995;13: 195–198.

129. Long L. Methotrexate-citrovorum factor individualized reduced dose therapy for ectopic pregnancy: report of 20 cases. *Chung Hua Fu Chan Ko Tsa Chih* 1993;28:402–404,441–442.

130. Lund J. Early ectopic pregnancy. *J Obstet Gynaecol Br Emp* 1955;62: 70–78.

131. Lundorff P, Thorburn J, Hahlin M, Kallfelt B, Lindblom B. Laparoscopic surgery in ectopic pregnancy: a randomized trial versus laparotomy. *Acta Obstet Gynecol Scand* 1991;70:343–348.

132. Lundorff P, Thorburn, Lindblom B. Fertility outcome after conservative surgical treatment of ectopic pregnancy: evaluation in a randomized trial. *Fertil Steril* 1992;57:998–1002.

133. Majmudar B, Henderson PH, Semple E. Salpingitis isthmica nodosa: a high-risk factor for tubal pregnancy. *Obstet Gynecol* 1983;62:73–78.

134. Makinen JI, Salmi TA, Nikkanen VP, Juhani Koskinen EY. Encouraging rates of fertility after ectopic pregnancy. *Int J Fertil* 1989;34:46–51.

135. Marcus SF, Brinsden PR. Analysis of the incidence and risk factors associated with ectopic pregnancy following *in vitro* fertilization and embryo transfer. *Hum Reprod* 1995;10:199–203.

136. Marshall RL, Jebson PJ, Davie IT, et al. Circulatory effects of carbon dioxide insufflation of the peritoneal cavity for laparoscopy. *Br J Anaesth* 1972;44:680–684.

137. Martinez F, Trounson A. An analysis of factors associated with ectopic pregnancy in a human *in vitro* fertilization program. *Fertil Steril* 1986:45:79–87.

138. Maruri F, Azziz R. Laparoscopic surgery for ectopic pregnancies: technology assessment and public health implications. *Fertil Steril* 1993; 59:487–498.

139. Mashiach S, Carp HJ, Serr DM. Nonoperative management of ectopic pregnancy: a preliminary report. *J Reprod Med* 1982;27:127–132.

140. McBain JC, Evans JH, Pepperell RJ, Robinson HP, Smith MA, Brown JB. An unexpectedly high rate of ectopic pregnancy following the induction of ovulation with human pituitary and chorionic gonadotropin. *Br J Obstet Gynaecol* 1980;87:5–9.

141. McCausland A. Endosalpingosis ("endosalpingoblastosis") following laparoscopic tubal coagulation as an etiologic factor of ectopic pregnancy. *Am J Obstet Gynecol* 1982;143:12–24.

142. McCausland A. High rate of ectopic pregnancy following laparoscopic tubal coagulation failures. *Am J Obstet Gynecol* 1980;136:97–101.

143. Mecke H, Argiriou C, Semm K. Treatment of tubal pregnancy by pelviscopy—complications, pregnancy and recurrence rates. *Geburtshilfe Frauenheilkd* 1991;51:549–553.

144. Menard A, Crequat J, Mandelbrot L, Hauuy JP, Madelenat P. Treatment of unruptured tubal pregnancy by local injection of methotrexate under transvaginal sonographic control. *Fertil Steril* 1990;54:47–50.

145. Merz E, Bahlmann F, Weber G, et al. Unruptured tubal pregnancy: local low-dose therapy with methotrexate under transvaginal ultrasonographic guidance. *Gynecol Obstet Invest* 1996;41:76–81.

146. Mitchell DE, McSwain HF, Peterson HB. Fertility after ectopic pregnancy. *Am J Obstet Gynecol* 1989;161:576–580.

147. Miyazaki Y. Studies on non-surgical therapy of ectopic pregnancy. *Acta Obstet Gynecol Jpn* 1983;58:132–143.

148. Mol BWJ, Ankum WM, Bossuyt PMM, Van der Veen F. Contraception and the risk of ectoic pregnancy: a meta-analysis. *Contraception* 1995;52:337–341.

149. Mol BWJ, Hajenius PJ, Engelsbel S, et al. An economic evaluation of laparoscopy and open surgery in the treatment of tubal pregnancy. *Acta Obstet Gynecol Scand* 1997;76:1–5.

150. Mottla GL, Rulin MC, Guzick, DS. Lack of resolution of ectopic pregnancy by intratubal injection of methotrexate. *Fertil Steril* 1992;57: 685–687.

151. Murphy AA, Nager CW, Wujek JJ, Kettel LM, Torp VA, Chin HG. Operative laparoscopy versus laparotomy for the management of ectopic pregnancy: a prospective trial. *Fertil Steril* 1992;57:1180–1185.

152. National Center for Health Statistics. *Advance report of final mortality statistics, 1992.* Hyattsville, MD: US Department of Health and Human Services, Public Health Service, CDC, 1994. *Mon Vital Stat Rep* 1994;43(6)(suppl).

153. Nazari A, Askari HA, Check JH, O'Shaughnessy AO. Embryo transfer techniques as a cause of ectopic pregnancy in *in vitro* fertilization. *Fertil Steril* 1993;60:919–921.

154. Neiman RA, Fye KH. Methotrexate-induced false photosensitivity reaction. *J Rheumatol* 1985;12:354–55.

155. Nyberg DA, Filly RA, Laing FL, Marck LA, Zarutski PW. Ectopic pregnancy: diagnosis by sonography correlated with quantitative hCG levels. *J Ultrasound Med* 1987;6:145–150.

156. Nyberg DA, Hughes MP, Mack LA, Wany KY. Extrauterine findings of ectopic pregnancy at transvaginal US: importance of echogenic fluid. *Radiology* 1991;178:823–826.

157. Oelsner G, Admon D, Shalev E, Shalev Y, Kukia E, Mashiach SA. New approach for the treatment of interstitial pregnancy. *Fertil Steril* 1993;59:924–925.

158. **Ory HW. The Women's Health Study: ectopic pregnancy and intrauterine contraceptive devices: new perspectives. *Obstet Gynecol* 1981;57:137–144.**

159. Ory SJ, Nadi E, Herrmann R, O'Brien PS, Melton LJ III. Fertility after ectopic pregnancy. *Fertil Steril* 1993;60:231–235.

160. O'Shea RT, Thompson GR, Harding A. Intraamniotic methotrexate versus CO_2 laser laparoscopic salpingostomy in the management of tubal ectopic pregnancy—a prospective randomized trial. *Fertil Steril* 1994;62:876–878.

161. Ou CS. Laparoscopic management of ectopic pregnancy. *J Reprod Med* 1993;38:849–852.

162. Pansky M, Bukovsky J, Golan A, et al. Reproductive outcome after laparoscopic local methotrexate injection for tubal pregnancy. *Fertil Steril* 1993;60:85–87.

163. Pansky M, Bukovsky I, Golan A, et al. Local methotrexate injection: a nonsurgical treatment of ectopic pregnancy. *Obstet Gynecol* 1989;161: 393–396.

164. Pansky M, Golan A, Schneider D, et al. Tubal patency after local methotrexate injection for tubal pregnancy. *Obstet Gynecol* 1989;2: 967–968.

164a. Pisarska MD, Casson PR, Moise KJ, Jr, DiMaio DJ, Buster JE, Carson SA. Heterotopic abdominal pregnancy treated at laparoscopy. *Fertil Steril* 1998;70:159–160.

165. Ploman L, Wicksell F. Fertility after conservative surgery in tubal pregnancy. *Acta Obstet Gynecol Scand* 1960;39:143–152.

166. Porpora MG, Olive MM, De Cristofaro A, Montanino G, Cosmi EV. Comparison of local injection of methotrexate and linear salpingostomy in the conservative laparoscopic treatment of ectopic pregnancy. *J Am Assoc Gynecol Laparosc* 1996;3:271–276.

167. Pouly JL, Mahnes H, Mage G, Canis M, Bruhat MA. Conservative laparoscopic treatment of 321 ectopic pregnancies. *Fertil Steril* 1986;4: 1093–1097.

168. Prapas J, Prapas N, Prapas S, Papanicolaou N. Conservative treatment of ectopic pregnancy with intramuscular administration of methotrexate (MTX/CV). *Acta Eur Fertil* 1992;23:25–28.

169. Prevost RR, Stovall TG, Ling FW. Methotrexate for treatment of unruptured ectopic pregnancy. *Clin Pharmacol* 1992;11:529–532.

170. Pulkkinen MO, Talo A. Myoelectrical activity in the human oviduct with tubal pregnancy. *Am J Obstet Gynecol* 1984;148:151–154.

171. Pyrgiotis E, Sultan KM, Neal GS, Liu H-C, Grifo JA, Rosenwaks Z. Ectopic pregnancies after *in vitro* fertilization and embryo transfer. *J Assist Reprod Genet* 1994;11:79–84.

172. Quasim SM, Trias A, Sachdev R, Kenmann E. Evaluation of serum creatinine kinase levels in ectopic pregnancy. *Fertil Steril* 1996;65: 443–445.

173. Ransom MX, Garcia AJ, Bohrer M, Corsan GH, Kemmann E. Serum progesterone as a predictor of methotrexate success in the treatment of ectopic pregnancy. *Obstet Gynecol* 1994;83:1033–1037.

174. **Raziel A, Golan A, Pansky M, Ron-El R, Bukovsky I, Caspi E. Ovarian pregnancy: a report of twenty cases in one institution. *Am J Obstet Gynecol* 1990;163:1182–1185.**

175. **Reece EA, Petrie RH, Sirmans MF, Finster M, Todd WD. Combined intrauterine and extrauterine gestations: a review. *Am J Obstet Gynecol* 1983;146:323–330.**

176. Risquez F, Foreman R, Maleika F, et al. Transcervical cannulation of the fallopian tube for the management of ectopic pregnancy: prospective multicenter study. *Fertil Steril* 1992;58:1131–1135.

177. **Rojansky N, Schenker JG. Heterotopic pregnancy and assisted reproduction: an update. *J Assist Reprod Genet* 1996;13:594–601.**

178. Rottem S, Thaler I, Timor-Tritsch IE. Classification of tubal gestations by transvaginal sonography. *Ultrasound Obstet Gynecol* 199;1:197–201.

179. Russell JB. The etiology of ectopic pregnancy. *Clin Obstet Gynecol* 1987;30:181–190.

180. Russell JB, Cutler LR. Transvaginal ultrasonographic detection of primary ovarian pregnancy with laparoscopic removal: a case report. *Fertil Steril* 1989;51:1055–1056.

181. Russell SA, Filly RA, Damato N. Sonographic diagnosis of ectopic pregnancy with endovaginal probes: what really has changed? *J Ultrasound Med* 1993;3:145–151.

182. Sand PK, Stubblefield PA, Ory SJ. Methotrexate inhibition of normal trophoblasts *in vitro. Am J Obstet Gynecol* 1986;155:324–329.

183. Sauer MV, Gorrill MJ, Rodi IA, et al. Non-surgical management of unruptured ectopic pregnancy: an extended clinical trial. *Fertil Steril* 1987;48:752–755.

184. Schenker JH, Eyal F, Polishuk WZ. Fertility after tubal pregnancy. *Surg Gynecol Obstet* 1972;135:74–76.

185. Schiff E, Shalev E, Bustan M, Tsabari A, Mashiach S, Weiner E. Pharmacokinetics of methotrexate after local tubal injection for conservative treatment of ectopic pregnancy. *Fertil Steril* 1992;57:688–690.

186. Schoen JA, Nowak RJ. Repeat ectopic pregnancy: a 16-year clinical survey. *Obstet Gynecol* 1975;45:542–546.

187. Schoenfeld A, Mashiach R, Vardy M, Ovadia J. Methotrexate pneumonitis in the non-surgical treatment of ectopic pregnancy. *Obstet Gynecol* 1992;80:520–521.

188. Seifer DB, Guttmann JN, Grant WD, Kamps CA, DeCherney AH. Comparison of persistent ectopic pregnancy after laparoscopic salpingostomy versus salpingostomy at laparotomy for ectopic pregnancy. *Obstet Gynecol* 1993;81:378–382.

189. Shalev E, Peleg D, Bustan M, Romano S, Tsabari A. Limited role for intratubal methotrexate treatment of ectopic pregnancy. *Fertil Steril* 1995;63:20–24.

190. Shalev E, Peleg D, Tsabari A, Romano S, Bustan M. Spontaneous resolution of ectopic tubal pregnancy: natural history. *Fertil Steril* 1995;63:15–19.

191. Shalev E, Yarom I, Bustan M, Weiner E, Ben-Shlomo I. Transvaginal sonography as the ultimate diagnostic tool for the management of ectopic pregnancy: experience with 840 cases. *Fertil Steril* 1998; 69:62–65.

192. Sheikh HH, Yussman MA. Ruptured ectopic pregnancy after bilateral laparoscopic tubal fulguration. *Am J Obstet Gynecol* 1976;125:569–570.

193. Sherman D, Langer R, Sadovsky G, et al. Improved fertility following ectopic pregnancy. *Fertil Steril* 1982;37:497–502.

194. Sherman D, Langer R, Sadovsky G, Bukovsky I, Caspi E. Improved fertility following ectopic pregnancy. *Fertil Steril* 1982;37:497–502.

195. Shott RJ, Cook LN, Andrews BF. Intra-abdominal pregnancy: an unusual cause of fetal growth retardation. *Am J Dis Child* 1973;126: 361–362.

196. Silva PD. A laparoscopic approach can be applied to most cases of ectopic pregnancy. *Obstet Gynecol* 1988;72:944–947.

197. Silva PD, Schaper AM, Rooney B. Reproductive outcome after 143 laparoscopic procedures for ectopic pregnancy. *Obstet Gynecol* 1993;81: 710–715.

198. Soriano D, Yefet Y, Oelsner G, Goldenberg M, Mashiach S, Seidman DS. Operative laparoscopy for management of ectopic pregnancy in patients with hypovolemic shock. *J Am Assoc Gynecol Laparosc* 1997; 4:363–367.

199. Stevens CA. Malformations and deformations in abdominal pregnancy. *Am J Med Genet* 1993;47:1189–1195.

200. Stika CS, Anderson L, Frederiksen MC. Single-dose methotrexate for the treatment of ectopic pregnancy: Northwestern Memorial Hospital three-year experience. *Am J Obstet Gynecol* 1996;174:1840–1848.

201. Stovall TG, Ling FW. Single-dose methotrexate: an expanded clinical trial. *Am J Obstet Gynecol* 1993;168:759–772

202. Stovall TG, Bradham DD, Ling FW, Naughton M. Cost of treatment of ectopic pregnancy: single-dose methotrexate versus surgical treatment. *J Womens Health* 1994;3:445–450.

203. Stovall TG, Ling FW, Buster JE. Outpatient chemotherapy of unruptured ectopic pregnancy. *Fertil Steril* 1989;51:435–438.

204. Stovall TG, Ling FW, Carson SA, Buster JE. Serum progesterone and uterine curettage in differential diagnosis of ectopic pregnancy. *Fertil Steril* 1992;57:456–458.

205. Stovall TG, Ling FW, Carson SA, Buster JE. Nonsurgical diagnosis and treatment of tubal pregnancy. *Fertil Steril* 1990;54: 537–548.

206. Stovall TG, Ling FW, Cope BJ, Buster JE. Preventing ruptured ectopic pregnancy with a single serum progesterone. *Am J Obstet Gynecol* 1989;160:1425–1431.

207. Stovall TG, Ling FW, Gray LA. Single-dose methotrexate for treatment of ectopic pregnancy. *Obstet Gynecol* 1991;77:754–757.

208. Stovall TG, Ling FW, Gray LA, Carson SA, Buster JE. Methotrexate treatment of unruptured ectopic pregnancy: a report of 100 cases. *Obstet Gynecol* 1991;77:749–753.

209. Stromme WB. Salpingotomy for tubal pregnancy. *Obstet Gynecol* 1953;1:427.

210. Svensson L, Mardh P-A, Ahlgren M, et al. Ectopic pregnancy and antibodies to *Chlamydia trachomatis. Fertil Steril* 1985;44:313–317.

211. Tait RL. Five cases of extrauterine pregnancy operated upon at the time of rupture. *BMJ* 1884;i:1250.

212. Tanaka T, Hayashi H, Kutsuzawa T, Fujimoto S, Ichinoe K. Treatment of interstitial ectopic pregnancy with methotrexate: report of a successful case. *Fertil Steril* 1982;37:851–852.

213. Tancer ML, Delke I, Veridiano NP. A fifteen-year experience with ectopic pregnancy. *Surg Gynecol Obstet* 1981;152:179–182.

214. Timonen S, Nieminen U. Tubal pregnancy: choice of operative method of treatment. *Acta Obstet Gynecol Scand* 1967;46:327–339.

215. Timor-Tritsch IE, Meh MN, Peisner DB, Lesser KB, Slavik BA. The use of transvaginal ultrasonography in the diagnosis of ectopic pregnancy. *Am J Obstet Gynecol* 1989;161:157–161.

216. Timor-Tritsch IE, Monteagudo A, Mandeville EO, Peisner DB, Anaya GP, Pirrone EC. Successful management of viable cervical pregnancy by local, injection of methotrexate. *Am J Obstet Gynecol* 1994;170: 737–739.

217. Timor-Tritsch IE, Monteagudo A, Matera C, Veit CR. Sonographic evolution of cornual pregnancies treated without surgery. *Obstet Gynecol* 1992;79:1044–1049.

218. Togas T, Vilos G, Gomel V. Laparoscopic treatment of interstitial pregnancy. *Obstet Gynecol* 1995;85:465–467.

219. Trio D, Strobelt N, Picciolo C, Lapinski RH, Ghidini A. Prognostic factors for successful expectant management of ectopic pregnancy. *Fertil Steril* 1995;63:469–472.

220. Trout S, Kemmann E. Reversible alopecia after single-dose methotrexate treatment in a patient with ectopic pregnancy. *Fertil Steril* 1995; 64:866–867.

221. Tulandi T, Atri M, Bret P, Falcone T, Khalife S. Transvaginal intratubal methotrexate treatment of ectopic pregnancy. *Fertil Steril* 1992; 58:98–100.

222. Tuomivaara L, Kauppila A. Radical or conservative surgery for ectopic pregnancy? A follow-up study of fertility of 323 patients. *Fertil Steril* 1988;50:580–583.

223. Ushakov FB, Elchalal U, Aceman PJ, Schenker JG. Cervical pregnancy: past and future. *Obstet Gynecol* 1996;52:45–59.

224. Valle JA, Lifchez AS. Reproductive outcome following conservative surgery for tubal pregnancy in women with a single fallopian tube. *Fertil Steril* 1983;39:316–320.

225. Verco CJ. Nonlaser video laparoscopic surgery for ectopic gestation. *Aust N Z J Obstet Gynaecol* 1991;31:168–170.

226. Verhulst G, Camus M, Bollen N, Steirteghem AV, Devroey P. Analysis of the risk factors with regard to the occurrence of ectopic pregnancy after medically assisted procreation. *Human Reprod* 1993;8: 1284–1287.

227. Vermesh M, Presser SC. Reproductive outcome after linear salpingostomy for ectopic gestation: a prospective 3-year follow-up. *Fertil Steril* 1992;57:682–684.

228. Vermesh M, Silva PD, Rosen GF, Stein AL, Fossum GT, Sauer MV. Management of unruptured ectopic gestation by linear salpingostomy: a prospective, randomized clinical trial of laparoscopy versus laparotomy. *Obstet Gynecol* 1989;73:400–404.

229. Vessey M, Meisler L, Flavel R, et al. Outcome of pregnancy in women using different methods of contraception. *Br J Obstet Gynaecol* 1979,548 56.

230. Washington AE, Katz P. Ectopic pregnancy in the United States: economic consequences and payment source trends. *Obstet Gynecol* 1993;81:287–292.

231. Weckstein LN, Boucher AR, Tucker H, et al. Accurate diagnosis of early ectopic pregnancy. *Obstet Gynecol* 1985;65:393–397.

232. Westrom L. Effect of acute pelvic inflammatory disease on fertility. *Am J Obstet Gynecol* 1975;121:707–713.

233. Wolf GC, Witt BR. Outpatient laparoscopic management of ectopic pregnancy with a local methotrexate injection. *J Reprod Med* 1991; 36:489–491.

234. World Health Organization, Task Force on Intrauterine Devices for Fertility Regulation. A multinational case-control study of ectopic pregnancy. *Clin Reprod Fertil* 1985;3:131–143.

235. Yao M, Tulandi T. Current status of surgical and nonsurgical management of ectopic pregnancy. *Fertil Steril* 1997;67:421–433.

236. Yao M, Tulandi T, Kaplow M, Smith AP. A comparison of methotrexate versus laparoscopic surgery for treatment of ectopic pregnancy: a cost analysis. *Hum Reprod* 1996;11:2762–2766.

237. Yeko TR, Mayer JC, Parsons AK, Maroulis GB. A prospective series of unruptured ectopic pregnancies treated by tubal injections with hyperosmolar glucose. *Obstet Gynecol* 1995;85:265–268.

238. Yeko TR, Villa A, Parsons AK, Maroulis B. Laparoscopic treatment of ectopic pregnancy: resident's learning experience. *J Reprod Med* 1994;39:854–856.

239. Ylöstalo P, Cacciatore B, Korhonen J, et al. Expectant management of ectopic pregnancy. *Eur J Obstet Gynecol Reprod Biol* 1993;49:83–84.

240. Yovich JL, Turner SR, Murphy AJ. Embryo transfer technique as a cause of ectopic pregnancies in *in vitro* fertilization. *Fertil Steril* 1985; 44:318–321.

241. Zilber U, Pansky M, Bukovsky I, Golan A. Laparoscopic salpingostomy versus laparoscopic local methotrexate injection in the management of unruptured ectopic pregnancy. *Am J Obstet Gynecol* 1996; 175:600–602.

242. Zouves C, Erenus M, Gomel V. Tubal ectopic pregnancy after *in vitro* fertilization and embryo transfer: a role for proximal occlusion or salpingectomy after failed distal tubal surgery? *Fertil Steril* 1991;56: 691–695.

243. Zullo F, Pellicano M, Di Carlo C, De Stefano R, Mastrantonio P, Nappi C. Late complications after systemic methotrexate treatment of unruptured ectopic pregnancies: a report of three cases. *Eur J Obstet Gynecol Reprod Biol* 1996;70:213–214.

CHAPTER 12

Prenatal Diagnosis and Genetics

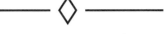

Kenneth Ward

Genetic screening has become a routine aspect of prenatal care. Widely available prenatal cytogenetic and molecular genetic tests sample chorionic villi, amniocytes, and fetal blood. The genes involved in mendelian conditions continue to be discovered at a rapid pace, and soon first-trimester DNA-based prenatal diagnosis will become possible for thousands of additional conditions. New technologies such as flow cytometry, fluorescent *in situ* hybridization, and DNA amplification with the polymerase chain reaction enable testing of a single cell for chromosomal or mendelian problems. This approach has already allowed prefertilization diagnosis of oocytes, preimplantation testing of embryos, and prenatal diagnosis using the small population of fetal cells present in the maternal circulation. During the next decade, gene therapy will be applied prenatally for the treatment of inborn errors and postnatally for the treatment of genetic diseases and cancer.

Genetic principles are central to understanding the pathophysiology of many of the conditions for which we provide care (Table 1). More than 20 million Americans have a diagnosed genetic disease. One percent of all newborns have a recognizable mendelian disorder, 0.5% have a chromosomal syndrome, and 2% have a polygenic, multifactorial disorder. Most pregnancy losses and most congenital anomalies have genetic causes. Genes also play an important role in many common gynecologic disorders, such as leiomyomata, endometriosis, gynecologic cancers, infertility, and abnormalities of sexual differentiation. Genetic variants are responsible for tendencies to have multiple gestations, preeclampsia, and gestational diabetes. Susceptibilities to infectious or teratogenic agents are genetically determined.

Recognizing that a condition is genetic enables prediction of its effect on the next generation. It also means that the gene responsible for the illness can be found, possibly leading to improved means of diagnosis, classification, and treatment. Correlation of the phenotype with the genotype often provides specific predictive insights. Because any DNA test can be performed prenatally, discovery of the gene that causes a particular disease can give at-risk couples the necessary information to prepare for having an affected child, to consider gene therapy if available, or to choose to end the pregnancy.

Patients often have genetic illnesses that will affect pregnancy or their gynecology care, illnesses that may remain undiagnosed unless physicians are thorough in their evaluation of unusual signs or symptoms. For example, a new obstetric patient presents with a wasted facial appearance, generalized weakness, and difficulty releasing her grip when shaking the physician's hand. She has the classic signs of myotonic dystrophy, an autosomal-dominant disorder. Formerly, myotonic dystrophy was a difficult diagnosis to establish in some patients, but the diagnosis can be made easily using DNA analysis of her blood. The physician and this woman need to know that she is at significant risk for developing polyhydramnios, which could result in preterm labor, that her fetus may have positional deformities and is at risk for a severe, often fatal, neonatal form of myotonia, and that her labor is likely to be prolonged and she may be unable to push in the second stage. If she requires cesarean section, she may have undiagnosed cardiac problems that place her at higher risk for anesthesia. If failure to recognize these risks results in a bad outcome, a lawsuit claiming negligence might be brought.

◊ PATTERNS OF INHERITANCE

Types of Birth Defects

There are many types of birth defects, and many of the terms that describe these defects are used in the discussion that follows (Table 2). *Deformation* is any abnormal form, shape, or position caused by mechanical forces. A *malformation* is a morphologic defect that results from abnormal development, and *disruption* is a morphologic defect that results from an extrinsic breakdown in or interference with normal development. An *anomaly* is a structural feature that departs from the normal form. A *syndrome* is a recognizable pattern of structural defects that often has a predictable natural history al-

TABLE 1. *The burden of genetic disease*

1 in 20 newborns has a detectable genetic defect at birth
Over 20 million Americans have a diagnosed genetic disease
Life years lost to genetic diseases are estimated to 6.5 times greater than years lost to heart disease—the nation's number 1 killer
30% of pediatric hospital admissions and 10% of adult admissions are for disorders that are wholly or partly genetic
All cancers have somatic or inherited genetic changes

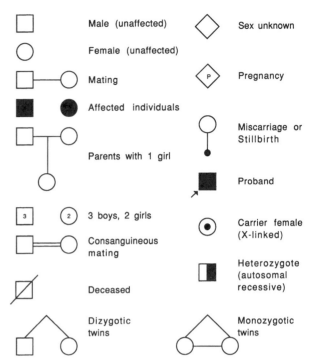

FIG. 1. Symbols used to draw a pedigree.

lowing diagnosis and classification. An *association* is a group of anomalies that frequently occur together but are not syndromes. A *sequence* is a pattern of defects that results from a single event early in pregnancy.

Single-gene (Mendelian) Disorders

The observation that "like begets like" has been stated throughout recorded history, but current theories describing how genetic traits and illnesses are inherited are just over 100 years old. In the late 1800s, Mendel described how individual genetic traits were passed on from generation to generation. Single-gene disorders (i.e., mendelian disorders) are conditions caused by a mutation at a single site in the DNA and inherited in the proportions predicted by Mendel's laws. These disorders can be dominant conditions, in which the phenotype is expressed even when only one chromosome of a pair has a defect, or recessive conditions, in which expression occurs only if the defect exists on both chromosomes. Classically, these different modes of inheritance are revealed by pedigree analysis (Figs. 1 and 2).

As we learn more about the tremendous variation that occurs at every loci, the distinctions between dominant and recessive conditions have become blurred. Dominance and recessiveness are attributes of the phenotype, not attributes of

TABLE 2. *Types of birth defects*

Anomaly	Structural feature that departs from the normal
Syndrome	Recognizable pattern of structural defects often with a predictable natural history that can be identified on several patients, thus allowing diagnosis and classification
Sequence	Pattern of defects that results from a single event early in pregnancy
Association	Grouping of anomalies that frequently occur together but are not actual syndromes
Malformation	Morphologic defect resulting from abnormal development
Disruption	Morphologic defect resulting from extrinsic breakdown or interference with normal development
Deformation	Abnormal form, shape, or position caused by mechanical forces

the gene or allele. They are empiric terms and depend on the sensitivity of the method used to describe the phenotype. The researchers must specify phenotypic features when describing inheritance. For instance, sickle cell anemia is a recessive disease only if the full-blown disease is considered, but it is a codominant condition if the hemoglobin is being analyzed by electrophoresis. The ABO blood group is an example of a trait in which both codominant and recessive inheritance are seen. The retinoblastoma gene is a recessive tumor-suppressor gene at the cellular level, but abnormalities in the gene are responsible for the autosomal-dominant tendency retinoblastomas and osteosarcomas to develop.

In autosomal-dominant conditions, the disease is expressed in persons who are heterozygous for the disease-causing mutation. McKusick's catalog of mendelian disorders describes more than 3000 dominant conditions. Marfan syndrome, myotonic dystrophy, neurofibromatosis, achondroplasia, and Huntington disease are examples of autosomal-dominant disorders. The probability of an affected person transmitting the abnormal gene to his or her progeny is 50% with each pregnancy. Typically, autosomal-dominant conditions have less than 100% penetrance, and fewer than 50% of the offspring show signs of the disorder. Male and female offspring are affected with equal frequency and severity. The trait passes through one parental line only, and father-to-son transmission can occur. For highly penetrant autosomal-dominant conditions, the gene is expressed in each generation (i.e., vertical transmission). New mutations are relatively common, and on average, paternal age is advanced when isolated, sporadic, or new mutation cases appear. Autosomal-

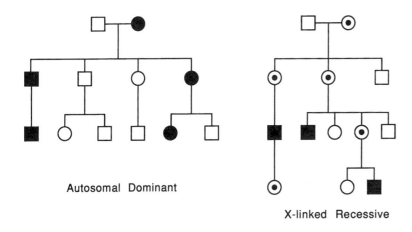

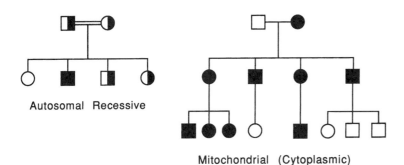

FIG. 2. Patterns of inheritance.

dominant phenotypes often involve isolated or multiple structural defects. They can be extremely variable, and the onset of clinical features is often age dependent. Dominant disorders tend to be less severe than recessive diseases, but they are usually lethal in the rare persons who are homozygous for a dominant disease.

Autosomal-recessive conditions are only expressed in persons in whom both versions (i.e., alleles) of the involved gene are abnormal. More than 1500 autosomal-recessive conditions have been described. Cystic fibrosis, sickle cell anemia, Tay-Sachs disease, and phenylketonuria are examples of autosomal-recessive disorders. Male and female offspring are affected with equal frequency and severity. Each parent is a heterozygous carrier, and abnormal genes are inherited from both parents. Each offspring of two carrier parents has a 25% chance of being affected, a 50% chance of being a carrier, and a 25% chance of being neither a carrier nor affected. If the recessive phenotype is extremely rare, consanguinity is usually found in the pedigree. Affected persons rarely have affected children; autosomal-recessive inheritance shows a horizontal pattern in a pedigree, with typically only a single generation of siblings affected. Affected persons who mate with unaffected persons who are not carriers have only unaffected, carrier offspring. Most autosomal-recessive phenotypes are biochemical or enzymatic in nature, and they tend to be less variable and more severe than dominant conditions.

X-linked inheritance occurs when a trait is carried on the X chromosome. Males are hemizygous for X chromosome genes, but females can be homozygous or heterozygous. Of the 300 recognized X-linked recessive diseases, the hemophilias and Duchenne muscular dystrophy are the best known. Characteristics of X-linked recessive inheritance include a higher incidence of the disorder in male than female offspring. The mutant gene or disease is never transmitted directly from father to son, and all the daughters of an affected man are carriers. The trait is transmitted through carrier females, and affected males in the same kindred are related to one another through the females. X-linked dominant diseases are much rarer; examples include Alport syndrome, vitamin D resistant rickets, and incontinentia pigmenti. They appear twice as often in female as in male offspring. All daughters of an affected man have the disorder, but no sons are affected. Heterozygous affected women transmit the mutant allele at a rate of 50% to progeny of both sexes. If the affected woman is homozygous, all of her children will be affected.

Y-linked or holandric inheritance occurs when a trait is carried on the Y chromosome. Only male offspring are affected, and there is only male-to-male transmission. There are no known disease genes that are inherited in this fashion, but genes for sex determination, tooth size, and height occur on the Y chromosome.

Mitochondrial inheritance, a more recently described type of inheritance, involves traits and disorders inherited through the mitochondrial chromosome. Mitochondria are inherited exclusively with the cytoplasm of the egg; a woman who carries a disease will pass the disease to 100% of her offspring. Male carriers will pass the disorder to none of their offspring. Leber optic atrophy and certain rare myopathies are inherited in this fashion.

Polygenic, Multifactorial Disorders

Multifactorial or polygenic inheritance is the most common form of inheritance. Even with classic mendelian disorders, there can be tremendous quantitative and qualitative differences in the phenotype between persons who have the same allele or the same genetic mutation. This variability can be evident as nonpenetrance of certain features or the entire phenotype and as differences in the severity of features, the frequency of cyclic or episodic events, or the age of onset of the first clinical sign of the disorder. Genetic variability can be caused by the underlying genetic background of the affected person or sex influences and limitations. The phenotype may be influenced by maternal factors such as cytoplasmic inheritance, the intrauterine environment, or imprinting. X-linked disorders can be altered by variations in X inactivation or lionization. Each genotype

undergoes subtle changes through somatic mutation, gene amplification, or transpositions and positional effects over time. Exogenous factors such as the environment, teratogens, medical intervention, and chance also influence variability.

Most congenital anomalies show multifactorial inheritance. A common error that some obstetricians make is to counsel a patient that rare conditions will not occur repetitively in her family. If the birth defect in question has a strong genetic component or if there is an identifiable environmental or teratogenic component that would recur in a subsequent pregnancy, the risks may remain high for that patient (Table 3). The rates may be even higher if a mendelian or chromosomal condition has gone unrecognized in the affected child. Before clinicians counsel patients about the recurrence risk of any birth defect, it is pertinent to review which syndromes are associated with that birth defect and ask whether any member of the family has those syndromes. When this requires skill or knowledge beyond the usual expertise of an obstetrician-gynecologist, referral to a medical geneticist is appropriate.

Multifactorial inheritance usually works according to a threshold model. Several factors must collaborate to cause a bodily function to go awry, and only after these factors reach some critical point is the phenotypic effect seen. Many different factors can affect the observed recurrence risk. The heritability of the condition is frequently the most important

TABLE 3. *Empiric recurrence risks for common congenital anomalies*

Anomalies	Normal parents, 1 affected child: risk subsequent children (%)	1 Affected parent: risk for first child (%)	Identical twin (%)	M:F ratio	Incidence
Cleft lip and palate	4, unilateral lip; 2.5, bilateral lip; 5.6, lip and palate	3.2	31	2:1	1/1000
Whites					1/750
Blacks					1/2500
Navajos					1/500
Japanese					1/600
Cleft palate alone	2	6	40	2:3	0.4/1000
Clubfoot	3	3	33	2:1	1.2/1000
Congenital heart disease					
Ventricular septal defect	4–5	3–4		1.3:1	5/1000
Patent ductus arteriosus	1–4	2.8		—	1/2000
Tetralogy of Fallot	2–3	1.6		—	—
Atrial septal defect	3	3.5		—	1/1000
Pulmonic stenosis	3	3		—	—
Aortic stenosis	3	—		—	—
Coarctation	2	—		—	—
Transposition	2	—		—	—
Arteriovenous canal	2–3	—		—	—
Neural tube defect	3 (U.S.A)	3	23	Varies with	1/700
(spinabifida/	5 (Great Britain)			defect	1/330
anencephaly)					
Whites					1/700
Jews					1/1200
Blacks					1/1500
Puerto Ricans					1/500
Congenital dislocation hip	3.5	3–5	35	1:7	2/1000
Pyloric stenosis	3.2 (if brother affected) 6.5 (if sister affected)	25.4 (if mother affected) 4.2 (if father affected)		4:1	1/250

factor. This is usually determined by examining whether monozygotic twins are concordant for a particular condition relative to dizygotic twins. For instance, neonatal seizures show a very high heritability rate, with 85% to 90% concordance in monozygotic twins verses 10% to 15% concordance in dizygotic twins. The population incidence of the condition is another important variable. The recurrence risk is higher for common disorders or within populations with a high incidence of the disorder. In disorders with a relatively high heritability, the recurrence risk of the disorder approximates the square root of the population incidence. There can be marked variation in the population frequency of different disorders and different ethnic groups. For instance, cleft lip occurs commonly in Native Americans, but African-Americans have a ninefold lower incidence of cleft lip than the general population.

If the incidence of a congenital anomaly shows a sex bias, the recurrence risk is higher in the offspring (and other relatives) if the parent is the less frequently affected sex. For example, pyloric stenosis affects five times as many male as female offspring, and empiric data show that there is a 25% chance of producing an affected child if the mother had pyloric stenosis at birth and only a 4% risk if the father is the affected parent. Similarly, the recurrence risk is higher when the sex of the affected child is the less frequently affected sex. Again, the risk of having another child with pyloric stenosis is 3.2% if the first affected sibling is male and 6.5% if the affected sibling is female. Hirschsprung disease, clubfoot, and cleft lip are examples of anomalies that are more common in male infants; cleft palate, anencephaly, hip dysplasia, and scoliosis are more common in female infants.

The number of affected individuals in a kindred can influence the recurrence risk. The greater the number of family members who have already been affected with a multifactorial condition, the more likely it is that the genetic background is favorable for expression of this condition. After a couple has one affected child with cleft lip and palate, there is a 4% empiric recurrence risk. After two affected children, the risk rises to 10%. Consanguinity also increases the risk of recurrence because of the greater likelihood of deleterious genes being shared, but a more distant relationship from an affected person decreases the risk of recurrence.

The severity of a disorder often predicts the recurrence risk. An illustration of this is found in Hirschsprung disease: The recurrence risk is proportional to the length of the aganglionic segment of the colon. Neural tube defects (NTDs) are the most notable exception to this rule because the recurrence risk for any NTD appears to be the same whether the first affected child had anencephaly or a small spina bifida lesion.

Cytogenetic Disorders

Cytogenetic disorders involve the loss or duplication of a large number of genes; multiple malformations and dysfunctions are observed. Some of the diagnostic clues for a cytogenetic disorder are subtle dysmorphic features, and others involve major structural malformations, particularly craniofacial, skeletal, cardiac, and genitourinary malformations. No individual anomaly is pathognomonic for a particular chromosomal syndrome; rather it is the pattern that can be distinctive. There is tremendous overlap between patterns, and because nonchromosomal syndromes can mimic chromosomal abnormalities, obtaining a karyotype is always necessary to confirm the diagnosis. Cytogenetic disorders are usually associated with some degree of mental retardation and growth deficiency. Most have an increased rate of perinatal loss and premature mortality of liveborn neonates. The rate of chromosomal abnormalities is at least 40% to 60% in first-trimester abortuses, and the rates of abnormalities are also elevated in fetal deaths and preterm and postterm deliveries (Tables 4 and 5). About 1 in 160 babies is born with a genetic defect detectable by ordinary cytogenetic means (Table 6).

Cytogenetic studies have been used clinically for approximately 35 years. In the late 1950s, it was determined that humans have 46 chromosomes and that many of the recognized birth defect syndromes, such as Down syndrome, Turner syndrome, and Klinefelter syndrome, have abnormalities of chromosome number or structure. Normally, the nucleus of most human cells contains two sets of chromosomes, with one set contributed by each parent. Each set has 22 autosomes and either an X or a Y sex chromosome (Fig. 3).

For at least 15 years, there was no easy way to differentiate chromosomes of similar sizes from one another, but in the 1970s modern banding techniques became available. Metaphase chromosome preparations can be prepared from any cell undergoing mitosis. Typically, to obtain adequate numbers of cells, mitosis is induced artificially using a mitogen such as phytohemagglutinin. The cells are then incubated in a dilute solution of an agent that poisons the mitotic spindle. The chromosomes are swollen using a hypotonic salt solution, fixed on a slide, and dried for staining. The stained chromosomes can be observed by light microscopy.

The dyes used to stain chromosome preparations reveal patterns of light and dark bands that reflect regional variations in the molecular composition of each chromosome. Giemsa is the most commonly used dye. Quinacrine (Q)-banding is a fluorescence technique that gives results similar to Giemsa

TABLE 4. *Incidence of chromosomal aberrations in pregnancy losses at various gestational ages*

Gestational age (wk)	With chromosomal abnormalities (%)
<8	72.1
8–11	53.5
12–15	47.9
16–19	23.8
20–23	11.9
24–27	13.2
Stillbirths	6.0
Neonatal deaths	5.5

(Data from Angel RR, Sandison A, Bain AD. Chromosome variation in perinatal mortality: a survey of 500 cases. *J Med Genet* 1984;21:39–44.)

TABLE 5. *Types of chromosomal abnormalities in spontaneous abortuses*

Type	Frequency (%)
Trisomy 14	3.7
Trisomy 15	4.2
Trisomy 16	16.4
Trisomy 18	3.0
Trisomy 21	4.7
Trisomy 22	5.7
Other Trisomies	14.3
45,X	18
Triploid	17
Tetraploid	6
Unbalanced translocations	3
Other	4

(Data from Carr and Gedeon, 1977.)

TABLE 6. *Incidence of chromosomal aberrations seen in newborn surveys*

Aberrations	Births
Sex chromosome abnormalities in males	
XYY	1/1000
XXY	1/1000
Other	1/3000
Sex chromosome abnormalities in females	
45,X	1/10,000
XXX	1/1000
Other	1/3000
Autosomal aberrations in babies	
+D(trisomy 13)	1/20,000
+E(trisomy 18)	1/8000
+G(nearly all trisomy 21)	1/800
Other trisomies	1/50,000
Rearrangements	
Balanced	1/500
Unbalanced	1/2000
Total chromosomal aberrations	1/160

(Data from Hook EB, Hamerton JL. In: Hook EB, Porter IH, eds: *Population cytogenetics: studies in humans.* New York: Academic Press, 1977.)

(G)-banding, while reverse (R)-banding gives a pattern opposite to that with G- or Q-banding. T-banding specifically stains the telemetric regions of chromosomes, which can help to screen for missing regions at the ends of chromosomes, and C-banding primarily stains the centromeric region of chromosomes.

Differences in the size of the chromosomes, the banding pattern, and the centromere position allow the 24 chromosomes to be differentiated from each other in an analysis called a karyotype. The most common features looked for on a karyotype include the presence of aneuploidy (i.e., abnormal number of chromosomes) or structural chromosomal abnormalities such as deletions, inversions, insertions, or translocations (Table 7) (Fig. 4).

Because the technology to study cytogenetic disorders is well established, there is greater experience with this than

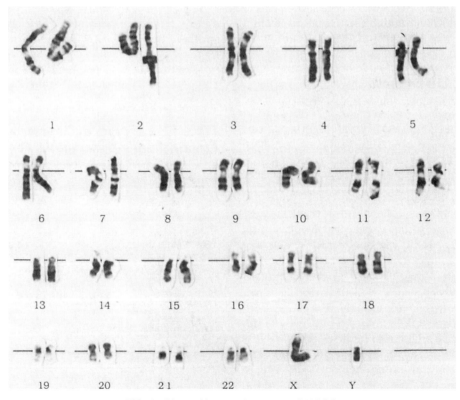

FIG. 3. Normal human karyotype (46,XY).

TABLE 7. *Chromosomal nomenclature*

p	Short ("petite") arm of a chromosome
q	Long arm of a chromosome
del	Deletion of a chromosomal segment
der	Derivative chromosome resulting from a structural rearrangement
dup	Duplication of a chromosome segment
i	Isochromosome
ins	Insertion of a chromosomal segment into another chromosome
inv	Inversion of a chromosomal segment
r	Ring chromosome
rob	Robertsonian translocation
t	Translocation
ter	Terminal segment of chromosome (pter=terminal short arm, qter=terminal long arm)
/	Diagonal hash-line indicates mosaicism (46XX/45X indicates a mosaic patient with cell lines containing 46 chromosomes and 45 chromosomes, respectively, i.e. mosaic Turner syndrome)
+ or −	When appearing before a chromosome, indicates the addition or loss of that whole chromosome (e.g., +21 indicates trisomy 21, Down syndrome). When appearing after a chromosome, indicates the addition or loss of a part of a chromosome (e.g., 8q− indicates the loss of part of the long arm of chromosome 8)

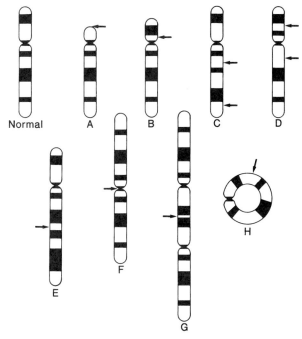

FIG. 4. Types of chromosomal abnormalities. **A:** Terminal deletion. **B:** Interstitial deletion. **C:** Paracentric inversion. **D:** Pericentric inversion. **E:** Translocation (additional material from a different chromosome). **F:** Isochromosome. **G:** Dicentric chromosome. **H:** Ring chromosome. The *arrows* indicate the sites of chromosomal breaks, where rearrangement occurs.

with other types of genetic testing. There are several well defined indications for obtaining a fetal karyotype (Table 8). Pregnant women who are 35 years old or older are routinely offered a fetal karyotype because trisomy tends to occur more commonly with advancing maternal age (Table 9). Other indications for obtaining a fetal karyotype include having a previous child with an abnormal karyotype, parental chromosomal rearrangements, unexplained intrauterine growth retardation, and an abnormally low level of maternal serum alpha-fetoprotein. In addition, many fetal anomalies associated with karyotypic abnormalities can now be visualized using high-resolution ultrasound (Table 10). A fetal structural abnormality detected by ultrasound is an indication for obtaining a fetal karyotype.

A variety of genetic defects, including the common trisomies and many chromosomal translocations, can be detected by routine karyotype analysis. Recent modifications, including chromosome painting that allows a particular chromosome to be identified directly and fluorescent *in situ* hybridization (FISH) that allows specific sites along the chromosome to be identified, have greatly extended the capabilities of the cytogenetics laboratory. However, there are molecular and single-gene rearrangements that cannot be observed by light microscopy and require molecular genetic technology for evaluation.

FISH is a cytogenetic technique in which a specific DNA probe with a fluorescent label is bound to homologous DNA in a clinical sample. FISH can be performed either on a metaphase chromosome spread to detect microdeletions and microduplications, or during interphase to detect a larger chromosomal region in a nondividing cell. Interphase FISH can be performed on cultured cells, tissue sections, and cytologic smears. It has been used to detect common aneuploidies, such as trisomy 21, trisomy 18, and trisomy 13, and the sex chromosome aneuploidies in prenatal diagnosis.

Because uncultured amniocytes can be used, the FISH technique can offer more rapid detection of chromosomal aneuploidies. In a recent report, FISH was performed as an adjunct to conventional cytogenetics in 4500 patients. Region-specific DNA probes to chromosomes 13, 18, 21, X, and Y were used to determine ploidy by analysis of signal number in hybridized nuclei. A sample was considered to be euploid when all autosomal probes generated two hybridization signals and when a normal sex chromosome pattern was observed in greater than or equal to 80% of hybridized nuclei. A sample was considered to be aneuploid when greater than or equal to 70% of hybridized nuclei displayed the same abnormal hybridization pattern for a specific probe. The accu-

TABLE 8. *Indications for a fetal karyotype*

Advanced maternal age
Previous child with an abnormal karyotype
Parental chromosome rearrangements
Fetal structural abnormality on ultrasound
Unexplained intrauterine growth retardation
Abnormally low maternal serum alpha-fetoprotein

TABLE 9. *Risk of karyotypic abnormalities related to maternal age at delivery*

Age (yr)	Trisomy 21		Any abnormality	
	Live birth	Amnio-centesis	Live Birth	Amnio-centesis
20	1/1734	1/1231	1/526	—
25	1/1250	1/887	1/476	—
30	1/965	1/685	1/385	—
31	1/915	1/650	1/385	—
32	1/794	1/563	1/322	—
33	1/639	1/452	1/286	—
34	1/496	1/352	1/238	—
35	1/386	1/274	1/192	1/83
36	1/300	1/213	1/156	1/76
37	1/234	1/166	1/127	1/67
38	1/182	1/129	1/102	1/58
39	1/141	1/100	1/83	1/49
40	1/100	1/78	1/66	1/40
41	1/86	1/61	1/53	1/32
42	1/66	1/47	1/42	1/26
43	1/52	1/37	1/33	1/21
44	1/40	1/29	1/26	1/19
45	1/31	1/22	1/21	1/15
46	1/24	1/17	1/16	1/12
47	1/19	1/13	1/13	1/20
48	1/15	1/10	1/10	1/18
49	1/11	1/8	1/8	1/16

(Data from Hook et al., 1983.)

TABLE 10. *Risk of a chromosome abnormality with selected sonographic findings*

Finding	Abnormal karyotype (%)[a]
Holoprosencephaly	40–60
Dandy-Walker malformation, cerebellar hypoplasia	↑
Isolated hydrocephalus	5–10
Spina bifida	1–5
Agenesis of the corpus callosum	↑
Choroid plexus cysts—large or associated with other abnormalities	1–2
Facial abnormalities	↑
Cystic hygroma	>60
Nuchal thickening	↑
Cardiac malformations	20–35
Duodenal atresia	30
Omphalocele	10
Hydrothorax	↑
Diaphragmatic hernia	↑
Genitourinary anomalies	4–10
Obstructive uropathy	↑↑
Renal cystic dysplasia with other abnormalities	↑
Clubfoot with other abnormalities	↑
Severe intrauterine growth retardation	↑
Polyhydramnios or oligohydramnios and other abnormalities	↑
Single umbilical artery with other anomalies	↑
Multiple placental cysts	↑
Nonimmune hydrops	10–20

[a]Values are provided only when there are a large enough experience and general consensus in the literature.

racy of all *informative* FISH results, euploid and aneuploid, was 99.8%, and the specificity was 99.9%. Current prenatal FISH protocols are not designed to detect all chromosomal abnormalities and should only be utilized as an adjunctive test to cytogenetics. FISH can provide rapid and accurate clinical information in pregnancies in which fetal abnormalities had been observed by ultrasound.

Future improvements are likely. FISH protocols under development would allow the simultaneous and unequivocal discernment of all human chromosomes. Each chromosome is labeled in a unique way using several different colors. A "spectral karyotype" can be generated, allowing visualization of a unique, defined emission spectra for each human chromosome. Computerized analysis may allow automatic and rapid analysis with resolution approaching routine G-banding.

Parent of Origin Effects

Genomic imprinting refers to the differential expression of genes based on the parent of origin of the gene. Imprinting is usually mediated by differential methylation of the alleles involved. Most experimental evidence regarding imprinting comes from animal studies, but some naturally occurring human analogs exist. The paternal genetic contribution appears to be essential for the development and function of the placenta and extraembryonic tissues, but the maternal contribution is required for embryonic development. Ovarian ter-

atomas, the most common benign pelvic tumor in women of reproductive age, are characterized by a diploid karyotype, in which both haploid sets of chromosomes are maternal in origin. Complete hydatidiform moles, which show failure of normal embryonic and fetal development, are usually diploid with two paternal haploid chromosome sets and no maternally derived chromosomes.

The differential function of parental chromosome contributions in development is also evident in the study of human triploidy. In an android conception (i.e., two paternal, one maternal chromosome sets), the fetus is severely growth retarded with a disproportionately large head and syndactyly of the digits of the hand. The placenta is usually very large and hydropic. Survival into the second trimester or occasionally into the third trimester is possible but usually requires the presence of mosaicism with a diploid cell line. When the chromosomal constitution is gynoid (i.e., two maternal, one paternal sets), the conceptus is underdeveloped and the placenta is small and cystic; such pregnancies rarely continue beyond the first trimester.

In some persons with an apparently normal karyotype, both versions of a pair of homologous chromosomes were inherited from one parent, a phenomenon called uniparental disomy. This can give rise to abnormalities if genomic imprinting causes regions of both chromosomes to be inactivated or overexpressed.

◊ MOLECULAR GENETICS REVOLUTION

In the mid 1950s, there were only two "facts" known about the human genome. It was thought that humans had 48 chromosomes and that X-chromosome inactivation in humans occurred by the same mechanism as that observed in fruit flies. Both of these observations have been proven to be in error. In the past few decades, there has been an explosion of knowledge about the human genome, largely attributed to advances in molecular biology.

Deoxyribonucleic Acid

Genes are the instructions required for building structural proteins, enzymes, and peptide hormones, and the complete set of genetic instructions for any organism is called its genome (Table 11). The human genome has 46 chromosomes, including 22 pairs of autosomes and two sex chromosomes. The genome consists of approximately 100,000 genes or 3 billion base pairs.

In 1944, Avery and colleagues demonstrated that DNA is the chemical that carries genetic instructions. Roughly equal parts of DNA and its supporting proteins make up the 46 chromosomes. If the strands of DNA in the nucleus of a single cell could be unwound and spliced together, the resulting DNA molecule would stretch more than 1.5 m long, but would be only 20 trillionths of a centimeter wide.

The genetic code is spelled out with the four nitrogenous bases: adenine, thymine, cytosine, and guanine (Fig. 5). The purine and pyrimidine bases are arranged in a ladder-like, double-helical arrangement that is very stable (i.e., theoretical dissociation constant = 10^{-23}). During cell division, DNA is duplicated with extremely high fidelity by synthesis of a new strand of one side of the molecular ladder.

Although the human genome consists of at least 100,000 genes, genes represent only one-tenth of the encoded information. Most of the genome is of unknown function, but it probably codes for the proper spacing, alignment, and punctuation of the genetic instructions. About 99.8% of the DNA sequence is identical from one person to the next. Stated another way, there are many minor differences between any two persons; on average, there is a variation of one nucleotide for every 200 to 500 base pairs. When these sequence differences occur within genes, they can lead to genetic diseases or ge-

DNA	CAG—CGG—GGT
RNA	GUC—GCC—CCA
Protein	Valine—Alanine—Proline

FIG. 5. Genetic code. The DNA code consists of four characters and is read three characters at a time. It is translated into a RNA message that instructs cells in how to assemble proteins from amino acid building blocks.

netic variation. Most of the minor differences have no observable effect, since they occur in the noncoding regions of the genome, regions of DNA that do not contain genes. These otherwise unimportant differences have been the basis of the current explosion of genetic knowledge, because much of our ability to study genes or diagnose genetic illness exploits differences (i.e., DNA sequence polymorphisms) in these regions to track or find neighboring genes.

The DNA sequence is read by cellular enzymes three bases at a time, and each triplet directs the positioning of a particular amino acid within the structure of a protein (see Fig. 5). The protein-coding instructions are transmitted to the cellular machinery through messenger ribonucleic acid (RNA), a transient, intermediary molecule similar to a single strand of DNA (Fig. 6). The RNA strand is transcribed from the DNA template in the nucleus and has an opposite or complementary genetic sequence. Messenger RNA moves from the nucleus into the cytoplasm, where the protein-manufacturing organelles build a protein. Analysis of messenger RNA molecules is extremely useful in the laboratory for detecting genes.

Approximately 5500 human genes have been cataloged. During the past decade, over 2000 human genes have been localized to their particular chromosomes, and roughly 600 have been characterized at the DNA level.

Several advances in molecular biology have enabled the molecular genetics revolution to take place. The first was the discovery of restriction enzymes, which are bacterial proteins that can cut DNA molecules at specific sites by recognizing the DNA sequence at those sites. Over 400 restriction enzymes have been discovered, many are commercially available, and about 25 are used commonly. Restriction fragment length polymorphisms (RFLPs) occur because of minor sequence changes (usually single base substitutions) that abolish or create a recognition site, altering the length of a digestion fragment. Restriction sites occur frequently, and several restriction sites can occur in the vicinity of any given gene. When these RFLPs are polymorphic, they become useful markers for linkage studies, diagnostic testing, and paternity testing (Fig. 7). RFLPs and other DNA polymorphisms provide the landmarks for genetic maps.

Scientists have gained a greater understanding of how to manipulate the physical conditions such as pH, salt concentration, and temperature of *in vitro* DNA reactions. These skills—combined with the use of restriction enzymes— allowed the development of recombinant DNA, or new com-

TABLE 11. *The human genome*

46 chromosomes including
22 pairs of autosomes
2 sex chromosomes
100,000 genes
3,000,000,000 base pairs

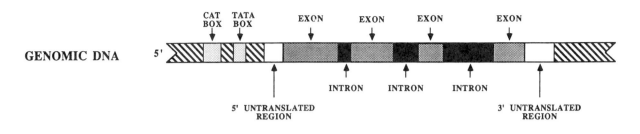

GENOMIC DNA

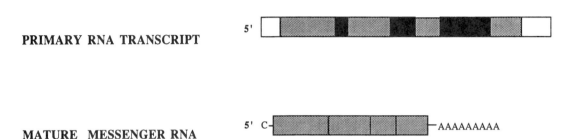

PRIMARY RNA TRANSCRIPT

MATURE MESSENGER RNA

FIG. 6. Anatomy of a gene. Regulatory regions are present in the 5′ region. Introns are spliced out of the final messenger RNA.

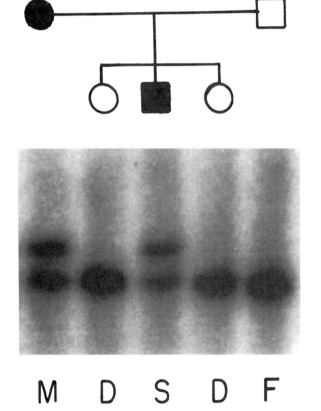

M   D   S   D   F

FIG. 7. Linkage study using restriction fragment length polymorphisms. Each lane represents the genotype of one family member: *M*, mother; *F*, father; *D*, daughter; *S*, son. In this example, the disease allele is associated with the upper band passed from the mother to the son.

binations of DNA engineered in the laboratory. Recombinant DNA technology has made possible the development of gene probes (pieces of DNA usually radioactively labeled) that recognize and bind specifically to a homologous sequence in another sample of DNA. These technologies also underlie cloning—the copying of DNA segments in lower animals and the manufacturing of human proteins using bacteria or cell cultures.

Various blotting technologies are commonly used to study DNA. With blotting, biologically relevant molecules undergo electrophoresis and are transferred to a stable membrane for repeated experiments. Blots are called Southern blots if DNA is being analyzed, Northern blots if RNA is analyzed, and Western blots if proteins are being analyzed.

DNA testing is clinically applicable to many disorders and can be performed in one of several ways (Table 12). When the molecular basis of a disease is known, direct mutation testing can provide a positive or negative answer on any DNA sample. For instance, in cystic fibrosis, hundreds of mutations have been discovered. A battery of mutations can be tested using a dot blot technique that is simple to interpret (Fig. 8).

Similarly, fragile X syndrome is usually the result of an expansion of a triplet sequence within the gene. Normal persons usually have only 5 to 50 copies of this triplet repeat, but affected patients have hundreds or thousands of copies of the triplet repeat. Similar triplet expansions cause myotonic dystrophy, Huntington disease, and Kennedy disease. The region containing the triplet can be amplified using the polymerase chain reaction (PCR). PCR produces millions of copies of the small region of DNA from the X chromosome that contains

TABLE 12. *Common conditions for which DNA testing is available*

Disease	Inheritance	Methodology used
Adult polycystic kidney disease	AD	Linkage analysis
Retinoblastoma	AD	Linkage analysis, sequencing
Myotonic dystrophy	AD	Direct mutation test (triplet expansion)
Huntington's chorea	AD	Direct mutation test (triplet expansion)
Sickle cell anemia	AR	PCR and ASO mutation detection
β-Thalassemia	AR	PCR and ASO mutation detection
α_1-Antitrypsin deficiency	AR	PCR then ASO mutation detection
Lesch-Nyhan syndrome	XLR	Multiplex PCR, then sequence
Ornithine transcarbamylase deficiency	XLR	PCR, then chemical cleavage
Fragile X syndrome	XLR	Direct mutation test (triplet expansion)
Hemophilia	XLR	Linkage analysis, mutation scanning, inversion test
Steroid sulfatase deficiency	XLR	Multiplex PCR for deletion detection
Duchenne muscular dystrophy	XLR	Multiplex PCR for deletion detection, linkage analysis

AD, autosomal dominant; AR, autosomal recessive; ASO, allele-specific oligonucleotide; PCR, polymerase chain reaction; XLR, X-linked recessive.

the fragile X repeat. Specificity is achieved by directing the reaction using two complementary primers on either side of the region of interest. Once amplified, the size of the product can be measured to evaluate the number of triplets, determining whether or not the mutation exists (Fig. 9).

For families with unusual mutations or with diseases for which the molecular basis is unknown, linkage testing can be performed. Linkage tests compare DNA polymorphisms close to the disease-causing gene in family members known to have or carry the disease with those of unaffected and at-risk family members. Indirect assessments can be made about whether or not at-risk persons have the disease allele. The accuracy of these predictions depends on correct diagnosis and relationships of the family members and the genetic distance between the polymorphism tested and the

disease allele. For some families, linkage testing can be uninformative (Fig. 10).

Human Genome Project

During the next decade, an international effort called the Human Genome Project will seek to define the complete set of genetic instructions of humans. The genome project is a joint venture of the National Institutes of Health, the U.S. Department of Energy, and many international organizations; it is the largest biologic research program ever attempted.

The project's first goal is to develop detailed genetic maps that depict the order in which genes, markers, and other landmarks occur along a chromosome. Scientists have already built a second-generation map with approximately 10,000 polymorphic markers that are sufficiently polymorphic and

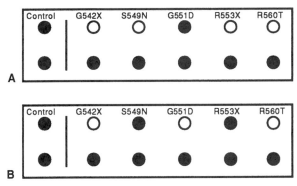

FIG. 8. Direct mutation diagram. Direct detection of cystic fibrosis mutations was made using the reverse dot blot technique. In this example, five mutations in exon 11 of the cystic fibrosis gene (G542X, S549N, G551D, R553X, and R560T) are tested for using a simple yes/no assay. Exon 11 is amplified using the polymerase chain reaction. The product of the reaction is labeled to allow its detection and placed on a membrane. The membrane has been prepared with oligonucleotide probes that detect either the normal or the abnormal sequence. Panel **A** is a result from a known cystic fibrosis carrier, and panel **B** is from a child with cystic fibrosis.

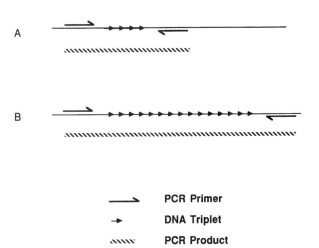

FIG. 9. Fragile X mutation detection. In patient *A*, a shorter polymerase chain reaction product corresponds with a smaller number of triplet repeats, while patient *B* exhibits an expanded number of repeats. Affected patients typically have hundreds or even thousands of copies of the triplet.

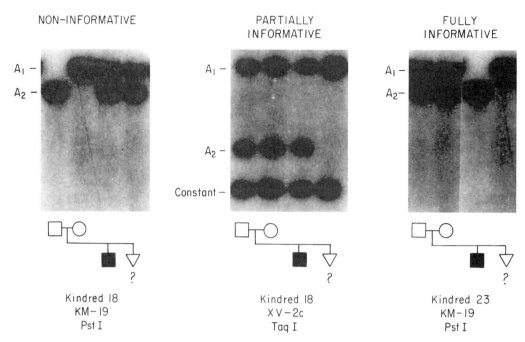

FIG. 10. Informativeness of linkage testing for cystic fibrosis. Marker KM-19 in kindred 18 is "not informative:" The disease alleles can not be distinguished in the parents.

roughly evenly distributed on all the chromosomes. There are two types of maps: linkage maps, which show the tendency for markers to be inherited together through different generations of a family, and physical maps, which depict actual measured distances along the chromosome. Although the tendency to show linkage is related to physical separation, there is not a one-to-one correlation between the molecular distances on linkage and physical maps.

Higher-resolution and better-quality maps can speed the search for disease-causing genes, especially genes for polygenic, multifactorial conditions. To find genes that cause a genetic disease, affected and normal persons from families with the disease under study are "typed" using genetic markers that have already been mapped to particular chromosomes. When affected persons from a family demonstrate a nonrandom tendency to have the same marker type, the likelihood that the disease gene is on the same chromosome and in the same region as the marker used can be computed. Additional markers from this region are then typed to add proof and to refine the localization. The region identified by the linkage analysis may contain hundreds or thousands of genes. Markers located on either side of the disease gene can be used as starting points to assemble cloned DNA fragments from the region into a contiguous representation of the entire region. DNA samples from patients with chromosomal deletions or translocations can be invaluable in determining relative locations of fragments from the region and eventually in locating the disease-causing gene.

The disease-causing gene is identified by looking for features in the DNA clones commonly seen in active genes. Finding a DNA sequence in other animal species or finding DNA fragments that are homologous to RNA from tissues involved in the disease helps to focus the search. Eventually, one gene is proven to be the disease-causing gene by finding mutations in the DNA sequence from patients and carriers. The identified mutations must cause biologically relevant disruptions in the predicted gene product. Various bioassays can be designed to prove that a particular gene defect can cause the phenotype in question. For instance, attempts are made to cause the disease in a transgenic animal by introducing the abnormal gene or to correct a mutant cell line by adding the normal gene.

A secondary objective of the genome project is to sequence the entire human genome over the next 7 years. This is an ambitious goal, considering that less than 1% of the genome has been sequenced. Twenty years ago, a researcher would have to work for 1 year to determine 10 to 20 bases of sequence, but some large laboratories can produce 50,000 base pairs of sequence per day. Even at that rate, it would take 200 years for a laboratory to sequence the entire genome!

At least 3% of the annual budget of the project is going to the ethical, legal, and social issues section of the enterprise. This amount of early attention to societal impact is unprecedented for a science and technology project. Grant-funded programs will examine privacy issues, genetic discrimination in insurance and employment, and the role of coercion. Genetic discoveries may challenge long-held beliefs about equality, predetermination, and free will as we learn about genes that have a major role in personality, creativity, intelligence, and mental illness. The safety, efficacy, and utility of new gene tests should be evaluated, especially before treatment is available.

◊ GENETIC EVALUATION

Genetic History and Physical Examination

Important details are being learned about many rare disorders that practitioners may see only once in their career. In the past, many practitioners have had a laissez faire attitude about genetic disorders, since "you can't do anything about your genes." However, it is important to detect genetic conditions so that patients can have adequate counseling about the condition and the risk to offspring. For severe conditions, patients are often interested in prenatal diagnosis, so they can consider pregnancy termination or prepare for the birth of an affected child. Our new predictive powers have led to an expanded medicolegal duty to warn patients of risks of which they may not have been aware. Failure to provide accurate and timely reproductive counseling has resulted in a host of lawsuits. Genetic diagnosis becomes even more critical as more treatment options become available for the child with a severe genetic disease.

In light of these expanding obligations to screen, what is expected of the general obstetrician-gynecologist? As with any medical diagnosis, the history is the most important part of the genetic evaluation. Important aspects of a genetic history such as the patient's age, menstrual history, and obstetric history are routinely queried as part of any routine obstetric or gynecologic history. In addition, it is important to ask about the ethnic background of both patients and their partners (Table 13). The family history should extend to third-degree relatives (i.e., cousins). A minimal familial history can usually be elicited using the following questions:

◊ Do you have a family history of diabetes, hypertension, cancer, or twins?

◊ Are there any diseases that seem to run in your family?

◊ Is there a history of genetic disease like cystic fibrosis, hemophilia, or muscular dystrophy?

◊ Is there anyone with mental retardation or any kind of birth defect?

◊ Have any of your sisters, cousins, or other relatives had problems with their pregnancies?

◊ Are your parents alive? Are they healthy?

◊ As far as you know, are you and your husband or partner related by blood?

◊ Do you know your ethnic background? (Do you know where your relatives are originally from?)

◊ Is there any reason you are especially concerned that you might have trouble with your pregnancy or that your baby may be born with a birth defect or other medical problem?

These questions take only a few minutes to ask a new patient. The final, open-ended question is often the most revealing. Alternatively, many practitioners find it helpful to ask similar questions using a patient-completed questionnaire. I use a form similar to the one suggested by the American College of Obstetricians and Gynecologists (Fig. 11). It is designed so that only "yes" responses need to be dealt with further. Including a form such as this one in the patient's chart clearly documents that a genetic history was obtained for medicolegal purposes.

TABLE 13. *Single gene disorders with an ethnic predilection*

Ethnic group	Disorder
Africans	Hemoglobinopathies, especially Hb S, Hb C, α- and β-thalassemia, persistent Hb F
	G6PD deficiency, African type
	Adult lactase deficiency
Ashkenazi Jews	Abetalipoproteinernia
	Bloom syndrome
	Dystonia musculorum deformans (recessive form)
	Familial dysautonomia
	Factor XI (PTA) deficiency
	Gaucher disease (adult form)
	Iminoglycinuria
	Niemann-Pick disease
	Pentosuria
	Spongy degeneration of brain
	Tay-Sachs disease
Chinese	α-Thalassemia
	G6PD deficiency, Chinese type
	Adult lactase deficiency
Eskimos	E_1^S (pseudocholinesterase deficiency)
Finns	Congenital nephrosis
	Aspartylglucosaminuria
Japanese	Acatalasia
	Oguchi disease
Mediterranean peoples (Italians, Greeks, Sephardic Jews)	Thalassemia (mainly β)
	G6PD deficiency, Mediterranean type
	Familial Mediterranean fever

G6PD, glucose-6-phosphate dehydrogenase.
(Adapted from McKusick, 1990.)

More than one-fifth of healthy obstetric patients affirmatively answer at least one important question on the form.

Physicians should suspect genetic factors if a patient presents with an unusual problem and other people in her family have the same disorder. Similarly, if a patient reports a positive family history, it is important to decide whether the patient unknowingly has the same disease. When a patient reports an unfamiliar genetic condition or a rare illness, the physician should seek out information about the genetics of this condition. Is she at risk of passing the condition to her offspring? Is prenatal diagnosis available? Is prenatal treatment available? For instance, a patient whose first child died of methylmalonicaciduria informed her obstetrician of this at the time of a subsequent pregnancy, and the obstetrician noted this history on prenatal record but did not inform the patient that there was a one in four risk that her current fetus could be affected. The obstetrician was unaware that prenatal diagnosis is available and, more important, that a simple treatment (i.e., giving the mother supplemental vitamin B_{12}) could prevent much of the morbidity of this particular form of methylmalonicaciduria. The child was born severely damaged and died at 2 years of age. The patient was very angry that she was not informed about prenatal therapy, and a law-

PRENATAL GENETICS SCREENING FORM

Last Name _____ First Name _____ Date _____

1. Will you be 35 years or older when the baby is due? Yes ____ No ____

Genetic Diseases Common to Certain Ethnic Groups

1. Are you or the baby's father of African descent? Yes ____ No ____
   If yes, have either of you been screened for sickle cell trait? Yes ____ No ____
2. Are you or the baby's father of Eastern European Jewish descent (Ashkenazi)? Yes ____ No ____
   If yes, have either of you been screened for Tay-Sachs disease? Yes ____ No ____
3. Do you or your partner have any close relatives from Italy, Greece, or other Mediterranean countries? Yes ____ No ____
   If yes, have either of you been screened for β-thalassemia? Yes ____ No ____
4. Do you or your partner have any close relatives from the Philippines or Southeast Asia? Yes ____ No ____
   If yes, have either of you been screened for α-thalassemia? Yes ____ No ____

Personal and Family Genetic History

1. Have you, the baby's father, or any member of your respective families ever had any of the following disorders:
   - Down syndrome (mongolism)? Yes ____ No ____
   - Other chromosomal abnormalities? Yes ____ No ____
   - Congenital heart defect? Yes ____ No ____
   - Hemophilia? Yes ____ No ____
   - Muscular dystrophy? Yes ____ No ____
   - Cystic fibrosis? Yes ____ No ____
   - Spina bifida (open spine), hydrocephaly (water on the brain) or anencephaly (absent brain)? Yes ____ No ____
   - A genetic disorder or birth defect not listed above? Yes ____ No ____
   - If yes, please list _____
   If a relative had any of the above, please indicate their relationship to you.
   _____
2. Do you or the baby's father have a birth defect? Yes ____ No ____
   If yes, please describe. _____
3. Have you ever had a baby who died in the womb or a baby with a birth defect? Yes ____ No ____
4. Have you had three or more first-trimester (first 12 weeks of pregnancy) miscarriages? Yes ____ No ____
5. Do you or the father of your baby have any relatives with mental retardation? Yes ____ No ____
6. Excluding iron or prenatal vitamins, have you taken any medications during pregnancy? Yes ____ No ____
   If yes please list. _____
7. Have you used any recreational drugs (e.g., alcohol, cocaine, speed) during pregnancy? Yes ____ No ____
   If yes, please list. _____
8. Is there any reason you are especially concerned about having a baby with a birth defect or problems with your pregnancy? Yes ____ No ____

FIG. 11. Genetic screening questionnaires.

suit was initiated. Obstetricians cannot be expected to be expert in every rare enzymopathy, but this case illustrates how important it is to seek out additional information about rare conditions through a literature search or by consultation with a genetics center. Fortunately, helpful computerized databases are available on the World Wide Web such as OMIM (Online Mendelian Inheritance in Man) (http://www.ncbi.nlm.nih.gov/omim) and HELIX, a directory of DNA diagnostic laboratories (http://www.helix.com).

The general physical examination may reveal dysmorphic features or a distinctive physical finding that is frequently associated with genetic problems. For instance, a dislocated lens found on funduscopic examination is a distinctive feature consistent with Marfan syndrome or homocystinuria. If the patient has no history of severe ocular trauma, she probably has one of these conditions. Obstetricians cannot be as good at detecting such clues as an expert medical geneticist, because "the eye cannot see what the mind does not know."

Genetic Counseling

Genetic counseling is a communication process that deals with the occurrence or risk of occurrence of a genetic disorder in a family. As our abilities to learn about the fetus have increased, more couples have an indication for prenatal diagnosis or a need to discuss reproductive options. Although every obstetrician has a role in providing genetic counseling, many practitioners find that genetic counselors—persons with advanced degrees who are specially trained in the educational, psychologic, and administrative aspects of medical genetics—are helpful consultants. Genetic counselors are experienced in obtaining and interpreting a thorough family history; often counselors are involved in the establishment or confirmation of a diagnosis. When presented with a prenatal diagnosis, they can obtain and interpret the history of a current pregnancy, explaining fetal risks and discussing the options available. Genetic counselors can provide the detailed counseling that is necessary regarding fetal chromosomal abnormalities of consanguinity, recurrence risks of multifactorial disorders, fetal abnormalities identified by ultrasound, or infertility and habitual abortion. They are extensively trained about genetic screening for diseases that are common in various ethnic groups. Genetic counselors play a central role in the discussions regarding the option of aborting a genetically abnormal fetus. This type of counseling is traditionally informational and nondirective.

Pregnancy Termination

Pregnancy terminations for genetic reasons can be particularly heart-wrenching for a couple because the pregnancy usually is a desired pregnancy. Patients should be encouraged to involve their physician, genetic counselor, clergy, other support persons, and family in these difficult decisions.

It is the physician's responsibility to explain the fetal diagnosis and prognosis. If a woman decides to terminate a pregnancy, the physician should explain the termination procedure, options if there are any, and the relative risks of the different procedures. The cost of the procedure is discussed and whether the procedure is covered by public funding or insurance. The physician should explain the benefits of diagnostic examination of the fetus by DNA, metabolic, or chromosomal analysis or by dysmorphologic examination. The disposition of the fetal remains should be discussed. The possibility that a fetus may live for a short period after induced labor termination is discussed. Whenever possible, patients are encouraged to see or hold the baby, and to name the baby.

Patients are advised that lactation may occur after the delivery, and they are told about the options available to reduce lactation. With late terminations, the option of having a memorial service or in some way commemorating the baby's existence should be discussed. Physicians and counselors help couples decide what information to tell other children and family members, friends, and acquaintances.

It is important to reinforce the fact that the genetic defect is not caused by the patient. The woman who is carrying the pregnancy and undergoes the termination may grieve in different ways from the father of the baby. Referral to local support groups and counselors is often appreciated. In 6 to 8 weeks after the procedure, a follow-up visit should be scheduled to summarize the diagnostic findings, review recurrence risks, and discuss prenatal diagnosis or therapy options for future pregnancies.

Laboratory Screening

Laboratory studies play an important role in the diagnosis of genetic disorders. A genetic illness is sometimes first discovered as an incidental finding on blood studies or an ultrasound examination. For instance, a low mean corpuscular volume on an automated complete blood count suggests thalassemia. In some instances, a positive family history prompts laboratory studies that clarify a patient's risk. Some programs have evolved to screen entire populations for genetic conditions using laboratory assays. Just as we currently perform a history and physical examination or a cholesterol screen to identify disease risk, soon there will be a DNA screen to detect mutations in dozens of important genes involved in cancer and cardiovascular and metabolic diseases.

Population screening is appropriate when a defined subset of the population is at risk, and an accurate and inexpensive heterozygote test is available (Table 14). It is optimal if

TABLE 14. *Population screening: frequency and incidence estimates for selected autosomal-recessive disorders in defined ethnic groups*

Disease	Ethnic group	Carrier frequency	Disease incidence in newborns	At-risk couple frequency[a]	Screening test
Sickle cell anemia	Blacks	0.08	1/600	1/150	Presence of sickle cell hemoglobin; confirmatory hemoglobin electrophoresis
Tay-Sachs disease	Ashkenazi Jews	0.032	1/3600	1/900	Decreased serum hexosaminidase-A
β-Thalassemia	Greeks, Italians	0.032	1/3600	1/900	Mean corpuscular volume <80%; confirmatory hemoglobin electrophoresis
α-Thalassemia	Southeast Asians and Chinese	0.04	1/2500	1/625	Mean corpuscular volume <80%; confirmatory hemoglobin electrophoresis
Cystic fibrosis	Northern Europeans	0.04	1/2500	1/625	Reverse dot blot for common mutations
Phenylketonuria	Europeans	0.016	1/16,000	1/4000	Newborn phenylalanine level

[a]Likelihood that both members of a couple are carriers, assuming nonconsanguinity, and that both are of the at-risk ethnic group.

prenatal diagnosis is available as well (e.g., sickle cell anemia, Tay-Sachs disease, thalassemia). The goals of screening programs are early diagnosis to allow better treatment of affected persons and identification of at-risk matings between persons who are heterozygotes or carriers of recessive disease. Neonatal screening programs for phenylketonuria, galactosemia, and hypothyroidism are carried out in most states. Successful carrier screening for Tay-Sachs disease has been achieved in several Jewish populations. The cost-effectiveness of the screening program is often a primary concern in deciding whether or not to proceed with population screening. Equally important issues include the ability to manage minor variants that do not require action, stigmatization of carriers, and responsibility for decisions not to screen.

◊ PRENATAL DIAGNOSIS

Limited but important information about the fetus can be gained using the traditional diagnostic techniques of history, auscultation, and palpation. It is important to consider the onset of fetal movement and the assumption of the vertex position as developmental milestones that the fetus does or does not achieve. Experienced examiners can assess fetal size, size or dates discordance, fetal positioning, and fetal heart rate abnormalities.

Maternal Serum Screening

Screening for fetal genetic conditions can be achieved by testing maternal serum. The first such program involved the use of maternal serum α-fetoprotein (MSAFP) levels to test for NTDs, an etiologically heterogeneous group of conditions characterized by failure of embryonic closure of the neural tube. A cause for a NTD can be identified in only 5% to 20% of cases, and most cases are thought to be polygenic or multifactorial. Between 90% and 95% of all infants with NTDs are born to women with no previous history of a child with a NTD.

There is substantial evidence for genetic predispositions to NTDs, including racial and ethnic variations in incidence, the increased incidence when consanguinity exists, sex bias, and increased monozygotic twin concordance. There is also strong evidence for environmental factors, including maternal folate deficiency, previous spontaneous abortion or stillbirth, and the seasonal incidence. Mendelian disorders associated with NTDs include Meckel syndrome, in which affected individuals have a posterior encephalocele. Chromosomal syndromes such as trisomy 18, trisomy 13, and triploidy and sporadic syndromes such as OEIS complex (i.e., omphalocele, exstrophy, imperforate anus, spinal defect) can result in NTDs. Other well described environmental causes of NTDs include amniotic band disruption sequence, maternal diabetes, maternal use of valproic acid (Depakene), and hyperthermia. Forty-five percent of fetuses with NTDs have anencephaly, 45% have spina bifida, 5% an encephalocele, the remaining 5% iniencephaly or exencephaly.

The incidence of NTDs is high (approximately 1%) in Ireland, Wales, Alexandria (Egypt), and the Punjab. The rate is 1 in 1000 to 2000 in the United States. Across the United States, the incidence is higher in the east than in the west, and highest in the Appalachian region. In addition, if a person has previously had one child with a NTD, the recurrence risk is 2% to 3%. If there have been two affected children, it is 6.4%, and as high as 25% with three affected children. For patients at high risk for a NTD, prenatal diagnosis can be performed by a targeted ultrasound and an amniocentesis for amniotic fluid AFP and acetylcholinesterase (AChE) at approximately 16 weeks' gestation. The peak concentration of AFP in the amniotic fluid occurs between 12 and 14 weeks, the widest margin between abnormal and normal distributions at approximately 16 to 18 weeks. A cut-off of 2.5 multiples of the median again yields a 98% detection rate with a 0.8% false-positive rate. AChE level determinations do not depend on gestational age. The 5% to 10% of NTDs that are closed will have normal amniotic fluid AFP and AChE levels. Other open fetal defects such as omphalocele and gastroschisis can cause a rise in amniotic fluid AFP.

MSAFP screening was introduced for screening women with no known risk factors for NTDs in the 1980s. As with all screening tests, its predictive value depends on the population prevalence and particular cut-off used for setting the limits of normal and abnormal. In the United States, a cut-off of 2.5 multiples of the median is frequently used, meaning that 5% of those tested will have positive results. With this cut-off, more than 95% of anencephalic fetuses, 80% of fetuses with open spina bifida, and approximately 5% of fetuses with closed spina bifida are detected, for an overall detection rate of approximately 64%. MSAFP screening is most accurate between weeks 16 and 18. MSAFP starts to increase at approximately 13 weeks and peaks at 32 weeks. An inaccurate gestational age is the most common reason for an abnormal MSAFP screen.

It is important to correct MSAFP values for maternal weight, race, diabetes, and multiple gestation. There is a negative correlation between maternal weight and MSAFP. Blacks have approximately 1.1 times the MSAFP level of whites, and Asians have an intermediate level between blacks and whites. In insulin-dependent diabetics, the MSAFP level is approximately 60% of nondiabetic controls, and it is inversely correlated with the hemoglobin A_{1C} levels. Between 1% and 2% of infants of diabetic mothers have babies with NTDs. In multiple gestation, the median twin MSAFP level between 16 and 20 weeks is about 2.5 multiples of the median for a singleton pregnancy.

Low MSAFP levels have been associated with Down syndrome. One-fifth to one-third of Down syndrome fetuses exhibit low MSAFP levels, with a median MSAFP of 0.7. Additional assays, such as unconjugated estriol, can provide more information about risk. Estradiol levels are low in cases of trisomy 21, very low in trisomy 18, and normal with spina bifida. Human chorionic gonadotropin (hCG) levels are high in trisomy 21, very low in trisomy 18, and low in anencephaly.

For some couples, MSAFP screening raises anxiety, as the results are available around the time when they feel that miscarriage is not going to occur and after the pregnant woman already feels fetal movement. In the counseling of patients about MSAFP screening, it is important to stress that it is a screening rather than a diagnostic test. The physician should explain the possible reasons for a high or low result, discuss the evaluation that would be recommended in that case, and stress that most babies with an abnormal screening result are normal. Frequently, discussions about AFP screening bring out other issues that the couple are worried about with respect to birth defects. This discussion is also an opportunity to educate the couple about the background incidence of birth defects.

The search is on for new biochemical markers that would improve the sensitivity and specificity of maternal serum screening. Retrospective studies suggest that maternal serum levels of dimeric inhibin A may be highly predictive. When the fetus is affected by Down syndrome, the maternal serum inhibin A concentrations are 2.1 times the median value in controls. Serum concentrations of inhibin A in Down syndrome pregnancies do not rise above normal until the end of the first trimester. The levels were not significantly different in women with fetuses affected by trisomy 18.

Small retrospective studies have also examined the feasibility of *first-trimester* screening for Down syndrome. Earlier screening for Down syndrome would allow more time for intervention in the event of a positive test. For women who choose pregnancy termination, the procedure can be carried out at a time when it is medically, psychologically, and perhaps morally less problematic. On the other hand, earlier tests will find many Down syndrome fetuses that would have spontaneously aborted. The follow-up diagnostic tests carry a greater risk of miscarriage (of normal pregnancies) at these earlier gestational ages. Screening for NTDs is impossible.

Initial studies show that maternal serum free β-hCG and pregnancy-associated plasma protein A are useful markers. The free β-hCG levels are approximately half the median, and pregnancy-associated plasma protein A levels are twice the median control levels in Down syndrome pregnancies. Urinary markers are also being evaluated. Large prospective studies are needed to further assess first-trimester screening. Eventually, sorting fetal cells from maternal blood may prove to be the most sensitive and specific screening test.

Fetal Imaging

For many years, the fetus could only be seen before birth using x-ray films. X-ray examinations have limited prenatal indications because of concerns about fetal radiation exposure and because of the limited information obtainable by radiographs (i.e., inspection of calcified structures). Today, fetal radiography is used mostly for the differential diagnosis of skeletal dysplasias in the third trimester. In the past, attempts to gain information about the fetal soft tissues involved injecting a water-soluble dye into the amniotic fluid

to outline the fetal gastrointestinal tract or a fat-soluble dye to outline the fetal skin. Modern high-resolution ultrasound has revolutionized fetal imaging, giving clinicians a noninvasive way to get information about the internal and external features of the fetus.

Newer imaging methods serve as a useful adjunct to ultrasound examination for the prenatal diagnosis of certain conditions. Computed tomography (CT) uses low doses of radiation and computerized processing to obtain cross-sectional images. Magnetic resonance (MR) imaging is based on detection of moving hydrogen atoms when tissues are subjected to a strong magnetic field. Both methods are expensive, but they are noninvasive and do not exhibit the shadowing phenomena seen with ultrasound. CT and MR imaging are most useful for suspected central nervous system anomalies, particularly if ultrasound imaging is limited by reverberation artifacts caused by the fetal skull. They are also useful for cases of oligohydramnios; decreased amniotic fluid makes ultrasound imaging difficult, but the condition holds the fetus still for CT or MR imaging.

Fetal movement is a major limiting factor with CT and MR imaging, but the newer, ultrafast CT scanners can produce an image within fractions of a second, with slightly lower resolution but an even lower dose of radiation compared with conventional CT. Another advantage of CT is the ability to use contrast agents. For instance, CT amniography can differentiate cystic adenomatoid malformation of the lung and diaphragmatic hernia by demonstrating the location of the fetal stomach and small bowel.

The scan speed of MR imaging scanners is improving and prenatal studies do not necessarily require maternal sedation or fetal paralysis with an intrauterine intramuscular injection of a muscle relaxant, such as curare. MR imaging allows differentiation in tissue densities and is exceptionally useful for differentiating white and gray matter in the central nervous system, fat, and flowing blood. MR imaging computers can construct images in any plane desired. Although there are no known biologic hazards with MR imaging, there are also no clear indications for use of MR imaging in the first trimester. Because the teratogenic risk is unknown, MR imaging use should be limited to the second and third trimesters.

Direct visualization of the fetus is indicated only in certain clinical situations and can be performed using a small-bore, fiberoptic endoscope. The trocar for the most commonly used fetoscope is 2.2 mm in diameter; the scope itself is 1.7 mm in diameter. The narrow field of view and the short focal length give a limited view of a small portion of the fetus. Fetoscopy may reemerge as an important adjunct to amniocentesis and fetal blood sampling as narrower scopes are developed. Scopes small enough to fit through the shaft of a 20-gauge needle have been developed, but it is not yet possible to get enough light inside the uterus to allow visualization with such a narrow scope. Embryoscopy has been used in the first trimester to visualize the embryo or early fetus through the membranes. This is accomplished by passing the endoscope through the cervix and up against the membranes. Neither fetoscopy nor embryoscopy may be possible in many cases because of the placental position or cloudy amniotic fluid.

Fetal Sampling for Prenatal Diagnosis

Amniocentesis

Amniocentesis was introduced to the United States in the 1960s, and it is the most extensively used fetal sampling technique. Genetic amniocentesis is routinely performed at approximately 15 weeks of gestation when the amniotic fluid volume is approximately 200 ml. At this gestational age, ultrasound examination cannot detail all of the fetal anatomy, but it can reliably ascertain dates and rule out multiple gestation. Typically, 30 ml of fluid is removed with a 20- to 22-gauge needle using a transabdominal approach with ultrasound guidance (Fig. 12). Biochemical testing can be performed on the fluid as indicated. Amniotic fluid AFP levels are routinely obtained to screen for open fetal defects, and fetal cells can be grown for karyotype determination or for DNA assays. DNA assays that use the PCR technique to amplify small amounts of DNA allow direct analysis of amniotic fluid. Roughly one-third of amniocenteses must be performed transplacentally. In most operators' experience, this has not been associated with substantially increased risk if care is taken to avoid major fetal vessels. The transplacental approach is associated with a slightly higher incidence of Rh sensitization. With either approach, it is imperative that Rh-negative women who may be carrying an Rh-positive fetus receive Rh_0 (D) immune globulin.

With multiple gestations, it is usually possible to sample each of the gestations present. Indigo carmine dye can be placed in the sac after the amniocentesis is completed to prevent tapping the same sac twice. Biochemical assays of amniotic fluid are somewhat harder to interpret in multiple gestations because many biologic molecules can diffuse from one sac into the other.

Few women describe amniocentesis as terribly painful. Those who do frequently experience a uterine contraction at the time the needle is inserted. It is not unusual to have some cramping or a bruised feeling at the site after the procedure. Vaginal spotting or amniotic fluid leakage occurs in 1% to 2% of cases. After a routine amniocentesis, the fluid usually stops leaking within 2 to 3 days. Even when the amniotic fluid volume becomes markedly decreased, miscarriage is not inevitable because the amniotic fluid can reaccumulate within a week, allowing the pregnancy to progress normally.

As ultrasound equipment has improved, the maternal risk incurred with amniocentesis has decreased. Symptomatic amnionitis occurs in less than 1 of 1000 patients. Serious maternal bowel or vascular injuries are extremely rare. The procedure-related rate of fetal loss after amniocentesis is generally quoted as 0.5% (1 in 200), but many centers are reporting lower rates.

Chorionic Villus Sampling

Chorionic villus sampling (CVS) is a diagnostic technique that was introduced to the United States in the mid-1980s. With this technique, a small sample of the chorionic villi is taken for examination of chromosomal status, biochemical assays, or DNA tests. Assays depending on analysis of amniotic fluid, such as AFP, cannot be performed on a CVS sample.

CVS usually is accomplished by the transcervical or transabdominal route. Occasionally, a transvaginal CVS is performed with the uterus extremely retroflexed. A transcervical CVS is usually performed between 9 and 12 weeks of gestation, at which time a plastic catheter, approximately 1.5 mm in diameter, is passed through the cervix and then directed toward the placental mass under continuous ultrasound guidance (Fig. 13). Between 10 and 20 mg of villi are aspirated through this catheter by negative pressure using a syringe. Transabdominal CVS is performed using an 18- to 20-gauge spinal needle passed into the thickest portion of the placenta that is readily assessible (Fig. 14). Villi are aspirated into a syringe. This procedure can be performed throughout gestation.

Transabdominal CVS is considered easier to learn and safer, but patient acceptance appears to be lower. Theoretically, transcervical CVS has a greater risk of infection, although this has not been borne out by large surveys. In most series, a larger sample is obtained with transcervical CVS, but more passes are required to obtain this sample. Transcervical procedures require more uterine manipulation, and patients have a greater frequency of bleeding or leakage of fluid during and after the procedure. Most laboratories report a greater level of maternal cell contamination with transcervical CVS, although this is rarely a clinically important issue. Those performing CVS should be facile with both techniques because patient anatomy frequently dictates which is the optimal technique. CVS compares favorably with amniocentesis with regard to safety. Two large National Institutes

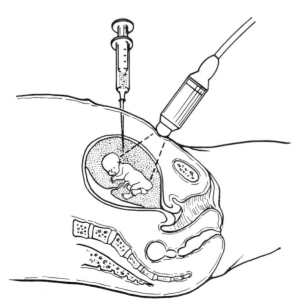

FIG. 12. Amniocentesis.

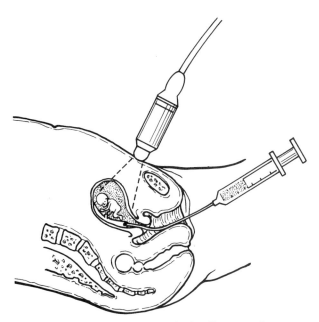

FIG. 13. Transvaginal chorionic villus sampling.

of Health cooperative trials found a procedure-related loss rate of approximately 0.8%.

In approximately 2% of first-trimester chorionic villus samples, a discrepancy is found between the cytogenetic analysis of the placenta and that of the fetus. Frequently, a second invasive procedure, usually amniocentesis or fetal blood sampling, is required to determine whether or not the fetus is affected. This phenomenon is called confined placental mosaicism (CPM). Pregnancies in which CPM is found by CVS may be at risk for spontaneous abortion, peri-

natal loss, or intrauterine growth retardation. The reported rates of loss have ranged from 3.6% to 16.7%. In chromosomally abnormal conceptuses, the presence of a mosaic normal cell line in the placenta may be the factor that allows prolonged survival of aneuploid fetuses. Kalousek et al. (1987) studied 14 placentas from liveborn or terminated pregnancies with trisomy 13 or 18 and found the placentas were all mosaic for or contained only diploid cells.

There have been several reports of increased incidence of limb anomalies when fetuses have undergone very early CVS using the transabdominal approach. These reports are of concern because the affected children have a relatively distinctive pattern of malformation, and it is biologically plausible that their anomalies may be related to CVS. The absolute number of fetuses with this problem is small, but the publicity regarding these findings has caused many women to avoid CVS.

The Centers for Disease Control and Prevention (CDC) performed a multistate case–control study to assess and quantify the risk for specific limb deficiencies associated with CVS. Between 1988 and 1992, 131 infants with nonsyndromic limb deficiency, born to mothers 34 years of age or older, were reported in seven population-based birth defect surveillance programs. Control subjects were 131 infants with other birth defects. They found that exposure to CVS was associated with a sixfold increase in risk for transverse digital deficiency (odds ratio: 6.4; 95% confidence interval, 1.1 to 38.6). The data showed a significant trend toward increased risk with earlier gestational exposure. The CDC estimates that the absolute risk for transverse digital deficiency in infants after CVS is approximately 1 in 3000. Further studies are needed to determine whether the problem is specific to CVS or whether the same risk applies to invasive first-trimester diagnostic manipulations.

Fetal Blood Sampling and Fetal Biopsy

Originally, fetal blood was sampled by inserting a needle into the placenta; the blood obtained was usually a mixture of fetal and maternal blood, which limited its usefulness. In 1977, fetoscopy came into use, allowing a needle to be placed into a cord vessel under direct sonographic visualization. Pure fetal samples could be obtained, but fetoscopy requires special equipment and expertise, and the procedure-related loss rate is between 3% and 7%. With improvement in ultrasound imaging during the mid-1980s, cordocentesis can be performed in a manner similar to amniocentesis (Fig. 15).

A transplacental route usually is preferred, and a spinal needle is advanced under ultrasound guidance into a vessel with cord insertion into the placenta. Cordocentesis is usually not performed until after 17 weeks. Depending on the indication, procedure-related loss rates of as low as 1% have been reported with no observed increase in the rate of preterm delivery. Typically, no maternal sedation or antibiotics are required. In most cases, a fetal sample can be obtained on the first attempt, usually in less than 10 minutes, and any substance

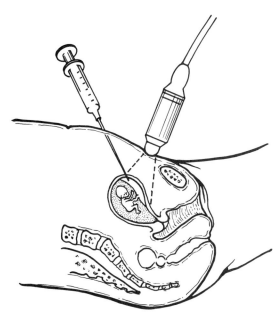

FIG. 14. Transabdominal chorionic villus sampling.

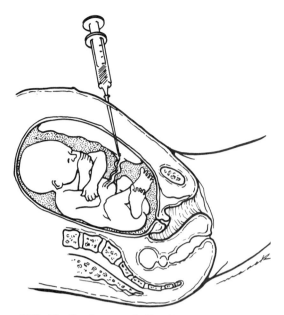

FIG. 15. Cordocentesis (fetal blood sampling).

measurable in adult blood can be assayed in fetal blood. Most cordocenteses are performed to obtain a fetal karyotype because of fetal anomalies or to determine the fetal hematocrit in the setting of isoimmunization or severe fetal anemia. Fetal platelet counts, acid-base status, antibody levels, and blood chemistries can be assayed as indicated. Hematologic values are routinely checked (particularly the mean corpuscular volume) to be certain that the blood obtained is fetal. A Kleihauer test can be performed to check for maternal blood contamination.

A variety of other tissues, particularly fetal skin, liver, and muscle, have been sampled prenatally to diagnose a genetic disorder using either electron microscopy or biochemical analysis. Such biopsies are necessary if a genetic abnormality is only expressed in certain tissues and the causative gene is unknown. Now that the molecular basis of many of these disorders is known, simpler DNA assays using villi, amniocytes, or blood usually obviate the need for tissue biopsy. Initially, fetal biopsies were performed using fetoscopy, but they are now performed under ultrasound guidance. Typically, local anesthesia, maternal sedation (with or without fetal paralysis), and prophylactic antibiotics are used for tissue biopsy procedures. As with any invasive procedure, Rh_0 (D) immune globulin is necessary for the nonsensitized Rh-negative mother who may be carrying an Rh-positive fetus.

Early Amniocentesis

Early amniocentesis is similar to amniocentesis at the "traditional" gestational age, except that the procedure is performed at 10 to 12 weeks' gestation. Early amniocentesis has been proposed as an alternative first-trimester prenatal diagnostic technique, but its safety is unproven. The largest reported experience is from the University of California, Davis, with 936 patients who had amniocentesis performed before 13 weeks' gestation. These amniocenteses were performed by a single operator, and smaller volumes of fluid (10 to 18 ml) were taken. Patients who were very obese or had a severely retroflexed or retroverted uterus were not offered early amniocentesis. In addition, patients who had prominent amnion chorion separation, intervening bowel or bladder, or decreased amniotic fluid volume were not studied. In this series, 0.7% of the fetuses were lost within 2 weeks of the procedure. This number included 4 of the 10 fetuses whose mothers experienced a leakage of fluid. The total loss rate after the procedure through 28 weeks was 2.9%, a figure that is comparable to the CVS experience. Several smaller studies of early amniocentesis have shown a much higher rate of fetal loss.

Despite the smaller volume of amniotic fluid obtained, it has not been a problem to culture cells for karyotype determination. Accurate standards do not exist for testing amniotic fluid AFP levels in early gestation, and it is reasonable to assume that AFP and AChE are less predictive in the early amniocentesis group.

Preimplantation Diagnosis

Various methods of diagnosis before a pregnancy is formally established are becoming available in the 1990s. Someday, these extremely early diagnoses may be necessary to allow initiation of genetic therapy treatments. For many couples, preimplantation diagnosis provides an alternative to selective pregnancy termination, allowing them to avoid the moral issues and the psychologic trauma that accompanies termination of a wanted pregnancy.

For most genetic conditions, carriers have both normal and abnormal gametes, and chance determines whether an abnormal gamete is incorporated into the conceptus. Aided by the rapid progress in assisted reproductive technologies and molecular diagnostics, it has become possible to test gametes *in vitro* and select healthy gametes for fertilization. Sperm sorting has been accomplished using molecular probes tagged with laser-activated dyes and using separation techniques such as flow cytometry, but current approaches usually cause unacceptable damage to the sperm. Greater success has been possible in genotyping oocytes, which are larger and more resistant to damage. Oocyte diagnosis takes advantage of the unique properties of female meiosis; unlike sperm, oocytes conveniently discard their unused genetic material in the form of polar bodies. For a heterozygous woman, the discarded genetic material can be tested to see whether it contains the abnormal allele. If it does, then the oocyte must contain the normal allele. Conversely, if the polar body tests positive for the normal allele, the oocyte must contain the abnormal allele. Only the normal oocytes are then fertilized. Contamination with cumulus cells adherent to the exterior surface of the zona pellucida can lead to errors.

Polar body biopsy can only be performed in conjunction with *in vitro* fertilization. The first polar body has no essential function and contains no embryonic material; they are small and relatively easy to remove using micromanipulation techniques (Fig. 16). Theoretically, DNA testing results can be obtained before fertilization, leaving a long period for confirmatory studies before implantation. Aneuploidy screening can also be incorporated, at least for maternal meiosis I nondisjunction. The main disadvantages are that polar body biopsy is an indirect assay of the oocyte and that it can be used only for maternal carriers. In addition, the farther away from the centromere the gene is located, the more likely recombination is to occur, making polar body biopsy indeterminate. Polar bodies that are heterozygous need to be discarded or the oocytes biopsied again to remove the second polar body.

Initial success has been greater with "selective implantation" protocols, in which the diagnosis is made during the first week after fertilization but before implantation. Preimplantation embryos can be grown *in vitro* and biopsied after the first few cleavage divisions. There is much experience with this technique in animal research, and embryo splitting at this stage has been used extensively for diagnosis in the cattle and sheep industry. The eight-cell preembryo is probably the ideal stage for biopsy. Cells are still independent and totipotent, they have not developed gap junctions that will make them adherent, and damage is tolerated relatively well. By this stage, some of the embryonic genes have begun to function, and it may become possible to perform some biochemical microassays. This technique is limited by the difficulty in removing blastomeres, which are larger than a polar body, and the short time to work with the sample before the chance of successful implantation begins to lessen. It has proved difficult to freeze spare embryos after biopsies, and as with other preimplantation techniques, there is the possibility of sperm or cumulus cell contamination.

Attempts have also been made to perform testing 5 days after fertilization, when the preembryo has reached the blastocyst stage. The blastocyst consists of roughly 120 cells that are mostly trophoblastic tissue, but the inner cell mass that eventually becomes the embryo is clearly visible. Only the best laboratories have had any success culturing human preembryos to this developmental stage *in vitro*. As an alternative, investigators have tried to lavage naturally conceived blastocysts from the uterus during the 2 to 3 days when the conceptus is normally free-floating in the endometrial cavity before implantation. Unfortunately, it has proved exceedingly difficult to obtain multiple blastocysts by lavage after superovulation.

Various methods of sampling blastocyst cells have shown success in animal models, including bisection, aspiration of the cavity, and excision of cells herniating through the zona pellucida. The latter is achieved after mechanical disruption of the zona to cause premature herniation or after spontaneous hatching. The advantages of blastocyst biopsy include the relative differentiation of the cells, greater cell number, better transfer efficiency, and self-selection of the healthiest embryos. Lavage of naturally conceived blastocysts offers a potentially "low-tech" approach to preimplantation diagnosis. Perhaps contrary to expectations, disruption of zona pellucida may enhance hatching. Technical limitations include the small number of blastocysts available and their limited incubation time. The cells are very adherent to each other, increasing the risk of damage to the inner cell mass. As with CVS mosaicism, there is the possibility that the trophectoderm does not reflect the fetal karyotype or biochemical status.

Fetal Cells in Maternal Circulation

The newest fetal sampling technique that shows promise involves separating fetal cells that occur naturally in the maternal circulation. Nucleated erythrocytes, fetal leukocytes, and syncytiotrophoblast cells are found in the maternal circulation during most pregnancies from as early as 6 weeks' gestation. It is possible to use a separation technique, such as flow cytometry, to establish an enriched population of fetal cells and then assay these cells for fetal mutations using a technique such as DNA amplification. Certain cell types have a long life span in the maternal circulation, allowing persistence of cells from prior pregnancies, and confusing results could result. "Vanished" abnormal cotwins can lead to diagnostic errors. Ultimately, this method may provide a noninvasive, reliable screen for aneuploidy that is inexpensive enough to use for low-risk populations.

◇ PRENATAL TREATMENT AND GENE THERAPY

As we begin to understand the molecular mechanisms by which genes cause disease, we will have the opportunity to design and apply preventive, health-maintaining measures. Some genetic conditions can be treated by giving patients the

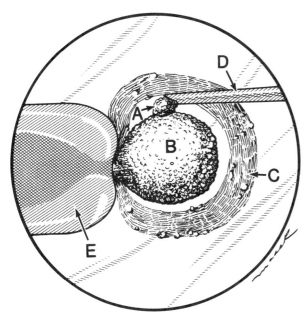

FIG. 16. Polar body biopsy is performed in conjunction with in vitro fertilization. (A, first polar body; B, oocyte nucleus; C, zona pellucida; D, glass biopsy needle; E, glass holding pipet.)

protein they are missing or by stimulating a function that is not performing properly (e.g., growth hormone deficiency, diabetes).

More sophisticated gene therapies are being tested. Finding the cystic fibrosis gene enabled cystic fibrosis to be "cured" in the test tube and improved in animal models. Scientists may be able to design proteins or antisense RNAs that can be used as a drug to block the effect of abnormal genes or kill cancer cells. Modified viruses may be used to insert corrected genetic instructions. Prenatal gene therapy with stem cell transplantation has been attempted for severe combined immunodeficiency with some preliminary success.

Many genetic conditions need to be treated prenatally. Although *in utero* treatment is experimental, prenatal treatment of disorders with vitamin-dependent or -responsive cofactors has been successful. For instance, prenatal diagnosis and treatment of the vitamin B_{12}-responsive form of methylmalonicacidemia by administration of 10 mg per day of vitamin B_{12} has successfully improved the biochemical defect. Similarly, infants with biotin-responsive multiple carboxylase deficiency have been aided by maternal biotin supplementation. In these rare disorders, prenatal treatment can mean the difference between life and death for affected infants. Dietary restriction of galactose in mothers who are at risk of delivering a galactosemic infant, and dietary restriction of phenylalanine in mothers who themselves have phenylketonuria are helpful means of preventing the devastating effects of these metabolic conditions. The era of gene therapy and prenatal tissue transplantation is likely to rapidly expand the therapeutic options for treating and preventing metabolic disease.

◊ GENETICS IN GYNECOLOGIC DISORDERS

Genes play an important role in the pathogenesis of many common gynecologic disorders. Information about two areas that are undergoing intensive study—sexual differentiation and gynecologic cancer—are summarized.

Sexual Differentiation

Molecular genetic investigations of persons with gonadal dysgenesis and pseudohermaphroditism have defined many aspects of sexual differentiation. Because it is the smallest chromosome, the Y chromosome became the first human chromosome to be completely mapped. Cytogenetic studies reveal that 46,XY persons with small deletions of Yp can sometimes have a female appearance and mixed gonadal dysgenesis. Some girls with the "normal" 46,XY karyotype were characterized and found to have molecular deletions on Yp as well. These observations led to the discovery of the *SRY* gene in the deletion region. *SRY* is the gene required for testicular development.

If a testis develops, Leydig cells then make androgens that stabilize development of the wolffian ducts and direct formation of the vasa deferentia, epididymides, and seminal

vesicles. Androgens need to be converted to dihydrotestosterone by 5-α-reductase to allow virilization of the external genitalia. Sertoli cells produce a glycoprotein called antimüllerian hormone (AMH) that causes regression of the müllerian duct. The gene for AMH has been localized to chromosome 19.

In the absence of a Y chromosome, the indifferent gonad develops into an ovary. Girls with the 45,X karyotype develop abnormally shaped streak ovaries, but they have normal formation of oocytes. Accelerated attrition of the oocytes occurs for unknown reasons, causing most women with Turner syndrome to be infertile. Detailed analysis of patients with partial deletions of the X chromosome proves that genes on the long and the short arm of X are involved in ovarian development. Autosomal loci are also important for normal ovarian development.

Gynecologic Cancers

Most cancers are clonal in origin; that is, they arise from a single aberrant cell. Cytogenetic or molecular alterations are uniformly observed in malignant cells. Although some of these changes appear to be random events occurring in rapidly dividing cells, other, specific genetic changes play an etiologic role in development of certain cancers.

Theoretical models assume a multistep process for the production of malignancy. Several mutations are required in the individual cell that first shows the malignant phenotype. Particular mutations may be either germinal (i.e., inherited) or somatic (i.e., acquired). Either can be seen in familial cancer clusters: germinal because of segregation within the family of a cancer-causing mutation and somatic because of shared environmental exposures to carcinogens. Mendelian transmission of cancer predisposition is usually observed as multifocal and early-onset disease. Typically, cancer-predisposing mutations are found to overexpress protooncogenes that normally drive important cell functions or to inactivate tumor suppressor genes that normally exert a protective effect.

Ovarian epithelial cancers are an example of a gynecologic cancer for which genetic predispositions have been assumed for some time. Racial variations in incidence occur; for instance, the incidence of ovarian cancer is lower in Japanese than in other Asian populations. Many family studies have shown that first-degree relatives are at increased risk. There are strong associations of ovarian malignancies with breast, endometrial, and colon cancer in the same patient or within a family. Lynch estimates that at least 5% to 10% of ovarian cancers are attributable to a major gene.

Various cytogenetic and molecular derangements occur in ovarian tumors. Specific translocations of chromosomes 6 and 14 occur. At a molecular level, 10% to 15% of tumors have changes in the *KRAS* oncogene, and others show amplification of the *NEU* oncogene. Some tumors show allelic loss at the retinoblastoma gene, *RB1,* and others have tumor-specific mutations in *p53* gene, a gene involved regularly in the pathogenesis of colon cancer. After we understand the pathophysiology of a disease such as ovarian cancer at the molecular level, it will be easier to devise rational treatments and perhaps a cure. *In vitro* experiments have successfully used antisense RNA to block expression of abnormal genes to reverse the malignant phenotype.

◊ TRENDS

The Human Genome Project promises to provide the most important information in human biology. Technologies developed for the genome project and the genomic sequence itself will provide the basis for much of biomedical research in the next century. The possibilities for understanding normal development, disease predisposition, and cancer are staggering. The ability to obtain an accurate prenatal diagnosis will expand exponentially over the next few decades. Gene therapy is becoming a reality faster than anyone thought possible. The challenge is for the obstetrician-gynecologist to stay abreast of all these developments and to educate patients about developments that can influence their care.

◊ RECOMMENDED READINGS

Aitken DA, Wallace EM, Crossley JA, et al. Dimeric inhibin A as a marker for Down's syndrome in early pregnancy. *N Engl J Med* 1996;334:1231–1236.

Baker V. Oncogenes in gynecologic malignancy. *Curr Opin Obstet Gynecol* 1992;4:75–80.

Bates A, Howard PJ. Distal long arm deletions of the X chromosome and ovarian failure. *J Med Genet* 1990;27:722–723.

Behzadian MA, Tho SP, McDonough PG. The presence of the testicular determining sequence, SRY, in 46,XY females with gonadal dysgenesis (Sawyer syndrome). *Am J Obstet Gynecol* 1991;165:1887–1890.

Buyse ML, ed. *Birth defects encyclopedia.* Cambridge: Blackwell Scientific Publications, 1990.

Callan NA, Blakemore KJ, Kan JS. Counseling in congenital heart defects. *Obstet Gynecol Surv* 1991;46:651–655.

Carr DH, Gedeon M. Population cytogenetics of human abortuses. In: Hook EB, Porter IH, eds. *Population cytogenetics.* New York: Academic Press, 1977:1–9.

Chueh J, Golbus MS. The search for fetal cells in the maternal circulation. *J Perinat Med* 1991;19:411–420.

Elias S, Annas GJ, Simpson JL. Carrier screening for cystic fibrosis: implications for obstetric and gynecologic practice. *Am J Obstet Gynecol* 1991;164:1077–1083.

Gadow EC, Lippold S, Otano L, Serafin E, Scarpati R, Matayoshi T. Chromosome rearrangements among couples with pregnancy losses and their adverse reproductive outcomes. *Am J Med Genet* 1991;41:279–281.

Gilbert F, Marinduque B. DNA prenatal diagnosis. *Curr Opin Obstet Gynecol* 1990;2:226–235.

Forest JC, Masse J, Moutquin JM. Screening for Down syndrome during first trimester: a prospective study using free beta-human chorionic gonadotropin and pregnancy-associated plasma protein. *A Clin Biochem* 1997;30:333–338.

Green ED, Waterston R. The Human Genome Project: prospects and implications for clinical medicine. *JAMA* 1991;266:1966–1975.

Grifo JA, Boyle A, Tang YX, Ward DC. Preimplantation genetic diagnosis: *in situ* hybridization as a tool for analysis. *Arch Pathol Lab Med* 1992;116:393–397.

Haddow JE, Palomaki GE, Knight GJ, et al. Prenatal screening for Down's syndrome with use of maternal serum markers. *N Engl J Med* 1992;327:588–593.

Hall JG. Genomic imprinting and its clinical implications. *N Engl J Med* 1992;326:827–829.

Hallak M, Johnson MP, Pryde PG, Isada NB, Zador IE, Evans MI. Chorionic villus sampling: transabdominal versus transcervical approach in more than 4000 cases. *Obstet Gynecol* 1992;80:349–352.

Hanson FW, Tennant F, Hune S, Brookhyser K. Early amniocentesis: outcome, risks, and technical problems at ≤12.8 weeks. *Am J Obstet Gynecol* 1992;166:1707–1711.

Hardy K, Handyside AH. Biopsy of cleavage stage human embryos and diagnosis of single gene defects by DNA amplification. *Arch Pathol Lab Med* 1992;116:388–392.

Holzgreve W, Miny P. Genetic aspects of fetal disease. *Semin Perinatol* 1989;13:260–277.

Hook EB. Rates of chromosome abnormalities at different maternal ages. *Obstet Gynecol* 1981;58:282–285.

Hook EB, Cross PK, Schreinemachers DM. Chromosomal abnormality rates at amniocentesis and in live-born infants. *JAMA* 1983;249:2034–2038.

Hurley PA, Rodeck CH. Fetal therapy. *Curr Opin Obstet Gynecol* 1992;4:4–9.

Jackson LG, Zachary JM, Fowler SE, et al. A randomized comparison of transcervical and transabdominal chorionic-villus sampling. *N Engl J Med* 1992;327:594–598.

Jones KL. *Smith's recognizable patterns of human malformation*, 4th ed. Philadelphia: WB Saunders, 1988.

Kalousek DK, Dill FJ, Pantzar T, McGillivray BC, Yong SL, Wilson RD. Confined chorionic mosaicism in prenatal diagnosis. *Hum Genet* 1987;77:163–167.

Langer A, Kudart E. Construction of a family pedigree in genetic counseling before amniocentesis. *J Reprod Med* 1990;35:715–718.

Krantz DA, Larsen JW, Buchanan PD, Macri JN. First-trimester Down syndrome screening: free beta-human chorionic gonadotropin and pregnancy-associated plasma protein A. *Am J Obstet Gynecol* 1996;174:612–616.

Mark HF, Jenkins R, Miller WA. Current applications of molecular cytogenetic technologies. *Ann Clin Lab Sci* 1997;27:47–56.

McGowan KD, Blakemore KJ. Amniocentesis and chorionic villus sampling. *Curr Opin Obstet Gynecol* 1991;3:221–229.

McKusick VA. *Medelian inheritance in man*, 9th ed. Baltimore: The Johns Hopkins University Press, 1990.

Nyberg DA, Mahony BS, Pretorius DH. *Diagnostic ultrasound of fetal anomalies: text and atlas.* Chicago: Year Book Medical Publishers, 1990.

Olney RS, Khoury MJ, Alo CJ, et al. Increased risk for transverse digital deficiency after chorionic villus sampling: results of the United States Multistate Case-Control Study, 1988–1992. *Teratology* 1995;51:20–29.

Pachi A, Maggi E, Giancotti A, Torcia F, Giampa G, Forleo S. Ultrasound and genetic counselling in the prenatal diagnosis of fetal malformations. *J Perinat Med* 1991;19:50–61.

Price JO, Elias S, Wachtel SS, et al. Prenatal diagnosis with fetal cells isolated from maternal blood by multiparameter flow cytometry. *Am J Obstet Gynecol* 1991;165:1731–1737.

Romero R, Pilu G, Jeanty P, Ghidini A, Hobbins JC. *Prenatal diagnosis of congenital anomalies.* Norwalk, CT: Appleton & Lange, 1988.

Rossiter BJF, Caskey CT. Molecular studies of human genetic disease. *FASEB J* 1991;5:21–27.

Sanders RC. Prenatal diagnosis of structural abnormalities. *Curr Opin Obstet Gynecol* 1991;3:259–265.

Schrock E, du Manoir S, Veldman T, Schoell B, et al. Multicolor spectral karyotyping of human chromosomes. *Science* 1996;273:494–497.

Scriver CR, Beaudet AL, Sly WS, Valle D. *The metabolic basis of inherited disease*, 7th ed. New York: McGraw-Hill, 1994.

Simpson JL, Golbus MS. *Genetics in obstetrics and gynecology*, 2nd ed. Philadelphia: WB Saunders, 1992.

Simpson JL, Mills J, Rhoads GG, Cunningham GC, Conley MR, Hoffman HJ. Genetic heterogeneity in neural tube defects. *Ann Genet* 1991;34:279–286.

Skinner MA, Iglehart JD. The emerging genetics of cancer. *Surg Gynecol Obstet* 1989;168:371–379.

Viscarello RR, Gollin YG, Hobbins JC. Alternate methods of first-trimester diagnosis. *Obstet Gynecol Clin North Am* 1991;18:875–890.

Wald NJ, Kennard A. Prenatal biochemical screening for Down's syndrome and neural tube defects. *Curr Opin Obstet Gynecol* 1992;4:302–307.

Ward BE, Gersen SL, Carelli MP, et al. Rapid prenatal diagnosis of chromosomal aneuploidies by fluorescence *in situ* hybridization: clinical experience with 4500 specimens. *Am J Hum Genet* 1993;52:854–865.

Watson JD. The Human Genome Project: past, present, and future. *Science* 1990;248:44–49.

CHAPTER 13

Teratology and Drugs in Pregnancy

◇

Jennifer R. Niebyl

◇ PRINCIPLES OF TERATOLOGY

Drugs ingested during pregnancy can affect the fetus. The term *placental barrier* is a contradiction because the placenta allows many drugs and dietary substances to cross. Patients should be educated about methods other than drugs to cope with tension, aches and pains, and viral illnesses during pregnancy. Drugs should be used only when necessary. The risk–benefit ratio should justify the use of any drug, and the minimal effective dose should be employed. Patients should be educated about the risks of recreational drug exposure. Because the long-term effects of drugs *in utero* may not be revealed for many years, caution is warranted for the use of any drug during pregnancy.

Passage of drugs across the placenta is influenced by several factors. Lipid-soluble substances readily cross the placenta, and water-soluble substances pass less well because of their greater molecular weight. The degree to which a drug is bound to plasma protein influences the amount of drug that is free to cross. Virtually all drugs cross the placenta to some degree, with the exception of large organic ions such as heparin and insulin.

Developmental defects may have genetic or environmental causes or interactions of both. Drug exposure can explain only 2% to 3% of birth defects. Approximately 25% of defects are genetic, but the cause is unknown for most defects.

The incidence of major malformations in the general population is usually quoted as 2% to 3%. A major malformation is defined as one that is incompatible with survival, such as anencephaly, or one that requires major surgery for correction, such as cleft palate or congenital heart disease. If all minor malformations are included, such as ear tags or extra digits, the rate may be as high as 7% to 10%. The risk of malformation after exposure to a drug must be compared with this background rate.

There is a marked species specificity in drug teratogenicity. For example, thalidomide was not found to be teratogenic in lower species, but it is a potent human teratogen. In certain strains of mice, corticosteroids produce a high percentage of offspring with cleft lip, although no studies have shown these drugs to be teratogenic in humans. Testing in subhuman primates may give the most predictive information.

The Food and Drug Administration (FDA) lists five categories of labeling for drug use in pregnancy:

Category A. Controlled studies in women fail to demonstrate a risk to the fetus in the first trimester, and the possibility of fetal harm appears remote.

Category B. Animal studies do not indicate a risk to the fetus, and there are no controlled human studies or animal studies to show an adverse effect on the fetus, but well-controlled studies in pregnant women have failed to demonstrate a risk to the fetus.

Category C. Studies have shown the drug to have animal teratogenic or embryocidal effects, but there are no controlled studies in women or no studies are available in animals or women.

Category D. Positive evidence of human fetal risk exists, but benefits in certain situations (e.g., life-threatening situations or serious diseases for which safer drugs cannot be used or are ineffective) may make use of the drug acceptable despite its risks.

Category X. Studies in animals or humans have demonstrated fetal abnormalities, or there is evidence of fetal risk based on human experience, or both, and the risk clearly outweighs any possible benefit.

The classic teratogenic period is from about day 31 after the last menstrual period in a 28-day cycle to 71 days from the last period (Fig. 1). This is the critical period of organogenesis, and teratogens may cause malformations that are usually recognized at birth. The timing of exposure is important. Administration of drugs early in this period affects the organs developing at that time, such as the heart or neural tube. Closer to the end of the classic teratogenic period, the ear and palate are forming and may be affected by a teratogen taken then. If not urgently needed, drug therapy should

197

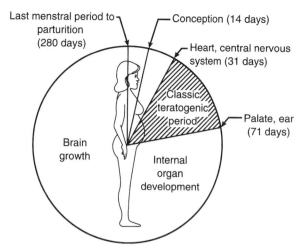

FIG. 1. The gestational clock shows the classic teratogenic period. (Adapted from Niebyl JR. *Drug use in pregnancy, 2nd ed.* Philadelphia: Lea & Febiger, 1988:2.)

be postponed until after this critical period of organ development has been completed.

Before the period of organogenesis, exposure to a teratogen usually causes an all-or-none effect. With exposure around conception, the conceptus does not survive or survives without anomalies. If a few cells do not survive at this time, the rest of the cells are totipotent with respect to later organogenesis.

The sensitive serum pregnancy tests can diagnose pregnancy as early as 1 week after conception. If there is any question about a possible pregnancy, these tests should be employed.

Fetal development continues in the second and third trimesters of pregnancy. Some of the anomalies of the uterus from diethylstilbestrol exposure occurred in the second trimester and were not recognized until after puberty. The brain continues to develop throughout pregnancy and the neonatal period. Fetal alcohol syndrome (FAS) may occur with chronic exposure to alcohol in the later stages of pregnancy. Drugs may affect the fetus in later pregnancy, although the effects may not be recognized until later in life.

Most drug therapy does not require cessation of nursing because the amount excreted into breast milk is small enough to be pharmacologically insignificant.

DRUGS IN PREGNANCY

Vitamin A Derivatives

Isotretinoin

Isotretinoin (Accutane) is a significant human teratogen. This drug is marketed for treatment of cystic acne and has been taken inadvertently by teenagers who were not planning pregnancy. When the drug was first marketed, it contained warnings that it had been shown to be teratogenic in subhuman primates and was contraindicated in pregnancy (i.e., FDA category X). Of 154 exposed human pregnancies, there

have been 21 reported cases of birth defects, 12 spontaneous abortions, 95 elective abortions, and 26 normal infants of women who were taking isotretinoin during early pregnancy. The actual risk of anomalies in patients studied prospectively is estimated to be about 25%, and an additional 25% are later recognized to have mental retardation.[1]

The malformed infants had a characteristic pattern of craniofacial, cardiac, thymic, and central nervous system (CNS) anomalies. They included microtia or anotia, micrognathia, cleft palate, heart defects, thymic defects, retinal or optic nerve anomalies, and CNS malformations, including hydrocephalus.

Unlike vitamin A, isotretinoin is not stored in tissue, and an exposure before pregnancy should not be a risk because the drug would not be detectable in serum 5 days after ingestion. Topical tretinoin (Retin-A) has not been associated with any teratogenic risk.

Etretinate

Etretinate (Tegison) is used in psoriasis and may well have a teratogenic risk similar to that of isotretinoin. Case reports of malformations, especially in the CNS, have appeared, but the absolute risk is unknown. The half-life of several months makes levels cumulative, and the drug carries a warning to avoid pregnancy within 6 months of use.

Vitamin A

There is no evidence that vitamin A itself in normal doses is teratogenic. Large doses ($\geq 25,000$ IU/day) should be discouraged during pregnancy because of the possibility of effects similar to those of isotretinoin and etretinate. Eighteen cases of birth defects have been reported after exposure to 25,000 IU or more of vitamin A during pregnancy. Although one study showed a risk at a level of 10,000 to 15,000 IU per day, this has not been confirmed.[18,23]

Antineoplastic Drugs and Immunosuppressants

Methotrexate, a folic acid antagonist, appears to be a human teratogen, although experience is limited. Three women who received methotrexate in the first trimester of pregnancy had infants with multiple congenital anomalies, including cranial defects and malformed extremities. Eight normal infants were delivered to seven women treated with methotrexate in combination with other agents after the first trimester.

Azathioprine (Imuran) has been used in patients with renal transplants and systemic lupus erythematosus. There was no documented increased incidence of anomalies in women treated in the first trimester. Some infants had leukopenia or were small for gestational age.

Four cases have been reported in which cyclosporin A was used for immunosuppression in renal transplant recipients. Cord blood levels that were 34% and 57% of maternal levels of cyclosporin A were found at delivery. The infants had no adverse effects.

Eight malformed infants have resulted from first-trimester exposure to cyclophosphamide (Cytoxan), but these infants were also exposed to other drugs or radiation. Low birth-weight may be associated with use after the first trimester, but this may also reflect the underlying medical problem.

Chloroquine is safe in doses used for malarial prophy-laxis, and there was no increased incidence of birth defects among 169 infants exposed to 300 mg once weekly. How-ever, after exposure to larger antiinflammatory doses (250 to 500 mg/day), congenital defects were reported, including two cases of cochleovestibular paresis.

Anticonvulsants

Epileptic women taking anticonvulsants during pregnancy have approximately double the general population risk of mal-formations. The general risk is 2% to 3%, and for epileptic women on anticonvulsants, the risk of major malformations is about 5%, especially cleft lip with or without cleft palate and congenital heart disease. Because valproic acid and carba-mazepine carry approximately a 1% risk of neural tube defects and possibly other defects, an alpha-fetoprotein screening is appropriate for these patients.[22] In addition, the offspring of epileptic women have approximately five times the general risk of epilepsy, making their risk 2% to 3%.

For any drug claimed to be a teratogen, it is possible to raise the issue of whether the disease for which the drug was prescribed in some way contributed to the defect. Women with a convulsive disorder have an increased risk of birth defects, even when they take no anticonvulsant drug.

The possible causes of malformations in epileptic women taking anticonvulsants include the disease itself, a genetic predisposition to epilepsy and malformations, genetic dif-ferences in drug metabolism, effects of the medications, and deficiency states such as decreased serum folate induced by drugs. Phenytoin decreases the absorption of folate and low-ers the serum folate, a condition that has been implicated in birth defects. A combination of more than three drugs or a high daily dose increases the chance of malformations.

Approximately 5% to 10% of offspring show the fetal hydantoin syndrome. This consists of microcephaly, growth deficiency, developmental delays, mental retardation, and dysmorphic craniofacial features.

A fetal genetic predisposition to phenytoin-induced birth defects has been documented. Several anticonvulsant med-ications have metabolites usually eliminated by the enzyme epoxide hydrolase. Of 19 fetuses studied by amniocentesis, four had low enzyme activity in amniocytes and were affected fetuses. The 15 fetuses with normal amniotic fluid levels of epoxide hydrolase did not have the characteristics of the fetal hydantoin syndrome.

Carbamazepine is frequently used as primary anticonvul-sant therapy. Jones et al. described a fetal carbamazepine syndrome similar to that observed with other anticonvulsants such as hydantoin. Both drugs are metabolized through sim-ilar pathways, raising the possibility that the epoxide inter-mediate may be the teratogenic agent. Fetal dysmorphic syn-dromes have now been described from exposure to the most commonly used anticonvulsants. If a patient is well con-trolled on one of these drugs, there may be no fetal benefit to switching to another anticonvulsant.

In a follow-up study of long-term effects of antenatal ex-posure to phenobarbital and carbamazepine, anomalies were not related to specific maternal medication exposure. There were no neurologic or behavioral differences between the two groups.

Some women may be taking anticonvulsant drugs without reevaluation of the need for continuation of the drugs. It has been shown that if the patient with idiopathic epilepsy has been seizure-free for 2 years and has a normal electroen-cephalogram (EEG), it may be safe to attempt a trial of with-drawal of the drug before pregnancy. The type of seizure, EEG findings, and age at onset of the seizures predict the like-lihood of recurrence. If the patient has not been taking her drug regularly, a low blood level may demonstrate her lack of compliance. If she has not had seizures, she may not need the drug.

There is insufficient information about the new antiepilep-tic drugs, such as lamotrigine, in pregnancy. Two of 47 infants exposed in the first trimester were malformed in the *Lamo-trigine Registry.*

Most authorities agree that the benefits of anticonvulsant therapy during pregnancy outweigh the risks of discontinua-tion of the drug if the patient is first seen during pregnancy. The blood level of the drug should be monitored to ensure a therapeutic level but minimize dosage. Neonatologists need to be aware that the patient is on anticonvulsants because these drugs can affect vitamin K–dependent clotting factors in the newborn. Some studies suggest that oral vitamin K supple-mentation in the last month of pregnancy may be beneficial.

Anticoagulants

Warfarin (Coumadin) has been associated with chondrodys-plasia punctata, similar to the genetic Conradi-Hunerman syndrome. This syndrome includes nasal hypoplasia and bone stippling evident on x-ray films, and it may include oph-thalmologic abnormalities, including bilateral optic atrophy, and mental retardation. These abnormalities are presumably caused by microhemorrhages during development. Even with use only after the first trimester, the ophthalmologic abnor-malities and mental retardation may occur. Fetal and mater-nal hemorrhage have also been reported in pregnant women on warfarin, although the incidence can be lowered with care-ful control of the prothrombin time.

The alternative drug, heparin, is a large molecule with a strong negative charge and does not cross the placenta. Be-cause it does not have an adverse effect on the fetus when given in pregnancy, this should be the drug of choice for patients requiring anticoagulation. However, some evidence suggests that therapy with 20,000 U/day for longer than 20 weeks may be associated with bone demineralization,[12] and the drug should be used for prolonged periods only when clearly necessary.

The risks of full anticoagulation during pregnancy are not justified in patients with only a history of thrombosis. Conservative measures should be recommended, such as elastic stockings and avoidance of prolonged sitting or standing. In patients with cardiac valve prostheses, full anticoagulation is necessary because low-dose heparin resulted in three valve thromboses, 2 of which were fatal, among 35 mothers so treated.

Low-molecular-weight heparins may have substantial benefits over standard unfractionated heparin.[19] The molecules are still relatively large and do not cross the placenta. The half-life is longer, allowing for once daily administration. They have a much more predictable dose–response relationship obviating the need for monitoring. There is less risk of heparin-induced thrombocytopenia and clinical bleeding at delivery, but studies suggesting less risk of osteoporosis are preliminary. The cost is substantially higher than that of standard heparin.

Lithium

In the *International Register of Lithium Babies,* 217 infants had been exposed at least during the first trimester of pregnancy, and 25 (11.5%) were malformed.[30] Eighteen had cardiovascular anomalies, including six cases of the rare Ebstein anomaly. However, two other reports suggest that there might have been some bias of ascertainment of the registry and that the risk of anomalies is much lower than previously thought. A case–control study of 59 patients with Ebstein anomaly showed no difference in the rate of lithium exposure in pregnancy from a control group of 168 children with neuroblastoma. A prospective study of 148 women exposed to lithium in the first trimester showed no difference in the incidence of major anomalies compared with controls. One fetus in the lithium-exposed group had Ebstein anomaly, and one infant in the control group had a ventricular septal defect. The researchers concluded that lithium is not a major human teratogen, but they recommended that women exposed to lithium be offered ultrasound and fetal echocardiography. The 60 unaffected infants who were followed until 5 years of age had no increased mental or physical abnormalities compared with unexposed siblings.

Because lithium is excreted more rapidly in pregnancy, serum lithium levels should be monitored. The perinatal effects of lithium have included hypotonia, lethargy, and poor feeding. Complications similar to those seen in adults on lithium have occurred in newborns, including goiter and hypothyroidism.

Two cases have been reported of polyhydramnios associated with maternal lithium treatment. Because nephrogenic diabetes insipidus has been reported in adults taking lithium, the presumed mechanism of this polyhydramnios is fetal diabetes insipidus. Polyhydramnios may be a sign of fetal lithium toxicity.

It is usually recommended that drug therapy be changed for pregnant women on lithium to avoid fetal drug exposure. However, discontinuing lithium is associated with a 70% chance of relapse of the affective disorder within 1 year, compared with a relapse rate of 20% for those who are kept on lithium.

Antidepressants

Imipramine (Tofranil) was the original tricyclic antidepressant claimed to be associated with cardiovascular defects, but the number of patients studied remains small. Of 75 newborns exposed in the first trimester, six major defects were observed, three of them cardiovascular.

Amitriptyline (Elavil) has been more widely used, and the majority of the evidence supports its safety. In the Michigan Medicaid study, 467 newborns had been exposed during the first trimester, with no increased risk of birth defects.

Fluoxetine (Prozac) is being used with increasing frequency as an antidepressant. No increased risk of major malformations or language or behavioral development has been found.[13,20] One study suggested increased minor anomalies and perinatal complications but did not control for the severity of psychiatric illness.

Thyroid and Antithyroid Drugs

Propylthiouracil (PTU) and methimazole (Tapazole) cross the placenta and may cause fetal goiter. However, the thyroid hormones T_3 and T_4 cross the placenta poorly, and fetal hypothyroidism produced by antithyroid drugs cannot be corrected satisfactorily by administration of thyroid hormone to the mother. The goal of antithyroid therapy during pregnancy is to keep the mother slightly hyperthyroid and minimize fetal drug exposure. Because methimazole has been associated with scalp defects in the infants and has more side effects, PTU is the drug of choice.

Radioactive iodine administered for thyroid ablation or for diagnostic studies is not concentrated by the fetal thyroid until after 12 weeks of pregnancy. With inadvertent exposure around the time of missed menses, there is no specific risk to the fetal thyroid from ^{131}I or ^{125}I administration.

The need for thyroxine increases in many women with primary hypothyroidism when they are pregnant, as reflected by an increase in serum thyrotropin concentrations. It is prudent to monitor thyroid function throughout pregnancy and to adjust the thyroid dose to maintain a normal thyrotropin level.

Tranquilizers

Conflicting reports have appeared about the possible teratogenicity of the various tranquilizers, including meprobamate (Miltown) and chlordiazepoxide (Librium), but in prospective studies, no teratogenicity has been found. A fetal benzodiazepine syndrome has been reported in seven infants of 36 mothers who regularly took benzodiazepines during pregnancy. There was growth retardation, dysmorphism, and CNS dysfunction in these infants. However, the abnormalities occurred with concomitant alcohol and substance abuse and may not be caused by the benzodiazepine exposure. In most clinical situations, the risk–benefit ratio does not justify the use of benzodiazepines in pregnancy. Perinatal use of diazepam has been associated with hypotonia, hypothermia, and respiratory depression.

Antiemetics

Whenever a drug is used in the first trimester, there is a risk that it will be blamed medically and legally if a malformation occurs. Nausea and vomiting in pregnancy should first be treated with nonpharmacologic remedies, such as eating crackers at the bedside on first awakening in the morning, omitting iron tablets, having frequent small meals, and eating protein snacks at night. However, approximately 10% of pregnant women have enough nausea that they request pharmacologic measures (Fig. 2).

Bendectin contained 10 mg of doxylamine and 10 mg pyridoxine (vitamin B_6). The incidence of congenital malformations in the general population is 2% to 3%, and it is not surprising that sporadic cases were reported of infants with malformations who were exposed to Bendectin in early pregnancy. In some retrospective studies, teratogenicity was claimed, but this was not confirmed in several large, prospective, controlled trials containing a total of more than 6000 exposed infants and more than 6000 controls.

Vitamin B_6 has been reported in two randomized, placebo-controlled trials to be effective therapy for nausea and vomiting in early pregnancy.[25] Doxylamine is available over the counter as Unisom (25 mg), and a combination similar to Bendectin can be made. Vitamin B_6 (50 mg, one-half tablet) and doxylamine (25 mg) at bedtime, one-half of each in the morning, and one-half of each in the afternoon is an effective combination.

Ginger is successful for treating hyperemesis. Hyperemesis was defined as vomiting during pregnancy that was severe enough to require hospital admission. A significantly greater relief of symptoms was found after ginger treatment than with placebo. The patients took 250-mg capsules containing ginger as powdered root four times a day. Although there are no teratogenic effects known for other antiemetics, much less information is available about them.

In a small, randomized, placebo-controlled study, meclizine (Bonine, Antivert) produced significantly better results than placebo. Prospective clinical studies have provided no evidence that meclizine is teratogenic in man. In 1014 patients in the Collaborative Perinatal Project and an additional 613 patients from the Kaiser Health Plan, no teratogenic risk was found.

No teratogenicity has been demonstrated for fetuses exposed to dimenhydrinate (Dramamine), but a 29% failure rate and a significant incidence of side effects, especially drowsiness, have been reported for the mothers.

The infants of the 595 patients treated with diphenhydramine (Benadryl) in the Collaborative Perinatal Project showed no signs of teratogenicity.

Trimethobenzamide is an antinauseant that is not classified as an antihistamine or a phenothiazine. The data that have been collected for a small number of patients are conflicting. In the Kaiser Health Plan Study, 193 patients were exposed to trimethobenzamide, and there was a suggestion of excess

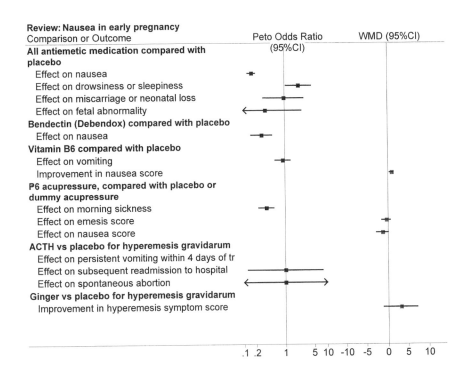

FIG. 2. Nausea in early pregnancy—comparison or outcomes.

of congenital anomalies ($p < 0.05$), but no concentration of specific anomalies was observed in these children, and some of the mothers took other drugs as well. For 340 patients in the Collaborative Perinatal Project, no evidence was found for an association between this drug and malformations.

Chlorpromazine is effective in treating hyperemesis gravidarum, and the most important side effect is drowsiness. Teratogenicity does not appear to be a problem with the phenothiazines as a group. In the Kaiser Health Plan Study, 976 patients were treated, and in the Collaborative Perinatal Project, a total of 1309 patients were treated, with no evidence of association between these drugs and malformations. In one study, chlorpromazine (Thorazine) seemed to be associated with an increased risk of malformations ($p < 0.01$) in the offspring of 133 exposed mothers. For 55 mothers exposed to promethazine (Phenergan) and 48 mothers exposed to prochlorperazine (Compazine), no increased risk of malformations of their offspring was found.

Antihistamines and Decongestants

No increased risk of anomalies has been associated with most of the commonly used antihistamines, such as chlorpheniramine. However, in the Collaborative Perinatal Project, the risk of malformations increased after exposure to brompheniramine (10 infants), an effect that was not found for other antihistamines. Terfenadine (Seldane) did not increase the risk for defects in 105 exposed pregnancies.[24]

Patients should be educated that these drugs represent symptomatic therapy for the common cold and have no influence on the course of the disease. Other remedies should be recommended, such as use of a humidifier, rest, and fluids. If medications are necessary, combinations with two drugs should not be used if only one drug is necessary. If the situation is truly an allergy, an antihistamine alone suffices. If decongestion is necessary, topical nasal sprays result in a lower dose to the fetus than systemic medication. Although there is no known teratogenic effect of these drugs, use of over-the-counter drugs for trivial indications should be discouraged because the long-term effects, especially of chronic use, are unknown.

Analgesics

Patients should be encouraged to use nonpharmacologic remedies for aches and pains during pregnancy, such as local heat and rest.

Aspirin

There is no evidence of any teratogenic effect of aspirin taken in the first trimester in human beings. However, aspirin does have significant perinatal effects because it inhibits prostaglandin synthesis. Uterine contractility is decreased, and patients taking aspirin in analgesic doses have delayed onset of labor, longer duration of labor, and an increased risk of prolonged pregnancy.

Aspirin causes decreased platelet aggregation, which contributes to increased risk of antepartum bleeding and bleeding at delivery. Platelet dysfunction has been described in newborns 5 days after ingestion of aspirin by the mother. Aspirin causes permanent inhibition of prostaglandin synthetase in platelets, and the only way for adequate clotting to occur is for more platelets to be produced in the bone marrow.

Multiple organs may be affected by chronic aspirin use. Prostaglandins mediate neonatal closure of the ductus arteriosus, and one case has been reported in which taking aspirin close to the time of delivery was related to closure of the ductus arteriosus *in utero*.

Other NSAIDs

No evidence of teratogenicity has been reported for other nonsteroidal anti-inflammatory drugs, e.g., ibuprofen, (Motrin, Advil), naproxen (Naprosyn), and short courses up to 48 hours would be apropriate if indicated for pain such as toothache or fractures. Chronic use may lead to oligohydramnios and constriction of the fetal ductus arteriosus.

Acetaminophen

Acetaminophen (Tylenol, Datril) has shown no evidence of teratogenicity. With acetaminophen, inhibition of prostaglandin synthesis is reversible, and after the drug has cleared, platelet aggregation returns to normal. The bleeding time is not prolonged in pregnant patients taking acetaminophen, unlike aspirin, and the drug is not toxic to the newborn. If a mild analgesic or antipyretic is indicated, acetaminophen is preferred to aspirin. The absorption and disposition of acetaminophen in normal doses are not altered by pregnancy.

Propoxyphene

Propoxyphene (Darvon) is an acceptable alternate mild analgesic with no known teratogenicity. However, it should not be used for trivial indications because it has potential for narcotic addiction. Evidence of risk in late pregnancy comes from case reports of infants of mothers who were addicted to propoxyphene and had typical narcotic withdrawal in the neonatal period.

Codeine

In the Collaborative Perinatal Project, no increased relative risk for malformations was observed among 563 codeine users. Codeine can cause addiction and newborn withdrawal symptoms if used to excess in the perinatal period.

Antibiotics and Antiinfective Agents

Because pregnant patients are particularly susceptible to vaginal yeast infections, antibiotics should be used only when clearly indicated. Therapy with antifungal agents may be necessary after the course of antibiotic therapy.

Penicillins

Penicillin derivatives, including amoxicillin and ampicillin, are apparently safe in pregnancy, as are erythromycin and the cephalosporins.

Sulfonamides

Sulfonamides have not been associated with any particular risk except when given to premature infants, in whom the drugs compete with bilirubin for albumin binding sites and contribute to an increased risk of hyperbilirubinemia in newborns. They are not the first choice in the third trimester, especially if the mother is at risk for preterm labor.

Trimethoprim

Trimethoprim is often given with sulfa in treatment of urinary tract infections. Two trials including 131 women failed to show any increased risk of birth defects after first-trimester exposure. However, in 2296 Michigan Medicaid recipients, first-trimester trimethoprim exposure was associated with a slightly increased risk of birth defects, particularly cardiovascular, and in a retrospective study the odds ratio was 2.3.[11]

Sulfasalazine

Sulfasalazine is used for treating ulcerative colitis and Crohn disease because of its relatively poor oral absorption. However, it does cross the placenta to the fetal circulation, with fetal concentrations approximately the same as maternal concentrations, although both are low. Neither kernicterus nor severe neonatal jaundice has been reported after maternal use of sulfasalazine, even when the drug was given up to the time of delivery.

Tetracyclines

In 341 infants exposed to tetracycline in the first trimester, no teratogenic effect was observed. However, the tetracyclines bind to developing enamel, discoloring the teeth. The drug affects deciduous teeth between approximately 26 weeks of pregnancy and 6 months of age in the infant, but it only affects the permanent teeth if given in childhood from approximately 6 months to 5 years of age. There is no teratogenic risk of first trimester exposure to doxycycline. Because the tetracyclines deposit in developing osseous sites and inhibit bone growth, alternative drugs are recommended in pregnancy.

Nitrofurantoin

No risk of birth defects has been correlated with exposure to nitrofurantoin (Macrodantin). It can induce hemolytic anemia in glucose-6-phosphate dehydrogenase–deficient patients, and because the newborn's red blood cells are deficient in reduced glutathione, the label carries a warning against use of the drug at term. However, hemolytic anemia in the newborn after exposure before birth has not been reported.

Aminoglycosides and Other Antituberculosis Drugs

Among 135 infants exposed to streptomycin during the first trimester, no teratogenic effects were observed. Transplacental passage has been demonstrated, and a rate of ototoxicity of 3% to 11% among children of mothers who received prolonged streptomycin or kanamycin treatment for tuberculosis during pregnancy has been reported. If these drugs are required for serious infections, their use should be restricted to a short course, and maternal serum levels should be monitored to minimize fetal exposure.

There is no evidence of any teratogenic effect of isoniazid, paraminosalicylate, rifampin, or ethambutol.

Quinolones

The quinolones (e.g., ciprofloxacin, norfloxacin) have a high affinity for bone tissue and cartilage and may cause arthropathies in children. However, no malformations or musculoskeletal problems were noted in 38 infants exposed *in utero* in the first trimester.[5] The manufacturer recommends against use in pregnancy and in children.

Metronidazole

Studies have failed to show any increase in the incidence of congenital defects among the newborns of mothers treated with metronidazole during early or late gestation. A recent metaanalysis confirmed no teratogenic risk.[6]

Metronidazole remains the most effective drug for trichomoniasis. Because of the past controversy surrounding this drug, deferring therapy until after the first trimester is probably wise. Treatment of bacterial vaginosis with metronidazole and erythromycin has resulted in reduced rates of premature delivery.

Acyclovir

Acyclovir (Zovirax) has resulted in no fetal abnormalities in 601 exposures reported.[3] The Center for Disease Control and Prevention recommends that pregnant women with disseminated infection, e.g., herpes, hepatitis, or varicella pneumonia, be treated with acyclovir.

Lindane

Toxicity in humans after the topical use of a 1% solution of lindane (Kwell) has been observed almost exclusively after misuse and overexposure to the agent. However, after application of lindane to the skin, about 10% of the dose used can be recovered in the urine. Although there is no evidence of specific reproductive damage attributable to lindane, the manufacturer recommends that its use during pregnancy be limited to two doses. Pregnant women should be cautioned about shampooing their children's hair, because absorption could occur across the skin of the mother's hands. Alternate treatments for lice during pregnancy are usually recommended, specifically pyrethrins with piperonyl butoxide (Rid), permethrin 1% (Nix), and, for scabies, permethrin 5% (Eliminate).

Antiasthmatics

Epinephrine

Minor malformations have been reported after first-trimester exposures to sympathomimetic amines, usually in commercial preparations used to treat upper respiratory infections. The rate of malformations in the infants of mothers who received epinephrine in the first trimester was not increased.

Terbutaline

Terbutaline (Brethine) is more rapid in onset and has a longer duration of action than epinephrine and is often preferred for treating asthma in the pregnant patient. No risk of birth defects has been reported. Long-term use has been associated with an increased risk of glucose intolerance.

Cromolyn Sodium

Cromolyn sodium may be administered in pregnancy, and the systemic absorption is minimal. Teratogenicity has not been reported in humans.

Isoproterenol and Albuterol

When isoproterenol (Isuprel) and albuterol (Ventolin) are given as topical aerosols in the treatment of asthma, the total dose absorbed is usually not significant. However, with oral or intravenous doses, their cardiovascular effects may cause decreased uterine blood flow. No teratogenicity has been reported.

Corticosteroids

Inhaled corticosteroids are effective therapy, and very little drug is absorbed. When prednisone or prednisolone is maternally administered it is inactivated by the placenta, and the concentration of active compound in the fetus is less than 10% of that in the mother. These are, therefore, the drugs of choice for treating medical diseases such as asthma. When corticosteroid effect is desired in the infant, such as for lung maturity, betamethasone and dexamethasone are preferred because they are minimally inactivated by the placenta.

There is no evidence that corticosteroids are teratogenic in humans. For a group of 145 infants exposed to corticosteroids in the first trimester, the rate of abnormalities was not increased.

Cardiovascular Drugs

Digoxin

No teratogenic effects of digoxin have been reported. Blood levels should be monitored in pregnancy to ensure adequate therapeutic levels. Digoxin-like immunoreactive substances may be mistaken in assays for fetal concentrations of digoxin. In one study of fetuses with cardiac anomalies, there was no difference in the immunoreactive digoxin levels whether or not the mother had received digoxin. In hydropic fetuses, digoxin may not easily cross the placenta.

Antihypertensive Drugs

α-Methyldopa (Aldomet) has been widely used for treating chronic hypertension in pregnancy. Although postural hypotension may occur, no unusual fetal effects have been observed. Hydralazine (Apresoline) may be used in pregnancy but is usually reserved for treatment of severe preeclampsia. These antihypertensive drugs have shown no teratogenic effects.

Angiotensin-Converting Enzyme Inhibitors

Angiotensin-converting enzyme inhibitors such as enalapril (Vasotec) and captopril (Capoten) can cause fetal renal tubular dysplasia in the second and third trimesters, leading to oligohydramnios, fetal limb contractures, craniofacial deformities, and hypoplastic lung development.[14] Fetal skull ossification defects have also been described. Pregnant women on these medications should be switched to other agents.[9]

Sympathetic Blocking Agents

Propranolol (Inderal) is a β-adrenergic blocking agent in widespread use for a variety of indications. No evidence of teratogenicity has been found. Bradycardia has been reported in the newborn as direct effect of a dose of the drug given to the mother within 2 hours of delivery of the infant.

Several studies of propranolol use in pregnancy appear to show an increased risk of intrauterine growth retardation or at least a skewing of the birth-weight distribution toward the lower range. Ultrasound monitoring of patients on this drug is prudent. Studies from Scotland suggest improved outcome with the use of atenolol to treat chronic hypertension during pregnancy (see Chapter 22).

Drugs for Ovulation Induction

In more than 2000 exposures, no evidence of teratogenic risk for clomiphene has been found, and the percentage of spontaneous abortions is close to the expected rate. Infants are often exposed to bromocriptine in early pregnancy. No teratogenic effects have been observed in over 1400 exposed pregnancies.

Estrogens and Progestins

Oral contraceptives and other hormones given in the first trimester of pregnancy have been blamed for a variety of birth defects, but studies have not confirmed a teratogenic risk for these drugs.

A study of 2754 infants born to mothers after bleeding in the first trimester suggested no increased risk of first-trimester exposure to progestins. In the study group, 1608 newborns had been exposed to progestogens (i.e., medroxyprogesterone acetate, 17α-hydroxyprogesterone caproate), and 1146 infants were delivered from untreated mothers. There was no difference in the rate of anomalies in any anatomic system in the two groups. In the Collaborative Perinatal Project, there was no evidence for teratogenicity of 17α-hydroxyprogesterone caproate (Delalutin) in 162 infants or in 253 exposed to progesterone. It appears that there is little or no risk to using oral contraceptives or progestins in the first trimester. Because of the medicolegal climate and the conflicting literature, it is wise to do a sensitive pregnancy test before prescribing these medications for a patient with amenorrhea.

Androgens

Androgens may masculinize a developing female fetus. Progestational agents, most often the synthetic testosterone derivatives, may cause clitoromegaly and labial fusion if given before 13 weeks of pregnancy. Danazol has been reported to cause mild clitoral enlargement and labial fusion when given inadvertently at a dosage of 800 mg/day for the first 10 to 12 weeks after conception.

Spermicides

An increased risk of abnormal offspring in mothers who used spermicides for contraception has not been confirmed. The consensus of the scientific community is that vaginal spermicides are not associated with increased malformations when women use them immediately before or during pregnancy.

◊ SOCIAL DRUG EXPOSURE

Smoking

Smoking is associated with decreased birthweight and increased prematurity. Abortions associated with maternal smoking tend to have a higher percentage of normal karyotypes and occur later than those with chromosomal aberrations. There is an increased risk of abruptio placentae, placenta previa, and premature and prolonged rupture of membranes. Risks of complications and of the associated perinatal loss increase with the number of cigarettes smoked. Discontinuation of smoking or reduction in the number of cigarettes smoked during pregnancy can reduce the risk of complications and of perinatal mortality, especially in women at high risk for other reasons. There is a positive association between smoking and sudden infant death syndrome. In this case, it is not possible to differentiate between the effects of maternal smoking during pregnancy and smoking after pregnancy, but both may play a role in increasing the risk.

Alcohol

Fetal alcohol syndrome has been reported in offspring of chronically alcoholic mothers and includes the features of gross physical retardation that begins prenatally and continues after birth. The Fetal Alcohol Study Group of the Research Society on Alcoholism has proposed strict criteria for the diagnosis. These criteria state that at least one characteristic from each of the following three categories must be present for a valid diagnosis of the syndrome:

1. Growth retardation before or after birth.
2. Facial anomalies, including small palpebral fissures, indistinct or absent philtrum, epicanthic folds, flattened nasal bridge, short length of nose, thin upper lip, low-set, unparallel ears, and retarded midfacial development.
3. Central nervous system dysfunction, including microcephaly, various degrees of mental retardation or other evidence of abnormal neurobehavioral development, such as attention deficit disorder with hyperactivity.

None of these features is individually pathognomonic for fetal alcohol exposure. The individual anomalies are nonspecific and may be seen even in the absence of maternal drinking. Confirmatory evidence for this diagnosis is a history of heavy maternal drinking during pregnancy.

In one study, 23 chronically alcoholic women were matched with 46 controls, and the pregnancy outcomes of the two groups were compared. Among the alcoholic mothers, perinatal deaths were about eight times more frequent. Growth retardation, microcephaly, and IQ scores below 80 were considerably more frequent findings for the offspring of alcoholic mothers than among the controls. The overall outcome was abnormal for 43% of the offspring of the alcoholic mothers and for 2% of the controls.

Another study addressed the risks of smaller amounts of alcohol: 9% of infants of abstinent or rare drinkers were categorized as having some abnormality, and 14% of infants of moderate drinkers were abnormal, which was not statistically significantly different. In heavy drinkers (i.e., average daily intake of 3 oz or more of 100 proof liquor), 32% of the infants had anomalies. Overall, including anomalies, growth retardation, and abnormal neurologic examination, 71% of the children of heavy drinkers were abnormal, which was twice the frequency of abnormality found in the moderate and rarely drinking groups. It appeared that an increased frequency of abnormality was not found until 45 ml of ethanol (equivalent to three drinks) daily was exceeded. Total malformation rates are not significantly higher among offspring of women who had an average of less than one drink daily or one to two drinks daily than among nondrinkers. Genitourinary malformations increased with increasing alcohol consumption, and the possibility remains that no safe drinking level exists for some malformations.

Heavy drinking remains a major risk to the fetus, and reduction even in midpregnancy can benefit the infant. An occasional drink during pregnancy carries no known risk, but no level of drinking is known to be safe.

Caffeine

There is no evidence of any teratogenic effect of caffeine in humans. The Collaborative Perinatal Project found no increased incidence of congenital defects in 5773 women taking caffeine in pregnancy, usually in combined analgesic medications. Early uncontrolled trials suggested that heavy ingestion of caffeine was associated with increased pregnancy complications such as low-birth-weight infants, spontaneous abortions, prematurity, and stillbirths. However, these studies were not controlled for use of tobacco and alcohol. In a subsequent study that was controlled for smoking, other habits, demographic characteristics, and medical history, no relation was found between low birthweight or short gestation and heavy coffee consumption. One study suggested an increase in term low birthweight infants (<2500 g at >36 weeks of gestation), with more than a 300-mg daily caffeine intake. Concomitant consumption of caffeine with cigarette smoking may increase the risk of low birthweight. Maternal coffee intake decreases iron absorption and may increase the chance of anemia.

Aspartame

Aspartame (NutraSweet) is metabolized into three products: aspartic acid, methanol, and phenylalanine. Aspartic acid does not readily cross the placenta. The amount of methanol from an aspartame-sweetened beverage is generally less than the content recorded for fruit juices and other natural food sources.

Phenylalanine is concentrated on the fetal side of the placenta. Sustained high blood levels of phenylalanine in the fetus associated with maternal phenylketonuria (PKU) are associated with mental retardation in the infant. However, when women ingest aspartame in pregnancy, even at high levels, the phenylalanine levels achieved in the blood are far below the neurotoxic levels achieved in mothers with PKU. This has also been studied in women known to be carriers of PKU, and the levels are still far below those associated with mental retardation. It seems unlikely that the use of aspartame in pregnancy causes fetal problems.

Narcotics

Menstrual abnormalities, especially amenorrhea, are common in heroin users, although they are not associated with the use of methadone. The goal of methadone maintenance is to bring the patient to a level of approximately 20 to 40 mg daily. The dose should be individualized at a level sufficient to minimize the use of supplemental illicit drugs because they represent a greater risk to the fetus than the higher doses of methadone required by some patients. Manipulation of the dose in women maintained on methadone should be avoided in the last trimester because of an association with increased fetal complications and fetal deaths *in utero,* attributed to fetal withdrawal *in utero.* Because management of narcotic addiction during pregnancy requires a host of social, nutritional, educational, and psychiatric interventions, these patients are best managed in specialized programs. The infant of the narcotic addict is at increased risk of abortion, prematurity, and intrauterine growth retardation. Withdrawal should be watched for carefully in the neonatal period.

Marijuana

No teratogenic effect of marijuana use during pregnancy has been documented. In a prospective study of marijuana use in 35 pregnancies, infants born to users (57%) exhibited significantly more meconium staining than those of nonusers (25%). However, users tended to come from lower socioeconomic backgrounds than nonusers. Most adverse outcomes of pregnancy were too infrequent to allow reliable comparisons between the groups.

In the 19th century, hashish was reported to stimulate uterine activity, and it has been used to hasten delivery. In one study, 29% of the marijuana users had an increased incidence of precipitous labor (<3 hours total), compared with 3% of controls.

In another population in which the users and nonusers of marijuana (19 patients in each group) were similar in general health, ethnic background, nutritional habits, and use of tobacco, these differences were not confirmed. In this same group of patients, an average use of marijuana six or more times per week during pregnancy was associated with a reduction of 0.8 weeks in the length of gestation, although no reduction in mean birthweight was observed. One study suggested a mean 79 g decrease in birthweight with marijuana use when urine assays were performed rather than relying on self-reporting.

Cocaine

Cocaine is a CNS stimulant and has local anesthetic and marked vasoconstrictive effects. Studies of cocaine use have consistently documented placental abruption. Less clear evidence links cocaine with spontaneous abortion, prematurity, small-for-gestational-age infants, microcephaly, and pregnancy-induced hypertension because these risks are confounded by reporting bias and socioeconomic variables.[16]

Several studies have suggested an increased risk of congenital anomalies after first-trimester cocaine use. In one study, the malformation rate was 10% among the offspring of cocaine users, 4.5% for those of polydrug users, and 2% for those of controls. The risk appears particularly significant for urinary tract defects, and dysmorphic features and neurobehavioral abnormalities are also seen.

In addition to causing congenital anomalies in the first trimester, cocaine can cause fetal disruption, presumably as a result of vascular insufficiency. Bowel infarction has occurred with unusual ileal atresia and bowel perforation. Limb infarction has resulted in missing fingers in a distribution different from the usual congenital limb anomalies.

Central nervous system bleeding *in utero* may result in porencephalic cysts.

◊ DRUGS IN BREAST MILK

Many drugs can be detected in breast milk at low levels, which are not usually of clinical significance to the infant. The rate of transfer into milk depends on the lipid solubility, molecular weight, degree of protein binding, degree of ionization of the drug, and the presence or absence of active secretion. Nonionized molecules of small molecular weight such as ethanol cross easily. If the mother has unusually high blood concentrations, as with increased dosage or decreased renal function, drugs may appear in higher concentrations in the milk. Nursing mothers should take the minimal effective dose of any drug necessary for therapy.

The amount of drug in breast milk is a variable fraction of the maternal blood level, which is proportional to the maternal oral dose. The dose to the infant is usually subtherapeutic, approximately 1% to 2% of the maternal dose on average. This amount is usually so trivial that no adverse effects occur. In the case of toxic drugs, however, any exposure may be inappropriate. Long-term effects of even small doses of drugs may yet be discovered. Drugs are eliminated more slowly in the infant with immature enzyme systems. The benefits of breast-feeding are well known, and the risk of drug exposure must be weighed against these benefits.

During the first few days after delivery and before lactation is fully established, the infant receives only a small volume of colostrum, and little drug is excreted with milk at this time. The physician should allay fears of patients undergoing cesarean sections by explaining that analgesics or other drugs administered at the time of surgery have no known adverse effects on the infant. For drugs requiring daily dosing during lactation, knowledge of pharmacokinetics in breast milk may minimize the dose to the infant. For example, nighttime dosing after nursing decreases the exposure if the infant is nursing less frequently overnight. In general, medications should be taken after breast-feeding.

Drugs Contraindicated During Breast-Feeding

The American Academy of Pediatrics has reviewed drugs taken during lactation and categorized the drugs as listed in the next few sections.[2] Drugs of abuse such as amphetamines, cocaine, heroin, marijuana, phencyclidine, and nicotine are all contraindicated during breast-feeding.

Cytotoxic Agents

Cytotoxic agents used for cancer chemotherapy may cause immunosuppression in the infant, although data are limited for these drugs. The potential risks of these drugs probably outweigh the benefits of continuing nursing.

After oral administration to a lactating patient with choriocarcinoma, methotrexate was found in milk in low but detectable levels. Most mothers would elect to avoid any exposure to the infant of this drug, but in environments in which bottle feeding is rarely practiced and presents practical and cultural difficulties, therapy with this drug would not in itself appear to constitute a contraindication to breast-feeding.

Bromocriptine

Bromocriptine is an ergot alkaloid derivative. Because it has an inhibitory effect on lactation, it should be avoided. However, in one report, a mother taking 5 mg/day for a pituitary tumor was able to nurse her infant.

Ergotamine

Ergotamine in the doses used in migraine medications has been associated with vomiting, diarrhea, and convulsions in the infant and should be avoided. However, if a patient requires ergot in the postpartum period for uterine contractility, it does not contraindicate nursing.

Lithium

Lithium (Eskalith, Lithobid) reaches one-third to one-half the therapeutic blood concentration in infants, who might develop lithium toxicity, with hypotonia and lethargy.

Radiopharmaceuticals

Radiopharmaceuticals require variable intervals of interruption of nursing to ensure that no radioactivity is detectable in the milk. The standard interval for gallium 67 is 2 weeks; for iodine 131, 2 to 14 days; for radioactive sodium, 4 days; and for technetium 99, 24 hours to 3 days. The milk may be tested for radioactivity before nursing is resumed for reassurance.

Drugs Whose Effect on Nursing Infants Is Unknown But May Be of Concern

Psychotropic drugs, including antianxiety, antidepressant, and antipsychotic drugs, may be of concern when given to nursing mothers for long periods. The effect of even small doses on the developing nervous system is unknown. Fluoxetine (Prozac) is excreted in low levels in breast milk.[8]

For metronidazole therapy, a single dose is preferred, and the mother may interrupt nursing for 12 to 24 hours to allow elimination of the drug.

Drugs Usually Compatible with Breast-Feeding

Narcotics, Sedatives, and Anticonvulsants

No evidence of adverse effects to the infant from nursing occurs with most of the sedatives, narcotic analgesics, and anticonvulsants. Patients may be reassured that, in normal doses, carbamazepine, phenytoin, magnesium sulfate, codeine, alphaprodine (Nisentil), morphine, and meperidine do not cause any obvious adverse effects in nursing infants. This is because the dose detectable in the breast milk is approximately 1% to 2% of the mother's dose, which is sufficiently low to have no significant pharmacologic activity.

With diazepam, the milk–plasma ratio at peak dose is 0.68, with only small amounts detected in the breast milk. In two patients who took carbamazepine while nursing, the concentration of the drug in breast milk at 4 and 5 weeks after delivery was similar, about 60% of the maternal serum level. No adverse effects were observed in either infant.

In studies in which phenobarbital and phenytoin levels were measured, only small amounts of the drug were detected in the breast milk. Because phenobarbital and diazepam are eliminated slowly by the infant, accumulation may occur. Women consuming barbiturates or benzodiazepines should observe the infants for sedation. Accumulation does not seem to occur with carbamazepine.

In 10 preeclamptic patients receiving magnesium sulfate intravenously at a dosage of 1 g/hr for 24 hours after delivery, the magnesium levels in breast milk were 64 µg/ml, compared with 48 µg/ml in controls. Breast milk calcium levels were not affected by magnesium sulfate therapy.

Analgesics

Aspirin is transferred in small amounts into breast milk. Salicylates are usually found in low concentrations because transport from plasma into milk is not favored; acids exist primarily in the ionized form. The risk is related to dosages greater than 16 300-mg tablets per day in the mother; at this level, the infant may achieve serum levels high enough to affect platelet aggregation. No harmful effects of acetaminophen have been documented. In one study, 3 mg/dl was detected in breast milk. In one patient taking propoxyphene in a suicide attempt, the level in the breast milk was one-half that of the serum. A breast-feeding infant could theoretically receive up to 1 mg of propoxyphene each day if the mother were to continually consume the maximal dose. One nursing infant had poor muscle tone when the mother was taking propoxyphene every 4 hours.

Antihistamines and Phenothiazines

Although the studies on these drugs are not extensive, no harmful effects have been observed for antihistamines or phenothiazines, and they have not been found to affect milk supply. Decongestants should be avoided in women who are having trouble producing an adequate milk supply.

Antihypertensives

After a single 500-mg oral dose of chlorothiazide, no drug was detected in breast milk at a sensitivity of 1 µg/ml. In one mother taking 50 mg of hydrochlorothiazide daily, the peak milk levels were about 25% of maternal blood levels. The drug was not detectable in the nursing infant's serum, and the infant's electrolyte levels were normal. Thiazide diuretics may decrease milk production during the first month of lactation.[2]

Propranolol is excreted in the breast milk, with milk concentrations after a single 40-mg dose less than 40% of the peak plasma concentrations. In one patient taking 40 mg four times daily, the plasma and breast milk concentrations peaked 3 hours after dosing, and the peak breast milk concentration of 42 ng/ml was 64% of the corresponding plasma concentration. After a 30-day regimen of 240 mg/day of propranolol, the predose and 3-hour postdose propranolol concentrations in breast milk were 26 and 64 ng/ml, respectively. An infant ingesting 500 ml/day of milk would ingest a maximum of 21 µg in 24 hours at a maternal dose of 160 mg/day and a maximum of 32 µg in 24 hours at a maternal dose of 240 mg/day. This would represent a dose to the infant of approximately 1% of the therapeutic dose. This amount of drug is unlikely to cause any adverse effect.

Atenolol is concentrated in breast milk to about three times the plasma level. However, the plasma concentration in the infant after a peak-level feeding is less than 10 ng/ml, which is not associated with side effects in the infant. The total infant dose is about 1% of the maternal therapeutic dose. Clonidine concentrations in milk are almost twice maternal serum levels. The neurologic and laboratory parameters of the infants of treated mothers were similar to those of untreated mothers.

Anticoagulants

Most mothers requiring anticoagulation may continue to nurse their infants with no problems. Heparin does not cross into milk and is not active if taken orally. At a maternal dose of warfarin of 5 to 12 mg/day in seven patients with maternal plasma concentrations of 0.5 to 2.6 µg/ml, no warfarin was detected in breast milk or infant plasma at a sensitivity of 0.025 µg/ml. This is probably because warfarin is 98% bound to protein. At maximal levels, 1 liter of milk would contain 20 µg of the drug, an insignificant amount unable to produce anticoagulation. Another report confirmed that warfarin appears only in insignificant quantities in breast milk. With careful monitoring of maternal prothrombin time so that the dosage is minimized and of neonatal prothrombin times to ensure lack of drug accumulation, warfarin may be safely administered to nursing mothers.

The oral anticoagulant bishydroxycoumarin (Dicumarol) has been given to 125 nursing mothers with no effect on the infants' prothrombin times and no hemorrhages. This level of safety does not apply to all oral anticoagulant drugs. In one case in which phenindione, which is not used in the United States, was being taken by a nursing mother, the infant underwent surgical repair of an inguinal hernia at 5 weeks of age. He developed a large hematoma, and his prothrombin time was elevated.

Corticosteroids

In one patient requiring corticosteroids, breast milk was obtained 2 hours after an oral dose of 10 mg of prednisone. The levels in the milk were 0.1 µg/100 ml of prednisolone and

2.67 µg/100 ml of prednisone. An infant taking 1 liter of milk would obtain 28.3 µg of the two steroids, an amount unlikely to have any deleterious effect.

MacKenzie and colleagues administered 5 mg of radioactive prednisolone to seven patients and found 0.14%, a negligible quantity, of the tag was secreted in the milk in the subsequent 60 hours. Breast-feeding is not contraindicated for the mother taking corticosteroids. Even at 80 mg/day, the nursing infant would ingest less than 0.1% of the dose, which is less than 10% of the infant's endogenous cortisol.

Digoxin

After a maternal dose of 0.25 mg, the peak breast milk levels of 0.6 to 1 ng/ml occur, and the milk–plasma ratio at the 4-hour peak is 0.8 to 0.9. This represents a small amount because of significant binding by maternal proteins. In 24 hours, an infant would receive about 1% of the maternal dose. No adverse effects have been reported in nursing infants.

Antibiotics

Penicillin derivatives are safe in nursing mothers. In the usual therapeutic doses of ampicillin, the mother's milk–plasma ratios are less than 0.2, and no adverse effects are observed in the infants. In susceptible persons or with prolonged therapy, diarrhea and candidiasis are theoretical concerns.

Dicloxacillin is 98% bound to protein. If this drug is used to treat breast infections, little contaminates the breast milk, and nursing may be continued.

Cephalosporins appear only in trace amounts in milk. After 500 mg of cefazolin given intramuscularly three times daily in one study, no drug was detected in breast milk. After 2 g of cefazolin given intravenously at the 3-hour peak level, 1.51 µg/ml was detected, for a milk–plasma ratio of 0.023. The infant was exposed to only 0.075% of the maternal dose.

Tooth staining and delayed bone growth from tetracycline have not been reported after the drug was taken by a breast-feeding mother. This is probably because of the high rate of binding of the drug by calcium and protein, limiting absorption from the milk. Because the amount in the milk is about one-half the level in the mother's plasma, the amount of free tetracycline available is too small to be significant.

Sulfonamides appear in small amounts in breast milk and are not contraindicated during nursing. However, during the first 5 days of life or in premature infants immediately after delivery, when hyperbilirubinemia may be a problem, the drug is best avoided because it may displace bilirubin from binding sites on albumin. In one study of sulfapyridine, the drug and its metabolites were detected in plasma and milk at levels of 4 to 7 µg/ml, and the infant would receive less than 1% of the maternal dose. Urine samples from the infant showed 50% of the delivered dose, and this does not appear to be hazardous to the infant. When a mother took 500 mg of sulfasalazine (Azulfidine) every 6 hours, the drug was undetectable in all milk samples.

There are no reported adverse effects on the infant of isoniazid administered to nursing mothers, and its use is considered compatible with breast-feeding.[2] Acyclovir concentrations in one nursing mother revealed a milk–serum ratio of 3.24 and a half-life of 2.8 hours for elimination from breast milk. The amount of acyclovir to which the infant would be exposed in a mother taking 1000 mg/day would be less than 1 mg/day, a very low dose.

Oral Contraceptives

Combined estrogen and progestin oral contraceptives cause dose-related suppression of the quantity of milk produced, although most studies used 50-µg preparations. The use of combined estrogen and progestin oral contraceptives during lactation has been associated with shortened duration of lactation, decreased milk production, decreased infant weight gain, and decreased composition of nitrogen and protein content of the milk. However, the composition and volume of breast milk varies considerably even without birth control pills. Lactation is inhibited to a lesser degree if the pill is started after the immediate postpartum period, and 3 weeks after delivery is recommended. In malnourished mothers, infant weight gain should be monitored. Because of this suppressant effect, the mother may terminate lactation because of decreased milk supply. However, if the patient persists in taking birth control pills while nursing, there is no documented adverse effect of the practice.

Studies indicate that an infant consuming 600 ml of breast milk daily from a mother using an oral contraceptive containing 50 µg of ethinylestradiol receives a daily dose in the range of 10 ng of the estrogen. The amount of natural estradiol received by infants who consume a similar volume of milk from mothers not using oral contraceptives is estimated at 3 to 6 ng during anovulatory cycles and 6 to 12 ng during ovulatory cycles. No consistent long-term adverse effects on children's growth and development have been described. Evidence indicates that D-norgestrel is metabolized rather than accumulated by the infants, and no adverse effects have been identified as a result of progestational agents taken by the mother. Progestin-only contraceptives do not alter breast milk composition or volume. Progestin-only pills are ideal for use in the breast-feeding mother.

Alcohol

Alcohol levels in breast milk are similar to maternal blood levels. One report has appeared of intoxication in an infant whose mother ingested 750 ml of port wine in 24 hours. If a moderate social drinker had two cocktails or two to three glasses of wine and had a blood alcohol concentration of 50 mg/100 ml, the nursing infant would receive about 82 mg of alcohol, which would produce insignificant blood concentrations.

Even this small amount may have an effect on the infant. One study suggested that ethanol ingested through breast milk has a slight but significant detrimental effect on motor development, but not mental development, in breast-fed infants. Another study showed that short-term alcohol consumption by lactating women significantly affected the odor of the milk and that the infants consumed significantly less milk, correlating with the alcohol concentration in the milk.[17]

Propylthiouracil

Propylthiouracil (PTU) is found in breast milk in small amounts. If the mother takes 200 mg PTU three times daily, the child could receive 149 µg daily or the equivalent of a 70-kg adult receiving 3 mg daily. One infant was studied until 5 months of age and exhibited no changes in thyroid parameters including thyroid-stimulating hormone. Lactating mothers on PTU can continue nursing with close supervision of the infant.[10]

Caffeine

Caffeine has had no adverse effects in nursing infants, even after the mother consumes several cups of strong coffee. In one study, the milk contained 1% of the total dose 6 hours after coffee ingestion, which is not enough to affect the infant. If a mother drinks excessive amounts of caffeine, and caffeine accumulates in the infant, the infant may show signs of caffeine stimulation such as wakefulness. It is recommended that nursing mothers limit their intake to a moderate level.

Smoking

Nicotine can enter the milk, but it reaches relatively low levels of 0.01 to 0.05 mg/100 ml if 20 cigarettes are smoked each day. Because nicotine is not readily absorbed by the infant's intestinal tract, signs of nicotine intoxication are unlikely to result from breast-feeding. The infant may have risks from passive smoking.

◊ RADIATION

Diagnostic Radiation

Diagnostic radiation at the levels currently employed is not teratogenic. An exposure of less than 5 to 10 cGy is incapable of producing any detectable teratogenic effect in humans or animals.[7] Diagnostic imaging exposes the fetus to small doses of radiation:

Maternal chest radiograph: 0.008 cGy
Intravenous pyelogram: 0.4 cGy
Computed tomography scan: 0.250 cGy per slice
Upper gastrointestinal series: 0.550 cGy
Barium enema: 1 cGy
Technetium 99m scan: 1 to 3 cGy
Thallium 201 scan: 0.5 to 1.0 cGy

If at any time during pregnancy an x-ray film is indicated to diagnose maternal illness, there should be no hesitation in obtaining the radiograph. It is possible that fetal irradiation in doses of as low as 2 cGy is associated with 1.3- to 1.8-fold increases in the risk of childhood leukemia in the exposed fetus.

No untoward effects of diagnostic ultrasound have been demonstrated in humans despite many studies to address such effects. Magnetic resonance imaging involves no ionizing radiation and holds great promise in the future for evaluating maternal and fetal abnormalities, but the data are still insufficient to evaluate its safety and efficacy in pregnancy.

Therapeutic Radiation

Only the therapeutic levels used to treat malignancy are teratogenic. During the preimplantation phase from fertilization to implantation, the most likely consequence of exposure to therapeutic radiation is spontaneous abortion, although no effect may be seen. The period of organogenesis in the first trimester is the most sensitive time for the fetus with regard to injury. The major effects are microcephaly and mental and growth retardation. However, the CNS, the eyes, and the hematopoietic system remain sensitive to the effect of radiation throughout pregnancy.

Video Display Terminals

In the 1980s, a cluster of cases of birth defects in the offspring of workers exposed to video display terminals (VDT) was reported. The defects were different in each affected child, with no consistent syndrome. Subsequent epidemiologic studies have not shown any higher risk of spontaneous abortions or birth defects among terminal users than among controls.[4] It seems likely that the initial clusters reported were encountered by chance.

The ionizing radiation generated by the VDT consists of x-rays, but the x-rays emitted by the cathode ray tube are entirely absorbed by the glass screen. Several studies could not detect measurable radiation from VDTs, and this was also the case in the reported clusters for which the involved VDTs were tested.

Among the types of nonionizing radiation, light and heat are emitted from VDTs at lower levels than that of the environment. Microwaves and radio frequencies emitted are in the same range as that given off by most home electrical appliances, which is two orders of magnitude less than the background. There is no need for concern or a change in working conditions for pregnant women working at VDTs.

Hyperthermia

Animal studies have shown that heat can be a significant teratogen. Some retrospective human studies suggested that fever in the first trimester might be associated with neural tube defects and dysmorphic syndromes, but a prospective trial did not confirm this. Finnish women have a low incidence of anencephaly (0.32/1000 births) despite regular use of saunas during pregnancy.

The teratogenic level suggested by animal studies is a core temperature of over 38.9°C, and the usual use of hot tubs is unlikely to raise a woman's body temperature to that level. It is recommended that pregnant women using a hot tub at 40°C stay in for less than 10 minutes.[21]

SUMMARY POINTS

◊ Infants of epileptic women taking anticonvulsants have double the rate of malformations of unexposed infants. The risk of fetal hydantoin syndrome is less than 10%.

◊ The risk of malformations after exposure *in utero* to isotretinoin is 25%, and an additional 25% of infants have mental retardation. Vitamin A itself in large doses may be teratogenic.

◊ Angiotensin-converting enzyme inhibitors can cause fetal renal failure in the second and third trimesters, leading to oligohydramnios, craniofacial deformities, and hypoplastic lungs.

◊ Aspirin in analgesic doses inhibits platelet function and prolongs bleeding time. Thus, alternate analgesics are recommended in pregnancy, preferably acetaminophen.

◊ Most drugs are safe during lactation as subtherapeutic amounts appear in breast milk, approximately 1% to 2% of the maternal dose. One notable exception is lithium.

Web Site

◊ Organization of Teratogen Information Services: http://orpheus.ucsd.edu/ctis

Computer Data Bases

◊ MICROMEDEX, Inc., 6200 South Syracuse Way, Suite 300, Englewood, CO 80111-4740.

◊ Reproductive Toxicology Center, REPROTOX, Columbia Hospital for Women Medical Center, 2440 M Street, NW, Suite 217, Washington, DC 20037-1404.

◊ Teratogen Information Service, TERIS, University of Washington, Office of Technology Transfer, 4225 Roosevelt Way, NE, Suite 301, Seattle, WA 98105.

◊ REFERENCES

1. Adams J. High incidence of intellectual deficits in 5-year-old children exposed to isotretinoin *in utero*. *Teratology* 1990;41:614.
2. American Academy of Pediatrics, Committee on Drugs. The transfer of drugs and other chemicals into human milk. *Pediatrics* 1994;93:137.
3. Andrews EB, Yankaskas BC, Cordero JF, et al. Acyclovir in pregnancy registry: Six years' experience. *Obstet Gynecol* 1992;79:7.
4. Bentur Y, Koren G. The three most common occupational exposures reported by pregnant women: an update. *Am J Obstet Gynecol* 1991;165:429.
5. Berkovitch M, Pastuszak A, Gazarian M, et al. Safety of the new quinolones in pregnancy. *Obstet Gynecol* 1994;84:535.
6. Bertin P, Taddio A, Ariburnu O, et al. Safety of metronidazole in pregnancy: a meta-analysis. *Am J Obstet Gynecol* 1995;172:525.
7. Brent RL. The effect of embryonic and fetal exposure to x-ray, microwaves, and ultrasound: counseling the pregnant and nonpregnant patient about these risks. *Semin Oncol* 1989;16:347.
8. Burch KJ, Wells BG. Fluoxetine/norfluoxetine concentrations in human milk. *Pediatrics* 1992;89:676.
9. Centers for Disease Control. Postmarketing surveillance for angiotensin-converting enzyme inhibitor use during the first trimester of pregnancy—United States, Canada, and Israel, 1987–1995. *MMWR* 1997; 46:240. *JAMA* 1997;277:1193.
10. Cooper DS. Antithyroid drugs: to breast-feed or not to breast-feed. *Am J Obstet Gynecol* 1987;157:234.
11. Czeizel A. A case-control analysis of the teratogenic effects of cotrimoxazole. *Reprod Toxicol* 1990;4(4):305.
12. Dahlman T, Lindvall N, Hellgren M. Osteopenia in pregnancy during long-term heparin treatment: a radiological study postpartum. *Br J Obstet Gynaecol* 1990;97:221.
13. Goldstein DJ, Corbin LA, Sundell KL. Effects of first-trimester fluoxetine exposure on the newborn. *Obstet Gynecol* 1997;87:713.
14. Hanssens M, Keirse MJNC, Vankelecom F, et al. Fetal and neonatal effects of treatment with angiotensin-converting enzyme inhibitors in pregnancy. *Obstet Gynecol* 1991;78:128.
15. Jacobson SJ, Jones K, Johnson K, et al. Prospective multi-centre study of pregnancy outcome after lithium exposure during first trimester. *Lancet* 1992;339:530.
16. Lutiger B, Graham K, Einarson TR, et al. Relationship between gestational cocaine use and pregnancy outcome: a meta-analysis. *Teratology* 1991;44:405.
17. Mennella JA, Beaucham GK. The transfer of alcohol to human milk: effects on flavor and the infant's behavior. *N Engl J Med* 1991;325:981.
18. Mills JL, Simpson JL, Cunningham GC, et al. Vitamin A and birth defects. *Am J Obstet Gynecol* 1997;177:31.
19. Nelson-Piercy C, Letsky EA, deSwiet M. Low-molecular-weight heparin for obstetric thromboprophylaxis: Experience of sixty-nine pregnancies in sixty-one women at high risk. *Am J Obstet Gynecol* 1997; 176:1062.
20. Nulman I, Rovet J, Stewart DE, et al. Neurodevelopment of children exposed *in utero* to antidepressant drugs. *N Engl J Med* 1997;336:258.
21. Ridge BR, Budd GM. How long is too long in a spa pool? *N Engl J Med* 1990;323:835.
22. Rosa FW. Spina bifida in infants of women treated with carbamazepine during pregnancy. *N Engl J Med* 1991;324:674.
23. Rothman KJ, Moore LL, Singer MR, et al. Teratogenicity of high vitamin A intake. *N Engl J Med* 1995;333:1369.
24. Schick B, Ham M, Librizzi R, et al. Terfenadine (Seldane) exposure in early pregnancy. *Teratology* 1994;49:417.
25. Vutyavanich T, Wongtra-Rjan S, Ruangsri R. Pyridoxine for nausea and vomiting of pregnancy: A randomized double-blind placebo-controlled trial. *Am J Obstet Gynecol* 1995;173:881.

CHAPTER 14

Ultrasound in Obstetrics

◇

Roya Sohaey
D. Ware Branch

◇ ULTRASOUND PHYSICS, EQUIPMENT, AND SAFETY

In the early 1900s, ultrasound was first used to detect submarines. Initially, ultrasound was a classified military tool, and the military term *SONAR* is an abbreviation for sound navigation and ranging. After declassification, the medical imaging capabilities of ultrasound technology quickly became apparent. In the past 40 years, ultrasound has become a fundamental part of obstetric care.

Ultrasound Physics and Instrumentation

Ultrasound is produced by the vibration of a synthetic piezoelectric crystal, which expands and contracts in response to rapidly alternating electrical potential, located in the transducer of an ultrasound machine. The transducer is capable of converting electrical energy to mechanical energy (ultrasound) and *vice versa.*

Like all energy waves, ultrasound waves have a wavelength and frequency. The wavelength is the distance between two consecutive wave peaks or valleys, and the frequency is the number of waves (or cycles) per second. Frequency is reported in hertz (Hz), named in honor of a German physicist. One cycle per second is 1 Hz, 1000 cycles per second is 1 kHz (kilohertz), and 1 million cycles per second is 1 MHz (megahertz). Most diagnostic ultrasound is performed in the 2 to 10 MHz range. For obstetric examinations, abdominal transducers with a 2 to 5 MHz range and vaginal transducers with 5 to 7 MHz are most commonly used. Appropriate selection of scanhead (another term frequently used for transducers) is imperative. As the transducer frequency range increases, image resolution increases but at a cost to the ability to visualize deeper structures (due to attenuation). For example, a linear-array 7-MHz transducer would not be able to penetrate deep enough to visualize a first-trimester gestational sac through a full maternal bladder. However, with vaginal

sonography, 5- and 7-MHz transducers work quite well because the distance between the transducer and the gestational sac is greatly decreased. As a general rule, the sonographer tries to use the transducer with the highest frequency possible and is always balancing resolution and attenuation to obtain the best images.

The type of ultrasound technology most commonly used in medical imaging is termed *pulse–echo sonography*—the transducer both sends and receives ultrasound waves. The piezoelectric crystal produces brief pulses of ultrasound and then spends the majority of its time "listening" for reflected sound. The listening period is about 1000 times longer than the sending period. Transit time is the time it takes for the ultrasound wave to travel from the transducer to the target (referred to as the reflector) and back to the transducer. Sound travels at 1540 meters per second through the tissues of the body. Sound is reflected back to the transducer only at boundaries between tissues with different acoustic properties (e.g., the fetal skin and amniotic fluid can be thought of as two structures with vastly different acoustic properties). At the boundary between the two, ultrasound waves are reflected back, and this allows visualization of the embryo or fetus within amniotic fluid.

Echo strength is determined by at least four important factors. The difference in acoustic properties of adjacent tissues is called *acoustic impedance mismatch* and determines the amount of echoes reflected back to the transducer. If the acoustic mismatch is great (i.e. at a soft tissue–bone interface), almost all of the ultrasound energy is reflected, resulting in an echogenic (bright) structure with distal acoustic shadowing (no echoes deep to the structure). The sonographer will note the shadowing from the fetal femur, especially when the femur is positioned parallel to the transducer, with the ultrasound waves reflecting perpendicular to its long axis. Another factor that determines echo strength is the angle at which the ultrasound beam strikes a reflecting interface. When the *angle of incidence* is 90 degrees (reflector is perpendicular to the ultrasound beam), maximum reflection occurs. The *strength* of the ultrasound beam also determines the strength of the reflected ultrasound echo. Weak beams do not reflect well. Using very powerful ultrasound beams, however, results in heating and damage of tissues. For this reason, ultrasound power must be carefully monitored, particularly for obstetric imaging. In addition, if echoes are too strong, they will result in poor image quality. Another factor that determines the appearance of structures is the *size of the reflector*. A large reflector (e.g., the fetal femur) will result in a sharp echogenic line and best demonstrate the outline of the structure, whereas small reflectors (e.g., biliary structures within the fetal liver) scatter the ultrasound beam and give the image a textured quality, called speckle. Figure 1 demonstrates some echo strength characteristics.

Standard ultrasound images are called B mode (brightness-mode display) and are directly related to the echo strength information received through the transducer. The stronger the reflected echo, the brighter the pixel will be on an ultrasound monitor (and subsequently on film or videotape documentation). Two-dimensional (2-D) (width and height) images are obtained by B-mode sonography. Unlike 2-D ultrasound, M-mode ultrasound supplies information about one series of points over time. This results in a wavy pattern in the presence of motion. M mode is used mostly to study the fetal heart, particularly fetal cardiac arrhythmia. Today's ultrasound machines are capable of showing the sonographer both the 2-D and the M-mode images simultaneously.

Doppler ultrasound has gained increasing popularity in obstetric imaging and deserves special discussion. The Doppler effect is the change in frequency and wavelength that occurs when an ultrasound wave is reflected from a moving object.

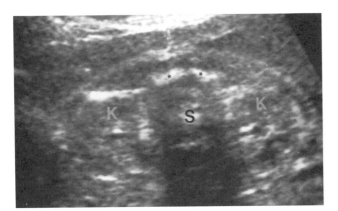

FIG. 1. Example of echo strength concepts. A transverse view of the abdomen at the level of the fetal kidneys *(K)* shows that the ultrasound beam angle of incidence is 90 degrees on the fetal spine *(S)*. Maximum reflection occurs from the spine, resulting in the echogenic appearance of the posterior elements *(asterisks)*. The acoustic impedance mismatch between the bone and the fetal skin is also great, resulting in further reflection of the ultrasound beam. The strong reflection of the ultrasound beam resulted in a lack of echoes deep to the spine, called acoustic shadowing. Smaller reflectors, such as the renal pelvises and renal parenchyma, scatter the ultrasound beam less and help provide anatomic detail and a textured appearance.

The frequency difference between the incident wave (the beam from the transducer) and the reflected wave (from the moving object, e.g., red blood cells in the umbilical artery) is the Doppler shift. The velocity of the object is directly related to the magnitude of the Doppler shift. Doppler ultrasound provides information about both direction and velocity of blood flow. Continuous wave Doppler technique samples all moving targets within the beam path, while pulsed Doppler (used more commonly in obstetrics) targets a more focal region of blood flow. Color flow Doppler simply converts velocity information into color on a 2-D ultrasound image. Direction of flow is represented by a color hue chosen by the operator (e.g., red is toward the transducer, blue is away from the transducer). The velocity of flow is represented by the shade of the color (light red is slower than dark red).

Appropriate scanhead (or transducer) selection is crucial for optimal image acquisition. Different scanhead choices include linear-array transducers, curvilinear transducers, and sector transducers. All are array transducers that contain multiple crystal elements activated singly or in groups. Electronic manipulation of ultrasound crystal "firing" allows ultrasound beam formation, steering, and focusing. Focusing of the ultrasound beam is operator controlled, and the area of interest should be within the chosen focal zone for optimal resolution. Linear-array transducers, as the name indicates, have a series of elements that are arranged in a linear manner. The elements repeatedly fire from one end to the other. Linear transducers provide the best inherent resolution but are often cumbersome to operate. Most obstetric imaging is performed with curvilinear or sector transducers. The shape of these scanheads permits imaging of a larger area of anatomy seen from a smaller contact zone with the patient. As mentioned previously, the sonographer is always balancing attenuation (ability to scan deeper structures) with resolution. Therefore, different scanheads may be necessary for a given examination. As a rule, the highest frequency that allows appropriate attenuation of the region of interest should be used. In general, obstetric ultrasound is performed with 3- to 5-MHz curvilinear and sector transducers. In obese patients, 2- to 2.5-MHz transducers may be necessary. Some scanheads function at several different frequencies (e.g., 2.5 MHz, 3.5 MHz, and 5 MHz), and thus the sonographer may not need to switch transducers as frequently. Most vaginal transducers are specialized sector transducers with 5- to 7-MHz frequencies.[24]

Ultrasound Artifacts

Artifacts are common in ultrasound and can be helpful or detrimental in interpreting an examination. Examples of four common artifacts—acoustic shadowing, enhanced through-transmission, lateral edge shadows, and reverberation artifacts—are shown in Figures 1 and 2. Artifacts such as enhanced through-transmission and acoustic shadowing actually help the sonographer determine the nature of the tissues being studied. Enhanced through-transmission is the phenomenon in which the ultrasound beam travels through a very homoge-

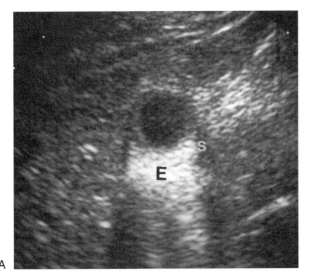 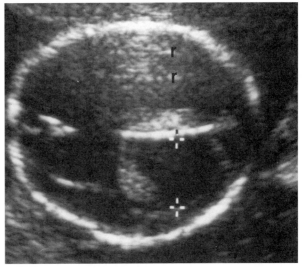

A   B

FIG. 2. Ultrasound artifacts: enhanced through-transmission, lateral edge shadows, and reverberation. **A:** The ultrasound beam travels through the fluid-filled gallbladder without impedance and is therefore enhanced *(E)* (bright echoes seen deep to the gallbladder). Lateral edge shadows *(S)* occur as the ultrasound beam is both reflected and refracted at the margin of the gallbladder. **B:** Reverberation occurs when the ultrasound beam reflects back and forth between reflecting surfaces. In this case, fetal hydrocephalus is present, and the ultrasound beam is reflecting between the margins of the near lateral ventricle (*r*, echogenic lines caused by reverberation). Note that the near field is usually more difficult to see, and therefore the ventricle farther from the transducer is usually seen better than the closer ventricle.

neous structure with low attenuation of the ultrasound beam (e.g., the fetal bladder filled with urine). The beam travels through the structure without impedance, and thus the echoes deep to the structure are amplified and much brighter than echoes otherwise at that depth. The ultrasonographic identification of fluid-filled structures relies on enhanced through-transmission. Acoustic shadowing is the opposite phenomenon. The ultrasound beam strikes an object that almost completely reflects the beam. The result is an echogenic outline of the surface of the structure and a shadow (absence of information about structures deep to the structure).

Ultrasound Safety

As mentioned previously, the ultrasound beam can heat and destroy tissue. The power of the ultrasound beam can be adjusted by the sonographer and is regulated by the U.S. Food and Drug Administration. Interestingly, output power from ultrasound machines vary greatly, and not all machines are required to display output power values. Sector scanners require higher power than linear arrays, and Doppler applications require the most power output. In recent years, newer ultrasound machines are operating at greater power settings than previously, and this has raised concern regarding the safety of ultrasound. The recognized upper limit of power considered safe is 1000 mW/cm^2.[13] In the interest of safety, ultrasound should be used judiciously during the periods of embryogenesis and organogenesis, and early-pregnancy Doppler interrogations should be limited or avoided.

◊ GENERAL OBSTETRIC GUIDELINES

A list of common problems for which obstetric ultrasound may be indicated is provided in Table 1. Whatever the indication, the importance of performing an adequate obstetric ultrasound examination cannot be overstated. To standardize the examination, specific guidelines have been established by leaders in the field of obstetric imaging and are endorsed by

TABLE 1. *Common indications for the use of ultrasound during pregnancy*

Uncertain menstrual dates
Determination of fetal size, growth, and weight
Number of gestations
Fetal presentation and lie
Vaginal bleeding
Pregnancy location
Uterus small or large for clinical dates
Pelvic pain
Suspected amniotic fluid abnormalities
Suspected uterine or adnexal abnormalities
Premature labor
Adjunct to procedures such as amniocentesis
Abnormal maternal serum screening values
  (i.e., alpha-fetoprotein)
History of congenital anomalies
Follow-up of previously identified abnormalities
  (i.e., anomalies, placenta previa)
Suspected fetal demise
Biophysical evaluation after 28 weeks

several professional organizations, including the American Institute of Ultrasound in Medicine (AIUM), the American College of Obstetrics and Gynecology (ACOG), and the American College of Radiology (ACR). These guidelines are updated every 3 to 5 years. Practicing ultrasound physicians should follow established guidelines. Currently, the AIUM and the ACR offer voluntary certification for ultrasound departments, and mandatory certifications may be instituted in the future. The 1994 AIUM guidelines[2] for the performance of the antepartum ultrasound examination are reviewed in Table 2, and examples of expected normal images are shown with expanded figure legends in Figures 3 to 11. The AIUM guidelines are emphasized in this chapter; they are nearly identical to the guideline recommended by the ACOG and the ACR. The AIUM is composed of a variety of practitioners of ultrasound, including radiologists, obstetricians, and sonographers.

First Trimester

The first trimester is defined as the first 13 weeks following the first day of the last normal menstrual period. With the advent of high-resolution ultrasound transducers (particularly vaginal transducers), early-pregnancy anatomy is well seen. Part II of the AIUM guidelines addresses evaluation of the first trimester. Table 3 and Figure 3 review normal first-trimester ultrasound features. Ultrasonographic findings related to pregnancy failure in the first trimester are reviewed below.

Poor Growth: Failure to Reach Expected Landmarks

Gestational sac and embryonic growth in the first trimester is predictable. Table 4 compares menstrual age with mean gestational sac diameter, embryo crown-rump length, and human

---

TABLE 2. *Summary of the AIUM's 1994 guidelines for the performance of the antepartum obstetrical ultrasound evaluation*

I: Equipment and documentation
Equipment
  Real-time equipment
  Transducers: 3–5 MHz abdominal, 5–7.5 MHz vaginal
Documentation
  Permanent record of images
  Labeled images: date, patient identification, image orientation (when necessary)
  Report of findings in the medical record
  Retention of images (per local and legal requirements)

II: First-trimester sonography
Technique
  Abdominal, vaginal, or both methods
Gestational sac (GS)
  Document GS location (uterine or adnexal)
  Document presence or absence of an embryo
  Document presence of yolk sac (if no embryo seen)
  Measure GS mean diameter (if measurable embryo not seen)
Embryo
  Document the embryo crown-rump length (CRL)
  Cardiac activity
  Demise: only if CRL is > 5 mm and no cardiac activity
Multiple gestations
  Document multiple embryos (multiple fluid collections may not be multiple pregnancies)
Uterus, adnexal structures, and cul-de-sac
  Document myomas: location, size
  Document adnexal masses
  Cul-de-sac scanned for presence or absence of fluid

III: Second- and third-trimester sonography
Document fetal life, number, presentation, and activity
Multiple pregnancies
  Number of gestational sacs
  Number of placentas
  Presence or absence of a dividing membrane
  Fetal genitalia

  Comparison of fetal size
  Comparison of amniotic fluid on each side of the membrane
Estimate amniotic fluid volume
  Report if normal, increased, or decreased
Placenta and umbilical cord
  Document placenta location, appearance, relationship to internal os
Gestational age assessment: fetal biometry measurements
  Done best at initial scan and not accurate in the third trimester
  Cranial measurements
    Biparietal diameter (BPD): an axial image that includes the thalamus
    Head circumference (HC): outer perimeter measurement at BPD level
  Abdominal and limb measurements
    Abdominal circumference (AC): transverse view at junction of the portal veins
    Femur length (FL): longest obtainable diaphyseal measurement of the near-field femur
Fetal weight and growth assessment: late second and third trimester
  Estimate fetal weight (using biometric data)
  Compare fetal weight with appropriate gestational age
  If previous studies have been done, estimate interval growth
Uterus (including cervix) and adnexal structures
  Presence, location, and size of myomas
  Adnexal masses
  Cervical assessment: may need vaginal or transperineal scanning
Fetal anatomic evaluation (minimal requirements)
  Cerebral ventricles
  Cerebral posterior fossa (cerebellar hemispheres and cisterna magna)
  Four-chamber view of heart
  Spine
  Stomach
  Urinary bladder and kidneys
  Umbilical cord insertion site

(Data from ref. 2.)

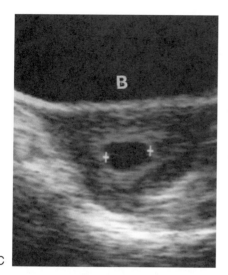
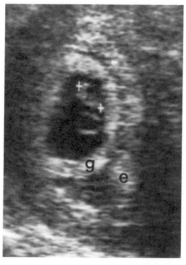
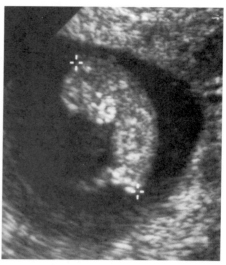

A-C

FIG. 3. Normal first-trimester features. **A:** The gestational sac (+ calipers) is located eccentrically within the uterine cavity and is round or oval and surrounded by an echogenic ring. The echogenic ring is within a larger echogenic ring formed by the decidual reaction of the endometrium. This ring-within-a-ring appearance is called a double decidual sac and helps the sonographer confirm that an intrauterine fluid collection is a gestational sac and not a pseudosac or endometrial fluid collection that can be seen in ectopic pregnancies. **B:** An embryo (calipers measure the length of the embryo, called the crown-rump length) and a yolk sac (thin-walled circle adjacent to the embryo) are seen within a gestational sac. A double decidual sac sign is also present (*g*, decidual reaction around the gestational sac; *e*, decidual reaction of the endometrium). **C:** As the embryo grows, a discernible crown (the superior caliper) and rump (the inferior caliper) can be seen, and a true crown-rump length can be measured.

chorionic gonadotropin (hCG) levels. Significant deviation from expected measurements reflects one of two situations: either the menstrual data are inaccurate, or the pregnancy has failed. In early pregnancy, repeat examination in 3 to 7 days can usually resolve the dilemma. Expected landmarks include visualization of (1) a yolk sac when the mean gestational sac diameter is greater than 10 mm (by transvaginal technique) and (2) an embryo when the mean gestational sac diameter is greater than 18 mm (by transvaginal technique).[18] When pregnancy failure is suspected on the basis of concerns about intrauterine gestational sac or embryonic growth, a conservative approach is recommended and may include the prudent use of short-term follow-up ultrasound examination (in 3 to 7 days) to evaluate interval growth.

Anembryonic Pregnancy (Blighted Ovum)

An anembryonic gestational sac, also referred to as a blighted ovum, is a common presentation of failed pregnancy. In this situation, an intrauterine gestational sac is seen, but an embryo is not present (Fig. 12). The examiner must make sure that an empty gestational sac is not the result of poor visualization or of a pregnancy too early for sonography to detect an embryo. A gestational sac greater than 20 mm (with vaginal scanning) or 25 mm (by transabdominal technique) should contain an embryo. With anembryonic pregnancy, an empty amnion or embryo remnants may be seen, but a living embryo is not present.[16]

Embryonic Demise

Embryos that measure greater than 5 mm should consistently demonstrate cardiac activity, indicating embryonic life. Spontaneous abortion rates decrease steadily for living embryos as the gestational age increases. The demise rate for living embryos between 6 and 10 mm in length is only 0.5%[9] versus almost 25% for all first-trimester pregnancies. The diagnosis of embryonic demise should be made with care. Observation of the embryo by two experienced clinicians (usually sonographer and physician) for several minutes is prudent. If there is any doubt, a repeat examination in 3 days should be performed. An embryonic heart rate of less than 90 beats per minute in embryos that are less than 8 weeks is associated with an 80% rate of eventual demise (Fig. 13).[5]

Perigestational Hemorrhage

In most cases, bleeding in early pregnancy comes from the chorionic frondosum (site of the future placenta). Blood that does not pass through the cervix may accumulate adjacent to the gestational sac and appear as a perigestational or subchorionic fluid collection (Fig. 14). Up to 20% of women with symptoms of a threatened abortion will demonstrate a subchorionic hematoma with ultrasound examination. Acute hemorrhages will be more echogenic than older collections of blood. Large perigestational hemorrhages are associated

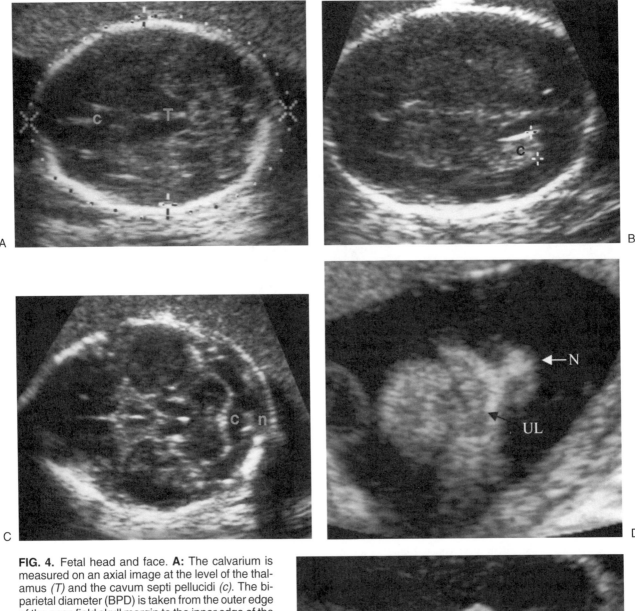

FIG. 4. Fetal head and face. **A:** The calvarium is measured on an axial image at the level of the thalamus *(T)* and the cavum septi pellucidi *(c)*. The biparietal diameter (BPD) is taken from the outer edge of the near-field skull margin to the inner edge of the far skull margin (+ calipers). The head circumference (HC) is a perimeter measurement along the outer calvarium (X calipers). **B:** The cerebral ventricles are evaluated on an axial scan of the fetal head superior to the BPD/HC view. The choroid plexus *(c)* fills the lateral ventricle at the atria (+ calipers). In normal fetuses, this measurement remains under 10 mm throughout pregnancy. **C:** The posterior fossa and nuchal skin are seen best by angling the transducer 10 to 15 degrees caudal to the standard BPD/HC view. From anterior to posterior, the bilobed cerebellum, the cisterna magna *(c)*, and the nuchal skin *(n)* are well seen. The cisterna magna is fluid-filled and should measure between 3 and 10 mm during the second and third trimesters. The nuchal skin (measured from the outer calvarium to the outer skin margin) should measure less than 6 mm between 16 and 21 weeks. **D, E:** Images of the fetal face are not required views for standard ultrasound examinations; however, they are often desirable views for parents. The coronal image through the fetal nose *(N)* and lips helps identify an intact upper lip *(UL)*, while sagittal images show features consistent with a normal face.

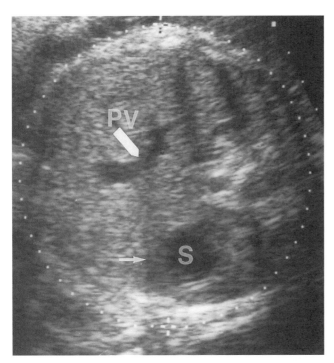

FIG. 5. Abdominal circumference (AC). The standard AC measurement is obtained on a transverse image of the upper abdomen at the level of the fluid-filled stomach fundus *(S)* and at the junction of the left and right portal veins *(PV)*. The abdomen should be round, and the outer perimeter of the abdomen, including the subcutaneous fat, is measured.

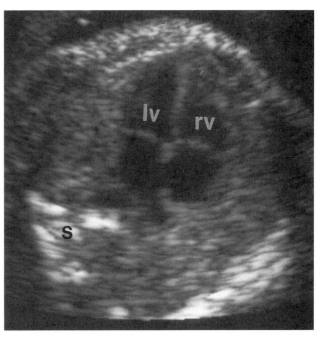

FIG. 7. Four-chamber heart. An axial scan of the chest demonstrates four cardiac chambers. The right *(rv)* and left *(lv)* ventricles should be roughly the same size, and the right and left atria should also be symmetric. The right ventricle (RV) often lies in contact with the anterior chest wall and contains the moderator band (seen as a medium echogenic structure at the apex of the RV).

with a higher pregnancy loss rate, even in the presence of a living embryo, whereas most small perigestational hemorrhages resolve without sequelae. A perigestational hemorrhage is considered large if it significantly misshapes the gestational sac or the chorionic frondosum is significantly lifted away from the uterus by the hemorrhage.

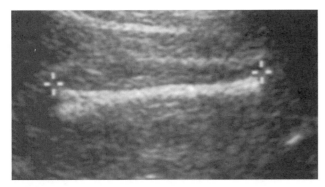

FIG. 6. Femur length (FL). The longest measurement of the femur located closest to the transducer should be obtained (calipers). The long axis of the femur should be parallel to the transducer (perpendicular to the ultrasound beam). Only the femoral diaphysis should be measured. An echogenic line from the femoral epiphysis may be seen but should not be included in the measurement.

Ectopic Pregnancy

The incidence of ectopic pregnancy is rising in the United States. Women with a history of pelvic inflammatory disease, previous ectopic pregnancy, intrauterine contraceptive device use, or artificial insemination are at increased risk for an ectopic pregnancy. The most common site for ectopic pregnancies is within the fallopian tube. Nontubal sites are rare and include the cervix, uterine cornua, ovary, and abdomen. Ultrasound, particularly transvaginal imaging, can detect greater than 90% of ectopic pregnancies and should be routinely used to evaluate any pregnancy that may be at risk for an ectopic gestation.[3,18]

Patients suspected of having an ectopic pregnancy may have a variety of ultrasound findings (Fig. 15). Imaging with high-resolution transvaginal transducers gives the sonographer the best opportunity to diagnose or rule out an ectopic pregnancy. The most reassuring ultrasound finding is the presence of a normal intrauterine pregnancy; the risk for a concurrent ectopic pregnancy is 1 in 30,000 for low-risk patients and 1 in 5000 for high-risk patients.

In the presence of an ectopic pregnancy, the most frequent ultrasound features are visualization of an empty uterus (usually with a prominent but empty decidual reaction) and the presence of an adnexal mass shown to be separate from the ovary. In two-thirds of cases, the adnexal mass resembles a gestational sac (with an adnexal echogenic ring), while in

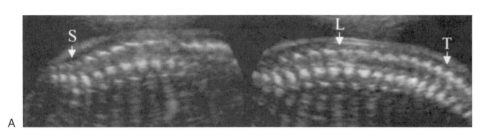
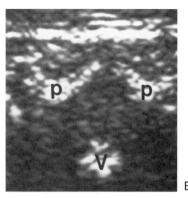

A

B

FIG. 8. Fetal spine. **A:** Coronal view through the posterior elements of the thoracic *(T)*, lumbar *(L)*, and sacral *(S)* spine shows the normal spine curvature and the distal point of the sacrum. **B:** A transverse view through one spinal vertebra shows the vertebral body ossification center *(v)* anteriorly and the paired posterior ossification centers *(p)*. The normal posterior elements may be parallel or convergent (as seen here) but should never diverge. The spine should be evaluated in both coronal and transverse planes.

one-third of cases it is a nonspecific complex mass representing an adnexal hematoma. A living ectopic embryo is seen in 17% of cases. The ectopic pregnancy is almost always on the same side as the ovarian corpus luteum, which can usually be seen with ultrasound. The corpus luteum is usually round and hypoechoic and can resemble an ectopic gestational sac except for the important distinction that it is intraovarian, while ectopic pregnancies are usually tubal. It is very important for the sonographer not to mistake the corpus luteum for an ectopic gestational sac.

In the setting of ectopic pregnancy, an intrauterine fluid collection (usually blood) may be mistaken for an intrauter-ine gestational sac. The normal gestational sac is covered by the decidual capsularis and is embedded within the decidual parietalis. This appearance has been called the "double decidual sac sign" (resembling a sac within a sac). The pseudo-gestational sac of an ectopic pregnancy demonstrates a single layer of decidual reaction around a fluid collection. Features of the normal gestational sac are reviewed in Figure 3.

In the very early stage of an ectopic pregnancy (at the lowest maternal serum hCG levels), the only sonographic finding may be echogenic fluid (representing blood) within the fallopian tube or free within the peritoneal space. The posterior cul-de-sac is well seen with vaginal ultrasound, and the

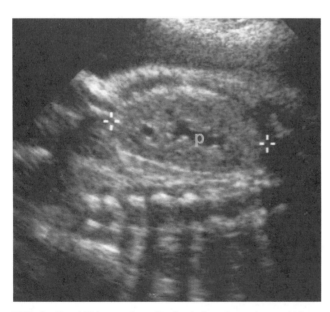

FIG. 9. Fetal kidneys. Longitudinal view through one kidney (calipers) shows that the renal parenchyma is usually hypoechoic relative to other abdominal structures. A small amount of fluid can normally be seen in the renal pelvis *(p)*. (See Fig. 1 for a transverse view through fetal kidneys.)

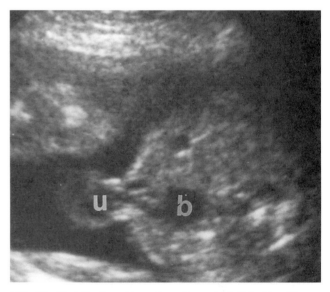

FIG. 10. Umbilical cord insertion site and fetal bladder. Transverse view of the lower abdomen shows a normal umbilical cord insertion site *(u)*. The intact skin at the cord insertion site is clearly seen. A fluid-filled urinary bladder *(b)* is also present. After 13 weeks, a fluid-filled urinary bladder is almost always seen.

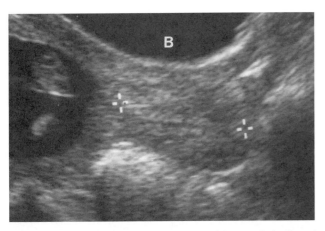

FIG. 11. Cervix. A midline sagittal image of the cervix (calipers) is obtained through a full maternal bladder *(B)*. The internal cervical os (near the left-sided caliper) is clear of placental tissue. Cervical length was normal.

presence of blood in the peritoneal space may be the only ultrasound finding in 15% of ectopic pregnancies. Nonclotted blood is faintly echogenic at high gain settings, while large hemorrhages will clot and have the sonographic appearance of a complex or septated mass. Normal pregnancies also may demonstrate peritoneal fluid, but usually this fluid is serous in nature and on ultrasound evaluation contains few to no internal echoes. The presence of echogenic fluid in the cul-de-sac should alert the sonographer to the probable presence of an ectopic pregnancy.

The use of Doppler techniques can increase the sensitivity of ultrasound for detecting ectopic pregnancies.[22] Color Doppler helps identify the sometimes subtle echogenic ring of an ectopic gestational sac as it lights up with color. Investigators have found that without the use of color Doppler, 2% to 16% of ectopic pregnancies may be overlooked.[19] Pulsed Doppler interrogation reveals a high-velocity (peak frequencies of 2 to 4 kHz), low-resistive (resistive indices of 0.18 to

TABLE 3. *Normal first-trimester ultrasound features*

Gestational sac (GS)
  Round or oval
  Located within fundus or body of uterus
  Echogenic borders
  Eccentric position within endometrium
  Can be seen as early as 4.5 weeks' menstrual age
Yolk Sac
  First structure seen within GS
  Seen transvaginally when GS measures > 10 mm
  Measures < 6 mm
  Round or slightly oval
Embryo
  Seen transvaginally when GS measures > 20 mm
  Cardiac activity seen if embryo measures > 5 mm
  Heart rate should be > 80 beats per minute
  Unique anatomic features: rhombencephalon, physiologic
    bowel herniation

TABLE 4. *Combined data comparing menstrual age with mean gestational sac diameter, crown-rump length, and serum hCG levels*

Menstrual age		Gestational sac size (mm)	Crown-rump length (cm)	hCG Level (first IRP), mean IU/l
Days	Weeks			
30	4.3	—	—	—
31	4.4	—	—	—
32	4.6	3	—	1710
33	4.7	4	—	2320
34	4.9	5	—	3100
35	5.0	5.5	—	4090
36	5.1	6	—	5340
37	5.3	7	—	6880
38	5.4	8	—	8770
39	5.6	9	—	11,040
40	5.7	10	0.2	13,730
41	5.9	11	0.3	15,300
42	6.0	12	0.35	16,870
43	6.1	13	0.4	20,480
44	6.3	14	0.5	24,560
45	6.4	15	0.6	29,110
46	6.6	16	0.7	34,100
47	6.7	17	0.8	39,460
48	6.9	18	0.9	45,120
49	7.0	19	0.95	50,970
50	7.1	20	1.0	56,900
51	7.3	21	1.1	62,760
52	7.4	22	1.2	68,390
53	7.6	23	1.3	73,640
54	7.7	24	1.4	78,350
55	7.9	25	1.5	82,370
56	8.0	26	1.6	85,560
57	8.1	26.5	1.7	—
58	8.3	27	1.8	—
59	8.4	28	1.9	—
60	8.6	29	2.0	—
61	8.7	30	2.1	—
62	8.9	31	2.2	—
63	9.0	32	2.3	—
64	9.1	33	2.4	—
65	9.3	34	2.5	—
66	9.4	35	2.6	—
67	9.6	36	2.8	—
68	9.7	37	2.9	—
69	9.9	38	3.0	—
70	10.0	39	3.1	—
71	10.1	40	3.2	—
72	10.3	41	3.4	—
73	10.4	42	3.5	—
74	10.6	43	3.7	—
75	10.7	44	3.8	—
76	10.9	45	4.0	—
77	11.0	46	4.1	—
78	11.1	47	4.2	—
79	11.3	48	4.4	—
80	11.4	49	4.6	—
81	11.6	50	4.8	—
82	11.7	51	5.0	—
83	11.9	52	5.2	—
84	12.0	53	5.4	—

hCG, human chorionic gonadotropin.

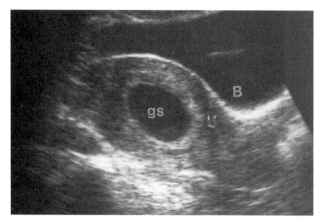

FIG. 12. Anembryonic gestational sac (blighted ovum). A large intrauterine gestational sac *(gs)* is present without any internal structures. A gestational sac greater than 25 mm (by transabdominal scanning) should contain a living embryo (*U,* uterus; *B,* maternal bladder).

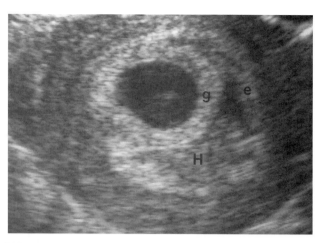

FIG. 14. Perigestational hemorrhage. A moderately echogenic hemorrhage *(H)* is seen adjacent to an early gestational sac *(g)* (*e,* endometrial decidual reaction).

0.58) blood flow pattern in the trophoblast or peritrophoblast tissue[22] (Fig. 16). However, Doppler criteria alone may be misleading, since the ovarian corpus luteum may also demonstrate a low-resistive (albeit usually not high-velocity) waveform pattern.

Gestational Trophoblastic Disease

With the use of serum hCG blood tests and early monitoring of pregnancy, molar pregnancies are most commonly detected in the first or early second trimester. Ultrasound intrauterine findings vary. An empty gestational sac (anembryonic pregnancy or blighted ovum) is frequently seen. An enlarged uterus filled with a multicystic mass represents the

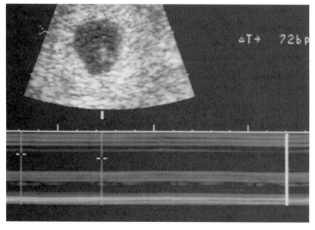

FIG. 13. Embryo bradycardia. M-mode interrogation of the heart rate in this asymptomatic early pregnancy showed a heart rate of only 72 beats per minute (normal is greater than 90). Five days later, the patient returned for a follow-up examination, and no cardiac activity was seen.

classic molar pregnancy finding (Fig. 17). Rarely, a fetus is seen in conjunction with an abnormal-appearing placenta, and this usually represents a coexistent molar pregnancy (complete mole and normal twin) or a partial molar pregnancy (triploidy karyotype).

Fetal Biometry and Growth

Fetal Biometry

Fetal biometry refers to the comparison of measured fetal biometric parameters to established normal data to determine the gestational age or to assess fetal growth. The most sensitive measurement for determining gestational age is the crown-rump length obtained during the first trimester. After the first trimester, the fetus is too large to measure in its entirety; therefore, selected structures are measured. A variety of structures could be measured, but four standard measurements are routinely performed and have been found to correspond well with menstrual age in normal fetuses. The four measurements routinely obtained are the biparietal diameter (BPD), the head circumference (HC), the abdominal circumference (AC), and the femur length (FL). Figures 4 to 6 show examples of these measurements. Table 5 compares biometric data with specific menstrual ages. In general, fetal measurements are obtained and then averaged to determine the ultrasonographic estimate of the fetal age.

Normal fetuses vary in size at the same gestational age. This variability in fetal size increases with increasing gestational age, and thus the ability of ultrasound measurements to accurately date a pregnancy decreases as a pregnancy advances. The effects of fetal biometric variability can be reduced by averaging fetal biometric data. This practice, however, does not eliminate variability. Early in the second trimester (12 to 18 weeks), the estimated gestational age determined by fetal biometric measurements is accurate to within 1 week of the true gestational age, while late in the

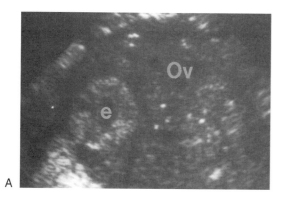

A

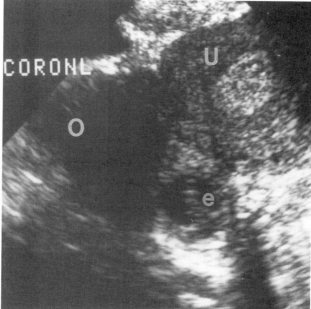

B

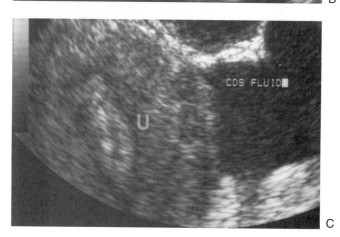

C

FIG. 15. Ectopic pregnancy: ultrasound findings in three cases. **A:** An ectopic gestational sac can resemble an intrauterine gestational sac. In this case, a small echogenic ring-like mass *(e)* adjacent to but separate from the ovary *(ov)* proved to be a nonruptured ectopic pregnancy. **B:** A normal-appearing yolk sac and a living embryo were seen in this ectopic gestational sac *(e)*. A prominent uterine decidual reaction *(U)* can be seen, and the ectopic gestation is usually on the side of the ovary *(o)* containing the corpus luteum. **C:** Echogenic cul-de-sac fluid may be the only ultrasound finding when an ectopic pregnancy is present. The fluid usually contains diffuse low- or medium-level echoes and represents nonclotted blood.

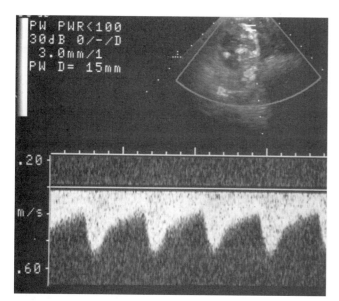

FIG. 16. Doppler interrogation of ectopic pregnancy. A high-velocity and low-impedance blood flow pattern is most typical of the trophoblastic or peritrophoblastic tissue surrounding an ectopic gestational sac. Color Doppler can help identify small ectopic gestational sacs that are difficult to see with gray imaging alone.

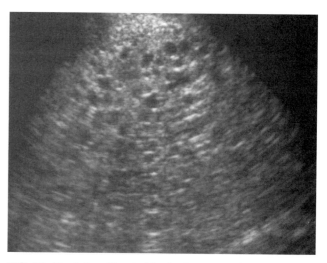

FIG. 17. Gestational trophoblastic disease (molar pregnancy). The uterus is enlarged, and the uterine cavity is filled with innumerable tiny cysts.

TABLE 5. *Predicted fetal measurements at specific menstrual ages*

Menstrual age (wks)	Biparietal diameter (cm)	Head circumference (cm)	Abdominal circumference (cm)	Femur length (cm)
12.0	1.7	6.8	4.6	0.7
12.5	1.9	7.5	5.3	0.9
13.0	2.1	8.2	6.0	1.1
13.5	2.3	8.9	6.7	1.2
14.0	2.5	9.7	7.3	1.4
14.5	2.7	10.4	8.0	1.6
15.0	2.9	11.0	8.6	1.7
15.5	3.1	11.7	9.3	1.9
16.0	3.2	12.4	9.9	2.0
16.5	3.4	13.1	10.6	2.2
17.0	3.6	13.8	11.2	2.4
17.5	3.8	14.4	11.9	2.5
18.0	3.9	15.1	12.5	2.7
18.5	4.1	15.8	13.1	2.8
19.0	4.3	16.4	13.7	3.0
19.5	4.5	17.0	14.4	3.1
20.0	4.6	17.7	15.0	3.3
20.5	4.8	18.3	15.6	3.4
21.0	5.0	18.9	16.2	3.5
21.5	5.1	19.5	16.8	3.7
22.0	5.3	20.1	17.4	3.8
22.5	5.5	20.7	17.9	4.0
23.0	5.6	21.3	18.5	4.1
23.5	5.8	21.9	19.1	4.2
24.0	5.9	22.4	19.7	4.4
24.5	6.1	23.0	20.2	4.5
25.0	6.2	23.5	20.8	4.6
25.5	6.4	24.1	21.3	4.7
26.0	6.5	24.6	21.9	4.9
26.5	6.7	25.1	22.4	5.0
27.0	6.8	25.6	23.0	5.1
27.5	6.9	26.1	23.5	5.2
28.0	7.1	26.6	24.0	5.4
28.5	7.2	27.1	24.6	5.5
29.0	7.3	27.5	25.1	5.6
29.5	7.5	28.0	25.6	5.7
30.0	7.6	28.4	26.1	5.8
30.5	7.7	28.8	26.6	5.9
31.0	7.8	29.3	27.1	6.0
31.5	7.9	29.7	27.6	6.1
32.0	8.1	30.1	28.1	6.2
32.5	8.2	30.4	28.6	6.3
33.0	8.3	30.8	29.1	6.4
33.5	8.4	31.2	29.5	6.5
34.0	8.5	31.5	30.0	6.6
34.5	8.6	31.8	30.5	6.7
35.0	8.7	32.2	30.9	6.8
35.5	8.8	32.5	31.4	6.9
36.0	8.9	32.8	31.8	7.0
36.5	8.9	33.0	32.3	7.1
37.0	9.0	33.3	32.7	7.2
37.5	9.1	33.5	33.2	7.3
38.0	9.2	33.8	33.6	7.4
38.5	9.2	34.0	34.0	7.4
39.0	9.3	34.2	34.4	7.5
39.5	9.4	34.4	34.8	7.6
40.0	9.4	34.6	35.3	7.7

menstrual age is between 18.5 to 21.5 weeks. Table 6 reviews the practice of averaging biometric data and summarizes the expected fetal measurement variability seen at different gestational ages.

Establishing the gestational age by ultrasound measurements pertains to normal fetuses, but distinctly abnormal measurements should not be averaged away. For example, a markedly short femur should not be included in the average of the measurements obtained. Instead, the physician should be concerned about the possibility of a skeletal dysplasia. Another special circumstance involves measurements of the fetal head. The BPD may be an inaccurate measurement when the fetal head is dolichocephalic (long and narrow) or brachycephalic (round and broad). If the sonographer is unsure as to whether the head shape is normal, the cephalic index can be easily computed. The occipitofrontal distance is divided by the BPD (both are taken as outer calvarial measurements), and this value is multiplied by 100. The normal cephalic index is 78.3 ± 4.3. If the cephalic index is abnormal, the HC, not the BPD, should be used in estimating menstrual age.

Fetal Growth

Fetal growth can be evaluated only when there is an accurate estimate of fetal age. The objective standard for evaluating fetal growth is based on the calculation of a fetal weight percentile (based on known, previously established gestational age). Fetal weight percentiles can be obtained by following a three-step process:

1. Determine the fetal age based on confident recount of the first day of the last normal menstrual period (LNMP) or based on prior ultrasound examinations (the earliest ultrasound examination should be used).
2. Estimate the fetal weight. Many formulas exist for the estimation of fetal weight, and most ultrasound equipment includes computer software that calculates an estimated fetal weight based on biometric data. The formula of Had-

TABLE 6. *Variability of ultrasound measurements in predicting menstrual age*

Criterion	Trimester	Variation
Last menstrual period	—	3 wk
Crown-rump length	1	5 d
Biparietal diameter (BPD)/ head circumference (HC)	1–2	10 d
BPD/HC	3	2–3 wk
Femur length (FL)	1–2	10 d
Femur length	3	3 wk
Abdominal circumference (AC)	1–2	12–14 d
Abdominal circumference	3	2–3 wk
Averaging of measurements: BPD/HC/AC/FL	1–2	7–10 d
Averaging of measurements: BPD/HC/AC/FL	3	2.3–2.4 wk

third trimester variability approaches 2.5 weeks. Therefore, if in the midthird trimester the sonographically determined gestational age is 34 weeks (based on the average of fetal biometric data), the actual menstrual age is between 31.5 to 36.5 weeks, whereas if in the midsecond trimester the sonographically determined gestational age is 20 weeks, the actual lock et al.[11] uses all fetal biometric data (BPD, HC, AC, and FL) and is log 10 weight = $1.5662 - 0.0108$ (HC) + 0.0468 (AC) + 0.171 (FL) + 0.00034 (HC)(HC) $- 0.003685$ (AC $\times$ FL). This formula is sensitive to 7.5% of actual fetal weight (1 SD) and obviously is used most readily with the help of a computer.

3. Compare the estimated fetal weight to the range of normal fetal weights for gestational age to determine a fetal weight percentile. Fetal weight percentiles for given gestational ages are shown in Table 7. It is generally accepted that normal fetal weight should be between the 10th and the 90th percentiles. Since abnormally small or large fetuses are at an increased risk for a poor outcome, their identification *in utero* is very important.

A fetus with estimated weight less than the 10th percentile is considered small for gestational age (SGA). In turn, this diagnosis may be due to intrauterine growth restriction (IUGR) or to the fetus simply having reached its hereditary growth potential. Many practitioners and investigators use the two terms, SGA and IUGR, synonymously. IUGR can result from many maternal or fetal causes, as outlined in Table 8. Placental insufficiency, either primary or secondary, is the most common cause of IUGR. Two different patterns of IUGR—

TABLE 8. *Intrauterine growth restriction: causes and ultrasound patterns*

Causes	Classic ultrasound growth pattern
Primary placental insufficiency	Late onset Asymmetric growth restriction (abdominal circumference and femur length affected most severely)
Maternal and secondary placental causes (hypertension, collagen vascular disease, renal disease, uterine anomalies or myomas, poor nutrition, smoking, excessive alcohol consumption, chronic placental abruption)	Late onset Asymmetric growth restriction
Intrauterine infection	Early onset Symmetric growth restriction (all biometric measurements equally affected)
Fetal chromosome anomaly (trisomy 18, trisomy 13, triploidy)	Early onset Symmetric growth restriction (may be asymmetric but severe with triploidy)

symmetric and asymmetric—have been described. With the symmetric pattern, the fetus measures SGA with regard to all biometric parameters (fetal head, abdomen, femur), while with the asymmetric pattern, the fetal head is spared. The symmetric pattern is associated with a worse prognosis; the asymmetric pattern usually is associated with late second- or third-trimester placental insufficiency. IUGR may also be classified as either early or late in gestational age of onset. The early onset of IUGR is associated with a more dismal prognosis. Table 8 compares the classic patterns of IUGR.

Amniotic Fluid and Fetal Well-being

Assessment of amniotic fluid should be performed at every second- and third-trimester ultrasound examination. There are several ways that this can be achieved. Subjective assessment of amniotic fluid relies on the ability of the sonographer to sense the overall amount of amniotic fluid present during the real-time examination. Experienced sonographers use this technique with reasonable accuracy. Early in the second trimester, the volume occupied by the fetus is about equal to the volume of amniotic fluid. The fetus does not appear confined within the uterus and is seen to move freely in a bath of fluid. Throughout the second and third trimesters, the volume of the fetus increases in comparison to the volume of fluid, and late in pregnancy the amount of fluid appears small in comparison with the fetus.

Objective methods for measuring amniotic fluid should be used when fluid abnormalities are suspected or when an

TABLE 7. *Estimated fetal weight percentiles*

Menstrual week	Percentiles (g)				
	3rd	10th	50th	90th	97th
10	26	29	35	41	44
11	34	37	45	53	56
12	43	48	58	68	73
13	55	61	73	85	91
14	70	77	93	109	116
15	88	97	117	137	146
16	110	121	146	171	183
17	136	150	181	212	226
18	167	185	223	261	279
19	205	227	273	319	341
20	248	275	331	387	414
21	299	331	399	467	499
22	359	398	478	559	598
23	426	471	568	665	710
24	503	556	670	784	838
25	589	652	785	918	981
26	685	758	913	1068	1141
27	791	876	1055	1234	1319
28	908	1004	1210	1416	1513
29	1034	1145	1379	1613	1724
30	1169	1294	1559	1824	1649
31	1313	1453	1751	2049	2189
32	1465	1621	1953	2285	2441
33	1622	1794	2162	2530	2703
34	1783	1973	2377	2781	2971
35	1946	2154	2595	3036	3244
36	2110	2335	2813	3291	3516
37	2271	2513	3028	3543	3785
38	2427	2686	3236	3786	4045
39	2576	2851	3435	4019	4294
40	2714	3004	3619	4234	4524

inexperienced sonographer is performing the examination. Two routinely used objective methods for measuring amniotic fluid are (1) measurement of a maximum vertical pocket (MVP) of fluid and (2) calculation of the amniotic fluid index (AFI). The MVP is obtained by measuring the anteroposterior dimension (depth) of the largest pocket of amniotic fluid that is void of fetal parts or umbilical cord. A pocket measuring 2 to 8 cm is considered normal. The AFI is calculated by dividing the uterus into four equal segments and measuring the largest pocket of fluid (anteroposterior measurement excluding fetal parts and umbilical cord) in each quadrant and then adding the four numbers together (Fig. 18). The AFI varies with gestational age, but as a rule of thumb, the normal AFI falls between 10 and 24 cm after 30 weeks' gestational age.

Oligohydramnios and Polyhydramnios

Oligohydramnios is defined as a deficiency in amniotic fluid and occurs in 0.5% to 5.5% of all pregnancies. Severe oligohydramnios, defined as an AFI of less than 2, carries with it a perinatal mortality rate 40 to 50 times greater than that of normal pregnancies (Fig. 19). Causes of oligohydramnios are summarized in Table 9. The most common cause of oligohydramnios is premature rupture of the membranes. Ultrasound can help identify fetal causes, such as renal agenesis and severe placental insufficiency.

Polyhydramnios, defined as an excess of amniotic fluid, complicates 1% to 4% of all pregnancies. It is associated with significant maternal and fetal morbidity. Table 10 summarizes the causes of polyhydramnios. The vast majority of

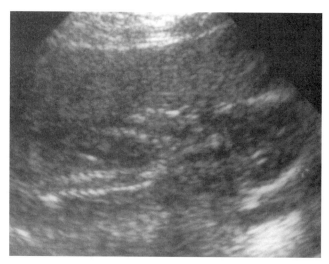

FIG. 19. Severe oligohydramnios. No amniotic fluid surrounds the fetus (skeletal structures seen). In this case, oligohydramnios was secondary to renal agenesis.

cases of polyhydramnios are mild in nature and of uncertain cause (idiopathic). However, idiopathic polyhydramnios should always be considered a diagnosis of exclusion. Ultrasound can be used to identify fetal anomalies and sequelae of infections that may explain moderate or severe polyhydramnios (Fig. 20).

Fetal Well-being: Biophysical Profile Test

Ultrasound can be used to assess the fetal biophysical state as it reflects fetal well-being or fetal distress due to hypoxemia and acidosis. The best known method is the biophysical profile test (Table 11).[14] Five variables are assessed: amniotic fluid volume, fetal movement, fetal tone, fetal breathing, and heart rate variability. Ultrasound is used for four of the variables, while the nonstress test (see Chapter 15) assesses heart rate variability. A score of 2 is given if

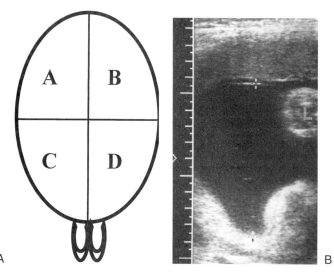

FIG. 18. Amniotic fluid index (AFI) calculation. **A:** The uterus is divided into four equal quadrants, and the largest vertical pocket of fluid in each quadrant is measured in centimeters (A, B, C, D). The sum of the four measurements is the AFI. **B:** The largest measurable vertical pocket in each quadrant should be void of fetal parts or umbilical cord (L, limb).

TABLE 9. *Common causes for oligohydramnios*

Pregnancy related
   Premature rupture of membranes
   Postdate pregnancy
   Intrauterine infection
   Placental insufficiency or abruption
Fetal genitourinary anomalies
   Renal atresia
   Bilateral renal anomalies
   Bladder outlet obstruction
   Posterior urethral valves
Fetal chromosome anomalies
Intrauterine growth restriction
Pharmaceutical causes
   Prostaglandin synthetase inhibitors
   Angiotensin-converting enzyme inhibitors
Idiopathic

TABLE 10. *Common causes for polyhydramnios*

Idiopathic: 60%–70%
Fetal macrosomia: with or without maternal diabetes
Maternal diabetes mellitus
Intrauterine infection
Twin-twin transfusion
Fetal anomalies
   Central nervous system disorders affecting fetal swallowing
   Gastrointestinal atresia and obstruction
   Fetal masses
   Cardiovascular anomalies
   Hydrops fetalis of any cause
   Musculoskeletal anomalies affecting fetal movement

TABLE 11. *Biophysical profile test: ultrasound parameters*

Fetal parameter: 30-minute observation	Score of 2 or 0
Amniotic fluid	2 = at least one pocket of fluid measuring 2 cm in perpendicular planes
	0 = failure to meet criterion for score of 2
Fetal movement	2 = at least three discrete gross body movements (limb and/or trunk)
	0 = failure to meet criterion for score of 2
Fetal tone	2 = at least one episode of limb extension (from flexion) with return to flexion
	0 = failure to meet criterion for score of 2
Fetal breathing	2 = at least one episode of breathing lasting 30 seconds without interruption
	0 = failure to meet criterion for score of 2

the fetus meets established criteria for a given variable, and a score of 0 is given if the fetus fails to meet the criteria for the variable. The final biophysical profile score is the sum of the individual variables, and it may be 0, 2, 4, 6, 8, or 10. The fetus is allowed 30 minutes to achieve the established criteria. The goal of the test is to identify the fetus at risk for *in utero* compromise or demise for whom intervention is possible.

Fetal Anatomy and Common Anomalies

As shown in Figures 4 through 10, certain fetal anatomic structures are routinely documented as recommended by published ultrasound guidelines. Some of the key required ultrasound views and some common anomalies are discussed below.

Fetal Neural Tube: Normal Anatomy and Neural Tube Defects

Neural tube defects (NTDs) are common, occurring in 1 in 500 to 600 live births and in 3% of all spontaneous abortions. With the widespread use of maternal serum alpha-fetoprotein

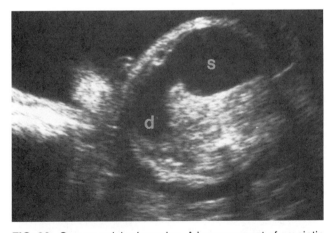

FIG. 20. Severe polyhydramnios. A large amount of amniotic fluid is present anterior to the gravity-dependent fetus. Visualization of a dilated fetal stomach and duodenum enabled the sonologist to correctly identify duodenal atresia as the cause of the severe polyhydramnios.

screening and high-resolution ultrasound, nearly all NTDs can be detected prenatally. NTDs are usually sporadic, and multiple factors have been cited as potential causes. Maternal causes of NTDs include diabetes mellitus and maternal use of valproic acid (Depakene) for seizure disorders. Chromosomal abnormalities associated with NTDs include trisomy 18, trisomy 13, and triploidy. The recurrence risk is estimated at 3% to 5%, although the use of folic acid supplementation prior to and during early pregnancy reduces the recurrence risk by 50%. The three major types of NTDs are spina bifida, anencephaly, and encephalocele.

Normal Calvarium and Spine Anatomy

As shown in Figure 4, three standard views are obtained through the fetal head.[8] In the first view, the BPD and HC measurements are obtained on an axial image through the calvarium at the level of the thalamus and the cavum septi pellucidi. This view is often called the transthalamic view. On this image, the frontal horns of the lateral ventricles are also seen. On the second standard view, the lateral cerebral ventricles are visualized on an axial view superior to the transthalamic view. On this view, the echogenic choroid plexus is seen filling most of the lateral ventricles. However, the choroid plexus is not present in the frontal or occipital horns of the lateral ventricles. Standard measurement of the diameter of the lateral ventricle can be performed on this view and is generally less than 10 mm (see Fig. 4B). The third standard view through the fetal calvarium is the posterior fossa view (see Fig. 4C). By angling the transducer 10 to 15 degrees caudal to the transthalamic view (in the direction of the posterior fossa), the sonographer obtains an image (from anterior to posterior) of the midbrain, cerebellum, cisterna magna, posterior skull, and the nuchal skin.

The fetal spine is a complex three-dimensional structure that presents a unique ultrasonographic challenge. Visualization of the fetal spine depends on the presence of ossification centers. The three ossification centers, one anterior and paired dorsal centers, start to ossify at 8 weeks menstrual age. The paired dorsal ossification centers may be positioned parallel to each other or converge toward the midline, but they should never diverge. The spine should always be imaged in two planes (see Fig. 8). Longitudinal views (coronal or sagittal) through the spine provide the best overview of the spine; however, transverse views are best for visualizing the posterior elements.

Neural Tube Defects: Spina Bifida, Anencephaly, Exencephaly

Almost all cases of spina bifida are manifested by the Arnold-Chiari II malformation syndrome, and therefore abnormalities are seen both in the calvarium and the spine. Before 24 weeks, the spinal dysraphism may be difficult to detect, while the cranial abnormalities are more obvious and are present in 99% of cases.[23] Interestingly, the severity of cranial findings does not reflect the severity of spinal dys-

raphism. The three classic findings in the fetal head associated with spina bifida are (1) obliteration of the cisterna magna with possible associated compression of the cerebellum, (2) ventricular dilatation, and (3) concave deformity of the frontal bones (Fig. 21). Of the three signs, the most important and sensitive for spina bifida is the obliteration of the normal cisterna magna.

The cisterna magna is a fluid-filled structure located posterior to the normally bilobed cerebellum and should measure between 3 and 10 mm in anteroposterior dimension after 15 weeks (see Fig. 4C). When an open spina bifida is present, compressive forces on the posterior fossa cause caudal displacement of the cerebellum and obliteration of the cisterna magna. With severe compression, the cerebellum may lie against the occiput of the skull and assume a crescentic ("banana") configuration. It is important to stress that cisterna magna obliteration is almost always present with spina bifida but the "banana" sign is not.

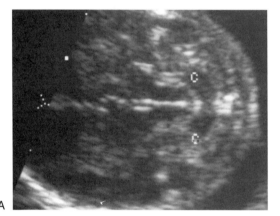

A

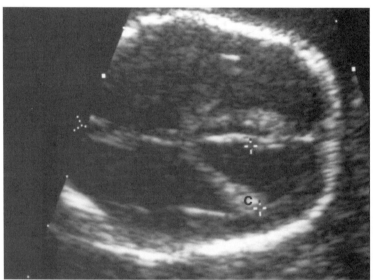

B

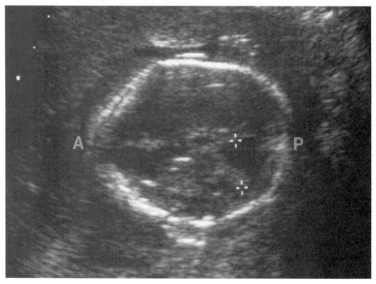

C

FIG. 21. Cranial findings in spina bifida. **A:** The cerebellum (c) is compressed against the occipital bone and assumes a crescent shape ("banana sign"). The normally seen fluid-filled cisterna magna is obliterated. (Compare with Fig. 4C, a normal posterior fossa view.) **B:** The lateral ventricles are dilated (+ calipers), and the choroid plexus (c) hangs away from the midline. **C:** Mild concavity of the frontal bones is also seen ("lemon sign"), but this finding can be normal in the second trimester and tends to resolve in the third trimester even when spina bifida is present (A, anterior skull; P, posterior skull).

Enlargement of the cerebral ventricles and frontal bone concavity are nonspecific signs that often are associated with spina bifida. Ventriculomegaly is best detected on the axial image at the level of the atria of the ventricles. The ventricle should not measure greater than 10 mm in transverse dimension on the standard image obtained at this level. The most common cause for fetal ventriculomegaly is spina bifida, and 75% of fetuses with spina bifida have some degree of ventriculomegaly. Frontal bone concavity, however, is not specific for spina bifida and may occur in up to 1% of normal fetuses. When present, the convex frontal deformity gives the skull a lemon configuration. Of the three described cranial findings, convex frontal deformity is the least sensitive and specific for spina bifida, and care should be taken not to misdiagnose normal mild frontal concavity as anomalous.

Sonographic evaluation of the fetal spine is more challenging than that of the fetal head. Coronal views through the posterior elements show focal widening of the normally parallel line of posterior ossification centers, while the transverse view confirms the divergent or U-shaped configuration of the posterior elements (Fig. 22). Sagittal views are least helpful but together with the transverse views may confirm the presence or absence of a meningocele fluid-filled sac. Open spina bifida by definition implies that a skin defect is present posterior to the spinal dysraphism, but a meningocele or meningomyelocele sac may or may not be seen. The extent of spinal dysraphism can usually be determined prenatally. Sonographic landmarks helpful in determining the level of the defect include the twelfth rib, associated with the T-12 level, and the top of the iliac wing, associated with the S-1 level. Fetuses with spina bifida are

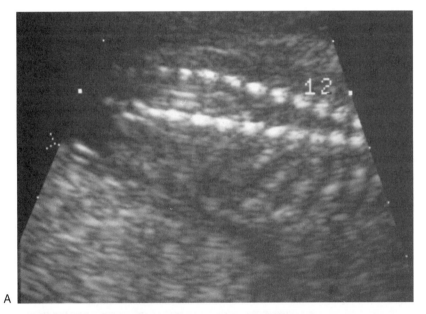

A

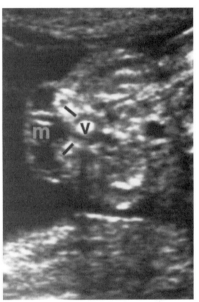

C

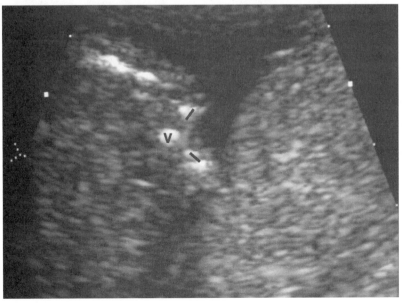

B

FIG. 22. Spina bifida. **A:** Coronal view through the lumbar and sacral spine shows divergence of the normally converging posterior elements. The twelfth rib is identified, and therefore the sonographer can estimate the level of involvement (all of lumbosacral spine in this case). **B:** Transverse view confirms the findings seen on the coronal view. The posterior elements are divergent *(black lines)*, and there is no skin covering the back of the sacrum. **C:** Transverse view of another fetus with spina bifida shows the presence of a meningocele sac *(m)* (*V*, vertebral body ossification center).

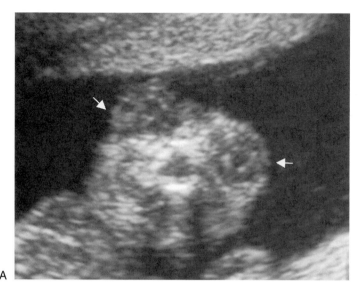
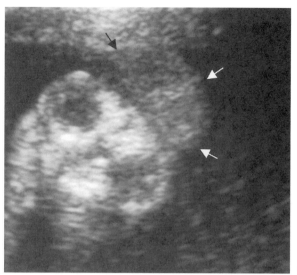

A

B

FIG. 23. Anencephaly. **A:** Frontal view of the fetal head demonstrates the distinct absence of a bony calvarium superior to the fetal orbits *(arrows)*. **B:** The dysplastic calvarial tissue superior to the orbits *(arrows)* is called angiomatous stroma.

at an increased risk for chromosomal anomalies (trisomy 18, trisomy 13, and triploidy), and chromosome analysis should be considered.

Two other NTDs are anencephaly and encephalocele. Anencephaly occurs with nearly equal frequency as spina bifida, whereas encephalocele is more rare, affecting 1 in 2000 to 10,000 newborns. Anencephaly is four times more common in female than male fetuses, is virtually 100% detectable with prenatal ultrasound, and is uniformly fatal. In this condition, failure of rostral neuropore closure leads to absence of a calvarium. The brain is thus exposed to amniotic fluid and repeated trauma, a noxious environment that eventually leads to brain destruction. The midbrain, skull base, fetal face, and brain stem are usually minimally impacted. The sonographic hallmark of anencephaly is the absence of a cranial vault superior to the orbits (Fig. 23). Dysplastic brain tissue (called angiomatous stroma) can be seen. While early diagnosis of this devastating anomaly is possible, care should be taken not to attempt diagnosis of calvarial absence prior to calvarial ossification (about 13 weeks' menstrual age).

Encephalocele describes protrusion of brain and/or meninges containing cerebrospinal fluid through a cranial defect. Occipital encephalocele is most common in the United States, accounting for 70% of all cases. Defects in the parietal bone, frontal bone, and skull base may also occur. Associated central nervous system anomalies are common and include hydrocephalus, spina bifida, and facial clefts. Meckel-Gruber syndrome is an autosomal-recessive disorder characterized by occipital encephalocele, renal cystic dysplasia, and polydactyly. Ultrasound features of encephalocele depend on the neural components involved and the site of the cranial defect (Fig. 24). The cranial defect should be

seen with confidence in order to accurately diagnose this anomaly. Rarely, a large scalp hemangioma (a relatively benign disorder with normal brain anatomy and an intact calvarium) may mimic an encephalocele.

Fetal Heart

The four-chamber view of the fetal heart is currently considered an adequate screening view for cardiac anomalies. It can be obtained in 95% of fetuses between 18 and 40 weeks. Any abnormality observed on the four-chamber view that cannot be fully explained should be investigated with a complete

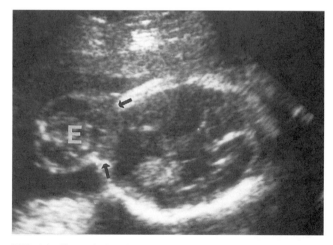

FIG. 24. Encephalocele. A posterior calvarial defect *(arrows)* is present, and brain tissue surrounded by cerebrospinal fluid is seen projecting outside of the confines of the calvarium *(E, encephalocele)*.

fetal echocardiogram. The normal four-chamber heart should show the following ultrasound features (see Fig. 7):

◊ Cardiac axis is to the left (usually at 45 degrees).
◊ Right ventricle and left ventricle are approximately the same size.
◊ Right atrium and left atrium are approximately the same size.
◊ Ventricular septum is intact.
◊ Atrial septum contains the foramen ovale flap that moves from right to left.
◊ Tricuspid valve is slightly inferior to the mitral valve.
◊ Right ventricle contacts the anterior chest wall.
◊ Right ventricle contains a prominent muscular band, called a moderator band, near the apex.

The approach to the abnormal four-chamber view of the heart is reviewed by McGahan[15] and involves a six-step approach that helps characterize the vast majority of cardiac defects. The following six questions should be asked about the abnormal-appearing heart:

◊ *Is the heart in a normal position?* An abnormal cardiac axis is associated with a 50% to 80% fetal mortality rate. Dextrocardia is defined as malposition of the cardiac apex to the right and can be caused by inversion of the normal ventricular relationship or rotation of the heart (dextroversion). The moderator band helps identify the right ventricle in these cases. Alternatively, the heart

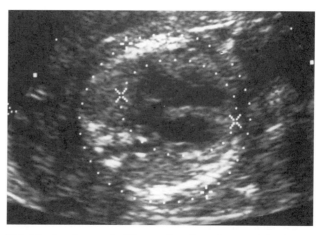

FIG. 26. Cardiomegaly. The cardiac circumference (X calipers) measured greater than 50% of the thoracic circumference (+ calipers). Hydrops fetalis and severe fetal anemia from homozygous α-thalassemia was the cause for heart failure in this case.

may be displaced but otherwise appear normal. The most common cause of cardiac malposition is the presence of a diaphragmatic hernia (Fig. 25).
◊ *Is the heart size normal?* Cardiac circumference can be compared with the chest circumference on the standard four-chamber view. The cardiac circumference should be 50% or less of the chest circumference. An abnormal cardiothoracic ratio (Fig. 26) may result from cardiomegaly, a small chest, or a combination of both.
◊ *Are the ventricles equal in size?* A small left ventricle may be secondary to a variety of hypoplastic left heart syndromes (Fig. 27), or it may be a secondary sign of coarctation of the aorta. Hypoplastic right heart is a complex cardiac anomaly that can be associated with pulmonary artery atresia. A single left or right ventricle may be present if an associated ventricle is atretic.

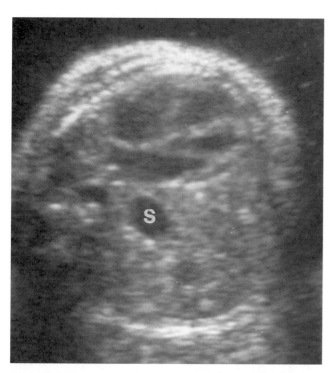

FIG. 25. Abnormal cardiac axis: diaphragmatic hernia. The heart is displaced into the right chest secondary to a left-sided, large diaphragmatic hernia. The fetal stomach *(S)* is seen adjacent to the heart.

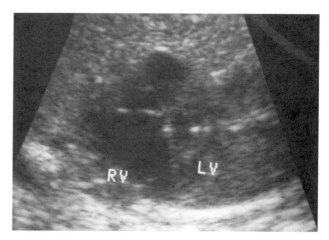

FIG. 27. Hypoplastic left heart. The left ventricle and left atrium are atretic and echogenic, compared to the right ventricle and right atrium.

◊ *Is there a septal defect?* Large ventricular septal defects (VSDs) may be detected with ultrasound, although small to moderate-sized VSDs may be difficult to visualize. VSDs may be associated with other cardiac anomalies, such as tetralogy of Fallot or truncus anomalies (Fig. 28). Atrial septal defects are even more difficult to identify *in utero,* in part because the normal atrial septum is interrupted by the normal foramen ovale flap. Complete atrioventricular septal defect (endocardial cushion defect) is almost always detected with the four-chamber view, and fetuses with this anomaly are at an increased risk for trisomy 21.

◊ *Are the atrioventricular valves in a normal position?* The tricuspid valve is normally located slightly inferior to the mitral valve. Abnormal inferior displacement of the septal leaflet of the tricuspid valve into the right ventricle is a feature of Ebstein anomaly (Fig. 29). Massive right atrial dilatation usually occurs in response to the faulty tricuspid valve. Mitral valve anomalies are infrequently identified *in utero.*

◊ *Is there any abnormality of the endocardium, myocardium, or pericardium?* Focal tiny echogenicities can occur normally in the ventricles, but a large echogenicity should raise the suspicion of a cardiac tumor, such as rhabdomyoma. A small amount of pericardial fluid is usually a normal finding (Fig. 30), but pericardial fluid collections measuring greater than 2 mm in width may be pathologic.

The sensitivity of the four-chamber view for detecting congenital heart disease (CHD) is debatable. Some investigators have shown that only 63% of CHDs are diagnosed with the use of the four-chamber view only. Meanwhile, the sensitivity for detecting CHD increases to 83% with the addition of great vessel outflow tract views. Future published guidelines

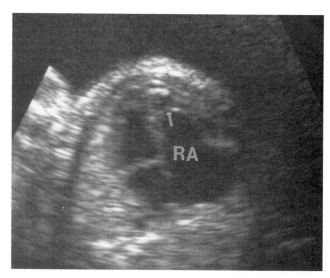

FIG. 29. Ebstein anomaly. The right atrium *(RA)* is enlarged and the right ventricle is small secondary to displacement of the tricuspid valve *(arrow)* toward the ventricular apex.

may recommend the routine evaluation of outflow tracts. Normal right ventricular and left ventricular outflow tract views are demonstrated in Figure 31.

Fetal Abdomen and Pelvis

The routine views through the fetal abdomen and pelvis (see Figs. 1, 5, 9, and 10) should measure and document the following: (1) the AC, (2) the fluid-filled gastric fundus (usually seen on the AC view), (3) the umbilical cord insertion site, (4) the kidneys, and (5) the urinary bladder. If these four images are routinely obtained, the sonologist can detect 96% of

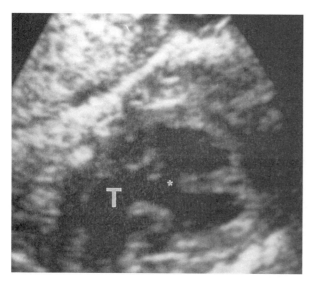

FIG. 28. Ventricular septal defect (VSD) with truncus anomaly. A membranous VSD *(asterisk)* is seen, and a single outflow vessel *(T)* was identified.

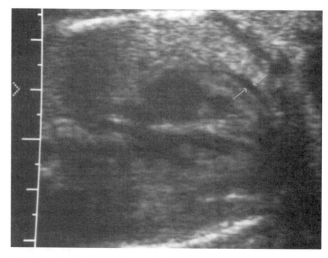

FIG. 30. Small pericardial effusion. A small amount of pericardial fluid *(arrows)* can normally be seen and usually measures less than 2 mm.

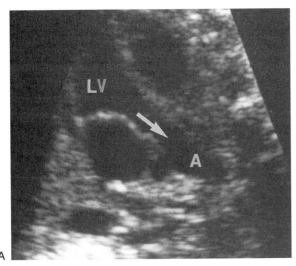
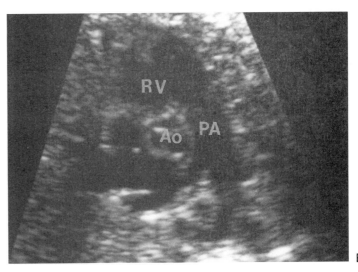

A   B

FIG. 31. Ventricular outflow tracts. **A:** Long-axis view of the left ventricular outflow tract shows that the aorta *(A)* arises from the left ventricle *(LV)*. **B:** Short-axis view of the right ventricular outflow tract shows the pulmonary artery *(PA)* arising from the right ventricle *(RV)*. The pulmonary artery is positioned anterior to the aorta *(Ao)*.

abdominal and pelvic anomalies.[12] Measurement of the fetal AC should be performed using a round-shaped transverse image obtained at the level of the fluid-filled gastric fundus and junction of the left and right portal veins. The subcutaneous tissues should be included in the measurement. Visualization of the umbilical cord insertion site should be obtained in the transverse plane, and care should be taken to visualize the skin margins on either side of the cord insertion since gastroschisis defects are usually periumbilical and small. The fetal bowel is seen on this view as well and should be isoechoic or slightly echogenic, compared to the fetal liver. Small bowel rarely contains fluid prior to the third trimester; in later pregnancy, fluid-filled bowel should not measure greater than 6 mm in diameter. Large bowel may contain meconium in the third trimester and should not be mistaken for a mass. The fetal kidneys are best seen on a transverse view through the fetal flank. Kidneys are usually slightly hypoechoic in comparison to bowel. The fetal renal pelvis may contain a small amount of urine normally. The fetal bladder is best seen on a transverse view through the pelvis (this view can be combined with a cross-sectional sacrum image).

Abdominal Wall Defects

Common abdominal wall defects include omphalocele and gastroschisis. The sonographer should be able to consistently detect these anomalies and differentiate between them. Both occur in approximately 1 in 4000 live births and carry an excellent prognosis when they occur as isolated defects.

 With an omphalocele, herniation of abdominal contents (usually liver with or without bowel and, rarely, only bowel) occurs into the base of the umbilical cord (Fig. 32). The umbilical cord inserts on the omphalocele, usually at the apex

but sometimes eccentrically. A membrane covers the omphalocele but may not be visible in the absence of fetal ascites. The membrane is composed of two layers (an inner peritoneal membrane and an outer amnion). An omphalocele containing only bowel may be mistaken for gastroschisis.

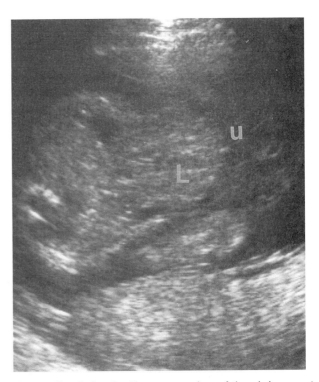

FIG. 32. Omphalocele. Transverse view of the abdomen at the level of the cord insertion site shows a large abdominal wall defect involving most of the liver *(L)*. The umbilical cord *(u)* inserts on the large omphalocele.

Overall, fetuses with omphalocele are at an increased risk for other anomalies and chromosomal abnormalities (occurring in 33% to 50% of cases), and therefore amniocentesis should be considered in all cases of omphalocele. Omphaloceles containing only bowel are associated with a higher rate of chromosomal abnormalities. Survival rates for uncomplicated omphalocele approach 90%, but the survival drops to 20% to 30% if other anomalies or chromosomal abnormalities are detected.

Gastroschisis results from a small paraumbilical abdominal wall defect. The defect is most commonly right-sided and measures less than 2 cm in size. In a typical case, only bowel is herniated, and since there is no enclosing membrane, the loops of bowel float freely in the amniotic fluid (Fig. 33). Since the extruded bowel is exposed to amniotic fluid, the bowel wall will often thicken, and bowel dilatation may occur. Intraabdominal bowel dilatation from obstruction may also occur. Fetuses with gastroschisis are at a higher than normal risk for IUGR. Decisions about early delivery should not be based on the sonographic appearance of the bowel. Fetuses with gastroschisis are not at increased risk for chromosomal abnormalities or other anomalies. The survival rate for these fetuses is greater than 90% when delivered at a tertiary care center.

Fetal Hydronephrosis

Minimal dilation of the renal pelvis is a common ultrasonographic finding representing a normal, physiologic condition. The normal fetal renal pelvis usually measures less than 5 mm in anteroposterior diameter prior to 20 weeks' gestation, less than 8 mm between 20 and 30 weeks, and less than 10 mm after 30 weeks. Measurements greater than these suggest congenital hydronephrosis that may be clinically significant (Fig. 34). Dilated calyces and ureters suggest a more severe obstruction. Serial examinations may be necessary to document whether the initial findings are persistent or progressive. Progressively worsening hydronephrosis is associated with a more unfavorable outcome.[1] In addition, the renal parenchyma should be carefully investigated when hydronephrosis is present. The presence or development of renal parenchymal cysts (postobstructive renal dysplasia) also implies severe obstruction. The most common reason for hydronephrosis is obstruction (usually at the ureteropelvic junction, less commonly at the ureterovesical junction), but dilatation may also occur from vesicoureteral reflux.

Hydrops Fetalis

Hydrops fetalis is a serious condition characterized by excessive fluid accumulation within extravascular sites. Fetal skin edema, ascites, pleural effusion, pericardial effusion, placental edema, and polyhydramnios are the hallmarks of hydrops fetalis and are easily seen by ultrasound (Fig. 35). Hydrops fetalis can be caused by immunologic and nonimmunologic factors.

Immune hydrops fetalis is caused by the transplacental passage of maternal antierythrocyte antibodies with subsequent destruction of fetal red blood cells. In the past, most cases of immune hydrops fetalis were due to anti-Rh(D) antibodies (Rh disease). The highly effective prevention of maternal Rh alloimmunization using $Rh_0(D)$ immune globulin has greatly decreased the incidence of Rh disease, and most cases of immune hydrops fetalis seen today are due to alloimmunzation to antigens other than Rh(D).

The majority of hydrops fetalis cases are nonimmune in origin. Nonimmune hydrops can be caused by infection (e.g., cytomegalovirus, syphilis, rubella, parvovirus B19), cardiovascular abnormalities (e.g., tachyarrhythmia, dysrhythmia, heart block, congenital cardiac anomalies), chromosomal anomalies (e.g., trisomy 21, Turner syndrome), skeletal dysplasias (e.g., thanatophoric dwarfism, arthrogryposis multi-

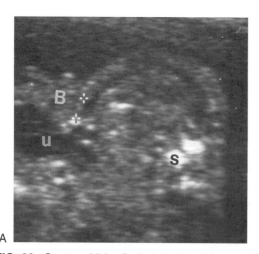
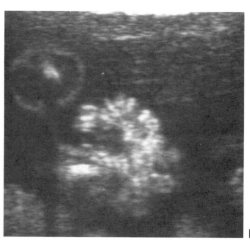

FIG. 33. Gastroschisis. **A:** A right-sided paraumbilical small abdominal wall defect is seen (calipers). Extracorporeal bowel *(B)* is present, and the umbilical cord inserts normally on the abdominal wall *(u)* (*s*, spine). **B:** The bowel floats freely in amniotic fluid and is not encapsulated by a membrane.

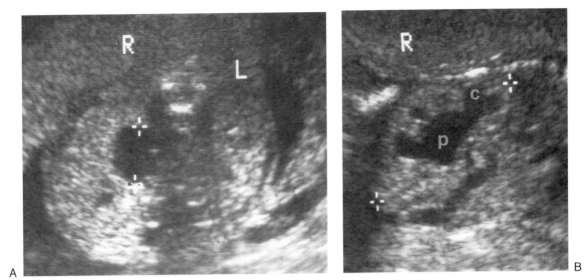

FIG. 34. Congenital hydronephrosis: ureteropelvic junction obstruction. **A:** Transverse view through the abdomen shows a dilated right renal pelvis (calipers). The left kidney and amniotic fluid volume were normal. **B:** Longitudinal views confirm the presence of renal pelvic dilatation *(p)*, as well as calyceal dilatation *(c)*.

plex congenita, osteogenesis imperfecta), twin transfusion syndrome, hematologic anomalies (e.g., α-thalassemia), genitourinary anomalies, pulmonary anomalies (e.g., lung mass, diaphragmatic hernia), gastrointestinal anomalies, placenta–umbilical cord anomalies (e.g., chorioangioma), and miscellaneous (e.g., congenital lymphedema, fetal tumors). In North American and northern European populations, the major cause of nonimmune hydrops fetalis is cardiac arrhythmia and cardiac structural abnormalities (20% to 76%). Since fetal arrhythmia is among the most treatable cause of nonimmune hydrops fetalis, sonographers should pay careful attention to the heart (including obtaining M-mode tracings) when hydrops fetalis is first diagnosed. In Taiwan, over 50% of nonimmune hydrops fetalis cases are secondary to homozygous α-thalassemia.

Prenatal ultrasound can detect hydrops fetalis, but unless accompanying fetal anomalies are seen, ultrasound cannot differentiate between nonimmune and immune hydrops. The ultrasound hallmarks of hydrops fetalis include skin thickening (usually greater than 5 mm), placental enlargement (usually greater than 4 cm), ascites, pericardial effusion, pleural effusion, and polyhydramnios. The diagnosis of hydrops

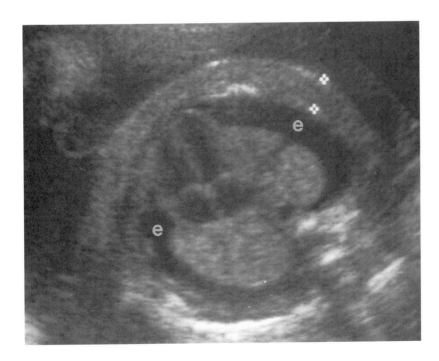

FIG. 35. Hydrops fetalis. Transverse view through the fetal chest shows bilateral pleural effusions *(e)* and anasarca (calipers measure skin thickness).

fetalis should be made with caution if only one abnormality is seen (e.g., isolated ascites may be secondary to an obstructed and decompressed urinary tract). Usually, visualization of effusion in two body cavities (e.g., ascites and pleural effusion) or effusion in one body cavity in addition to anasarca (skin thickening and ascites) is more typical for hydrops fetalis.

Ultrasound Evaluation of the Placenta: Normal Appearance, Placenta Previa, and Placental Abruption

The placenta should be assessed routinely. The placenta is homogeneously echogenic (compared to the hypoechoic myometrium and the anechoic amniotic fluid) and of uniform thickness (Fig. 36). The size or volume of the placenta is difficult to measure with ultrasound; however, placental thickness can easily be measured (distance between the placenta–myometrium interface and the placenta–amnion interface) and compared to the menstrual age. As a rule of thumb, the placenta grows approximately 1 mm per week after 10 weeks; thus, the normal placental thickness at 10 and 20 weeks' gestation is 10 mm and 20 mm, respectively. At term, the placenta measures approximately 30 mm in thickness. Placental thickness greater than 4 to 4.5 cm is considered abnormal at any time. Excessively large placentas are associated with maternal diabetes, maternal or fetal anemia, chronic infection, and hydrops fetalis. Unusually small placentas are difficult to diag-

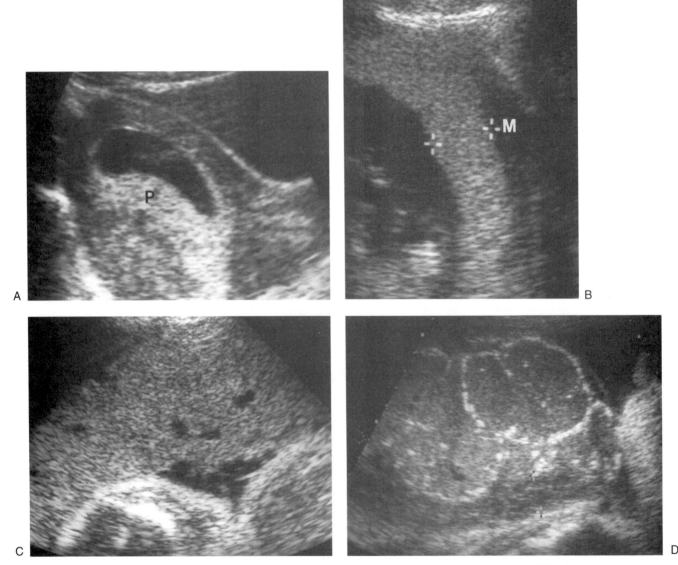

FIG. 36. Normal placenta. **A, B:** During the early and midsecond trimester, the placenta *(P)* is homogeneously echogenic, compared to the myometrium *(m)*, and measures approximately 10 to 20 mm in thickness (calipers). **C:** Small hypoechoic lesions in the placenta are commonly seen and are usually of no clinical concern. Numerous lesions or lesions seen early in pregnancy may be associated with placental insufficiency. **D:** The mature placenta (grade III) may calcify in a compartmental or cotyledon pattern.

nose prenatally but are associated with maternal hypertension, preeclampsia, polyhydramnios, and fetal IUGR.

After 25 weeks, cystic, calcific, and hypoechoic areas can be seen in the normal placenta (see Fig. 36C,D). The observation of numerous placental lesions (more than four or five), large lesions (greater than 30 mm), and lesions seen prior to 20 to 25 weeks should alert the sonographer to the possibility of placental dysfunction or insufficiency. Placental calcifications occur normally as the placenta ages. Attempts have been made to correlate the amount and distribution of placental calcifications with fetal lung maturity. Placental grading won popularity in the 1970s and 1980s; however, today experts agree that placental maturity does not correlate well with fetal lung maturity. The observation of abundant placental calcifications prior to 36 weeks is associated with IUGR, maternal hypertension, and oligohydramnios.

The location of the placenta and its relationship to the internal cervical os should be documented in every second- and third-trimester pregnancy evaluated with ultrasound. A placenta that appears to be low-lying or partially covering the internal cervical os in the second trimester may have migrated away from the cervix by the late second or early third trimester. In the vast majority of cases, the sonographer can adequately visualize the placenta and the internal cervical os by scanning the lower uterine segment in the sagittal plane through a partially filled maternal urinary bladder (see Fig. 11). Sometimes,

however, fetal parts, a myometrial contraction, or the maternal bladder (too full or too empty) hinders visualization of the cervix and lower edge of the placenta. In these cases, transperineal (translabial) or transvaginal imaging may be necessary. Transperineal ultrasound is a technique in which a sector transducer is covered and placed on the perineum. Using the vagina as an acoustic window, the sonographer can obtain unsurpassed images of the cervix and the internal os (Fig. 37).

Placenta previa is characterized as complete or marginal. With complete previa, the entire internal cervical os is covered by the placenta. The placenta may be centrally or eccentrically implanted on the os, but in such cases it rarely resolves prior to term. Ultrasound can easily identify complete previas (Fig. 38). Marginal previas, on the other hand, present a greater diagnostic and management challenge. With marginal previa, the placenta lies close to but does not completely cover the internal cervical os (Fig. 39). A recent study showed that an os-to-placenta distance measurement of greater than 20 mm is associated with a high likelihood for safe vaginal delivery. In contrast, only 1 of 11 patients with an os-to-placenta distance of less than 10 mm was able to deliver vaginally.[6] Translabial ultrasound is helpful in visualizing and measuring the os–placenta relationship. Obviously, the clinical presentation is most important for managing placenta previa, but ultrasound may help predict outcome, especially in asymptomatic cases.

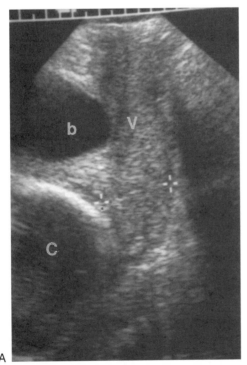 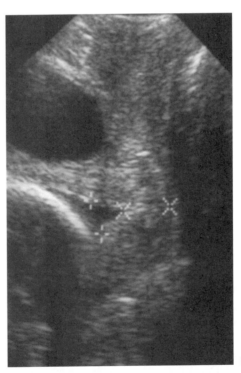

A   B

FIG. 37. Cervical evaluation: translabial technique. **A:** Translabial image shows the normal sagittal orientation of the vagina *(V)*, cervix (calipers), and maternal bladder *(b)*. The fetal calvarium *(c)* is seen against the internal cervical os. **B:** In translabial visualization of premature internal os dilatation in another patient, the + calipers measure the amount of internal os dilatation, while the X calipers delineate the portion of the cervix that remains closed (approximately 50%).

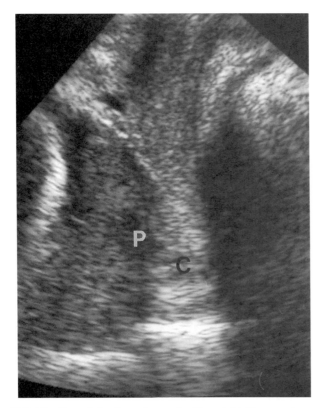

FIG. 38. Complete placenta previa. Translabial image shows that the internal os of the cervix *(c)* is completely covered by the placenta *(p)*.

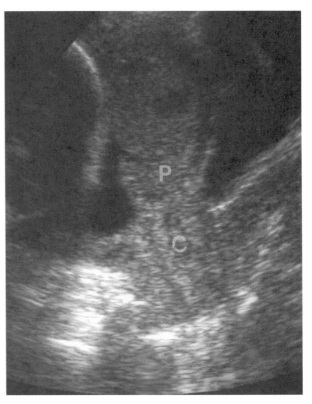

FIG. 39. Marginal placenta previa. Transabdominal sagittal view of the lower uterine segment shows that the inferior edge of the anterior placenta *(P)* is located at the cervical internal os.

Placental abruption is defined as premature separation of the placenta from the uterus. A spectrum of ultrasound findings associated with abruption has been described. The appearance of a placental hemorrhage depends on the location and the age of the hemorrhage. Acute hemorrhages are hyperechoic and can be isoechoic to the placenta. An acute placental hemorrhage may appear simply as placental thickening. Within the first week, blood becomes hypoechoic in relationship to the placenta, and by 2 to 3 weeks blood becomes almost anechoic. Three placental abruption locations have been described with ultrasound: periplacental, preplacental, and retroplacental. Most placental abruptions are periplacental (also called marginal or subchorionic) (Fig. 40), while preplacental (between the placenta and its covering membranes on the amniotic fluid side of the placenta) and retroplacental abruptions are more rare and carry the worst prognosis. With periplacental abruption, the sonographer may or may not be able to visualize the detached placental edge. In many instances, a woman with second- or third-trimester bleeding will have a normal ultrasound examination. In these cases, an abruption is probably present but not seen with ultrasound. The blood may be isoechoic with the placenta, or a small marginal abruption has occurred and most of the blood has passed through the cervix. These sonographically silent abruptions carry a better prognosis than those that are not.

Ultrasound Screening for Chromosomal Anomalies

The role of ultrasound as a screening tool for chromosomal anomalies is controversial. Table 12 lists the anomalies that have been found to be associated with trisomy 21 (Down syndrome), trisomy 18, trisomy 13, and 45,X (Turner syn-

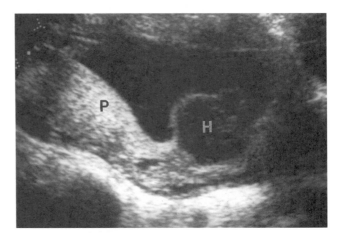

FIG. 40. Marginal placenta abruption. Sagittal view of the uterus shows that the inferior edge of the posterior placenta *(P)* is slightly lifted, and periplacental hematoma *(H)* is present in the subchorionic space.

TABLE 12. *Anomalies associated with common chromosome abnormalities*

Trisomy 21 (Down syndrome)
Often a normal fetal ultrasound
Major anomalies
    Cardiovascular malformation (endocardial cushion defect)
    Duodenal atresia
    Cystic hygroma
    Hydrocephalus (rare, usually mild)
Markers (minor findings often seen in normal fetuses also)
    Nuchal fold thickening (> 6 mm between 16 and 21 wk)
    First trimester nuchal lucency (>3 mm)
    Mild long-bone shortening
    Mild renal pelviectasis
    Hyperechoic bowel
    Fifth finger clinodactyly
    Sandle gap foot deformity
    Intracardiac echogenic focus

Trisomy 18
Rarely a normal fetal ultrasound
Major anomalies
    Early and symmetric intrauterine growth restriction
    Cardiac defects in 90%, often complex
    Microcephaly
    Nonspecific central nervous system anomalies
    Gastrointestinal system anomalies: omphalocele
    Nonspecific genitourinary tract anomalies
Markers
    Clenched hands with overlapping fingers
    Choroid plexus cysts
    Micrognathia
    Two-vessel umbilical cord
    Rocker-bottom feet

Trisomy 13
Rarely a normal fetal ultrasound
Major anomalies
    Holoprosencephaly
    Cardiovascular anomalies
    Renal cystic dysplasia
    Omphalocele
    Facial anomalies: hypotelorism, cyclopia, cleft lip/palate
Markers
    Polydactyly
    Two-vessel umbilical cord
    Rocker-bottom feet

Turner syndrome (45X)
May have a normal fetal ultrasound
Major anomalies
    Cystic hygroma
    Hydrops fetalis
    Cardiovascular malformation: coarctation of the aorta
    Renal agenesis
Markers
    Nuchal thickening
    Long-bone shortening
    Horseshoe kidneys

drome). The anomalies are characterized as major anomalies and minor anomalies or markers. While major structural anomalies have a clear association with chromosomal abnormalities (e.g., endocardial cushion defect of the heart and trisomy 21, holoprosencephaly and trisomy 13), minor anomalies represent subtle changes from normal anatomy that may or may not be associated with chromosomal abnormalities (e.g., choroid plexus cyst and trisomy 18). Advising parents with regard to isolated minor anomalies observed during routine obstetric ultrasound becomes a complicated and anxiety-provoking experience for the sonologist and patient alike. Meanwhile, the list of minor anomalies associated with chromosomal anomalies (particularly trisomy 21) has grown in recent years. In general, the more that minor anomalies are seen in a screening ultrasound, the greater is the risk for a chromosomal anomaly. One group of investigators produced a weighted scoring system for the following ultrasound markers:

◇ Femur and humerus bone length (1 point if shortening is present),
◇ Renal pyelectasis (1 point if the renal pelvis measures greater than 4 mm),
◇ Bowel echogenicity (1 point if hyperechoic bowel is present),
◇ Choroid plexus cysts (1 point if present),
◇ Nuchal thickness (2 points if present),
◇ Major abnormalities (2 points if present).[4]

According to their findings, if amniocentesis is performed when the fetal marker score is 2 or greater, 77% of fetuses with trisomy 21, trisomy 18, or trisomy 13 will be detected. Of the trisomy 21 fetuses in this series, 73% scored 2 or greater. Basically, the more markers present, the greater risk is for chromosomal anomalies. The two markers that deserve special attention are choroid plexus cysts and nuchal translucency/thickness.

Cysts of the choroid plexus are seen in approximately 1% of normal fetuses before 20 weeks (Fig. 41), usually resolve by 26 weeks, and are of no clinical significance in the vast majority of cases. However, 50% of fetuses with trisomy 18 have choroid plexus cysts raising the concern that these cysts may be a marker for trisomy 18. The majority of fetuses with trisomy 18, however, demonstrate other major malformations, and the association between isolated choroid plexus cysts and chromosomal anomalies is controversial. In the setting of isolated choroid plexus cysts, some investigators found a 9.5% rate of fetal chromosomal anomalies, and others rates as low as 0.75%. A metaanalysis by Gross et al.[10] suggested that the risk is as low as 1 in 374. Certainly, a targeted fetal ultrasound examination and frank discussion of the implications of the finding are warranted when choroid plexus cysts are seen in a low-risk patient. The fetal heart and hands are scanned carefully, since almost all trisomy 18 fetuses demonstrate overlapping fingers and complex cardiac defects. The number and size of choroid plexus cysts and

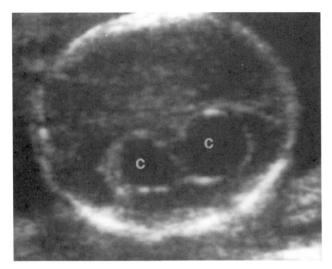

FIG. 41. Choroid plexus cysts. Axial image through the lateral ventricles shows two choroid plexus cysts in the far-field ventricle *(c)*. These cysts resolved 6 weeks later, and the fetus was normal at birth.

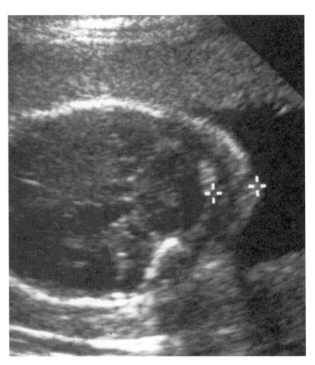

FIG. 42. Nuchal thickening. Prominent posterior nuchal skin is seen (calipers measured the skin at 7.5 mm). The nuchal skin is measured on the routine posterior fossa image and should measure less than 6 mm between 16 and 21 weeks. (Compare with Fig. 4C.)

whether or not they are bilateral are of debatable significance with regard to trisomy 18.

Anomalies of the posterior fetal neck are strong markers for chromosomal abnormalities. Increased nuchal translucency, increased nuchal skin thickness, and cystic hygroma are the common abnormalities seen. The routinely obtained posterior fossa view allows adequate evaluation of the posterior fetal neck (see Fig. 4C). Increased nuchal skin thickness is generally defined as a skin-width measurement of 6 mm or greater at 16 to 21 weeks' menstrual age (Fig. 42). Fetuses with second-trimester nuchal skin thickening are at an increased risk for trisomies, usually trisomy 21. Even as an isolated finding, second-trimester nuchal thickening is the most specific ultrasound finding for the detection of trisomy 21, and most investigators report a 20% to 30% risk for trisomy 21. Cystic hygroma is a larger cystic collection at the posterior fetal neck that usually contains septations (Fig. 43). Approximately two-thirds of fetuses with cystic hygroma will have a chromosomal anomaly, usually Turner syndrome (XO).

Increased nuchal translucency and cystic hygroma may also be seen in the first and early second trimester (Fig. 44). Taipale et al.[21] recently studied the significance of increased fetal nuchal translucency detected by transvaginal ultrasound between 10 and 16 weeks' menstrual age. Increased fetal nuchal translucency in this age group is defined as a skin-width measurement greater than 3 mm. In 76 fetuses with nuchal abnormalities (0.8% of the 10,010 patients prospectively studied), 18 (24%) had an abnormal karyotype. The most common chromosomal abnormality detected was trisomy 21. They concluded that transvaginal ultrasonography can be a sensitive tool for detecting fetal aneuploidy and can be done earlier than serum screening.

Umbilical Cord Doppler Interrogation

Doppler interrogation of the fetal–placental circulation is receiving a great deal of attention in the literature, and normal waveform patterns of maternal, placental, and fetal vessels have been described in detail. A complete discussion of Doppler evaluation of pregnancy is beyond the scope of this chapter, and therefore we will limit our discussion to the umbilical artery Doppler examination.

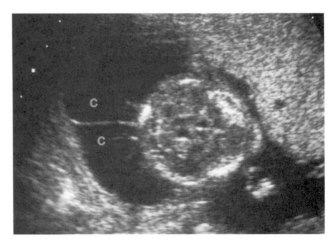

FIG. 43. Cystic hygroma. A large septated cystic mass is seen posterior to the fetal head and neck (*C*, fluid-filled cysts).

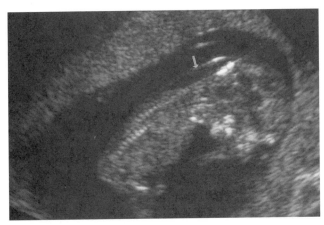

FIG. 44. First-trimester nuchal lucency. Sagittal view of a 12-week fetus shows a focal posterior nuchal fluid collection *(arrow)*. This fetus was diagnosed with an unbalanced translocation, but most fetuses with aneuploidy and increased nuchal lucency (greater than 3 mm) have trisomy 21.

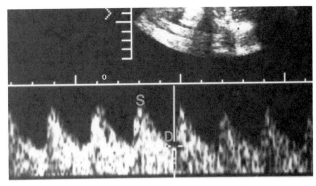

FIG. 45. Normal umbilical artery Doppler waveform. Doppler interrogation of a free loop of umbilical cord shows a normal arterial waveform. The peak systolic–end diastolic (S/D) ratio is calculated by dividing the frequency value at peak systole *(S)* by the frequency value at end diastole *(D)*. After 30 weeks, the S/D ratio is usually less than 3.0.

Umbilical artery Doppler interrogation can be used to screen for fetal acidosis. With advancing gestational age, blood flow resistance in the placental circulation decreases, and as a result a low resistive umbilical artery pattern emerges. Since the umbilical artery is tortuous, umbilical artery waveform analysis is usually limited to systolic and diastolic ratios and not angle-dependent velocity readings (Fig. 45). The peak systolic–end diastolic (S/D) ratio is easily calculated and can be compared with the gestational age. After 30 weeks, the S/D ratio should be less than 3. A free loop of cord (not near the cord origin or insertion and not compressed) should be sampled during a fetal quiet time (not during active breathing or movement).

An abnormal umbilical artery Doppler examination in a high-risk pregnancy identifies an increased risk for complica-

tions related to fetal hypoxia, and absent or reversed diastolic flow in the umbilical artery suggests a particularly high-risk circumstance (Fig. 46). In one series, absent end-diastolic flow was associated with a 16% mortality rate, and reversed diastolic flow with a 50% mortality rate. Cord Doppler assessment can be a valuable complement to an equivocal biophysical profile examination and in cases of suspected IUGR.

Efficacy of Routine Ultrasound in Pregnancy

At least eight prospective, controlled trials have been performed to assess whether or not the use of routine (screening) ultrasound in early pregnancy improves outcome, compared with the selective use of fetal ultrasound evaluation for specific clinical reasons. The most recent and best known study in the United States was a multicenter trial, known as the

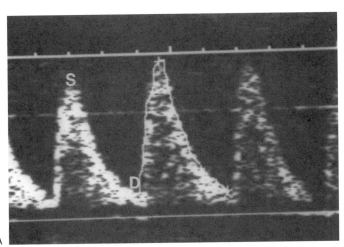
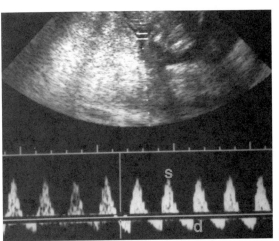

FIG. 46. Abnormal umbilical arterial cord Doppler waveforms. **A:** End-diastolic flow *(D)* is markedly diminished, and therefore the peak systolic–end diastolic ratio is elevated. This high-resistive pattern is often seen in association with intrauterine growth restriction. **B:** Reversal of diastolic flow is an ominous finding and suggests the presence of fetal hypoxia (*d*, blood flow seen below the baseline during diastole).

RADIUS trial, involving over 15,000 women. Patients randomized to the routine ultrasound group had a sonographic fetal evaluation at 15 to 22 weeks' gestation and again at 31 to 35 weeks' gestation; women randomized to the control group underwent fetal sonography only for medical indications identified by their physicians[7]. There were no differences in the rates of fetal death, neonatal death, or significant neonatal morbidity between the groups. The overall rate of any adverse perinatal outcome for each group was similar (5% versus 4.9%). Moreover, the maternal outcomes, including the rates of induced abortion and amniocentesis, were similar for each group.

The RADIUS trial has been criticized for the relatively low rate of detection of fetal anomalies in the routine ultrasound group (17% before 24 weeks' gestation). In turn, critics suggest that a higher rate of anomaly detection would have allowed an impact on fetal outcome, most significantly through termination of pregnancy in cases of serious or lethal abnormalities. There are two explanations for the low rate of detection of fetal anomalies. First, and most important, the neonatal follow-up evaluation in the RADIUS trial was systematic and thorough, identifying virtually all anomalies and thus increasing the denominator against which prenatal detection of anomalies was judged. Other studies have not been so thorough. A possible second explanation is that a sizable proportion of the routine ultrasounds were performed by personnel who did not have a focused interest in obstetric imaging and who may not have sought to identify anomalies as completely as personnel with a special obstetric-imaging interest. It remains, however, that the contribution of this possible problem to the overall perinatal and maternal outcomes is uncertain.

Neilson[17] performed a metaanalysis of the prospective, controlled trials of routine fetal ultrasound in pregnancy for the Cochrane Collaboration. He identified eight controlled trials and found that routine ultrasound results in earlier diagnosis of twin pregnancies and reduction in the rate of induction for apparent postterm pregnancy. Overall, the data indicate that routine ultrasound does not alter perinatal mortality or any of a number of perinatal morbidities. In one trial, a committed encouragement for pregnancy termination when serious or lethal fetal anomalies were found resulted in a reduction in the perinatal mortality rate.[20] However, the large difference in the rates of detection of fetal anomalies between the two centers in this trial serves to emphasize the importance of expertise in the performance of fetal ultrasonography.

◊ REFERENCES

1. Anderson N, Clautice-Engle T, Allan R, et al. Detection of obstructive uropathy in the fetus: predictive value of sonographic measurements of renal pelvic diameter at various gestational ages. *AJR* 1995;164: 719–723.
2. American Institute of Ultrasound in Medicine. *1994 Guidelines for performance of the antepartum obstetrical ultrasound examination.* Laurel, MD: American Institute of Ultrasound in Medicine, 1994.
3. Atri M, Leduc C, Gillet P, et al. Role of endovaginal sonography in the diagnosis and management of ectopic pregnancy. *Radiographics* 1996; 16:755–774.
4. Benacerraf BR. Use of sonographic markers to determine the risk for Down syndrome in second trimester fetuses. *Radiology* 1996;201:619–620.
5. Benson CB, Doubilet PM. Slow embryonic heart rate in early first trimester: indication of poor pregnancy outcome. *Radiology* 1994;192:343–344.
6. Dawson WB, Dumas MD, Romano WM, et al. Translabial ultrasonography and placenta previa: does measurement of the os–placenta distance predict outcome? *J Ultrasound Med* 1996;15:441–446.
7. Ewigman BG, Crane JP, Frigoletto FD, LeFevre ML, Bain RP, McNellis D. Effect of prenatal ultrasound screening on perinatal outcome. RADIUS study group. *N Engl J Med* 1993;329:821–827.
8. Filly RA, Cardoza JD, Goldstein RB, et al. Detection of fetal central nervous system anomalies: a practical level of effort for a routine sonogram. *Radiology* 1989;172:403–408.
9. Goldstein SR. Embryonic death in early pregnancy: a new look at the first trimester. *Obstet Gynecol* 1994;84:294–297.
10. Gross SJ, Shulman LP, Tolley EA, et al. Isolated fetal choroid plexus cysts and trisomy 18: a review and meta-analysis. *Am J Obstet Gynecol* 1995;172:83–87.
11. Hadlock FP, Harrist RB, Carpenter RJ, et al. Sonographic estimation of fetal weight: the value of femur length in addition to head and abdomen measurements. *Radiology* 1984;150:535–540.
12. Levine D, Callen PW, Goldstein RB, et al. Imaging the fetal abdomen: how efficacious are the AIUM/ACR guidelines? *J Ultrasound Med* 1995;14:335–341.
13. Lizzi F, Mortimer A, Miller M, et al. Bioeffect considerations for the safety of diagnostic ultrasound. *J Ultrasound Med* 1988;7-9(suppl):1–38.
14. Manning FA. Dynamic ultrasound-based fetal assessment: the fetal biophysical profile score. *Clin Obstet Gynecol* 1995;9:144–150.
15. McGahan JP. Sonography of the fetal heart: findings on the four chamber view. *AJR* 1991;156:547–553.
16. McKenna KM, Feldstein VA, Goldstein RB, et al. The "empty amnion": a sign of early pregnancy failure. *J Ultrasound Med* 1995;14:117–121.
17. Neilson JP. Routine ultrasound in early pregnancy. Cochrane Review. In: The Cochrane Library, Update Software, 1996.
18. Nyberg DA, Hill LM, Bohm-Velez M, Mendelson EB, eds. *Transvaginal ultrasound.* St. Louis, MO: Mosby–Year 1992.
19. Pellerito JS, Taylor KJW, Quedens-Case C, et al. Ectopic pregnancy: evaluation with endovaginal color flow imaging. *Radiology* 1992;183:407–411.
20. Saari-Kemppainen A, Karjalainen O, Ylostalo P, Heinonen OP. Ultrasound screening and perinatal mortality: controlled trial of systematic one-stage screening in pregnancy. The Helsinki Ultrasound Trial. *Lancet* 1990;336:387–391.
21. Taipale P, Hiilesmaa V, Salonen R, Ylostalo P. Increased nuchal translucency as a marker for fetal chromosomal defects. *N Engl J Med* 1997;337:1654–1658.
22. Taylor KJW, Ramos IM, Geyock AL, et al. Ectopic pregnancy: duplex Doppler evaluation. *Radiology* 1989;173:93–97.
23. Watson WJ, Chescheir NC, Katz VL, et al. The role of ultrasound in evaluation of patients with elevated maternal serum alpha-fetoprotein: a review. *Obstet Gynecol* 1991;78:123–128.
24. Zweibel WJ. Image optimization, ultrasound artifacts, and safety considerations. In: Zweibel WJ, Sohaey R, eds. *Introduction to ultrasound.* Philadelphia: WB Saunders, 1998;18–30.

CHAPTER 15

Antepartum–Intrapartum Fetal Monitoring

◇

David A. Miller
Richard Paul

The concept of the fetus as a patient is fundamental to the contemporary practice of obstetrics. In historical context, however, this philosophy is relatively new. It has evolved over the course of the 20th century as a product of improved safety of cesarean section and enhanced ability to monitor the condition of the fetus. In the early 1800s, cesarean-related maternal mortality exceeded 75%, and the operation rarely was performed for the sole benefit of the fetus. During the late 1800s, advances in surgical technique made cesarean section much safer, but 10% maternal mortality continued to limit its use. Throughout the 20th century, improvements in anesthesia, blood banking, transfusion techniques, antibiotic therapy, and general medical care have yielded dramatic reductions in cesarean-related mortality. By 1970, the maternal mortality rate of cesarean section was 113.8 per 100,000 deliveries, and the current rate is estimated to be as low as 20 to 25 per 100,000. The precipitous decline in maternal risk has led to more liberal use of cesarean section, including increased acceptance of operative intervention on behalf of the fetus. In fact, as maternal mortality has continued to fall, the percentage of cesareans performed for "fetal distress" has risen more than 10-fold from 0.8% in the mid-1930s to 9.2% in 1991.

Auscultation of the fetal heart was first reported in the Western medical literature by Mayor in 1818. In 1822, Le Jumeau proposed that auscultation of the fetal heart sounds could be useful in judging the state of fetal health or disease. Using only the stethoscope (mediate auscultation) or the ear of the examiner placed directly on the maternal abdomen (immediate auscultation), Kennedy, Schwartz, Winckel, and others described the fetal heart rate (FHR) changes resulting from umbilical cord compression, head compression, and "asphyxial intoxication." In 1917, Hillis described the modified stethoscope known today as the DeLee-Hillis fetoscope.

In 1906, Cremer recorded the first fetal electrocardiogram (ECG). By placing one electrode on the maternal abdomen above the fundus and another in the vagina, he was able to detect small fetal electrical impulses among the higher-voltage maternal signals. The concept of direct application of the ECG electrode to the fetus *in utero* was introduced in the 1950s, and the first practical electronic FHR monitor became available in the United States in 1968. Electronic fetal monitoring gained widespread acceptance and by 1993 was employed in 79% of all pregnancies in the United States.

Since its inception, the primary objective of FHR monitoring has been to identify the fetus in distress so that measures might be taken in time to avert permanent fetal damage or death. However, a clear consensus regarding the definition of "fetal distress" has not been established. It has been described as "a condition in which fetal physiology is so altered as to make death or permanent injury a probability within a relatively short period of time," and is usually considered to denote disruption of normal fetal oxygenation, ranging from mild hypoxia to profound fetal asphyxia. The term *hypoxia* refers to the reduction of tissue oxygen supply below physiologic levels. Asphyxia, derived from the Greek word meaning "a stopping of the pulse," implies a combination of hypoxia and metabolic acidosis. Historically, the clinical diagnosis of birth asphyxia has been based on findings such as meconium-stained amniotic fluid, abnormal FHR patterns, low Apgar scores, abnormal blood gases, and neonatal neurologic abnormalities. When present together, these findings are highly suggestive of a recent asphyxial insult. Isolated abnormalities, however, correlate poorly with birth-related asphyxia and subsequent neurologic impairment. In 1989, Gilstrap and co-workers recommended that the diagnosis of birth asphyxia be reserved for infants who are severely depressed (5-minute Apgar score less than 3) and acidotic (pH less than 7.0) at birth, require resuscitation, and have seizures in the first day of life. In 1991, the American College of Obstetricians and Gynecologists Committee on Obstetrics, Maternal and Fetal Medicine stated that

> . . . a neonate who has had severe hypoxia close to delivery that is severe enough to result in hypoxic encephalopathy will show other evidence of hypoxic damage including all of the following: (1) a profound umbilical artery metabolic or mixed acidemia (pH less than 7.00), (2) persistence of an Apgar score of 0–3 for longer than 5 minutes, (3) neonatal neurologic sequelae such as seizures, coma and/or hypotonia, and (4) multiorgan system dysfunction (cardiovascular, gastrointestinal, hematologic, pulmonary, or renal).

At the cellular level, asphyxia triggers a cascade of events, including membrane depolarization, disruption of energy metabolism, altered neurotransmission, ion shifts, protease activation, free radical production, and phospholipid degradation. Profound and prolonged asphyxia may result in cell death and, eventually, death of the organism. Sublethal asphyxia may lead to multiorgan system dysfunction. In the newborn, asphyxial cardiac injury may result in conduction defects, myocardial dysfunction, and congestive heart failure. Manifestations in the gastrointestinal tract include hypoxic-ischemic mucosal injury, stress ulcers, hepatic injury, and necrotizing enterocolitis. In the lungs, asphyxial sequelae include meconium aspiration syndrome, persistent pulmonary hypertension, impaired surfactant production, and respiratory distress syndrome. Asphyxial renal injury may lead to renal insufficiency or acute renal failure. Hematologic manifestations include neutropenia, thrombocytopenia, and disseminated intravascular coagulation. In the central nervous system (CNS), disruption of membrane depolarization and neurotransmission may lead to seizures and respiratory depression. Impairment of CNS water-regulating mechanisms and disruption of the blood–brain barrier may result in cerebral edema and neuronal necrosis. Severe asphyxial brain injury may lead to long-term neurodevelopmental impairment.

Cerebral palsy (CP) is a major disorder of neurodevelopment, defined as "a chronic disability, characterized by aberrant control of movement and posture, appearing early in life and not the result of recognized progressive disease." It may be accompanied by mental retardation (41%), seizures (23%), or cortical visual impairment. The insult responsible for the development of CP may occur at any time during the prenatal, perinatal, or postnatal periods. Unlike in other major neurodevelopmental disorders, the relationship between CP and abnormal or difficult birth has long been recognized.

In 1862, William John Little, an orthopedic surgeon, presented a treatise to the Obstetrical Society of London, "On the influence of abnormal parturition, difficult labours, premature birth and asphyxia neonatorum, on the mental and physical condition of the child, especially in relation to deformities." Upon reviewing the birth histories of children with spastic rigidity and observing a high incidence of preterm delivery, breech presentation, prolonged labor, late onset of crying and respiration, and neonatal convulsions and stupor, he concluded that infantile spastic palsies could be caused by virtually nothing other than abnormalities of the birth process. Subsequently, Schreiber, Lilienfeld, Eastman, and others reported similar observations, lending support to Little's hypothesis.

Animal data further implicated fetal asphyxia as a cause of neurologic injury. In 1943, Windle demonstrated clinical and histopathologic evidence of neural damage in experimentally asphyxiated fetal guinea pigs. He later reported the effects of prolonged anoxia on fetal rhesus monkeys. Total anoxia for less than 8 minutes did not produce consistent injury, whereas anoxia for more than 10 minutes invariably resulted in neuropathology. There were no survivors beyond 20 to 25 minutes of anoxia. The pattern of injury produced by prolonged anoxia included neuronal necrosis in the brain stem, thalamus, and basal ganglia, with relative sparing of the cerebral cortex. However, these observations did not correlate with the cerebral injury, mental retardation, and spasticity seen in CP. Myers (1972) demonstrated that, unlike total anoxia, prolonged partial asphyxia in monkeys produced acidosis, late FHR decelerations, and neuropathologic defects consistent with the findings in the common forms of CP. In addition to lesions in the thalamus and basal ganglia, prolonged partial asphyxia caused generalized cerebral necrosis or focal necrosis in the parasagittal regions and the border zones between the parietal and occipital lobes.

Although early studies created and fostered the assumption that birth-related asphyxia was the primary cause of CP, recent evidence challenges this assumption. In 1986, Nelson and Ellenberg reported a multivariate analysis of risk in 189 cases of CP. After accounting for major congenital malformations, low birthweight, microcephaly, and alternative explanations for the disorder, they were able to attribute only 9% of CP cases to birth asphyxia. In 1988, Blair and Stanley reached very similar conclusions in a study of 183 CP cases and 549 matched controls. Although birth asphyxia nearly tripled the odds of developing CP, only 8.2% of CP cases were potentially attributable to birth asphyxia.

As early as the 19th century, researchers using auscultation recognized that certain FHR patterns were associated with adverse perinatal outcome. In 1833, Kennedy commented on the poor prognosis associated with a FHR deceleration that exhibited "slowness of its return when a contraction is passing on." In 1838, Schwartz implicated "asphyxic intoxication" as a cause of alterations in the "individual normal frequency" of the fetal heart sounds, noting that "in those cases in which the heart sounds returned slowly to their earlier rhythm, or when the attenuations persisted or deteriorated during the pauses, the result would be a weak, moribund or dead fetus." The introduction of direct electronic fetal monitoring and fetal scalp blood sampling in the 1960s provided additional tools for evaluating the fetus. In 1967, Hon and Quilligan proposed a classification system for FHR decelerations. In 1969, Kubli and associates demonstrated the correlation between

FHR decelerations and fetal acidosis, reporting that fetuses with no decelerations, early decelerations, or mild variable decelerations had average scalp pH values greater than or equal to 7.29, whereas those with severe variable or late decelerations had pH values less than or equal to 7.15. In 1975, Paul and associates reported significantly higher scalp pH values in fetuses with normal FHR variability than in those with decreased variability. Kubli and Hammacher noted that the absence of FHR accelerations correlated with poor perinatal outcome. Later, Clark and co-workers (1984) and Smith and colleagues (1986) demonstrated that the presence of FHR accelerations predicted normal scalp pH values. With the development of indirect monitoring techniques, the experience derived from direct intrapartum monitoring became applicable to the antepartum period, leading to the development of antepartum testing.

◊ FETAL MONITOR

The fetal monitor tracing is a continuous paper strip composed of two Cartesian graphs. The FHR tracing is displayed on the upper graph, with time on the x-axis and heart rate on the y-axis (range 30 to 240 beats per minute [beats/min]). Uterine activity is displayed on the lower graph, with time on the x-axis and pressure on the y-axis (range 0 to 100 mm Hg). Heart rate and uterine activity are plotted separately on the heat-sensitive paper by two thermal pens. On both grids, fine vertical lines represent 10-second intervals, and heavy lines denote 1-minute intervals. In the United States, the standard paper speed is 3 cm per minute.

◊ DIRECT FETAL HEART RATE AND UTERINE ACTIVITY MONITORING

Direct transcervical application of an ECG electrode to the fetus requires dilatation of the cervix, rupture of the membranes, and access to the fetal presenting part. These prerequisites limit the use of direct monitoring to the intrapartum period. When applied to the fetal presenting part, the ECG electrode detects electrical impulses originating in the fetal heart (Fig. 1A). Amplified signals are processed by a cardiotachometer, comparing each incoming fetal QRS complex to the one immediately preceding it. The interval between the two complexes is used to calculate a heart rate that is plotted as a point on the paper chart. This process is repeated with each cardiac cycle (approximately 120 to 160 times each minute), yielding a graphic beat-to-beat display of the FHR. Direct assessment of uterine activity employs a thin, flexible intrauterine pressure catheter (IUPC) placed transcervically into the amniotic cavity. Intrauterine pressure is transmitted from the amniotic fluid through the fluid-filled IUPC to a pressure transducer. The transducer converts pressure measurements into electrical signals, and continuous pressure readings are displayed on the uterine activity graph.

◊ INDIRECT FETAL HEART RATE AND UTERINE ACTIVITY MONITORING

Indirect monitoring does not require the transcervical placement of electrodes or catheters and therefore can be performed at any time during pregnancy. This technique employs an ultrasound transducer that is applied to the maternal abdomen (Fig. 1B). Ultrasound waves originating from the transducer penetrate the tissues and are reflected by tissue interfaces. Waves reflected from the moving structures of the fetal heart return to the transducer and are translated into electrical signals. In a process similar to that used in direct monitoring, these signals are converted into a graphic display of the FHR. Indirect assessment of uterine activity is performed with a pressure transducer (tocodynamometer) applied tightly to the maternal abdomen over the uterine fundus. Uterine contractions exert pressure on the abdominal wall that is transmitted to the tocodynamometer. Changes in pressure are converted into electrical signals and are plotted on the uterine activity graph.

◊ INTERPRETATION OF THE FETAL MONITOR STRIP

Analysis of the fetal monitor strip requires a systematic approach. First, uterine activity is evaluated with attention to the frequency, duration, and strength of contractions, as well as the baseline uterine tone between contractions. Next, the FHR is analyzed with respect to (1) the baseline heart rate, (2) variability in the FHR, and (3) periodic patterns, including FHR accelerations and decelerations. This approach is summarized in Table 1.

Uterine Activity

The normal frequency of uterine contractions during labor is every two to three minutes; however, cervical change may result from contractions occurring less frequently. In most cases, five to seven uterine contractions within a 15-minute period reflect adequate uterine activity. Increased contraction frequency is termed *uterine tachysystole* and is defined by six or more uterine contractions within a 10-minute window for two consecutive windows. Tachysystole may be seen in cases of placental abruption or hyperstimulation of the uterus by oxytocin or prostaglandin cervical-ripening agents. Normal uterine contractions last approximately 40 to 60 seconds. Prolonged contractions may result from "coupling" of contractions, uterine hyperstimulation, or acute complications such as placental abruption or uterine rupture. The normal baseline uterine pressure between contractions is approximately 10 mm Hg. Abnormally high baseline pressures in excess of 20 mm Hg may result from hyperstimulation or occasionally from overdistention of the uterus by excessive amnioinfusion, polyhydramnios, or fetal macrosomia. During contractions, normal uterine pressure ranges from 30 to 80 mm Hg, although pressures in excess of 80 mm Hg may be observed during the second stage

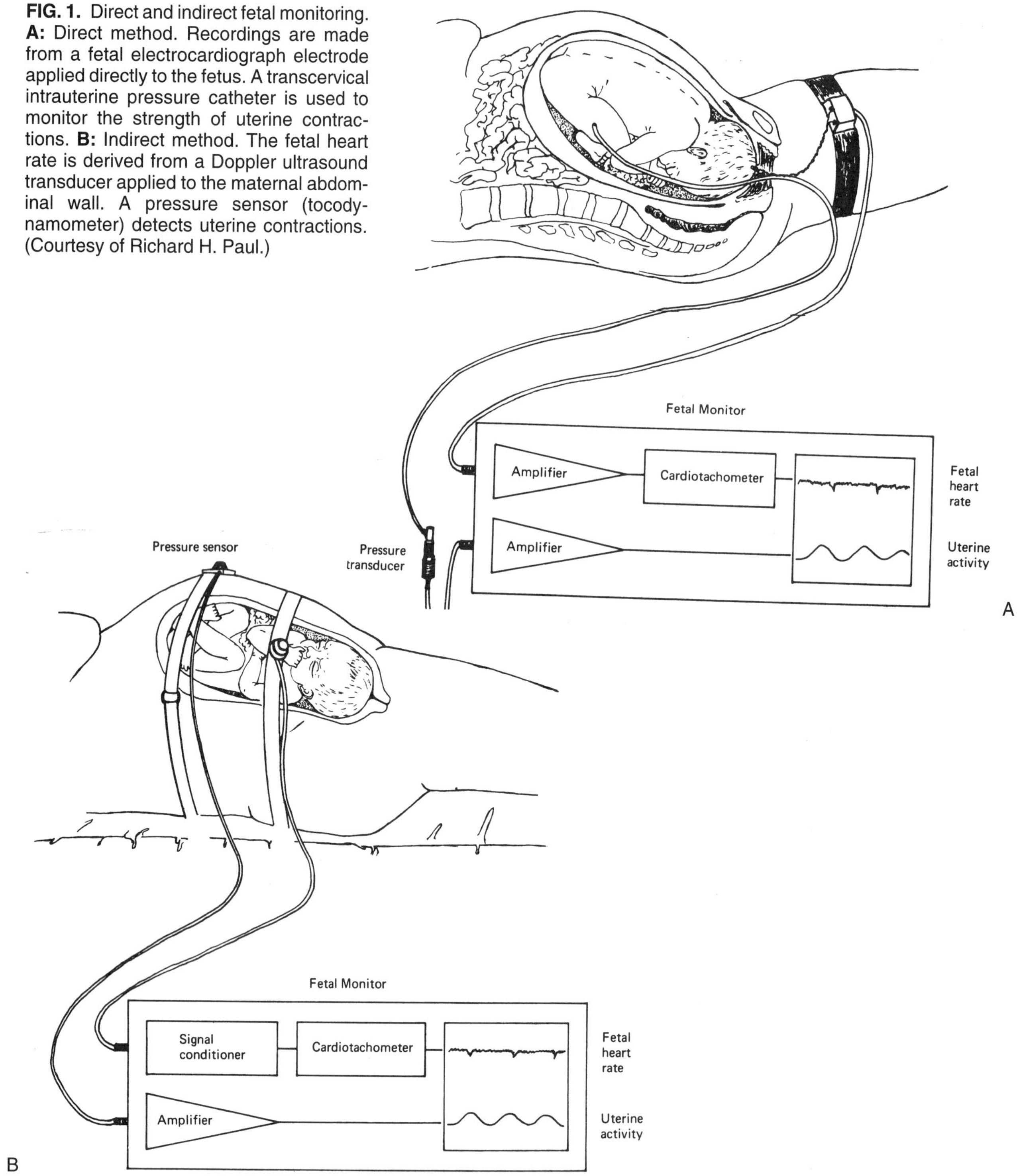

FIG. 1. Direct and indirect fetal monitoring. **A:** Direct method. Recordings are made from a fetal electrocardiograph electrode applied directly to the fetus. A transcervical intrauterine pressure catheter is used to monitor the strength of uterine contractions. **B:** Indirect method. The fetal heart rate is derived from a Doppler ultrasound transducer applied to the maternal abdominal wall. A pressure sensor (tocodynamometer) detects uterine contractions. (Courtesy of Richard H. Paul.)

of labor. In 1957, Caldeyro-Barcia proposed a method of quantitating uterine activity by calculating the contraction pressure (peak minus baseline) of each uterine contraction during a 10-minute window. The sum of the contraction pressures is expressed in Montevideo units. For example, four contractions in a 10-minute window, each 50 mm Hg above the baseline, would yield 200 Montevideo units. Montevideo units in excess of 180 to 200 usually are considered to reflect adequate uterine activity.

Baseline Fetal Heart Rate

The normal FHR baseline ranges from 120 to 160 beats/min. Early in pregnancy, it is closer to 160 beats/min, declining as

TABLE 1. *Fetal monitor interpretation*

Uterine activity assessment
    Contraction frequency
    Contraction duration
    Baseline uterine tone
    Contraction strength
Fetal heart rate assessment
    Baseline rate
        Tachycardia
        Bradycardia
        Sinusoidal pattern
    Variability
        Increased variability
        Average or normal variability
        Decreased variability
        Absent variability
    Periodic patterns
        Accelerations
        Decelerations
            Early decelerations
            Variable decelerations
            Late decelerations

gestational age advances. Likewise, the FHR may decrease gradually toward 120 beats/min during the course of labor. A FHR baseline below 120 beats/min is termed *bradycardia,* and a rate in excess of 160 beats/min is termed *tachycardia.* Abnormalities in the FHR baseline may have very different causes and consequences. It is important therefore to characterize the underlying etiology as accurately as possible and to institute appropriate therapy at the earliest possible time.

Bradycardia

Bradycardia is defined as an abnormally low baseline FHR (less than 120 beats/min) and must be differentiated from the episodic FHR changes characteristic of decelerations. Although FHR decelerations are very common, true fetal bradycardia is not. A bradycardic FHR baseline between 100 and 120 beats/min observed in association with otherwise reassuring FHR patterns probably represents a normal variant. Rarely, fetal bradycardia may be seen in association with maternal beta-blocker therapy, hypothermia, hypoglycemia, hypothyroidism, or fetal cardiac conduction defects (congenital atrioventricular block). Documentation of fetal heart block should prompt a search for structural fetal cardiac abnormalities, which may be present in 20% of cases. Other causes of heart block include viral infections (e.g., cytomegalovirus) and damage to the cardiac conduction system by transplacental passage of maternal anti-Ro (anti–SS-A) antibodies. Most congenital causes of fetal bradycardia do not present as abrupt changes in the FHR and rarely require emergency intervention. Any abrupt decline in the FHR below 120 beats/min more likely represents a deceleration than a change in the baseline, and should be considered pathologic until proven otherwise.

Tachycardia

Fetal tachycardia has many possible etiologies. Most often, it is the result of decreased vagal and/or increased sympathetic outflow, associated with fever, infection, fetal anemia, or fetal hypoxia. Other causes include maternal hyperthyroidism, sympathomimetic medications (e.g., ritodrine [Yutopar], terbutaline), parasympatholytic medications (e.g., atropine, phenothiazines), and fetal tachyarrhythmias (e.g., paroxysmal supraventricular tachycardia, atrial fibrillation, atrial flutter, and ventricular tachyarrythmias).

Sinusoidal Pattern

The sinusoidal FHR pattern is an uncommon FHR baseline abnormality. It has the appearance of a smooth sine wave with an amplitude of 5 to 15 beats/min and a frequency of 2 to 5 cycles per minute. There is little beat-to-beat variability, and accelerations are absent. Although the pathophysiologic mechanism is unclear, this pattern classically is associated with hypoxia and severe fetal anemia secondary to Rh isoimmunization. Additionally, it has been reported in association with fetomaternal hemorrhage, chorioamnionitis, fetal sepsis, and administration of narcotic analgesics. A persistent sinusoidal pattern that is not attributable to medications is a concerning finding and demands immediate evaluation.

Fetal Heart Rate Variability

Variability in the FHR results from constant interplay between the sympathetic and parasympathetic arms of the fetal autonomic nervous system. Modulation of vagal tone occurs in response to changes in blood pressure detected by baroreceptors in the fetal aortic arch. Oxygen and carbon dioxide fluctuations, detected by chemoreceptors in the carotid bodies, similarly influence vagal outflow. In the absence of stress, sympathetic outflow is thought to be relatively tonic. Continual adjustments in vagal tone are manifested in the FHR tracing as "short-term" (beat-to-beat) variability superimposed on broader, cyclical fluctuations of 3 to 5 cycles per minute, referred to as "long-term" variability. As demonstrated in Figure 2, a FHR tracing should not be considered normal unless both short-term and long-term variability are present. In clinical use, the term *FHR variability* refers to the composite of short-term and long-term variability and is quantitated by measuring the difference between the peaks and troughs of the long-term fluctuations. FHR variability is considered normal or average when both short-term and long-term variability are present, and the difference between the peaks and troughs of the long-term fluctuations is 6 to 25 beats/min. Average variability reflects a nonacidotic vagal connection between the fetal CNS and the cardiac conduction system. Increased variability (more than 25 beats/min), or *saltatory* FHR pattern, is uncommon and most often represents an exuberant autonomic response of a normal fetus. On occasion, it may reflect increased catecholamine release in the early stages of fetal hypoxia. Careful evaluation of the associated

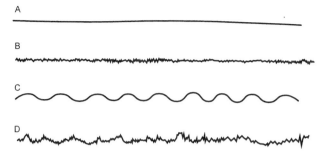

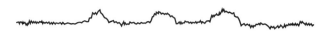

FIG. 2. Fetal heart rate variability. **A:** Short-term variability absent, Long-term variability absent—Abnormal. **B:** Short-term variability present, Long-term variability absent—Abnormal. **C:** Short-term variability absent, Long-term variability present—Abnormal. **D:** Short-term varibility present, Long-term variability present—Normal.

FHR findings should help to clarify such cases. Decreased (3 to 5 beats/min) or absent (0 to 2 beats/min) FHR variability reflects diminished fetal CNS activity, usually attributable to fetal sleep cycles or to medications administered to the mother (e.g., analgesics, magnesium sulfate, benzodiazepines, phenothiazines, atropine). Persistently decreased variability, however, may signal fetal acidosis. This is particularly true in the presence of other FHR findings suggestive of hypoxia, including tachycardia, loss of reactivity, or repetitive decelerations.

Periodic Patterns

The FHR baseline is frequently interrupted by accelerations and/or decelerations in rate. These periodic patterns have important clinical implications regarding the well-being of the fetus.

Accelerations

Accelerations in the FHR occur with 90% of fetal movements as early as the second trimester, probably as a result of increased catecholamine release and decreased vagal stimulation of the heart. A typical acceleration pattern is displayed in Figure 2. By 32 weeks' gestation, nearly all normal fetuses will have 15 to 40 spontaneous accelerations per hour, reflecting normal oxygenation of the CNS–cardiac axis. The frequency and amplitude of accelerations may be diminished by fetal sleep states, medications (narcotics, magnesium sulfate, atropine), prematurity, or fetal acidosis. Often, fetal scalp stimulation or vibroacoustic stimulation will provoke fetal movement and FHR accelerations. If these measures fail to induce FHR accelerations, hypoxia should be suspected, particularly if other FHR characteristics are not reassuring.

Decelerations

Decelerations in the FHR are most commonly encountered during the intrapartum period. They are divided into three categories: early, variable, and late decelerations (Fig. 3).

FIG. 3. Fetal heart rate accelerations.

Classification is based on the characteristic appearance of the deceleration and its temporal relationship to the onset of a uterine contraction.

Early Decelerations

Early decelerations are typically uniform, shallow dips in the FHR (rarely below 100 beats/min) that mirror uterine contractions, beginning when the contraction begins and ending when the contraction ends. They are thought to result from fetal head compression, transient elevation of intracranial pressure, and reflex augmentation of vagal tone. Early decelerations classically appear during labor when the cervix is dilated 4 to 6 cm. Perinatal outcome is not adversely affected by these decelerations, and they are considered clinically benign.

Variable Decelerations and Prolonged Decelerations

Variable decelerations result from umbilical cord compression. They are abrupt and angular in appearance and have a variable temporal relationship to uterine contractions. As the umbilical cord is compressed, the thin-walled, compliant umbilical vein is the first vessel occluded, resulting in decreased fetal venous return, relative hypovolemia, and a reflex increase in the FHR. This observation often is termed a "shoulder." Further compression of the umbilical cord leads to occlusion of the umbilical arteries, removing the low-resistance placenta from the circuit and dramatically increasing fetal peripheral resistance. This leads to elevation of the fetal blood pressure and a baroreceptor-mediated slowing of the FHR in an attempt to return the blood pressure to normal. Maximum vagal tone may result in a junctional or idioventricular escape rhythm that appears as a relatively stable rate of 60 to 70 beats/min at the nadir of the deceleration. As cord compression is relieved, this sequence of events occurs in reverse, at times resulting in transient tachycardia or "overshoot" at the end of the deceleration. Variable decelerations are classified as

◊ Mild—duration less than 30 seconds, depth greater than 70 beats/min,
◊ Moderate—duration 30 to 60 seconds, depth less than 80 beats/min, or
◊ Severe—duration greater than 60 seconds, depth less than 70 beats/min.

Isolated, infrequent variable decelerations have little clinical significance. Repetitive severe variables, however, may not allow sufficient fetal recovery between decelerations, resulting in persistent hypoxemia, hypercapnia, and respiratory acidosis. Prolonged tissue hypoperfusion may lead to metabolic acidosis and, ultimately, fetal death. In animal models, Clapp reported that frequent episodes of hypoxemic stress, produced by intermittent umbilical cord occlusion over a period of hours, produced fetal injury even in the absence of acidosis. When repetitive, severe variable decelerations are present, prolapse of the umbilical cord must be excluded. Other causes include nuchal cord, uterine rupture, placental abruption, uterine hypertonus, and tachysystole. Occasionally, variable decelerations fail to return promptly to the baseline and may more accurately be termed *prolonged* decelerations. Prolonged decelerations usually result from umbilical cord compression (cord prolapse, nuchal cord) or other acute interruption of uteroplacental transfer of oxygen (tetanic contraction, uterine rupture, maternal hypotension, maternal apnea, placental abruption).

Late Decelerations

Late decelerations reflect inadequate uteroplacental transfer of oxygen during contractions. Typically, they are smooth, uniform decelerations that begin after the onset of a contraction and end after the contraction ends. During uterine contractions, decreased maternal perfusion of the uteroplacental unit causes a decline in fetal PO_2. Fetal PO_2 levels below a critical threshold of 15 to 18 mm Hg trigger a complex chemoreceptor- and baroreceptor-mediated reflex. Initially, centralization of blood volume (favoring perfusion of the brain, heart, and adrenals) occurs via vasoconstriction in the vascular beds of the limbs and gut. The resulting increase in peripheral resistance provokes a reflex deceleration in the FHR. Isolated late decelerations within an otherwise normal tracing have little clinical significance. However, repetitive hypoxemia and centralization of blood volume, as evidenced by repetitive late decelerations, may force hypoperfused tissues to convert from aerobic to anaerobic metabolism. Organic acid byproducts of anaerobic metabolism (pyruvate, lactate) diffuse slowly across the placenta and may accumulate in the fetus, leading to metabolic acidosis, asphyxia and possibly death. Late decelerations may be caused by any factor that (1) reduces the normal placental transfer of oxygen or (2) increases the fetal oxygen demand beyond the available supply. Such factors include uterine hypertonus or tachysystole (oxytocin, prostaglandins, uterine rupture, placental abruption), maternal hypertension (chronic hypertension, preeclampsia, collagen vascular disease, renal disease, diabetes), suboptimal maternal cardiac output (cardiac disease, hypovolemia, supine hypotension, sympathetic blockade from regional anesthesia, sepsis), maternal hypoxia (apnea, cardiac disease, pulmonary disease), reduced oxygen-carrying capacity of maternal blood (anemia, hemoglobinopathy), and fever (increased fetal metabolism and increased oxygen consumption).

◊ ANTEPARTUM TESTING

Early in its development, electronic FHR monitoring required direct access to the fetus and was limited to the intrapartum period. Later, Doppler ultrasound technology made it possible to monitor the FHR before labor. The experience gained from intrapartum monitoring was applied to the antepartum period and led to the development of antepartum testing. The goals of antepartum testing are (1) to identify fetuses in jeopardy so that permanent injury or death might be prevented and (2) to identify healthy fetuses so that unnecessary intervention might be avoided. The key measure of the effectiveness of an antepartum test is the false-negative rate, defined as the incidence of fetal death within 1 week of a normal antepartum test. Reported false-negative rates range from 0.4 to 1.9 per 1000 with current testing methods. Another important measure is the false-positive rate. A false-positive test may be defined as an abnormal test that prompts delivery but is not associated with evidence of acute fetal compromise (e.g., meconium-stained amniotic fluid, intrapartum fetal distress, or low Apgar scores) or chronic fetal compromise (e.g., fetal growth retardation of less than the 10th percentile for gestational age). False-positive rates range from 30% to 90% with current testing methods.

Antepartum testing is used primarily in patients who are considered to be at increased risk for fetal hypoxia or asphyxia secondary to suboptimal uteroplacental transfer of oxygen. Common obstetric and medical indications for antepartum testing are summarized in Table 2. The optimal gestational age at which to begin antepartum testing is not known. However, for most medical indications, testing is initiated by 32 to 34 weeks. Table 3 summarizes the usual timing of antepartum testing for obstetric indications. Initiating testing prior to 32 weeks might be expected to prevent more fetal deaths. However, fetal death resulting from uteroplacental insufficiency is uncommon prior to 32 to 34 weeks. Moreover, in view of the high false-positive rates of most testing protocols, earlier initiation of testing should be expected to increase the incidence of unnecessary intervention and iatrogenic prematurity, with its attendant complications.

TABLE 2. *Indications for antepartum testing*

Obstetric indications	Medical indications
Postterm pregnancy	Diabetes mellitus
Intrauterine growth retardation	Chronic hypertension
	Cardiac disease
Previous stillbirth	Renal disease
Decreased fetal movement	Thyroid disease
Pregnancy-induced hypertension	Collagen vascular disease
	Antiphospholipid syndrome
Premature rupture of membranes	Substance abuse
Multiple gestation	
Rh isoimmunization	
Oligohydramnios	

TABLE 3. *Antepartum testing for obstetric indications*

Indication	Initiation
Postterm pregnancy	41 wk
Cholestasis of pregnancy	32–34 wk
Previous stillbirth	32–34 wk[a]
Multiple gestation	32–34 wk
Decreased fetal movement	Diagnosis
Pregnancy-induced hypertension	Diagnosis
Premature rupture of membranes	Diagnosis
Rh isoimmunization	Diagnosis
Intrauterine growth retardation	Diagnosis
Oligohydramnios	Diagnosis

[a] Or 1 week earlier than previous loss.

Contraction Stress Test and Oxytocin Challenge Test

The first antepartum testing technique, the contraction stress test (CST) or oxytocin challenge test (OCT), arose from intrapartum observations linking late FHR decelerations with poor perinatal outcome. The test sought to identify uteroplacental insufficiency by demonstrating late decelerations in fetuses exposed to the stress of spontaneous (CST) or induced (OCT) uterine contractions. Kubli and associates (1969) found that late decelerations occurring during spontaneous uterine contractions were associated with increased rates of fetal death, growth retardation, and neonatal depression. Similar observations were made by other investigators using oxytocin or nipple stimulation to provoke uterine contractions. The CST is performed weekly and is considered negative if there are at least three uterine contractions in a 10-minute period with no late decelerations on the tracing. Failure to produce three contractions within a 10-minute window or inability to trace the FHR results in an unsatisfactory test. Prolonged decelerations, variable decelerations, or late decelerations occurring with fewer than half of the contractions constitute a suspicious or equivocal test. Unsatisfactory, suspicious, or equivocal tests require repeat testing the following day. The CST or OCT is considered positive when at least half of the contractions during a 10-minute window are associated with late decelerations. Freeman and colleagues (1982) tested more than 4600 women with the CST and reported a false-negative rate of 0.4 per 1000. When the last test before delivery was a reactive, negative CST, the perinatal mortality rate was 2.3 per 1000, compared to a mortality rate of 176.5 per 1000 when the last test was a nonreactive, positive CST. Reported false-positive rates for the CST range from 8% to 57%, with an average of approximately 30%. Principal advantages of this form of testing include excellent sensitivity and a weekly testing interval. Limitations include a high rate of equivocal results requiring repeat testing, increased expense and inconvenience (particularly if oxytocin is required), and increased time requirement compared to nonprovocative tests. Additionally, use of the CST is contraindicated in several clinical settings, including preterm labor, placenta previa, vasa previa, cervical incompetence, multiple gestation, and previous classical cesarean section.

Nonstress Test

FHR accelerations occurring in association with fetal movements form the basis of the nonstress test (NST). Although many criteria have been reported, a normal or "reactive" NST usually is defined by two accelerations in a 10- to 20-minute period, each lasting at least 15 seconds and peaking at least 15 beats/min above the baseline. In most institutions, the test is repeated once or twice weekly. Boehm and colleagues (1986) reported that the latter approach yielded a threefold reduction in the incidence of fetal death, although the difference was not statistically significant. Freeman and co-workers (1982) reported a false-negative rate of 1.9 per 1000 among 1542 women tested weekly with the NST. Manning and associates (1983) reported an average false-negative rate of 6.4 per 1000 among nine large clinical trials using the NST as the primary method of surveillance. Assessment of FHR characteristics other than reactivity (baseline rate, variability, decelerations) may improve the sensitivity of the test. Phelan and colleagues (1984) noted variable decelerations in 33% of 239 postterm patients undergoing weekly NSTs. Compared to nonreactive tests, reactive NSTs within 1 week of delivery were associated with significantly lower rates of meconium passage and low Apgar scores, as well as a trend toward fewer cesarean sections. However, when reactive tests were accompanied by variable decelerations, the rates of meconium passage and cesarean procedures for fetal distress were similar to those encountered with nonreactive tests. The authors concluded that FHR decelerations during the NST, regardless of reactivity, warrant consideration of delivery. Reported false-positive rates of the NST vary widely, with an average rate of approximately 50%. When performed twice weekly and interpreted in the context of associated FHR patterns, the NST alone appears to be an acceptable, though not optimal, method of antepartum testing. Advantages include ease of use and interpretation, low cost, and minimal time requirement. The chief disadvantages include a high false-positive rate and a higher false-negative rate than achieved with other methods.

Biophysical Profile

The biophysical profile (BPP), as described by Manning and associates (1980, 1985), assesses five biophysical variables. FHR reactivity, fetal movement, tone, and breathing reflect acute CNS function, while amniotic fluid volume serves as a marker of the longer-term adequacy of placental function. Two points are assigned for each normal variable and zero for each abnormal variable for a maximum score of 10. A BPP score of 8 to 10, with normal amniotic fluid volume, is considered normal. A score of 6 is considered suspicious, and testing usually is repeated the following day. Scores less than 6 are associated with increased perinatal morbidity and mortality and usually warrant hospitalization for further evaluation or delivery. Among 12,620 women tested weekly using the BPP, Manning and co-workers reported a false-negative rate of 0.6 per 1000. Johnson and colleagues (1986) reported significantly lower rates of cesarean delivery for fetal distress (3% versus 22%), low 5-minute Apgar scores (1.6% and 3.2% versus 12.5%), and meconium aspiration syndrome when the last BPP score before delivery was normal than when it was abnormal. The false-positive rate of the BPP varies with the score of the last test prior to delivery. Manning and co-workers reported a false-positive rate of 0% among 11 patients in whom the last BPP score before delivery was 0, compared to a false-positive rate greater than 40% among 182 patients with a last BPP score of 6. The BPP is a reliable predictor of fetal well-being. The false-negative rate is superior to that of the NST alone and compares favorably with the false-negative rate of the CST. Advantages of BPP include excellent sensitivity, a weekly testing interval, a low false-negative rate, and improved detection of structural fetal anomalies. The primary limitation is the requirement for personnel trained in sonographic visualization of the fetus. Additionally, although the duration of ultrasound observation is less than 10 minutes in the majority of cases, the complete BPP is more time-consuming than other noninvasive tests. However, Manning and associates reported that when all ultrasound variables were normal, addition of the NST did not alter the discriminative accuracy of the test. Omission of the NST shortens testing time considerably.

Modified Biophysical Profile

The modified biophysical profile (MBPP) combines the strengths of the NST (ease of use, low cost) and the complete BPP (improved sensitivity, low false-negative rate), while minimizing the requirement for additional training in sonographic visualization of the fetus. The test is performed once to twice weekly and utilizes the NST as a short-term marker of fetal status and the amniotic fluid index (AFI) as a marker of longer-term placental function. Interpretation of the NST incorporates assessment of reactivity, baseline rate, variability, and FHR decelerations (Fig. 4). Late, prolonged, or significant variable decelerations, particularly in the setting of borderline amniotic fluid volume (AFI 5 to 10 cm), are considered abnormal. Regardless of reactivity, oligohydramnios (AFI less than 5 cm) constitutes an abnormal test. Bochner reported an increased incidence of cesarean section for fetal distress if either the NST or the amniotic fluid volume was abnormal. Clark reported no unexpected fetal deaths in 2628 pregnancies tested with the MBPP as the primary method and the CST as the backup test. Nageotte and co-workers (1994) evaluated 2774 high-risk pregnancies with twice weekly MBPPs and reported one unexplained fetal death within 1 week of a normal test result, for a false-negative rate of 0.36 per 1000. Miller and colleagues (1996) reported 54,617 MBPPs in 15,482 high-risk pregnancies. Antepartum testing in high-risk pregnancies yielded a fetal death rate that was nearly sevenfold lower than that in the untested, low-risk population. The overall false-negative rate of the MBPP was 0.8 per 1000, and the false-positive rate was 60%. Abnormal test results prompted inter-

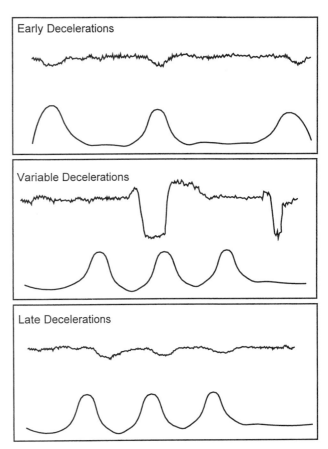

FIG. 4. Fetal heart rate decelerations.

vention in 15.5% of the tested population; however, iatrogenic prematurity occurred in only 1.5% of women tested before 37 weeks. When the MBPP is used as described by Miller, Nageotte, and associates, the AFI is repeated twice weekly. Recent studies by Lagrew and Wing and associates (1996) suggest that weekly AFI determinations may be reasonable prior to 41 weeks, provided that the AFI remains greater than 8 cm. Beyond 41 weeks, oligohydramnios may develop more rapidly, and the AFI should be assessed twice weekly. Large reports reveal the false-negative rate of the MBPP to be similar to those of the CST and the complete BPP. Additionally, it is easier to perform and less time-consuming than the CST or the complete BPP. The sensitivity of the MBPP is superior to that of the NST alone. Limitations include the need for backup testing in 10% to 50% of patients, a high false-positive rate, and a twice weekly testing interval.

Fetal Movement Counts

Maternal perception of normal fetal movement has long been recognized as a reliable indicator of fetal well-being. Conversely, prolonged absence of fetal movement may signal fetal death. Cessation of fetal movement in response to hypoxia has been demonstrated in animal studies; however, controlled data in human fetuses are lacking. Nevertheless, any acute decrement in the number or strength of fetal movements should raise the suspicion of fetal compromise and should prompt further evaluation. Many clinicians recommend routine fetal movement counting, particularly in patients who are considered high-risk. A common approach is to recommend daily counting of fetal movements for 1 hour. Ten fetal movements in a 1-hour period are considered reassuring. If fewer than 10 movements are appreciated, counting is continued for another hour. Fewer than 10 movements in a 2-hour period should alert the patient to contact her physician for further evaluation. Another protocol calls for movement counting two to three times daily for 30 minutes. With this approach, further evaluation is recommended if there are fewer than four strong movements in a 30-minute period.

Although controlled trials in low-risk patients have not demonstrated a significant benefit of formalized movement counting over routine questioning during prenatal visits, evidence from one study using nonconcurrent controls suggests a lower rate of fetal death and a higher incidence of intervention for fetal distress in patients using a formalized protocol of fetal movement counting. Fetal movement counting is an inexpensive method of involving the patient in her own care and may be a valuable adjunct to routine prenatal care, regardless of risk category. Some fetal monitors have the capability to display a Doppler-detected fetal movement profile. This technology may aid the clinician in determining the true baseline FHR and has been shown to reduce the incidence of nonreactive NSTs by half.

Doppler Velocimetry

Doppler velocimetry of fetal, umbilical, and uterine vessels has been the focus of intensive study in recent years. This technology utilizes systolic-to-diastolic flow ratios and resistance indices to estimate blood flow in various arteries. Recent studies have shown statistically significant improvement in perinatal outcome with the use of Doppler ultrasonography in pregnancies complicated by fetal growth restriction. Although severe restriction of umbilical artery blood flow, as evidenced by absent or reversed flow during diastole, has been correlated with fetal growth restriction, acidosis, and adverse perinatal outcome, the predictive values of less extreme deviations from normal remain undefined. In conditions other than fetal growth restriction, Doppler velocimetry does not appear to be a useful screening test for the detection of fetal compromise and is not recommended for use as a screening test in the general obstetric population. Doppler velocimetry is used in some settings as an adjunct to standard methods of fetal assessment but should not be considered a replacement for traditional fetal monitoring.

OTHER METHODS OF FETAL ASSESSMENT

Fetal Scalp Blood Sampling

In 1961, Saling introduced fetal scalp blood sampling as a method of determining the fetal acid–base status during labor.

The technique requires dilatation of the cervix, rupture of the membranes, and access to the fetal presenting part. A lighted plastic endoscopic cone is inserted into the vagina and through the cervical os so that it rests against the fetal presenting part. Care should be taken to ensure that it is not placed over a fontanelle. The area to be sampled is dried with a sponge and coated with a thin layer of silicone to facilitate the formation of a blood globule. The scalp is then punctured with a microscalpel, and blood is collected by capillary action in a heparinized capillary tube. After the sample is mixed, it is transported on ice to the laboratory for blood gas analysis. During labor, a normal scalp blood pH is 7.25 to 7.35. A fetal scalp pH of greater than or equal to 7.25 provides evidence of a nonacidotic fetus. In the presence of a persistently nonreassuring FHR tracing, the pH should be repeated every 30 to 60 minutes. A scalp pH of 7.20 to 7.25 is considered suspicious, and sampling should be repeated within 30 to 60 minutes.

Historically, pH values less than 7.20 have been considered acidotic; however, minor deviations below normal correlate poorly with perinatal outcome. Because abnormal perinatal outcome has not been consistently observed with values greater than 7.0, there is debate regarding the specific pH value that should be considered acidotic. In light of the technical difficulty of the procedure and the uncertainty regarding interpretation of results, many centers have reduced their reliance on fetal scalp blood sampling. Goodwin reported that the elimination of fetal scalp blood sampling at Los Angeles County–University of Southern California resulted in no significant increase in cesarean section for fetal distress, birth asphyxia, or low Apgar scores. Many proponents of FHR monitoring contend that fetal status can be assessed accurately with the FHR tracing alone and that fetal scalp blood sampling is needed only rarely, particularly when fetal scalp stimulation and/or fetal vibroacoustic stimulation are used to clarify difficult cases.

Fetal Scalp Stimulation and Fetal Vibroacoustic Stimulation

In 1984, Clark reported that FHR accelerations of 15 beats/min for 15 seconds in response to fetal scalp stimulation predicted a scalp pH greater than or equal to 7.19. Among fetuses without an acceleratory response to scalp stimulation, 39% were considered acidotic (pH less than 7.19). Smith and colleagues (1986) reported a similar relationship between fetal scalp pH and the FHR response to vibroacoustic stimulation with an artificial larynx applied to the maternal abdomen over the fetal head for 1 to 3 seconds. Among 30 fetuses with FHR accelerations in response to this stimulus, all had scalp pH values greater than or equal to 7.25. Half of the fetuses that did not respond to acoustic stimulation had pH values less than 7.25. FHR accelerations in response to external stimuli are thought to have the same predictive value as spontaneous accelerations. Fetal stimulation is used in antepartum testing to shorten the time of the NST and in the intrapartum period to confirm fetal well-being when spontaneous accelerations are absent. There is no evidence in humans of adverse long-term effects of vibroacoustic stimulation.

Amniocentesis

Amniocentesis is a technique by which a fine needle is placed transabdominally into the amniotic cavity under ultrasound guidance, and a small amount of amniotic fluid is removed for analysis (Fig. 5). Early in pregnancy, amniocentesis may be performed for prenatal diagnosis. Fetal squamous cells shed into the amniotic fluid are cultured for use in karyotype analysis and other genetic tests. In Rh-sensitized pregnancies, amniotic fluid bilirubin levels are used to estimate the severity of fetal hemolysis and the need for intervention. Later in pregnancy, amniocentesis is used most often to assess fetal lung maturity prior to delivery. As the fetal lungs mature,

type II pneumocytes secrete increasing quantities of surfactant into the alveoli, and the net outward flow of pulmonary fluid permits the detection of surfactant in the amniotic fluid. Surfactant is a mixture of proteins and lipids that reduces the surface tension of the alveoli and prevents them from collapsing during expiration. In the absence of surfactant, the lungs remain stiff and noncompliant, requiring high pressures to maintain alveolar expansion. Resultant respiratory distress syndrome may require prolonged intubation, leading to barotrauma and bronchopulmonary dysplasia. Pulmonary maturity tests are based on the quantitation of surfactant in the amniotic fluid. As surfactant increases, the risk of respiratory distress syndrome decreases. One of the major components of surfactant, lecithin, increases substantially in the amniotic fluid to maturity at 35 weeks' gestation. Sphingomyelin is a cell membrane lipid that is present in the amniotic fluid

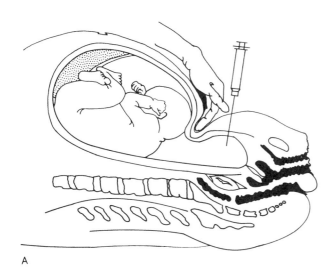

A

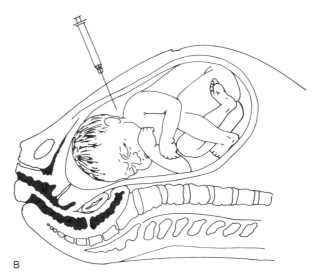

B

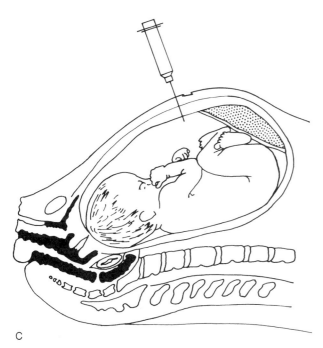

C

FIG. 5. Amniocentesis performed **(A)** by suprapubic approach, **(B)** at a site behind the nape of the fetal neck, and **(C)** in the area of fetal small parts. (Courtesy of Richard H. Paul.)

throughout gestation. The ratio of lecithin to sphingomyelin (L/S ratio) is used to assess the increase in lecithin production and predict the likelihood of respiratory distress syndrome. In general, a L/S ratio of 2.0 or greater is associated with a low incidence of respiratory distress syndrome and is considered mature. A L/S ratio of 1.5 to 1.9 is considered transitional, and a ratio less than 1.0 is immature. These values and their interpretation may vary significantly, depending on laboratory technique, prevalence of respiratory distress syndrome in the population, and diabetic status. Therefore, decisions should be based on cut-off levels established by the reference laboratory performing the test.

Phosphatidylglycerol (PG) is another component of surfactant that is detected in increasing concentrations in the amniotic fluid beyond 35 weeks' gestation. Levels of PG greater than 3% correlate with pulmonary maturity.

Percutaneous Umbilical Blood Sampling

Electronic FHR monitoring, ultrasound, and fetal scalp blood sampling can provide useful information regarding the acid–base status of the fetus. Occasionally, however, direct access to circulating fetal blood is necessary. A classic example is the fetus with severe anemia secondary to Rh-isoimmunization. In this condition, maternal antibodies directed against fetal red blood cell antigens cross the placenta and bind to fetal red blood cells, resulting in hemolysis. At term, suspected fetal anemia can be managed by delivery and treatment of the neonate. Earlier in pregnancy, however, it may be preferable to delay delivery by assessing the fetal hematocrit and, if necessary, performing intrauterine blood transfusion. Percutaneous umbilical blood sampling (PUBS) is a procedure that affords direct access to fetal venous blood. Using sterile technique and direct ultrasound guidance, a fine needle is passed transabdominally into the umbilical vein. Once fetal blood samples have been obtained, medications or blood may be infused through the needle. Other indications for PUBS include suspected antibody-mediated fetal thrombocytopenia and fetal cardiac arrhythmias requiring assessment of fetal drug levels or direct fetal administration of antiarrhythmic agents.

◊ MANAGEMENT OF INTRAPARTUM FETAL DISTRESS

Timely diagnosis and appropriate management of intrapartum fetal distress remain among the most challenging tasks facing the obstetrician. A clear understanding of the pathophysiology of FHR abnormalities is essential to optimal management. In general, fetal distress is a state in which deterioration of fetal status is anticipated within a relatively short time. It results most often from acute or chronic disruption of uteroplacental blood flow or oxygen delivery. Other etiologies include worsening fetal cardiac arrhythmias, hydrops fetalis, fetomaternal hemorrhage, fetal sepsis, and

severe fetal anemia. Deteriorating fetal status may be reflected in the FHR by tachycardia, a sinusoidal FHR pattern, loss of variability, loss of reactivity, repetitive severe variable or late decelerations, or prolonged decelerations.

In the presence of persistent fetal tachycardia, potential sources of infection must be excluded. Intraamniotic infection requires intrapartum antibiotic therapy. Possible causative medications should be discontinued, and maternal hyperthyroidism should be excluded. Fetal cardiac arrhythmias may require sonographic evaluation to exclude structural abnormalities and cardiac failure. Antiarrhythmic medications may be instituted, if deemed necessary. Tachycardia alone does not constitute fetal distress. However, tachycardia often occurs in association with other FHR patterns suggestive of hypoxia. In such cases, consideration should be given to fetal scalp pH determination or delivery. A more practical and less invasive approach employs fetal scalp stimulation or vibroacoustic stimulation. If fetal stimulation fails to provoke FHR accelerations, delivery should be considered.

A true, persistent sinusoidal pattern that is not attributable to medications is a concerning finding. Evaluation should be undertaken to exclude Rh-isoimmunization, fetomaternal hemorrhage, fetal anemia, and intraamniotic infection. If the pattern does not resolve, consideration should be given to scalp pH determination or delivery.

Loss of FHR variability and reactivity must be considered in the context of the clinical setting and other FHR findings. These changes may be explained by the administration of narcotic analgesics, magnesium sulfate, or other CNS depressants. Pathologic loss of variability and reactivity rarely evolves in a previously normal tracing without intervening FHR abnormalities. If, however, loss of variability and reactivity are preceded by decelerations or other evidence of hypoxia, they should be considered to reflect fetal acidosis until proven otherwise. Normal scalp pH values or accelerations provoked by manual or vibroacoustic fetal stimulation argue against significant acidosis.

Repetitive severe variable decelerations require immediate attention. Umbilical cord prolapse must be excluded. Cord compression may be relieved by changes in maternal position. Uterine hypertonus or tachysystole may be treated by discontinuing oxytocin, administering uterine relaxants (e.g., magnesium sulfate, terbutaline), or both. Restoration of normal amniotic fluid volume with amnioinfusion in patients with oligohydramnios has been demonstrated in randomized trials to reduce the frequency and severity of variable decelerations, as well as the incidence of cesarean section for fetal distress. The results of these studies are summarized in Figures 6 and 7. In cases of thick meconium, instillation of fluid into the amniotic cavity has been shown to reduce the severity of meconium aspiration syndrome. Transcervical amnioinfusion of 250 ml of normal saline should increase the AFI by 4 cm. Ideally, an AFI of at least 10 cm should be maintained. Repetitive severe variable decelerations that persist despite these maneuvers must be evaluated in the context of the associated FHR patterns. In the absence of reassuring

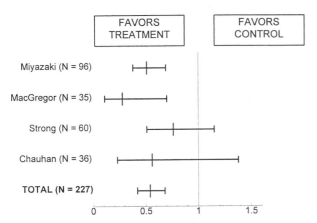

FIG. 6. Results of randomized trials of amnioinfusion for the treatment of persistent variable decelerations.

FHR findings or normal scalp pH values, delivery should be expedited.

Prolonged decelerations usually reflect acute events. Umbilical cord prolapse, uterine rupture, and placental abruption must be considered. Maternal positional changes and/or manual elevation of the fetal head may relieve cord compression, if present. Acute maternal hypotension, observed often in association with sympathetic blockade from regional anesthesia, may respond to positional changes, intravenous fluids, and ephedrine. Tetanic uterine contractions are treated by discontinuing oxytocin and administering uterine relaxants (e.g., magnesium sulfate, terbutaline), as needed. Supplemental oxygen is administered by facemask. If the above measures fail to result in resolution of the prolonged deceleration, rapid delivery is indicated.

The goal in treating late decelerations is to improve uteroplacental perfusion and oxygen delivery to the fetus. Usual measures include (1) left lateral decubitus position to improve maternal venous return and cardiac output, (2) supplemental oxygen by facemask, (3) intravenous fluid bolus of 250 to 500 ml of crystalloid to restore the maternal intravascular volume and improve cardiac output, and (4) discontin-

uation of oxytocin. If repetitive late decelerations do not respond to these measures, consideration should be given to scalp pH determination or delivery.

◊ CONCLUSION

Our ability to assess the condition of the fetus has improved dramatically over the past 40 years. While diagnostic precision is enhanced by electronic FHR monitoring, ultrasound technology, and direct access to amniotic fluid and fetal blood, room for improvement remains. Electronic FHR monitoring is a very sensitive tool for the detection of fetal compromise; truly compromised fetuses rarely fail to exhibit abnormal FHR patterns. The converse, however, is not true. Abnormal FHR patterns frequently are observed in the absence of fetal compromise. The limited positive predictive value is the principle shortcoming of FHR monitoring. Accuracy may be improved by combining FHR analysis with assessment of biophysical variables such as amniotic fluid volume, fetal movement, breathing, tone, and blood flow characteristics. Other variables under investigation include continuous intrapartum fetal pulse-oximetry, Doppler-detected fetal movement assessment, and fetal ECG interpretation. To date, the most effective combination of variables has not been defined, and no one approach to fetal surveillance has demonstrated clear superiority over the others. Yet, despite the limitations, antepartum testing in "high-risk" pregnancies has been reported to yield a fetal death rate nearly seven times lower than that in untested, "low-risk" pregnancies. If this observation is substantiated, future investigation will be needed to address the role of antepartum fetal surveillance in uncomplicated, low-risk pregnancies.

◊ RECOMMENDED READINGS

History of Fetal Monitoring
Goodlin R. History of fetal monitoring. *Am J Obstet Gynecol* 1979;133:325.
Gültekin-Zootzmann B. The history of monitoring the human fetus. *J Perinat Med* 1975;3:135.
Fetal Distress
Gilstrap LC, Leveno KJ, Burris J, Williams ML, Bertis BL. Diagnosis of birth asphyxia on the basis of fetal pH, Apgar score, and newborn cerebral dysfunction. *Am J Obstet Gynecol* 1989;161:825.
Asphyxia and Cerebral Palsy
Blair E, Stanley FJ. Intrapartum asphyxia: a rare cause of cerebral palsy. *J Pediatr* 1988;112:515.
Myers RE. Two patterns of perinatal brain damage and their conditions of occurrence. *Am J Obstet Gynecol* 1972;122:246.
Nelson KB, Ellenberg JH. Antecedents of cerebral palsy: multivariate analysis of risk. *N Engl J Med* 1986;315:81.
Windle WF, Becker RF. Asphyxia neonatorum: an experimental study in the guinea pig. *Am J Obstet Gynecol* 1943;45:183.
Fetal Heart Rate Monitoring
Hammacher K. The clinical significance of cardiotography. In: Huntingford P, Hunter M, Saling E, eds. *Perinatal Medicine*. New York: Academic Press, 1970:80.
Hon EH, Quilligan EJ. The classification of fetal heart rate. *Conn Med* 1967;31:779.
Kubli FW, Hon EH, Khazin AF, Takemura H. Observations on heart rate and pH in the human fetus during labor. *Am J Obstet Gynecol* 1969;104:1190.
Paul RH, Suidan AK, Yeh S, Hon EH. The evaluation and significance of intrapartum baseline FHR variability. *Am J Obstet Gynecol* 1975;123:206.

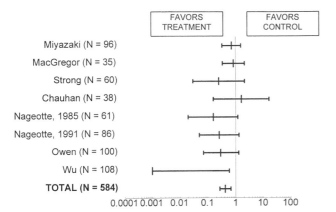

FIG. 7. Results of randomized trials of the effect of amnioinfusion on the incidence of cesarean section for fetal distress.

Fetal Scalp Stimulation/Vibroacoustic Stimulation

Clark SL, Gimovsky ML, Miller FC. Fetal heart rate response to scalp blood sampling. *Am J Obstet Gynecol* 1984;144:706.

Clark SL, Gimovsky ML, Miller FC. The scalp stimulation test: A clinical alternative to fetal scalp blood sampling. *Am J Obstet Gynecol* 1984; 148:274.

Smith CV, Nguyen HN, Phelan JP, Paul RH. Intrapartum assessment of fetal well-being: a comparison of fetal acoustic stimulation with acid-base determinations. *Am J Obstet Gynecol* 1986;155:726.

Prolonged Decelerations in FHR baseline

Clapp JF, Peress NS, Wesley M, Mann LI. Brain damage after intermittent partial cord occlusion in the chronically instrumented fetal lamb. *Am J Obstet Gynecol* 1988;159:504.

Contraction Stress Test/Oxytocin Challenge Test

Freeman RK, Anderson G, Dorchester W. A prospective multi-institutional study of antepartum fetal heart rate monitoring. II. Contraction stress test versus nonstress test for primary surveillance. *Am J Obstet Gynecol* 1982;143:778.

Ray M, Freeman RK, Pine S, et al. Clinical experience with the oxytocin challenge test. *Am J Obstet Gynecol* 1972;114:1.

Nonstress Test

Boehm FH, Salyer S, Shah DM, Vaughn WK. Improved outcome of twice weekly nonstress testing. *Obstet Gynecol* 1986;67:566.

Manning FA, Lange IR, Morrison I, Harman CR. Determination of fetal health: methods for antepartum and intrapartum fetal assessment. *Curr Probl Obstet Gynecol* 1983;7:3.

Phelan JP, Platt LD, Yeh S-Y, et al. Continuing role of the non-stress test in the management of post-dates pregnancy. *Obstet Gynecol* 1984;64:624.

Biophysical Profile

Johnson JM, Harman CR, Lange IR, et al. Biophysical profile scoring in the management of postterm pregnancy: an analysis of 307 patients. *Am J Obstet Gynecol* 1986;154:269.

Manning FA, Morrison I, Lange I, et al. Fetal assessment based upon fetal BPP scoring: experience in 12,620 referred high-risk pregnancies. I. Perinatal mortality by frequency and etiology. *Am J Obstet Gynecol* 1985; 151:343.

Manning FA, Platt LD, Sipos L. Antepartum fetal evaluation: development of a fetal biophysical profile. *Am J Obstet Gynecol* 1980;136:787.

Modified Biophysical Profile

Bochner CJ, Medearis AL, Davis J, Oakes GK, Hobel CJ, Wade ME. Antepartum predictors of fetal distress. *Am J Obstet Gynecol* 1987;157:353.

Clark SL, Sabey P, Jolley K. Nonstress testing with acoustic stimulation and amniotic fluid assessment: 5973 tests without unexpected fetal death. *Am J Obstet Gynecol* 1989;160:694.

Lagrew DC, Pircon RA, Nageotte M, Freeman RK, Dorchester W. How frequently should the amniotic fluid index be repeated? *Am J Obstet Gynecol* 1992;167:1129.

Miller DA, Rabello YA, Paul RH. The modified biophysical profile: antepartum testing in the 1990's. *Am J Obstet Gynecol* 1996;174:812.

Nageotte JP, Towers CV, Asrat T, Freeman RK. Perinatal outcome with the MBPP. *Am J Obstet Gynecol* 1994;170:1672.

Wing DA, Fishman A, Gonzalez C, Paul RH. How frequently should the amniotic fluid index be performed during the course of antepartum testing? *Am J Obstet Gynecol* 1996;174:33.

Fetal Scalp Blood Sampling

Goodwin TM, Milner-Masterson L, Paul RH. Elimination of fetal scalp blood sampling on a large clinical service. *Obstet Gynecol* 1994;83:971.

Amnioinfusion

Chauhan SP, Rutherford SE, Hess LW, Morrison JC. Prophylactic intrapartum amnioinfusion for patients with oligohydramnios: a prospective randomized study. *J Reprod Med* 1992;37:817.

MacGregor SN, Banzhaf WC, Silver RK, Depp R. A prospective randomized evaluation of intrapartum amnioinfusion. *J Reprod Med* 1991;36:69.

Macri CJ, Schrimmer DB, Leung A, Greenspoon JS, Paul RH. Prophylactic amnioinfusion improves outcome of pregnancy complicated by thick meconium and oligohydramnios. *Am J Obstet Gynecol* 1992; 167:117.

Miyazaki FS, Nevarez F. Saline amnioinfusion for relief of repetitive variable decelerations: a prospective randomized study. *Am J Obstet Gynecol* 1985;153:301.

Nageotte MP, Bertucci L, Towers CV, Lagrew DL, Modanlou H. Prophylactic amnioinfusion in pregnancies complicated by oligohydramnios: a prospective study. *Obstet Gynecol* 1991;77:677.

Nageotte MP, Freeman RK, Garite TJ, Dorchester W. Prophylactic intrapartum amnioinfusion in patients with preterm premature rupture of membranes. *Am J Obstet Gynecol* 1985;153:557.

Owen J, Henson BV, Hauth JC. A prospective randomized study of saline solution amnioinfusion. *Am J Obstet Gynecol* 1990;162:1146.

Strong TH, Hetzler G, Sarno AP, Paul RH. Prophylactic intrapartum amnioinfusion: a randomized clinical trial. *Am J Obstet Gynecol* 1990;162:1370.

Wu BT. Intrapartum amnio-infusion in patients with oligohydramnios. *Chung Hua Fu Chan Ko Tsa Chih* 1989;24:2.

Doppler Ultrasound

Alfirevic Z, Neilson JP. Doppler ultrasonography in high-risk pregnancies: systematic review with meta-analysis. *Am J Obstet Gynecol* 1995;172:1379.

Maulik D. Doppler ultrasound in obstetrics. In: Cunningham G, MacDonald P, Gant N, Leveno K, Gilstrap L, eds. *Williams' obstetrics supplement.* Stanford, CT: Appleton & Lange, 1996:1.

CHAPTER 16

Preterm Labor

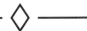

Michael T. Parsons
William N. Spellacy

Preterm delivery is a serious perinatal event occurring in about 8% of pregnancies. An infant is classified as preterm if the delivery occurs before 37 weeks' gestation. An infant weighing less than 2500 g at birth is low-birthweight. Whereas previously all infants born weighing less than 2500 g were labeled premature, premature versus small term infants can usually be differentiated with more accurate measurement of gestational age. Of all infants born with birth weights less than 2500 g, about one-third are mature but growth-retarded, and have different and unique problems (see Chapter 18).

The definition of labor has two components: (1) regular uterine contractions, usually at least three in 30 minutes, and (2) changes in the cervix, including effacement and dilation. Despite great effort to prevent preterm delivery, the incidence has actually increased over the past 20 years. This chapter reviews the following aspects of preterm labor: mechanisms of labor onset, etiology of preterm labor, identification of high-risk patients, prenatal care for high-risk patients, management of preterm labor, and controversies regarding preterm labor.

◇ SIGNIFICANCE OF PRETERM BIRTH

Although about 8% of infants are born at less than 37 weeks' gestation, complications in these infants account for greater than 70% of nonanomalous neonatal deaths and much morbidity, including respiratory distress syndrome, intraventricular hemorrhage, bronchopulmonary dysplasia, patent ductus arteriosus, retinopathy of prematurity, sepsis, necrotizing enterocolitis, apnea, hyperbilirubinemia, hypoglycemia, visual and hearing impairment, cerebral palsy, chronic lung disease, and, in later years, poor school performance. The smaller the infant is, the greater are the risks.

◇ MECHANISMS OF LABOR ONSET

Labor occurs when mechanisms are present that convert the uterus from a state of containment to an environment that at-

tempts to expel the fetus. This expulsion of the fetus requires a coordination of myometrial contractility and cervical softening and dilation. Most animals reach a point in pregnancy at which the mechanisms that produce labor override those that maintain the pregnancy. In women with singleton pregnancies, the time of labor is considered normal if gestation is between 37 and 42 completed weeks since the start of the last menstrual period. Lack of understanding of the initiation of labor has hampered the ability to develop therapies to prevent or stop it. Once a thorough understanding of labor in term pregnancies is obtained, there may be better management approaches to preterm labor.

Animal models have helped in understanding labor. Important findings in animal labor models include an increase in oxytocin receptors present in the myometrium, gap junctions developing between myometrial cells, an increased response to agents capable of producing contractions in the uterus, and physical and biochemical changes of the cervix resulting in a softened consistency. Uterine smooth muscle contractility is produced by the actin–myosin interaction, following myosin light chain phosphorylation, which is controlled by kinase. Myosin light chain kinase is activated by calcium as a calmodulin–calcium complex. Cyclic adenosine monophosphate (cyclic AMP) also regulates kinase by inhibiting phosphorylation. Many factors are involved in this control. Some of the proposed theories of labor will be discussed.

Hormonal

Alteration in systemic or local levels of steroid hormones is an initiating factor of labor in some animals. The understanding of their possible role in human labor has been continuously evolving. The withdrawal of the uterine inhibitor hormone progesterone has been shown to play a major role in many animals (e.g., sheep, rats, rabbits). In sheep, this withdrawal seems to be caused by increased responsiveness of

257

fetal adrenal cells to adrenocorticotropic hormone (ACTH) that results in increased production of cortisol. Through several steps, cortisol redirects placental steroid biosynthesis and decreases progesterone secretion. The decreased circulating progesterone in the sheep permits increased myometrial gap junction formation, an increase in prostaglandin formation, and increased response of the uterus to agents capable of producing contractions. In this sheep model, fetal ACTH secretion has control of the onset of labor.

Major differences exist, however, between sheep hormonal status and that of primates, including humans. In humans, there is no great increase in cortisol from the fetal adrenal gland before labor, nor has a dramatic decrease in progesterone been consistently demonstrated. Progesterone, however, is important in human pregnancy, and numerous studies have examined the its role or the progesterone-to-estrogen ratio before the onset of labor. In the 1974, Turnbull et al. demonstrated a significant fall in serum progesterone levels and a rise in estrogen levels in many women before entering labor. Other studies failed to consistently find these changes. Estriol may be a signal from the fetus indicating that it is mature and ready for delivery. Production of estriol increases during the last month of pregnancy. In the large amounts produced, estriol is as active as estradiol in stimulating uterine growth. There are reports of an elevation in estradiol/progesterone in amniotic fluid, estriol/progesterone in saliva, and possibly elevated plasma estriol/progesterone or estradiol/progesterone at the end of pregnancy.

Administration of progesterone has not been demonstrated to delay term or preterm labor in primates. The antiprogesterones—RU 486 or mifepristone and ZK 98299 or onapristone—in humans and other primates can enhance the responsiveness of the uterus and induce cervical change within 12 to 48 hours, again suggesting a role for progesterone in preventing labor onset.

Oxytocin

It is well known that oxytocin produces uterine activity when administered to pregnant women. The role of endogenous oxytocin as an initiator of term or preterm labor is less well defined. Some reasons to suspect that oxytocin is a universal initiator of labor are its ability to induce labor when given exogenously and the increase in blood levels that accompanies labor in most species. Because of the pulsatile manner of oxytocin release and the difficulty in measuring the hormone, its precise role in humans has been difficult to ascertain. Compared with oxytocin levels in nonlaboring patients, levels appear to be significantly increased during the first stage of labor and increased to a greater amount during the second stage of labor. Oxytocin levels are higher in umbilical artery blood than in umbilical vein or maternal blood. This finding suggests a fetal source for early labor oxytocin. It is clear that the uterus becomes more sensitive to oxytocin in the days preceding labor. The number of myometrial cell membrane oxytocin receptors greatly increases as pregnancy advances, with a further increase during labor itself. In women as well as in other species, the concentration of oxytocin receptors is a major reason for increased contractility of the uterus. The increase in oxytocin receptors is the result of increased estrogen levels.

Prostaglandins

Another important part of the parturition model is the synthesis and release of prostaglandins E_2 and $F_{2\alpha}$. This is supported by an increase in prostaglandins or metabolites in the amniotic fluid, endometrium, decidua, myometrium, and blood at the time of labor, the administration of prostaglandins inducing labor, and inhibitors to prostaglandin synthesis delaying labor. It is likely that the prostaglandins have a role in parturition originating from the decidua and myometrium. Oxytocin has the ability to stimulate prostaglandin release through the decidual receptors. In addition, infection of the membranes can release prostaglandins and may be an initiating factor in many cases of preterm labor.

The bacterial products may be directly responsible for the stimulation of prostaglandin release in the following ways: Bacterial phospholipase releases the precursor arachidonic acid from the amnion, leading to increased prostaglandin synthesis. Gram-negative organisms may be able to produce prostaglandins through endotoxin stimulation of the decidua or membranes. Gram-positive organisms may also have prostaglandin-stimulating abilities through peptidoglycans. Phospholipase A_2 is contained within the lysosome of the fetal membranes. As phospholipase A_2 is released from the lysosome, prostaglandin may be synthesized, resulting in uterine contractions.

Cytokines

Cytokines are substances secreted by a person's immune system in response to infection. There is recent interest in the role of cytokines and growth factors (e.g., epidermal growth factor, insulin-like growth factors 1 and 2) as potential initiators of labor. The cytokines interleukin (IL)-1β, IL-6, and tumor necrosis factor (TNF) stimulate the amnion and decidua to produce prostaglandins and increase at time of labor, while transforming growth factor (TGF)-β inhibits prostaglandin production by other cytokines and may have antiprogestin properties. Cytokines found in the amniotic fluid of patients with preterm labor are IL-1β, TNF, and macrophage colony-stimulating factor.

Other Factors

Endothelins are potent vasoconstrictors in the sarafotixin-like family. Some isoforms of endothelins are potent uterotonins. Although endothelin does not appear to increase at time of labor, uterine sensitivity and endothelin-receptor number do increase in the pregnant uterus. There is some decrease of endothelin 1 in the amniotic fluid of patients in labor, but this may be a consequence rather than an initiator of labor. Nitric oxide, produced from L-arginine by the enzyme nitric oxide synthase (NOS), mediates relaxation of vascular smooth muscle. It has been shown in various animal tissues, including human, that the NOS enzyme decreases in myometrial tissue at term. Thus, nitric oxide may have a role in maintaining a quiescent uterus.

It can be hypothesized that parturition is a development of an estrogen environment. This estrogen environment promotes changes in the maternal pituitary with increased oxytocin synthesis and release. Estrogen may also be acting on the placenta and cervix. As the antiestrogen progesterone decreases, estrogen can act to increase oxytocin receptors, prostaglandin production, and gap junction number and size. As the cervix ripens, the underlying membranes and decidua become exposed to the vaginal bacteria, triggering an inflammatory response with release of cytokines and prostaglandins. At this point, the paracrine events take dominance over the endocrine effects. Some conditions, such as infection, can overwhelm the endocrine phase of parturition.

◊ RISKS FOR PRETERM LABOR

Approximately two-thirds of preterm deliveries are due to preterm labor or rupture of the membranes, with the majority of the others due to medical complications such as hypertension or placental hemorrhage. It is important to identify women at risk for preterm labor early in pregnancy if prevention/treatment is to be successful. These risk factors are discussed below.

Age and Race

Patients in the extremes of age have an increased incidence of preterm labor. However, the risk may not be age itself but rather confounding factors associated with age. For example, young women have more sexual partners and vaginal infections, while older women may have more uterine irregularities, such as myomas. Patients of lower economic means, as well as patients with inadequate prenatal care, are at increased risk for preterm labor. Race has been found in several series to be an independent risk factor for preterm deliveries. Some studies have shown that blacks have a shorter gestational period and their infants are of lower weight per week of age. Virji and Cottington (1991) found a twofold increased rate of preterm delivery among black women. The higher rates of both preterm labor and low-birth-weight infants in black women are independent of economic status.

Prior Preterm Delivery

If a patient's first pregnancy results in preterm delivery, she has a twofold increased incidence of preterm delivery with subsequent pregnancies. If her first two pregnancies resulted in preterm deliveries, she has a threefold increased chance of delivering preterm during her third pregnancy. Conversely, successful completion of a pregnancy at term reduces the incidence of preterm delivery with subsequent pregnancies. While the history of a prior preterm birth is one of the most consistent and accepted risk factors, its relative risk is only 2; therefore, only 16% of all preterm births will be identified by this information. The role of a prior induced abortion in future risk of preterm labor is less clear. Some investigators found that the risk of preterm labor increased with each additional induced abortion, while other investigators found no association between spontaneous or induced abortions and the risk of preterm labor.

Infection

Non–Genital Tract Infections

Maternal infection predisposes a pregnancy to preterm labor and delivery. Many studies over the years have suggested an association between asymptomatic bacteriuria and preterm labor, and a metaanalysis of these data by Romero et al. (1989) reaffirmed this strong association. Patients with asymptomatic bacteriuria have almost twice the risk of entering preterm labor and delivering preterm as patients without bacteria in their urine. Untreated acute pyelonephritis can result in a 30% risk of preterm labor. Other infectious diseases can also lead to an increased incidence of preterm labor. Patients with pneumonia have a 25% incidence of preterm labor. Rarer systemic infections, such as malaria and typhoid fever, have been associated with high preterm labor rates, greater than 50% in some series.

Genital Tract Infections

Many organisms have been implicated in preterm labor, but few have been proved causes. There is little question that infection with *Treponema pallidum* is a strong factor in the production of uterine contractility and premature birth. Patients with untreated primary or secondary syphilis have up to a 50% prematurity rate compared with an 8% rate in control groups. Gonococcal infection has also been shown to be associated with an increased incidence of preterm delivery. This may be a marker for other sexually transmitted bacterial infections, however. With routine culture early in pregnancy and treatment of those with positive results, the role of this infection as a causative agent may be greatly reduced.

In their analysis, Romero et al. (1989) reviewed the literature for group B streptococcus (GBS) and found that the association between colonization with GBS in the cervix and vagina and prematurity could be demonstrated in only one out of seven studies. Their conclusion was that GBS colonization of the genital tract was not associated with preterm delivery in the absence of asymptomatic bacteriuria or ruptured membranes.

Chlamydia trachomatis has been associated with preterm labor in some studies, but most investigators found that, like GBS, it is associated with preterm delivery only in the setting of preterm premature rupture of the membranes (PROM). The role of *Ureaplasma urealyticum* in preterm birth is also controversial. In a review by Gibbs et al. (1992) of infection in premature birth, no evidence was found that *U. urealyticum* had a role. McGregor et al. (1990) found that the presence of *Mycoplasma* increased the risk of preterm labor with a relative risk factor of 1.8. Krohn et al. (1991), however, did not find *M. hominis* to be associated with an increased preterm delivery rate. Some studies indicated that *Trichomonas vaginalis* is associated with increased preterm delivery, whereas others suggested that this finding is controversial. Minkoff et al. (1984) identified *Bacteroides* infection as a cause of preterm birth. Krohn et al. found that the presence of *Bacteroides bivius* in the vagina of pregnant women increased the preterm delivery rate by a relative risk of 2.0.

Bacterial vaginosis, a condition occurring when the normal predominant *Lactobacillus* vaginal flora is replaced with *Gardnerella vaginalis, Mobiluncus* species, *Mycoplasma* species, and other gram-negative anaerobic bacteria, is associated with increased preterm delivery. This flora alteration causes a rise in the vaginal pH to greater than 4.5, and therefore vaginal pH becomes a risk factor for preterm labor.

The organisms discussed thus far have been associated with vaginal or cervical infection. The role of infection in the amniotic fluid with intact membranes has also been extensively investigated in patients with preterm labor. Multiple studies found that the normally sterile intraamniotic cavity can be colonized and infected by various organisms. In series in which amniocentesis was performed in patients with preterm labor and intact membranes, positive cultures for organisms were found in 15% to 30% of cases. Bacteria, either in the amniotic fluid or perhaps in the decidual tissue lining the membranes, appear capable of eliciting contractions through the release of endogenous cell mediators, cytokines, or the inflammatory response.

Preterm Premature Rupture of Membranes

PROM is a common cause of preterm labor and delivery (see Chapter 17).

Pregnancy Complications

Uterine size is a contributing factor in the timing of the initiation of labor. A uterus distended beyond its normal size has an increased risk of starting to contract spontaneously before term. The uterus can be distended because of a multiple gestation or an increased amount of amniotic fluid. Women with twins have a 50% preterm delivery rate. Uterine distention is associated with an increase in gap junction formation, which in turn causes the uterus to have an increased synchronous contractile mechanism at an earlier than normal gestational age. Abnormalities of the placenta and of placental implantation may increase the risk of preterm labor and delivery. Abruptio placentae causes increased uterine irritability and

contractions, which often lead to preterm labor. Some studies indicated that placenta previa also predisposes to early contractions. Surgical procedures, especially in proximity to the uterus such as appendectomy and in adnexal cases, increase the risk of uterine irritability and contractions.

Cervical incompetence contributes to increased preterm labor, as well as to earlier, painless pregnancy loss. This may be caused by exposure of the membranes to the vaginal flora, initiating an infectious process. Some uterine anomalies have a strong association with preterm delivery. With a bicollis bicornuate uterus, for example, the incidence of preterm labor may be as high as 80%. A complete septate uterus carries a much smaller risk. The presence of myomata, uterine anomalies (together with incompetent cervix or T-shaped endometrial cavity) caused by intrauterine diethylstilbestrol exposure, also increases the risk of preterm delivery.

Sexual activity and orgasm increase contractions, breast nipple stimulation releases oxytocin and results in contractions. Both orgasm and coitus have been studied as possible causes of preterm labor. Coitus can cause contractions because of the high concentration of prostaglandins in semen, which are absorbed vaginally. In addition, coitus may increase the number of bacteria present in the vaginal vault. Although some studies in the 1970s linked coitus to increases in preterm labor, studies in the 1980s did not find the same association. In normal pregnancies, the overall evidence does not seem to place women at risk for preterm labor after coitus. Many physicians, however, request that their patients at high risk for preterm labor or PROM restrict their sexual activity.

Fibronectin

An extracellular glycoprotein, fibronectin is produced by many cell types in the body in different molecular forms and functions to bind cells together. Fetal fibronectin (fFN) seems to play a part in the intercellular adhesion and maintenance of the placental attachment to the decidua. It is normally found in the cervical vaginal fluid during the early part of pregnancy, decreases in amount so that none is found after 20 weeks, but then reappears as labor approaches; it is in high concentration in the amniotic fluid. Damage to fetal membranes can release fFN into the vagina, as can separation of the chorion from the decidua. Lockwood et al. (1991) reported that increasing amounts of fFN in cervicovaginal secretions can be a marker for preterm labor. Values greater than 50 ng/ml are considered positive. Several investigators were able to identify patients who will deliver preterm with a sensitivity of about 70% to 80% and a specificity of about 80% to 90%. Thus, if the test is positive, the relative risk of preterm delivery is three to seven times normal. In several reports, the negative predictive value of fFN for perterm labor was greater than 95%. Thus, in the absence of fFN in the cervical vaginal secretion, there is a less than 5% chance that delivery will occur in the next 7 days. This impressive negative predictive value may prove useful in the number of pa-

TABLE 1. *Risk factors for preterm delivery*

Factor	Approximate relative risk
Twin pregnancy	6–7
Uterine anomalies	2–10
Vaginal fibronectin	3–7
Black race	2
Prior preterm delivery	2
Urinary tract infection	2
Bacterial vaginosis	2
Vaginal pH >4.5	2

tients treated for questionable preterm labor. In taking a cervicovaginal sample, care must be taken not to contaminate it with amniotic fluid or maternal blood.

The relative risk for preterm labor for many of these factors is summarized in Table 1.

Prenatal Care for High-risk Women

Women identified as being at increased risk for preterm labor should be triaged to a special prenatal program. They must be taught to recognize the early signs of preterm labor, such as an increase and change in vaginal discharge, a bloody show, increased uterine contractions and pelvic cramps, leakage of amniotic fluid, and pelvic fullness or backache (Table 2). If any of these signs develops, the woman must contact her health care provider for evaluation. This early symptom recognition education program is important and should be reinforced at each prenatal visit, so that women in preterm labor present early. Because breast stimulation releases oxytocin, orgasm causes uterine contractions, and seminal fluid has a high concentration of prostaglandins, at-risk women should be encouraged to decrease sexual stimulation during pregnancy. They should also avoid strenuous exercise or work and should increase their resting time.

Although the goal of preterm labor treatment is to prevent preterm delivery, much can be achieved in terms of reducing neonatal morbidity by short gains of time *in utero*. In the critical period from 22 to 32 weeks' gestation, a 1-week delay in delivery could reduce morbidity and mortality by as much as 15%. Neonatal morbidity and mortality are reduced by glucocorticoid treatment of the preterm fetus prior to delivery. Studies have shown that there are great reduction in perinatal mortality if the fetus reaches a weight of 1600 g and in perinatal morbidity if the fetus reaches 1900 g.

During the 10-week window from 22 to 32 weeks' gestation, high-risk women should be seen every 1 to 2 weeks. At their visits, the routine prenatal care evaluations of weight,

TABLE 2. *Signs of preterm labor*

Uterine contractions/cramps
Vaginal discharge
Bleeding
Backache
Leaking amniotic fluid

blood pressure, urine glucose and albumin levels, uterine fundal height measurements, and fetal heart rate should be done. In addition, patients should be reminded of the signs of preterm labor and counseled on good nutritional intake. A vaginal examination is important to assess any cervical change or vaginal infection. A test of vaginal pH and cervicovaginal FN levels may also be done.

◊ **EVALUATION OF PRETERM LABOR**

The diagnosis of preterm labor requires the simultaneous finding of regular uterine contractions and cervical changes occurring in a woman between 20 and 37 weeks' gestation. Preterm labor symptoms are often nonspecific. Contractions may be painful or painless but are persistent. The number of contractions per hour varies significantly in women, and patients differ in their ability to perceive contractions. In a study by Beckmann et al. (1996), an analysis was made of over 700 women receiving home uterine activity monitoring to determine how often they could detect contractions using self-palpation versus the recording by the tocodynamometer. Overall, the patients missed an average of 85.7% of their contractions and perceived contractions that were not present an average of 40.3% of the time.

Most will agree that a patient at less than 37 weeks' gestation with regular contractions and cervical dilation of 3 cm and effacement of 80% should be considered in preterm labor without waiting for further cervical change. The more difficult diagnosis involves patients having regular contractions but only minimal cervical dilation. These women need serial examinations to determine whether or not cervical change occurs. The rate of false-positive diagnoses is high, and as many as 50% of placebo-treated patients diagnosed with preterm labor go on to delivery at term. On the other hand, if the diagnosis of preterm labor is missed, an early delivery could occur without treatment. The earlier the patient is in gestation, the more aggressive one should be in evaluation and treatment.

If there is doubt about the gestational age, an ultrasound examination may be helpful. If there is concern that the fetus might be mature but growth-retarded, amniocentesis can be done to measure lung maturity. The ultrasound scan may also detect the presence of fetal breathing, which usually indicates that the contractions are false labor and of less concern. In true labor, the fetus usually stops breathing, presumably because of elevated serum prostaglandin concentrations.

◊ **MANAGEMENT OF PRETERM LABOR**

Not all preterm labors are treated. If the fetus is dead or has major congenital anomalies incompatible with life, or if the mother has medical problems such as severe preeclampsia requiring early delivery and the fetus is already viable (e.g., weight 2000 g), then the labor is not treated and the infant is delivered. If no contraindication to continuing the pregnancy exists and the infant is expected to survive, an attempt is made to stop the premature labor.

The patient population suitable for medical management is small. Excluded from it are (1) women with PROM (about 35% of preterm labor), (2) women with serious maternal or fetal diseases, such as abruption, chorioamnionitis, preeclampsia–HELLP syndrome (hemolysis, elevated liver enzymes, and low platelets), fetal distress, and major congenital anomalies incompatible with life (about 20%), (3) and women who present in advanced labor with more than 5 cm of cervical dilation (about 20%). The resulting population suitable for medical management is thus only about 25% of the total patients with preterm labor, or about 2% of all pregnancies. The steps in management of preterm labor are listed in Table 3 and will be discussed in detail.

Bed Rest and Hydration

The first therapeutic approach to diagnosed preterm uterine labor is admission to the hospital to attempt to increase uterine blood flow and improve the intrauterine environment, quieting the uterus. This is done by using two measures: bed rest on the side and maternal hydration. Uterine blood flow is greatly affected by the mother's position, and maximum uterine blood flow is achieved with the woman lying on her side. Uterine blood flow is also greatly affected by the maternal blood volume, and dehydration reduces both. Animal studies have found that rapid fluid administration blocks the posterior pituitary release of antidiuretic hormone. A woman in preterm labor can be quickly hydrated with a bolus of 500 ml of balanced electrolyte solution, such as Ringer's lactate, administered intravenously over a 30-minute period. Hydration is continued at a rate of at least 125 ml per hour. While uterine contractions frequently stop, recent studies question the efficacy of these treatments in preventing preterm delivery.

Tocolysis

Many tocolytic drugs have been developed and used, and several experimental drugs are being evaluated. Intravenous alcohol was one of the first drugs found to successfully decrease uterine activity. It is infrequently used today because of the difficulty in managing the patient, who becomes intoxicated. Alcohol blocks the release of the posterior pituitary hormones vasopressin and oxytocin. Other earlier therapies included some form of progestin administration. The

TABLE 3. *Treatment of preterm labor*

Bed rest
Hydration
Tocolytics (e.g., magnesium sulfate or ritodrine [Yutopar])
Glucocorticoids
Group B streptococcus culture and prophylactic treatment
Transfer to perinatal center
Atraumatic delivery

two most frequently used tocolytics are intravenous magnesium sulfate and the β-mimetic drugs.

Magnesium Sulfate

High concentrations of magnesium sulfate have been shown to decrease uterine activity with an efficacy comparable to that of intravenous alcohol. The drug is administered first as a bolus to achieve high blood concentrations and then as a maintenance infusion. The bolus usually consists of 6 g of intravenous magnesium sulfate administered in 250 ml of solution over a 30-minute period; the infusion is then maintained at 2 to 4 g per hour. Because 90% of magnesium sulfate is excreted by the kidneys and women in preterm labor usually have normal, pregnancy-increased renal clearance, these women need more magnesium to achieve therapeutic blood levels than women being treated for preeclampsia. Blood levels of 6 to 8 mg/dl are optimal. Although the exact mechanism of action of magnesium sulfate is unknown, it likely decreases the free calcium ion concentration in the intracellular compartment of the uterine myometrial myosin light chains, which blocks kinase phosphorylation and therefore decreases the electrical potential of the cell.

Although magnesium sulfate is widely used, its true efficacy in decreasing preterm delivery has not been proven. A study by Cox et al. (1990) randomized 156 patients with preterm labor to treatment with magnesium sulfate versus saline. Using infusions to raise the maternal plasma magnesium concentration to 5.5 mg/dl did not improve outcome compared to saline. Critics felt that the 4 g loading dose and the 5.5 mg/dl concentration were suboptimal for tocolytic effects.

The disadvantages of magnesium sulfate include the potential for toxic levels, which can cause apnea or cardiac arrest, and blockage of myoneural conduction, which leads to the absence of shivering and a resultant decrease in maternal body temperature. The latter could impair early recognition of intrauterine infection. The patient's reflex activity should be frequently tested because it is a reliable index of plasma magnesium concentrations. In the absence of reflex activity, plasma magnesium concentrations should be determined. If there is any evidence of decreased maternal renal function, either with elevated creatinine levels or oliguria, magnesium sulfate must be used cautiously. One contraindication is myasthenia gravis. Short-term neonatal effects include hypotonia and respiratory depression. There have been a few cases of bony abnormalities due to calcium loss and decreased mineralization detected in infants that had long-term exposure *in utero*.

Maternal magnesium treatment may also be associated with some neonate advantages. Several studies found that premature infants delivered to women treated with magnesium sulfate had a reduced incidence of cerebral palsy. It is hypothesized that magnesium sulfate may help prevent hemorrhage in the germinal matrix of the preterm infant. Others found a decreased incidence of interventricular hemorrhage in very low-birthweight infants born to mothers who received antepartum magnesium. Because of obstetricians' familiarity with magnesium sulfate as a therapy in preeclampsia and because of this agent's low toxicity rate compared to other tocolytics, magnesium sulfate has become a popular choice for initial therapy.

β-*Mimetic Drugs*

There are two types of β-mimetic receptors: β_1 receptors affect the cardiac rate and glycogen breakdown; β_2 receptors relax smooth muscle of the bronchial tree, blood vessels, and uterus. No drug exists that has unique β_1 or β_2 activity; rather all β-mimetic drugs have a mixed pattern of action. Uterine relaxation is caused by a drug's effect in increasing cyclic AMP in the myometrial cell, causing calcium binding to the intracellular sarcoplasmic reticulum. This lowers the intracellular free calcium concentration, which in turn decreases the electrical potential of the cell. The U.S. Food and Drug Administration has approved the use of ritodrine (Yutopar) as a β-mimetic tocolytic. The literature is replete with reports of other β-mimetics, such as terbutaline, used as tocolytics Thus, the choice of a β-mimetic depends on the obstetrician's familiarity with the drug. Although the package insert suggests an upper dosage limit of administration for these drugs, they must in fact be given in a dosage that is adequate to produce a biologic effect without toxicity, and the ultimate concentration needed cannot be totally predicted. The physician needs to administer enough medication to achieve either complete absence of uterine activity or significant maternal side effects to contraindicate increasing the dosage. The maternal pulse rate closely mirrors the blood concentration of the drug; therefore, the pulse rate can be used to clinically assess the adequacy of the dosage. Because the drugs freely cross the placenta, the increased heart rate is seen both in the fetus and in the mother. If maternal tachycardia is not achieved, then drug blood levels are subtherapeutic. These drugs are administered intravenously and slowly titrated upward until a response is achieved. For ritodrine, the recommended beginning dosage is 100 µg per minute intravenously, with increases of 50 µg per minute every 10 minutes to a maximum of 350 µg per minute.

A significant risk involved in the use of these drugs is the development of pulmonary edema. There are several predisposing factors for this complication. The presence of significant cardiopulmonary disease is a contraindication to the use of these drugs. Another risk factor is maternal tachycardia greater than 120 beats per minute sustained for long periods. If uterine activity continues and the maternal pulse rate is less than 120 beats per minute, the infusion rate may be increased until this level of tachycardia exists. Three other risk factors recognized for pulmonary edema are twin pregnancy, maternal infection at the time of treatment, and use of intravenous drug infusions beyond 24 hours.

Other problems with the drugs include their β_1 metabolic effects. During the early minutes of infusion, the blood glucose concentration increases as glycogen is broken down by the drug's cyclic AMP–stimulating effect. In normal women, this results in a simultaneous increase in insulin secretion from the beta cells of the pancreas, and there is then a gradual lowering of the blood glucose level toward normal. Women with diabetes may develop severe hyperglycemic ketoacidosis. If chest pain, premature ventricular contractions, or atrial fibrillation occur with use of a β-mimetic agent, the drug should be discontinued and oxygen administered. Finally, use of these drugs has been associated with an increased frequency of neonatal intraventricular hemorrhage, which may be due to an increased cardiac output in the infant secondary to placental transmission of the drug causing fetal tachycardia.

β-mimetic drugs have a double exponential disappearance curve, giving them a prolonged half-life of more than 12 hours. This means that good blood levels persist for hours after the infusion is stopped. In practice, the drugs are administered intravenously to a concentration that stops uterine activity. That dosage is then maintained for an additional 6 to 12 hours, and the infusion is then discontinued.

A study published in 1992 from the Canadian Preterm Labor Investigators Group demonstrated that the use of ritodrine in 352 patients versus placebo in 356 controls significantly delayed delivery for 48 hours, but there were no differences in the incidence of delivery before 37 weeks, infants weighing less than 2500 g, or other measures of neonatal morbidity. While 48-hour delivery delay seems small, it is enough time to transfer the mother to a tertiary hospital and give the fetus glucocorticoid treatment.

If significant uterine activity is not detected the next day, the patient can be allowed some ambulation (e.g., bathroom privileges). After the tocolytic agent has been discontinued and the patient observed for another day with no significant uterine activity, she can usually be discharged home. Some patients may benefit from prolonged hospitalization, such as those with a very immature fetus and advanced cervical dilation.

At home, the patient should be instructed to maintain good hydration and to limit her activity, with the preference being bed rest. She should not return to work until the fetus is mature. She must be made aware of the symptoms of recurrent labor. Use of an oral tocolytic on an ambulatory basis is of little help. This is probably because the tachyphylactic effect of the drugs in the β-mimetic group prevents this chronic oral therapy from achieving blood concentrations that are adequate to affect the uterus. Indeed, subtherapeutic drug levels have been found in most studies reported in an ambulatory setting. This is also clinically evident during monitoring of maternal pulse rates, because they usually show little effect with oral treatment.

Despite the extensive use of β-mimetic and magnesium sulfate tocolytics during the 1980s in the United States, the frequency of preterm delivery has not decreased. In addition, large, randomized, placebo-controlled trials and metaanalyses of smaller studies have failed to show much success beyond delaying delivery for 48 hours. As a result, several newer tocolytic agents are being investigated. These include prostaglandin synthetase inhibitors, calcium channel blockers, oxytocin antagonists, nitric oxide, and combinations of drugs. In preliminary studies, each of these groups has demonstrated tocolytic activity, but they have also shown potential adverse secondary effects.

Prostaglandin Synthetase Inhibitors

Nonsteroidal antiinflammatory drugs (NSAIDs) reduce the synthesis of prostaglandins by inhibiting cyclooxygenase, thereby preventing the conversion of arachidonic acid to prostaglandin. An unpublished review by Panter et al. found some benefit of indomethacin (Indocin) in prolonging pregnancy by 48 hours. One dosing protocol calls for indomethacin, 50 mg orally or 100 mg per rectum, followed by 25 mg orally every 4 to 6 hours up to 48 hours. Maternal side effects of NSAIDs include nausea, heartburn, and gastric bleeding, as well as alterations in bleeding time, thrombocytopenia, and asthma in susceptible patients. Fetal ductal constriction may occur because of inhibition of prostacyclin and prostaglandin E_2. The incidence of ductal constriction is increased after 32 weeks' gestation, with rates of up to 50% in some series. Ductal constriction is usually transient and resolves after discontinuation of the medication. Other reported side effects include oligohydramnios from decreased renal blood flow, primary pulmonary hypertension, necrotizing enterocolitis with small bowel perforation, acute renal failure, and intracerebral hemorrhage in the newborn. Other prostaglandin inhibitors such as sulindac (Clinoril) and ketorolac (Toradol) have been used for attempted tocolysis. Initially thought to have fewer severe side effects than indomethacin because of less placenta transfer, sulindac has been found to decrease fetal urine output and produce ductal constriction.

Calcium Channel Blockers

Calcium channel blockers, including nifedipine, nicardipine, and verapamil, have been used for preterm labor, based on the hypothesis that reducing intracellular free calcium concentration will inhibit contractions. A prospective randomized study by Papatsonis et al. (1997) determined that nifedipine was superior to ritodrine in prolonging pregnancy and had fewer side effects. The side effects of these drugs include maternal headache, flushing, and nausea. Currently, nifedipine is most often used as a tocolytic agent. Dosage regimens vary from 10 to 20 mg every 4 to 6 hours orally, while others use up to 40 mg (10 mg every 15 minutes) sublingually in the first hour, followed by 60 to 160 mg per day of slow-release nifedipine.

Oxytocin Antagonists

Oxytocin antagonists, which competitively bind to oxytocin receptors, decrease uterine activity in the baboon preterm labor model. Goodwin et al. (1994) demonstrated a decrease in uterine contractions with administration of the oxytocin antagonist atosiban to women with early preterm labor. Because of fewer side effects, such compounds may offer sig-nificant advantages over other tocolytic agents of equal efficacy, when used early in preterm labor. One concern is their potential to block antidiuretic hormone with subsequent water-electrolyte disturbances.

Nitric Oxide

Nitric oxide, a smooth muscle relaxant, is being investigated for a role in the prevention of preterm labor. A nitric oxide donor, glyceryl trinitrate, stopped preterm labor in 13 women. In addition, L-arginine infusion to produce nitric oxide has been used to transiently decrease myometrial activity.

Combined Agents

There is a paucity of published studies using combined tocolytic agents, and thus there are few data to suggest that use of multiple agents has a clear benefit over a single agent. Caution is usually expressed about combining magnesium sulfate and calcium channel blockers because of their similarity of action. Because infection may be a causative factor in many patients with preterm labor, several groups have attempted to administer an antibiotic along with a tocolytic agent. No significant advantages have been reported.

The anticipated success rate for these treatments depends on the stage of labor at which they are administered. The earlier in labor tocolytic agents are begun, the better their apparent success rate will be. The reason for this may in part be that very early labor is often false labor and will stop with no therapy. Various success definitions have been used, including delay of delivery for 48 hours, delay for 7 days, and delay until the fetus has achieved at least 2500 g in birthweight or 37 weeks' gestation. In most studies with early labor (i.e., cervical dilation of less than 2 cm at the time of treatment), bed rest and hydration achieved a 50% success rate in stopping uterine activity. This success is improved to about 75% with the administration of a tocolytic agent. Tocolytic agents therefore appear to have about 25% efficacy in decreasing uterine activity. Uterine activity in some patients can be stopped even late in labor, and therefore most therapies are started or continue until the cervix is dilated 5 cm.

Maternal Transport

Because therapy fails in about 25% of all patients, the mother should be treated in a center with a neonatal intensive care unit (NICU) capable of managing premature neonates. After stabilization in a level I unit, she should be transported to a level II or III center, depending on the gestational age of the fetus. The advantage of delivering very low-birthweight infants at a tertiary care hospital with a neonatal intensive care unit has been demonstrated in many studies showing decreased neonatal morbidity and mortality. If the labor cannot be stopped or a transfer is unsafe for the mother, then the neonatal transfer team should be present at the delivery for resuscitation and then transfer of the neonate to the NICU.

Glucocorticoids

Liggins and Howie (1972) first demonstrated a reduction of respiratory distress syndrome in preterm infants of mothers who were administered betamethasone (Celestone). Many other studies have substantiated this finding. The mechanism by which corticosteroids decrease lung disease is enzyme induction in type II pneumocytes of increased production of surfactant, which in turn reduces alveolar surface tension. A metaanalysis by the National Institutes of Health (1995) found that corticosteroids reduce respiratory distress and neonatal mortality by 50%. In addition to the pulmonary status of newborns, corticosteroids were found to decrease the incidence of intraventricular hemorrhage, probably by promoting maturation of the germinal matrix and reducing necessary respirator pressure.

All women between 24 and 34 weeks of pregnancy at risk for preterm delivery are candidates for antenatal corticosteroid therapy. Treatment should consist of either two doses of 12 mg of betamethasome intramuscularly 24 hours apart or 4 doses of 6 mg of dexamethasome intramuscularly 12 hours apart. Some benefit begins at 24 hours, with maximum benefit at 48 hours after initiation of therapy and lasting for 7 days. Treatment is given weekly until fetal maturity. Reported maternal problems include pulmonary edema, elevated white blood cell counts to 18,000/mm³, and more difficult glucose control. Another concern is that weekly administration of steroids can impair adrenal response in the newborn or the mother. The risk of infection in the mother and newborn after steroid administration does not seem to be a problem in the presence of intact membranes. While earlier studies suggested that thyrotropin-releasing hormone might benefit the preterm fetal lung, subsequent studies show no efficacy.

Group B Streptococcus Treatment

Premature infants are very susceptible to early GBS infections. The Center for Disease Control and Prevention and the American College of Obstetricians and Gynecologists (ACOG) recommend the use of prophylactic antibiotics (e.g., penicillin) for patients in preterm labor until the GBS carrier status is known. Rectovaginal cultures for GBS should be obtained, and the antibiotic can be discontinued when the cultures come back negative.

Atraumatic Delivery

One objective in the delivery of a preterm infant is to minimize the potential for trauma. Preterm infants in vertex presentations can be safely delivered vaginally. If the infant encounters significant resistance from the perineum, an episiotomy is indicated. Data indicate that a cesarean delivery is of benefit to the small breech infant to avoid the trauma of a vaginal delivery and the possibility of an entrapped head in the incompletely dilated cervix. If a cesarean delivery is performed to avoid trauma, the uterine incision should be generous enough to facilitate atraumatic delivery. If the lower uterine segment is not well developed, then a vertical incision may be needed.

Difficult decisions are often required regarding the expected viability of a preterm infant. Smith and Bottoms (1993) demonstrated that femur length less than 40 mm and a biparietal diameter less than 54 mm were reflective of the lower limits of neonatal survival. These two measurements may be helpful in making treatment decisions for the very immature fetus. Improvements in neonatal care in recent years, such as surfactant administration, have significantly improved survivability of smaller infants. Survival of infants weighing less than 550 g is rare, however, and morbidity is high.

Controversies with Preterm Labor

Several controversies exist in the literature regarding management programs and their application in perinatal medicine. This results from a failure to study the program in a scientifically valid, randomized, controlled protocol. These controversies include home tocolytic agents, home uterine monitoring, risk scoring systems and amniocentesis.

Home Tocolytic Agents

As described earlier, use of oral tocolytic agents offers no prophylactic advantage after the acute parenteral treatment of preterm labor with tocolytic agents. The most probable reason for their failure is that the blood concentration of the drug seldom achieves therapeutic levels.

Rust et al. (1996) compared oral terbutaline, oral magnesium chloride, and placebo to prevent recurrent preterm labor after hospital treatment. There was no difference among the 3 groups in perinatal outcome. They concluded that maintenance oral tocolytic therapy did not decrease uterine activity, reduce the rate of recurrent preterm labor or preterm birth, or improve perinatal outcome.

Subcutaneous administration of low-dose terbutaline via pump has been used as an expensive yet unproved method to attempt to delay preterm delivery. Complications, including newborn cardiac disease and maternal sepsis and death, have been described in patients using these pumps.

Home Uterine Monitoring

A combination of recorded uterine activity monitoring at home transmitted by telemetry to central review stations with daily telephone calls from a health care provider has been proposed to decrease preterm labor and delivery by the early recognition of preterm labor. Uterine monitoring is often done for 1 hour or longer per day. Several nonrandomized studies suggested that this management scheme allowed the identification of women with early signs of preterm labor, such that subsequent management then reduces the frequency of preterm delivery. However, in most randomized, controlled studies, home uterine monitoring and provider-initiated contact have not proved to be useful. Home uterine monitoring has not been endorsed by the ACOG, whose Committee Opinion number 172 (May, 1996) states:

> The available data do not support the effectiveness of HUAM (home uterine monitoring) for the prevention of preterm births. Well designed, prospective, randomized clinical studies of sufficient power are still needed to establish the benefit, if any, of HUAM for the prevention of preterm delivery or for the prevention of associated adverse neonatal outcomes. Data are insufficient to support a benefit from HUAM in preventing preterm birth. Therefore, the American College of Obstetricians and Gynecologists do not recommend the use of this system of care.

An area that should be studied for predictive value is the pattern of uterine contractions in the weeks leading up to delivery. In humans, as in the baboon model, there is a diurnal uterine activity pattern with increased contractions in the early evening hours. A study by Germaine et al. (1993) observed that women who delivered preterm had a loss of the expected diurnal pattern of contractions. This may indicate that patients are not subject to hormonal control but other influences on uterine activity might override the natural factors.

Risk Scoring Systems

Several prenatal risk scoring systems have been developed to identify women at increased risk for having preterm labor. The most notable among these is the system developed by the Collaborative Group on Preterm Birth Prevention (1993) and popularized by the March of Dimes organization. Although this scoring system has had a significant impact in reducing preterm labor in the hospital setting, where it was developed, it has not been helpful in other trials at local, state, and regional levels. The most significant risk in this scoring system is the history of a prior preterm delivery, a factor applicable only for multiparous women. A second consistent risk factor in the score is multiple pregnancy. The third is known uterine or cervical anomalies.

Amniocentesis

Although most investigators agree that some patients (i.e., perhaps as many as 15%) with preterm labor have an infectious etiology, there are few data to support the routine use of amniocentesis in preterm labor with intact membranes and no clinical signs of infection. If an amniocentesis is used to diagnose intraamniotic infection, a negative Gram stain to exclude bacteria is most sensitive in ruling out infection prior to obtaining the culture results. Other tests to diagnose infection include elevated amniotic fluid white blood cell counts, low glucose levels of 10 mg/dl or less, and high interleukin levels. There is a higher yield for positive amniotic fluid infection at earlier gestational ages in preterm labor. There may be a role for amniocentesis in individual patients with preterm labor when gestational age is unsure and growth retardation

may be suspected, when there is clinical suspicion of intrauterine infection, or if aggressive efforts are being made to maintain the fetus *in utero* and the risk–benefit ratio for allowing delivery needs to be assessed.

Cerclage

With the suggestion that some cases of incompetent cervix allow bacteria to enter the intrauterine environment and result in preterm labor, the idea of prophylactic cerclage to prevent preterm labor has been advanced. There are few data at this time to support this as a preventive measure of preterm labor and preterm birth. One study by the Medical Research Council of the Royal College of Obstetricians and Gynaecologists (1993) suggested that there is a decrease in delivery at less than 33 weeks' gestation (17% to 13%) in patients who underwent a prophylactic cerclage for prior preterm delivery.

Phenobarbital and Vitamin K

Another fetal treatment used with mixed success is phenobarbital or vitamin K administration to the mother to prevent neonatal intraventricular hemorrhage and jaundice. Phenobarbital therapy improves liver glucuronyl transferase activity so that better neonate bilirubin clearance can be achieved. This potentially reduces the severity of neonatal jaundice.

Thorpe et al. (1994) failed to substantiate previous reports that treatment with phenobarbitol and vitamin K reduced the incidence of neonatal intracranial hemorrhage. Although Shankaran et al. (1997) found that antenatal phenobarbital therapy significantly decreased moderate and severe intracranial hemorrhages (1.6% vs. 9.4%), a subsequent, larger study by the same investigators reversed these findings, showing no decrease in the incidence of hemorrhages (risk ratio: 1.0).

SUMMARY POINTS

◊ Preterm delivery is a significant contributor to neonatal morbidity and mortality.

◊ The mechanisms for the onset of preterm labor are not completely understood, and this limits the development of effective therapies.

◊ Woman at risk for this problem include those of black race or those with prior preterm deliveries, multiple fetuses, uterocervical anomalies, or vaginal infections.

◊ Treatment includes rest, hydration, tocolytics, GBS prevention, and fetal glucocorticoid administration.

◊ Maternal transfer to a tertiary care center for delivery is important.

◊ RECOMMENDED READINGS

Beckmann CA, Beckmann CR, Stanziano GJ, et al. Accuracy of maternal perception of preterm uterine activity. *Am J Obstet Gynecol* 1996;174:672.

Canadian Preterm Labor Investigators Group. Treatment of preterm labor with the beta-adrenergic agonist ritodrine. *N Engl J Med* 1992;327:308.

Collaborative Group on Preterm Birth Prevention. Multicenter randomized, controlled trial of a preterm birth prevention program. *Am J Obstet Gynecol* 1993;169:352.

Cox SM, Sherman LM, Leveno KJ. Randomized investigation of magnesium sulfate for prevention of preterm birth. *Am J Obstet Gynecol* 1990:163:767.

Dyson DC, Danbe KH, Bamber JA, et al. Monitoring women at risk for preterm labor. *N Engl J Med* 1998;338:15.

Germain AM, Valenzuela GJ, Ivankovic M, et al. Relationship of circadian rhythms of uterine activity with term and preterm labor. *Am J Obstet Gynecol* 1993;168:1271.

Gibbs RS, Romero R, Hillier SL, et al. A review of premature birth and subclinical infection. *Am J Obstet Gynecol* 1992:166:1515.

Goodwin TM, Paul R, Silver H. The effect of the oxytocin antagonist atosiban on preterm uterine activity in the human. *Am J Obstet Gynecol* 1994;170:474.

Hillier SL, Nugent RP, Eschenbach DA, et al. Association between bacterial vaginosis and preterm delivery of a low-birth-weight infant. *N Engl J Med* 1995;333:1737.

Krohn MA, Hillier SL, Lee ML, et al. Vaginal *Bacteroides* species are associated with an increased risk of preterm delivery among women in preterm labor. *J Infect Dis* 1991:164:88.

Liggins GC, Howie RN. A controlled trial of antepartum glucocorticoid treatment for prevention of the respiratory distress syndrome in premature infants. *Pediatrics* 1972;50:515.

Lockwood CJ, Senyei AE, Dische MR, et al. Fetal fibronectin in cervical and vaginal secretions as a predictor of preterm delivery. *N Engl J Med* 1991;325:669.

McGregor JA, French JI, Richter R, et al. Antenatal microbiologic and maternal risk associated with prematurity. *Am J Obstet Gynecol* 1990;163:1465.

Minkoff H, Grunebaum AN, Schwarz RH, et al. Risk factors for prematurity and premature rupture of membranes: a prospective study of the vaginal flora in pregnancy. *Am J Obstet Gynecol* 1984;150:965.

MRC/RCOG Working Party on Cervical Cerclage. Final report of the Medical Research Council/Royal College of Obstetricians and Gynaecologists multicentre randomized trial of cervical cerclage. *Br J Obstet Gynaecol* 1993;100:516.

Murtha AP, Greig PC, Jimmerson CE, Herbert WN. Maternal serum interleukin-6 concentration as a marker for impending preterm delivery. *Obstet Gynecol* 1998;91:161.

Naef RW, Allbert JR, Ross EL, Weber BM, Martin RW, Morrison JC. Premature rupture of membranes at 34 to 37 weeks' gestation: aggressive versus conservative management. *Am J Obstet Gynecol* 1998;178:126.

NIH Consensus Development Panel on the Effect of Corticosteroids for Fetal Maturation on Perinatal Outcomes. Effect of corticosteroids for fetal maturation on perinatal outcomes. *JAMA* 1995;273:413.

Papatsonis DNM, VanGeijn HP, Ader HJ, et al. Nifedipine and ritodrine in the management of preterm labor: a randomized multicenter trial. *Obstet Gynecol* 1997;90:230.

Romero R, Mazor M, Oyarzun E, et al. Is there an association between colonization with group B streptococcus and prematurity? *J Reprod Med* 1989;34:797.

Romero R, Oyarzun E, Mazor M, et al. Meta-analysis of the relationshp between asymptomatic bacteriuria and preterm delivery/low birth weight. *Obstet Gynecol* 1989;73:576.

Rust OA, Bofill JA, Arriola RM. The clinical efficacy of oral tocolytic therapy. *Am J Obstet Gynecol* 1996;175:838.

Shankaran S, Papile L, Wright LL, et al. The effect of antenatal phenobarbital therapy on neonatal intracranial hemorrhage in preterm infants. *N Engl J Med* 1997;337:466.

Smith RS, Bottoms SF. Ultrasonographic prediction of neonatal survival in extremely low-birth-weight infants. *Am J Obstet Gynecol* 1993;169:490.

Thorp JA, Parriott J, Ferrette-Smith D, et al. Antepartum vitamin K and phenobarbital for preventing intraventricular hemorrhage in the premature newborn: a randomized double-blind, placebo-controlled study. *Obstet Gynecol* 1994;83:70.

Turnbull AC, Patten PT, Flint AP, et al. Significant fall in progesterone and rise in oestradiol levels in human peripheral plasma before the onset of labor. *Lancet* 1974;i(848):101.

Virji SK, Cottington E. Risk factors associated with preterm deliveries among racial groups in a national sample of married women. *Am J Perinatol* 1991;8:347.

Wilson L Jr, Parsons MT, Flouret G. Inhibition of spontaneous uterine contractions during the last trimester in pregnant baboons by an oxytocin antagonist. *Am J Obstet Gynecol* 1990;163:1875.

Zeeman GG, Khan-Dawood FS, Dawood MY. Oxytocin and its receptor in pregnancy and parturition: current concepts and clinical implications. *Obstet Gynecol* 1997;89:873.

CHAPTER 17

Premature Rupture of Membranes

◇

Michael T. Parsons
William N. Spellacy

◇ INTRODUCTION

Premature rupture of the membranes (PROM) is the spontaneous rupture of fetal membranes before the onset of labor at any gestational age. Preterm PROM occurs earlier than 37 weeks of gestation. The incidence of PROM in all pregnancies is approximately 8%, most occurring at term. Preterm PROM occurs about 2% of the time.

The amniotic fluid surrounding the developing fetus is produced primarily from umbilical cord transfer and transudation though the fetal skin in early pregnancy and from fetal urine and lung fluid later in gestation. Throughout gestation there is a continued turnover of the fluid with a half-life of about 3 hours. The fluid surrounding the fetus is important for the development of the fetal lungs, limb movement, heat exchange, and protection of the umbilical cord and infant from compression. If the fetal membranes rupture, these protective mechanisms may be compromised if the fluid is lost. In addition, a portal is established for entry of bacteria from the vagina, thus producing a risk for chorioamnionitis and fetal infection. Finally, rupture often leads to the onset of labor. Thirty-five percent of preterm neonates are the result of preterm PROM.

This chapter reviews PROM in terms of etiology, diagnosis, complications, and management.

◇ ETIOLOGY OF PROM

Membranes

The fetal membranes consist of the amnion and the chorion. The amnion is the inner layer, which, although thinner, is of greater strength than the chorion. The chorion is attached at its outer surface to the decidua capsularis. The balance of intrinsic factors regulates the connective tissue synthesis and degradation in the amnion and chorion. There are enzymes called metalloproteinases that cannibalize the extracellular matrix components. There are also inhibitors of these enzymes. Toward term the proteolytic metabolism of the amnion and chorion extracellular matrix predominates, the concentration of collagen in the membranes decreases, weakening the membranes. Membranes that rupture prematurely seem to be focally rather than generally weakened or thinned. Under investigation as etiologic factors of rupture of membranes are bacterially produced phospholipase A_2, collagenase, other proteases, and changes in pH. In other studies, changes in the elasticity of the membranes felt to be secondary to a decrease in specific collagen makeup have been found.

Risk Factors

Several clinical factors place a pregnant patient at increased risk of preterm premature rupture of membranes, and these are listed in Table 1.

◇ RISK FACTORS FOR PROM

The risk for preterm PROM is increased two- to fourfold in women who experienced preterm PROM in a previous pregnancy. In addition, patients with previous preterm delivery with or without PROM have an increased risk (odds ratio 2.8). Several studies have found that women with either first or second trimester bleeding are at significantly increased risk. The bleeding may be a result of abnormal placentation or abruption. Previous cervical surgery, including conization, cervical incompetence, and two or more elective terminations of pregnancy, all increase risk. The NICHD preterm prediction study found that a short cervical length (2.5 cm or less with transvaginal ultrasound) was the best predictor of preterm PROM. Overdistention of the uterus from multiple gestations

TABLE 1. *Risk factors for PROM*

Prior PROM
Short cervix < 2.5 cm
Prior preterm delivery
Cervical incompetence, damage
Hydramnios
Twins
Smoking
Infection
Early pregnancy bleeding

or polyhydramnios increases the risk. The only connective tissue disease associated with increased preterm PROM is Leisch-Nyhan.

The risk for preterm PROM is increased up to two times in women who smoke during pregnancy, and this risk appears to be increased in a dose-dependent manner. There are reports that zinc and ascorbic acid deficiency increase the risk, but most studies have failed to find a consistent pattern of nutritional risk factors.

It is controversial whether routine digital examinations at term contribute to rupture of membranes. A study by Lenihan found that weekly cervical examinations increased the risk of PROM from 6% to 18%. In contrast, McDuffie found that weekly cervical examinations from 37 weeks until delivery had no significant effect on the frequency of PROM.

Infectious Causes

Lower genital tract infections have been associated with increased preterm PROM, including group B *Streptococcus, Chlamydia trachomatis, Neisseria gonorrheae,* and bacterial vaginosis.

The effects of group B *Streptococcus* (GBS) on PROM seem to relate to the number of bacteria present. The presence of group B *Streptococcus* in the vagina on routine culture does not increase the risk of preterm PROM, but heavy vaginal colonization (growth on primary plates) and GBS bacteriuria have been associated with preterm PROM. A large study by Regan et al. of over 13,000 women reported that GBS carriage was not a risk factor for preterm PROM.

There are conflicting data on the role of *Chlamydia* in preterm PROM. Several studies have implicated *Chlamydia* as an etiologic factor for preterm PROM. Alger et al. in 1988 found significantly more chlamydial cultures positive if preterm PROM was present (44% vs. 15%). Sweet et al. in 1987 found that preterm PROM was not more common with positive chlamydial cultures, but preterm PROM was more common if there was positive serum IgM (19% vs. 8%). Other studies with chlamydia have not found this association. In a case–control study, Ekwo found that women positive for gonorrhea were 7.6 times more likely to have preterm PROM, but there was not an increased risk for women with *Chlamydia.*

Other genital tract pathogens that alter the vaginal environment and pH include *Bacteroides fragilis* and other anaer-obes, *Trichomonas vaginalis,* and bacterial vaginosis. If a pregnant woman has repeated vaginal pH values determined, and all are less than or equal to 4.0, the incidence of preterm PROM is 8%. If at least one value is greater than 4.5, the incidence of preterm PROM is 19%. If all are greater than 4.5, the incidence of preterm PROM is 47%. The NICHD preterm prediction study found a relationship between the acquisition but not initial presence of bacterial vaginosis between 24 and 28 weeks of gestation and preterm birth secondary to preterm PROM (odds ratio 1.8).

There are several mechanisms by which bacteria could increase the incidence of PROM. Bacteria can produce protease and phospholipase, which may weaken the membrane. Activated neurophils have been shown *in vitro* to reduce the bursting tension and elasticity of the membranes. In addition, the host-mediated response of cytokines may play an etiologic factor. Gomez and Romero concluded that the pathogenesis of preterm PROM and preterm labor can be considered expressions of the same basic phenomenon, activation of the host defense macrophage system. They hypothesize that if the host response results in preferential activity leading to the secretion of uterotonic agents such as prostaglandins, preterm labor will result. If, however, the activation of the host response results mainly in the production of proteases, patients are more likely to have PROM.

◊ COMPLICATIONS

Maternal

The maternal complications of PROM are listed in Table 2. Maternal infection or chorioamnionitis, in which the bacteria invade and cause inflammation of the membranes before delivery, is common. Organisms present in chorioamnionitis include those commonly found in the vagina, including the aerobic and anaerobic streptococci, aerobic coliform gram-negative bacteria, and other anaerobes including *Bacteroides* and *Fusobacterium.* Clinical chorioamnionitis occurs in approximately 10% to 20% of patients with preterm PROM. However, if an amniocentesis is performed, positive amniotic fluid cultures in patients with preterm PROM range in various series from 14% to more than 43%. Centers that culture for *Mycoplasma* and *Ureaplasma* as well as for bacteria report the higher positive culture rate. It is not clear if the genital mycoplasmas represent mere colonization or true infection. Another maternal complication of preterm PROM is postpartum endometritis, which may or may not be preceded by chorioamnionitis.

TABLE 2. *Maternal complications of PROM*

Labor
Infection: chorioamnionitis, endometritis
Cesarean delivery
Abruption

In a series by Cox et al., the risk of cesarean delivery in patients with preterm PROM was nearly 40%. The most common reasons for the increased cesarean delivery rate included variable decelerations of the fetal heart rate and an increased incidence of malposition of the fetus. Anath et al. conducted a metaanalysis of published studies on placental abruption. They found that abruption was three times more likely to occur in pregnancies complicated by preterm PROM.

Infant

The length of the latency period until labor after PROM is inversely related to the gestational age at rupture. At term, 90% of patients are in labor within 24 hours. Between 28 and 34 weeks of gestation, 50% of patients are in labor within 24 hours, and 80% are in labor within 1 week. At 24 to 26 weeks of gestation, only 50% are in labor within 1 week.

The complications of PROM for the infant are listed in Table 3. Infection is a major cause of neonatal morbidity, with the most frequent bacterial causes of sepsis being group B *Streptococcus* and *Escherichia coli.*

Fetal distress may be a result of abruptio placenta, umbilical cord prolapse, or umbilical cord compression. The incidence of prolapsed umbilical cord in preterm PROM is estimated at 2% and depends on the presentation of the fetus. Vertex presentations have the lowest risk. Umbilical cord compression can also occur with prolapse of the cord or secondary to oligohydramnios. The incidence of fetal distress in labor leading to cesarean delivery is over three times greater in patients with preterm PROM than with preterm labor and intact membranes and most commonly is associated with severe variable decelerations from cord compression.

A study by Kilbride et al. evaluated singleton pregnancies at less than 29 weeks of gestation complicated by preterm PROM. He found that both duration of severe oligohydramnios (less than 1 cm vertical pocket) and gestational age at time of PROM were independent significant predictors of increased neonatal risk. Severe oligohydramnios for more than 14 days at less than 25 weeks of gestation has a predicted neonatal mortality greater than 90%. Dysmorphic compression deformities and pulmonary hypoplasia are serious problems of prolonged rupture of the membranes. A study by Rotschild determined that if rupture of membranes occurred at 19 weeks of gestation or earlier, 50% of infants had pulmonary hypoplasia, but this fell to about 10% with preterm PROM at 26 weeks of gestation. The proposed mechanisms for pulmonary hypoplasia include compression of the infant's thorax and restriction of fetal fluid breathing. Another proposed mechanism is that the increased net outflow of lung fluid removes the intraalveolar stenting property with the resultant collapse of alveoli.

It has been difficult to predict which infants will develop pulmonary hypoplasia after preterm PROM. Ultrasound studies have indicated that the absence of fetal breathing on a single exam is not predictive, although persistent absence may be. Other measurements that may be helpful include the thoracic circumference, lung length, thoracic circumference/abdominal circumference ratio, thoracic area/heart ratio, perinatal flow, and inhibition of breathing-related modulation of blood flow in the ductus.

◊ EVALUATION

Diagnosis

When a woman thinks she has ruptured her membranes, she should be seen by a health professional for an examination to make the diagnosis. The diagnostic studies for PROM are listed in Table 4.

The differential diagnosis of rupture of membranes includes loss of mucus plug, vaginal discharge associated with infection, and urinary incontinence. In making the diagnosis of PROM, the history of leaking fluid by the patient is correct over 90% of the time. The initial evaluation may reveal a moist perineum. If the patient is not going to be delivered immediately, then a digital exam should not be done, as it can introduce bacteria into the uterus and shorten the latent phase. A sterile speculum exam may demonstrate pooling of fluid in the posterior vaginal vault. Direct observation of fluid leaking from the cervical os is proof of ruptured membranes. The normal pH of the vagina is between 4.5 and 6.0 in pregnancy, whereas the pH of the amniotic fluid is 7.1 to 7.3. Nitrazine paper changes to a dark blue from yellow with a pH above 6.5. Nitrazine paper to diagnose amniotic fluid in the vagina has an overall accuracy of approximately 93%, but false positive results can result from blood, semen, alkaline urine, and vaginal infections. If there is prolonged rupture of membranes and minimal amniotic fluid present, a false-negative result may be obtained.

TABLE 3. *Infant complications of PROM*

Prematurity
Infection: pneumonia, meningitis, bacteremia
Pulmonary hypoplasia
Limb and body deformities
Prolapsed cord
Cord compression (oligohydramnios)
Abruption

TABLE 4. *Diagnostic studies for PROM*

History
Vaginal pooling
pH >7.0 (nitrazine paper)
Ferning
Fetal products (cells, fat, fibronectin, AFP, hPr)
Dye injections

The diagnosis of PROM could also be confirmed by observing arborization or "ferning" of the amniotic fluid on a slide. Fluid from the vagina is placed on a slide, allowed to dry and observed under a microscope. The crystallization of sodium chloride gives the familiar ferning pattern of an evergreen. This method has an overall accuracy of diagnosis of PROM of approximately 96%. False positives are rare but have been reported with contamination with semen and cervical mucus. In addition, fingerprints on the slide have been misdiagnosed as a ferning pattern. False negatives can result from a dry swab, contamination with blood at a 1 : 1 dilution, or not allowing sufficient time for the fluid to dry on the slide. Amniotic fluid arborization is unaffected by meconium at any concentration and is unaffected by pH alteration.

Other substances that have been tested in vaginal secretions to demonstrate the presence of amniotic fluid include fetal squamous cells, fat, prolactin, diamine oxidase, α-fetoprotein, and fetal fibronectin. The use of maternal orally administered phenazopyridine (Pyridium) for a change in color of amniotic fluid and secretions into the vagina is not useful.

When the diagnosis of ruptured membranes is unclear by these tests, a transabdominal dye injection is sometimes performed. A dye such as indigo carmine blue is injected into the amniotic fluid, and a sponge is placed into the vagina and later inspected for the dye. Methylene blue should not be used because of reported methemoglobinemia in the fetus. This test is invasive, and the accuracy of diagnosis is not established. An unpublished study by Kalter and Parsons found that an observation time no longer than 2 hours is sufficient to identify patients with ruptured membranes using dye injection.

Fetal Maturity

Determination of the fetal age and maturity status is useful in developing a treatment plan. The patient's history and early milestones of the pregnancy should be used. Ultrasound examination of the fetus can be difficult because of the decreased fluid surrounding the fetus. Some investigators have reported less accurate sonographic measurements, especially of the abdomen and head. Amniocentesis is sometimes used for lung maturity testing as part of the overall decision process as to delivery. Vaginal pool collection is less accurate for L/S ratio determination.

Cervical Status

In addition to documentation of ruptured membranes, the sterile speculum exam can evaluate the amount of cervical dilation and can exclude the possibility of a fetal extremity or umbilical cord prolapsing through the cervix. Endovaginal ultrasound can apparently be used with safety in patients who have preterm PROM. Carlan et al. evaluated the role of endovaginal ultrasound by performing weekly exams versus a control group that did not receive vaginal ultrasound evalua-

tion. There was no difference in latency period from rupture to delivery nor in the incidence of chorioamnionitis, endometritis, or neonatal infection.

Infection

When the diagnosis of PROM is made, lower vaginal–perianal cultures should be taken for group B *Streptococcus* studies, and antibiotics should be given until these culture results return as negative.

All patients with preterm PROM should be evaluated for possible chorioamnionitis. Physical exam includes palpation of the uterus for tenderness and visualization of the cervix for purulent discharge. Fetal tachycardia is an early ominous sign. Temperature elevation is often a late sign of chorioamnionitis, as are maternal leukocytosis and elevated C-reactive protein levels. An amniocentesis is sometimes indicated to evaluate for an intrauterine infection. Analyses of amniotic fluid for possible infection before the culture report returns include positive Gram stain for bacteria, white blood cells, and glucose concentration less than 10 mg/dl. Gram stain does not identify *Mycoplasma* colonization, and the amniotic white blood cells may not be accurate because of contamination from the vagina. Studies have also shown elevated interleukin 6 (IL-6) in infected amniotic fluid. There is a higher incidence of nonreactive NSTs in patients with intrauterine infection, but the test is not sensitive. A biophysical profile of 6 or less has been shown in several studies to correlate with intrauterine infection, but this may be a better prediction of fetal infection than of chorioamnionitis. Most fetuses that are present in an environment with chorioamnionitis do not become infected. However, they do show a higher frequency of cerebral palsy (relative risk 7–9×).

◊ MANAGEMENT

Management is generally focused on the risks for the infant. The risk of staying in the uterus is infection, and the risks in delivery are those of prematurity. In general, fetuses at 34 weeks of gestation or more or those where the mother has clinical chorioamnionitis need delivery. For the fetus of less than 34 weeks' gestation, expectant management *in utero* to gain organ maturity is best. If the patient has a cervical cerclage in place, it should be removed, as increased maternal infection and death are reported where the cerclage was left in place.

Steroids

There have been several studies indicating that the rupture of membranes itself has an accelerating action on fetal lung maturity. Berkowitz et al. demonstrated in 1978 that the time factor of at least 16 hours of ruptured membranes helped to mature the lungs of the fetus. One of the proposed mechanisms is a release of fetal or maternal glucocorticoids as a stress reaction to the preterm PROM. Bauer et al. found that neonatal cortisol levels were increased in correlation with the duration of ruptured membranes in a PROM relative to a control group, whereas maternal cortisol levels were not as elevated. This theory of accelerated lung maturation with preterm PROM has recently been challenged by Hallak and Bottoms. They found that of the 1395 women studied retrospectively who delivered between 24 and 35 weeks of gestation, PROM did not decrease the risk of respiratory distress syndrome.

The use of corticosteroids in patients with preterm PROM continues to be controversial. Although steroids in patients with preterm labor and intact membranes have been shown to be advantageous and to decrease the incidence of RDS and intraventricular hemorrhage, the data on patients with preterm PROM have not been as clear. Possible disadvantages include increasing the infectious morbidity of the mother and neonate.

Two metaanalyses on the role of corticosteroids reach different conclusions. A review by Ohlsson in 1989 found that metaanalysis of five randomized controlled trials demonstrated a reduction in respiratory distress syndrome in the steroid treatment group ($p = 0.001$). However, after one study, which was considered of lowest quality because of the patient randomization by medical record number, was excluded, no significant reduction in RDS ($p = 0.286$) was found. There was a significant increase in endometritis and a trend toward an increase in neonatal infections and cesarean delivery rates with treatment. Crowley performed a metaanalysis of eight randomized trials from 1977 to 1991 and found that antenatal corticosteroid therapy in patients with PROM substantially reduced the incidence of RDS (odds ratio 0.44). No increase in perinatal infection was evident. The study that was removed from Ohlsson's analysis was included in this analysis. The majority of the studies in these metaanalyses did not include the use of antibiotics.

A recent study by Lewis et al. assessed the efficacy of steroids in patients with preterm PROM after treatment with ampicillin–sulbactam. After 12 hours of treatment with antibiotics, patients were randomized into two groups. One group received 12 mg betamethasome intramuscularly, repeated in 24 hours, while the other group did not receive steroid therapy. Antibiotics were continued for 7 days, and steroids were repeated weekly. The study was not blinded nor placebo controlled. There was a significant reduction in the incidence of RDS in the steroid group (18.4% vs. 43.6%, $p = 0.03$). There was no statistical difference in the latency period of 14.7 days versus 15.8 days in the control group. The neonatal and maternal infectious morbidities were similar. The authors concluded that this study provides preliminary data that treating patients with preterm PROM with a broad-spectrum antibiotic before corticosteroids decreases respiratory distress syndrome without any increase in adverse outcome and that future efforts should address this in a double-blind, placebo-controlled design.

The portion of the 1994 ACOG Committee Opinion No. 147 regarding corticosteroid therapy includes the following NIH recommendation: "Antenatal corticosteroid use is recommended in women with preterm PROM at less than 30–32 weeks of gestation in the absence of clinical chorioamnionitis because of the high risk of IVH at these early gestational ages." However, the ACOG conclusion to this NIH report states "The College's Committee on Obstetric Practice supports the conclusions of the NIH consensus conference with the exception of the recommendations for treatment of women with preterm PROM. The Committee believes that further research is needed to evaluate the risks and benefits of using corticosteroids in women who have preterm PROM." This view that "More data are needed regarding the risks and benefits of antenatal corticosteroid therapy in the presence of preterm PROM" is reiterated in the 1997 guidelines for *Prenatal Care, 4th edition,* cooperatively published by The American College of Obstetricians and Gynecologists and the American Academy of Pediatrics.

Antibiotics

Prophylactic antibiotics are widely used in asymptomatic patients to treat occult infections and/or prevent subsequent infections from occurring. The possible advantages include reducing maternal infection, reducing neonatal infection, prolonging the latency period, and early treatment of group B *Streptococcus* while awaiting culture results. Some disadvantages include the side effects of antibiotics, the cost of the antibiotics, and increasing resistant organisms.

Antibiotics administered intravenously reach significant concentrations in amniotic fluid within minutes and can surpass maternal serum levels within 2 to 4 hours. In 1988 Amon et al. randomized patients with preterm PROM to expectant management versus treatment with ampicillin. They demonstrated a significant decrease in neonatal infection in the ampicillin group (17% vs. 2%, $p < 0.04$) and a prolongation of the latency period. There have been several recent studies and metaanalyses supporting the use of antibiotics.

A metaanalysis by Egarter et al. of seven randomized trials with 657 patients evaluated the role of antibiotic treatment in preterm PROM on neonatal morbidity. They found that antibiotic therapy significantly reduced the risk of neonatal sepsis by 68% (odds ratio 0.32) and reduced intraventricular hemorrhage by 50% (odds ratio 0.50). In their review, there was no significant effect of antibiotics on respiratory distress syndrome, necrotizing enterocolitis, or mortality.

A metaanalysis by Mercer et al. in 1995 of 13 trials including 1594 women demonstrated that antibiotic treatment after preterm PROM did reduce the incidence of women delivering within 1 week (62% vs. 76%, odds ratio 0.51) as well as maternal morbidity including chorioamnionitis (12% vs. 23%, odds ratio 0.45), postpartum infection (8% vs. 12%, odds ratio 0.63), neonatal sepsis (5.1% vs. 8.7%, odds ratio 0.51), and intraventricular hemorrhage (9.4% vs. 13.8%, odds ratio 0.7) but no decrease in maternal postpartum infection, RDS, or neonatal death.

Lovett et al. evaluated the role of antibiotic prophylaxis in women with preterm PROM who received antenatal corticosteroids. In an attempt to reduce neonatal infection and improve outcome, in addition to corticosteroids patients received either

(1) ampicillin–sulbactam for 72 hours followed by amoxicillin–clavulanate, (2) ampicillin for 72 hours followed by amoxicillin, or (3) placebo. There were significantly better outcomes in the groups that received antibiotics versus the placebo group ($p = 0.03$). They concluded that antibiotic prophylaxis in combinations with corticosteroids in preterm PROM significantly lowered the frequency of neonatal mortality, sepsis, respiratory distress syndrome, and increased the birthweight compared to corticosteroids alone.

The NICHD Maternal Fetal Medicine Network performed an 11-center study comparing (1) expectant management and placebo versus (2) expectant management and antibiotics (intravenous ampicillin, 2 g every 6 hours, and intravenous erythromycin, 250 mg every 6 hours for 48 hours followed by oral amoxicillin 250 mg every 8 hours and erythromycin base 333 mg every 8 hours for 5 days) for women with preterm PROM between 24 and 32 weeks of gestation. The results indicated that if patients were GBS negative, there was a prolonged median time to delivery (6.1 vs. 2.9 days, $p < 0.001$), an increase in latency at 2, 7, 14, and 21 days, and an increased birthweight (1549 vs. 1457 g) in the antibiotic group. In the total patient population, there was a decreased relative risk of chorioamnionitis (23% vs. 32.5%, $p = 0.04$), respiratory distress syndrome (40.5% vs. 48.7%, $p = 0.04$), and necrotizing enterocolitis (2.3% vs. 5.8%, $p = 0.03$) in the antibiotic group.

Antibiotic regimens that have been used vary greatly from ampicillin, ampicillin–sulbactam, ampicillin plus erythromycin, or a cephalosporin. The duration of antibiotic treatment has varied from the return of negative cervical/vaginal cultures to treatment for 5 to 7 days to continuing antibiotic treatment until delivery. Prolonged therapy does have the risk of neonatal infection with resistant pathogens. A review by Gibbs and Eschenbach recommends the 7-day regimen described in the NICHD Maternal Fetal Medicine Network Study. If bacterial vaginosis is suspected, clindamycin can be substituted for erythromycin. At a minimum, the group B streptococcal prevention protocol (ACOG Committee Opinion #173, June, 1996) should be followed.

Herpes Simplex

When a patient with preterm premature rupture of membranes has an active herpes lesion in the genital area, there is additional concern regarding the virus causing intrauterine infection of the fetus. Major et al. reviewed 18 cases of preterm PROM from 24 to 32 weeks of gestation with associated recurrent genital herpes. Six of these 18 patients were treated with antenatal acyclovir. Expectant management was performed in all patients, and the latency period until delivery ranged from 12 hours to 5 weeks. Three women had more than one recurrence subsequent to membrane rupture. Eight women were delivered by cesarean because of the presence of lesions at the time of delivery. There was no evidence of neonatal herpes infection in any of the 18 infants. The data on use of acyclovir during pregnancy are limited, but there are over 270 reported cases of exposure during pregnancy with no adverse effects. There are reported cases that acyclovir in primary herpes infections decrease the fetal exposure. Cesarean section delivery should be done if PROM occurs at term when active herpes lesions are present.

Tocolytics

Tocolytic agents are discussed in depth in Chapter 16. Their use in patients with preterm PROM has been limited. Possible advantages of using tocolytic agents in patients with preterm PROM include prolonging the pregnancy to obtain greater maturity and for a short time gain if steroids are chosen. Possible disadvantages include the increased risk of infection and the side effects of the tocolytics. Studies by Garite in 1987 and Weiner in 1988 did not demonstrate an advantage in using tocolysis in patients in PROM for prolonging the pregnancy for 48 hours. Although each case must be handled individually, at this point studies have not demonstrated much benefit of tocolytics, and they are not widely used with ruptured membranes.

Delivery

A major decision remaining is when to deliver patients with preterm PROM. Advantages of early timed delivery include avoiding infection, cord accident, distress, and fetal dysmorphic changes. Possible disadvantages include the prematurity and the costs/risks of induction and/or cesarean section.

Mercer et al. examined the value of performing amniocentesis to document maturity and then delivery in patients with preterm PROM between 32 and 36 weeks of gestation. Of 164 women with preterm PROM, 13 had immature studies, 4 had chorioamnionitis, and 12 had unsuccessful amniocentesis. Ninety-three patients who agreed to participate had mature amniotic fluid. These 93 patients with mature fluid were randomized to expectant management versus induction of labor. Induction of labor was associated with a shorter latency period to delivery, shorter hospitalization of the infant, decreased antepartum chorioamnionitis (0% vs. 14.9%, $p = 0.01$), and a trend toward decrease in total chorioamnionitis (10.9% vs. 27.7%, $p = 0.06$). There was no difference in the incidence of cesarean delivery (8.7% vs. 6.4%) and no difference in neonatal sepsis (4.4% vs. 6.8%). Using 34 weeks of gestation or 2000 g estimated weight seems reasonable for the decision point on delivery versus expectant management.

If the mother has clinical chorioamnionitis, delivery should be by induction of labor if possible to avoid peritoneal contamination at cesarean.

Midtrimester PROM

The most difficult cases are those in whom rupture occurs very early in pregnancy. Midtrimester premature rupture of the membranes, as defined by Moretti and Sibai, occurs between 16 and 26 weeks of gestation. This is uncommon, occurring in approximately 0.7% of pregnancies. A 1996 paper by Schucker and Mercer summarized 14 years of studies of patients with midtrimester PROM. They found that approximately 57% of patients delivered within 1 week and 78% delivered within 1 month of membrane rupture. In patients who underwent conservative management after midtrimester PROM, the fetal death rate was 15%, and neonatal death rate was 40%, for an overall survival rate of just 45%. Long-term sequelae including chronic lung disease, developmental and neurologic abnormalities; hydrocephalus and cerebral palsy were found in 31% of the infants discharged from the hospital. The chance of neonatal survival with rupture of membranes before 24 weeks was approximately 30%. In pregnancies with PROM at less than 20 weeks of gestation, there was approximately a 16% chance for intact neonatal survival.

There are factors that influence outcome in the very early preterm PROM, most notably the amount of amniotic fluid remaining and the presence of infection. Hadi and Hodson summarized 11 articles published between 1984 and 1995 on PROM during the second trimester. They found the overall incidence of chorioamnionitis to be 38% in patients with PROM between 20 and 25 weeks of gestation. In addition, they found a direct relationship between reduced amniotic fluid volume and chorioamnionitis. Chorioamnionitis occurred in 24% of pregnancies with an amniotic fluid pocket greater than 2 cm and in 69% of pregnancies with inadequate amniotic fluid. The overall perinatal survival rate was approximately 55%. If delivery occurred before 25 weeks of gestation, only 7% of the neonates survived. Pregnancies that had adequate amniotic fluid volume that continued beyond 25 weeks had an 89% survival rate, whereas those with inadequate amniotic fluid had a perinatal survival rate of 31%. The overall incidence of long-term chronic lung disease, neurologic abnormalities, and cerebral palsy in survivors was 39%.

The prognosis should be discussed with the patient. Expectant management with a previable fetus is sometimes carried out as an outpatient with frequent observation for infection. Many patients elect to undergo induction of labor.

Decreased Amniotic Fluid

If, on initial evaluation of the patient with ruptured membranes, a decreased amount of amniotic fluid is detected, additional problems present. Vintzeleos demonstrated in an article in 1985 that when no amniotic fluid could be detected on ultrasound, the incidence of severe variable decelerations increased to 63%, the cesarean section rate was 68%, there was over a 30% incidence of Apgar scores less than 7, and 3 out of 19 incidents of perinatal death. Several series have reported that decreased amniotic fluid volume correlates with a decreased number of days gained *in utero* before the onset of labor.

Maternal intravenous hydration and bed rest may help improve the amniotic fluid index. In a study by Chelmow et al., it was found that in nonlaboring patients at 24 to 37 weeks of gestation with documented PROM, hydrating patients with 1 liter of normal saline over a 30-minute period increased the

AFI by 5.1 cm versus the control group of 0.6 cm ($p < 0.008$). They concluded that the AFI is sensitive to maternal hydration in patients with preterm rupture of membranes and can be increased with IV fluid bolus. Drugs that alter urine output such as lithium and vasopressin have also been tried in research studies, with variable success. Amnioinfusion at time of labor should be considered with oligohydramnios or variable fetal heart rate decelerations.

Post-Genetic-Amniocentesis PROM

The outcome of pregnancies that have leakage of amniotic fluid after the performance of a genetic amniocentesis is much better than the previously discussed spontaneous preterm PROM in early pregnancy. A study by Gold reported that of 603 second trimester amniocenteses, 7 (1.2%) had midtrimester PROM. The fluid leakage resolved in all seven patients and 6 of the 7 patients went on to have an uncomplicated term delivery. Other series have reported iatrogenic PROM after second trimester genetic amniocentesis occurring approximately 0.2% of the time with usually successful pregnancy outcomes.

Home Management

A controversial issue in the management of patients with preterm PROM, especially as cost concerns become a larger issue, is that of home management. Obstetricians have very strong opinions on the risk of sending patients home versus the cost of keeping them in the hospital at bed rest, based mostly on individual experiences. A prospective randomized study performed by Carlan et al. evaluated the role of home management of patients with preterm PROM. They studied 67 patients with singleton fetuses in cephalic presentation with adequate amniotic fluid and without advanced cervical dilation (<4 cm) at the end of 72 hours of hospital observation. They were randomized to (1) home management with frequent monitoring of temperature and pulse every 6 hours, fetal movement chart, bed rest, NST and CBC two times per week, and ultrasound and speculum exam every week, versus (2) continued hospitalization. Only a small proportion of patients with preterm PROM (18%) could meet the safety criteria for inclusion in the study. The patients who were entered into this study had similar perinatal outcomes, length of latency period, and gestational age at delivery. Two perinatal deaths did occur in the home management group, both less than 600 g, and there was one early neonatal death in the hospital group of a 694-g infant. As expected, there was a significant decrease in the days of maternal hospitalization and maternal hospital expenses in the home group. There may be role for selected women with early PROM who are not infected after several days and who stop leaking fluid and have adequate fluid on ultrasound examination and a cervix less than 2 cm to go home on bed rest with home nurse monitoring.

Term PROM

Studies by Galask and co-workers have demonstrated that amniotic fluid inhibits bacterial growth for about 24 hours, mainly through its zinc content. As a result, a period of observation at term with PROM should have limited infection risk. Rupture of membranes before the onset of labor at term occurs in approximately 6% to 8% of pregnancies. Treatment plans vary from immediate induction to expectant management for the onset of labor. As opposed to preterm PROM, prematurity and compression anomalies are not the risk; infection of the patient or the neonate and the avoidance of cesarean delivery are the main challenges. It has been the impression of many clinicians that if immediate induction of labor is undertaken in all patients at term with rupture of membranes, the cesarean delivery rate may be increased. On the other hand, expectant management may increase the infection rate.

Kappy et al. published a retrospective study of patients with term PROM who were treated with either induction of labor or expectant management. In their series, they found a significant decrease in the incidence of cesarean delivery in the group that was expectantly managed (33% vs. 47%). The same author published a follow-up study several years later adding additional support to the role of expectant management. They had no increase in the risk of neonatal infection.

Hannah et al. also evaluated the induction of labor versus expectant management for PROM. Over 5000 women were enrolled in a study comparing (1) the induction of labor with intravenous oxytocin, (2) the induction of labor with vaginal prostaglandin E_2 gel, or (3) expectant management followed by induction with oxytocin or prostaglandin gel if labor did not ensue within 4 days. They found no significant difference in the rate of neonatal infection or in cesarean delivery among the three groups. However, clinical chorioamnionitis was less likely to develop in women in the induction with oxytocin group than those in the expectant management group (4% vs. 8.6%, $p < 0.001$). In addition, women in the study expressed a greater preference for induction of labor over expectant management. Criticism of the study included the large number of patients with favorable Bishop scores who were left alone, no cervical examination reported in many, and the lack of detail on GBS prophylaxis.

In a metaanalysis performed by Mozurkewich, 23 articles were reviewed examining the outcome of PROM at term by (1) immediate oxytocin induction, (2) conservative management, or (3) vaginal or endocervical prostaglandin E_2. The main outcome variables were cesarean birth, chorioamnionitis, endometritis, and serious neonatal infections. There were no statistically significant differences in cesarean deliveries or neonatal infections noted among the management schemes. Immediate oxytocin induction resulted in fewer cases of chorioamnionitis (odds ratio 0.67) and endometritis (odds ratio 0.71) compared to conservative management. Vaginal prostaglandin induction resulted in more chorioamnionitis compared to the use of oxytocin (odds ratio 1.55) but less chorioamnionitis than in the conservative management group (odds ratio 0.68).

Because 90% of women at term will spontaneously begin labor within 24 hours of PROM, it seems reasonable to observe no longer than 12 to 24 hours and to begin an oxytocin induction if no labor has started.

SUMMARY POINTS

◊ Premature rupture of the membranes (PROM) contributes 35% of preterm births.

◊ PROM increases risks of maternal and infant infection, especially important is neonatal Group B Streptococcus infection.

◊ Chorioamnionitis increases infant cerebral palsy risks 7–9 times.

◊ PROM before 24 weeks gestation increases infant limb deformities, lung hypoplasia, cord compression and death.

◊ PROM at 24–34 weeks needs conservative management if not infected and 5–7 days of antibiotic treatment improves outcomes.

◊ In conservative management the vaginal examinations should be by sterile speculum only.

◊ PROM at term needs labor induction after a 12–24 hour latent period if contractions are absent.

◊ RECOMMENDED READINGS

Alger LS, Lovchik JC, Hebel JR, et al. The association of *Chlamydia trachomatis, Neisseria gonorrhea,* and group B streptococci with preterm rupture of the membranes and pregnancy outcome. *Am J Obstet Gynecol* 1988;159:397–404.

Amon E, Lewis SV, Sibai BM, Villar MA, Arheart KL. Ampicillin prophylaxis in preterm premature rupture of the membranes: a prospective randomized study. *Am J Obstet Gynecol* 1988;159:539–543.

Anath CV, Savitz DA, Luther ER. Maternal cigarette smoking as a risk factor for placental abruption, placenta previa and uterine bleeding in pregnancy. *Am J Epidemiol* 1996;144:881–889.

Bauer CR, Stern L, Colle E. Prolonged rupture of membranes associated with a decreased incidence of respiratory distress syndrome. *Pediatrics* 1974;53:7–12.

Berkowitz RL, Kanter RD, Beck GJ, et al. The relationship between premature rupture of the membranes and the respiratory distress syndrome. An update and plan of management. *Am J Obstet Gynecol* 1978;131: 503–508.

Carlan SJ, O'Brien WF, Parsons MT, et al. Preterm premature rupture of the membranes: a randomized study of home versus hospital management. *Obstet Gynecol* 1993;81:61–64.

Carlan SJ, Richmond LB, O'Brien WF. Randomized trial of endovaginal ultrasound in preterm premature rupture of membranes. *Obstet Gynecol* 1997;89:458–461.

Chelmow D, Baker ER, Jones L. Maternal intravenous hydration and amniotic fluid index in patients with preterm ruptured membranes. *J Soc Gynecol Invest* 1996;3:127–130.

Cox SM, Williams ML, Leveno KJ. The natural history of preterm ruptured membranes: What to expect of expectant management. *Obstet Gynecol* 1988;71:558–562.

Crowley PA. Antenatal corticosteroid therapy: a meta-analysis of the randomized trials, 1972 to 1994. *Am J Obstet Gynecol* 1995;173:322–335.

Ekwo EE, Gosselink CA, Woolson R. Risk for premature rupture of amniotic membranes. *Int J Epidemiol* 1993;22:495–503.

Egarter C, Leitich H, Karas H, et al. Antibiotic treatment in preterm premature rupture of membranes and neonatal morbidity: a meta analysis. *Am J Obstet Gynecol* 1996;174:589–597.

Galask RP, Snyder IS. Bacterial inhibition by amniotic fluid. *Am J Obstet Gynecol* 1968;102:949–955.

Garite TJ, Keegan KA, Freeman RK, et al. A randomized trial of ritodrine tocolysis versus expectant management in patients with premature rupture of membranes at 25 to 30 weeks of gestation. *Am J Obstet Gynecol* 1987;157:388–393.

Gibbs RS, Eschenbach DA. Use of antibiotics to prevent preterm birth. *Am J Obstet Gynecol* 1997;177:375–380.

Gold RB, Goyert GL, Schwartz DB, et al. Conservative management of second trimester post amniocentesis fluid leakage. *Obstet Gynecol* 1989;74:745–747.

Gomez R, Romero R, Edwin SS, et al. Pathogenesis of preterm labor and preterm premature rupture of membranes associated with intraamniotic infection. *Infect Dis Clin North Am* 1997;11:135–176.

Hadi HA, Hodson CA, Strickland D. Premature rupture of the membranes between 20 and 25 weeks' gestation: role of amniotic fluid volume in perinatal outcome. *Am J Obstet Gynecol* 1994;170:1139–1144.

Hallak M, Bottoms SF. Accelerated pulmonary maturation from preterm premature rupture of membranes: a myth. *Am J Obstet Gynecol* 1993;169:1045–1049.

Hannah ME, Ohlsson A, Farine D, et al. Induction of labor compared with expectant management for prelabor rupture of the membranes at term. TERMPROM Study Group. *N Engl J Med* 1996;334:1053–1054.

Kappy KA, Cetrulo CL, Knuppel RE, et al. Premature rupture of the membranes: a conservative approach. *Am J Obstet Gynecol* 1979;134:655–661.

Kilbride HW, Yeast J, Thibeault DW. Defining limits of survival: lethal pulmonary hypoplasia after midtrimester premature rupture of membranes. *Am J Obstet Gynecol* 1996;175:675–681.

Lenihan JP Jr. Relationship of antepartum pelvic examinations to premature rupture of the membranes. *Obstet Gynecol* 1984;63:33–37.

Lewis DE, Brady K, Edwards MS, et al. Preterm premature ruptured membranes: a randomized trial of steroids after treatment with antibiotics. *Obstet Gynecol* 1996;88:801–805.

Lovett SM, Weiss JD, Diogo MJ, Williams PT, Garite TJ. A prospective double-blind, randomized, controlled clinical trial of ampicillin–sulbactam for preterm premature rupture of membranes in women receiving antenatal corticosteroid therapy. *Am J Obstet Gynecol* 1997;176: 1030–1038.

Major CA, Towers CV, Lewis DF, et al. Expectant management of patients with both preterm premature rupture of membranes and genital herpes. *Am J Obstet Gynecol* 1991;164:248 (abst 16).

McDuffie RS Jr, Nelson GE, Osborn CL, et al. Effect of routine weekly cervical examinations at term on premature rupture of the membranes: a randomized controlled trial. *Obstet Gynecol* 1992;79:219–222.

Meis PJ, Goldenberg RL, Mercer B, et al. The preterm prediction study: significance of vaginal infections. National Institute of Child Health and Human Development Maternal-Fetal Medicine Units Network. *Am J Obstet Gynecol* 1995;173:1231–1235.

Mercer B, Miodovnik M, Thurnan G, et al. Antibiotic therapy for reduction of infant mortality after preterm premature rupture of the membranes. A randomized controlled study. *JAMA* 1997;278:989–995.

Mercer BM, Arheart KL. Antimicrobial therapy in expectant management of preterm premature rupture of membranes. *Lancet* 1995;346:1271–1279.

Mercer BM, Crocker LG, Boe NM, et al. Induction versus expectant management in premature rupture of the membranes with mature amniotic fluid at 32 to 36 weeks: a randomized trial. *Am J Obstet Gynecol* 1993;169:775–782.

Moretti M, Sibai BM. Maternal and perinatal outcome of expectant management of premature rupture of membranes in the midtrimester. *Am J Obstet Gynecol* 1988;159:390–396.

Mozurkewish EL, Wolf FM. Premature rupture of the membranes at term: a meta analysis of three management schemes. *Obstet Gyneol* 1997;89: 1035–1043.

Ohlsson A. Treatment of preterm premature rupture of the membranes: a meta-analysis. *Am J Obstet Gynecol* 1989;160:890–906.

Regan JA, Klebanoff MA, Nugent RP, et al. Colonization with group B streptococci in pregnancy and adverse outcome. VIP Study Group. *Am J Obstet Gynecol* 1996;174:1354–1360.

Rotschild A, Ling EW, Puterman ML. Neonatal outcome after prolonged preterm rupture of the membranes. *Am J Obstet Gynecol* 1990;162: 46–52.

Schuker JL, Mercer BM. Midtrimester premature rupture of the membranes. *Semin Perinatol* 1996;20:389–400.

Sweet RL, Landers DV, Walker C, et al. *Chlamydia trachomatis* infection and pregnancy outcome. *Am J Obstet Gynecol* 1987;156:824–833.

Vintzileos AM, Campbell WA, Nochimson DJ, et al. Degree of oligohydramnios and pregnancy outcome in patients with premature rupture of the membranes. *Obstet Gynecol* 1985;66:162–167.

Weiner CP, Renk K, Klugman M. The therapeutic efficacy and cost-effectiveness of aggressive tocolysis for premature labor associated with premature rupture of the membranes. *Am J Obstet Gynecol* 1988;159: 216–222.

CHAPTER 18

Fetal Growth Retardation

◇

William N. Spellacy

Only recently have perinatologists become concerned about fetal growth disturbances, despite the discrepancies in fetal growth patterns that have always occurred. A major difficulty with the clinical management of these conditions is that their diagnosis requires two pieces of data, gestational age and fetal weight, neither of which is precisely or easily obtained during the perinatal period. Excessive fetal growth produces large-for-gestational-age, or macrosomic, infants, defined both as more than 4000 g and as more than 4500 g in birthweight, whose major problems have been dystocia and trauma during delivery. Small-for-gestational-age, or intrauterine growth-retarded or growth-restricted (IUGR), infants are those in the lower 10% of weight for age. Other definitions have been used, such as the ponderal index (weight divided by the length squared), but since length is difficult to measure in neonates, this index is often unreliable. With about 4 million births per year in the United States, this means that more than 400,000 cases of IUGR occur per year. IUGR infants are at high risk for fetal and neonatal problems, including death. The management of many high-risk conditions has improved to the point that normal perinatal outcomes are expected, for example, with Rh sensitization and treatment of the pregnant patient with diabetes. As a result, other high-risk conditions, such as fetal growth retardation, have become more frequent perinatal problems. IUGR now commands the prime attention of researchers and clinicians alike. The results of studies have helped in the recognition, understanding, and management of IUGR. This chapter reviews the data available on IUGR in terms of the control of normal fetal growth, the cause of IUGR, useful tests for detecting abnormal fetal growth, the clinical importance of the problem, and the management of this type of high-risk pregnancy.

◇ CONTROLLING FETAL GROWTH

In normal pregnancy, the fetus and placenta grow at different rates. The placenta expands early and develops into a large tertiary villus structure, with its maximum surface area for ex-

change normally peaking at about 37 weeks' gestation, when it reaches about 11 m². This placental development seems to be in response to the environment of oxygenated maternal blood bathing the cotyledons from open uterine spiral arteries whose ends have been replaced by trophoblast cells. At 37 weeks, the placental weight is about 500 g. From then until delivery, there is a slight decline in its surface area as microinfarctions occur. It is of interest that many parameters of pregnancy also peak at 37 weeks, including amniotic fluid volume and maternal blood human placental lactogen (hPL) levels, suggesting a peak in placental function at that time as well. The placenta partially regulates fetal growth. The fetal growth curve continues throughout pregnancy. In the last few weeks of gestation, beginning at about the 36th week, the rate of weight increase per week begins to slow. The fetus is then normally depositing fat in the form of 16-carbon palmitate derived from the two carbon acetate segments that result from glucose metabolism. Because fat has a high caloric content (9 calories per gram) compared with carbohydrates and proteins (4 calories per gram), the accumulation of calories in the fetus continues to increase rapidly in normal pregnancy until term, despite the reduced absolute fetal weight gain in the last 4 weeks. As a result of this high metabolic activity, the fetus' temperature is about 0.5°C above that of the mother. This excess heat is transferred by blood back to the mother, who dissipates it through her skin. After delivery, it is common for mothers to shiver as a compensation for losing this heat source.

The fetus requires three major forms of substrate for its growth. First, it receives glucose freely across the placenta from the maternal blood by facilitated diffusion. In a steady state, the maternal and fetal blood glucose levels are similar, with the fetal level being about 80% of the maternal level. Because this form of transfer requires a coupling mechanism at the placental–membrane border, an elevation of the maternal level above fasting results in a widening of the maternal–fetal gradient. All maternal amino acids are actively transported to the fetus and thus are in higher concentration in fetal than in maternal blood. This active transport process for amino acids seems to be under the control of the syncytiotrophoblast cyclic adenosine monophosphate concentration. Finally, oxygen crosses from the maternal blood to the fetal blood by simple diffusion, and the transfer depends on blood flow rates through the uterus and placenta and the concentration gradients, as noted in the Fick principle. Although many other, minor ingredients are necessary for fetal metabolism, these three are key.

In utero, glucose is burned with oxygen to produce energy in the form of adenosine triphosphate. The energy is used to convert amino acids into protein, and the result is a growing intrauterine infant. Regulation of this growth rate depends not only on the placental transfer of these substrates but also on fetal hormones such as insulin, insulin-like growth factors, and insulin-like growth factor–binding proteins. Fetal leptins may also be involved. Fetal pituitary growth hormone does not seem to be needed because, congenitally, growth hormone–deficient infants (i.e., ateliotic sexual dwarfs) are of normal size at birth. An excess or a deficiency of substrates and growth factors leads to overgrowth (i.e., macrosomia) or undergrowth (i.e., IUGR), respectively.

◊ CAUSES OF FETAL GROWTH RETARDATION

The causes of IUGR can be conveniently grouped into three broad categories relating to the substrate: (1) maternal-substrate availability, (2) placental-substrate transfer, and (3) fetal-substrate utilization. These categories vary in frequency and also in their potential for fetal damage. Thus, although maternal causes such as poor nutrition are common, they rarely do more than produce small infants. Placental and fetal causes are infrequent, but they contribute significantly to infant morbidity and mortality. It is therefore important to determine the cause of IUGR, as it will determine the level of concern and need for treatment.

Within each category, there are important subgroups. For example, the maternal grouping requires that the critical substrate—glucose, amino acids, and oxygen—be in the blood. Maternal nutrition before and during pregnancy is important in terms of fetal growth. Although most average-size mothers gain about 25 to 35 lb (11.4 to 15.9 kg) in pregnancy, good fetal outcome requires a larger weight gain in a thin woman than in an obese woman. Thus, most malnourished women who become pregnant deliver smaller-than-normal infants. These infants develop normally. Abnormalities may also occur if the mother has a chronic lung disease such as asthma, cyanotic heart disease (i.e., low blood oxygen), a malabsorption syndrome (i.e., gastrointestinal bypass procedures), or an abnormal bowel syndrome manifested by low, flat glucose tolerance curves. Women in the latter group may consume a good diet, but because it is poorly absorbed, they do not have an adequate substrate level in their blood. Some patients consume little food because they use their social resources for other things, such as buying street drugs (e.g., cocaine). Alcohol and especially beer consumption may also adversely affect fetal growth. The maternal group is the most frequent cause of IUGR, but it is also the least serious. Although the infants are small, most do not have altered perinatal mortality or long-term morbidity.

The placenta group includes those women with poor uterine blood flow or a small placental surface area. If there is maternal vascular disease, such as hypertension with abnormal spiral arteries, then the growth phase of the placenta may stop early, resulting in a smaller placenta that not only weighs less but also has a reduced surface area for exchange. The uterine blood flow can be reduced by diseased blood vessels or vessels that are in spasm.

A close relation exists between placental surface area and fetal weight. A good example of this is shown in Figure 1. In this instance, a twin dizygotic pregnancy had marked dis-

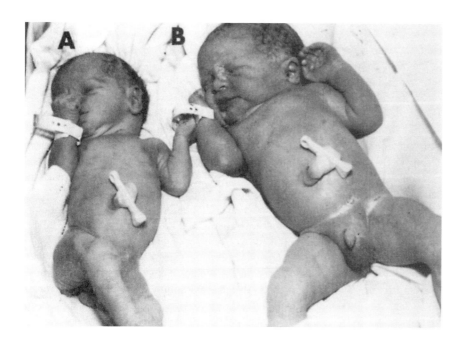

FIG. 1. Twins demonstrating a difference in growth for the same gestational age. Baby girl *A* weighed 1824 g, and baby boy *B* weighed 3150 g, a difference of 1326 g, or 42% of the boy's weight.

crepancy in infant weights at birth (1824 g and 3150 g). The placental surface area for the smaller infant was only about one-fourth the total placenta, showing how a lack of placental tissue results in fetal failure to grow (Fig. 2).

The mother's inability to recognize and accept fetal antigens could establish an immunologic host defense that would alter placental growth or function and produce an IUGR fetus. Smoking can also affect this area because it causes the release of both epinephrine and norepinephrine, which can result in uterine blood vessel spasm and reduced uterine blood flow. In addition, the fetal vessel endothelial layer produces less prostacyclin if the mother smokes, which can also reduce fetal blood flow. Many studies have shown that the infants of smokers weigh 150 to 300 g less than those of non-smokers. Maternal smoking has it greatest impact in older mothers and has little impact in teenage mothers. Controlled studies of mothers who smoke but stop during their pregnancy have shown that the infants of these mothers grow larger than the infants of mothers who continue to smoke. The most common clinical symptom of constricted uterine blood vessels is maternal hypertension; it is also the most common maternal factor associated with IUGR. The small placenta in hypertensive women is a serious problem because it can result in fetal hypoxia, organ damage, and death.

An unusual problem is confined placental mosiacism. In this case, the fetus has a normal karyotype and IUGR. The placenta has an abnormal karyotype, is usually small, and has a limited surface area.

The fetal group includes those pregnancies in which the substrate is not used normally by the fetus, although it is in the mother's blood and crosses the placenta. Two general conditions are responsible for this. The first is major congenital anomalies. Although cardiovascular anomalies are the most common, the severe forms are often associated with even more serious problems, such as trisomy 13 or trisomy 18. The second fetal problem group is accelerated fetal metabolism caused by infection with any of the TORCH agents. These include toxoplasma, rubella, cytomegalovirus, herpes simplex, and others, such as human immunodeficiency virus. About one-third of TORCH-affected infants are growth-retarded. If this is a possibility, a blood TORCH titer screen is needed.

◊ DIAGNOSIS OF FETAL GROWTH RETARDATION

The diagnosis of IUGR depends first on a simple, inexpensive clinical screen and then on more expensive laboratory tests to confirm or refute the diagnosis. Several risk scoring systems have been developed that identify a population to be concerned about. Most risk scoring systems include the uterine fundal height measurements. Clinical palpation for fetal size is known to be inaccurate. The serial measurement of uterine fundal height, from the symphysis across the uterus to the top of the fundus, is a useful index of fetal growth. Many factors can affect the result, including the correct placement of the tape and changes in fetal engagement and position, urine bladder volume, amniotic fluid volume, maternal obesity, and fetal weight. The test must be done in the same way by each examiner and at a time when the maternal bladder is empty. Several studies reported an accuracy of about 75% in diagnosing IUGR with this test, and there is no increased cost. The routine measurement of uterine fundal height at each prenatal visit, as well as the plotting of this measurement on a graphic chart, is a key to early diagnosis. An example of such a chart that can become part of the prenatal record is shown in Figure 3.

Confirmation of the clinical suspicion of IUGR can be done with more sophisticated and expensive tests. The first group of tests are biophysical. The ultrasonographic visual-

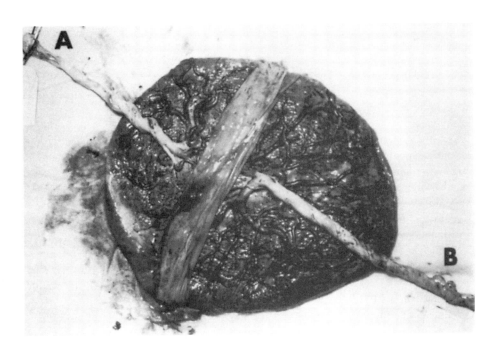

FIG. 2. The dizygotic twins' placenta weighed 1010 g. Twin A has a much smaller portion of the placenta.

Name:

Number:

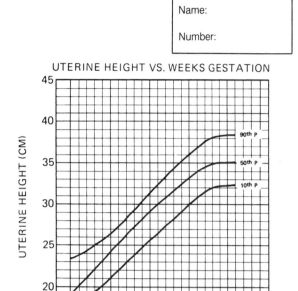

UTERINE HEIGHT VS. WEEKS GESTATION

By_____
Signature

FIG. 3. Uterine fundal height chart for fetal growth retardation diagnosis.

ization of the intrauterine cavity has greatly assisted in the diagnosis. The first studies were of fetal head size, but their accuracy was only about 50%. This is not too surprising, since nature allows the brain to continue to grow under the most adverse circumstances as a natural protection for central nervous system (CNS) function. Thus, the brain is the last organ affected in IUGR, yielding the brain-sparing effect. This is accomplished in the fetus by catecholamine release and the redistribution of blood flow toward critical organs, such as the brain, heart, and adrenals. The storage organs, such as the liver, are early affected in their growth patterns and therefore are much better indices of fetal nutrition. A more important ultrasound measurement is the abdominal circumference, for which the scan is taken across the umbilical vein as it enters the fetal liver. In addition, fetal bone growth (i.e., femur length and biparietal diameter [BPD]) and amniotic fluid volume determinations may be helpful ultrasound examinations.

Other studies that can be useful include measurements of placental and fetal biochemical factors present in the maternal circulation and related to fetal or placental weight. These include estriol, hPL, and SP$_1$ protein. Amniotic fluid levels of the C peptide fragment of proinsulin and of glucose are also of assistance in the diagnosis. With IUGR, all these biochemical markers tend to be low.

Several studies of maternal serum alpha-fetoprotein (AFP) levels early in pregnancy (i.e., 16 weeks) showed that high unexplained levels greater than 2 times the multiple of the median are often associated with preterm labor or the later development of IUGR. These studies may represent cases in which placental disruption occurs early (i.e., 16 weeks), resulting in leakage of fetal AFP into the maternal blood to give the high levels. These placental breaks may inhibit the later development of a large normal placenta for transfer, and fetal growth is then affected.

A final diagnostic test that is useful involves measurement of uterine and umbilical artery blood waveforms using Doppler flow instrumentation. An abnormal umbilical artery systolic–end diastolic ratio (i.e., more than 3.0) suggests placental vascular resistance. Comparison studies, however, show that ultrasound has a higher predictive accuracy than Doppler blood flow for diagnosing IUGR.

◊ COMPLICATIONS OF FETAL GROWTH RETARDATION

The complications of IUGR are principally those affecting the infant. Although the mother may have problems that cause growth retardation, such as hypertension or asthma, the most serious problems are for the infant. By definition, its size will be small for gestational age. If the condition has been present for a relatively short time, the CNS may continue to grow while other systems, such as the abdomen and especially its storage organ, the liver, will not. This gives the clinical picture of asymmetric IUGR with normal head size and small trunk. If, however, the process has been going for a long time, then even brain growth may be adversely affected; this presents as symmetric growth retardation, in which both the body and the head are small for the infant's age. The latter type is more severe because of its long-standing state and often represents conditions present from the first trimester, such as anomalies, including the trisomies, and congenitally infected infants (TORCH). Because the placenta is often small in cases in which it is responsible for the problem, the respiratory reserve of these fetuses is marginal. Umbilical blood samples obtained before labor often show fetal hypoxia and sometimes acidosis. Umbilical erythropoietin levels are elevated, demonstrating chronic hypoxia in many fetuses. These infants do not tolerate uterine contractions well. Indeed, in about 30% of IUGR cases, the results of an oxytocin contraction stress test (i.e., oxytocin challenge test) are positive, and about 50% develop fetal hypoxia or acidosis during labor, when uterine activity is much stronger. The latter problem may be associated with the passage of meconium and its aspiration, leading to respiratory difficulties in the nursery. In addition, probably because of the marginal oxygenation *in utero* plus the low amniotic fluid volume, many of these fetuses develop variable fetal heart rate decelerations in nonstress types of testing, suggesting umbilical cord compression patterns. The loss of amniotic fluid and the development of oligohydramnios can be a serious problem for the fetus, one in which movement can suddenly compress the umbilical cord, causing death. At first, the fetus may attempt to compensate for the poor placental transfer of oxygen by developing a marked polycythemia in response to its high erythropoietin (i.e., hyperviscosity syndrome), with hematocrits greater than 65%; then, after birth, it can have problems of multiorgan thrombosis, heart failure, and hyperbilirubinemia. Because little fat is deposited on these fetuses, most develop hypoglycemia early in neonatal life if they are not fed because they cannot mobilize glucose from glycogen and free fatty acids from fat for metabolism; instead, they use all their blood glucose for neonatal fuel. Depending on the cause, there may be other problems, too, for example, anomalies, signs of intrauterine infections (e.g., rubella, cytomegalovirus, or herpes simplex), and drug withdrawal.

It is not surprising, then, that both fetal and neonatal death rates are significantly increased; their levels depend on the severity of the problem. The overall perinatal mortality for the IUGR infant is six to eight times higher than that observed in normal pregnancies, and this problem clearly represents one of the most serious high-risk gestations that needs to be managed.

A final concern is the development of infants who survive. Many studies have been done longitudinally to investigate this aspect of the problem. During the first 10 years, these children remain physically small, compared with matched controls. They are lighter and shorter, and the circumferences of their organs, such as their heads and chests, are reduced. Their neurologic evaluation indices are also significantly reduced, suggesting lower intelligence levels. School performance can be subnormal because of their inability to maintain long attention spans. Thus, deficits in areas such as reading and mathmatics occur. In twin studies in which one twin is growth-retarded, long-term follow-up has shown reduced intelligence in that infant group as well.

◊ MANAGEMENT

Because of the many serious problems that can occur in the growth-retarded fetus or neonate, some pregnancies need to be managed by an experienced perinatal team in a tertiary referral center. The management of these pregnancies depends on the following general principles:

◊ Early detection (e.g., high-risk groups, testing);
◊ Elimination of contributing factors (e.g., diet, smoking, drugs);
◊ Increase uterine blood flow (e.g., bed rest, hydration);
◊ Serial fetal surveillance (e.g., weekly nonstress tests, oxytocin contraction tests, ultrasound, Doppler blood flow studies, cordocentesis);
◊ Early delivery in a perinatal center.

To introduce some management program, the cases first need to be detected. Early diagnosis is best because it provides time for intervention before fetal damage occurs. Clinicians must therefore be aware of the problem and be testing for it, especially in pregnancies at risk, such as in women who are hypertensive, who smoke, who demonstrate poor nutrition or little weight gain, or who have a history of IUGR deliveries, because the problem does recur. The use of aspirin as preventive therapy has shown promise in a metaanalysis.

Second, the contributing factors must be eliminated. These include poor dietary intake, smoking, and drug abuse. The diet of a pregnant woman should contain about 300 calories per day more than the diet of a nonpregnant woman; therefore, all pregnant women should be instructed to eat a diet of about 2100 to 2300 calories per day. The composition of the diet is less important than the number of calories it contains. Nonetheless, a protein content of 1.3 to 1.5 g/kg per day is recommended. Women on this diet gain differently, depending on their prepregnancy weights and size. Normal-weight women gain about 25 to 35 lb (11.4 to 15.9 kg), whereas thin women gain more and obese women gain less. No studies after early pregnancy have shown a clear need for prenatal vitamin supplementation if the diet is adequate, although additional exogenous iron is recommended. All women should be encouraged to stop smoking and stop drinking alcohol during pregnancy; if the patient is a substance abuser, she should be rehabilitated, for example, in a methadone program. Other identifiable causes should be corrected, if possible. For example, strenuous work and physical activity should be avoided by women with a poor vascular system evidenced by hypertension. Intrauterine feeding of the fetus has been tried but is still experimental; further studies in these areas may prove rewarding. Continuous oxygen therapy may be needed for women with cardiac or lung disease, and total parenteral nutrition has been used successfully in mothers with severe gastrointestinal disease inhibiting normal absorption.

Uterine blood flow is directly related to maternal blood pressure in a maximally dilated vascular system. For this reason, the third principle of management—to increase uterine blood flow as much as possible—does not mean lowering maternal blood pressure in the patient with hypertension, unless the blood pressure is considered a serious risk to the mother's health. Another important point is to have the woman remain on bed rest, optimally on her left side, where uterine blood flow is maximal. Although exercise and physical activity do not seem to present a problem in terms of the infant in normal pregnancies, they are contraindicated in high-risk pregnancies. The problem of women who continue to work during pregnancy arises here. If the pregnancy is normal and the work is not strenuous, then a 6-week window of leave is usual, with 2 weeks off before delivery and 4 weeks off after delivery. If the woman has problems, such as hypertension and IUGR, bed rest for extended periods may be necessary, and standing or physical work is contraindicated.

Before an intensive fetal surveillance program is begun, a fetal karyotype should be done if there is a serious risk of trisomy in the normally pregnant woman with severe symmetric fetal growth retardation. Either amniotic fluid or umbilical blood can be used. The antepartum surveillance program should be started as soon as something can be done about an abnormal result. Because most perinatal centers have normal survivors at about 24 weeks' gestation, this is about the time to start the studies if the diagnosis of IUGR has been made. The diagnosis, however, usually is not made until much later in a pregnancy. The following evaluation tests must be done serially until the pregnancy is terminated:

◊ Nonstress tests: fetal heart rate monitor;
◊ Amniotic fluid volume: ultrasound;
◊ Head growth (BPD): ultrasound.

If the weekly nonstress test is nonreactive (i.e., failure to have two or more heart rate accelerations of 15 beats per minute for 15 seconds each in a 20-minute strip), then it must be followed by a contraction stress test (CST). In this test, dilute intravenous oxytocin is administered until the uterus contracts three times in 10 minutes, and late-type decelerations of fetal heart rate are looked for. These tests detect placental insufficiency. Some have used the ultrasound biophysical profile or umbilical artery Doppler blood flow studies to evaluate these fetuses. Cordocentesis and fetal blood gas studies may be useful in severe cases. The second test must be the weekly ultrasound assessment of amniotic fluid volume. A useful test has been the four-quadrant assessment of the amniotic fluid index, which normally is greater than 6 cm. A third weekly test is done to determine fetal brain growth by ultrasound measurements of BPD.

Because intrauterine monitoring is not perfect and because some infants are damaged or die with this problem, it seems reasonable to deliver these babies early. If all surveillance tests are normal, then the optimal time for delivery appears to be about the 38th week of gestation, if the cervix is favorable for an induction of labor. If the surveillance tests become abnormal before that time, then an assessment of fetal maturity needs to be done; this often involves the use of amniocentesis with measurements of the fetal lung surfactant content, usually using a test like the lecithin–sphingomyelin ratio. The indications for delivery before 38 weeks with fetal maturity are a positive result in the CST with late decelerations, loss of amniotic fluid with resulting oligohydramnios, and ultrasound studies showing failure of head growth (i.e., BPD), an indication that the brain may also be affected. The latter subgroup is at high risk for developing CNS dysfunction.

Continuous assessment of fetal well-being during labor is important because many fetuses develop hypoxia. Such assessment is most easily accomplished by continuous electronic monitoring of fetal heart rates, for which an internal fetal scalp electrode is used when technically feasible. Oligohydramnios may result in cord compression and variable fetal heart rate decelerations. These can be treated by amnioinfusion. An alteration in basal fetal heart rate or pattern or in short-term variability that suggests fetal hypoxia and acidosis should be confirmed with fetal scalp blood sampling, if possible. If the alteration is confirmed (i.e., fetal scalp blood pH is less than 7.2), then the fetus needs intrauterine resuscitation and rapid delivery, usually by cesarean section. Fetal resuscitation can be done by initiating maternal hydration, positioning the mother on her left side, raising the presenting part, administering oxygen, and stopping uterine activity with a uterine tocolytic agent such as a β-mimetic (e.g., terbutaline, 0.25 mg subcutaneously). After delivery, the umbilical cord should be clamped quickly so as not to transfuse more red blood cells into the neonate with possible polycythemic hyperviscosity syndrome. Umbilical artery blood gases should be measured.

Caring for the growth-retarded neonate is equally important. If meconium has been passed, then immediate suctioning of the respiratory tract when only the head is out, followed by neonatal intubation to remove the meconium from the airway, is necessary to minimize the amount of meconium pulled down into the lungs. These measures may not prevent meconium aspiration, but they reduce the severity. If the neonate is hypoxic and depressed, it needs rapid resuscitation with measures such as intubation, artificial breathing assistance, oxygen, cardiac massage, hydration, and occasionally drugs such as epinephrine and sodium bicarbonate. Assessment for causative factors such as congenital anomalies and intrauterine infections must be done rapidly, and these conditions must be managed appropriately if detected. A hematocrit can identify hyperviscosity syndrome, and therapy may require phlebotomy or plasma exchange. Blood glucose level monitoring in the early hours of life is important to detect and treat hypoglycemia. If the blood glucose level falls below 40 mg/dl, parenteral glucose needs to be administered. Monitoring and maintaining body temperature at about 35°C minimizes the metabolic rate, and therefore oxygen consumption. If the mother was normal, the infant appears normal but small for its age, and the placenta is small, then confined placental mosaicism should be suspected and a placental karyotype obtained. Finally, long-term follow-up of these children is important to assess the success of the treatment program.

SUMMARY POINTS

◊ Intrauterine growth retardation occurs in an infant whose birthweight is in the lower 10th percentile for its gestational age. About 400,000 such infants are born in the United States each year.

◊ The condition may be caused by maternal, placental, or fetal factors. Early diagnosis is important, and clinically small uterine fundal height growth patterns suggest a need for appropriate ultrasound testing.

◊ Because infant morbidity and mortality are so significantly elevated in some of these pregnancies, special care needs to be taken. Therapy includes good nutrition, avoidance of confounding factors such as smoking and drugs, and sometimes bed rest to improve uterine blood flow.

◊ Fetal health must be serially monitored with tests such as a weekly nonstress test and ultrasound measurement of amniotic fluid volumes and fetal head size.

◊ Early timed and monitored delivery in a tertiary center where appropriate neonatal intensive care is available is critical. Long-term follow-up is important for survivors.

◊ RECOMMENDED READINGS

Basso O, Olsen J, Knudsen LB, Christensen K. Low birth weight and preterm birth after short interpregnancy intervals. *Am J Obstet Gynecol* 1998;178:259.

Battaglia C, Artini PG, A'Ambrogio G, et al. Maternal hypertension in the treatment of intrauterine growth retardation. *Am J Obstet Gynecol* 1992;167:430.

Berkowitz GS, Mehalek KE, Chitkara U, et al. Doppler umbilical velocimetry in the prediction of adverse outcome in pregnancies at risk for intrauterine growth retardation. *Obstet Gynecol* 1988;71:742.

Bossak WS, Spellacy WN. Accuracy of estimating fetal weight by abdominal palpation. *J Reprod Med* 1972;9:58.

Busacca M, Balconi G, Pietra A, et al. Maternal smoking and prostacyclin production by cultured endothelial cells from umbilical arteries. *Am J Obstet Gynecol* 1984;148:1127.

Freeman RK, Anderson G, Dorchester W. A prospective multi-institutional study of antepartum fetal heart rate monitoring. II. Contraction stress test versus nonstress test for primary surveillance. *Am J Obstet Gynecol* 1982;143:778.

Jazayeri A, Tsibris JCM, Hunt LT, Spellacy WN. Umbilical plasma erythropoietin correlations with blood gases and gestational age in appropriately grown infants. *Am J Perinatol* 1996;13:227.

Jones MD Jr, Battaglia FC. Intrauterine growth retardation. *Am J Obstet Gynecol* 1977;127:540.

Leitich H, Egarter C, Husslein R, et al. A meta-analysis of low-dose aspirin for the prevention of intrauterine growth retardation. *Br J Obstet Gynaecol* 1997;104:450.

Lin CC, Evans MI. *Intrauterine growth retardation: pathophysiology and clinical management.* New York: McGraw-Hill, 1984.

Low JA, Handley-Derry MH, Burke SO, et al. Association of intrauterine fetal growth retardation and learning deficits at age 9 to 11 years. *Am J Obstet Gynecol* 1992;167:1499.

Matsuda T, Nakano Y, Nishikawa Y, Yamaguchi R. Fetomaternal amino acid patterns and cyclic AMP in the human placenta with abnormal pregnancies, particularly with SFD. *Tohoku J Exp Med* 1977;121:253.

Miller JM Jr, Gabert HA. Comparison for dynamic image and pulsed Doppler ultrasonography for the diagnosis of the small-for-gestation-age fetus. *Am J Obstet Gynecol* 1992;166:1820.

Nicolaides KH, Campbell S, Bradley RJ, et al. Maternal oxygen therapy for intrauterine growth retardation. *Lancet* 1987;i:942.

Nuget FW, Rajala M, Olshea RA, et al. Total parenteral nutrition in pregnancy: conception to delivery. *J Parenter Enteral Nutr* 1987;11:424.

Pardi G, Buscaglia M, Ferrazi E, et al. Cord sampling for the evaluation of oxygenation and acid-base balance in growth-retarded human fetuses. *Am J Obstet Gynecol* 1987;157:1221.

Pazos R, Vuolo K, Aladjem S, et al. Association of spontaneous fetal heart rate decelerations during antepartum nonstress testing and intrauterine growth retardation. *Am J Obstet Gynecol* 1982;144:574.

Pearce JM, Chamberlain GVP. Ultrasonically guided percutaneous umbilical blood sampling in the management of intrauterine growth retardation. *Br J Obstet Gynaecol* 1987;94:318.

Phillips OP, Tharapel AT, Lerner JL, et al. Risk of fetal mosaicism when placental mosaicism is diagnosed by chorionic villus sampling. *Am J Obstet Gynecol* 1996;174:850.

Rutherford SE, Phelan JP, Smith CV, Jacobs N. The four-quadrant assessment of amniotic fluid volume: an adjunct to antepartum fetal heart rate testing. *Obstet Gynecol* 1987;70:353.

Schubring C, Kiess, W, Englaro P, et al. Levels of leptin in maternal serum, amniotic fluid, and arterial and venous cord blood: relation to neonatal and placental weight. *J Clin Endocrinol Metab* 1997;82:1480.

Spellacy WN, Buhi WC, Birk SA. Human placental lactogen and intrauterine growth retardation. *Obstet Gynecol* 1976;47:446.

Stein Z, Susser M, Rush D. Prenatal nutrition and birth weight: experiments and quasi-experiments in the past decade. *J Reprod Med* 1978;21:287.

Susa JB, Widness JA, Hintz R, et al. Somatomedins and insulin in diabetic pregnancies: effects on fetal macrosomia in the human and rhesus monkey. *J Clin Endocrinol* 1984;58:1105.

Thompson ML, Theron GB, Fatti LP. Predictive value of conditional centile charts for weight and fundal height in pregnancy in detecting light for gestational age births. *Eur J Obset Gynecol Reprod Biol* 1997;72:3.

Wenstrom K, Andrews WW, Maher JE. Amnioinfusion survey: prevalence, protocols, and complications. *Obstet Gynecol* 1995;86:572.

CHAPTER 19

Postdate Pregnancy
◇

William N. Spellacy

The postdate pregnancy was described in a 1902 article by Ballantyne, who noted not only its occurrence but also its risks. By the 1950s, the syndrome was well recognized in the literature from Western Europe, where the condition was a frequent reason for the induction of labor. Clifford (1954), a pediatrician, was one of the first in the United States to recognize the significance of the problem, whereas most obstetricians did not consider it a serious or significant perinatal threat. Since the 1970s, many high-risk pregnancies have been studied. The introduction of regionalized care for high-risk obstetrics has moved complicated gestations such as preeclampsia, diabetes mellitus, and Rh sensitization from the physician's office practice to the perinatal center for care. This has left normal pregnant women in private obstetric practice. Many of these women go past their expected due dates for delivery and move to a postdate status. This becomes one of the most frequent problems remaining in obstetric practice. The definition of the postdate pregnancy is 42 or more weeks' (more than 294 days) gestation, and its frequency of occurrence has been reported to be between 3% and 12%. This chapter describes the accurate dating of gestation—which is essential to making the diagnosis—causes of postdate gestations, maternal and infant problems that accompany these pregnancies, and a management plan to provide optimal outcomes.

◇ DATING THE PREGNANCY

One of the most important aspects of early prenatal care is to accurately date the gestation and set the expected date of confinement (EDC). Few women know the date of their ovulation and many do not recall the exact date of their last menses. The accuracy of dating the pregnancy then depends on (1) seeing the pregnant woman early in her gestation and (2) performing several dating tests that all agree. Most calculations begin with the determination of the last menstrual dates. It is important to ask specifically for the date of the first day of the last normal menses, because the woman may

not realize the importance of this information and may provide the last day of flow, which would introduce an error of 2 to 7 days for the calculated EDC. Studies have determined the mean duration of gestation. Kortenoever (1950) reviewed 7054 pregnancies in Holland in which the last menses was known and considered normal and found that the mean duration was 282 days. In another study of 5596 singleton gestations exceeding 28 weeks in which the last menses was known, Nakano (1972) found the mean duration to be 278.5 days. Thus, the 280-day mean duration from last menses seems fairly reliable. Using Naegele's rule, the last menstrual date minus 3 months plus 7 days gives a reasonable estimate for the EDC. This calculation makes the assumption that ovulation occurs on the 14th day of the 28-day cycle. The follicular phase is the variable portion of the cycle; if ovulation is delayed and the follicular phase is prolonged, then this method of calculating the EDC will be in error. In a study by Saito et al. (1972), 15.5% of pregnancies reached 42 weeks by last menstrual period definition. However, when basal body temperature records in the same women were reviewed to determine the precise time of ovulation, no pregnancies exceeded 285 days from ovulation to delivery.

Many other clinical parameters are also useful in dating gestations. The size of the uterus on pelvic examination early in pregnancy is helpful. As the uterus grows into the abdomen, the fundal height measurements from the symphysis are also useful. The uterus reaches the umbilicus at about 17 weeks, and the fundal height is about 20 cm at 20 weeks' gestation. Jimenez et al. (1983) found that the mother's perception of first fetal movements was not different for primigravida and multigravida and that the movements occurred on average at 17 weeks' gestation (range, 12 to 21 weeks). Others, however, have noted that multigravidas feel fetal movement earlier than primigravidas. In addition, fetal heart tones can first be heard with a stethoscope at a mean time of 17 weeks (range, 14 to 19 weeks). Thus, patients should be seen frequently during the critical early weeks if there is uncertainty about the pregnancy duration, so that the clinical parameters can be recorded as precisely as possible.

Several laboratory studies can help date a gestation. Serum levels of placental hormones, such as human chorionic gonadotropin (hCG) and human placental lactogen (hPL), rise linearly in early pregnancy and have proved to be good indices of gestational age. The accuracy of dating with early-pregnancy hCG measurements has been accurate to ±3.2 days between 29 and 60 days' gestation. Pregnancy-specific proteins, such as SP_1 protein, can also be used as duration markers, but their accuracy is not significantly better than hPL levels. The EDC is usually predictable within ±7 days by hPL testing.

The use of ultrasound to determine gestational age is now well accepted. There are limitations to this method, however. First, most tables of measured fetal part versus gestational age were developed from studies done on women who did not know the precise date of their ovulation, and this error is therefore built into the tables. Second, not all fetuses are the same size and grow at the same rate, and thus this variation exists in the normal tables. Third, male and female fetuses grow at different rates, but most tables are not specific for fetal sex or race. Finally, the precision of placing the cursors on the ultrasound image varies with sonographers, and this introduces error. It is important to understand the limitations of ultrasound dating of pregnancies. Just because a computer prints out a precise date, such as 26⅔ weeks, it does not mean that that level of accuracy has been achieved. It is better to round off these determinations to the nearest week. In the early gestational weeks, from week 5 through week 10, one can measure the gestational sac diameter. This measurement has a standard error of ±0.64 for predicting the weeks. From weeks 12 to 23, however, the fetal head biparietal diameter is accurate for dating and has a prediction error of 6.3 days. Other fetal bone studies, such as femur length, can also be used, and O'Brien et al. (1981) found an accuracy of dating with this method of ±6.7 days between weeks 12 and 23. Chervenak et al. (1986) found ultrasound crown-rump length measurements to be the most accurate method and superior to using serum hCG levels early in pregnancy. The accuracy of ultrasound dating decreases as the pregnancy advances because there is more variation in fetal size with age. Thus, this method is reliable only if the examinations are done before week 25.

After the 26th week of pregnancy, the clinician must not reset the EDC but must manage the pregnancy according to the date on the record, even if it is inaccurate.

◊ CAUSES OF POSTDATE PREGNANCY

The most frequent cause of postdate gestation is inaccurate pregnancy dating because of the failure to have a regular ovulation pattern. This is a double problem. First, it causes a large number of pregnancies to be labeled high risk and therefore to receive more intensive management. Such management means more expensive tests and possibly more op-

erative intervention with induction of labor or cesarean section, and increases the costs for patients and the work effort for the health care providers. Second, it falsely categorizes many normal gestations as high risk, and their obvious good outcomes dilute the importance of the syndrome and lull obstetricians into believing that the postdate pregnancy is not serious. The diagnosis is common when menstrual cycles are irregular with delayed ovulations or when last menstrual dates are recalled inaccurately and early prenatal dating is not established with ultrasound examinations. This is demonstrated by one study that showed that 7.5% of women were postdate by their menstrual history. In the same group, only 2.6% were postdate by ultrasound examinations. If both menstrual dates and ultrasound examinations were used, only 1.1% were postdate. Another contributing factor is if a woman became pregnant shortly after discontinuation of oral contraceptives. Delays in ovulation by 2 or more weeks in the first few spontaneous cycles after oral contraceptive use are common, so the last menses is a poor criterion for dating those pregnancies.

Less common contributors are unusual problems such as anencephaly of the fetus or sulfatase deficiency in the placenta. The fetus with anencephaly can deliver early as well as late, but the pregnancy with sulfatase deficiency, which is an X-linked problem, routinely delivers the male fetus in the postdate period. This condition prevents the conversion of androgens (dehydroepiandrosterone sulfate) to estrogens, which are important to labor onset.

Most true postdate gestations are of unknown cause. It is accepted that prostaglandins produced in the uterus play a key role in starting labor. It is also common for the postdate gestation to have an unripe cervix as it enters this period. Many studies have shown that the cervix can rapidly be changed by the local application of prostaglandins. These data suggest that the cause may be either a deficiency in prostaglandin production or a refractoriness of the cervix to respond to endogenous prostaglandins. Further research in this area should be rewarding in terms of a better understanding of the problem, as well as more effective therapy. Clinically, one should remember that the condition of the cervix is not useful in dating the pregnancy.

◊ MATERNAL PROBLEMS

The woman who goes past her EDC by 2 or more weeks faces several problems. The first is the emotional strain of apprehension, expectation, and anxiety produced by her not starting labor on time. She has focused on her due date for many months; to pass that date and then to continue pregnancy with no signs of labor leave her frustrated, worried, and concerned. The second problem, already alluded to, relates to the medical intervention in terms of assessments and attempted delivery. The many additional tests and visits to the physician's office, as well as attempts at labor induction or cesarean section, increase her anxiety, cause inconvenience, and raise the cost of medical care. The final potential problem is the physical trauma that can be experienced in the delivery of a macrosomic infant. Vaginal and cervical lacerations complicate the immediate delivery, as well as creating potentially long-term problems such as cervical incompetence, pelvic relaxation, and stress urinary or fecal incontinence. Although all maternal problems are important, none is life-threatening for the woman.

◇ INFANT PROBLEMS

The four problems for the infant in a postdate gestation are much more serious than those for its mother. The first problem is oligohydramnios with acute cord compressions, which can occur when the amniotic fluid volume decreases to a low level. Cord accidents frequently cannot be predicted, although variable fetal heart rate decelerations on continuous monitoring and the disappearance of amniotic fluid on real-time ultrasound scanning are clues to this problem. All postdate pregnancies must be evaluated for oligohydramnios.

A second problem is macrosomia. In the past, this was defined as a birthweight greater than 4000 g but is now defined as a birthweight greater than 4500 g. It results from continued growth over an extra 2 or more weeks *in utero*. The possibility of this problem occurring increases if the mother is obese or has diabetes mellitus. The consequences of macrosomia include obstructed labor and, more important, birth trauma, especially shoulder dystocia and brachial nerve injury or hypoxia. Prediction of the macrosomic infant is often possible by ultrasound assessment of fetal weight and uterine fundal height measurements. The ultrasound estimates are best done by abdominal circumference (AC) scans. Although the AC is one of the most difficult measurements on ultrasound, it is the most important in predicting macrsosomia. An AC greater than 36 cm suggests macrosomia. Ultrasound scans have an error of about 10%, so most macrosomic infants can be identified. A uterine fundal height measurement greater than 40 cm in a nonobese woman suggests macrosomia.

Meconium aspiration is a third and important problem. The fetus seldom passes meconium before 32 weeks' gestation; after that, the frequency of meconium passage progressively increases as the fetus grows older. Some fetuses pass meconium in response to hypoxia. In postdate pregnancies, the incidence of meconium passage exceeds 25%. An associated complication is that as the volume of amniotic fluid decreases postdate, the passed meconium is less likely to be well diluted, resulting in a thicker meconium being available for aspiration by the fetus. The thicker the meconium is, the more likely the respiratory passages will be obstructed if the meconium is carried deep into the lung structure. In addition, meconium blocks the action of alveolar surfactant to reduce surface tension and thus interferes with lung function.

The fourth problem for the infant is placental insufficiency. The placenta reaches its maximum size and surface area at about 37 weeks' gestation; all its functions usually peak at that time as well. After that point, surface area and function gradually reduce. If the infant continues to grow, then the placenta–infant ratio decreases, and the transfer of critical substrate may reach a point at which intrauterine existence is compromised. Fetal erythropoietin, which is released in response to hypoxia, is elevated in many postdate pregnancies. To survive in the uterus under these abnormal conditions, the fetus can decrease its energy requirements in two ways. First, the fetus may decrease its growth rate, which also leads to a loss of deposited fat and glycogen. It then shows signs of fetal growth retardation and dysmaturity, with wrinkled and peeling skin and long digit nails. Second, it can stop moving. The fetus may demonstrate hypoxia at rest, but more often it occurs after the stress of uterine contractions, especially if they are strong enough to dilate the cervix, as in labor. In many of these compromised infants, fetal bradycardia with hypoxia and acidosis develop during labor. The compromised placental reserve can then present with a wide spectrum of changes, including poor fetal growth, loss of fetal fat and glycogen, meconium passage, decreased fetal movement, loss of amniotic fluid, nonreactive fetal heart rates, late-type fetal heart rate decelerations with uterine contractions, hypoxia and acidosis, low Apgar scores, central nervous system damage, and death.

◇ MANAGEMENT OF POSTDATE PREGNANCY

Because the incidence of postdate complications rises significantly after 42 weeks' gestation, these pregnancies must be identified by 41 weeks so that they can be managed appropriately from the beginning of the 42nd week. Low levels of vaginal fetal fibronectin at 41 weeks predict postdate pregnancies well. The principal concepts in management are as follows:

◇ Only normal pregnancies should be allowed to go past the EDC.
◇ Terminating the pregnancy will correct the problem.
◇ The *in utero* environment must be monitored for the risks of oligohydramnios and placental insufficiency.
◇ Delivery problems of shoulder dystocia with macrosomic infants, meconium aspiration, and hypoxia/acidosis must be avoided.

The specific plan for management is outlined in the following sections.

Weekly Vaginal Examinations

The patient must have weekly vaginal examinations to assess the condition of the cervix. When the cervix reaches a dilation and effacement at which induction of labor will be easy and probably successful, the woman should be admitted to the hospital for the procedure. Usually, this is safely accomplished if the cervix is dilated 3 cm or more. If the vertex is at station 0, induction can be started by amniotomy; an intravenous oxytocin infusion may also be needed. Induction of labor in these cases decreases the need for cesarean section. The use of locally applied prostaglandin gel in changing the cervix from unfavorable to favorable is safe. Use of misoprostol (Cytotec), a synthetic analog of prostaglandin E₁ in the vaginal fornix has proven very effective, safe, and inexpensive.

Weekly Real-time Ultrasound Scans

A physiologic change accompanying the maturation of a pregnancy is the gradual reduction of the amniotic fluid volume. The fluid usually reaches its maximum volume of 1000 ml at about 37 weeks' gestation and then decreases to 800 ml by 40 weeks and to 250 ml by 42 weeks. The gradual and continual loss of amniotic fluid creates the ominous oligohydramnios environment in which fetal compression of the umbilical cord becomes a serious risk. Because cord compression is usually not predictable, occurs abruptly, and can result in sudden fetal damage or death, it must be a major concern to the obstetrician. In some cases, the amniotic fluid volume can disappear rapidly, but most studies report a decrease in volume of about 25% per week.

Many studies have demonstrated a significant increase in perinatal mortality with oligohydramnios. The uterus should thus be scanned with real-time ultrasound on a weekly basis to assess amniotic fluid volume. A useful measurement is the amniotic fluid index (AFI). The AFI is determined by scanning all four quadrants of the uterus, determining the largest pocket of fluid in each, and measuring its vertical diameter. The sum of these should be greater than 6 cm. The lower abdominal quadrants are more predictive than the upper ones. The placental grade is of little additional help.

The ultrasound diagnosis of oligohydramnios should be an indication to proceed to delivery. If induction of labor is attempted, the fetal heart rate must be continually monitored electronically to detect signs of cord compression in the form of variable decelerations. Variable decelerations can be treated during labor with amnioinfusions of saline solution. An infusion of 250 ml increases the amniotic fluid index by about 4–6 cm. The risks of amnioinfusion include infection, uterine rupture, and amniotic fluid emboli. The ultrasound examination can also estimate fetal weight to determine whether or not the fetus is becoming macrosomic. If the fetus is approaching macrosomic size and the cervix is favorable, labor can be induced.

Weekly Fetoplacental Function Tests

As the pregnancy progresses, there is a gradual decrease in the functional surface area of the placenta for transfer and a gradual growth of the fetus, producing more fetal requirements for transfer. Thus, the fetoplacental reserve gradually is reduced, and at some point it will be below the limit of adequacy for normal intrauterine existence. This change occurs slowly, and, as a result, most tests provide a long enough lead time to be clinically useful. Many tests can be applied to these pregnancies to assess the fetal risks. Those that have been well studied include the following.

Estriol

The amount of estriol in the maternal blood and urine depends on the size of the placenta and fetus and their functional state. As the placenta decreases its function for a given gestational age, estriol production gradually decreases, and many studies have demonstrated that this is a useful biochemical marker of fetoplacental compromise in the postdate gestation. Most laboratories use plasma free estriol as the test because the assay systems are easy to perform and the problems of 24-hour urine collection are eliminated. The test is not used much today.

Human Placental Lactogen

Serum hPL is a useful marker of the functional mass of the placenta. Levels decrease as placental function decreases and are related to placental mass. Accordingly, the test has been used as an adjunct marker of placental reserve. Studies of postdate gestations have shown some predictability of intrauterine compromise with the test but not enough to be able to use it as the only assessment of the intrauterine environment. The test is not used much today.

Antepartum Fetal Heart Rate Monitoring

Both the nonstress test (NST) and the contraction stress test (oxytocin challenge test [OCT]) have been used in many studies to assess the fetal risks in postdate pregnancies, and they both seem to provide valid assessments. The OCT seems more sensitive, however, because it results in a lower perinatal mortality. Because of safety and convenience, the weekly NST is the most frequently used. Two accelerations of the heart rate of 15 beats per minute for 15 seconds in a 20-minute period are considered reactive. Oligohydramnios and cord compression are always potential risks; for this reason, the fetal heart rate strips should be carefully reviewed for evidence of variable decelerations because they may be predictive of that problem and are associated with a significant increase in perinatal mortality. The fetal heart rate and ultrasound studies have been combined into a biophysical profile assessment, which also includes evaluations of fetal tone, movement, and breathing. There are few data in randomized, controlled studies, however, to suggest that improved perinatal outcomes result from such monitoring. Likewise, umbilical and uterine artery Doppler blood flow studies have added little in this condition. When they are used, the umbilical artery systolic/diastolic ratio upper normal level should be 2.4.

The fetus in postdate pregnancies is clearly mature. If it is delivered healthy and does not have congenital anomalies, it will do well in the nursery and survive. Thus, if any test shows that the risk for the fetus is increasing, it must be acted on immediately by proceeding to delivery. Use of these tests is shown in Figure 1.

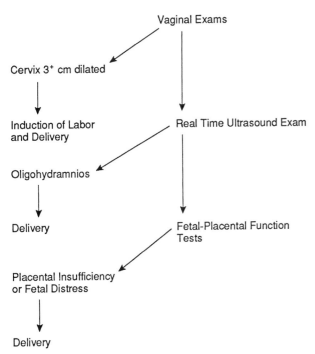

FIG. 1. Management of postdate pregnancies includes weekly examination and testing.

Delivery

Once the decision has been made to deliver or the patient spontaneously begins labor, there are several significant problems that need to be guarded against.

Labor Dysfunction—Shoulder Dystocia

The incidence of shoulder dystocia is significantly increased in postdate pregnancies in which the fetus has reached macrosomic size. Serious shoulder dystocia can result in arm and clavicle fracture, brachial plexus injuries, or/and hypoxia. Fortunately, only about 10% of the nerve injuries are permanent. The fetus must be screened for this problem with ultrasound assessment of fetal weight. If the estimate reaches 5000 g, an elective cesarean section should be considered because there is a 10% error in the estimate that makes the likelihood of a fetus' weighing 4500 g good. If vaginal delivery is attempted, an adequate bony pelvis and pubic arch are needed. The obstetrician must be familiar with the techniques to free an impacted shoulder if it occurs, including episiotomy, McRobert's manuever, suprapubic pressure, woodscrew maneuver, and delivery of the posterior arm. Uterine fundal pressure should not be used.

Meconium Aspiration

Passage of meconium is frequent in the postdate pregnancy, with usual incidences in excess of 25%. This suggests that fetal hypoxia is more common in postdate pregnancies. The major problem for the infant is that when meconium is deeply aspirated into the respiratory tract, it plugs the airway and causes respiratory distress, pneumothorax, and neonatal death. Attempts have been made to reduce these problems by aspirating the respiratory tract with a DeLee suction trap before the chest is delivered and then immediately intubating the neonate and suctioning below the vocal cords. Studies have shown that even this aggressive approach does not prevent all serious neonatal problems. Although about 2% of neonates still have meconium aspiration syndrome, the severity of their respiratory problems is significantly reduced by this approach. Amnioinfusion may help by diluting the thick meconium. Prevention of fetal hypoxia is important because it causes gasping, which pulls meconium deep into the lungs and damages the lung tissue directly. Finally, some respiratory difficulty in the neonate from meconium aspiration can be secondary to fetal hypoxia and the shunting of blood away from the lung, which causes direct lung tissue damage.

Fetal Distress

The postdate fetus is in double jeopardy for distress in labor because of associated oligohydramnios with common cord compression accidents and placental insufficiency. Thus, when these infants are in labor, they must be continuously and carefully assessed. This is best done with continuous electronic fetal heart rate monitoring. The information derived from this source is better with internal monitoring, so this should be done as soon as obstetrically feasible. If ominous signs of potential fetal hypoxia are present late in labor, a fetal scalp blood sample can be obtained to determine the pH level. This test reduces the number of unnecessary cesarean sections done for heart rate changes. There must be the capability of performing a rapid emergency cesarean section if fetal distress develops. This means a decision-to-delivery time of less than 30 minutes for small level I obstetric units and 15 minutes for larger level II and III units. During the preparation time, an attempt should be made to resuscitate the fetus. This is best carried out by administering oxygen to the mother, moving her to her left side and adequately hydrating her, elevating the presenting fetal part, and stopping uterine activity with a tocolytic drug such as terbutaline (0.25 mg subcutaneously).

SUMMARY POINTS

◊ The problem of postdate pregnancy is compounded by inaccurate pregnancy dating. Biochemical and biophysical assessments of gestational age in the first half of pregnancy are needed when menstrual data are unreliable. The EDC should not be changed after 26 weeks of pregnancy.

◊ The causes of true postdate (42+ weeks) pregnancies are usually unknown. The maternal problems include anxiety, apprehension, and

continues

summary points continued

possibly traumatic birth of a large infant. The infant problems include oligohydramnios with acute cord compression, meconium passage and aspiration, macrosomia with labor problems or shoulder dystocia, and placental insufficiency with dysmaturity, hypoxia, organ damage, acidosis, and death.

◊ Management includes weekly vaginal cervical examinations, real-time ultrasound assessment of amniotic fluid volume and fetal size, and fetoplacental function tests such as weekly fetal heart rate monitoring (i.e., NST).

◊ Delivery should be accomplished if the cervix is favorable, the amniotic fluid is lost, the fetus is macrosomic, or fetal distress occurs. The outcome for these infants should be excellent, and normal mental development is expected.

◊ RECOMMENDED READINGS

Ballantyne JW. The problem of the postmature infant. *J Obstet Gynecol Br Emp* 1902;2:23.

Boyd ME, Usher RH, McLean FH, Kramer MS. Obstetrics consequences of postmaturity. *Am J Obstet Gynecol* 1988;158:334.

Chervenak FA, Brightman RC, Thornton J, et al. Crown-rump length and serum human chorionic gonadotropin as predictors of gestational age. *Obstet Gynecol* 1986;67:210.

Clifford SH. Postmaturity with placental dysfunction—clinical syndrome and pathologic findings. *J Pediatr* 1954;44:1.

Davis RO, Philips JB III, Harris BA Jr, et al. Fetal meconium aspiration syndrome occurring despite airway management considered appropriate. *Am J Obstet Gynecol* 1985;151:731.

Dyson DC, Miller PD, Armstrong MA. Management of prolonged pregnancy: induction of labor versus antepartum fetal testing. *Am J Obstet Gynecol* 1987;156:928.

Ecker JL, Greenberg JA, Norwitz ER, et al. Birth weight as a predictor of brachial plexus injury. *Obstet Gynecol* 1997;89:643.

Eden RD, Seifert LS, Winegar A, Spellacy WN. Perinatal characteristics of uncomplicated postdate pregnancies. *Obstet Gynecol* 1987;69:296.

Fischer RL, Kuhlman KA, Depp R, Wapner RJ. Doppler evaluation of umbilical and uterine arcuate arteries in the postdate pregnancy. *Obstet Gynecol* 1993;78:363.

Grubb DK, Rabello YA, Paul RK, et al. Post-term pregnancy: fetal death rate with antepartum surveillance. *Obstet Gynecol* 1992;79:1024.

Hannah ME, Hannah WJ, Hellman J, et al. Induction of labor as compared with serial antenatal monitoring in post-term pregnancy—a randomized controlled trial. *N Engl J Med* 1992;326:1587.

Jazayeri A, Tsibris JCM, Spellacy WH. Elevated umbilical cord plasma erythropocetin levels in prolonged pregnancies. *Obstet Gynecol* 1998;92:61.

Jimenez JM, Tyson JE, Reisch JS. Clinical measures of gestational age in normal pregnancies. *Obstet Gynecol* 1983;61:438.

Kortenoever ME. Pregnancy of long duration and postmature infant. *Obstet Gynecol Surv* 1950;5:812.

Lagrew DC, Freeman RK. Management of postdate pregnancy. *Am J Obstet Gynecol* 1986;154:8.

Lockwood CJ, Moscarelli RD, Wein R, et al. Low concentrations of vaginal fetal fibronectin as a prediction of deliveries occurring after 41 weeks. *Am J Obstet Gynecol* 1994;171:1.

Lykkesfeldt G, Nielsen MD, Lykkesfeldt AE. Placental steroid sulfatase deficiency: biochemical diagnosis and clinical review. *Obstet Gynecol* 1984;64:49.

Marks AD, Divon MY. Longitudinal study of amniotic fluid index in postdate pregnancy. *Obstet Gynecol* 1992;79:229.

Matthews TG, Warshaw JB. Relevance of the gestational age distribution of meconium passage *in utero*. *Pediatrics* 1979;64:30.

Nakano R. Post-term pregnancy: a five-year review from Osaka National Hospital. *Acta Obstet Gynecol Scand* 1972;51:217.

O'Brien GD, Queenan JT, Campbell S. Assessment of gestational age in the second trimester by real-time ultrasound measurement of the femur length. *Am J Obstet Gynecol* 1981;139:540.

Pollack RN, Hauer-Pollack G, Divon MY. Macrosomia in postdate pregnancies: the accuracy of routine ultrasonographic screening. *Am J Obstet Gynecol* 1992;167:7.

Rutherford SE, Phelan JP, Smith CV, Jacobs N. The four-quadrant assessment of amniotic fluid volume: an adjunct to antepartum fetal heart rate testing. *Obstet Gynecol* 1987;70:353.

Saito M, Yazawa K, Hashiguchi A, et al. Time of ovulation and prolonged pregnancy. *Am J Obstet Gynecol* 1972;112:31.

Sanchez-Ramos L, Kaunitz AM, Wears RL, et al. Misoprostol for cervical ripening and labor induction: a meta-analysis. *Obstet Gynecol* 1997;89:633.

Shime J, Librach CL, Gare DJ, Cook CJ. The influence of prolonged pregnancy on infant development at one and two years of age: a prospective controlled study. *Am J Obstet Gynecol* 1986;154:341.

Spellacy WN, Miller S, Winegar A, Peterson PQ. Macrosomia—maternal characteristics and infant complications. *Obstet Gynecol* 1985;66:158.

Wenstrom K, Andrews WW, Maher JE. Amnioinfusion survey: prevalence, protocols, and complications. *Obstet Gynecol* 1995;86:572.

Yeh SY, Read JA. Management of post-term pregnancy in a large obstetric population. *Obstet Gynecol* 1982;60:282.

CHAPTER 20

Multiple Pregnancies

◇

William N. Spellacy

◇ TWIN GESTATION

Twin pregnancies have been an interest of the lay and obstetric communities for centuries. After years of investigation and modifications in the management programs, they still represent a high-risk pregnancy condition. At delivery, twins represent about 1% of births and 2% of infants, but they contribute 12% to the United States' overall perinatal mortality rate of about 10 per 1000 births. Overall, the fetal mortality rate for twins is increased fourfold, the neonatal mortality rate is increased sixfold, and the perinatal mortality rate is increased tenfold over the rates for singletons. On a weight basis, the overall mortality rate for twins is increased by a factor of 1.5. For infants weighing less than 2500 g, twins have a better survival rate than singletons. For infants weighing more than 2500 g, singletons fare better.

Etiology and Epidemiology

The overall incidence of twins at delivery is approximately 1%. There are two types of twins, monozygotic and dizygotic, depending on how many ova are released. Monozygotic twinning is a chance occurrence and is little affected by other parameters. It occurs in approximately 3 to 4 of 1000 births throughout the world. Rates increase slightly with delayed implantation, as occurs with *in vitro* fertilization. The occurrence seems to be related to a defective zona pellucida that allows ovum cleavage.

The frequency of dizygotic twinning does vary throughout the world and has several factors affecting its incidence. Heredity is one important factor. If the mother's first-degree relatives have had twins, the chance of her carrying twins is increased. If the mother has already had one set of dizygotic twins, her chance of repeating in a subsequent pregnancy is increased twofold. There is no hereditary effect contributed by the father's side of the family.

Maternal race can affect the frequency of twinning. Monozygotic twinning frequency is unaffected by race, but dizygotic twinning occurs in approximately 7 to 10 per 1000 births for whites, 10 to 40 per 1000 births for persons of African descent, and 3 per 1000 births for Asians. Maternal age and size also influence the rate, with the highest frequency of dizygotic twinning occurring in mothers more than 35 years of age and in women who are obese.

Use of certain drugs in the preovulatory phase of the cycle increases the frequency of dizygotic twinning. These drugs include opiates and those for ovulation induction. For example, the frequency of twinning with the use of clomiphene or gonadotropin-releasing hormone (Gn-RH) is 10%, but with menotropins-induced (follicle-stimulating hormone [FSH]) cycles, it is 30% to 50%. Alterations in gonadotropin levels can produce multiple ovulations. Women who have spontaneously had dizygotic twins have been studied for their cyclic gonadotropin levels, but the results were inconsistent. In a few studies, preovulatory FSH levels have been found to be elevated. Because inhibin levels were normal, it was suggested that the Gn-RH may be increased in the cycles in which spontaneous multiple ovulations occur. However, many other studies have failed to find gonadotropin level alterations in women who previously had twin pregnancies. Few studies have been done of the cycle of the twin fertilization.

Placentation

In dizygotic twinning, two individual placental units are produced, and the membrane between these two have amnion and chorion layers from each infant. Thus, the central membrane between the infants has two amnion layers and two chorion layers, a situation always seen with dizygotic twins. In monozygotic twins, the placentation depends on the time at which the twin division occurs, because the amnion and chorion form at different times in gestation. If division of the zygote occurs in less than 3 days, two independent placental units are formed, and the central membrane contains two amnion and two chorion layers, the same as for dizygotic twins. The chorion forms by day 3, and if the division occurs between days 3 and 8, the placenta has two amnion membranes and only one chorion, and the central membrane between the infants is thin, because it does not contain chorionic tissue; this is called a monochorionic placenta. The amnion forms by day 8, and if the division occurs between days 8 and 13 of gestation, no central membrane develops, and a monoamniotic monochorionic twin placenta occurs. These types of development are illustrated in Figure 1. If the division occurs after day 13, the result is a physical attachment of the twin bodies, producing conjoined twins.

Examination of the placenta and a detailed description of its central membrane are critical for determining the zygosity of the infants. The microscopic appearance of the central membrane containing two or four layers is seen in Figure 2. If the infants are of opposite sex, the pregnancy is dizygotic. If the central membrane contains only amnion, the infants are monozygotic. If the central membrane has two amnion and two chorion layers (i.e., dichorionic) and the infants are the same sex, the twins may be dizygotic or monozygotic. The identification of zygosity in twin pairs of same-sex infants is difficult if the central membrane is dichorionic; they could be monozygotic or dizygotic twins. A specific diagnosis can sometimes be made by blood or HLA typing, but in other cases the only sure way of identification is by skin graft testing. Twin infants have shorter umbilical cords than singletons. In monozygotic twins, cord lengths are usually equal.

Diagnosis

Twins are diagnosed by clinical, biochemical, and biophysical methods. The clinical examination revels a uterine fundal height growing at a greater rate than expected for a singleton pregnancy at that time. Later in gestation, two fetuses may be palpated, and two different heart rates may be detected. Using only these clinical parameters, approximately one-third of all twin pregnancies are missed and diagnosed only at delivery. Biochemical tests may demonstrate higher levels of fetal or placental substances in the maternal circulation than those found during a singleton pregnancy. Higher levels of maternal serum alpha-fetoprotein (AFP), human chorionic gonad-otropin (hCG), human placental lactogen, and estriol suggest a twin gestation.

The definitive diagnosis is made with a biophysical test. In the past, x-ray diagnoses confirmed a twin gestation. Modern ultrasound studies can outline the twin pregnancy (Fig. 3), its placentation, the structure of the central membrane, and the fetal sexes. Errors in ultrasound diagnosis are most common when more than two fetuses are present. When a patient is sent for confirmation of a twin pregnancy and the ultrasonographer scans and finds two fetuses, the examination may then stop, although more infants may be present. All patients with a twin pregnancy should have a thorough uterine examination to rule out the possibility of three or more fetuses.

Maternal Complications

The physiologic changes occurring in the mother with a twin gestation are an exaggeration of what occurs in a singleton pregnancy. She has a greater increase in blood volume, pulse, cardiac output, and weight gain. The average weight gain for a normal-sized woman with twins is 35 to 45 lb (15.9 to 20.4 kg) for the gestation. The eight medical problems that are significantly increased in women carrying a twin gestation are listed in Table 1.

Preterm Labor

Two large studies of twin pregnancies by Potter and Guttmacher demonstrated that the mean delivery time for twins was 37 weeks' gestation (256 and 258 days). Preterm labor for twin gestations is increased seven to ten times above singleton rates. It is a significant contributor to perinatal morbidity and mortality.

Hypertension

Women with a twin pregnancy have a twofold to fivefold increased frequency of hypertension complicating their preg-

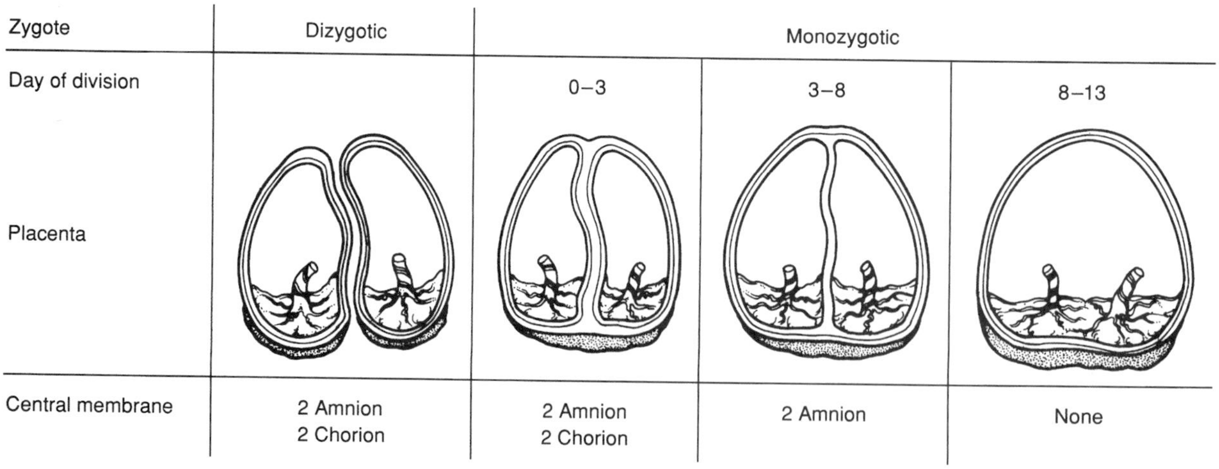

Zygote	Dizygotic	Monozygotic		
Day of division		0–3	3–8	8–13
Placenta				
Central membrane	2 Amnion 2 Chorion	2 Amnion 2 Chorion	2 Amnion	None

FIG. 1. Types of placentation in monozygotic and dizygotic twinning.

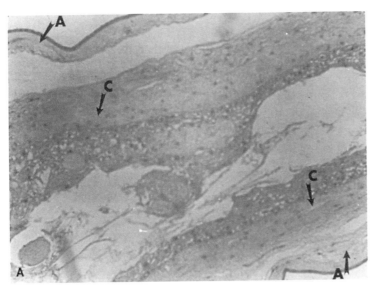
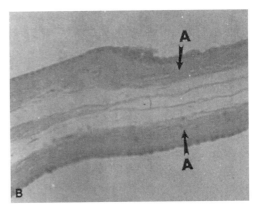

FIG. 2. In monozygotic twinning, the central membrane contains **(A)** four layers or **(B)** two layers (*A*, amnion; *C*, chorion).

nancy. This includes pregnancy-induced hypertension and preeclampsia with the accompanying proteinuria.

Abruption

Twin pregnancies have a threefold increased frequency of abruption, even when controlling for maternal hypertension. Although abruption occurs most frequently in the third trimester, it is also a significant risk immediately after vaginal delivery of the first infant, because the uterus changes its shape and sometimes shears off the placenta.

Anemia

The expanded maternal blood volume, together with the increased demand by the fetus for two essential nutrients, folic acid and iron, contributes to the increased frequency of anemia. Women with twin pregnancies have two to three times the risk of developing anemia (hemoglobin less than 10 g/dl) during their pregnancy. These women should receive supplements of folic acid (1 mg/day) and elemental iron (60 mg/day) during pregnancy.

Hydramnios

Hydramnios occurs in 2% to 5% of twin gestations, and twin pregnancies account for approximately 8% to 10% of all cases of hydramnios. Acute hydramnios may accompany these pregnancies, particularly if there is a twin-to-twin transfusion with subsequent growth discordance. Medical management of these cases of hydramnios may be successful with drugs such as indomethacin (Indocin), 100 to 150 mg per day. In the acute cases, aggressive removal of fluid with multiple amniocenteses may be necessary.

Urinary Tract Infection

Women with multiple gestations have a 1.4-fold increased risk of developing urinary tract infection during pregnancy.

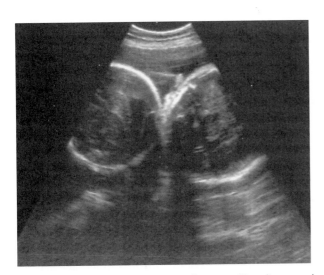

FIG. 3. Twin pregnancies can be diagnosed by ultrasound.

TABLE 1. *Maternal complications with twin pregnancies*

Problems	Increased likelihood over singleton pregnancy
Preterm labor	7–10
Hypertension	2–5
Abruption	3
Anemia	2–3
Hydramnios	3–5
Urinary tract infection	1.4
Postpartum hemorrhage	2–4
Cesarean section	2–3

This is usually a lower tract infection, because the incidence of pyelonephritis is not significantly increased. Preventive management involves urine cultures performed routinely during the gestation: one at the first prenatal encounter and the second at approximately 32 weeks' gestation. Any time that a woman is symptomatic for a urinary tract infection, an additional urine culture is necessary.

Postpartum Hemorrhage and Other Maternal Complications

Overdistention of the uterus frequently causes it to not contract well in the postpartum period. Approximately 10% of women delivering twins have postpartum uterine atony. Because postpartum bleeding is controlled by uterine muscle contraction, the atony may contribute to postpartum hemorrhage. Approximately 5% of women delivering twins have acute postpartum hemorrhage, which affects the management of the delivery. Blood may be made available before delivery, especially if the patient is anemic, and aggressive use of postpartum oxytocic drugs and uterine massage can be used to minimize bleeding.

Other maternal complications have been suggested but are not routinely found. Placenta previa is occasionally listed as a problem, but in most large series it has not been significantly increased in twin pregnancies. Diabetes is not increased in twin pregnancies. Glucose tolerance tests in women with twins show a lower maternal glucose level than that seen in women with singletons, and no more glucose screening is necessary for twin pregnancies than for singleton pregnancies.

Because of the frequent nonvertex presentation of one or more infants during labor, the use of cesarean section for delivery is increased.

Infant Complications

Ten infant complications occur in twin pregnancies (Table 2), and they all increase the risk of perinatal mortality.

Prematurity

Because the average time to delivery of twin gestations is 37 weeks, the frequency of preterm delivery is 50%. This is a

TABLE 2. *Infant complications with twin pregnancies*

Prematurity
Congenital anomaly
Discordance
Vanishing twin
Monoamniotic cord entanglement
Dead fetus syndrome
Locking twins
Combined pregnancy
Mole and fetus
Delayed delivery of second infant

major contributor to neonatal morbidity and mortality. Most animal species have a maturation of their pulmonary function at approximately 85% of their average gestational age. Singleton infants have mature lungs at approximately 34 to 35 weeks' gestation, but twins reach this stage at 31 to 32 weeks' gestation. As a consequence, small infants weighing less than 2500 g from a twin pregnancy fare better in the nursery and have lower mortality rates than comparable-weight infants from singleton pregnancies. Fetal growth slows earlier in twins than in singletons, so the diagnosis of growth retardation by ultrasound cannot accurately be made using singleton growth curves.

Congenital Anomalies

The frequency of congenital anomalies is increased two to three times in twins, and this increase is mostly confined to monozygotic infants who share the same karyotype. Because the anomalies are often accompanied by a two-vessel umbilical cord, they can be screened for during the antepartum period with routine ultrasound examinations.

Discordance

Discordance is defined as a significant difference in the weight of the two infants, variously set at more than 20% or 25% by different investigators, and the condition occurs in about 10% of twin pregnancies. Two major contributors are known for discordance. The first is a significant difference in placental surface area for the two infants. The infant with the smaller placenta experiences growth retardation and near the end of gestation has a high likelihood of demonstrating placental insufficiency. The second, more common cause for discordance is twin-to-twin transfusion. In about 85% of monochorionic placentas, there is an anastomosis of the vessels between the two fetuses, but severe blood shunting occurs in less than 5% of cases. The risk for the twin-to-twin transfusion problem occurs with monochorionic placentas, especially if there is a velamentous cord insertion. With the shunting of blood, one infant is a donor, and the other is a recipient. The donor infant is small, pale, and anemic, may have an accompanying oligohydramnios, and can have heart failure as a neonate. The recipient infant is be large, plethoric, and polycythemic, has polyhydramnios, and can develop heart failure and hyperbilirubinemia as a neonate. The recipient twin has more vascular coils in its umbilical cord, which may assist in pumping blood from the placenta. Both infants are at significant risk from this problem, and it represents an extremely high-risk perinatal event.

The diagnosis at birth can be confirmed by a discrepancy between cord blood hemoglobin levels of greater than 5 g/dl. During the antepartum period, when discordance of growth is suspected, ultrasound examinations can be performed. A difference in biparietal diameter of more than 5 mm or a difference of estimated fetal weight by ultrasound examination of more than 25% suggests discordance. Confirmation is suggested if Doppler studies of umbilical artery flow show large differences. Twin-to-twin transfusions can be excluded if a diagnosis of dichorionic placenta is made. This can be determined using ultrasound and the rule of two (Scardo et al., 1995): finding two infants of different sexes, two separate placentas, or a central membrane more than 2-mm thick. Each of these methods has been used in the antepartum diagnosis to judge the potential risk. Early-pregnancy ultrasound scans at the placenta–membrane junction can show a "twin peak" or lambda sign with dichorionic placentas.

If acute polyhydramnios occurs with twin-to-twin transfusion, the prognosis for fetal survival is poor, but the best management approach for this problem is aggressive mechanical reduction of the hydramnios by repeated amniocenteses.

Vanishing Twin

The vanishing twin syndrome refers to seeing twins on an early ultrasound examination but delivering only a singleton infant. With routine ultrasound studies in early pregnancy, it appears that the twin pregnancy frequency is close to 2%. Because only 1% of deliveries are twins, approximately one-half of all twin pregnancies vanish. Most of the early gestations that are lost show a gestational sac without a fetal pole on ultrasound scans. An episode of early-pregnancy vaginal bleeding usually accompanies the pregnancy loss. Serial studies of hCG levels show that they are lower in vanishing twin gestations than in normal twin pregnancies. After delivery of the surviving infant, the placenta frequently shows a whitish plaque on the membranes, which is the remnant of the other gestational sac. No harm is apparent for the mother or the surviving infant.

Monoamniotic Twin Pregnancy

If the monozygotic conceptus divides between days 8 and 13 of gestation, no central membrane is formed. This occurs in 2% of twin pregnancies. The risk in these pregnancies is cord entanglement with fetal movement, which can lead to obstruction of blood flow and fetal death (Fig. 4). Most fetuses that die are less than 32 weeks' gestation. The diagnosis can be suspected by being unable to find a central membrane on the ultrasound scan. The scan in Figure 5 shows a central membrane, ruling out this problem. The suspected diagnosis could be confirmed with an amniogram. After a gestation has passed 32 weeks, the risks for the infant is minimal, because its movement is limited and further entanglement is unlikely, so management can be expectant. Before that time, drugs such as sulindac (Clinoril) may help by reducing amniotic fluid and the chance of fetal turning.

Dead Fetus Syndrome

Approximately 2% to 7% of twin pregnancies result in the death of one of the fetuses during the second half of gestation. If this occurs, it is extremely unlikely that maternal problems will result, because rarely has significant hypofibrinogenemia been documented. Maternal fibrinogen levels decrease, but they usually plateau at about 150 mg/dl. Although some investigators have given mothers heparin as prophylaxis, others have achieved equally good results with no treatment.

There is a potential problem for the surviving infant. If the placenta is a dichorionic type, no vascular anastomosis exists, and the surviving fetus should fare well. However, with a monochorionic placenta, there is a high likelihood of vascular communication between the two twins. As soon as the first twin dies, there are vascular products that flow into the live twin. These may produce acute disseminated intravascular coagulation with multiple organ damage, particularly in the renal and central nervous system areas. Renal cortical cysts and multiple cystic lesions in the brain, known as multicystic encephalomalacia, are common. Approximately 25% of these infants die *in utero*, and as many as 50% of survivors

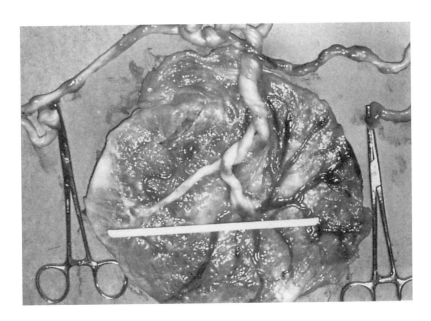

FIG. 4. In monozygotic monoamniotic twins with no central membrane, cord entanglement can occur with fetal movement, leading to obstruction of blood flow and possible death of the fetuses.

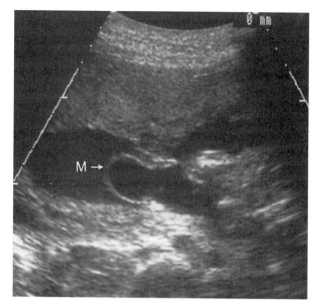

FIG. 5. Abdominal ultrasound shows a central membrane in this monozygotic twin gestation.

have brain damage. Because the process is rapid, management should be immediate delivery if the surviving infant has reached a viable gestational age, although even with rapid delivery some survivors are damaged.

Locking Twins

If twins are delivered vaginally and the first infant is breech with the second infant vertex, the two twins' heads can be interlocked with a chin-to-chin approximation. This is an infrequent complication with an incidence of about 1 in 90,000 pregnancies. It can be managed by turning the heads. It has been suggested that the infants can be placed back into the uterus, followed by a cesarean section delivery, although few cases have been reported.

Combined Pregnancy

The problem of a combined pregnancy occurs in approximately 1 in every 30,000 pregnancies. One conceptus is in the uterus, and the other is in an ectopic position. Operative management of the ectopic pregnancy is needed early in pregnancy.

Mole and Fetus

Rarely, a twin pregnancy may have one placenta developing into a hydatidiform mole and the other conceptus developing as a normal fetus and placenta. Ultrasound studies can diagnosis this type of problem.

Delayed Delivery

Long intervals between infant deliveries have been reported for some pregnancies. This is important to remember if the first de-

livery occurs at a previable time. Delays of 21 to 143 days have been reported, and such a delay could be long enough for the second twin to reach a viable stage of maturation.

Management

Antepartum Period

During the antepartum period, the emphasis should be on the prevention of recognized potential problems. The major problem of preterm labor can often be predicted by regular vaginal examinations using the cervical score. The cervical score represents the centimeters of thickness of the cervix (i.e., effacement) minus the centimeters of dilation. Little risk exists of premature delivery in the next 7 to 14 days, until the cervical score is more than 0.

Most controlled studies on the use of bed rest during the pregnancy to prevent preterm labor in a twin gestation found no significant effect. However, many of these were started late in the pregnancy, when rest was begun at 32 to 34 weeks' gestation. A few studies suggested some benefit in terms of lengthening gestation and increasing the weight of infants if the bed rest was introduced from week 24 of gestation and maintained through week 34 of gestation. Although hospital bed rest does not seem justified in terms of the cost, the use of home rest during this period does seem reasonable. It adds little cost to the pregnancy management, other than the loss of the mother's income. The patient could have some limited activities, such as bathroom privileges and sit-up eating, which improves compliance. Prophylactic tocolytics have been of no proven value in twin pregnancies. Although home uterine monitoring to detect uterine activity has proven unsuccessful in singleton pregnancies, the approach may be helpful in twin gestations.

If premature labor begins, the patient needs hospitalization with acute parenteral tocolytic management (see Chapter 16). β-mimetic tocolytics have a higher risk for pulmonary edema complications in twin than in singleton gestations, particularly if prolonged for more than 24 hours. If there is a question about maturation of the fetus, pulmonary maturation can be assessed with amniotic fluid studies such as the lecithin–sphingomyelin ratio. The results are identical in the two twins if they are not discordant. If discordance exists, both sacs need to be tapped. Use of a glucocorticoid such as betamethasone (Celestone) to accelerate fetal lung maturation has not shown success in twin pregnancies.

Another problem that can be prevented is maternal anemia. Because women carrying twins require higher concentrations of folic acid and iron, they need daily supplements of 1 mg of folic acid and 60 mg of elemental iron. There is no evidence that other prenatal vitamins are of any help.

Because twin discordance results from twin-to-twin transfusions, establishing the type of placentation early in pregnancy is important. If a dichorionic placenta is established by the ultrasound rule of two, surveillance for this problem is not necessary. If there is a monochorionic placentation, serial ultrasound assessments for discordance are needed.

Prenatal genetic testing is important because of the increased frequency of congenital anomalies among twins. It appears that the risk for chromosomal abnormalities is higher in twin gestations, and genetic analysis by means of amniocentesis or chorionic villus sampling should be recommended for a twin gestation if the mother is 31 years of age, compared with 35 years of age for a singleton. Maternal serum AFP levels are elevated in twin gestations, and the median level for twins at 16 weeks' gestation is 2.5 times the multiple of the median, compared with 2 times for singletons. If genetic analysis using amniocentesis is required, both sacs should be tapped. Using a glucometer and glucose as a marker, the examiner can identify quickly that independent sacs have been tapped. Use of colored dye as a marker should be avoided; methylene blue, for example, has been implicated in causing fetal hematolytic anemia and jejunal atresia.

If hypertension or other problems that increase the risk for the fetus occur, serial fetal surveillance should be performed. This can be adequately done using fetal heart rate monitoring and doing weekly nonstress tests on each infant. A nonreactive test needs follow-up with a contraction stress test. If preterm labor has already threatened the pregnancy, a biophysical profile could be substituted. Good perinatal mortality data have resulted from such testing. Regular ultrasound examinations should also be done to verify adequate growth rates for each infant. The ultrasound examination should document fetal growth, amniotic fluid volume, the central membrane, and anomalies. Because the average delivery time for twins is 37 weeks' gestation, the physician may assume a twin gestation is in the postdate period after it has reached 39 or more weeks' gestation. Appropriate surveillance testing should be started at that time.

Intrapartum Period

Studies performed during early labor show that approximately one-half of twin infants will be vertex presentations and that the other one-half will be breech or transverse-lie presentations. If both infants are vertex, most obstetricians allow normal labor and delivery of each infant. Before electronic fetal heart rate monitoring began in the 1950s, it was shown that the optimal time for vaginal delivery between the two infants was 5 to 15 minutes. With continuous heart rate monitoring of the second infant after the first is delivered, there appears to be no optimal time for delivery, and no operative intervention is necessary if labor is progressing. If contractions do not occur after the first twin delivers, an oxytocin infusion can be started.

During labor, both fetuses should be monitored with electronic continuous heart rate recordings. Early cord clamping is important after the first delivery because excessive bleeding of the cord could exsanguinate the second twin if a monochorionic placental vascular anastomosis exists. The risk of abruption increases with the delivery of the first infant, and this situation must be monitored carefully. If vaginal delivery is attempted, the delivery room should be set up for a possible emergency cesarean section of the second infant. An ultrasound machine should be available to determine the presentation of the second infant immediately after delivery of the first. Support staff, including an anesthesiologist and neonatologist, should be present. Cord hematocrits should be obtained if same-sex twins are delivered, and these blood samples should be sent to the laboratory immediately because they may disclose a twin-to-twin transfusion problem.

If the first twin presents vertex and the second presents breech, many obstetricians deliver the first infant vaginally and attempt an external version on the second infant to allow it to deliver vaginally with a vertex presentation. Because obstetricians often deliver breeches by cesarean section, many twin presentations in which the second infant is not in a vertex position in early labor undergo elective cesarean section for both. Sometimes, cesarean section is only done for the second twin if it cannot be converted to a vertex presentation or if fetal distress occurs. The overall cesarean section rate for twins is about 75%.

Postpartum Period

Because of the potential risk for uterine atony and postpartum hemorrhage, the mothers should be closely monitored during the first 3 hours after delivery of twins. Adequate oxytocics should be administered, and the uterine fundus should be regularly massaged to be certain that good uterine tone exists. An intravenous access line must be in place, and if the mother began labor with anemia, blood products should be available in case of significant acute hemorrhage. The maternal task of caring for twin infants is often overwhelming. Dialogue with and support for the mother in the early weeks after delivery are important. Postpartum depression is more common in women delivering twins.

◊ TRIPLETS

The spontaneous occurrence of triplets can be predicted by the Hellin rule: If the frequency in a population of twins is n, then that for triplets is n^2. In the 1990s, when assisted reproductive technologies are commonly used and induction of ovulation is frequent, multiple ovulations and pregnancies with two to eight fetuses are not uncommon. Although the spontaneous frequency of triplets is approximately 1 in 10,000 pregnancies, the actual frequency is much higher.

Little is known is about triplet pregnancies because few large series have been described. The usual maternal weight gain is approximately 45 to 50 lb (20.5 to 23 kg). The usual spontaneous time for delivery is 32 to 34 weeks, and the average infant weight is 1800 to 1900 g. Fetal growth is normal in the first two trimesters but begins to slow, compared with singletons, by 27 weeks' gestation. For twins, the slow down occurs at about 30 weeks' gestation.

Discordance among triplets is much more common, with approximately 30% of these pregnancies having a weight discordance of at least 25%. In twin gestation, approximately

10% have that degree of weight discordance. Studies have shown that an early-pregnancy reduction of fetuses from three to two does not increase survival rates, and no such attempt is recommended. The perinatal mortality rate for triplets is similar to that for twins.

The maternal complications and infant complications are similar to those for twins. Most obstetricians deliver triplets by cesarean section because of the likelihood that one or more of the infants will be in a nonvertex presentation.

◊ QUADRUPLETS OR MORE

When a women has four or more infants *in utero,* the overdistention of the uterus leads to much earlier preterm labor. Most of these pregnancies are the result of ovulation induction or *in vitro* fertilization. For quadruplets, the average maternal weight gain is about 50 to 55 lb (23 to 25 kg), and the average time for delivery is 30 to 31 weeks. The average infant weight is approximately 1200 to 1500 g. A reduction in fetal numbers during the first trimester has been successful in bringing the number of infants to two or three and in improving the perinatal survival rate.

Although many quintuplets have been delivered and survived successfully, there is only one case where seven fetuses survived.

◊ RECOMMENDED READINGS

Andrews WW, Leveno KJ, Sherman ML, et al. Elective hospitalization in the management of twin pregnancies. *Obstet Gynecol* 1991;77:826.

Bahado-Singh R, Schmitt R, Hobbins JC. New technique for genetic amniocentesis in twins. *Obstet Gynecol* 1992;79:304.

Brown JE, Schloesser PT. Pregnancy weight status, prenatal weight gain, and the outcome of term twin gestation. *Am J Obstet Gynecol* 1990; 162:182.

Carlson NJ, Towers CV. Multiple gestation complicated by the death of one fetus. *Obstet Gynecol* 1989;73:685.

Elster AD, Bleyl JL, Craven TE. Birth weight standards for triplets under modern obstetric care in the United States, 1984–1989. *Obstet Gynecol* 1991;77:387.

Giles WB, Trudinger BJ, Cook CM, et al. Umbilical artery flow velocity wave forms and twin pregnancy outcome. *Obstet Gynecol* 1988;72:894.

Guttmacher AF. Clinical aspects of twin pregnancy. *Med Clinic No Am* 1939;23:427.

Johnson JM, Harman CR, Evans JA, et al. Maternal serum α-fetoprotein in twin pregnancy. *Am J Obstet Gynecol* 1990;162:1020.

Kohl SG, Casey G. Twin gestation. *Mt Sinai J Med* 1975;42:523.

Lambalk CB, Boomsma DI, De Boer L, et al. Increased levels and pulsatility of follicle-stimulating hormone in mothers of hereditary dizygotic twins. *J Clin Endocrinol Metab* 1998;83:481.

MacGillivray I, Nylander PPS, Corney G. *Human multiple reproduction.* Philadelphia: WB Saunders, 1975.

Meyers C, Adam R, Dungan J, Prenger V. Aneuploidy in twin gestations: when is maternal age advanced? *Obstet Gynecol* 1997;89:248.

Newman RB, Godsey RK, Ellings JM, et al. Quantification of cervical change: relationship to preterm delivery in the multifetal gestation. *Am J Obstet Gynecol* 1991;165:264.

Peek MJ, McCarthy A, Kyle P, et al. Medical amnioreduction with sulindac to reduce cord complications in monoamniotic twins. *Am J Obstet Gynecol* 1997;176:334.

Porreco RP, Burke S, Hendrix ML. Multifetal reduction of triplets and pregnancy outcome. *Obstet Gynecol* 1991;78:335.

Potter EL, Fuller H. Multiple pregnancies at the Chicago Lying-in Hospital, 1941–1947. *Am J Obstet Gynecol* 1949;58:139.

Saunders NJ, Snijders RJM, Nicolaides KH. Therapeutic amniocentesis in twin-twin transfusion syndrome appearing in the second trimester of pregnancy. *Am J Obstet Gynecol* 1992;166:820.

Scardo JA, Ellings JM, Newman RB. Prospective determination of chorionicity, amnionicity, and zygosity in twin gestations. *Am J Obstet Gynecol* 1995;173:1376.

Spellacy WN. Antepartum complications in twin pregnancies. *Clin Perinatol* 1988;15:79.

Spellacy WN, Buhi WC, Birk SA. Carbohydrate metabolism in women with a twin pregnancy. *Obstet Gynecol* 1980;55:688.

Spellacy WN, Buhi WC, Birk SA. Human placental lactogen levels in multiple pregnancies. *Obstet Gynecol* 1978;52:210.

Spellacy WN, Cruz AC, Buhi WC, et al. Amniotic fluid L/S ratio in twin gestation. *Obstet Gynecol* 1977;50:68.

Spellacy WN, Handler A, Ferre CD. A case-control study of 1253 twin pregnancies from a 1982–1987 perinatal data base. *Obstet Gynecol* 1990; 75:168.

Spellacy WN, Kalra PS, Buggie J, et al. Gonadotropin responses to graded GNRF injections in women with prior twin pregnancies. *J Reprod Med* 1982;27:435.

Strong TH Jr. The umbilical pump: a contributor to twin-twin transfusion. *Obstet Gynecol* 1997;89:812.

Tchabo JG, Tomai T. Selected intrapartum external cephalic version of the second twin. *Obstet Gynecol* 1992;79:421.

Tessen JA, Zlatnik F. Monoamniotic twins: a retrospective controlled study. *Obstet Gynecol* 1991;77:832.

Wittmann BK, Farquharson D, Wong GP, et al. Delayed delivery of second twin: report of four cases and review of the literature. *Obstet Gynecol* 1992;79:260.

CHAPTER 21

Diabetes Mellitus and Pregnancy

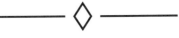

William N. Spellacy

Reproduction in women with diabetes mellitus before the discovery of insulin was almost nonexistent. This was because most women died before puberty or were so hyperglycemic after that time that they had amenorrhea and were infertile. When a pregnancy occasionally did occur, it usually ended as a disaster, with the mother or infant, or both, dying. In 1921, Banting and Best discovered insulin, and it soon became available as a therapy for the disease. Since then, a great deal has been learned about diabetes mellitus as a complication of pregnancy, and, by using that information, women with diabetes mellitus can now expect normal pregnancy outcomes.

◊ CARBOHYDRATE METABOLISM DURING NORMAL PREGNANCY

Blood glucose levels change in women when they become pregnant. The major alteration is a lowering of fasting levels; in addition, there is a prolonged rise in glucose values after a meal or oral glucose challenge. The lowered fasting levels are thought to occur because there is a constant drain of glucose into the uterus. Glucose is transported across the placenta easily by facilitated diffusion, where the fetus uses it as its major fuel. The prolonged elevation of the glucose tolerance curve is thought to be caused by delayed emptying of the gastrointestinal tract as a result of smooth muscle relaxation. The overall profile shows that blood glucose levels fall to their lowest point at 20 weeks of gestation and that glycosylated hemoglobin (HgbA$_{1c}$) falls to its lowest point at 24 weeks.

Another major change is that the beta cells of the maternal pancreas hypertrophy and secrete two to three times as much insulin late in pregnancy compared with the nonpregnant state. This change begins at the end of the first trimester and peaks near term. Insulin does not cross the placenta. The major alterations in insulin levels compared with the minor alterations in glucose levels demonstrate that pregnancy is a condition of insulin resistance. This finding can be confirmed by performing insulin tolerance tests during pregnancy, which show that a dose of insulin injected into a term pregnant woman produces only a slight decrease in glucose compared with the same per-kilogram dose injected before or after pregnancy. The physiological insulin resistance of pregnancy is caused by a complex of metabolic functions carried on by the placenta, including its production of progesterone and estrogens, its alteration of cortisol dynamics, its degradation of insulin with insulinase, and its production of prolactin, placental lactogen, and growth hormone. These changes do little to the tissue insulin receptors, and thus, the resistance is mainly a postreceptor phenomenon. The altered carbohydrate metabolism changes back quickly after the placenta is delivered.

◊ SCREENING FOR DIABETES DURING PREGNANCY

The insulin resistance caused by pregnancy places a stress on the beta cells, making this an ideal time to detect subtle abnormalities in their capacity to secrete insulin. Some women have normal test results during early pregnancy, but because of a limited ability to produce insulin, they become insulin-deficient late in pregnancy and, as a result, have hyperglycemia until delivery. This condition is termed gestational diabetes. Immediately postpartum, the test results of these women can return to normal, but as the women are followed for long periods postpartum, a significant number eventually develop overt diabetes. In one study, O'Sullivan noted this development in 60% of women studied for 16 years postpartum. The more severe her diabetes during pregnancy, the more likely she will have diabetes by 5 years postpartum.

Women who are at high risk for having diabetes (e.g., their parents or siblings have it, or they demonstrate glucosuria) should be screened when they are first seen. All women, regardless of risk, should be screened at the end of the second trimester (i.e., 26 weeks). If new data develop, such as late-pregnancy macrosomia or glucosuria, they should be screened again. The screening test is to administer a 50-g oral glucose load and obtain a plasma glucose value 1 hour later. The dividing point is 140 mg/dl; values less than that are normal. If the value is over 140 mg/dl, the woman needs an oral glucose tolerance test (OGTT). If the screen is over 200 mg/dl, she probably does not need an OGTT and should be next followed with a fasting glucose test. If the result of that test is significantly elevated (>140 mg/dl), the diagnosis of diabetes can be made. Although the screen has fewer false-positive results if it is performed in a fasting state, that often is not practical.

The OGTT should be started in the morning after 3 days of a good diet, including 250 g of carbohydrates per day. The woman should fast for at least 10 hours before the test. During the test, she should remain inactive. Urine tests for glucose should not be done because they are almost always positive and because no one makes the diagnosis of diabetes in pregnancy by the presence of glucosuria. After a fasting blood sample is drawn, the woman should drink a solution containing 100 g of glucose. Repeat blood samples for glucose values should be obtained at 1, 2, and 3 hours. The upper limits for these values are shown in Table 1. If all values are below these limits, the test is normal, and no further testing needs to be done unless something changes, such as, the woman develops glucosuria. If two or more values are elevated, the woman has gestational diabetes. If only one value is elevated, she is borderline abnormal and should have a repeat OGTT done in about 1 month. Because of the progressively increasing insulin resistance of pregnancy, some of these borderline tests will become frankly abnormal. If the OGTT cannot be done on a woman, for example, because the glucose load makes her nauseated, then an intravenous glucose tolerance test using a 25-g glucose load (i.e., 50 ml of 50% glucose) can be substituted.

◊ GESTATIONAL DIABETES

Gestational diabetes is the most common type of diabetes complicating pregnancy, and it is only a medium-risk complication. Many of these women are obese. The woman with gestational diabetes has a normal OGTT when she is not pregnant, so her disease usually is mild. The perinatal risks of this condition are low, especially if the woman is young (i.e., younger than 25 years of age). The major risk for the fetus is the development of macrosomia (the two definitions being greater than 4000 or 4500 g). Most of these women can be managed with diet treatment alone, unless their fasting glucose values are elevated. The diet should be about 35 calories per kilogram ideal weight (i.e., about 300 calories more than her stable-weight nonpregnant diet). If the glucose levels cannot be normalized with this treatment, then insulin needs to be added. Several studies have shown that the routine use of prophylactic insulin decreases the frequency of macrosomia but does not eliminate it. The pregnancy usually can be allowed to go to term but seldom beyond. Monitoring can be done with fasting and 1-hour glucose values every 2 to 3 weeks. A HgbA$_{1c}$ level once per month is helpful. Nonstress tests may be done once per week beginning at about week 39. Amniocentesis seldom is needed. Ultrasound studies may be useful if there is concern about macrosomia, hydramnios, or anomalies. Vaginal delivery usually can be expected. The major risk is that the mother will later develop diabetes, and she should be tested periodically for this. Another risk for the mother is polycystic ovarian disease (PCO).

◊ INSULIN-DEPENDENT DIABETES

Many serious problems affect women who have insulin-dependent diabetes complicating their pregnancies. Because diabetes also affects the vascular system and the extent of this effect relates most closely to the duration of the disease, the duration of the disease also relates to the pregnancy outcome. In the past, this concept was used by White in setting up her classification of diabetes in pregnancy (i.e., White's classes A through F) to predict outcomes. Thus, class A patients have gestational diabetes; class B patients have had their disease for less than 10 years; class C patients have had their disease for 10 to 20 years; and class D patients have had their disease for more than 20 years. With modern management, the predictive values of White's classification are less precise, but the system is still important in providing the health-care team with an estimate of the degree of difficulty that can be expected, especially with vascular complications.

Maternal Problems

The following are the most common problems a woman experiences when diabetes mellitus complicates pregnancy:

◊ Hypoglycemia,
◊ Hyperglycemia,
◊ Urinary tract and other infections,
◊ Hypertension,
◊ Hydramnios,
◊ Retinopathy.

TABLE 1. Pregnancy oral glucose tolerance test using a 100-g load

Sample	Upper limits for normal glucose levels (mg/dL)			
	Fasting	1 h	2 h	3 h
Blood	90	165	145	125
Plasma	105	190	165	145

Hypoglycemia

Maternal hypoglycemia usually occurs during the first half of pregnancy. There is a slightly increased sensitivity to insulin in the early weeks of gestation, but this usually is not enough to explain the problem. More commonly, the woman enters the gestation controlled on a fixed insulin injection and a fixed caloric intake. When human chorionic gonadotropin levels rise, she develops anorexia, nausea, and sometimes even vomiting. The caloric intake then decreases, and if she keeps her insulin injections constant, she is prone to develop hypoglycemia. There is little evidence that this harms the pregnancy. It must be dealt with by decreasing the insulin dose to fit the caloric load and, if needed, by using antiemetics.

Hyperglycemia

Maternal hyperglycemia tends to occur during the second half of pregnancy. The insulin resistance of pregnancy makes the injected insulin less effective at that time, and as a result, the woman develops hyperglycemia unless she increases her daily insulin dose. Most—if not all—of the infant problems are caused by excess glucose exposure *in utero,* so this is a serious problem. As the insulin resistance develops, the blood glucose level must be evaluated frequently so that the insulin dose can be increased appropriately to maintain euglycemia. The major increase in needed insulin typically occurs between weeks 20 and 30 of gestation. A decreased need for insulin late in pregnancy can also occur, but it is an ominous sign because it usually means that the placenta is failing to function and that the insulin resistance is disappearing. Placental insufficiency in terms of oxygen transport may also be occurring. After delivery of the placenta, there is a sharp decrease in the need for insulin, and the usual dose on day 1 postpartum is only one-half of that at term.

Urinary Tract and Other Infections

Estrogen dilates blood vessels, and in the kidney, this causes increased renal blood flow and glomerular filtration during pregnancy. As a result, the filtration of glucose also increases. This glomerular glucose load exceeds the proximal and distal tubules' ability to extract it, so all normal pregnant women have glucosuria of up to 300 mg/day. Women with elevated blood glucose levels have even more glucose in their urine. The most common mechanism for bacteria to enter a woman's urinary tract is during sex, when the colonized urethral organisms, usually *E. coli* from the stool, are massaged into the bladder. The relaxation of the urinary tract muscle during pregnancy causes ureteral reflux and dilation of the collection tract. The glucose substrate for bacterial growth plus urine retention put these women at high risk for infection. This situation is present in about 20% of pregnant women with diabetes. Urine cultures should be obtained at the first visit and again at 32 weeks of gestation, as well as if symptoms of infection develop. The presence of a single type of organism at concentrations of 10,000/mL or higher must be treated. Treatment of asymptomatic bacteriuria can reduce the development of pyelonephritis from 25% to 2.5%.

Other infections (e.g., wound infections after cesarean section) are also more common in diabetics because of the patients' high tissue glucose levels. All women with diabetes who have a cesarean section require prophylactic antibiotic treatment.

Hypertension

The abnormal blood vessels of pregnant women with diabetes can lead to the development of hypertension in the later weeks of gestation. This condition is found in about 20% of such women. Increasing duration of disease increases the risk for hypertension.

One theory for this condition is that the woman's abnormal endothelium cannot produce enough prostacyclin to antagonize the elevated angiotensin II vasopressor levels. The blood pressure must be closely monitored in the latter one-third of gestation; if it becomes abnormal, bed rest should be the first line of therapy. Antihypertensive drugs such as α-methyldopa (Aldomet) may be needed if the fetus is still immature.

Hydramnios

Excess amounts of amniotic fluid (i.e., >2000 ml) can occur with diabetes, especially if glucose is poorly controlled. The frequency of this condition has been reported to be between 10% and 20%. One theory is that maternal hyperglycemia produces fetal hyperglycemia and fetal glucosuria. The increased amniotic fluid glucose that results is osmotically active and brings in the excess water. It also produces polyuria for the fetus. Another problem that must be considered is that a fetal anomaly that interferes with swallowing, such as anencephaly or a gastrointestinal obstruction, exists. Ultrasound is helpful in making these diagnoses.

Retinopathy

The severity of diabetic retinopathy mainly depends on the duration of disease and the extent of vessel involvement. During pregnancy, about 15% of women experience some exacerbation. The serious problem is with proliferative retinopathy. These new vessels are stimulated by several growth factors, which are increased in pregnancy. In these cases, there is about an 85% chance of exacerbation during the gestation, and some progress to the point of blindness. If these proliferative lesions are treated with laser coagulation, they can be controlled. The lesions are no longer a medical reason for pregnancy termination. The pregnant woman with diabetes should have an ophthalmologic consultation in each trimester and, if needed, laser therapy.

Infant Problems

Infants of diabetic mothers (IDMs) face a number of problems, including the following:

◊ Spontaneous abortion,
◊ Congenital anomalies,
◊ Respiratory distress,
◊ Hypoglycemia,
◊ Macrosomia,
◊ Hypocalcemia,
◊ Hyperbilirubinemia,
◊ Perinatal mortality.

Abortion

The overall frequency of spontaneous abortion is not increased in diabetic pregnancies if glucose control is good. However, with poor control in the first trimester, there is an increased frequency of abortion. Thus, hyperglycemia in the first half of pregnancy increases the spontaneous abortion rate.

Congenital Anomalies

Most large clinical studies have reported a threefold increase in anomalies for the IDM. The anomalies can be in any system, but the cardiovascular and nervous systems are most frequently affected. One that is infrequent yet unique is sacral agenesis. The mothers of all infants with this anomaly should be tested for diabetes. Large studies of anomalous IDMs have suggested that the time in gestation when the insult occurs is restricted to weeks 3 to 6. Miller and associates measured the $HgbA_{1c}$ levels in women with diabetes at the end of their first trimester and found that only pregnancies with elevated $HgbA_{1c}$ levels had an increased frequency of anomalies. These findings suggested that hyperglycemia early in pregnancy (i.e., weeks 3 to 6 of gestation) produced the anomalies and that the test could also be used for genetic counseling. In addition, it suggested that good glucose control early in pregnancy could help to prevent anomalies for IDMs. Other studies supported this finding. More recent animal studies suggest that the altered substrate results in an excess of free oxygen radicals in the fetus, causing anomalies. The use of scavenger enzymes or antioxidants prevented these anomalies. Prospective studies have shown that preconception glucose control significantly lowers IDM anomaly rates. If the woman comes for preconception counseling, another helpful point is to teach her to document ovulation. This can be done with simple tests such as daily basal body temperature recordings. Such records firmly date the gestation.

Respiratory Distress

The frequency of respiratory distress for the IDM is increased sixfold for all gestational ages of birth. Many factors are involved in neonatal breathing, and it relates to more than the lung type II pneumocytes' production of surfactant. Animal data suggest that fetal hyperinsulinemia, which accompanies hyperglycemia, can interfere with the ability of cortisol to accelerate surfactant production. An inverse relationship exists between maternal glucose levels and amniotic fluid lecithin–sphingomyelin (L/S) ratios.

Neonatal Hypoglycemia

Neonatal hypoglycemia is common in the IDM in the first hours of life. When a fetus is exposed to high glucose levels coming across the placenta from a hyperglycemic mother, it reacts by producing large amounts of insulin in an attempt to reduce the glucose. Despite the high blood insulin levels, there is little down-regulation of insulin receptors; thus, these infants are at high risk for developing hypoglycemia. As soon as the umbilical cord is clamped at delivery, the source of blood glucose is greatly reduced, but if the pancreas is still producing the excess insulin, hypoglycemia results. Good maternal glucose control can prevent the problem. The blood glucose levels of the IDM must be frequently monitored, and the concentration should stay above 40 mg/dl. If hypoglycemia occurs, oral or parenteral glucose treatment must be started to maintain an adequate blood glucose concentration, which is an important fuel for the neonate's central nervous system. Prolonged and severe neonatal hypoglycemia can cause permanent brain damage. The IDM gradually reduces its insulin output, and normal glucose levels result.

Macrosomia

The hyperglycemic fetus releases large amounts of insulin, uses the glucose for energy to grow, and deposits calorie stores in glycogen and fat sites. Such an infant becomes macrosomic. Macrosomia has been defined in two ways: as infants weighing more than 4000 g and as infants weighing more than 4500 g. This high birthweight causes several problems. First, birth trauma, especially shoulder dystocia, can occur when a large infant is delivered vaginally. Brachial plexus injuries are common in these cases but are usually transient. Macrosomic IDMs have larger shoulder diameters, and the incidence of dystocia in these infants is twice as high as that in equal-weight infants from mothers who do not have diabetes. This complication can be avoided by closely controlling maternal glucose prenatally and can be predicted by ultrasound assessments of fetal size before vaginal delivery. Ultrasound assessments of fetal weight have an error rate of about 10%. If macrosomia of >4500 g is confirmed, cesarean delivery should be considered. If vaginal delivery is attempted, the obstetrician must be certain that the bony pelvis is adequate and must be prepared to carry out the appropriate maneuvers to release an impacted shoulder. Fat neonates tend to develop into obese adults with all the associated health risks. Avoidance of macrosomia is, therefore, important.

Hypocalcemia

The IDM often shows some signs of irritability and even tetany that may be related to low blood calcium levels. No clear explanation exists as to why this problem is more frequent in these neonates. If hypocalcemia is present, it can be quickly reversed with exogenous calcium therapy.

Hyperbilirubinemia

Neonatal jaundice is more common in the IDM than in the normal infant. It probably results from a higher hematocrit developed *in utero,* especially if oxygen availability is decreased. The jaundice usually is mild and can be treated with hydration and ultraviolet lamp exposure.

Perinatal Mortality

The fetus may experience sudden death, especially if severe hyperglycemia occurs. Of the fetuses whose mothers develop ketoacidosis, about 50% die. The exact mechanism involved is not known, but acute oxygen deprivation caused by glucose binding to hemoglobin or sudden shifts in water and electrolytes with glucose movements have been suspected. All fetal well-being studies lose their validity if maternal hyperglycemia occurs.

Management

The key factors involved in the successful management of these high-risk pregnancies are good glucose control, monitoring, and early delivery.

Glucose Control

The blood glucose levels of a woman who is not diabetic are lower during pregnancy. The same levels should be obtained for the woman who is diabetic. The purpose of this goal is not to improve the course of the mother's pregnancy but to reduce the likelihood of the fetus developing complications. Control is obtained by monitoring the mother's diet, insulin dose, and glucose levels.

Diet

Glucose control requires that the woman consume the same caloric load every day at the same times. This is an important contribution of the mother to her care. She should be instructed on this at her first prenatal visit. If she is already on a diet that maintains her at a stable weight, she needs only to increase this by about 300 calories per day. If she is not on a special diet, one should be started, using about 35 calories per kilogram of ideal weight per day and including 1.3 g of protein and 250 g of carbohydrates.

Insulin Dose

The woman must use enough insulin to keep her blood glucose level normal. Because insulin has a molecular weight of 6000, it does not cross to the fetus. The dose used is unimportant as long as it is enough. The beginning dose is higher in late pregnancy; therefore, the physician can start with 0.5 units/kg in the first half of gestation and go to 0.7 units/kg in the second half. Some obese patients need large amounts of insulin per day. In general, insulin needs increase twofold to threefold during the 20- to 30-week period. Split injections maybe necessary, and the total dose usually can be given as follows: two-thirds in the morning (as two-thirds long-acting and one-third short-acting) and one-third in the evening (as one-half long-acting and one-half short-acting). When the insulin requirements are increasing, it is good to consider a total theoretical dose at 15 to 20 units/day higher, to calculate the ideal distribution of long- and short-acting morning and evening insulin and then to increase slowly toward this ideal. The insulin should be injected 30 minutes before meals. Although portable insulin pumps are now being used by many people with diabetes, they have not proved to be superior to multidose insulin therapy during ambulatory care in pregnancy. When the woman is hospitalized, for example, at the time of delivery, it often is easier to control glucose with an intravenous insulin infusion. Most women with diabetes are well controlled if they receive 1 unit of insulin per hour and 125 ml of 5% dextrose per hour. Slight adjustment of the glucose or insulin infusion rate may be necessary.

Oral hypoglycemic agents should not be used during pregnancy for several reasons. First, a significant number of users break away from their control and develop severe hyperglycemia during pregnancy; this is a serious risk for the fetus. Second, prolonged neonatal hypoglycemia has been associated with their use. Finally, it has been suggested that they might increase fetal anomaly rates, although these data are not firm.

Glucose Levels

To be certain that the fetus is exposed to normal glucose levels, maternal glucose profiles must be monitored. Several parameters should be studied.

Home Blood Glucose Monitoring. Maternal blood glucose values are the best index of control, and reliable data can be obtained by the patient using a home glucose monitoring unit. The woman should be taught to measure and record glucose levels and to bring the results to each visit. Important daily determinations should include fasting, a pre–major meal, peak levels 1 hour after a major meal, and at bedtime. After a major meal, the blood glucose level rises 40 to 50 mg/dl. The fasting values should be 70 to 80 mg/dl, and the peak 1 hour after meals should be less than 140 mg/dl. If values over 160 are obtained, the woman should call the physician immediately. Because home glucose monitoring uses blood rather than plasma, the values are lower by about 15%.

Twenty-Four-Hour Urine Glucose. The amounts of total glucose spilled per day give a good index of the blood glucose profile. A normal pregnant woman excretes 300 mg/day, whereas a pregnant woman with diabetes who is poorly controlled may excrete more than 30 g/day. The patient should collect a 24-hour urine specimen the day of each physician visit and bring this with her. It can be dipped for glucose content in the office and be used as a check on the home blood glucose values. With good control, urine values are trace to 1+. If, however, urine values are running 3+ to 4+ glucose, then hyperglycemia is occurring, and the accuracy or timing of the patient's blood glucose sampling needs to be verified. If the values are accurate, then other time points need to be evaluated, such as the middle of the night. The urine can be discarded, and there is no increased cost to the patient.

Office Visits. When the patient comes for prenatal care, fasting and 1-hour-past-meal glucose levels should be determined.

Hemoglobin A_{1c}. If blood glucose concentrations rise above normal, the glucose covalently couples to proteins. On hemoglobin, glucose binds to valine on the β chain. The glucose remains there for the life of the red blood cell. The glucose-labeled protein is detectable by its altered electrophoretic mobility. Depending on the half-life of the protein, that glycosylated product tells about the blood glucose profiles in the past. Glycosylated albumin describes the glucose profiles for the past 1 to 2 weeks, and glycosylated hemoglobin ($HgbA_{1c}$) tells about the prior 4 to 5 weeks. It is useful to determine $HgbA_{1c}$ levels each month during the pregnancy as another index of glucose control. Because hemoglobin F has a similar electrophoretic mobility, it may interfere with some assays. The $HgbA_{1c}$ levels typically decrease about 1% during pregnancy and reach their low point at 24 weeks of gestation.

Amniotic Fluid Glucose. Glucose is transferred to the amniotic fluid during maternal hyperglycemia, and it is slow to move out of that compartment. Thus, amniotic fluid glucose levels reflect the prior 7 days of maternal blood levels. Amniotic fluid glucose levels commonly decrease as pregnancy advances, and in the last month of gestation, they tend to be less than 20 mg/dl. If an amniocentesis is done for some reason, such as for fetal maturity studies, a glucose level should be obtained as well. The amniotic fluid glucose level provides more information about the adequacy of glucose control and also gives the physician information about the infant. Neonates delivered from amniotic fluids with high glucose levels are depressed and have lower Apgar scores.

Fetal Monitoring

The high-risk fetus needs careful serial monitoring during pregnancy. The best monitor is that of glucose control. Other well-being tests also need to be done. Although daily plasma free estriol levels have proved useful, they are expensive, difficult to do, and not widely used. Electronic monitoring of the fetal heart rate is the most widely used test. For this high-

risk condition, the contraction stress test (i.e., oxytocin challenge test) gives the best perinatal survival results. This testing should be started at about 32 weeks of gestation unless maternal hypertension is present, in which case it should be started earlier. The ominous late deceleration is looked for, and most authorities agree that a negative window is three contractions in 10 minutes. Although the nonstress test has also been used, it does not seem to be as sensitive. Performing the nonstress test more often than once per week may improve its sensitivity, but these data have not yet been reported. Few data are available on the nipple stimulation test for women with insulin-dependent diabetes. Clearly, it is not as accurate as the oxytocin challenge test in terms of producing controlled and physiological uterine activity. Data on the use of the biophysical profile with women who are diabetic are also limited. The changes in amniotic fluid volume that are associated with diabetes and the effects of glucose change on fetal breathing, movement, and tone may affect interpretation, but these have not been well studied.

Early Delivery

Fetal Maturity Testing

With good glucose control and fetal monitoring studies, diabetic pregnancies have been carried to later periods of gestation than in the past. Because the condition *in utero* cannot be completely predicted, and because the infant will do well if delivered with mature lungs, delivery usually is accomplished at week 38 of gestation. For this peculiar high-risk condition, fetal lung maturation is better predicted by the amniotic fluid phosphatidylglycerol (PG) content than by the L/S ratio. Indeed, IDMs with respiratory distress can have amniotic fluid evaluations with mature L/S ratios but be deficient in PG. The first ultrasound-guided amniocentesis is, therefore, usually done at 37 to 38 weeks of gestation. When PG is present, delivery is planned.

Delivery

Unless there is an obstetric contraindication, induction of labor and vaginal delivery are the choice. Fetal macrosomia should be ruled out with an ultrasound examination. If the ultrasound estimate of fetal weight is 4500 g or more, elective cesarean section should be considered. During labor, continuous electronic fetal heart rate monitoring should be used, and as soon as it is possible, this should be accomplished with an internal electrode. If oxytocin is administered, it is best to monitor amniotic fluid pressure with a fluid-filled catheter. Low amounts of oxytocin are all that are needed to stimulate good contractions, and infusion rates should not be increased rapidly for fear of producing uterine hyperstimulation and fetal distress. High oxytocin schedules produce more hypertonic contractions, which might not be tolerated by this high-risk fetus. Contraction strength must reach about 200 Montevideo units to achieve good labor. At the time of delivery at the perinatal center, a team should be present to resuscitate and care for the neonate.

◊ POSTPARTUM FAMILY PLANNING

After delivery, the diabetic woman should be counseled about future reproduction. These patients should not delay having additional children because their best reproductive years occur during their youth. Between pregnancies, diabetic women will need some method of contraception that will not have any potential adverse effects on the disease. These women should be informed about barrier contraception including diaphragms and condoms. The intrauterine device is also a good method with minimal adverse effects. Concern was once raised about the risk of infection in a woman with diabetes who uses an intrauterine device, but studies to date have not shown this to be true. If the woman elects to use oral contraceptives, the low-dose combination types with low progestin are best. Her glucose control should be monitored during their early use.

After the woman with diabetes has completed her family, sterilization should be offered because this eliminates the risks and failures of the contraceptive methods.

◊ RECOMMENDED READINGS

Coustan DR, Reece A, Sherwin RS, et al. A randomized clinical trial of the insulin pump vs intensive conventional therapy in diabetic pregnancies. *JAMA* 1986;255:631.

Cruz AC, Buhi WC, Birk SA, Spellacy WN. Respiratory distress syndrome with mature lecithin/sphingomyelin ratios: diabetes mellitus and low Apgar scores. *Am J Obstet Gynecol* 1976;126:78.

Cunningham MD, Desai NS, Thompson SA, Greene JM. Amniotic fluid phosphatidylglycerol in diabetic pregnancies. *Am J Obstet Gynecol* 1978;131:719.

Dibble CM, Kochenour NK, Worley RJ, et al. Effect of pregnancy on diabetic retinopathy. *Obstet Gynecol* 1982;59:699.

Ecker JL, Greenberg JA, Norwitz ER, et al. Birth weight as a predictor of brachial plexus injury. *Obstet Gynecol* 1997;89:643.

Feig DS, Chen E, Naylor CD. Self-perceived health status of women three to five years after the diagnosis of gestational diabetes: A survey of cases and matched controls. *Am J Obstet Gynecol* 1998;178:386–393.

Freeman RK, Anderson G, Dorchester W. A prospective multi-institutional study of antepartum fetal heart rate monitoring. II. Contraction stress test versus nonstress test for primary surveillance. *Am J Obstet Gynecol* 1982; 143:778.

Hallman M, Kulovich M, Kirkpatrick E, et al. Phosphatidylinositol and phosphatidylglycerol in amniotic fluid: indices of lung maturity. *Am J Obstet Gynecol* 1976;125:613.

Kitzmiller J, Gavin LA, Gin GD, et al. Preconception care of diabetes—glycemic control prevents congenital anomalies. *JAMA* 1991;265:731.

Miller E, Hare JW, Cloherty JP, et al. Elevated maternal hemoglobin A$_{1c}$ in early pregnancy and major congenital anomalies in infants of diabetic mothers. *N Engl J Med* 1981;304:1331.

Mills JL, Baker K, Goldman AS. Malformations in infants of diabetic mothers occur before the seventh gestational week. Implications for treatment. *Diabetes* 1979;28:292.

Ogata ES, Sabbagha R, Metzger B, et al. Serial ultrasonography to assess evolving fetal macrosomia—studies in 23 diabetic women. *JAMA* 1980;243:2405.

O'Sullivan JB, Mahan CM, Charles D, et al. Screening criteria for high-risk gestational diabetic patients. *Am J Obstet Gynecol* 1973;116:895.

Pedersen J. *The pregnant diabetic and her newborn, 2nd ed.* Baltimore: Williams & Wilkins, 1977.

Robert MF, Neff RK, Hubbell JP, et al. Association between maternal diabetes and the respiratory distress syndrome in the newborn. *N Engl J Med* 1976;294:357.

Siman CM, Eriksson UJ. Vitamin E decreases the occurrence of malformations in the offspring of diabetic rats. *Diabetes* 1997;46:1054.

Smith BT, Giroud CJP, Robert M, Avery ME. Insulin antagonism of cortisol action on lecithin synthesis by cultured lung cells. *J Pediatr* 1975;87:953.

Spellacy WN. Family planning and the diabetic mother. *Semin Perinatol* 1978;2:395.

Spellacy WN. Understanding and managing of pregnancy in women with diabetes mellitus. In: Gold JJ, Josimovich JB, eds. *Gynecologic endocrinology, 4th ed.* New York: Plenum Press, 1987;529.

Spellacy WN, Goetz FC. Plasma insulin in normal late pregnancy. *N Engl J Med* 1963;268:988.

Spellacy WN, Buhi WC, Cohn JE, Birk SA. Usefulness of rapid blood glucose measurements in obstetrics: Dextrostix/Reflectance Meter System. *Obstet Gynecol* 1973;41:299.

Spellacy WN, Miller S, Winegar A, Peterson PQ. Macrosomia—maternal characteristics and infant complications. *Obstet Gynecol* 1985;66:158.

Spellacy WN, Buhi WC, Bradley B, et al. Maternal, fetal and amniotic fluid levels of glucose, insulin and growth hormone. *Obstet Gynecol* 1973; 41:323.

Stamler EF, Crus ML, Mimouni F, et al. High infectious morbidity in pregnant women with insulin-dependent diabetes: an understated complication. *Am J Obstet Gynecol* 1990;163:1217.

Tsibris JCM, Raynor LO, Buhi WC, et al. Insulin receptors in circulating erythrocytes and monocytes from women on oral contraceptives or pregnant women near term. *J Clin Endocrinol* 1980;51:711.

White P. Diabetes mellitus in pregnancy. *Clin Perinatol* 1974;1:331.

CHAPTER 22

Hypertensive Disorders of Pregnancy

◇

D. Ware Branch
T. Flint Porter

The condition of marked edema during pregnancy, complicated by seizures in some cases, was recognized by the ancient Greeks. For over a century, the term toxemia was used to describe hypertensive disorders of pregnancy as well as various associated and poorly understood gestational complications. In modern obstetrics, hypertensive disorders of pregnancy are understood to encompass a clinical spectrum of abnormalities ranging from minimal elevations in blood pressure to severe hypertension with multiorgan dysfunction. Collectively, these disorders complicate 5% to 10% of all pregnancies, but up to 20% of nulliparas (National High Blood Pressure Education Program Working Group, 1990) and 40% of women with chronic renal disease or vascular disorders are affected. Hypertension in pregnancy remains a cause of significant maternal and fetal–neonatal morbidity and mortality. Fetal–neonatal jeopardy results primarily from compromised placental perfusion and the need for preterm delivery in severe cases. In developed countries, up to 25% of all perinatal deaths are attributable to hypertensive disease in pregnancy. The major maternal hazards are the consequences of severe hypertension, grand mal seizures (eclampsia), and damage to other end-organs. In many areas of the world, hypertensive disease in pregnancy is the single most common cause of maternal death. With modern management, preeclampsia can be ameliorated, and eclampsia largely prevented. Any physician who practices obstetrics must be familiar with this disorder.

◇ CLASSIFICATION AND DIAGNOSIS

A number of terms have been used to categorize the hypertensive disorders of pregnancy, and proposed categories are complicated and confusing. The following concise and clinically useful classification was recommended by the American College of Obstetricians and Gynecologists and has been endorsed by the National Institutes of Health Working Group on High Blood Pressure:

I. Preeclampsia and eclampsia: Maternal hypertension with proteinuria and/or pathologic edema. Eclampsia is the occurrence of convulsions precipitated by hypertensive disease of pregnancy.
II. Chronic hypertension of any etiology preceding pregnancy.
III. Chronic hypertension with superimposed preeclampsia or eclampsia.
IV. Transient hypertension: Elevated maternal blood pressure during pregnancy or in the first 24 hours postpartum without proteinuria or edema.

Some authorities group conditions identified as transient hypertension and preeclampsia and eclampsia together under the broader term *pregnancy-induced hypertension* (PIH), a term that is recognized by the American College of Obstetricians and Gynecologists (ACOG, 1996). Some physicians use the term pregnancy-induced hypertension as synonymous with transient hypertension, i.e., elevated maternal blood pressure during pregnancy or in the first 24 hours postpartum without proteinuria or edema. Others contend, however, that transient hypertension is a retrospective diagnosis, and there is no consensus regarding the best term for hypertension in pregnancy without proteinuria or pathologic edema. Even without proteinuria or pathologic edema, new-onset hypertension in the latter half of pregnancy should be managed as preeclampsia in the best interest of the mother and fetus. For this reason, the term *preeclampsia* is used throughout this chapter with the recognition that some women will not have proteinuria when they first present with hypertension. Other more complicated classification systems exist but have no apparent advantage over simpler classification systems.

Definition of Hypertension in Pregnancy

Hypertension in pregnancy is defined as either a systolic blood pressure of ≥140 mm Hg or an increase of ≥30 mm Hg from a baseline in the first half of pregnancy, or a diastolic blood pressure of ≥90 mm Hg or an increase of ≥15 mm Hg from a baseline in the first half of pregnancy. To meet strict criteria for hypertension in pregnancy, the elevated blood pressures must be observed on at least two occasions 6 hours apart.

The use of increments of ≥30 mm Hg systolic or ≥15 mm Hg diastolic to define hypertension in pregnancy has been criticized by some authorities as too liberally diagnosing hypertension, in part because maternal blood pressure normally falls during the second trimester, and the diastolic pressure of many primigravidas with otherwise normotensive pregnancies rises more than 15 mm Hg sometime during their pregnancies. On the other hand, clinicians must be aware that a woman with lower than average baseline blood pressure may develop hypertension in pregnancy without blood pressures reaching or exceeding 140/90 mm Hg. Nulliparas with increases of either ≥30 mm Hg systolic or ≥15 mm Hg diastolic have significantly higher rates of hypertensive disease in pregnancy than those without such increases in blood pressure.

One diagnostic difficulty encountered is the lack of universal agreement about the measurement of blood pressure during pregnancy. The use of the onset of Korotkoff phase V (i.e., disappearance of auscultated sound) is the most practical method and the one used by American obstetricians. It may also be useful to record phase IV in the 10% of women who demonstrate a large difference between muffling and disappearance. Subjective errors in blood pressure in women measured by sphygmomanometry can occur because of either cuff size or the circumference of the patient's arm. The average blood pressure in women also increases about 1.4% per year after 37 years of age.

Preeclampsia

Traditionally, preeclampsia has been defined as a syndrome of pregnancy-induced hypertension accompanied by proteinuria or edema. It is frequently accompanied by disturbances in other organ systems. It is unique to the pregnant human and most often occurs in primigravidas. Proteinuria has traditionally been defined as more than 300 mg of protein in a 24-hour urine specimen or, less accurately, more than 1+ protein (equivalent to approximately 100 mg/dl) on dipstick sampling of a random urine specimen. Proteinuria is a highly variable and usually late sign of preeclampsia that correlates with the glomerular lesion associated with preeclampsia (McCartney, 1971). Proteinuria can be influenced by such factors as contamination of the urine specimen with vaginal secretions, blood, or bacteria; urine specific gravity and pH; exercise; and posture.

Edema is subjectively estimated by the degree of swelling or excessive weight gain. However, many normal pregnant women have generalized edema late in pregnancy, and it is often difficult to distinguish this from the edema of preeclampsia. Thus, edema should be considered pathologic only if it is generalized and involves the hands, face, and legs. Note also that edema may be absent in patients with preeclampsia and eclampsia.

TABLE 1. *Criteria for severe preeclampsia*

Blood pressure consistently > 160 mm Hg systolic or > 110 mm Hg diastolic

New onset of proteinuria > 2 g in a 24-hr urine collection or > 3+ in a randomly collected specimen

Oliguria (< 400 ml in 24 hr) or increasing serum creatinine levels

Platelet < 100,000/μl, hemolytic anemia, or increase in lactic acid dehydrogenase and direct bilirubin levels

Headache, visual disturbances, or other cerebral signs

Epigastric or right upper quadrant pain

Cardiac decompensation, pulmonary edema, or cyanosis

Fetal growth retardation

Preeclampsia may be categorized as mild or severe, primarily on the basis of the degree of hypertension or proteinuria and whether or not other organ systems are involved (Table 1). Its unpredictable course, which ranges from slow to fulminant progression, makes even mild disease potentially dangerous. One deceptive variant, the HELLP syndrome—hemolysis (H), elevated liver enzymes (EL), and low platelet count (LP) (Weinstein, 1982)—has received considerable attention. It may present initially as minimal changes in blood pressure and more prominent findings of hemolysis, elevated levels in liver function tests, and thrombocytopenia.

Eclampsia

Eclampsia is a more severe form of preeclampsia in which generalized seizures or coma ensues. Convulsions usually are preceded by headaches, epigastric pain, hyperreflexia, and hemoconcentration, but at times, they occur suddenly and without warning in asymptomatic women with only mild hypertension disease of pregnancy. Neurologic disorders such as coincidental epilepsy or other causes of seizures must be excluded. Seizures first appear before labor in about 50% of cases, during labor in 25%, and early postpartum in the other 25%. Whether or not otherwise unexplained seizures occurring more than 48 hours after delivery represent postpartum eclampsia is debated, but there is no question that a rare patient with preeclampsia will have convulsions 2 days or more after delivery.

Chronic Hypertension

Chronic hypertension complicating pregnancy is distinguished from preeclampsia when the hypertension antedates pregnancy, appears before week 20 of gestation, or persists indefinitely after delivery. Most of these women have essential hypertension, which may be associated with superimposed preeclampsia, but more often the hypertension is mild, and the pregnancy is uncomplicated. Women with underlying diseases as the cause of their chronic hypertension are at greater risk for superimposed preeclampsia. Preeclampsia tends to recur in these patients, often earlier and more severely, in subsequent pregnancies. Sometimes it is difficult to be certain of a diagnosis of chronic hypertension because of changes in blood pressure that normally occur during midpregnancy. Women with mild hypertension may have a blood pressure within the normal range during the midtrimester, and many of these women show greater decreases in their blood pressure during pregnancy than do normotensive women (Sibai et al., 1983). Chronic hypertension is regarded as severe if the systolic blood pressure is more than 160 mm Hg or the diastolic is more than 110 mm Hg. Superimposed preeclampsia is defined as an exacerbation of hypertension with the development of proteinuria or generalized edema that was not previously present.

Transient Hypertension

Women with latent or transient hypertension during late pregnancy have no other signs of preeclampsia or preexisting hypertension and no evidence of pregnancy compromise. The blood pressure normalizes postpartum, but hypertension often recurs during subsequent pregnancies. This classification probably includes women with different etiologies of hypertension, and women with this diagnosis are likely to have essential hypertension later in life (Cunningham and Lindheimer, 1992).

◊ ETIOLOGY OF PREECLAMPSIA

In 1916, preeclampsia was called the disease of theories; almost a century later, this characterization is still accurate. Despite extensive interest and research, the cause of preeclampsia remains uncertain. There are, however, well-recognized predisposing factors (Table 2) as well as data to support contributions from several areas in the pathogenesis of the disease.

Immunogenetic Factors

Because preeclampsia most often occurs in first pregnancies, it is tempting to speculate that an aberrant immune reaction to foreign paternally derived antigens is responsible for the disease. Following this line of reasoning, the lower rates of preeclampsia in second pregnancies might imply a protective effect incurred by prior exposure to either paternal or an unknown placental antigen. Exposure to fetal antigen *per se* is not required to develop preeclampsia because the disease is a

TABLE 2. *Risk factors for preeclampsia*

Primigravid status
Family history of preeclampsia or eclampsia
Previous preeclampsia or eclampsia
New paternity
Extremes of maternal age (younger than 20 or older than 35 years of age)
Preexisting hypertensive vascular, autoimmune, or renal disease
Diabetes mellitus
Multiple gestation
Nonimmune or alloimmune fetal hydrops
Triploidy
Hydatidiform mole

well-recognized complication of hydatidiform mole. Two observations indirectly support an immunogenetic hypothesis. First, the rate of preeclampsia is increased in pregnancies conceived by a new reproductive partner or using donor insemination. Second, the rate of preeclampsia is increased in women becoming pregnant after using a birth control method that prevents semen exposure (Klonoff-Cohen et al., 1989) and is comparatively decreased by longer periods of cohabitation prior to pregnancy (Robillard et al., 1994).

Maternal tissues are in direct contact with two trophoblastic tissues: syncytiotrophoblast and extravillous cytotrophoblast. In terms of antigenicity, however, both syncytiotrophoblast and extravillous cytotrophoblast are remarkably inert, containing no classic major histocompatibility (MHC) antigens. Extravillous cytotrophoblast does, however, carry a nonclassic, truncated MHC I (class Ib) antigen known as HLA-G. HLA-G is selectively expressed at the interface of the placenta and mother and is minimally polymorphic. Elegant work by Munz and colleagues suggests that one of the primary functions of HLA-G is inhibition of natural killer cell activity through binding of the HLA-G molecule to natural killer cell surface receptors (Munz et al., 1997). Because cells that bear no MHC class I antigens are targeted by natural killer cells, the proven immunosuppression of natural killer cells by HLA-G would serve to promote trophoblast survival. Some investigators have found that trophoblastic cells from women with preeclampsia fail to express HLA-G mRNA or protein or have attenuated expression of HLA-G. Others have found that endovascular cytotrophoblast in the uteroplacental circulation of women with preeclampsia express HLA-DR antigens, perhaps rendering them susceptible to cytotoxic T cells.

A familial predisposition to preeclampsia is well established and may operate primarily as a single-gene recessive trait. Maternal genotype alone has been implicated because of the increased frequency of preeclampsia in the mothers, daughters, and granddaughters of women who have a history of eclampsia. Because women with preeclampsia are more likely to be positive for HLA-DR4 than normal women (Simon et al., 1988), it has been suggested that a defect could lie in a recessive immune response gene linked to HLA. However, one group found no association between HLA-A and -B and preeclampsia (Simon et al., 1988) (Fig. 1).

Assuming autosomal recessive inheritance, investigators failed to find a linkage using random DNA markers in families with preeclampsia (Hayward et al., 1992). In contrast, another group found that a molecular variant of the angiotensinogen gene (T235), known to be associated with essential hypertension, also is associated with primigravida preeclampsia (Ward et al., 1993). These investigators speculate that increased concentrations of tissue or plasma angiotensinogen leads to increased baseline concentrations or reactivity of angiotensin II and hence hypertension. More recently, Dizon-Townson and colleagues (1996) have found that nearly 10% of women with preeclampsia have the Leiden mutation of the factor V gene.

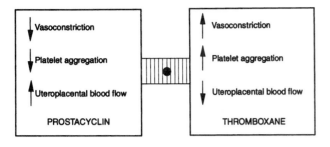

NORMAL PREGNANCY

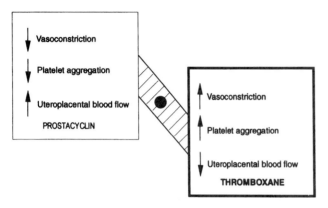

PREECLAMPSIA

FIG. 1. Physiological balance of prostacyclin and thromboxane in normal pregnancy and the proposed imbalance resulting in thromboxane dominance in preeclampsia.

An autoimmune connection to preeclampsia also is suspected. Some, but not all, investigators have found reduced circulating levels of complement factors (C3 and C4) in preeclamptic patients. Antiphospholipid syndrome, an autoimmune condition, is associated with particularly high rates of preeclampsia in women progressing beyond 15 to 20 weeks of gestation. Furthermore, approximately 15% of women with severe preeclampsia of onset before 34 weeks of gestation have significant levels of antiphospholipid antibodies (Branch et al., 1990).

Increased Vascular Reactivity and the Endothelial Injury

The underlying abnormality in preeclampsia involves increased vascular sensitivity to pressor hormones and eicosanoids and general arteriolar constriction. In turn, increased vasoconstriction results in increased blood flow resistance and arterial hypertension. As far as antecedent biophysical events are concerned, the loss of the usual pregnancy-associated refractoriness to arterial vasopressors precedes the clinical condition by days to weeks. In now classic studies, Gant and colleagues (1973) showed that women destined to develop preeclampsia had an increased vasopressor response to infused angiotensin

II well before hypertension could be detected (Fig. 2). The precursor to angiotensin II is angiotensinogen, a protein secreted by the liver and cleaved by renin to produce angiotensin I. Angiotensin I, which has little vasopressor activity, is then converted into biologically active angiotensin II by an angiotensin-converting enzyme bound to vascular endothelium. Circulating angiotensin II interacts with specific receptors to induce smooth muscle contraction, stimulate aldosterone production and sodium retention, facilitate norepinephrine release, inhibit norepinephrine reuptake by sympathetic nerve terminals, and potentiate vascular smooth muscle reactivity to norepinephrine.

Much subsequent investigation has focused on a role for vasoactive eicosanoids, and a considerable body of evidence indicates that preeclampsia is marked by deficient prostacyclin (PGI_2) activity and thromboxane A_2 (TxA_2) dominance. Prostacyclin is a potent vasodilator and inhibitor of platelet aggregation synthesized by the vascular epithelium and the renal cortex. Thromboxane A_2 is a potent vasoconstrictor and promoter of platelet aggregation produced primarily by platelets. The regulation of angiotensin II sensitivity appears to be closely linked to prostanoid synthesis. Prostaglandin synthetase inhibitors augment the pressor response to angiotensin II; the infusion of prostaglandin E_2, prostaglandin E_1, and PGI_2 reduces the pressor response to angiotensin II in pregnancy. Preeclampsia is characterized by a reduction in the biosynthesis of PGI_2 as marked by reduced renal excretion of PGI_2 metabolites. Moreover, this reduction precedes the development of clinical disease. Urinary excretion of TxA_2 metabolites appears to correlate with blood pressure

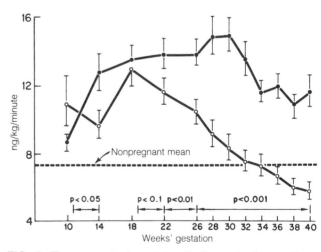

FIG. 2. The amount of angiotensin II required to evoke a pressor response during pregnancy in 120 primigravidas who remained normal *(black dots)* and in 72 primigravidas who developed pregnancy-induced hypertension *(open circles)*. *Vertical bars* represent the standard error of the mean. Differences between the two groups were highly significant after week 22 of gestation. (From Gant NF, Daley GL, Chand S, et al. A study of angiotensin II pressor responsiveness throughout primigravid pregnancy. *J Clin Invest* 1973;52:2682.)

and other clinical indices of preeeclampsia. Renal production of prostaglandin E_2 and PGI_2 also is reduced in preeclampsia.

Within the last several years, several groups of investigators have taken the view that the primary lesion in preeclampsia is at the level of the vascular endothelium (Roberts et al., 1991), a hypothesis that allows for the explanation of some other well-established observations. There is abundant evidence of endothelial cell activation or injury in preeclampsia, as indicated by decreased levels of PGI_2 (see above), elevated levels of factor VIII-related antigen, increased levels of fibronection and fibronectin-EDI+, and increased levels of plasminogen activator inhibitor I (PAI). Some investigators have identified antiendothelial antibodies in sera from women with preeclampsia. Others have shown that sera taken from preeclamptic women contain factor(s) that are either cytotoxic to monolayer cultures of endothelium or at least activate endothelial cells *in vitro*. Finally, others have found mitogenic factors in sera from women destined to become preeclamptic, yet another feature of endothelial injury. Candidate circulating factors that damage or activate the endothelium include tumor necrosis factor-α (TNF-α), interleukins (IL), and endothelin. Elevated circulating levels of TNF-α have been observed in women with preeclampsia, and this cytokine is known to activate endothelial cells as well as induce glomerular endothelial damage. Plasma levels of IL-1 receptor antagonist, which inhibits IL-1 action, are increased in women with preeclampsia. Endothelin is a potent vasoconstrictor and mitogen, and several groups have found increased circulating concentrations of endothelin-1 in women with preeclampsia, though not all investigators agree. Increased expression of endothelin-1 mRNA in placental villous tissue of preeclamptic patients has been documented. More recently, investigators have found increased levels of endothelial growth factor and platelet-derived growth factor in preeclamptic women; both of these factors might activate endothelial cells.

Endothelium-derived relaxing factor, now recognized to be nitric oxide, may be the primary mediator of vascular refractoriness to vasopressors in pregnancy. Alterations in its production or the response of vascular smooth muscle to nitric oxide could well play a role in preeclampsia, though Silver and colleagues (1996) found no relationship between plasma nitrite and nitrate concentrations and severe preeclampsia. Bradykinin-induced nitric oxide release from umbilical cord vessels is markedly reduced in tissues from women with preeclampsia. Higher concentrations of an inhibitor of nitric oxide synthesis have been found in women with preeclampsia.

Coagulation Abnormalities

A number of clotting abnormalities are associated with preeclampsia, and it is not surprising that some investigators hypothesize that a coagulopathy may be one of the primary events in the disease. Thrombocytopenia is relatively common. Most authorities hold that decreased platelet counts are secondary to endothelial cell injury, though the finding that platelet-associated IgG is found in many patients with preeclampsia raises the possibility of an immune-mediated mechanism. β-Thromboglobulin, released when platelets aggregate, is found in increased levels in the plasma of women with preeclampsia.

Increased levels of thrombin–antithrombin III complexes in the circulation of preeclamptic women indicate ongoing thrombin generation. Decreased levels of protein C and antithrombin III in preeclamptic women also indicate thrombin generation because these proteins are consumed in neutralizing thrombin. Fibrin degradation is increased in preeclampsia as evidenced by elevations of D-dimer concentrations.

Oxygen Free Radicals and Lipid Peroxidation

Some investigators believe that increased or dysregulated generation of oxygen free radicals with resultant plasma lipid peroxidation may be the underlying cause of endothelial damage and abnormal placental vascularization in preeclampsia (Walsh, 1994). Increased free radical formation in pregnancy is well documented and may be related to increased cell turnover at the placental–maternal interface or an alternation in endogenous free radical scavenging mechanisms. Plasma oxygen free radical formation is elevated in women with preeclampsia. Perhaps more importantly, increased levels of oxygen free radicals are detectable before the onset of preeclampsia in women destined to develop the disease. Lipid peroxidation is increased in preeclamptics (Uotila et al., 1993). Finally, lower serum antioxidant activity has been reported in patients with preeclampsia than in normotensive controls (Mikhail et al., 1994).

Abnormalities of Cytotrophoblastic Differentiation and Invasion

In normal pregnancy, extravillous cytotrophoblasts in anchoring chorionic villi invade the uterine wall and terminal portions of the spiral arteries, replacing the vascular endothelium as far as the distant third of the myometrial segments of the vessels. In doing so, invasive cytotrophoblasts not only anchor the placenta to the myometrium, they also alter the terminal portions of the spiral arteries. In the process, most of the muscular layer of the arterioles is replaced by fibrinoid material. This loss of musculature and elasticity is accompanied by a rather dramatic increase in the luminal width. As a result, the terminal portions of the arteries that feed the intervillous space of the placenta become nonelastic, "large-bore" vessels with greatly reduced resistance to blood flow. This important physiological alteration in the terminal portions of the spiral arteries is such that the entrance of maternal blood into the intervillous space is driven by the pressure differential between the mean maternal arterial blood pressure, the pressure inside the intervillous space, and the pressure in the veins draining the intervillous space. The entire system is a low-pressure, low-resistance circuit, and the reconstruction of the terminal portions of the spiral arteries by cytotrophoblasts plays an extremely important role in its development.

Investigators have shown that the process of cytotrophoblast invasion is accompanied by characteristic cellular changes, including up-regulated expression of type IV collagenase (Librach et al., 1991), HLA-G, and human placental lactogen. The invading cytotrophblasts express a variety of adhesion molecules involved in invasion of the decidual–myometrial interstitium and vasculature, including a decidual–endothelial cell cadherin, platelet–endothelial adhesion molecule-1, vascular endothelial cell molecule-1, $\alpha 1$ and $\alpha 4$ integrins, $\beta 1$ integrins, and angiogenesis-related $\alpha V \beta 3$ (Zhou et al., 1997b).

In preeclampsia, this invasion process is retarded to some degree, resulting in a relative (though not absolute) lack of physiological change in the spiral arteries. Placental bed biopsy studies show that the cytotrophblasts in preeclamptic pregnancies do not possess the characteristic invasion cell phenotype (Zhou et al., 1997a). These findings suggest that a primary defect of preeclampsia might be in the cytotrophoblasts themselves and their lack of invasive potential. Alternatively, an abnormal interaction of the cytotrophoblasts and maternal tissues may be at fault. In either case, one of the most popular current hypotheses regarding the pathogenesis of preeclampsia is that inadequate cytotrophoblast invasion with a resulting lack of physiological change in the spiral arteries is a primary event in the disease. The underperfused placenta or fetus then elaborates factor(s) into the maternal circulation that cause preeclampsia, perhaps through an effect on endothelium.

◊ MATERNAL AND FETAL COMPLICATIONS OF PREECLAMPSIA

Kidneys

A distinct kidney lesion identifiable by light and electron microscopy and characterized by swelling of glomerular capillary endothelial and mesangial cells is widely accepted as pathognomonic for preeclampsia (Fig. 3). The glomerulus enlarges, and the capillary lumen narrows, but the basement membrane, tubules, and vasculature usually are not altered. This histologic picture, which may be accompanied by subendothelial deposits of fibrin-like proteinaceous material, is termed glomerular capillary endotheliosis and seldom is seen in the absence of proteinuria.

Both renal blood flow and glomerular filtration are reduced in preeclampsia. In mild disease, this is likely because of reduced plasma volume. Plasma levels of creatinine and urea nitrogen are usually normal. However, plasma uric acid levels are elevated, and the degree of elevation roughly parallels the severity of disease. In more severe cases, renal ischemia from vasospasm may result in creatinine levels that are up to threefold elevated above normal. Renal ischemia also may result in oliguria, an indication of severe disease. Infrequently, acute tubular necrosis and renal failure may occur. Rarely, renal cortical necrosis ensues.

The glomerular damage of preeclampsia causes proteinuria in the form of leakage of large-molecular-weight proteins such as albumin, globulins, and transferrin into the urine. Pathologic proteinuria is defined as the presence of more than 300 mg of urinary protein in 24-hour urine collection. Proteinuria in severe preeclampsia is greater than 5 g of protein in 24 hours.

Liver

Periportal fibrin deposition and zonal necrosis often are found in fatal cases of eclampsia, but these are similar to lesions seen in the livers of pregnant women who died of shock associated with infections, placental abruption, or postpartum hemorrhage. Bleeding from periportal hemorrhagic necrosis may extend beneath the hepatic capsule to form a subcapsular hematoma. In rare cases, rupture of a subcapsular hematoma or frank intrahepatic hemorrhage may occur. This life-threatening situation usually presents with severe epigastric pain and evidence of blood loss.

Hepatic dysfunction as evidenced by elevated heptocellular enzyme levels is common in preeclampsia and contributes to the diagnosis of HELLP syndrome. These patients often present with an atypical clinical picture, and the signs and symptoms of preeclampsia may be overlooked because of conspicuous right upper quadrant pain, nausea, and vomiting (Table 3). The underlying problem may be attributed mistakenly to hepatobiliary disease or other gastrointestinal disorders, particularly by nonobstetric physicians less familiar with the manifestations of preeclampsia.

Placenta

As discussed above, many pregnancies complicated by preeclampsia fail to develop the normal physiological alteration of the terminal spiral arteries feeding the intervillous spaces. Instead, microscopic examination of the placenta bed often shows varying degrees of a spiral artery vasculopathy characterized by accumulation of lipid-laden macrophages in the intima, fibrinoid necrosis of the media, and intimal fibroblastic proliferation. A mononuclear infiltrate is often present. This lesion, which is often called "acute atherosis," is felt by many authorities to be the characteristic vascular lesion of preeclampsia (Fig. 4). The reduction in intervillous perfusion with subsequent inadequate oxygenation of the fetal–placental unit is the main cause of perinatal morbidity and mortality associated with preeclampsia. The clinical consequences may be fetal growth impairment, significant fetal hypoxia, or, in extreme cases, fetal death. The risk of placental abruption is also increased, depending on the severity of the disease.

Cardiopulmonary System

Hemoconcentration is common in women with severe preeclampsia or eclampsia, and the intravascular volume expansion that is normal for pregnancy is either not present or significantly reduced. Whether cardiac output is normal, decreased,

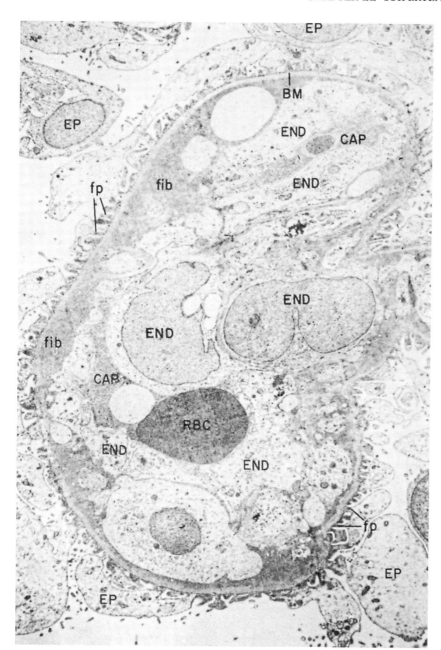

FIG. 3. Glomerular loop from a patient with preeclampsia. Pronounced swelling has greatly restricted the capillary lumen (CAP). Fibrinoid (fib) is present between the endothelium (END) and the basement membrane (BM; subendothelial location) and, to some extent, between endothelial cells (interendothelial location). Epithelial foot processes (fp) and basement membrane appear essentially normal (Original magnification × 11,500; EP, epithelium; RBC, red blood cell; from Hooper J, Fanquhar G, Yamauchi H, Mood MD, Page EW. *Obstet Gynecol* 1961;17:271.)

or increased in early preeclampsia remains a subject of controversy. In women with severe preeclampsia, invasive hemodynamic studies have found that the left ventricular stroke work index is elevated in most cases, reflecting a hyperdynamic state; however, it is variable from case to case. The systemic vascular resistance of women with severe preeclampsia is normal or elevated. Given the observed variations in cardiac output and systemic vascular resistance, pulmonary capillary pressures may be low, normal, or high. Frank cardiac failure is uncommon. When it occurs, circulatory collapse most often happens during labor or a few hours after delivery and in elderly multiparas whose hypertension is difficult to control.

Pulmonary edema is an infrequent complication of preeclampsia. Its cause in untreated patients with severe preeclampsia is uncertain but is probably multifactorial and includes altered capillary membrane permeability, reduced colloid osmotic pressure, and elevated pulmonary vascular hydrostatic pressures. Pulmonary edema more often is a complication of the treatment of severe preeclampsia. Protracted oxytocin administration, fluid administration to compensate for sympathetic blockade resulting from conduction anesthesia, and overreplacement of fluid losses are typical causes of iatrogenic intravenous fluid overload.

Hematologic System

Preeclampsia is associated with activation of the coagulation system. As discussed previously, one probable mechanism is endothelial injury in the microcirculation with resultant deposition of platelets and fibrin. The high fibronectin, low

TABLE 3. *Clinical features of six pregnant women with HELLP syndrome*

RUQ pain and N & V	AST (mg/dl)	Bilirubin (mg/dl)	Blood pressure	Proteinuria (dipstick)	Platelets/µl
++++	600	4.6	170/100	++	42,000
++++	240	1.7	150/98	+	15,000
++++	276	2.7	160/100	+	75,000
+++	975	8.3	140/100	+++	27,000
++	428	3.5	140/90	+++	30,000
++++	1450	1.3	190/95	+	29,000

antithrombin III, and increased β-thromboglobulin levels found in patients with preeclampsia are suggestive of endothelial injury with thrombin generation and platelet aggregation. The increase in fibronectin and another basement membrane glycoprotein, laminin 4, may antedate the appearance of hypertension by several weeks. Increased protein C inactivation by α_1-antitrypsin is found in preeclampsia. This may contribute to the increased levels of thrombin. In turn, thrombin consumes antithrombin III and results in fibrin deposition. Fibrinolysis is normal in women with preeclampsia, and not surprisingly, some investigators have noted increased levels of fibrin degradation products such as D-dimers and fibrinopeptide A in preeclamptic patients. Hypofibrinogenemia may occur in severe cases. Nonetheless, frank bleeding from a consumptive coagulopathy is distinctly rare in preeclampsia.

Evidence of increased platelet consumption is found frequently in preeclampsia, and a selective reduction in platelet count is the most common coagulation abnormality, with platelet counts <100,000/µl occurring in about 15% of patients. In spite of this, severe thrombocytopenia resulting in significant bleeding is fortunately infrequent.

Preeclampsia often is complicated by some degree of red cell destruction, and moderate to severe hemolytic anemia with hemoglobinuria may be present in severe cases. The schisto-cytes that may be seen in such cases are secondary to microangiopathic hemolysis and fragmentation of erythrocytes in the microcirculation from endothelial damage accompanied by platelet and fibrin deposition.

Central Nervous System

Although it is generally agreed that the central nervous system (CNS) changes in severe preeclampsia and eclampsia represent a form of hypertensive encephalopathy, the precise pathogenesis remains uncertain. In large autopsy series, the most common neuropathic changes in women with eclampsia are multifocal petechial hemorrhages at the gray matter–white matter junction (Fig. 5). However, these findings may not be representative of surviving patients. The CNS clinical manifestations in severe preeclampsia and eclampsia are most consistent with vasoconstrictive cerebral ischemia and resultant vasogenic edema. Cerebral blood flow and oxygen utilization are not markedly lower in eclamptic women than in normal or preeclamptic gravidas. Many patients with eclamptic seizures have nonspecific abnormalities in electroencephalograms, and the tracings usually return to normal by 3 months. Cranial computed tomographic (CT) scanning has revealed characteristic white matter hypodensities in up to 50% of eclamptic women,

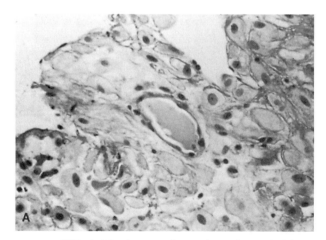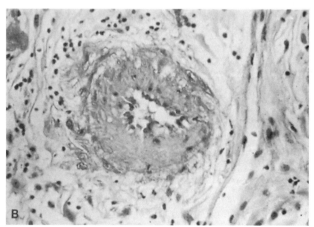

FIG. 4. The impact of preeclampsia on decidual spiral arterioles. **(A)** Photomicrograph of a spiral arteriole in the decidua of a normotensive primigravida who underwent cesarean section at term because of dystocia. **(B)** Photomicrograph of a spiral arteriole in the decidua of a primigravida with preeclampsia who underwent cesarean section in week 37 of pregnancy because of fetal distress. Note the considerable compromise in vascular lumen caused by prominent atherosis.

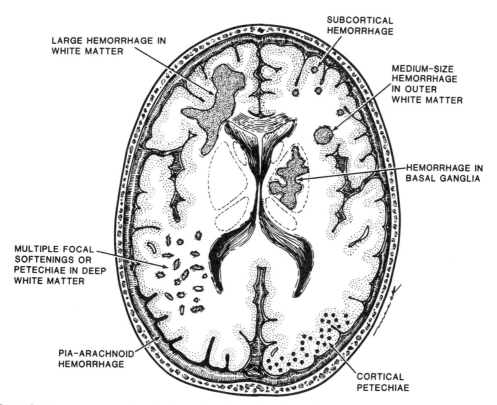

FIG. 5. Central nervous system findings at autopsy in eclampsia patients were compiled by Sheehan and Lynch. (From Digre KB, Varner MW, Osborn AG, Crawford S. Cranial magnetic resonance imaging in severe pre-eclampsia versus eclampsia. *Arch Neurol* 1993;50:399.)

most prominently in the occipital and parietal areas. The abnormal results in cranial magnetic resonance imaging (MRI) reported in 50% of patients with severe preeclampsia and 90% of patients with eclampsia suggest that MRI is a more sensitive imaging procedure for women with eclampsia (Fig. 6).

Visual disturbances are common features of severe preeclampsia. A small proportion of women with severe preeclampsia or eclampsia will develop blindness due to occipital cortical ischemia.

◊ MANAGEMENT

Preeclampsia is encountered by all physicians who practice obstetrics. Decisions regarding the proper management of preeclamptic patients are some of the most difficult in obstetrics and require astute clinical judgment and a thorough knowledge of the range of severity and natural progression of the disease. The most effective therapy for preeclampsia is delivery of the fetus and placenta. Therefore, in pregnancies at or near term in which the cervix is favorable, labor should be induced. Preeclampsia remote from term presents a much more difficult problem. The decision whether to intervene and deliver a preterm infant that may require prolonged intensive care or to institute and continue expectant management is determined by disease severity and the length of gestation (Table 4).

Mild Preeclampsia

Most patients with preeclampsia present with mild disease. Such patients are not candidates for delivery if the fetus is immature or the cervix is unfavorable for induction. Successful management, usually consisting of rest and observation, can be carried out with the patient at home or in the hospital. The goals of therapy in this situation are to monitor maternal and fetal parameters while allowing time for the fetus to mature and the cervix to ripen.

In this cost-conscious time, outpatient management of mild preeclampsia is popular and may be undertaken as long as the patient with stable disease is compliant. The prudent physician will establish a structured management approach that includes frequent evaluation of maternal and fetal well-being, usually including twice-weekly assessments of mother and fetus. A traditional cornerstone of management is maternal rest in the lateral decubitus position ("bed rest"). This minimizes vasopressor activity, maximizes uteroplacental blood flow, results in lower blood pressures, and promotes diuresis. Strict and continuous bed rest is seldom necessary and infrequently achieved in practice. It may be reasonable to advise pregnant women with elevated blood pressure to greatly limit their activities and set aside at least two 2- to 3-hour blocks of time each day when they can be off their feet. There is little to suggest, however, that this management alters the underlying pathophysiology of preeclampsia; rather, reduced activity and

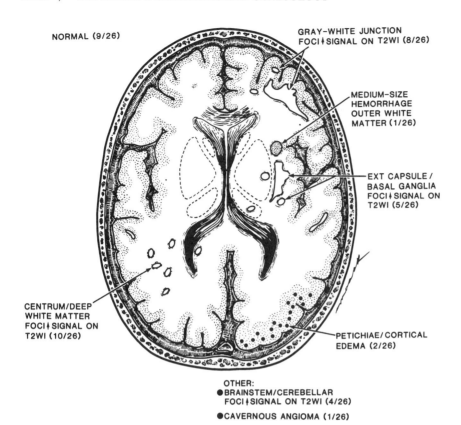

NORMAL (9/26)

GRAY-WHITE JUNCTION
FOCI↑SIGNAL ON T2WI (8/26)

MEDIUM-SIZE
HEMORRHAGE
OUTER WHITE
MATTER (1/26)

EXT CAPSULE /
BASAL GANGLIA
FOCI↑SIGNAL ON
T2WI (5/26)

CENTRUM/DEEP
WHITE MATTER
FOCI↑SIGNAL ON
T2WI (10/26)

PETICHIAE/CORTICAL
EDEMA (2/26)

OTHER:
● BRAINSTEM/CEREBELLAR
FOCI↑SIGNAL ON T2WI (4/26)
● CAVERNOUS ANGIOMA (1/26)

FIG. 6. Compilation of observed magnetic resonance imaging findings in 26 patients with severe preeclampsia or eclampsia. (From Digre KB, Varner MW, Osborn AG, Crawford S. Cranial magnetic resonance imaging in severe preeclampsia versus eclampsia. *Arch Neurol* 1993;50:399.)

bed rest are likely palliative and merely allow continuation of the pregnancy. Although home blood pressure monitoring would appear attractive, its use probably increases the cost of outpatient management and has not been shown to improve maternal or fetal outcome. Also, neither antihypertensives nor low-dose aspirin is beneficial in ameliorating the disease or in improving maternal or fetal outcome once mild preeclampsia is present. When women with preeclampsia are managed on an

outpatient basis, it is extremely important to advise them to immediately report to the hospital if they develop symptoms of severe preeclampsia. Any sign of disease progression should prompt hospitalization.

Patients who develop worsening proteinuria, worsening hypertension, or symptoms suspicious for severe preeclampsia should be considered for admission to the hospital and inpatient care. Appropriate assessments include (1) daily monitoring for symptoms of severe preeclampsia or reduced fetal movement, (2) maternal blood pressure determinations several times per day, (3) daily monitoring of maternal urine for worsening proteinuria, and (4) once- or twice-weekly fetal biophysical testing (e.g., nonstress tests) (Table 5). Preeclampsia does not invariably progress rapidly, and in many cases, the pregnancy can be managed expectantly until the fetus reaches maturity. If the patient definitely becomes normotensive after hospitalization and is remote from term with no evidence of fetal compromise, resumption of outpatient surveillance is appropriate in some cases. However, early and prolonged hospitalization for patients with preeclampsia improves perinatal survival, reduces maternal morbidity, and is cost effective (Gilstrap et al., 1978). For patients with mild disease, there are few maternal or fetal benefits achieved by expectant management beyond 34 to 36 weeks of gestation, and delivery should be accomplished in all cases by 37 to 38 weeks of gestation. Delay beyond this time risks worsening hypertensive disease, with its potential for adverse maternal and fetal outcomes, while providing little or no benefit to either mother or fetus.

TABLE 4. *Management of hypertension complicating pregnancy*

Clinical condition	Therapy
Preeclampsia or chronic hypertension when the fetus is mature	*Definitive* Prevent convulsions Control blood pressure Deliver fetus
Preeclampsia or chronic hypertension when the fetus is premature in the presence of severe preeclampsia	*Definitive* Prevent convulsions Control blood pressure Deliver fetus
Eclampsia, whether the fetus is mature or premature	*Definitive* Treat convulsions Control blood pressure Stabilize mother Deliver fetus
Preeclampsia or chronic hypertension when the fetus is preterm	*Expectant* Ambulatory treatment Hospitalization
Hypertension in the first 20 weeks of gestation	Depends on the severity of hypertension

TABLE 5. *Serial examinations recommended for preeclamptic hospitalized patients*[a]

Mother
Blood pressure (four times daily)
Assessment for proteinuria, edema, weight, hyperreflexia, headache, visual disturbance, epigastric pain (daily)
Hematocrit, platelet count (every 2 days)
Serum uric acid and creatinine levels, 24-hr urine for total protein and creatinine clearance (twice weekly)
Liver function tests[b] (weekly)

Fetus
Fetal movement record (daily)
Antepartum testing (nonstress test and amniotic fluid index) (twice weekly)
Ultrasound for fetal growth (every 2 to 3 weeks)

[a]Recommendations are for hospitilized patients from time of diagnosis to delivery. Frequency of evaluations can be increased or decreased, depending on severity of disease.

[b]Serum aspartate aminotransferase (formerly SGOT), lactic dehydrogenase, and serum bilirubin.

Severe Preeclampsia

Delivery is always appropriate therapy for the mother with severe preeclampsia but may pose significant risks to the premature fetus, especially for gestational ages less than 32 weeks. Maternal morbidity and mortality associated with severe preeclampsia result principally from severe hypertension, eclampsia, and the HELLP syndrome. Most serious maternal complications arise because of undiagnosed severe preeclampsia as a result of inadequate prenatal care or an inappropriate tendency to delay hospitalization or delivery in women with worsening disease.

With improvements in neonatal care resulting in improved neonatal outcome for premature infants, delivery is clearly indicated in women with severe preeclampsia beyond 32 weeks of gestation. When the clinical situation permits, glucocorticoid treatment to enhance fetal lung maturity should be used in cases >34 weeks of gestation. At the other extreme, immediate delivery also is indicated with women with previable or very premature fetuses (less than 24 weeks of gestation) because delaying delivery would appear to increase the risk of an adverse maternal outcome without substantially improving the fetal–neonatal outcome. Finally, immediate delivery is indicated at any gestational age in a patient with severe preeclampsia and evidence of rapidly worsening disease.

The most controversial aspect of severe preeclampsia management is the proposed expectant care of patients between 24 and 32 weeks of gestation who meet one or more criteria for the diagnosis of severe preeclampsia and who appear clinically stable without threat of immediate, serious maternal complications or fetal compromise. Even some patients with HELLP syndrome on admission show improvement after corticosteroid administration, thereby allowing enhancement of fetal lung maturity (Magann et al., 1994). Because of the substantial risks of neonatal death or serious neonatal morbidity as a result of complications of prematurity, some investigators have argued that neonatal outcome might be improved in such cases by delaying delivery by as little as a few days (Odendaal et al., 1990; Sibai et al., 1990, 1994). Figure 7 summarizes an analysis of expectant management in cases of severe preeclampsia remote from term. Both neonatal respiratory distress syndrome and total neonatal morbidity are reduced by expectant management. It must be emphasized that even the most ardent supporters of expectant management of severe preeclampsia in patients between 24 and 32 weeks of gestation proceed along very cautious lines, with strictly defined criteria for patient selection and meticulous observation to determine whether expectantly managed patients should be delivered because of maternal or fetal concerns. Women with severe preeclampsia between 24 and 32 weeks of gestation should receive glucocorticoid treatment to enhance fetal lung maturity.

Clinically significant levels of antiphospholipid antibodies are found in a small proportion of women with preterm severe preeclampsia (Branch et al., 1990). These should be identified because they constitute a population of women at increased risk of thrombotic disease. Though data from prospective trials are lacking, physicians should consider thromboprophylaxis through 6 weeks postpartum in this subset of patients. Screening all preeclamptic patients for antiphospholipid antibodies is not indicated because no association has been found between these autoantibodies and the usual type of preeclampsia that develops near term.

Treating Hypertension

Blood pressure that rapidly increases to 160/110 mm Hg or greater should be treated to avoid potential hypertension-related damage to the maternal central nervous system. The ideal drug in such situations is one that reduces blood pressure in a controlled manner, avoiding precipitous reductions that may compromise placental perfusion. The goal is to lower the blood pressure to a mildly hypertensive level (diastolic pressure between 90 and 100 mm Hg). Hydralazine is the preferred agent because of its effectiveness and safety. An initial dose of 5 mg given as an intravenous bolus is increased by 5 to 10 mg every 20 minutes until a suitable blood pressure is achieved. This is repeated whenever the diastolic blood pressure rises to 110 mm Hg. Because the drug has a duration of action of several hours, adequate control of severe hypertension often can be achieved after one or two intravenous treatments. Labetalol (20 to 50 mg intravenously) is a useful second-line drug for women whose hypertension is refractory to hydralazine.

Meticulous attention to fluid balance is an important aspect of managing severe preeclampsia. Input and output should be assessed hourly, and a Foley catheter should be inserted to permit accurate measurement of urine output. The aim is to maintain urine output at or above 30 ml/hr while avoiding fluid overload.

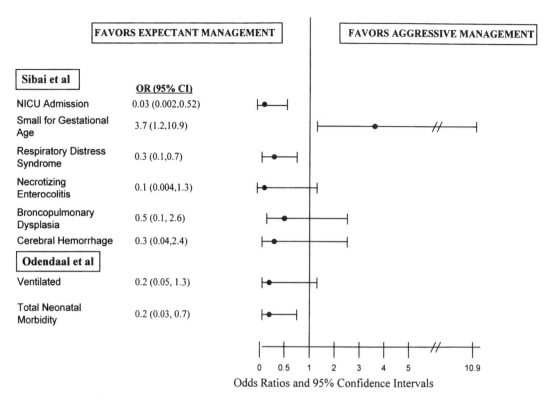

FIG. 7. Expectant versus aggressive management of severe preeclampsia.

Preventing Convulsions

Eclamptic seizures are a dreaded complication of preeclampsia because they are associated with unacceptably high mortality and morbidity rates. Predicting which patients with preeclampsia will have eclampsia has proven difficult. Certainly, the degree of blood pressure elevation does not correlate well enough for predictive purposes—20% of women with eclampsia have only a minimal rise in blood pressure, and many more have no more than a modest rise. For this reason, it is fortunate that magnesium sulfate ($MgSO_4 \cdot 7H_2O$), the drug of choice for the prevention of eclamptic seizures, has such an excellent therapeutic index. It is recommended that all preeclamptic women, even those with mild disease, be treated with magnesium sulfate for seizure prophylaxis during labor and for the first 24 hours postpartum. The drug can be administered by a continuous intravenous infusion pump in a loading dose of 4 g in 100 ml of fluid per hour followed by 2 to 3 g/hr as a maintenance dose. The infusion rate is adjusted to keep serum magnesium levels between 4 and 8 mg/dl. An intramuscular regimen consisting of a 10-g loading dose and 5 g every 4 hours is used less frequently because the painful injections are less acceptable to patients. In the therapeutic range, magnesium slows neuromuscular conduction and depresses CNS irritability. Loss of patellar reflexes occurs at serum magnesium levels of 8 to 10 mg/dl, respiratory depression at 10 to 15 mg/dl, and defective cardiac conduction at more than 15 mg/dl. Maternal urine output, respiratory rate, deep tendon reflexes, and level of consciousness must be fre-

quently monitored to avoid magnesium toxicity. If respiratory depression occurs, 1 g of calcium gluconate should be given intravenously over 3 minutes. Magnesium sulfate may also decrease beat-to-beat variability of the fetal heart rate.

Other anticonvulsant medications have been tried in pregnancy. However, evidence from randomized controlled trials indicates that magnesium sulfate is superior to both diazepam and phenytoin for the prevention of seizures in eclampsia (Lucas et al., 1995; Eclampsia Collaborative Trial Group, 1995) (Fig. 8).

Method of Delivery

For most patients with preeclampsia, induction with attempted vaginal delivery is preferable as long as there are no contraindications and should be carried out expeditiously once the decision to deliver is reached. In some patients, an unripe cervix will require ripening with prostaglandins. Induction of labor is established with intravenous oxytocin, and amniotomy is performed as soon as it is deemed safe. It is reasonable and prudent to formulate a clear endpoint, usually within 8 to 12 hours from initiation of oxytocin induction, when the patient will be delivered by cesarean section if labor is not established.

Blood loss can be great and may be tolerated poorly in the woman with severe preeclampsia compared to normal pregnancy because of contracted blood volume. In addition, magnesium sulfate inhibits uterine tone, placing the patient at greater risk for postpartum hemorrhage. For this reason, type-

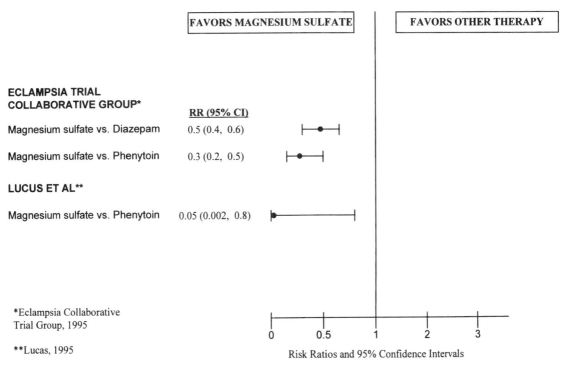

| | FAVORS MAGNESIUM SULFATE | FAVORS OTHER THERAPY |

**ECLAMPSIA TRIAL
COLLABORATIVE GROUP***

RR (95% CI)

Magnesium sulfate vs. Diazepam   0.5 (0.4, 0.6)

Magnesium sulfate vs. Phenytoin   0.3 (0.2, 0.5)

LUCUS ET AL**

Magnesium sulfate vs. Phenytoin   0.05 (0.002, 0.8)

*Eclampsia Collaborative
Trial Group, 1995

**Lucas, 1995

0   0.5   1   2   3

Risk Ratios and 95% Confidence Intervals

FIG. 8. Seizure prophylaxis using magnesium sulfate compared to other anticonvulsant therapy.

specific blood should be readily available. Epidural anesthesia is appropriate for most laboring preeclamptic patients. However, experienced judgment is required to identify patients in whom the use of regional anesthesia is considered unsafe for mother and fetus (see Chapter 7). Invasive hemodynamic monitoring may be useful and necessary in certain patients with severe preeclampsia or eclampsia based on specific indications (see Chapter 31).

Eclampsia

The incidence of eclampsia is about 0.2% of all deliveries. It is associated with multiorgan dysfunction and a wide spectrum of signs and symptoms ranging from isolated mild hypertension to extreme hypertension, hyperreflexia, proteinuria, and generalized edema. Whether eclampsia is totally preventable is controversial. Although the incidence can be significantly lowered by adequate antenatal care and the appropriate use of magnesium sulfate prophylaxis in labor and the postpartum period, some cases present with few warning signs or symptoms.

The protocol used to manage eclampsia is outlined in Table 6. Other anticonvulsants have been recommended and are used in other parts of the world. Magnesium sulfate has proved effective, and its success rate is better than that reported for either phenytoin or diazepam (Hutton et al., 1992; Dommise, 1990; Lucas et al., 1995; Eclampsia Trial Collaborative Group, 1995). Once convulsions have ceased, arterial blood gas measurements and a chest x-ray should be obtained to assess maternal oxygenation and exclude aspiration. Neither CT nor MRI

is essential in patients with a typical presentation for eclampsia because these tests seldom change management. Cranial imaging is indicated for patients with atypical eclampsia, focal neurologic deficits, or coma to search for possible intracranial hemorrhage and other serious abnormalities that require specific pharmacologic or surgical therapy.

Immediate delivery by cesarean section during or soon after an eclamptic seizure can be dangerous. It is virtually always better to stabilize the maternal condition, a task usually accomplished within several hours. It is then safe to proceed with definitive treatment, which is delivery. Induction of labor with oxytocin often is successful, particularly after 32 weeks of gestation. The fetal heart rate and uterine activity must be closely monitored. Fetal bradycardia is a common finding

---

TABLE 6. *Protocol for treating eclampsia*

1. Turn patient on her side
2. Establish airway and administer oxygen
3. Administer 4 to 6 g of magnesium sulfate intravenously over 10 to 15 min followed by 2 g/hr maintenance dose adjusted later based on patellar reflexes, urine output and serum magnesium levels
4. Obtain arterial blood gas measurement and chest x-ray
5. If convulsions are controlled and maternal condition is stable, initiate induction or delivery within 3 to 6 hr
6. Continue to administer magnesium sulfate for at least 24 hr after delivery or last convulsion
7. Obtain computed tomographic scan or magnetic resonance imaging if seizures are atypical or coma is prolonged

during an eclamptic seizure, but the rate usually returns to normal once convulsions cease and the mother is well oxygenated. If bradycardia persists or the uterus is hypertonic, placental abruption should be suspected. Eclampsia before 32 weeks of gestation is associated with a high incidence of fetal growth retardation, abruption, and intrapartum fetal distress, any of which may necessitate cesarean section.

Chronic Hypertension

Most patients with chronic hypertension have essential hypertension, and the increased morbidity and mortality in these patients are primarily related to the development of superimposed preeclampsia and placental abruption. Hypertension secondary to disorders such as renal disease, pheochromocytoma, endocrine disease, and coarctation of the aorta is relatively uncommon in pregnancy. Factors that place the patient at higher risk to develop superimposed preeclampsia are maternal age more than 40 years, hypertension for longer than 15 years, blood pressure higher than 160/110 mm Hg early in pregnancy, class B to F diabetes, cardiomyopathy, and renal or autoimmune disease. Appropriate evaluation necessitates a complete physical examination, including funduscopic examination. Recommended laboratory investigations include urinalysis and culture, 24-hour urine collection for total protein excretion and creatinine clearance, and assessment of electrolytes and renal chemistries. Some patients may require electrocardiography, chest radiography, and testing for antiphospholipid antibodies, antinuclear antibodies, urine catecholamines, or vanillylmandelic acid.

Daily sodium intake should be restricted to 2 g, and frequent rest periods encouraged. Patients are seen every 2 weeks until they reach 28 weeks of gestation, and thereafter are seen weekly until delivery. At each visit, systolic and diastolic blood pressure should be recorded, and the urine tested for the presence of glucose and protein. Depending on the clinical circumstances, additional evaluation of maternal status, including serial measurements of hematocrit, serum creatinine, serum uric acid, creatinine clearance, and 24-hour urinary excretion of protein, may be warranted. Prompt hospitalization is indicated if the hypertension worsens, proteinuria is significant, or uric acid levels are elevated. An elevation of uric acid to more than 6 mg/dl often is an early sign of superimposed preeclampsia.

There is considerable disagreement regarding the treatment of chronic hypertension in pregnancy, particularly about which drugs are most appropriate and at what level of blood pressure treatment should be started. Antihypertensive therapy usually is begun at diastolic pressures of more than 100 mm Hg. Methyldopa is the most commonly used antihypertensive agent and remains the drug of choice because of its long record of effectiveness and safety. Table 7 summarizes the clinical experience with other antihypertensive agents.

The rare case of maternal death associated with chronic hypertension in pregnancy usually is caused by a malignant rise in blood pressure with subsequent congestive heart fail-

TABLE 7. *Antihypertensive therapy for chronic hypertension in pregnant patients*

α_2-Adrenergic receptor agonists
Methyldopa is the antihypertensive drug used most extensively during pregnancy. The dosage is 250 to 500 mg every 6 hr. Its safety and efficacy are supported by randomized trials and a 7.5-year follow-up of children born to treated mothers.

α-Adrenergic receptor and β-adrenergic receptor antagonists
Labetalol appears to be as effective as methyldopa, but no follow-up studies of children born to mothers given labetalol have been conducted.

β-Adrenergic receptor agonists
These drugs, especially atenolol and metoprolol, appear to be safe and efficacious in late pregnancy, but fetal bradycardia has been reported. Fetal growth restriction has been reported when treatment was started in early gestation or midgestation.

Diuretics
Diuretic therapy begun before conception usually is continued during pregnancy.

Peripheral vasodilators
Hydralazine commonly is used as adjuvant therapy with methyldopa and β-adrenergic receptor antagonists. Calcium-channel blockers have been used, and no human neonatal problems have been demonstrated. The experience with minoxidil is limited, and this drug is not recommended.

Angiotensin-converting enzyme inhibitors
Angiotensin converting enzyme inhibitors have been associated with oligohydramnios and neonatal renal failure. They should not be used in pregnancy.

ure or cerebrovascular accidents. There is little evidence to suggest any maternal benefits from treating mild to moderate hypertension during pregnancy. Treatment of severe hypertension, on the other hand, is associated with a reduction in maternal morbidity and mortality (Redman, 1980). Perinatal outcome is closely linked to the incidence of superimposed preeclampsia and placental abruption, and antihypertensive therapy does not alter the incidence of these complications.

Women with chronic hypertension should undergo serial fetal surveillance and serial ultrasound measurements to detect evidence of placental insufficiency and fetal growth impairment (see Chapter 15). Many mildly hypertensive patients with no other problems can continue to near term with close monitoring. However, continuing the pregnancy beyond 38 to 39 weeks of gestation is imprudent because delay beyond this time risks worsening hypertensive disease, with its potential for adverse maternal and fetal outcomes, while providing little or no additional benefit to either mother or fetus. High-risk pregnancies and patients receiving antihypertensive drugs usually are delivered at 37 weeks of gestation or earlier. Complications such as superimposed preeclampsia, placental abruption, fetal growth retardation, and fetal distress may dictate delivery, regardless of gestation. In nonemergency situations wherein preterm delivery is contemplated, amniocentesis is performed, and antepartum corticosteroid therapy is initiated for fetal lung immaturity.

◊ PREDICTION OF PREECLAMPSIA

Numerous factors and clinical tests have been proposed as screening tests to predict the future development of preeclampsia. In a recent multicenter trial, investigators identified four risk factors that were predictive for the development of preeclampsia (Sibai et al., 1995). The three most predictive were a systolic blood pressure greater than 120 mm Hg during the first trimester, maternal weight greater than 20% above desirable weight, and smoking, but for each the predictive value was low. Conversely, a previous miscarriage or abortion lowered the risk of subsequent preeclampsia.

Assessment of difference in maternal diastolic blood pressure between the lateral decubitus and supine positions has modest predictive value in detecting patients destined to develop preeclampsia. Unfortunately, the test has a relatively high false-negative rate and takes approximately 10 minutes to perform properly. The angiotensin II infusion test has a better predictive value, but it is unsuitable clinically because it is invasive, time consuming, and not widely available. Changes in uteroplacental blood flow velocity measured by Doppler ultrasound eventually may prove helpful, but further assessment is necessary.

Few laboratory methods have proved useful in predicting preeclampsia. The maternal serum concentration of uric acid is elevated in virtually all women with preeclampsia, correlates well with disease severity, and may rise above control levels before the onset of clinical symptoms. However, this rise becomes significant only in the week before delivery, making this a rather late predictor. Elevated alpha-fetoprotein (AFP) measurements in the second trimester with no explainable cause have been associated with an increased risk of preeclampsia in the third trimester. However, discrepancies in the magnitude of risk between studies make it difficult to use AFP as an acceptable screening tool.

More recently, plasma fibronectins, a group of glycoproteins produced by many sources in the human body, have been found to be increased in women destined to become preeclamptic (Lockwood and Peters, 1990). A twofold increase in plasma fibronectin in patients with preeclampsia and in as many as 94% of subjects who eventually develop preeclampsia have been reported. In one study, this increase occurred in 75% of patients 1 month before the onset of hypertension (Lazarchick et al., 1986). Others have found that the type III domain of fibronectin, which is specific to vascular fibronectin, may be increased during the first trimester.

Patient and family history are as accurate as any other factors in predicting the likelihood of preeclampsia, and they cost nothing. Nulliparity itself has a minimal but real predictive value in that approximately 5% to 7% of women undergoing their first pregnancy will develop preeclampsia compared to <1% in normotensive multiparas. Among women with chronic hypertension, the rate of preeclampsia is at least 25% and approaches 75% in women with severe underlying hypertension. Black race has often been cited as a risk factor for the development of preeclampsia, but this has been refuted in recent studies (Sibai et al., 1995).

◊ PREVENTION OF PREECLAMPSIA

Although prenatal care has not been shown to prevent mild preeclampsia, it does reduce the incidence of severe disease and improve perinatal outcome. Preventive measures such as a low-salt diet, limitation of weight gain, nutritional supplementation, and diuretics have not proved beneficial. In addition, although bed rest may allow a patient with mild preeclampsia to continue her pregnancy, there is no evidence that prophylactic bed rest is beneficial in preventing disease (Mathews et al., 1982).

Low-Dose Aspirin

Aspirin binds irreversibly with the cyclooxygenase enzymes within platelets and inhibits TxA_2 synthesis. Although it also interferes with PGI_2 production by the vascular endothelium, the endothelial cell recovers the ability to produce PGI_2 within about 6 hours. These effects are largely dose dependent (Fig. 9). The selective inhibition of platelet TxA_2 synthesis by an intermittently administered low-dose aspirin may restore a more physiological PGI_2–TxA_2 balance in pregnant women with preeclampsia. This concept forms the rationale for clinical attempts at preventing preeclampsia with aspirin. Dipyridamole, another potentially beneficial drug, increases peroxidase activity within platelets, which indirectly increases PGI_2 production and inhibits platelet aggregation.

Initial clinical studies suggested that low-dose aspirin therapy was effective in reducing the risk of preeclampsia (Imperiale and Petulis, 1991; Beaufils et al., 1985; Wallenburg et al., 1986; Benigni et al., 1989; Schiff et al., 1989; McParland et al., 1990; Uzan et al., 1991). The published results of six randomized, controlled trials with a total of 326 treated and 240 untreated patients pooled by metaanalysis are summarized in Fig. 10. Most patients included in these trials were at moderate to substantial risk for preeclampsia based on a variety of factors. As shown, all outcomes studied occurred significantly less often in aspirin-treated pregnant women than in untreated controls. To the contrary, a larger, placebo-controlled trial in women at moderate to high risk for preeclampsia found no beneficial effect associated with low-dose aspirin (Caritis, 1997). This trial is particularly convincing in that it included over 1800 women with diabetes, chronic hypertension, or multifetal gestations.

Low-dose aspirin also has been studied in women at relatively low risk for preeclampsia. The largest study involved a multicenter, randomized trial in healthy nulliparous pregnant women and found no significant reduction in hypertensive disorders of pregnancy, including preeclampsia, associated with low-dose aspirin treatment. Investigators found, however, that

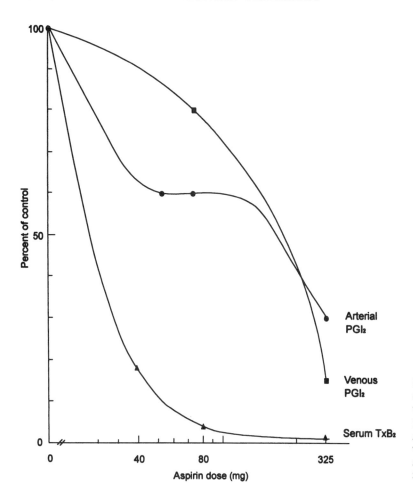

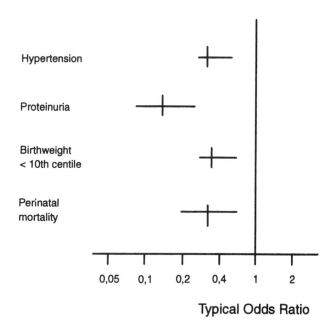

FIG. 9. Comparison of effects of aspirin ingestion on platelet production of thromboxane (TxB_2) and venous and aortic production of prostacyclin (PGI_2). (Adapted from Weksler BB, Pett SB, Alonso D, et al. Differential inhibition by aspirin of vascular and platelet prostaglandin synthesis in atherosclerotic patients. *N Engl J Med* 1983; 308:800.)

low-dose aspirin reduced the rate of preeclampsia in a subset of women whose systolic blood pressure was between 120 and 134 mm Hg at study entry (Sibai et al., 1993). A smaller, placebo-controlled trial noted that low-dose aspirin significantly reduced the rate of preeclampsia (Hauth et al., 1995). It is important to note, however, that low-dose aspirin did not alter the maternal or neonatal morbidity or mortality rates in either study of low-risk patients.

To summarize, available data regarding the efficacy of low-dose aspirin to prevent preeclampsia are conflicting, with the best studies finding either no effect on the rate of preeclampsia or no change in maternal or fetal morbidity or mortality.

Calcium

Diminished dietary calcium intake and hypocalciuria have been reported in patients with preeclampsia (Taufield et al., 1987). These findings have led to trials of calcium supplementation as a prophylactic measure. Initial studies were promising, with less preeclampsia in women treated with calcium in pregnancy (Belizan et al., 1991; Bucher et al., 1996; Lopez-Jaramillo et al., 1997). However, as with low-dose aspirin, a multicenter trial failed to find any difference in the rate of preeclampsia in low-risk women treated with calcium supplementation (Levine et al., 1997). In women at

FIG. 10. Graphic overview of odds ratios and 95% confidence intervals of the effects of low-dose aspirin on the occurrence of hypertension, preeclampsia, and fetal–neonatal sequelae from six randomized, controlled clinical trials. In patients at risk, all odds ratios are less than 1 in those who received low-dose aspirin. (Adapted from Bremer HA, Wallenberg HCS. Aspirin in pregnancy. *Fetal Matern Med Rev* 1992;4:37.)

high risk for preeclampsia, however, a randomized controlled trial found a significant reduction in the incidence of preeclampsia in calcium-supplemented patients (Sanchez-Ramos et al., 1994).

Other

Most pharmacologic attempts at preeclampsia prophylaxis have been unsuccessful. Diuretic agents have been used in women at high risk for the development of preeclampsia, but this practice has largely been abandoned, as no benefit could be found. The administration of other antihypertensives is usually reserved for women with diastolic blood pressures greater than 105 mm Hg. However, investigators in a recent randomized, controlled trial found a significant decrease in the development of preeclampsia in women treated with ketanserin, a serotonin-2-receptor blocker (Steyn and Odendaal, 1997). This drug is not available in the United States.

◊ PROGNOSIS

Preeclampsia typically resolves promptly after the infant and placenta are delivered. Even when the disease is severe, mother and child often can leave the hospital 2 to 3 days after vaginal delivery or at the customary time after cesarean section. Hypertension occasionally remains severe and difficult to control after delivery. In this situation, methyldopa or one of the agents discussed in Table 7 can be used as necessary. Asymptomatic women whose blood pressure remains elevated but is less than 160/100 mm Hg may be discharged without antihypertensive treatment as long as appropriate follow-up is planned. The blood pressure is monitored every week to make sure that the hypertension does not persist.

Preeclampsia and eclampsia do not contraindicate the use of oral contraceptives as long as the patient has become normotensive by the time the medication is prescribed, typically between postpartum weeks 3 and 6. Women who develop pill-induced hypertension after preeclampsia do so with about the same frequency as nonhypertensive women of comparable age. Pill-induced hypertension after preeclampsia often reflects underlying chronic vascular disease or essential hypertension.

In primigravidas with the typical mild form of preeclampsia, the disease usually does not recur in subsequent pregnancies. With severe preeclampsia, the recurrence rate is 30% to 50%. Most multiparous women who have had preeclampsia or eclampsia have some predisposing factor, commonly chronic hypertension. In these women, the recurrence of superimposed preeclampsia may be as high as 70% (Chesley, 1978). This does not invariably mean that a patient should not undertake another pregnancy; many women with recurrent mild forms of hypertension have little difficulty. The postpartum period is an ideal time for full investigation and preconceptional counseling regarding permanent sterilization or adequate preparation for the next pregnancy.

The patients perhaps most likely to seek counseling regarding the likelihood of preeclampsia are those who have suffered severe preeclampsia in a prior pregnancy. Investi-

gators have found that among young primigravidas with severe preeclampsia or eclampsia, 47% had preeclampsia in their second pregnancy, more than half of which were severe (Sibai et al., 1986). The same group has found that patients with severe preeclampsia in the second trimester of pregnancy have a 65% recurrence risk of preeclampsia in subsequent pregnancies (Sibai et al., 1991). Of those with preeclampsia, 32% developed the disease in the second trimester, and a similar proportion developed the disease between 28 and 36 weeks of gestation. Overall, severe preeclampsia complicated 21% of subsequent pregnancies in the second trimester. Another group found that 43% of women with HELLP syndrome would have preeclampsia in a subsequent gestation, and 27% would suffer recurrent HELLP syndrome (Sullivan et al., 1994).

◊ REFERENCES

American College of Obstetrics and Gynecology. Hypertension in pregnancy. *ACOG Tech Bull* 1996;219.

Beaufils M, Uzan S, Donsimoni R, Colau JC. Prevention of preeclampsia by early antiplatelet therapy. *Lancet* 1985;1:840–842.

Belizan JM, Villar J, Gonzalez L, et al. Calcium supplementation to prevent hypertensive disorders of pregnancy. *N Engl J Med* 1991;325:1399–1405.

Benigni A, Gregorini G, Frusca T, et al. Effect of low-dose aspirin on fetal and maternal generation of thromboxane by platelets in women at risk for pregnancy-induced hypertension. *N Engl J Med* 1989;321:357–362.

Branch DW, Andres R, Digre KB, et al. The association of antiphospholipid antibodies with severe preeclampsia. *Obstet Gynecol* 1990;73:541–545.

Bucher HC, Guatt GH, Cook RJ, Hatala R, Cook DJ, Lang JD, Hunt D. Effect of calcium supplementation on pregnancy induced hypertension and preeclampsia: a meta-analysis of randomized controlled trials. *JAMA* 1996;275:1113–1117.

Caritis SN. *Low-dose aspirin does not prevent preeclampsia in high risk women.* NICHD MFMU Network. Abstract 6. Paper presented at the Annual Meeting of the Society of Perinatal Obstetricians, January, 1997.

Chesley LC. *Hypertensive disorders in pregnancy.* New York: Appleton-Century-Crofts, 1978.

Cooper DW, Deane EM, Marshall P, Gallery EDM. C3 allotypes in pregnancy hypertension and eclampsia. *Hum Hered* 1988;38:52–55.

Cunningham FG, Lindheimer MD. Hypertension in pregnancy. *N Engl J Med* 1992;326:927–932.

Dizon-Townson D, Nelson L, Moline L, Easton K, Ward K. Severe preeclampsia is associated with the factor V Leiden mutation. *Am J Obstet Gynecol* 1996;174:343–346.

Dommise J. Phenytoin sodium and magnesium sulfate in the management of eclampsia. *Br J Obstet Gynaecol* 1990;97:104–109.

Eclampsia Trial Collaborative Group. Which anticonvulsant for women with eclampsia? Evidence from the Collaborative Eclampsia Trial. *Lancet* 1995;345:1455–1463.

Gant NF, Daley GL, Chand S, Whalley PJ, MacDonald PC. A study of angiotensin II pressor response throughout primigravid pregnancy. *J Clin Invest* 1973;52:2682–2689.

Gilstrap LC, Cunningham FG, Whalley PJ. Management of pregnancy-induced hypertension in the nulliparous patients remote from term. *Semin Perinatol* 1978;1:73.

Hauth JC, Goldenberg RL, Parker CR, et al. Low-dose aspirin therapy to prevent preeclampsia. *Am J Obstet Gynecol* 1993;168:1088–1093.

Hayward C, Livingstone J, Holloway S, Liston WA, Brock DJ. An exclusion map for preeclampsia: Assuming autosomal recessive inheritance. *Am J Hum Genet* 1992;50:749–757.

Hutton JD, James DK, Sirrat GM, et al. Management of severe pre-eclampsia and eclampsia by UK consultants. *Br J Obstet Gynaecol* 1992;99: 554–556.

Imperiale TF, Petulis AS. A meta-analysis of low-dose aspirin for the prevention of pregnancy-induced hypertensive disease. *JAMA* 1991;266: 260–264.

Klonoff-Cohen HS, Savitz DA, Cefalo RC, McCann MF. An epidemiologic study of contraception and preeclampsia. *JAMA* 1989;262:3143–3147.

Lazarchick J, Stubbs T, Romein L, VanDorsten JP, Loadholt CB. Predictive value of fibronectin levels in normotensive gravid women destined to become preeclamptic. *Am J Obstet Gynecol* 1986;154:1050–1052.

Levine RJ, Hauth JC, Curet LB, et al. Trial of calcium to prevent preeclampsia. *N Engl J Med* 1997;337:69–76.

Librach CL, Werb Z, Fitzgerald ML, et al. Ninety-two kilodalton type IV collegense mediates invasion of human cytotropholasts. *J Cell Biol* 1991; 113:437–439.

Lockwood CJ, Peters JH. Increased plasma levels of ED-1 cellular fibronectin precede the clinical science of preeclampsia. *Am J Obstet Gynecol* 1990; 162:358–362.

Lopez-Jaramillo P, Delgado F, Jacome P, Teran E, Ruano C, Rivera J. Calcium supplementation and the risk of preeclampsia in Ecuadorian pregnant teenagers. *Obstet Gynecol* 1997;90:162–167.

Lucas MJ, Leveno KJ, Cunningham FG. A comparison of magnesium sulfate with phenytoin for the prevention of eclampsia. *N Engl J Med* 1995; 333:201–205.

Magann EF, Bass D, Chauhan SP, et al. Antepartum corticosteroids: Disease stabilization in patients with the syndrome of hemolysis, elevated liver enzymes, and low platelets (HELLP). *Am J Obstet Gyncol* 1994;171: 1148–1153

Mathews DD, Agarwall V, Shuttleworth TP. A randomized control trial of complete bedrest versus ambulation in the management of proteinuric hypertension during pregnancy. *Br J Obstet Gynecol* 1982;89:128–131.

McCartney CP, Schumacher GF, Spargo BH. Serum proteins in patients with toxemic glomerular lesion. *Am J Obstet Gynecol* 1971;111:580–590.

McParland P, Pearce JM, Chamberlain GVP. Doppler ultrasound and aspirin in recognition and prevention of pregnancy-induced hypertension. *Lancet* 1990;1:1552–1555.

Mikhail MS, Anyaegbunam A, Garfinkel D, et al. Preeclampsia and antioxidant nutrients: decreased plasma levels of reduced ascorbic acid, alpha tocopherol, and geta carotene in women with preeclampsia. *Am J Obstet Gynecol* 1994;171:150–157.

Munz C, Holmes N, King A, Loke YW, Colonna M, Schild H, Rammensee HG. Human histocompatibility leukocyte antigen (HLA)-G molecules inhibit NKAT3 expressing natural killer cells. *J Exp Med* 1997;185: 385–391.

National High Blood Pressure Education Program Working Group. Report on high blood pressure during pregnancy. *Am J Obstet Gynecol* 1990; 163:1691–1712.

Odendaal HJ, Pattinson RC, Bam R, et al. Aggressive or expectant management for patients with severe preeclampsia between 28–34 weeks gestation: a randomized controlled trial. *Obstet Gynecol* 1990;76:1070–1075.

Redman CWG. Treatment of hypertension in pregnancy. *Kidney Int* 1980; 18:267–278.

Roberts JM, Taylor RM, Goldfein A. Clinical and biochemical evidence of endothelial cell dysfunction in the pregnancy syndrome preeclampsia. *Am J Hypertens* 1991;4:700–708.

Robillard PY, Hulsey TC, Perianin J, Janky E, Miri EH, Papiernik E. Association of pregnancy-induced hypertension with duration of sexual cohabitation before conception. *Lancet* 1994;344:973–975.

Sanchez-Ramos L, Briones D, Launitz A, Delvalle GO, Gaudier FS, Walker CD. Prevention of pregnancy induced hypertension by calcium supplementation in angiotensin II sensitive patients. *Obstet Gynecol* 1994;84:349–353.

Schiff E, Peleg E, Goldenberg M, et al. The use of aspirin to prevent pregnancy-induced hypertension and lower the ratio of thromboxane A$_2$ to prostacyclin in relatively high risk pregnancies. *N Engl J Med* 1989; 321:351–356.

Sibai BM, El-Nazer A, Gonzalez-Ruiz A. Severe preeclampsia–eclampsia in young primigravid women: subsequent pregnancy outcome and remote prognosis. *Am J Obstet Gynecol* 1986;155:1011–1016.

Sibai BM, Mercer BM, Schiff E, Friedman SA. Aggressive versus expectant management of severre preeclampsia at 28 to weeks gestation: a randomized controlled trial. *Am J Obstet Gynecol* 1994;171:818–822.

Sibai BM, Caritis SN, Thom E, et al: Prevention of preeclampsia with low-dose aspirin in healthy nulliparous pregnant women. *N Engl J Med* 1993;329:1213–1218

Sibai BM, Gordon T, Thom E, et al. Risk factors for preeclampsia in healthy nulliparous women: A prospective multicenter study. *Am J Obstet Gynecol* 1995;172:642–648.

Sibai BM, Adella TN, Anderson GD. Pregnancy outcome in 211 patients with mild chronic hypertension. *Obstet Gynecol* 1983;61:571.

Sibai BM, Akl S, Fairlie F, Moretti M. A protocol for managing severe preeclampsia in the second trimester. *Am J Obstet Gynecol* 1990;163: 733–738

Sibai BM, Mercer B, Sarinoglu C. Severe preeclampsia in the second trimester: Recurrence risk and long-term prognosis. *Am J Obstet Gynecol* 1991;65:1408–1412.

Silver RK, Kupferminc M, Russell T, et al. Evaluation of nitric oxide as a mediator of severe preeclampsia. *Am J Obstet Gynecol* 1996;175:1013–1017.

Simon P, Fauchet R, Pilorge M, et al. Association of HLA-DR4 with the risk of recurrence of pregnancy hypertension. *Kidney Int* 1988;34:S125.

Steyn DW, Odendaal HJ. Randomized controlled trial of ketanserin and aspirin in prevention preeclampsia. *Lancet* 1997;350:267–271.

Sullivan CA, Magann EF, Perry KG. The recurrence risk of the syndrome of hemolysis elevated liver enzymes, and low platelets (HELLP) in subsequent gestations. *Am J Obstet Gynecol* 1994;171:940–943.

Taufield PA, Ales KL, Resnick LM, et al. Hypocalciuria in preeclampsia. *N Engl J Med* 1987;316:715–718.

Uotila JT, Tuinaala RJ, Aarnis TM. Findings on lipid peroxidation and antioxidant function in hypertensive complications of pregnancy. *Br J Obstet Gynaecol* 1993;100:270–276.

Uzan S, Beaufils M, Breart G, et al. Prevention of fetal growth retardation with low-dose aspirin: findings of the EPREDA trial. *Lancet* 1991;337: 1427–1431.

Wallenburg HCS, Dekker GA, Mokovitz JW, Rotmans P. Low-dose aspirin prevents pregnancy-induced hypertension and preeclampsia in angiotensin-sensitive primigravidae. *Lancet* 1986;1:1–3.

Walsh SW. Lipid peroxidation in pregnancy. Hypertension in pregnancy. *World Rev Nutr Diet* 1994;76:114–118.

Ward K, Hata A, Jeunemaitre X, et al. A molecular variant of angiotensinogen associated with preeclampsia. *Nat Genet* 1993;4:59–61.

Weinstein L. Syndrome of hemolysis, elevated liver enzymes, and low platelet count: a severe consequence of hypertension in pregnancy. *Am J Obstet Gynecol* 1982;142:159–167.

Zhou Y, Damsky CH, Fisher SJ. Preeclampsia is associated with failure of human cytotrophoblasts to mimic a vascular adhesion phenotype. One cause of defective endovascular invasion in this syndrome? *J Clin Invest* 1997;99:2152–2164.

Zhou Y, Fisher SJ, Janatpour M, et al. Human cytotrophoblast adopt a vascular phenotype as they differentiate: a strategy for successful endovascular invasion? *J Clin Invest* 1997;99:2139–2151.

CHAPTER 23

Medical and Surgical Complications of Pregnancy

— ◊ —

Katharine D. Wenstrom
Maureen P. Malee

◊ HEMATOLOGIC DISEASE

Iron Deficiency Anemia

Anemia is defined as a hemoglobin (Hgb) concentration of less than 12 g/dl in nonpregnant women. During pregnancy, plasma volume expands proportionately more than Hgb or red cell volume, resulting in Hgb dilution. Anemia in gravid women is thus defined as a Hgb concentration of less than 10 g/dl. In addition to blood loss, anemia can result from decreased production or increased destruction of red blood cells. The initial workup consists of an examination of the red cell indices and a peripheral smear, with additional tests as indicated (Fig. 1).

Iron deficiency is the most common cause of anemia in gravid women, occurring in 15% to 25% of all pregnancies. Iron deficiency is suspected when the mean corpuscular volume (MCV) is less than $80/\mu m^3$, and is confirmed by demonstrating an elevated total iron-binding capacity (TIBC), a low serum iron, a serum iron–TIBC ratio less than 20%, and/or a low ferritin. Effects of iron deficiency on the fetus are usually minimal, although neonatal anemia is increased. Iron is actively transported across the placenta, and fetal iron and ferritin levels are three times higher than maternal levels. However, iron deficiency anemia has been weakly associated with preterm birth, and in the setting of severe maternal anemia (Hgb less than 6 g/dl), intrauterine growth restriction (IUGR) may occur. In pregnant women, iron deficiency can cause symptoms including fatigue, headache, lightheadedness, and reduced exercise tolerance. Blood loss at delivery may be tolerated poorly in anemic patients, and postpartum tissue healing may be compromised. For these reasons, treatment during pregnancy is recommended.

The total iron requirement of pregnancy is 1000 mg: 500 mg increases the maternal red blood cell mass, 300 mg is trans-ported to the fetus and placenta, and 200 mg compensates for blood loss at delivery. The iron requirements of pregnancy increase steadily toward term, but average 3.5 mg per day. Even though iron absorption efficiency increases during pregnancy, excess iron must be ingested to ensure sufficient dosing. The currently recommended supplementation for nonanemic gravidas is 300 mg of ferrous sulfate per day, which contains 60 mg of elemental iron. Anemic gravidas (Hgb of 8 or 9 g/dl) should take 300 mg ferrous sulfate twice or three times a day. Patients who cannot tolerate iron tablets may take an enteric-coated tablet or a liquid suspension (Table 1).

The severely anemic patient (Hgb less than 8 g/dl) may require parenteral therapy in the form of intramuscular or intravenous iron dextran. Because 0.2% to 0.3% of patients have an anaphylactic response to iron dextran, all patients should receive a small test dose 1 hour before the initiation of treatment, and therapy should be provided in an area with ready access to resuscitative medication and equipment. The total dose of iron required can be calculated using this formula:

Total dose of iron dextran (ml) = [0.0476 × body weight in kg × (desired Hgb concentration − observed Hgb concentration)] + 1 ml/5 kg of body weight up to a maximum of 14 ml

This dose can be given intramuscularly or intravenously (by slow push), 2 mg per day, until the total dose has been given, or the entire dose can be given diluted in 500 to 1000 ml of 0.9% saline and administered intravenously over 1 to 6 hours. Adequate parenteral therapy should result in a marked increase in the reticulocyte count within 7 to 14 days.

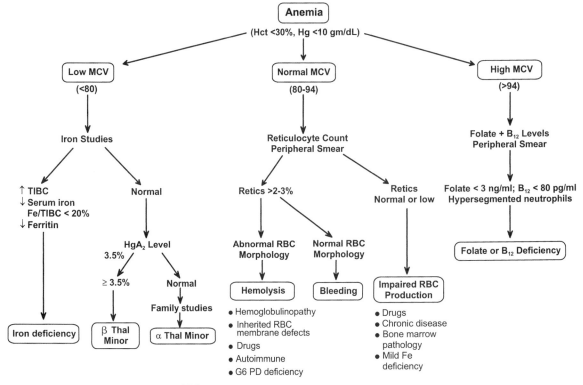

FIG. 1. Workup of anemia in pregnancy.

Megaloblastic Anemia

Megaloblastic anemia is characterized by red blood cells with increased MCV and white blood cells with altered morphology (hypersegmented neutrophils, anisocytosis, and poikilocytosis). It complicates up to 1% of pregnancies and is usually caused by folate deficiency, although it can occur after exposure to sulfa drugs or hydroxyurea or, rarely, because of vitamin B_{12} deficiency.

Folate deficiency can develop over a relatively short time because liver stores of folate are sufficient to meet the body's needs for only 1 to 2 months. Malnutrition (e.g., alcoholism), malabsorption, anticonvulsant therapy, oral contraceptive use, or pregnancy can rapidly deplete the body's folate stores. Hypersegmented neutrophils (more than 5% of neutrophils having five or more lobes) appear after 7 weeks of deficiency, red blood cell folate is reduced after 18 weeks, and anemia occurs after 20 weeks. The daily folate requirement for a nonpregnant individual is 50 to 100 µg; a pregnant woman needs 300 to 400 µg. This dose may be difficult to achieve through dietary manipulation because folate is

found primarily in fresh fruits and vegetables and is destroyed by cooking. As a separate issue, it now seems apparent that some women require excess folate to overcome a relative enzyme deficiency leading to high blood and amniotic fluid levels of homocysteine and an increased risk for fetal neural tube defects. For these reasons, women contemplating pregnancy should be advised to ingest a daily folic acid supplement (0.4 mg per day if there is no family history of neural tube defects; 4 mg per day if there is a family history), beginning before conception and continuing throughout the first trimester of pregnancy.

In contrast, *vitamin B_{12} deficiency* is rare because very little of the body's stores is used each day. Ingested vitamin B_{12} is bound to intrinsic factor produced by the parietal cells of the stomach and then absorbed through the mucosa of the distal ileum. Patients who have had a gastrectomy, ileitis, or ileal resection, or who have pernicious anemia, pancreatic insufficiency, or intestinal parasites may eventually become vitamin B_{12} deficient.

When megaloblastic anemia is suspected, the history should be reviewed for predisposing factors. The peripheral smear should be examined both to confirm altered cell morphology and to rule out a mixed (i.e., folate and iron) deficiency. Serum folate and vitamin B_{12} levels should be measured: A fasting folate level less than 3 ng/ml or a vitamin B_{12} level less than 80 pg/ml indicates deficiency. Folate deficiency responds to 0.5 to 1.0 mg folate orally per day, while a B_{12} deficiency requires vitamin B_{12}, 1 mg intramuscularly, per week for 6 weeks.

TABLE 1. *Iron preparations and dosages*

Preparations	Elemental iron content (%)	Dose containing 60 mg elemental iron (mg)
Ferrous fumarate	30	200
Ferrous gluconate	11	550
Ferrous sulfate	20	300

Thalassemia

Occasionally, a patient will have a microcytic anemia (MCV less than $80/\mu m^3$) without laboratory evidence of iron deficiency. In this situation, the Hgb concentration is low not because of insufficient substrate but because of a genetic defect in Hgb production called thalassemia. Thalassemia has a high incidence in certain ethnic groups, especially those originating in the Mediterranean basin, the Middle East, Africa, Asia, and India.

Hgb is a tetramer composed of two copies each of two different polypeptide chains; the identity of the chains determines the type of Hgb produced. During embryonic and fetal life, genes directing production of different types of polypeptide chains and thus different types of Hgb are switched on and then off sequentially. At birth, a normal individual produces α and β chains, along with very small quantities of δ and τ chains (Fig. 2). Normal adults produce primarily hemoglobin A (HgbA), composed of two α and two β polypeptide chains.

Two genes direct β-chain production, one on each copy of chromosome 11. Over 100 different gene mutations have been identified that prevent or reduce β-chain transcription; if one gene carries such a mutation, β-chain production will be reduced by half and abnormally low quantities of Hgb will be produced. This results in β-*thalassemia minor*. The excess α chains combine instead with δ chains, producing a molecule called HgbA₂, or with τ chains, producing hemoglobin F (HgbF). If β-thalassemia minor is suspected because the patient has microcytic anemia without iron deficiency, Hgb electrophoresis should be performed. Levels of HgbA₂ greater than 3.5% and HgbF greater than or equal to 2% confirm the diagnosis (Table 2). The gravid patient with β-thalassemia minor generally tolerates pregnancy well. She should receive folic acid supplementation, but not iron supplementation unless iron deficiency is also diagnosed.

TABLE 2. *Hemoglobin electrophoresis findings in various hemoglobinopathies*

Condition	HbA (%)	HbA₂ (%)	HbS (%)	HbF (%)	HbC (%)
Sickle cell trait	55–60	2–3	40–45	1	—
Sickle cell disease	0	2–3	85–95	5–15	—
Sickle cell/ β-thalassemia	10–20	3–5	60–80	10–20	—
Hemoglobin SC disease	0	2–3	45–50	1	45–50
β-thalassemia trait (β-thalassemia minor)	82–94	4–8	—	2–3	—
Normal	96–97	2–3	—	1	—

Patients with mutations preventing transcription of both β-chain genes have β-*thalassemia major* (β-thalassemia), or Cooley anemia. Erythropoiesis is ineffective because there is no β-chain production, and the α chains precipitate, causing red cell destruction. Occasionally, the mutations allow some β-chain production, resulting in a less severe reduction of Hgb synthesis (β⁺-thalassemia). Surviving women with this diagnosis are transfusion-dependent and often sterile.

An entity designated *thalassemia intermedia* has also been described, in which the clinical course is milder than with homozygous β-thalassemia. Some individuals with this condition produce large quantities of τ chains that combine with α chains to produce fetal Hgb; the presence of 17% to 35% fetal Hgb defines *hereditary persistence of HgbF*. Alternatively, these individuals may have some degree of α-thalassemia in addition to β-thalassemia, resulting in less α-chain precipitation and hemolysis. Patients with thalassemia intermedia have severe hemolytic anemia but generally are not transfusion-dependent.

Before genetic counseling is provided to the patient with β-thalassemia minor, MCV screening, followed by Hgb electrophoresis if the MCV is low, should be offered to the father of the fetus. If the father has normal Hgb, the fetus has a 50% chance to have β-thalassemia minor and a 25% chance to have normal Hgb. If the father has β-thalassemia minor, the fetus has a 50% chance to have β-thalassemia major, which is associated with increased morbidity and mortality. Prenatal testing of the fetus should be offered to high-risk women; at least 20% of β-chain mutations can be detected by chorionic villus sampling (CVS) or amniocentesis.

α-Chain production is directed by four genes, two on each copy of chromosome 16. Mutation of only one gene results in no clinical or laboratory abnormalities and is thus referred to as the silent carrier state. Mutations in two of the four genes results in α-*thalassemia minor*, a condition characterized by mild microcytic hypochromic anemia. Patients with α-thalassemia minor have a low MCV but normal levels of HgbA₂. The patient with these laboratory results should be referred for genetic evaluation and family studies to confirm the diagnosis.

Mutation of three of the four α genes results in *hemoglobin H (HgbH) disease*. Affected patients have some HgbA

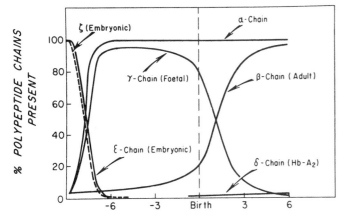

FIG. 2. Production of hemoglobin polypeptide chains in relationship to gestational age. (From Rucknagel DL, Laros RK. Hemoglobinopathies: genetics and implications for studies of human reproduction. *Clin Obstet Gynecol* 1969;12:4; with permission.)

and a large percentage of HgbH (four β-chains). The clinical course is characterized by chronic hemolytic anemia that may worsen in pregnancy. Loss of all four α-chain genes causes α-*thalassemia major*, resulting in fetal hydrops and perinatal death. As with β-thalassemia, testing of the father is crucial for accurate genetic counseling. Consideration of the patient's ethnic background is also important. Asians with α-thalassemia minor usually have the two mutant genes on the same chromosome (*cis* position), and thus have a 50% risk of passing on both affected genes with each conception. In contrast, patients of other ethnic origins usually carry the mutant genes on opposite chromosomes (*trans* position), so that only one affected gene can be transmitted with each conception. All forms of α-thalassemia can be detected by CVS or amniocentesis.

Hemoglobinopathies

Many Hgb gene mutations have been identified (over 400 to date) that alter polypeptide function, instead of preventing production. These Hgb variants generally have either reduced oxygen transport capabilities or cause hemolytic anemia. Hemoglobin S (HgbS) and hemoglobin C (HgbC) are the most frequent variants and can occur in association with thalassemia as well (Table 3).

A mutation causing a single amino acid substitution of valine for glutamic acid at position 6 on the β-chain changes normal Hgb to sickle Hgb. An individual who is homozygous for this mutation has *sickle cell anemia,* producing only HgbS and a small quantity of fetal Hgb (HgbF), but no HgbA. Sickle Hgb functions well in the oxygenated state but aggregates, forming rod-shaped polymers, in the deoxygenated state. Polymerized Hgb precipitates in the red blood cell, changing the cell from a biconcave disc to an elongated crescent or sickle shape. Sickled red blood cells are not deformable and cannot squeeze through the microcirculation; obstruction results in local hypoxia that leads to a vicious cycle of further sickling and obstruction. Localized ischemia and infarction cause tissue damage.

Patients with sickle cell anemia usually produce increased quantities of HgbF. HgbF is not distributed uniformly among all red cells but is present at levels of 0% to 20% per cell. In cells containing HgbF, restoration of normal oxygen tension may reverse the sickling and halt the destructive process. Cells containing little or no HgbF become irreversibly sick-

led and are rapidly cleared from the system in a process leading to hemolytic anemia; patients with homozygous HgbS typically have hematocrits of 20% to 30% and reticulocyte counts of 10% to 25%. Hydroxyurea therapy has been shown to increase both the number of red cells containing HgbF and the quantity of HgbF per cell. Unfortunately, there are few data regarding the safety of hydroxyurea use in pregnancy; it is a category D drug.

Any pathologic state causing acidosis, dehydration, or hypoxia can precipitate sickling, hemolysis, vasoocclusion, and infarction. Pregnancy is a time of stress and is often characterized by an increase in sickle crises and associated problems (e.g., pneumonia, pyelonephritis, pulmonary emboli, congestive heart failure) and by pregnancy complications such as IUGR, preterm birth, and preeclampsia. The goal of pregnancy management should be to maintain adequate oxygen delivery to the tissues and to avoid or rapidly control infections or other stressors that could precipitate a crisis.

Sickle cell anemia patients should ingest 1 mg of folate per day to support increased erythropoiesis in the face of chronic hemolysis, and should receive the polyvalent pneumococcal vaccine because chronic splenic infarction leads to functional asplenia by adulthood. Iron supplementation should not be given prophylactically but should be prescribed if there is laboratory evidence of iron deficiency anemia. All sickle cell patients should undergo a funduscopic examination, with laser therapy as needed, because they are at increased risk for proliferative retinopathy. Asymptomatic bacteriuria and other infections should be treated aggressively.

One controversy concerns the possible benefit of antepartum prophylactic exchange transfusions. A study by Cunningham et al. (1983) supports prophylactic transfusion. This group retrospectively compared the pregnancies of 24 women with sickle cell anemia who received prophylactic red blood cell transfusions initiated at or before midpregnancy, to the pregnancies of 24 sickle cell patients managed conventionally (blood transfusions performed only if indicated for clinical problems). In the prophylactic transfusion group, transfusions were initiated at or before midpregnancy and scheduled to maintain the hematocrit above 25% and the percentage of HgbA above 40%. The prophylactically transfused group required fewer antepartum hospitalizations, had less maternal morbidity, and experienced less perinatal morbidity and mortality than the conventionally managed group. However, some complications were associated with transfusion therapy. One woman developed anti-E alloimmunization, four women experienced accelerated destruction of donor red blood cells, and one patient suffering from iron overload attributed to the transfusions developed severe preeclampsia that precipitated heart failure and pulmonary edema, and subsequently died.

A study by Koshy et al. (1988) supports transfusion only for specific indications. In this prospective randomized trial, 36 patients received serial prophylactic transfusions beginning immediately upon entry into the study, and 36 received transfusions for medical or obstetric indications only. Although the

TABLE 3. *Frequency of sickle hemoglobinopathies in African-Americans*

Hemoglobinopathy	Frequency
Sickle cell trait (HbSA)	1:10
Sickle cell disease (HbSS)	1:400
Hemoglobin SC disease (HbSC)	1:800
Hemoglobin S / β-thalassemia	1:1250
Hemoglobin C trait (HbAC)	1:35
Hemoglobin C disease (HbCC)	1:4800

prophylactically transfused group did have fewer pain crises, other maternal morbidity and perinatal outcome was not significantly different between the groups. These results are hard to interpret, however, as sickle cell patients with neurologic dysfunction, nephrotic syndrome or renal failure, liver disease, lung disease, coagulopathy, or red cell antibodies were excluded from entry into the study. Additionally, 44% of the control patients received transfusions during their pregnancies.

One interpretation of the available data is that while some women with sickle cell anemia may escape prophylactic transfusion because they have no associated organ damage, very few crises, and a high percentage of HgbF, many sickle cell patients will require antepartum transfusion. Even those patients who avoid transfusion during pregnancy should be transfused prior to delivery, as the stresses of labor, anesthesia, operative delivery, and any associated complications (e.g., preeclampsia, chorioamnionitis) can precipitate a serious crisis. Transfusions should be planned to achieve a hematocrit above 30% and HgbA above 50%. Unless complications dictate otherwise, delivery can be at term, with cesarean section for obstetric indications only.

Substitution of lysine for glutamic acid at the sixth position of the β chain results in the production of HgbC. HgbC is less soluble than HgbA and can cause a mild hemolytic anemia, but it is more stable than HgbS under hypoxic conditions. Nonpregnant women who are compound homozygotes for HgbS and HgbC generally have less severe anemia and fewer pain crises than women with HgbSS, but under the stress of pregnancy they experience the same maternal morbidity and pregnancy complications. Additionally, severe bone pain frequently occurs in individuals with HgbSC, and acute respiratory compromise as the result of embolization of necrotic bone marrow has been reported. The antenatal management of women with HgbSC should be the same as that of women with HgbSS.

If one β-chain gene carries the sickle cell mutation and the other gene is functionally deleted, the patient has *sickle cell–β-thalassemia*. Pregnancy-related morbidity in these patients is the same as for sickle cell anemia, and they should be managed similarly. Patients with *HgbCC* or *C-β-thalassemia* have a very mild anemia and usually do not experience hemoglobinopathy-related pregnancy complications.

Heterozygotes for the sickle Hgb mutation have *sickle cell trait*. Individuals with sickle trait have red cells that sickle under conditions of markedly reduced oxygen tension (i.e., the sickle Dex test), but Hgb electrophoresis confirms the presence of 55% to 60% HgbA, in addition to 35% to 40% HgbS. Sickling does nor occur *in vivo*, except under conditions of severe stress and hypoxia. Because the renal medulla is especially sensitive to reduced oxygen tension, patients with sickle trait may have episodes of painless, self-limited hematuria. During pregnancy, they exhibit an increased susceptibility to urinary tract infections. There are also reports of increased preeclampsia in these patients. Sickle trait patients should be offered genetic counseling; the father of the fetus should be tested so that the precise risk to the fetus can

be provided. Prenatal diagnosis is possible by CVS or amniocentesis. No special therapy is generally required during labor and delivery.

Congenital Hemolytic Anemias

Hereditary Spherocytosis, Elliptocytosis, and Pyropoikilocytosis

Hemolytic anemia can occur for a variety of reasons. It may result from a hemoglobinopathy, may be autoimmune, drug-induced, or pregnancy-induced (very rarely), or may occur as the result of inherited red cell membrane abnormalities. Hereditary spherocytosis, elliptocytosis, and pyropoikilocytosis result from congenital defects of different red cell membrane proteins. All are autosomal-dominant disorders occurring at an incidence of 1 in 4000 to 5000. All result in variant red cell shapes, such that affected red cells cannot readily pass through the spleen. While trapped in the spleen, the cell membranes are damaged, leading to red cell lysis, hemolytic anemia, jaundice, and splenomegaly. Splenectomy is the treatment of choice and effectively eliminates the anemia. Most women of reproductive age will already have undergone splenectomy. Although the abnormality of red cell shape persists, affected women tolerate pregnancy, labor, and delivery well, with few associated problems. The rare patient who has not undergone splenectomy may experience hemolytic anemia sufficient to require red cell transfusions. All patients should receive the polyvalent pneumococcal vaccine and should ingest a folic acid supplement throughout pregnancy. Infection should be treated aggressively, as it may cause hemolysis. The offspring of affected individuals have a 50% chance of inheriting the condition. Affected neonates may experience severe neonatal jaundice requiring exchange transfusion or splenectomy.

Glucose-6-phosphate Dehydrogenase Deficiency

Glucose-6-phosphate dehydrogenase (G6PD) deficiency is an inherited defect of an enzyme essential to the hexose monophosphate shunt. Because of this defect, under oxidant stress Hgb sulfhydryl groups become oxidized, and Hgb precipitates in the red blood cell, leading to hemolytic anemia. The gene is most prevalent among individuals of African, Asian, Mediterranean, or Middle Eastern origin. Known stressors include viruses, bacteria, toxins, fava beans, and certain drugs such as antimalarials, sulfa drugs, and nitrofurantoin. Over 400 different gene mutations leading to G6PD deficiency have been described; the A variant is most common and is present in 1 in 20 black men and 1 in 10 black women in the United States. Although G6PD deficiency is X-linked and males are preferentially affected, women with this gene defect can be symptomatic; some heterozygotes have markedly reduced G6PD levels because unfavorable lyonization can lead to a large proportion of cells expressing the defect, and homozygosity for G6PD deficiency can occur (in at least 1 in 400 black women). Precipitating drugs should be avoided in known carriers.

Platelet Disorders

Thrombocytopenia, defined as a platelet count less than 150,000/mm³, occurs relatively frequently in pregnancy. Burrows and Kelton prospectively monitored 2284 pregnancies over 1 year and determined that 8.3% of normal gravidas have platelet counts of 97,000/mm³ to 150,000/mm³, without any associated maternal or fetal morbidity. The diagnosis of mild pregnancy-associated thrombocytopenia is one of exclusion, however, requiring that other pathologic forms of thrombocytopenia be ruled out. Thrombocytopenia in pregnancy can be caused by defective platelet production (bone marrow pathology such as leukemia, lymphoma, metastatic disease), sequestration (splenomegaly), or accelerated platelet destruction; accelerated destruction occurs most commonly. Destructive processes may be nonimmunologic and unique to pregnancy (e.g., preeclampsia, placental abruption), may occur as part of sepsis or disseminated intravascular coagulation, or may result from immune dysfunction (e.g., systemic lupus erythematosus, immune thrombocytopenic purpura). These causes of thrombocytopenia are discussed elsewhere.

Thrombotic Thrombocytopenic Purpura

Thrombotic thrombocytopenic purpura (TTP) is a disorder characterized by the pentad of thrombocytopenia, hemolytic anemia, fever, neurologic abnormalities, and renal failure. It is rare and of unknown etiology, and affects individuals of all ages, although most commonly young women. The untreated mortality rate exceeds 90%. Patients typically present with bleeding (uterine, gastrointestinal, or other) along with a mild Coombs-negative hemolytic anemia, thrombocytopenia, and mild jaundice. Hypertension and renal failure occur later in the course of the disease. All disease signs and symptoms result from microvascular damage caused by platelet thrombi, fibrin deposition, and microaneurysms in arterioles. Endothelial cell function, including prostaglandin production, is abnormal, although it is not known whether this causes TTP or results from it. Immune dysfunction may play a role.

When TTP manifests in the third trimester, it may be difficult to distinguish from preeclampsia or the syndrome of hemolysis, elevated liver enzymes, and low platelets (HELLP syndrome). One distinguishing feature is that tests of coagulation (prothrombin time, partial thromboplastin time, fibrinogen, fibrin dimers) are usually normal in TTP. The advent of a fever of unknown origin or transient neurologic symptoms, as well as nonspecific complaints of arthralgias, nausea, or abdominal pain, may aid in diagnosis. End-organ damage worsens as the disease persists. Delirium, seizures, hemiparesis, visual field defects, and coma indicate a very poor prognosis and an increased risk of mortality.

Distinguishing TTP from preeclampsia in its various forms is vital because TTP responds only to plasmapheresis or exchange transfusion, although delivery is eventually curative for preeclampsia. Steroids, heparin, splenectomy, and antiplatelet drugs have had only variable success in management of this disease. Plasmapheresis should be initiated as soon as the diagnosis is made, regardless of the clinical severity. If the patient is at or near term, magnesium sulfate therapy and delivery should also be initiated because of the possibility that the true diagnosis is preeclampsia. Cesarean delivery should be for obstetric indications only.

Hemolytic Uremic Syndrome

Hemolytic uremic syndrome (HUS) is similar to TTP, with similar microangiopathy, except that the kidneys are primarily affected. The patient usually presents with hemolytic anemia, thrombocytopenia, and oliguric renal failure; laboratory tests reveal a normal coagulation profile and hemoglobinuria. Most patients are hypertensive. The pathologic process is usually confined to the kidney, although some patients have mild neurologic symptoms. *Postpartum renal failure* is probably the same entity, except that the pregnancy has already ended. Treatment in both cases consists of dialysis and red blood cell transfusions to maintain the hematocrit above 20%. Maternal morbidity and mortality are significant, with death frequently resulting from uncontrollable hemorrhage.

◊ COAGULATION DEFECTS

Von Willebrand Disease

Von Willebrand disease is an inherited defect of von Willebrand factor (vWF), one of the proteins in the coagulation cascade. vWF is a large glycoprotein synthesized by endothelial cells and megakaryocytes and serves two functions: It is the plasma carrier for factor VIII, and it allows normal platelet aggregation at sites of endothelial injury. These two functions are directed by two different regions of the molecule, and several different mutations in both of these domains have been identified. There are three forms of von Willebrand disease.

Type I (approximately 75% of cases) and type II von Willebrand disease (25%) are inherited as autosomal-dominant traits. Affected individuals have one normal vWF gene in addition to the abnormal gene, and some normal vWF will therefore be produced. As a result, individuals with type I disease are usually mildly affected, exhibiting easy bruising or bleeding only after dental procedures. Individuals with type II disease usually experience more severe bleeding problems, such as menorrhagia or corpus luteum hemorrhage. Type III disease is autosomal-recessive and extremely rare and is usually associated with severe symptoms because affected patients have no normal allele and thus produce no vWF. Clinical manifestations are similar to those associated with hemophilia. The many different known mutations and heterozygosity in the majority of cases account for the variability observed in symptoms and in laboratory test results.

If the diagnosis is not made before pregnancy, it may be considered after excessive bleeding from a surgical or episiotomy site. In retrospect, the patient may describe easy bruising or heavy periods. The pedigree is likely to include other similarly affected family members. The diagnosis is confirmed by all or some combination of the following laboratory tests: a prolonged bleeding time, decreased vWF concentration, reduced ristocetin cofactor activity, and reduced factor VIII activity.

Women with von Willebrand disease usually tolerate pregnancy well, in large part because the production of all coagulation factors is increased and vWF factor levels can reach near-normal levels. Despite this, the bleeding time may still be prolonged, and treatment may be required. If the bleeding time is prolonged at term, levels of vWF must be increased so that postpartum or surgical hemorrhage can be avoided. One way to increase the vWF level is to administer desmopressin acetate for 48 hours prior to planned delivery. Patients with type I disease have the best response to desmopressin; those with type III disease usually do not respond at all. Alternatively, vWF replacement can be provided. Fresh frozen plasma contains all coagulation factors in equal proportions, cryoprecipitate contains factor VIII, vWF, and fibrinogen, and lyophilized factor VIII contains only that protein. For patients with von Willebrand disease, the recommended therapy is 15 to 20 U of cryoprecipitate given twice daily just prior to delivery and for 2 to 3 days afterward. Factor VIII concentrate can be administered instead. Effective treatment should normalize the bleeding time.

Women with type I or type II von Willebrand disease have a 50% risk of having an affected child; those with type III disease have minimal risk, unless they are related to their spouse. Prenatal diagnosis is possible but, unless termination is a consideration, is unlikely to affect labor and delivery management, as affected neonates experience minimal bleeding difficulties.

Hemophilias A and B

Hemophilias A and B result from X-linked deficiencies of two different coagulation proteins. Female carriers of hemophilia A have a mutation in one factor VIII gene, while carriers of hemophilia B have a mutation in one gene for factor IX; levels of these factors are thus reduced by half or more. These decreased factor levels are adequate for normal hemostasis, and carrier women are usually clinically unaffected. In rare circumstances, a woman may exhibit all the classic features of hemophilia (i.e., if she is homozygous for the mutation or if she is a carrier and has unfavorable lyonization leading to preferential expression of the X chromosome carrying the mutation); such patients benefit from factor replacement.

Carrier mothers should be offered genetic counseling. Half their daughters will be carriers, and half their sons will have hemophilia. Prenatal diagnosis is available. Knowledge of fetal hemophilia status allows consideration of pregnancy termination. In ongoing pregnancies, knowledge that a male fetus carries a hemophilia gene allows the obstetrician to plan to avoid a scalp electrode during labor and vacuum or forceps delivery. Cesarean delivery should be for obstetric indications only, as atraumatic spontaneous vaginal delivery does not entail additional risk for the affected fetus.

◊ GASTROINTESTINAL DISEASES

Nausea and Vomiting

Mild and self-limited nausea and vomiting in the first trimester of pregnancy occur in 60% to 80% of women. Chronic nausea and vomiting, or hyperemesis gravidarum, complicates 1 in 200 to 300 pregnancies. This disorder is characterized by dehydration, electrolyte imbalance, and nutrition depletion, and prompts medical intervention.

The etiology of hyperemesis is unclear. Theories have suggested the influence of human chorionic gonadotropin, the pituitary–adrenal axis, transient hyperthyroidism, and psychogenic factors. Regardless of the cause, intervention is appropriate, ranging from intravenous hydration and antiemetics (e.g., droperidol, metoclopramide, and prochlorperazine) to nasogastric enteral feeding and hyperalimentation. Pregnancies complicated by mild or severe hyperemesis are not at increased risk for growth abnormalities, congenital anomalies, or prematurity (Table 4).

Reflux Esophagitis

Half of all pregnant women complain of reflux esophagitis, or heartburn, sometime during pregnancy, particularly in the third trimester. Complaints include burning substernal discomfort with or without radiation, dysphagia exacerbated by meals, increased intraabdominal pressure, all worse in the recumbent position. The differential diagnosis includes angina, achalasia, and structural or functional causes of dysphagia.

Reflux esophagitis may result from decreased gastroesophageal sphincter tone, delayed gastric emptying, or mechanical displacement of intraabdominal viscera by the enlarging uterus. Treatment is similar to treatment of the nonpregnant population: antacids after meals and avoidance of overeating or eating at bedtime. In severe refractory cases, cimetidine and metoclopramide are appropriate therapeutic interventions.

Peptic Ulcer Disease

Gastric secretion and motility are reduced and mucus secretion is increased during gestation. As a result, peptic ulcer disease (PUD) is uncommon in pregnancy, and its complications, such as hemorrhage and perforation, quite rare. Patients with PUD often experience considerable improvement, if not remission, of disease in pregnancy; PUD recurs in most within 2 years of delivery.

Upper Gastrointestinal Bleeding

Hyperemesis can be accompanied by gastrointestinal (GI) bleeding. Although GI bleeding prompts a concern for PUD with hemorrhage, most pregnant women with hematemesis will prove to have Mallory-Weiss tears. These small, linear mucosal tears near the gastroesophageal junction respond to iced saline lavage, antacids, and intravenous cimetidine. Endoscopy can be performed in pregnancy and will detect esophageal rupture with bleeding (Boerhaave syndrome), a

TABLE 4. *Gastrointestinal disease in pregnancy*

Disorder	Frequency	Trimester	Symptomatology	Treatment	Perinatal outcome
Hyperemesis	Common	First	Nausea and vomiting	Antiemetics; nutrition support	Unaffected
Reflux esophagitis	Common	Third	Heartburn	Antacids	Unaffected
Peptic ulcer disease	Uncommon	—	—	—	Unaffected
Cholecystitis	Uncommon	Any	Postprandial pain, nausea, anorexia	Bowel rest; hydration; surgery	Unaffected
Pancreatitis	Uncommon	Any	Midepigastric pain, anorexia, nausea, emesis	Bowel rest; hydration; pain relief	Unaffected
Inflammatory bowel disease	Common	Any	Bloody diarrhea	Sulfasalazine; steroids; immunosuppressive drugs	Probably worsened
Hepatitis	Common	Any	Fever, nausea, emesis, fatigue, jaundice	Supportive	Vertical transmission
Acute fatty liver	Rare	Third	Malaise, nausea, vomiting, epigastric pain	Delivery; supportive	Unaffected if aggressive treatment of mother

much more serious diagnosis for which surgery and gastroenterology consultations are appropriate.

Cholelithiasis and Biliary Disease

Studies utilizing serial ultrasound examinations over the course of pregnancy confirm that the risk of gallstones is increased, to an incidence of 2% to 10%, because pregnancy is characterized by decreased gallbladder motility and increased biliary sludge. Many women with cholelithiasis are relatively asymptomatic during pregnancy and require no intervention. However, acute cholecystitis complicates about 1 in 1000 to 1600 gestations. It is heralded by postprandial pain in the right upper quadrant or epigastric area, with radiation to the back or shoulder. This type of pain, with anorexia, nausea, emesis, low-grade fever, and leukocytosis, suggests stone obstruction of a duct. Ultrasound examination is very helpful, detecting approximately 95% of stones.

Management is the same as in a nonpregnant individual. Three-fourths of patients with acute cholecystitis will respond to medical therapy consisting of bowel rest, nasogastric suction, intravenous hydration, antibiotics, and analgesics. The remainder will require surgical intervention for persistent pain, empyema, gangrene, or perforation. Open laparoscopic cholecystectomy during pregnancy is becoming more widely accepted. Although the second trimester is considered optimal for any surgical procedure, delay in treatment should be avoided regardless of gestational age.

Pancreatitis

Pancreatitis occurs with an incidence of 1 in 1500 to 4000 during pregnancy; most cases are due to cholelithiasis. Ethanol abuse, certain medications, trauma, and hypertriglyceridemia are etiologic far less often. Symptoms include midepigastric pain with back radiation, anorexia, nausea, and emesis. In normal pregnancy, serum amylase and lipase levels tend to increase only slightly with advancing gestation. The upper limits of normal for amylase and lipase in the first two trimesters are 100 U/dl and 200 U/dl, respectively. Significant elevations of these enzymes are therefore consistent with pancreatitis, although the degree of elevation does not correlate with disease severity. As in the nonpregnant population, pancreatitis is managed by bowel rest, nasogastric suction, analgesia, and intravenous hydration.

In most patients, inflammation subsides within 2 to 7 days. In the minority, abscess or pseudocyst formation prompts abdominal exploration. In this population, perinatal morbidity ranges from 5% to 15%, and perinatal mortality can be as high as 38%, most likely resulting from accompanying hypovolemia, hypoxia, and acidosis.

Inflammatory Bowel Disease

The term *inflammatory bowel disease* refers to two forms of intestinal inflammation, namely, Crohn disease and ulcerative colitis. These diseases share many features in common but can usually be differentiated. Their etiology is unclear, although there appears to be a genetic predisposition.

The effect of inflammatory bowel disease on perinatal outcome is unclear, as reports conflict regarding the coincidence of preterm labor and delivery or IUGR. The risk of preterm delivery may be increased as much as threefold, and IUGR twofold. Attention should be given to patient education and careful monitoring of fetal growth.

Ulcerative Colitis

Ulcerative colitis involves mucosal and submucosal layers of the rectum, extending without interruption proximally for a variable distance. Patients often complain of colicky abdominal pain and bloody diarrhea and may have arthritis, uveitis, or erythema nodosum. Colon cancer occurs in 1% per year. The clinical course is one of exacerbations and remissions. The most serious complication is toxic megacolon, which can necessitate an emergency colectomy. Medical management includes sulfasalazine (Azulfidine), mesalamine, and prednisone. If ulcerative colitis is quiescent at the time of conception, only one-third to one-half of patients will experience reactivation, often in the first trimester. Active disease at the time of conception has a worse prognosis. When the disease is active, aggressive medical management, including parenteral nutrition, is essential.

Crohn Disease

Crohn disease is different from ulcerative colitis in several respects. The degree of bowel involvement is greater and can be transmural. Both small and large bowel can be involved, and "skip" areas are common. Symptoms can include diarrhea but are more often obstructive in nature. Complications include toxic megacolon and fistula formation, which is problematic for vaginal delivery if the perineum is involved. As in ulcerative colitis, the patient may also have arthritis, and the risk of cancer is increased. Cancer risk correlates with the extent of mucosal pathology (pancolitis confers the highest risk) and the duration of the disease; in patients with long-standing disease, the risk exceeds 1% per year. Quiescent disease at conception carries a good prognosis. Prednisone, sulfasalazine, and immunosuppressant drugs help control disease activity. Surgery is necessary in about 5% of such pregnant patients.

Hepatitis

Acute viral hepatitis in pregnancy is a systemic illness with fever, nausea, emesis, and fatigue. Jaundice is common at presentation, and liver function tests are markedly elevated. With the exception of hepatitis E viral (HEV) infection, viral hepatitides do not occur more frequently or with greater severity in pregnancy. *HEV infection* is more dangerous in a pregnant patient, with a mortality of 15% to 20%. It is transmitted by the fecal–oral route and occurs most frequently in countries with poor sanitation (e.g., the Middle East, Africa, and India). Infection in the third trimester is often associated with fulminant hepatitis, as well as preterm delivery, neonatal death, and maternal death.

Hepatitis A

Hepatitis A virus (HAV) is a RNA virus, with fecal–oral transmission and an incubation period of 15 to 50 days. This highly contagious disease is self-limited, with resolution over 2 to 3 weeks. Acute HAV infection is confirmed by a positive anti-HAV IgM antibody test. There are no chronic sequelae, and HAV does not cross the placenta. A single dose of hepatitis immune globulin is recommended as soon as possible after exposure. If the exposed pregnant patient becomes in-fected, close contacts, including the neonate, should be offered passive immunotherapy.

Hepatitis B

Hepatitis B virus (HBV) is a double-stranded DNA virus. Its incubation period is 40 to 100 days, and it can be recovered from all body fluids, most importantly, blood, breast milk, and amniotic fluid. HBV surface antigen (HBsAg) and anti-HBc IgM antibody are seen in the early clinical phase of infection, before icteric changes or elevations in liver function tests; they indicate infectivity (Fig. 3). The presence of HBV e antigen (HBeAg) denotes active viral replication. While HBeAg usually indicates acute infection, its persistence correlates both with the chronic carrier state and with the ultimate development of hepatocellular carcinoma. The risk of maternal–fetal transmission increases with maternal viremia late in pregnancy and is thought to result from exposure of the fetus to infected tissues and blood at delivery or, rarely, from vertical transmission. If the mother develops HBV infection remote from delivery and has developed anti-HB antibodies, the risk of fetal or neonatal infection is less. Thus, if the pregnant patient contracts HBV in the second trimester, only 6% of neonates are seropositive; this increases to 67% in the third trimester and 100% immediately postpartum.

The absence of HBsAg excludes active or chronic infection, and there is no risk for neonatal transmission. In the at-risk patient who is HBsAg- and antibody-negative, HBV vaccination should be offered, as it is not contraindicated in pregnancy. If the patient is HBsAg-positive at delivery, the fetus is at high risk for acute infection; in the presence of HBeAg or anti-HBe antibody, the fetus is at increased risk of becoming a chronic carrier. The neonate's risk of active or chronic disease is significantly reduced by HB immune globulin and the HBV vaccine; these should be given at de-

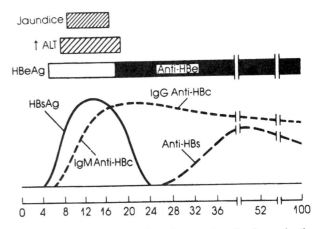

FIG. 3. Timing of hepatitis B antigen and antibody production in acute hepatitis B infection. (From Dienstag JL, Isselbacher KJ. Acute hepatitis. In: Isselbacher KJ, Braunwald E, Wilson JD, Martin JB, Fauci AS, Kasper DL, eds. *Harrison's principles of internal medicine,* 13th ed. New York: McGraw-Hill, 1994:1458; with permission.)

livery. The mother should be followed serially for the disappearance of HBsAg and the appearance of HBs antibody. Once HBs antibody appears, the baby is no longer at risk. Breast-feeding does not increase the risk of infection in these infants.

Hepatitis C

Hepatitis C virus (HCV) is the agent primarily responsible for non-A, non-B (posttransfusion) hepatitis. HCV is a single-stranded RNA virus. Principal risk factors for HCV transmission are blood product transfusion and intravenous drug use. Acute HCV infection follows an incubation period of 3 to 60 days, and only 25% of infected patients will be symptomatic. The presence of HCV antibody indicates chronic infection and does not confer immunity; approximately half of those infected develop chronic liver disease. No specific therapy has been shown to be efficacious in decreasing the morbidity of the disease. Coinfection with HCV and human immunodeficiency virus (HIV) is thought to accelerate the progression of hepatic injury.

Seroprevalence studies in pregnant patients in the United States indicate an incidence of hepatitis C of 2% to 4%. The maternal–fetal transmission rate is less than 5% with acute infection and 10% with chronic infection. Coinfection with HIV is associated with an increased rate of perinatal transmission to 23% to 44%. Breast-feeding in the HCV-positive patient is not contraindicated.

Hepatitis D

Hepatitis D virus (HDV) is a RNA virus that is dependent on coinfection with HBV for replication. HDV is acquired as a coinfection with HBV or as a superinfection in a chronic HBV carrier. Coinfection rarely leads to chronic disease, whereas superinfection is associated with an 80% likelihood of chronic hepatitis. Perinatal transmission of HDV can be prevented by the same immunoprophylaxis used for HBV.

Pregnancy following Liver Transplantation

Following liver transplantation, most authorities recommend that pregnancy be avoided for at least 12 months, so that graft viability can be assessed and immunosuppression can be achieved with the lowest possible medication doses. Thirty-eight percent of liver transplant patients are hypertensive; pregnancy does not increase this incidence or hasten graft rejection. The incidence of spontaneous abortion is similar to that of the general pregnant population, and the incidence of preeclampsia is 13.5%. Anemia complicates 31% of pregnancies in liver transplant patients, and rejection develops or worsens in 9%. Fifty-eight percent deliver at term, and the majority deliver appropriately grown babies vaginally.

Acute Fatty Liver

Acute fatty liver of pregnancy (AFLP) has an incidence of 1 in 13,000 deliveries. AFLP accounts for a large percentage of severe liver disease in pregnancy and is accompanied by a mortality of up to 25%. Primiparity, male fetal sex, and multiple gestation appear to confer a higher risk. The etiology is unknown, and liver biopsy reveals microvesicular fatty infiltrates.

Symptoms typically appear in the late third trimester and include malaise, persistent nausea, and vomiting. Right upper quadrant or epigastric pain is noted in 50% to 80%. Laboratory abnormalities include elevated liver function tests, increased ammonia and uric acid, hemolysis, hypoglycemia, and coagulopathy. Early recognition is essential; if untreated, AFLP progresses to multiorgan system failure and death. Once it is diagnosed, intensive supportive care is provided, and delivery is accomplished. Under these circumstances, maternal and fetal mortality are less than 20%. Survivors have no long-term sequelae, and recurrence in subsequent pregnancies is a rarity.

◊ CARDIOVASCULAR DISEASE

Physiologic Changes in Pregnancy

Normal pregnancy entails many physiologic changes that can stress the cardiovascular system. The plasma volume increases by 50%, while the red cell mass increases by only 25%, resulting in a physiologic anemia. Cardiac output increases by 30% to 50% during the first half of pregnancy (as the result of an increase in both stroke volume and heart rate), by a further 30% during active labor, and by 45% during pushing. Systemic vascular resistance decreases during pregnancy, with both systolic and diastolic blood pressures falling during the second trimester and then returning to prepregnancy values in the third trimester. During labor, each uterine contraction results in an autotransfusion of 300 to 500 ml of blood. Cardiac output during this time is influenced by maternal vascular volume, maternal position, pain, and the method of pain relief (epidural anesthesia, spinal anesthesia, or intravenous narcotics). Cardiac output rapidly increases at delivery, as the result of autotransfusion and relief of caval compression by the involuting uterus.

Women with cardiovascular disease may tolerate these physiologic changes poorly. Knowledge of the pregnancy-associated risks and complications associated with each type of heart disease allows the physician to choose management that optimizes the chances for a good pregnancy outcome. For each patient, the prepregnancy cardiovascular status should be established and used as a reference in assessing any pregnancy-related cardiac changes. The New York Heart Association (NYHA) classification scheme is useful for quantifying symptomatology:

◊ Class I—patients are asymptomatic in all situations;

◊ Class II—patients are symptomatic only with exertion;

◊ Class III—patients are symptomatic during activities of daily living;

◊ Class IV—patients are symptomatic at rest.

While useful for categorizing symptoms, this classification scheme does not necessarily predict pregnancy outcome. In one large retrospective study, for example, the majority of cases of pulmonary edema and maternal death occurred in women who were functional class I or class II. However, this scheme can be used to assess changes in cardiac function. Any change in cardiac classification during the pregnancy, even if only from class I to class II, can be ominous and should prompt a thorough evaluation and aggressive management; bed rest or hospitalization is often required.

Rheumatic Heart Disease

Approximately 4% of reproductive age women have heart disease. While this number has remained fairly constant, the relative incidence of the various forms of heart disease has changed dramatically in the last few decades. During most of the 20th century, the majority of heart disease resulted from rheumatic fever; the ratio of rheumatic heart disease to congenital heart disease was 20 to 1. In the last few decades, however, the prevalence of rheumatic heart disease has significantly decreased, while the number of adult survivors with congenital heart disease has increased; the ratio is now 3 to 1 or less. Nevertheless, rheumatic valvular disorders still account for a substantial proportion of heart disease in reproductive-age women.

Mitral Stenosis

Mitral stenosis is the most common form of rheumatic heart disease in women. Rheumatic fever typically occurs at ages 6 to 15 years. If myocarditis is present, mitral insufficiency will develop, followed in approximately 5 years by mitral stenosis. Symptoms usually do not begin for another 15 years after that, with severe complications such as right-sided heart failure occurring in another 5 to 10 years. The mean age for the initiation of symptoms is thus 31, with incapacity occurring at age 38 if the condition is untreated. Initial symptoms include fatigue and dyspnea on exertion, which progress to dyspnea at rest and hemoptysis. Atrial arrhythmias, infection, or pulmonary embolism can lead to heart failure.

The stenotic mitral valve impairs left ventricular filling and thus limits any increase in cardiac output. Pregnancy-mediated cardiovascular changes, especially increased intravascular volume and increased heart rate, can exacerbate the impaired filling and lead to decompensation during pregnancy and especially during labor, delivery, and the puerperium. Left atrial volume and pressure increase, pulmonary venous pressure increases, and eventually features of pulmonary hypertension and right ventricular hypertrophy and failure can develop. The goals of management are to optimize cardiac output by preventing rapid ventricular rates and avoiding decreases in systemic vascular resistance, and to reduce stress on the right ventricle by minimizing increases in blood volume and avoiding situations in which pulmonary artery pressure is increased (i.e., hypercarbia, hypoxia, or acidosis). Two serious complications associated with mitral stenosis are atrial fibrillation and pulmonary edema; both have been associated with maternal death.

During pregnancy, tachyarrhythmias should be treated because a rapid heart rate prevents adequate ventricular filling and decreases cardiac output. Beta-blockers should be considered for the patient with a heart rate above 90 beats per minute. Digoxin may be required for the patient with atrial fibrillation. During labor, pain must be managed effectively. Epidural anesthesia can be used if care is taken not to overload the patient with fluid beforehand and not to decrease systemic vascular resistance during the infusion. Fluid management must be meticulous, with extra attention given to the patient in the immediate postpartum period, when autotransfusion rapidly increases the central blood volume. Pulmonary function must be closely followed; a pulmonary catheter may assist in the management of patients with severe disease. Because the pulmonary capillary wedge pressure (PCWP) may not accurately reflect left ventricular filling pressure in the setting of severe mitral stenosis, the PCWP should be maintained in the high-normal to elevated range. If general anesthesia becomes necessary, agents that produce tachycardia (e.g., atropine, meperidine, ketamine) should be avoided. Rarely, surgery becomes necessary during the pregnancy to open the valve.

Although the American Heart Association recommends antibiotic prophylaxis only for women who have a vaginal delivery in the presence of an infection or who undergo urethral catheterization, many clinicians provide prophylaxis to all cardiac patients. Subacute bacterial endocarditis (SBE) prophylaxis usually includes ampicillin, 2 g, and gentamicin, 1.5 mg/kg intravenously, 30 minutes before delivery, and ampicillin, 1 g intravenously, or amoxicillin, 1 g orally, 6 hours after delivery. Penicillin-allergic patients should receive vancomycin, 1 g, before delivery and again 8 hours later, instead of ampicillin.

Mitral Insufficiency

Mitral insufficiency results in regurgitation of blood from the left ventricle back into the left atrium, with resulting left atrial enlargement. Most patients tolerate mitral insufficiency well and remain asymptomatic for 30 to 40 years. However, because pulmonary edema or embolism, atrial tachycardia, and infective endocarditis can occur during pregnancy, patients with mitral insufficiency should be closely monitored. Anything that stresses or impairs the function of the left ventricle should be avoided; increases in systemic vascular resistance, atrial fibrillation, bradycardia, or myocardial depressants can all result in left ventricular decompensation. During labor, pain should be treated effectively, and fluid management calculated to maintain left ventricular volume without increasing it. Epidural anesthesia can be very effective as long as preprocedure hydration is conducted cautiously. SBE prophylaxis should be given. Occasionally, surgical valve replacement is necessary during pregnancy.

Aortic Insufficiency

Aortic insufficiency (AI) usually occurs 7 to 10 years after an episode of rheumatic fever myocarditis and remains asymptomatic for another 7 to 10 years. The regurgitant valve causes a chronic increase in left ventricle volume, eventually leading to increased compliance, increased end-diastolic pressure, and pulmonary congestion and edema. Most pregnant women with AI are relatively asymptomatic. This is in part because the decreased systemic vascular resistance and increased heart rate typical of pregnancy tend to increase forward flow through the insufficient valve. However, cardiovascular changes occurring during labor and delivery can lead to decompensation, especially if intravascular volume is markedly increased or systemic vascular resistance is increased by pain or other stressors.

Epidural anesthesia is ideal for such patients because it eliminates pain and decreases systemic vascular resistance. However, care must be taken not to reduce diastolic blood pressure or provoke a bradycardic episode, as left ventricular output will decrease as a result. Myocardial depressants should be avoided, and fluids must be carefully managed to maintain adequate volume but not overload the left side of the heart. Frequent pulmonary examinations to rule out pulmonary congestion may be helpful. SBE prophylaxis should be given.

Aortic Stenosis

Aortic stenosis (AS) resulting from rheumatic fever rarely complicates pregnancy because the time lag between the rheumatic fever episode and the occurrence of stenosis is usually 35 to 40 years. However, AS can occur in reproductive-age women, with those who are symptomatic having the worst outcome.

The normal cross-sectional area of the aortic valve is 2.6 to 3.5 cm^2; an orifice less than 2.6 cm^2 is usually heralded by a loud systolic murmur, while an orifice less than 1 cm^2 produces symptoms of dyspnea, chest pain, and syncope. AS results in a relatively fixed stroke volume that is dependent on both adequate diastolic filling and heart rate. While some increase in heart rate helps to maintain an adequate cardiac output, tachycardia greater than 140 beats per minute, bradycardia, and decreased systemic vascular resistance are poorly tolerated.

For these reasons, epidural anesthesia may be a poor choice for pain relief during labor, and the patient should instead be managed with intravenous medications and paracervical or pudendal block. Fluid management must be meticulous, taking care to maintain an adequate intravascular and thus end-diastolic volume. A pulmonary artery catheter may be very helpful in directing fluid management. The PCWP should be maintained within a narrow range to avoid both pulmonary edema and hypotension; a slightly elevated PCWP (i.e., 16 mm Hg) is optimal.

Congenital Heart Disease

Congenital heart disease currently accounts for the majority of all heart disease in reproductive-age women. Many women now reach adulthood without surgical correction of their lesion, while for others early surgery has been life-saving. Women who have undergone surgical correction, have normal hemodynamics, and are completely asymptomatic generally tolerate pregnancy, labor, and delivery well without special considerations. Women with uncorrected lesions, however, require special management. The most common uncorrected heart abnormalities seen in pregnancy are atrial septal defect (ASD), patent ductus arteriosus (PDA), ventricular septal defect (VSD), pulmonic stenosis, congenital AS, coarctation of the aorta, and tetralogy of Fallot.

Both maternal and fetal outcomes depend on the nature of the cardiac lesion, the patient's functional capacity, the history of surgical repair (if any), and the presence or absence of pulmonary hypertension or cyanosis. In the presence of cyanosis, there is an increased risk of functional deterioration, congestive heart failure, maternal mortality, IUGR, preterm birth, miscarriage, and stillbirth. In one series, only 55% of pregnancies in cyanotic mothers resulted in a live birth.

Women with congenital heart disease should receive *genetic counseling* regarding the etiology of their lesion and risks to their fetus. Isolated congenital heart malformations are considered multifactorial in origin, and thus have a general recurrence risk of 3% in first-degree relatives. However, a more precise recurrence risk can be provided if the heart defect is categorized according to the aspect of cardiac development that went awry: cell migration abnormalities, defective cell death, extracellular matrix abnormalities, targeted growth defects, and blood flow–related lesions. Only flow-related heart defects have a significant risk of recurrence of approximately 11% to 13.5%. Many structural cardiac defects can be identified by second-trimester ultrasound examination or fetal echocardiogram.

Mitral Valve Prolapse

Mitral valve prolapse (MVP) is the most common congenital valvular lesion, with an incidence of 5% to 10% in the general population. The majority of patients with MVP are asymptomatic and tolerate pregnancy, labor, and delivery well. Occasionally, arrhythmias occur. Although the patient's cardiovascular status should be closely monitored, no special therapy is usually required, other than SBE prophylaxis.

Left-to-right Intracardiac Shunts

Left-to-right intracardiac shunts can result from *ASDs, VSDs,* or *PDA.* Small shunts are often well tolerated for many years. If there is no pulmonary hypertension and the patient is asymptomatic, pregnancy does not impose significant increased risk and may actually improve cardiac hemodynamics because the decreased systemic vascular resistance encourages forward flow. Increased systemic vascular resistance or increased maternal heart rate may increase the shunt and should be avoided; epidural anesthesia for labor and delivery can thus be very helpful. Patients with ASDs are at increased risk of developing supraventricular dysrhythmias that should be controlled with medication.

If, however, the shunt is substantial, resulting in many years of increased pulmonary blood flow, pulmonary hypertension and right heart failure can develop, and the shunt reverses. The combination of pulmonary hypertension and *right-to-left shunt* through any communication between the systemic and pulmonary circulation is known as *Eisenmenger syndrome*. This condition is life-threatening in the pregnant patient, with a maternal mortality of 40% to 60%. Death is due to congestive heart failure and thromboembolic phenomena. The outcome for the fetus is also exceptionally poor, with a perinatal mortality exceeding 28% and a 55% incidence of preterm birth. Women with Eisenmenger syndrome should be strongly discouraged from becoming pregnant or carrying a pregnancy. Management of the gravid patient with this condition includes hospitalization, oxygen therapy, prophylactic anticoagulation, and treatment of heart failure with digoxin and diuretics. Delivery usually requires pulmonary artery catheterization, careful epidural anesthesia, and shortening of the second stage of labor with forceps delivery.

Tetralogy of Fallot

Right-to-left shunting is also seen in tetralogy of Fallot. This term describes the combination of VSD, right ventricular outflow tract obstruction, right ventricular hypertrophy, and overriding aorta. The amount of right-to-left shunting is determined by both the size of the VSD and the degree of right ventricular outflow tract obstruction. Uncorrected tetralogy of Fallot is a cyanotic condition characterized by decreased arterial oxygen saturation and polycythemia. Pregnancy can cause further decompensation because the decreased systemic vascular resistance increases the right-to-left shunt; shunting is also increased by a rise in the pulmonary vascular resistance resulting from the stress of labor. With uncorrected tetralogy of Fallot, 40% of women develop heart failure during pregnancy, and 12% die; the fetal mortality rate is 36%. Pregnancy management includes bed rest, oxygen therapy, and inotropic support as necessary. Because any decrease in systemic vascular resistance can be life-threatening, epidural or spinal anesthesia should be avoided. Intravenous medication and paracervical or pudendal block can be utilized, and the second stage of labor should be shortened.

Congenital Aortic Stenosis

Congenital AS accounts for 5% of all congenital heart disease, with bicuspid aortic valve being the most common malformation. Many patients with bicuspid aortic valve are completely asymptomatic and tolerate pregnancy, labor, and delivery well. For those who are symptomatic, management considerations are the same as for AS resulting from rheumatic heart disease.

Coarctation of the Aorta

Coarctation of the aorta rarely complicates pregnancy because most affected women undergo surgical correction as children. Patients with uncorrected coarctation face an increased risk of aortic dissection and rupture during pregnancy, and thus an increased risk of maternal (up to 9%) and fetal (20%) death. Because the coarctation results in a fixed stroke volume, management is similar to that for AS.

Pulmonic Stenosis

Pulmonic stenosis can be either valvular, which usually does not progress until late in life, or subvalvular, which can become steadily worse during the reproductive years. The right ventricle hypertrophies to maintain output but eventually decompensates, leading to left ventricular failure as well. Right ventricular output is dependent on preload and heart rate, and systemic vascular resistance typically increases to compensate for any reduction in left ventricular output. During labor and delivery, fluids must be managed carefully so that preload is neither increased nor decreased, and bradycardia must be avoided. Because increased systemic vascular resistance is an important compensatory mechanism, epidural or spinal anesthesia should be used very cautiously, if at all.

Other Cardiac Abnormalities

Primary Pulmonary Hypertension

Primary pulmonary hypertension leads to right ventricular hypertrophy and eventually to right ventricular and then left ventricular failure. Pregnancy exacerbates this condition, resulting in a maternal mortality rate as high as 50%. Management is similar to that for Eisenmenger syndrome.

Hypertrophic Cardiomyopathy and Asymmetric Septal Hypertrophy

Hypertrophic cardiomyopathy and asymmetric septal hypertrophy are relatively well tolerated in pregnancy. The increased intravascular volume of pregnancy tends to distend the left ventricle and reduce the degree of outflow obstruction. However, decreased systemic vascular resistance may increase the left ventricular ejection force and thus increase outflow obstruction.

Management goals include avoiding significant increases or decreases in intravascular volume, avoiding tachycardia, avoiding any decrease in systemic vascular resistance, and avoiding anything that increases myocardial contractility. Pain relief during labor can best be provided with intravenous medication and paracervical or pudendal block.

Peripartum Cardiomyopathy

Peripartum cardiomyopathy is a global congestive heart failure characterized by dilatation of all four chambers of the heart, low cardiac output, and pulmonary edema. Arrhythmias may develop, along with pulmonary or systemic embolism. By definition, peripartum cardiomyopathy arises in the last month of pregnancy or in the first 5 months postpartum, and there is no other discernible etiology. The patient may complain of orthopnea, dyspnea, edema, weakness, and palpitations. The chest x-ray, echocardiogram, and electrocardiogram (ECG) are all consistent with cardiomegaly. The left ventricle and left atrium are enlarged, the ejection fraction is markedly reduced, and pulmonary congestion is often present.

Management consists of aggressive treatment of heart failure with digitalis, diuretics, and vasodilators as necessary, strict bed rest, and prophylaxis against thromboembolism. The prognosis is poor. If heart size and function do not return to normal within 6 months, the mortality rate is high (up to 85% in some series), and survivors are often left with a dilated cardiomyopathy that imposes significant morbidity. A proportion of patients experience a complete normalization of heart size and function within 6 months of the onset of disease and then remain NYHA cardiac functional class I or II. These patients should be counseled that the risk of recurrence of cardiomyopathy in future pregnancies approaches 50% and that complete recovery from a second episode cannot be assured.

Myocardial Infarction

The risk of myocardial infarction (MI) in a reproductive-age woman is low (1 in 10,000); contributing factors include atherosclerosis, thrombosis, coronary aneurysm, and dissection. The risk of death is highest at the time of the MI and is gestational-age dependent; maternal morality is approximately 23% in the first and second trimesters but 50% in the third. The risk of death is also high if delivery occurs within 2 weeks of the infarction.

A pregnant woman with MI should receive the same treatment as a nonpregnant individual. Every effort should be made to minimize cardiac workload and myocardial oxygen consumption; epidural anesthesia should be provided during labor and delivery, and oxytocin should be avoided because of its antidiuretic hormone–like properties. Patients should be advised not to become pregnant for at least 1 year after a MI, and then only if normal ventricular function is confirmed by echocardiography, coronary angiography, or radionuclide studies.

Thromboembolic Disease

Venous thromboembolism occurs in 1 in 1000 to 2000 pregnancies and is a leading cause of maternal mortality in the United States. Venous stasis, which is aggravated by uterine compression of the pelvic veins, is a major predisposing factor. Levels of coagulation proteins are also unfavorably altered in pregnancy: Factors II, VII, and X and fibrin increase, levels of protein S decrease, and the fibrinolytic system is inhibited. Years ago, when postpartum ambulation was discouraged, the majority of thromboses occurred after delivery.

Now, however, 50% or more of all thromboses occur in the antepartum period, making diagnosis and therapy a challenge.

Superficial Thrombophlebitis

Superficial thrombophlebitis involves only the superficial saphenous veins and is a relatively benign condition often associated with varicosities. It is treated symptomatically with analgesia, rest, and elastic support.

Deep Venous Thrombosis

Deep venous thrombosis (DVT) is a pathologic condition that can be life-threatening. It occurs most commonly in the iliofemoral region or in the veins of the calf and is characterized by edema and lower extremity aching and limb discoloration. Most DVT in pregnancy occurs on the left side. Because these symptoms may also be present in normal uncomplicated pregnancy, diagnosis requires a search for predisposing factors and a high index of suspicion. Most DVTs can be accurately diagnosed noninvasively. Impedance plethysmography is both highly sensitive and specific for identifying obstruction of the proximal veins (iliac, femoral, and popliteal). Likewise, real-time sonography and duplex Doppler sonography reliably detect proximal vein thrombosis, although they may fail to identify calf vein obstruction. During any examination after the late second trimester, the uterus should be displaced off the vena cava to prevent lower extremity engorgement leading to false-positive results. If ultrasound is properly performed, however, a positive result after any of these three tests should be considered confirmatory and sufficient to warrant the initiation of therapy. If these studies are equivocal or negative and suspicion is high, venography can be performed and is considered highly accurate. The amount of fetal radiation exposure associated with unilateral venography without an abdominal shield is 0.3 rad (0.003 Gy); a limited venogram requires less than 0.05 rad (0.0005 Gy).

Pulmonary Thromboembolism

Pulmonary thromboembolism (PTE) is characterized by dyspnea, tachypnea, tachycardia, pleuritic chest pain, cough, and anxiety. In pregnancy, PTE is usually caused by emboli from a DVT and appears to occur more frequently in the postpartum period. Arterial blood gases confirm hypoxemia and hypocapnia, the ECG shows tachycardia with right heart strain, and the chest x-ray reveals subsegmental atelectasis. If there is a strong clinical suspicion of PTE, intravenous heparin therapy should be immediately initiated. The patient is thus protected from further compromise, while awaiting confirmation of the diagnosis with a ventilation–perfusion (V/Q) scan. Perfusion defects that are unmatched by ventilation defects indicate a high probability of PTE, while a normal V/Q scan excludes the diagnosis. Intermediate results, however, do not rule out a PTE and must be resolved by pulmonary angiography. Pulmonary angiography can be performed while the patient is receiving heparin. As with DVT, necessary diagnostic procedures should not be withheld because the patient is pregnant. The combination of chest x-ray, V/Q scan, and pulmonary angiography exposes the fetus to a radiation dose of only 0.5 rad (0.005 Gy)

It is now clear that some individuals carry a gene mutation that predisposes them to a thromboembolic event. Women who are heterozygotes for *protein C* or *protein S deficiency* have an approximately 2% to 8% incidence of antepartum thromboembolism and an 11% to 20% postpartum incidence; heterozygotes for *antithrombin III deficiency* have a 12% to 48% incidence. A mutation in the gene for factor V—the *factor V Leiden mutation*—produces a single amino acid substitution that prevents factor V destruction and causes activated protein C resistance; women carrying this mutation have a 28% incidence of pregnancy-associated thromboembolism. These mutations are all dominant with variable expressivity. Most carriers have affected family members who display varying degrees of pathology.

Laboratory tests to diagnose all these deficiencies are available and should be considered in the workup of a patient with a history of thromboembolism, especially if there are a strong family history and no clear predisposing factors. Tests for protein C, protein S, and antithrombin III deficiencies cannot be performed while the patient is anticoagulated. Factor V Leiden mutation is identified by molecular analysis, however, and can thus be diagnosed at any time. While knowledge of such mutations would not affect management of an acute thromboembolic event, it would have a profound effect on the patient's future medical management; many authorities recommend continued anticoagulative prophylaxis once such mutations have been identified. While not related to a specific gene defect, antiphospholipid antibody syndrome also imposes an increased risk of both thromboembolism and pregnancy loss and should be considered in the workup for thromboembolic disease.

Treatment for PTE consists of intravenous heparin for 5 to 10 days followed by subcutaneous heparin every 12 hours or three times a day for the remainder of the pregnancy. Heparin is a large molecule that does not cross the placenta and has few reported side effects (mild thrombocytopenia or reversible osteoporosis after long-term therapy). The dose should be titrated to achieve a midinterval activated partial thromboplastin time (aPTT) 1.5 to 2.5 times normal or a plasma heparin level of 0.1 to 0.2 IU/ml within 24 hours of the acute event; failure to do so increases the risk of recurrent thromboembolism by a factor of 15. Most patients require a minimum of 24,000 IU per 24 hours (Table 5). Heparin can also be administered by continuous subcutaneous pump. Low-molecular-weight heparin has aroused interest because it has a longer half-life than ordinary heparin and thus can be administered once daily. However, its efficacy in pregnancy has not been established. Warfarin sodium derivatives are not recommended during pregnancy because they readily cross the placenta and have pathologic effects on the fetus. First-trimester exposure imposes the highest risk, resulting in some or all of the features of warfarin sodium embryopathy, including midfacial hypoplasia, central nervous system (CNS) abnormalities (e.g., microcephaly, hydrocephalus, or agenesis of the corpus callosum), optic atrophy, epiphyseal stippling, low birthweight, mental retardation, and seizures. Exposure beyond the first trimester may cause hemorrhage and secondary disruption of CNS and skeletal structures.

Heparin has a short half-life (60 to 90 minutes) and can be reversed with protamine sulfate. When delivery is planned or the patient enters labor, heparin should be discontinued and the aPTT checked. Most patients can undergo epidural anesthesia or cesarean section within 4 to 6 hours of their last heparin dose, and protamine can be administered if reversal of anticoagulation is required sooner. Heparin should be resumed 12 to 24 hours postpartum, depending on the type of delivery and the occurrence of any complications, with warfarin sodium administered simultaneously. Once therapeutic, warfarin alone should be continued for at least 6 weeks.

The recurrence risk of PTE in a subsequent pregnancy is 4% to 15%; the risk is much higher if the patient has a predisposing gene mutation or other risk factor. Prophylactic heparin therapy should therefore be provided in subsequent pregnancies, although the ideal heparin dose and duration of treatment remain to be determined. Some authors recommend a dose of 5000 to 10,000 IU every 12 hours, increasing as the pregnancy progresses, while others believe the dose should be adjusted to maintain a plasma heparin level of 0.1 to 0.2 IU/ml. Prophylactic heparin therapy is usually initiated in the midtrimester or earlier if the patient has a thrombophilic gene mutation.

TABLE 5. *Protocol for adjustment of intravenous heparin dose*

Activated partial thromboplastin time (sec)	Repeat bolus?	Stop infusion?	New rate of infusion	Repeat measurement of activated partial thromboplastin time
<50	Yes (5000 IU)	No	+3 ml / h (+2880 IU /24 h)	6 h
50–59	No	No	+3 ml / h (+2880 IU /24 h)	6 h
60–85	No	No	Unchanged	Next morning
86–95	No	No	−2 ml / h (−1920 IU / 24 h)	Next morning
96–120	No	Yes (for 30 min)	−2 ml / h (−1920 IU / 24 h)	6 h
>120	No	Yes (for 60 min)	−4 ml / h (−3840 IU / 24 h)	6 h

(From Toglia MR, Weg JG. Venous thromboembolism during pregnancy. *N Engl J Med* 1996;335:110; with permission.)

Mechanical Heart Valves

Women with mechanical heart valves also require therapeutic anticoagulation during pregnancy. As noted above, coumarin derivatives should be avoided during embryogenesis. Women with mechanical valves can be switched to therapeutic subcutaneous heparin before attempting conception or can be switched immediately after conception is verified (i.e., 1 to 2 weeks after the first missed period). The optimal agent for anticoagulation from 14 to 39 weeks is controversial. The advantages of heparin include its inability to cross the placenta and its rapid reversibility. Disadvantages include difficulty in maintaining a therapeutic dose and failure to prevent all valve thromboses. While coumarin may provide more consistent anticoagulation, its effects cannot be readily reversed and extend to the fetus. Consultation with the patient's cardiologist may be helpful.

◊ PULMONARY DISEASE

Asthma

Asthma manifests as a spectrum of illness from infrequent, spontaneously resolving symptoms to repetitive, severe, life-threatening attacks. Symptomatic asthma involves fluctuating degrees of wheezing, dyspnea, chest tightness, and/or cough associated with reversible obstructive airway disease or bronchial hyperreactivity. Reversibility is objectively defined as an increase in forced expiratory volume in 1 second (FEV_1) of 12% and at least 200 ml.

Pathophysiologic mechanisms suspected as causal in asthma include genetic predisposition and airway hyperreactivity with a tendency to bronchoconstriction, airway inflammation, and abnormal mucociliary function. Triggering factors include allergen exposure, respiratory infections, exercise, aspirin, and nonsteroidal antiinflammatory drugs (NSAIDs), and environmental irritants (e.g., tobacco smoke, pollutants).

Asthma may improve, worsen, or remain unchanged during pregnancy. Typically, the more severe the disease, the more likely it is to worsen. The course of asthma in a previous pregnancy is fairly predictive of the course in a subsequent pregnancy in about 60% of women. The peak incidence of asthma exacerbations is 24 to 36 weeks' gestation, with relative improvement during the last month of pregnancy. Severe or uncontrolled asthma is associated with an increased risk of preeclampsia and maternal mortality, as well as IUGR, preterm delivery, and perinatal mortality; potential mechanisms may include hypoxia and medication exposure. It is apparent that perinatal outcome is much improved when optimal control is achieved.

Therapy should include education in the use of a peak-flow meter, the importance of compliance with medications, and the avoidance of known triggers. Mild intermittent disease is treated with an inhaled β_2-agonist such as albuterol, two puffs every 4 hours, when needed. More severe or continuous symptoms are treated with regularly scheduled β-mimetics. Inhaled cromolyn sodium, a mast cell stabilizer, is added if symptoms persist. An inhaled glucocorticoid (e.g, beclomethasone dipropionate) is added next, at two to four puffs every 6 hours. Theophylline is no longer considered a first-line drug for chronic therapy. Instead, if inhaled therapy fails, oral prednisone, 40 to 60 mg per day, is recommended until acute symptoms resolve, followed by tapering for 10 to 14 days. Maintenance of inhaled beclomethasone while on oral steroids increases the risk of oral candidiasis.

Acute asthma attacks in pregnancy should prompt a thorough evaluation. Blood gas analysis in the normal pregnant woman typically reveals a pH of 7.35 and a higher Po_2 (102 to 106 mm Hg) and lower Pco_2 (28 to 30 mm Hg) than in nonpregnant patients. During the early stages of an asthma attack, the blood gas is often consistent with hyperventilation, with an even lower Pco_2 and an elevated pH. After a prolonged attack, the patient will tire and may eventually hypoventilate. Therefore, a Pco_2 greater than 35 mm Hg or a Po_2 less than 70 mm Hg indicates severe respiratory compromise.

In addition to arterial blood gases, the evaluation should include a complete blood cell count, electrolytes, spirometry, and a chest x-ray (Table 6). A respiratory therapist should be involved. Initial management consists of intravenous hydration and inhaled oxygen to maintain a Po_2 greater than 70 mm Hg and adequate urine output (in the face of alkalosis), followed by a nebulized β_2-agonist, such as albuterol, up to three doses in the first 60 to 90 minutes and then 1 to 2 hours thereafter. Next, intravenous methylprednisone, 1 mg/kg, every 6 to 8 hours is added, with tapering as clinical improvement occurs. Some clinicians also give intravenous aminophylline, 6 mg/kg loading dose and 0.5 mg/kg per hour maintenance dose, to keep blood levels between 8 and 12 mg/ml. Patients should receive intravenous antibiotics in the event that an infection is confounding. Finally, terbutaline, 0.25 mg per hour subcutaneously for three doses, is offered. In the absence of clinical response, transfer to an intensive care setting is considered because respiratory support may become necessary.

Antepartum management in patients with well controlled mild to moderate asthma should be like that of an uncomplicated pregnant patient. In those patients with poorly controlled severe asthma, however, the pregnancy should be monitored for IUGR and preeclampsia, and weekly tests of fetal well-being should be instituted if these complications

---

TABLE 6. *Treatment of acute asthma attack*

1. Arterial blood gas, complete blood cell count, electrolytes, peak flow meter, chest x-ray
2. Call respiratory therapy
3. IV hydration, supplemental oxygen therapy to maintain $Po_2>70$ mm Hg; monitor urine output
4. Albuterol, nebulized, 3 doses in initial 60–90 min
5. Methylprednisolone, 1 mg/kg IV q6h
6. Aminophylline, 6 mg/kg IV loading dose, then 0.5 mg/kg/h maintenance
7. Antibiotic IV 8. Terbutaline, 0.25 mg SC
9. Transfer to ICU for respiratory support in absence of improvement

occur. Of treated asthmatic women, 10% experience pulmonary symptoms in labor, in which case they are treated as outlined above. For those patients on a maintenance corticosteroid or those who received a steroid course during the pregnancy, supplemental hydrocortisone, 100 mg intravenously every 8 hours for three doses, is recommended.

Medications to be avoided in the asthmatic patient include beta-blockers, and prostaglandins. NSAIDs should be avoided in aspirin-sensitive patients. Magnesium sulfate and calcium channel blockers are well tolerated. Epidural anesthesia is preferred to general anesthesia.

Tuberculosis

Pregnancy does not worsen the course of tuberculosis (TB), and TB does not alter the overall outcome of pregnancy. However, it is important to diagnose and treat infected patients aggressively, as congenital TB can develop if a tubercular infection and bacteremia develop in a pregnant patient.

TB screening consists of the purified protein derivative (PPD) tuberculin test or Mantoux test. Forty-eight to 72 hours following intradermal injection, the presence or absence of induration at the injection site is determined. In patients with immunologic dysfunction (e.g., HIV infection), no reaction may be elicited. Therefore, a control skin test, such as for *Candida,* is also placed. Most women have been exposed, and those who are not anergic will react. Reaction at the site of the control, and not at the site of the PPD test, indicates a negative PPD. Induration greater than or equal to 5 mm is considered positive in an HIV-positive patient, in anyone in recent contact with an active TB case, and/or in anyone with clinical or radiologic evidence of TB. Induration greater than or equal to 10 mm is considered positive in health care workers, chronic alcoholics, or institutionalized individuals. Finally, induration greater than or equal to 15 mm on the PPD test is considered positive in all low-risk patients. When a skin test is positive, a chest x-ray should be done; with shielding, this procedure involves minimal fetal radiation exposure. If the chest x-ray is normal, or abnormal but inconsistent with TB, the patient is offered treatment to prevent disease development: isoniazid, 300 mg every day for 6 months. If the chest x-ray is consistent with old TB and further evaluation fails to reveal active TB, the patient should receive isoniazid, 300 mg every day for 12 months after delivery.

If the chest x-ray is consistent with TB, further workup to confirm the diagnosis is necessary. The workup should include a thorough history, physical examination, and a sputum smear and culture; the sputum tests confirm the diagnosis. Treatment for 6 to 9 months with two or more drugs is required, as in nonpregnant patients. Isoniazid and rifampin are the drugs of choice. If there is suspicion of drug resistance, ethambutol and pyrazinamide are considered. Household contacts of any patient with active TB should be identified, evaluated, and treated as necessary.

Maternal treatment does not treat the infant. Recognition of congenital TB can be difficult, and unrecognized active disease has significant mortality. Treatment in infants is similar to that in adults. Isolation of the uninfected infant from any potential close infectious contact is recommended until effective treatment is underway, although the infant may breast-feed.

Viral Pneumonia

Influenza Pneumonia

Influenza pneumonia is caused by myxoviruses. Previous reports of increased mortality in the pregnant population have not been substantiated in more recent studies. Treatment is supportive, as antiviral agents are not well studied in this population. Influenza is not associated with an increased incidence of congenital anomalies, and there is no indication for influenza vaccine in the low-risk population.

Varicella Pneumonia

Varicella pneumonia can complicate 0.3% to 50% of all primary varicella infections in adults. Pregnant women are at increased risk of this complication, which has a mortality of up to 40%. Respiratory symptoms typically develop 2 to 5 days after the onset of fever, rash, and malaise. The physical examination can be unimpressive. Any pregnant woman with varicella and respiratory symptoms should be thoroughly evaluated and hospitalized if pneumonia is suspected. Aggressive treatment with acyclovir (Zovirax), a DNA polymerase inhibitor, has decreased mortality in the pregnant population by 50%, without an increase in fetal anomalies.

Two to five percent of primary varicella infections occurring at less than 20 weeks' gestation are associated with congenital varicella syndrome. This syndrome includes microphthalmia, hypoplastic limbs, nasal hypoplasia, and skin lesions. Infants born within 5 days of the development of maternal rash can develop disseminated neonatal varicella, with a 60% to 70% morbidity rate and a 5% to 20% mortality rate. In such cases, delivery should be delayed, if possible, to allow maternal antibodies to reach the fetus.

Cystic Fibrosis

Experience with pregnant patients with cystic fibrosis (CF) is increasing, as the median age of survival is now 27 to 28 years. Most patients with CF have chronic obstructive pulmonary disease and pancreatic insufficiency, but this heritable, autosomal-recessive disorder has a broad spectrum of clinical manifestations. Progressive bronchopulmonary disease is the predominant cause of morbidity and mortality in CF. It is characterized by exacerbations of chronic endobronchial infection, bronchiectasis, and airway obstruction.

Prospective controlled studies of CF in pregnancy are lacking. Counseling regarding the effects of pregnancy on the disease process is therefore difficult. In general, progressive pulmonary deterioration with hypercapnia/hypoxemia and/or cor pulmonale or pulmonary hypertension contraindicate pregnancy. In the absence of these and in the presence of pancreatic sufficiency, the majority of women with CF deliver normal babies at term, with a maternal morbidity and mortality not unlike those of the nonpregnant CF population.

Sarcoidosis

Pulmonary sarcoidosis rarely complicates pregnancy. If it changes during pregnancy, it usually improves, although the disease can relapse or exacerbate postpartum. No special management is necessary for the pregnant patient with sarcoidosis. Angiotensin-converting enzyme levels do not vary with disease activity, so following such levels is without benefit. If an exacerbation occurs, such as worsening pulmonary symptoms, chest x-ray deterioration, CNS or ophthalmic involvement, or hypercalcemia, systemic steroids are recommended.

◊ RENAL DISEASE

Urinary tract infections are a common complication in pregnancy, occurring in 10% to 15% of women. Pregnancy-associated urinary stasis, glucosuria, and vesicoureteral reflux are predisposing factors. Responsible organisms include *Escherichia coli* (75% to 90%), *Klebsiella* (10% to 15%), and *Proteus* (5%) species. *Pseudomonas*, *Streptococcus*, and *Staphylococcus* species are present infrequently.

Renal Infections

Asymptomatic Bacteriuria

Asymptomatic bacteriuria (ASB) is defined as greater than 10,000 organisms per milliliter of urine in an asymptomatic woman. The incidence of ASB in the pregnant population is 6%, the same as in nonpregnant, sexually active women. The incidence is twice as high in women with sickle cell disease trait. Failure to identify and treat pregnant women with ASB will result in an incidence of pyelonephritis of 25% to 40%, but treatment reduces this 10-fold. Treatment typically consists of empiric antibiotic therapy, such as 10 to 14 days of ampicillin or nitrofurantoin, or therapy based on *in vitro* bacterial sensitivities. A repeat culture should be performed 1 week following therapy completion, as 30% of infections recur.

Cystitis

Cystitis is symptomatic bacteriuria without flank pain or fever. Urinary urgency, frequency, and dysuria are the most common complaints. Diagnosis and treatment do not differ from those of ASB. Occasionally, the same symptoms are associated with sterile urine; in this situation, the infecting agent is likely to be *Chlamydia trachomatis* and will respond to erythromycin therapy.

Pyelonephritis

Renal parenychmal infection, or pyelonephritis, complicates 1% to 3% of pregnancies. Patients with acute pyelonephritis are typically febrile; symptoms can include chills, urgency, dysuria, and nausea/vomiting. Other signs include costovertebral angle tenderness, pyuria, and/or bacteriuria. Most cases of pyelonephritis are right-sided or bilateral; disease limited to only the left side suggests an anatomic abnormality. Bacterial endotoxins and cytokines produced by activated macrophages are responsible for many of these symptoms. Hospitalization is routinely recommended, although outpatient management may be effective and safe in selected pregnant women. The risk of preterm labor is increased with pyelonephritis. Once a urine culture is obtained, intravenous antibiotic therapy and vigorous intravenous hydration are started. The antibiotic of choice is usually a cephalosporin, as a large proportion of *E. coli* strains are ampicillin-resistant. If the patient is afebrile within 24 hours, oral antibiotic treatment is started. If she remains afebrile for another 24 hours, she can be discharged home to complete a 10-day antibiotic course. If she remains febrile, changing or adding antibiotics to the regimen must be considered. If the urine culture and sensitivity results are available, they can be used to guide selection of drugs. If the organism is sensitive to the original antibiotic, gentamicin should be added. If no clinical improvement is seen, a renal ultrasound should be performed to rule out calculi or abscess.

Recurrent pyelonephritis occurs in 10% to 18% of patients. To reduce this risk, chronic suppressive therapy consisting of nitrofurantoin, 100 mg each night, is often recommended. Urine is obtained for culture and sensitivity every month, or with patient complaints. Documented recurrent infection is treated with a 10-day course of antibiotics. For the patient with recurrent or persistent disease, a urologic evaluation, including intravenous pyelogram and voiding cystogram, is recommended 3 months postpartum.

Urinary Calculi

Urinary calculi occur in 1 in 1000 pregnancies. Pregnancy does not affect the risk or severity of calculi formation. However, calculi do increase the incidence of urinary tract infections to 20% to 45%. Patients with known calculi are typically placed on suppressive nitrofurantoin therapy throughout the pregnancy. Urine cultures are performed every month, and infection is aggressively treated.

Urolithiasis should be suspected if the patient presents with colicky flank pain, tenderness, hematuria, or unresolved bacteriuria. The diagnosis can usually be made by ultrasound, as 90% of calculi contain calcium and are echodense. Acute urolithiasis is treated with analgesia and vigorous intravenous hydration; if infection is documented, antibiotic therapy is instituted. A ureteral stent or percutaneous nephrostomy may be required to relieve persistent obstruction.

Chronic Renal Disease

The effect of pregnancy on chronic renal disease varies with the degree of renal insufficiency. Mild renal insufficiency, defined as a serum creatinine less than 1.4 mg/dl, can be as-

TABLE 7. *Renal disease prognosis*

	Mild	Moderate	Severe
Creatinine (mg/dl)	<1.4	1.5–2.4	≥2.5
Disease course	Decline in pregnancy; return in prepregnancy function postpartum	Accelerated deterioration in renal function in 10%	30%–40% with decline in renal function to end-stage disease in 1–2 yr postpartum
Perinatal effect		Mortality 15% Preeclampsia 50% Preterm delivery 30%–80% Growth restriction 57%	

sociated with a decline in renal function, increased proteinuria, and hypertension. However, renal function typically returns to prepregnancy levels after delivery (Table 7).

Moderate renal insufficiency is defined as a creatinine greater than 1.4 mg/dl but less than 2.5 mg/dl. Several series suggest that 10% of women with moderate renal insufficiency experience accelerated deterioration of renal function during pregnancy; women whose prepregnancy creatinine is greater than 2 mg/dl are at greatest risk. Hypertension typically escalates, and its control is essential for good outcome. Although methyldopa is frequently prescribed, the lag between dose and effect may make it a suboptimal choice. Betablockers, such as labetalol, and calcium channel blockers, such as nifedipine, have been shown to be effective.

Less information is available regarding pregnant patients with severe renal insufficiency (creatinine greater than 2.5 mg/dl). Thirty to forty percent of these patients experience a decline in renal function to end-stage disease within 12 to 24 months postpartum.

Patients with renal insufficiency are at high risk of perinatal mortality (up to 15%), preeclampsia (more than 50%), preterm delivery (30% to 80%), and IUGR (up to 57%). Monitoring of baseline and subsequent laboratory values, routine urine cultures with prompt treatment for infection, serial ultrasound examinations for fetal growth, and formal tests of fetal well-being are indicated.

Acute Renal Failure

Acute renal failure is a rare but potentially devastating complication of pregnancy. It has many causes, including preeclampsia, hemorrhage, and placental abruption. Although typically characterized by persistent oliguria, diuretic therapy is not helpful, as it does not correct the cause of the renal failure. In the presence of azotemia and severe oliguria, dialysis is usually initiated and continued until renal function returns. Fortunately, morbidity and mortality from renal failure have decreased as obstetric recognition and intervention have become more prompt, and intensive supportive therapy has become more widely available.

Dialysis

Although most women with severely impaired renal function are infertile, chronic hemodialysis or peritoneal dialysis may make pregnancy possible. Hemodialysis is usually initiated earlier in the pregnant patient than in the nonpregnant, as the risk for intrauterine fetal demise increases at a blood urea nitrogen (BUN) above 80 mg/dl. The goal of dialysis is to maintain the BUN at 50 to 60 mg/dl, while limiting volume changes and episodes of hypotension. Peritoneal dialysis may be superior to hemodialysis because it minimizes fluid shifts and does not require maternal anticoagulation, although data to support its preferential use in pregnancy are limited. Because dialysis is often accompanied by contractions, magnesium sulfate can be added to the dialysate to maintain a serum level of 5 mEq/l. Increased hours on hemodialysis and increased frequency of treatments are recommended, as these improve management of weight and diet issues.

Renal Transplantation

Most pregnancies after renal transplantation are successful. Patients are typically advised to avoid pregnancy for 2 years following surgery to allow recovery, stabilization of graft function, and confirmation of graft survival on maintenance doses of immunosuppressive agents (prednisone, to up 15 mg/day; azathioprine, up to 2 mg/kg/day). Once pregnancy is achieved, suspicion of graft rejection is high in the presence of fever, oliguria, graft enlargement, tenderness, and decline in renal function. Because the differential diagnosis also includes severe preeclampsia, pyelonephritis, and recurrence of glomerulopathy, renal biopsy may be necessary to confirm rejection. The immunosuppressive agents typically prescribed, including prednisone, azathioprine, and cyclosporine, are considered to be safe in pregnancy.

◊ NEUROLOGIC DISORDERS

Neurologic diseases occur frequently in the general population (Table 8) and in reproductive-age women, and pregnancy can provoke or exacerbate certain neurologic abnormalities.

Headache

Headache is a common complaint during pregnancy. Tension headaches typically persist for hours and are characterized by a tight sore feeling in the back of the head and neck. The pain usually responds to rest, application of heat or ice packs to the neck, massage, antiinflammatory drugs, or a mild tranquilizer

TABLE 8. *Prevalence of neurologic disorders*

Disorder	Prevalence
Migraine	2000
Epilepsy	650
Cerebral palsy	250
Multiple sclerosis	100
Spinal cord injury	50
Subarachnoid hemorrhage	50
Myasthenia gravis	4
Genetic disorders (excluding congenital central nervous system malformations)	<10

(From Kurtzke JF. The current neurologic burden of illness and injury in the United States. *Neurology* 1982;32:1207; with permission.)

such as chlordiazepoxide. Strategies to relieve stress are important to prevent recurrence. Depression headaches usually occur in association with other symptoms of depression and respond to antidepressant medication and counseling.

Migraine Headache

Migraine headaches are commonly seen in pregnancy because migraines occur predominantly in women of childbearing age and the hormones of pregnancy may provoke an attack. Several studies have suggested a link between steroid hormone levels and migraine symptoms, although the relationship is unclear. While many women experience an exacerbation of symptoms or have their first migraine during pregnancy, 64% of women with a history of menstrual migraine headaches experience a dramatic improvement in symptoms during pregnancy.

There are at least four types of migraine headaches. *Common migraine* is characterized by a frequently unilateral headache lasting several hours, nausea and vomiting, and scalp tenderness. There is often a family history of similar headaches. *Classic migraine* has the same symptoms but is preceded by premonitory sensory phenomena, such as visual scotomas or hallucinations. *Basilar migraine* includes symptoms of vertigo, dysarthria, or diplopia, while *complicated migraine* involves more serious neurologic symptoms.

The diagnosis of new-onset migraine headaches during pregnancy is usually one of exclusion; other disorders such as brain tumor, stroke, and epilepsy need to be ruled out. The patient can undergo the same evaluation as a nonpregnant individual, usually consisting of a thorough history and neurologic examination and sometimes including computed tomography (CT) or magnetic resonance (MR) imaging or awake and asleep electroencephalograms. Acute treatment is also very similar in the pregnant patient and can include aspirin or acetaminophen with or without caffeine or butalbital, narcotics, phenothiazine antiemetics, or sumatriptan succinate (Imitrex). Ergotamine should not be given during pregnancy because it is a potent vasoconstrictor that can adversely affect uterine and placental blood flow. NSAIDs should also

be avoided in the third trimester. If headaches are chronic, the patient may benefit from amitriptyline or nortriptyline, propranolol, or verapamil. Valproic acid (Depakene) may be prescribed after the first trimester, when the fetal neural tube is completely formed.

Epilepsy

Epilepsy affects 0.5% to 2.0% of the population and complicates 1 in 200 pregnancies. Seizures are usually classified according to whether they are partial or generalized, as well as by a description of the seizure itself. Absent seizures, or petit mal, involve loss of consciousness alone without any accompanying motor activity. Although both progesterone and estrogen have been shown to influence seizure activity, the relationship of pregnancy and seizure activity is unclear; 46% of women experience no change in seizure frequency, 20% experience a reduction, and 34% experience an increase in seizure activity during gestation. Factors that increase the frequency of seizures during pregnancy include discontinuation of antiepileptic medication in the belief that it harms the fetus, subtherapeutic drug levels because the dose was not adjusted to compensate for expanding maternal vascular volume, inability to ingest medication because of nausea and vomiting, and lowering of the seizure threshold by sleep deprivation and stress.

The new onset of seizures during pregnancy is concerning. While gestational epilepsy is probably a distinct entity, it is a diagnosis of exclusion. A complete workup should be performed as for a nonpregnant individual. *Status epilepticus* is a medical emergency, and the pregnant woman should be treated in the same manner as a nonpregnant individual. The airway must be secured and protected, and intravenous fluids, together with a glucose bolus and thiamine, 100 mg, should be given; intravenous phenytoin, phenobarbital, or diazepam should be administered. If possible, a wedge should be placed under one hip to displace the uterus off the vena cava. Although fetal heart rate abnormalities may be present during the seizure, the mother should be stabilized before any intervention is contemplated; in most cases, resuscitation of the mother resuscitates the fetus. A thorough workup, including a toxicology screen and anticonvulsant drug levels, should be initiated.

Most epileptic women require seizure medication to remain seizure-free. For many anticonvulsant drugs, the benefit of preventing seizures outweigh any potential risks to the fetus. Other medications are clearly teratogenic and should be avoided, if possible; these include valproic acid before 8 weeks' gestation and trimethadione (Tridione). However, women with epilepsy are at increased risk for fetal malformations, whether or not they ingest anticonvulsant medication. Although women taking multiple medications are at highest risk, it is not clear whether the increased risk is due to fetal drug exposure or whether it correlates with severity of maternal disease. Fetal factors play a role as well; for example, fetuses with epoxide hydrolase deficiency are at high risk for fetal hydantoin syndrome. The epileptic gravida should be counseled that her disease increases the risk of birth defects from the background rate of 3% to approximately 7%.

The lowest medication dose associated with seizure prevention should be prescribed. Stressors should be minimized, and the patient should ingest a multivitamin with folate. Some authors advocate prescribing oral vitamin K in the last month of pregnancy to women taking phenytoin, but this is controversial, as it is not clear that vitamin K crosses the placenta and exposed fetuses are usually given vitamin K neonatally. A second-trimester targeted ultrasound examination, with other ultrasound examinations as needed to assess fetal growth, is warranted. During labor, antiseizure medications should be continued, and pain relief should be excellent so that hyperventilation with pain does not lead to a respiratory alkalosis that could lower the seizure threshold. The patient may breast-feed. The anticonvulsant content of breast milk is inversely proportional to the degree of protein binding. However, even drugs that are not highly protein-bound (e.g., carbamazepine, phenobarbital, primidone [Mysoline]) are present at low levels, so that the total dose ingested by the infant is usually negligible.

Subarachnoid Hemorrhage

Intracranial vascular anomalies can become symptomatic during pregnancy. Rupture of such malformations, resulting in subarachnoid hemorrhage, occurs in 1 in 75,000 pregnancies. Subarachnoid hemorrhage is heralded by sudden intense headache, visual changes or cranial nerve abnormalities, focal neurologic deficits, or an altered level of consciousness. In addition, the patient often complains of nausea, vomiting, and photophobia. The examination reveals signs of meningeal irritation, tachycardia, hypertension, slight fever, and mild leukocytosis and proteinuria. Subarachnoid hemorrhage may result from a ruptured *cerebral angioma, saccular aneurysm,* or *arteriovenous malformation* (AVM); aneurysm rupture reportedly occurs three times more often than rupture of an AVM. The mortality rate is been reported to be as high as 35%.

If intracranial hemorrhage is suspected during pregnancy, the patient should undergo a CT scan to confirm the hemorrhage and localize the bleeding. If the CT scan is normal but hemorrhage is strongly suspected, examination of the cerebrospinal fluid (CSF) to confirm the presence of blood followed by angiography to locate the lesion may be indicated. Treatment consists of bed rest, sedation, and analgesia; surgical correction is often recommended. Aneurysms that have bled once are very likely to bleed again within weeks of the first bleed, and 5% to 7% of AVMs bleed again in the first year. Therapy should not be withheld from the patient because she is pregnant. Hypothermia during neurosurgery is usually well tolerated by the fetus, although hypotension should be avoided if at all possible. If the patient requires neurosurgery near term, cesarean section just prior to the craniotomy may avoid fetal compromise, if the fetus is mature. Otherwise, there is usually no maternal benefit to terminating the pregnancy. Patients who experience an intracranial hemorrhage within 2 months of delivery or who have an unrepaired aneurysm should not undergo the Valsalva maneuver during labor; epidural anesthesia and forceps delivery are indicated.

Ischemic (Thrombotic) Stroke

Ischemic (thrombotic) stroke is uncommon in reproductive-age women, occurring in 1 in 7000 to 11,000 pregnancies; however, it can occur in association with hypertension, diabetes, hyperlipidemia, antiphospholipid antibody syndrome, sickle cell disease, rheumatic heart disease, septicemia, and smoking. *Cerebral artery thrombosis* is most often associated with atherosclerosis and may be preceded by transient ischemic attacks. *Cerebral artery embolism* is usually associated with cardiac arrhythmia. In either case, the affected patient presents with the sudden onset of severe headache, hemiplegia or other neurologic deficits, or new-onset seizures. A thorough workup should be performed, including complete blood cell count, sedimentation rate, serum lipid profile, ECG or echocardiogram, and head CT scan or cerebral angiography, as necessary. Therapy includes rest, analgesia, aspirin, and heparin. Heparin may be discontinued prior to vaginal delivery and restarted postpartum; cesarean section should be for obstetric indications.

Cerebral Venous Sinus Thrombosis

Cerebral venous sinus thrombosis is usually a puerperal complication, occurring in association with preeclampsia, sepsis, or a coagulation defect. The patient complains of severe headache, drowsiness, and confusion and may have convulsions, focal neurologic deficits, hypertension, or papilledema. The diagnosis is made by CT scan or angiography. Treatment consists of mannitol or dexamethasone to reduce intracranial edema, together with antiepileptic medication if seizures have occurred. Heparin may be given if hemorrhage has been ruled out. If sepsis is a cofactor, the source must be identified, and the infection treated aggressively. The mortality rate can be as high as 30%; poor prognostic factors include obtundation, coma, accompanying subarachnoid hemorrhage, or rapid deterioration. However, the prognosis for survivors is excellent.

Malignancy

Primary CNS malignancies occur in 3 to 5 per 100,000 people per year; although pregnancy does not alter this incidence, intracranial malignancies account for 10% of all maternal deaths. The malignancy may arise during pregnancy, or the physiologic changes of pregnancy may induce symptoms in a previously asymptomatic tumor. Symptoms typically include headache, vomiting, altered levels of consciousness, seizures, and hypertension. The presence of papilledema helps to distinguish intracranial pathology from other entities such as preeclampsia. Diagnosis is by CT or MR imaging. If an operable tumor of high malignant potential is suspected (e.g., high-grade gliomas, choroid plexus papillomas, posterior fossa tumors) or if there are significant neurologic complications such as seizures or progressive hydrocephalus, surgery should be performed without delay. Intraoperative hypothermia is usually well tolerated by the fetus, although hypotension should be avoided if possible. In contrast, minimally symptomatic lesions of low malignant potential (e.g., meningioma) may be followed and definitively treated postpartum.

It should be kept in mind that a proportion of intracranial malignancies are metastatic from other sites, primarily breast, lung, or gastrointestinal or genitourinary tracts. A complete history and physical examination is therefore crucial. Choriocarcinoma may present with intracranial findings, and pituitary tumors may become symptomatic in pregnancy.

If intracranial malignancy is diagnosed early in pregnancy, pregnancy termination is not routinely indicated but might be appropriate in patients with uncontrollable seizures or progressive loss of consciousness. Patients who have undergone craniotomy within 2 months of delivery should not undergo the Valsalva maneuver during labor; epidural anesthesia and forceps delivery are indicated. Cesarean section should be for obstetric indications only.

Pseudotumor Cerebri

Pseudotumor cerebri is defined by increased intracranial pressure, papilledema, and headache without focal neurologic abnormalities. The etiology is unknown. Although pregnancy does not increase the incidence, the majority of cases occur in obese women of reproductive age. Pregnancy complications experienced by such women are likely to be related to their obesity and not their neurologic diagnosis. Women with pseudotumor cerebri should be followed with serial visual-field and acuity testing. Treatment typically consists of repeated lumbar punctures, shunting, corticosteroids, or acetazolamide (Diamox); all can be safely used in pregnancy. Although weight loss and diuretics may also be helpful, they should be deferred until postpartum.

Multiple Sclerosis

Multiple sclerosis (MS) is a multifocal demyelinating disease of CNS white matter, characterized by chronic inflammation, selective demyelination, and scarring. The etiology is unknown but may involve virally triggered autoimmune phenomena in a genetically susceptible individual. There are three forms of MS: *relapsing MS,* which is defined by recurrent attacks of neurologic abnormality followed by greater or lesser degrees of recovery; *chronic progressive MS,* which gradually worsens from the onset without remission; and *inactive MS,* in which patients have fixed neurologic deficits that neither progress nor resolve. Because it is most commonly seen in 20- to 40-year-old white women and does not

impair fertility, MS can occur coincidently with pregnancy. Symptoms and signs include weakness, hyperreflexia, paresthesia, hypesthesia, ataxia, visual loss resulting from optic neuritis, diplopia, facial nerve palsy, vertigo, urgency, or incontinence; none of the symptoms or signs can be explained by a single anatomic lesion. The diagnosis is one of exclusion, with MS confirmed by CSF abnormalities and MR imaging. In many patients, MS has been diagnosed before conception, and medical therapy in the form of adrenocorticotropic hormone (ACTH) and glucocorticoids has been instituted. Patients with chronic progressive MS or severe relapsing MS may require more aggressive therapy with immunosuppressive drugs such as cyclosporine, azathioprine, or cyclophosphamide. All these drugs may be continued in pregnancy, if there is clear maternal benefit. Affected patients may also require an antispasmodic, urinary tract infection prophylaxis, and physical therapy.

Women with MS should be counseled that pregnancy increases the likelihood of urinary tract infections and constipation and may exacerbate fatigue and mobility problems. Women with para- or quadriplegia are at risk for unmonitored, precipitous delivery. Women with a lesion at or above T-6 are at risk for autonomic dysreflexia. Although some women experience relatively little symptomatic progression during pregnancy, flares are common in the first 3 postpartum months. Breast-feeding may have to be discontinued, and the patient may require assistance with infant care.

Myasthenia Gravis

Myasthenia gravis is a chronic autoimmune neuromuscular disease characterized by easy fatigability of facial, oropharyngeal, extraocular, and limb muscles. The primary defect is IgG-mediated destruction of striated muscle acetylcholine receptors. The diagnosis is made with the edrophonium chloride test (edrophonium inhibits acetylcholinesterase, which allows acetylcholine levels to increase and improves strength in myasthenic muscles), nerve stimulation tests, and measurement of acetylcholine receptor antibodies. The incidence of myasthenia gravis is 1 in 10,000; women are affected more often than men and experience a peak occurrence in their 20s and 30s. Symptoms typically wax and wane and are not altered by pregnancy, although postpartum exacerbation is common. Thymectomy is usually performed shortly after diagnosis because it results in symptomatic improvement and may ultimately eliminate the need for medical therapy.

Pregnant women with mild disease usually require only adequate rest and the avoidance of strenuous activities. More seriously affected women require medical therapy in the form of pyridostigmine bromide or neostigmine bromide, glucocorticoids, or immunosuppresive drugs. Plasmapheresis can relieve acute symptoms by mechanically removing the pathologic antibodies and can be performed in pregnancy, if care is taken not to cause maternal hypotension or hypovolemia. Because the disease does not affect smooth muscle, labor and delivery proceed normally. The patient may receive oxytocin and analgesics, but care should be taken to avoid extensive regional blocks that could compromise maternal respiration. Certain drugs are tolerated poorly and should be avoided; these include magnesium sulfate, aminoglycosides, certain antiarrhythmics (e.g., quinine, quinidine, and procaine), procaine anesthetics, curare, succinylcholine, and large doses of narcotics. Because the antireceptor IgG antibody easily crosses the placenta, the neonate will be transiently symptomatic in approximately 10% of cases and require tertiary care.

Myotonic Dystrophy

Myotonic dystrophy is an autosomal-dominant, multisystem disease characterized by muscle stiffness (myotonia), progressive dystrophic changes in muscles of the face, neck, and distal limbs, and posterior subcapsular cataracts. It occurs in 3 to 5 per 100,000 individuals and is usually diagnosed in late childhood or early adulthood with the development of progressive muscle weakness and atrophy. Affected patients have characteristic facies (drooping eyelids, bitemporal wasting, and weakness with diminished expressivity of the mouth), weakness and atrophy of small hand muscles, and respiratory and gastrointestinal difficulties. Although menstrual irregularities and infertility are common, affected patients can become pregnant. Such patients are at increased risk for pregnancy complications, including polyhydramnios, preterm labor, dysfunctional labor, and postpartum hemorrhage. Maternal deaths related to aspiration pneumonia or cardiac failure have been reported. Symptoms are usually worse in the last half of pregnancy and often improve after delivery.

The molecular defect is a region of CTG trinucleotide repeats in the myotonin gene on the long arm of chromosome 19. The number of repeats in this region determines the severity of the symptoms; expansion of the region, along with an increase in symptom severity, can occur with each generation. The fetus of an affected mother is thus at risk of inheriting an expanded form of the gene and having the severe congenital form of the disease. Affected infants are floppy at birth, have diminished suck and cry reflexes, and have serious respiratory compromise. Prenatal diagnosis is available. Severely affected women and their affected infants usually require tertiary care.

Spinal Cord Injury

Spinal cord injury resulting in para- or quadriplegia occurs in 1 in 10,000 individuals per year in the United States. Reproductive-age women with spinal cord injuries generally tolerate pregnancy well, although pregnancy may exacerbate bowel dysfunction or pressure necrosis of the skin and may increase the incidence of urinary tract infections. Women with lesions below T10-12 feel uterine contractions normally. Women with lesions above this level, however, usually do not feel their contractions and are at risk for a precipitous unattended delivery. Such women should be taught to palpate their uterus for contractions on a regular basis during the third trimester.

Women whose lesion is above T-6 are at risk for autonomic hyperreflexia. In this condition, any number of stimuli (labor, urethral catheterization, cervical or rectal examination) can provoke afferent nerve impulses that enter the cord and initiate focal segmental reflexes that are not modulated or inhibited by higher centers, resulting in stimulation of the sympathetic nervous system. Symptoms include pilomotor erection, excessive sweating, facial flushing, dilated pupils, severe headache, paroxysmal hypertension, and bradycardia. Epidural anesthesia can prevent or control such sympathetic stimulation and is therefore a crucial part of labor management. Vaginal delivery is possible for some spinal cord injury patients because the expulsive forces of the uterus are sufficient to bring down the fetal head for a forceps delivery. If cesarean section is required, regional anesthesia is ideal.

◊ ENDOCRINE

Pituitary Tumors

The pituitary gland normally enlarges by 30% during pregnancy, and compression of the optic chiasm infrequently results in bitemporal hemianopsia. Pituitary secretions are altered by pregnancy: Follicle-stimulating hormone and luteinizing hormone levels are decreased, and ACTH and prolactin are increased; thyroid-stimulating hormone (TSH) concentrations, however, vary with gestational timing.

Pituitary adenomas are benign neoplasms of anterior pituitary cells. Adenomas can secrete hormones, such as prolactin or ACTH, and cause hypopituitarism and/or headache or visual problems. They are classified by size as micro- or macroadenomas, with microadenomas being less than 10 mm. They can also be classified by the hormone they secrete, with prolactin-secreting adenomas being the most prevalent at 26%. Diagnosis is confirmed by MR imaging or CT scan. Hyperprolactinemia can manifest as galactorrhea, menstrual disorders, infertility, hirsutism, headache, and visual field defects.

Treatment options include medical, surgical or radiation therapy. Medical treatment is with the dopamine agonist parlodel, which decreases prolactin levels to normal in up to 90% of treated patients. Bromocriptine is not known to be teratogenic, but treatment during pregnancy is typically discontinued. As the normal pituitary enlarges during pregnancy, the potential for enlargement of an adenoma exists as well. Pregnant women should be educated about and monitored for the signs of expansion, such as headaches and visual field changes. This occurs infrequently, as only 2% of microadenomas and 15% of macroadenomas show signs or symptoms of tumor growth in pregnancy. Serial visual field examinations are usually done each trimester. Surgery and radiation are alternative treatment modalities for adenomas, with surgery reserved for patients with very large tumors in whom medical therapy fails. Breast-feeding is unaffected by hyperprolactinemia. Bromocriptine is reinstituted at its completion.

Diabetes Insipidus

Diabetes insipidus (DI) involves water loss secondary to inadequate renal tubule reabsorption. Polyuria, polydipsia, and excessive thirst are characteristic. There are three causes of DI (Table 9). *Hypothalamic (central) DI* results from inadequate arginine vasopressin (AVP) secretion in response to stimuli and can be genetic (rare) or acquired. Acquired central DI occurs as the result of tumor, trauma, infection, Sheehan syndrome, or autoimmune disease. *Nephrogenic DI* results from decreased renal sensitivity to normal or elevated AVP levels and can be familial or acquired; lithium also causes this type. Primary polydipsia, typically psychogenic in origin, involves excessive fluid intake and AVP suppression.

DI is diagnosed with a water deprivation test. In a pregnant patient with a viable fetus, this test is performed with continuous fetal monitoring. Dehydration in DI will be accompanied by rising serum osmolality and an inability to concentrate the urine. Intranasal administration of desmopressin acetate prompts urine concentration and confirms the diagnosis. Its use is not associated with maternal or fetal complications.

Thyroid Disease

Maternal Thyroid Function during Normal Pregnancy

Normal pregnancy results in modest thyroid enlargement, detectable on physical examination. Serum levels of TSH and thyroid-releasing hormone (TRH) are the same in the pregnant patient as in the nonpregnant, while levels of thyroid-binding globulin (TBG) increase due to estrogen-enhanced hepatic production. Because total thyroxine (T_4) and tri-iodothyronine (T_3) are also increased, free biologically active T_3 and T_4 concentrations are unchanged in normal pregnant women. Human chorionic gonadotropin has the same α chain as TSH, so there is an inverse relationship between these hormone levels during pregnancy.

Maternal Hypothyroidism

Most pregnant patients treated for hypothyroidism during pregnancy are diagnosed before pregnancy and are already on replacement therapy; in these patients, the dosage should initially be maintained. A patient may also develop hypothyroidism during pregnancy. The most common cause of hypothyroidism is *Hashimoto thyroiditis*, which is confirmed by demonstrating the presence of circulating antithyroglobulin and antimicrosomal antibodies. Women who have undergone thyroid ablation for Graves disease and are inadequately re-

placed may also be hypothyroid. Symptoms include excessive fatigue, dry skin, cold intolerance, constipation, bradycardia, and irritability. Myxedema is rare. Laboratory evaluation reveals low free T_4 and high TSH. The goal of therapy is to provide enough T_4 to normalize the TSH and the pulse rate, which should be checked every 2 to 3 weeks. A typical replacement dosage is 150 μg of levothyroxine per day. At least 75% of all hypothyroid patients will require a higher dose during pregnancy; the dose is typically increased in 50 μg increments.

Maternal Hyperthyroidism

Hyperthyroidism complicates 1 in 500 pregnancies. Causes include Graves disease, acute or subacute thyroiditis, toxic nodular goiter, toxic adenoma, and gestational trophoblastic disease (Table 10). Patients with Hashimoto thyroiditis may also exhibit signs of hyperthyroidism if they make antithyroid antibodies (a combination of Graves disease and Hashimoto thyroiditis, or "Hashitoxicosis") or if they make anti-TSH receptor antibodies.

The most common cause of hyperthyroidism in pregnancy is *Graves disease*. The diagnosis is based on a triad of manifestations, including hyperthyroidism with diffuse goiter, ophthalmopathy (particularly exophthalmos), and dermopathy. Graves disease is an autoimmune disorder in which circulating thyroid-stimulating immunoglobulins (TSIs) bind to thyroid follicular cell TSH receptors, stimulating excess thyroid hormone synthesis and secretion. The patient may have other autoimmune diseases, including systemic lupus erythematosus, myasthenia gravis, and immune thrombocytopenia.

The diagnosis of hyperthyroidism can be difficult, as the patient may report symptoms that are commonly seen in a normal pregnancy. These include shortness of breath, palpitations, and heat intolerance. Signs and symptoms of hyperthyroidism that are not typical of pregnancy and thus aid in its diagnosis include weight loss or poor weight gain and increased bowel frequency. Laboratory evaluation confirms the diagnosis. Free T_4 is high in hyperthyroid patients. Rarely (in 3% to 5%), T_4 may be normal and free T_3 elevated.

Hyperthyroidism can be treated with antithyroid medications, surgery, or radioactive sodium iodine (^{131}I). All medications have some contraindications in pregnancy. Propylthiouracil (PTU) and methimazole (Tapazole) are trionamides that inhibit thyroid hormone biosynthesis. PTU lowers T_4 levels faster than methimazole, giving it an advantage for therapy. The recommended dose of PTU is 300 to 450 mg initially, followed by a 50- to 300-mg daily maintenance dose,

TABLE 9. *Causes of diabetes insipidus*

| Hypothalamic |
| Genetic |
| Acquired |
| Nephrogenic |
| Primary polydipsia |

TABLE 10. *Causes of hyperthyroidism*

| Graves disease |
| Acute (subacute) thyroiditis |
| Hashimoto disease |
| Toxic nodular goiter |
| Toxic adenoma |
| Gestational trophoblastic disease |

usually divided into a three-times-a-day dosage regimen. Both PTU and methimazole cross the placenta and can have inhibitory effects on fetal thyroid function. Once a high-normal free T_4 level has been achieved, the PTU dose should be reduced to the smallest dose that maintains this level, thus decreasing the risk of fetal hypothyroidism. During therapy, maternal thyroid function should be evaluated every 3 to 4 weeks to guide dosage adjustments.

Before initiation of therapy, a baseline white blood cell count and differential should be obtained. Adverse reactions to PTU include skin rash (2% to 8%), bronchospasm, drug fever, hepatitis, oral ulcers, and idiopathic agranulocytopenia. Idiopathic agranulocytopenia usually occurs during the first 3 months of therapy (1 in 500 patients) and is reversible after stopping the PTU. An adverse reaction to one thionamide does not necessarily predict a similar reaction to another.

Both PTU and methimazole are taken up by the fetal thyroid gland after the first trimester. At PTU doses of 300 mg or greater daily, fetal goiter and hypothyroidism have been reported; at doses lower than 300 mg daily, fetal clinical outcome is usually improved, and at doses lower than 200 mg daily, fetal T_4 levels can be normal. Aplasia cutis has been described in some fetuses exposed to methimazole, which may make PTU preferable during pregnancy. After birth, women taking these antithyroid medications may pass physiologically significant doses of the medication into their milk. If women on antithyroid medications choose to nurse, the infant's thyroid function should be checked periodically to prevent undiagnosed neonatal hypothyroidism.

Beta-blockers may be useful in decreasing the sympathetic-like symptoms of hyperthyroidism, while thyroid hormone levels are being reduced by other forms of therapy. In addition, propranolol has an inhibitory effect on the peripheral conversion of T_4 to T_3 and thus lowers circulating thyroid hormone levels. This action is additive to the effects of the thionamides. The recommended propranolol dose for this indication is 20 to 40 mg orally three to four times a day.

Surgical thyroid ablation, or thyroidectomy, may be necessary during pregnancy if very high doses of PTU (greater than 300 mg daily) are chronically needed to control maternal hyperthyroidism. Medical thyroid ablation with ^{131}I should not be considered during pregnancy because of the possibility of simultaneous fetal thyroid ablation. Antenatal treatment with ^{131}I at the usual dose results in 0.75 to 1.5 rad (0.0075 to 0.015 Gy) of fetal radiation exposure. Patients with inadvertent first-trimester exposure can be reassured that the fetal thyroid does not begin concentrating iodine until 10 to 12 weeks' gestation, and maternal thyroid ablation before this time would not be expected to affect the fetus. Exposure after 12 weeks' gestation, however, may result in congenital hypothyroidism. Theoretically, 10 days of maternal PTU administration after accidental exposure may benefit the fetus by decreasing uptake of ^{131}I iodine into the fetal thyroid.

The patient with the most serious complication of Graves disease, *thyroid storm* or *crisis*, can present with tachycardia,

TABLE 11. *Treatment of thyroid storm*

Propylthiouracil: 600 mg PO (NG), then 300 mg q6h
Sodium iodide: 1g/500 empc IV qd
Propranolol: 40–60 mg Po q 4–6h
Dexamethasone: 1 mg Po IM q6h
Oxygen, acetaminophen, fluid replacement

NG, nasogastric tube administration.

hyperpyrexia, circulatory collapse, and death. Thyroid storm involves a massive release of thyroid hormones and is often precipitated by a stressor, such as infection (e.g., pyelonephritis), thyroid gland palpation, or labor and delivery. Thyroid storm is an emergency and must be treated aggressively to prevent maternal decompensation. Treatment may require the administration of multiple agents for up to 1 to 2 weeks (Table 11). PTU should be given in high doses: 600 mg orally initially followed by 300 mg orally every 6 hours. The thionamides can be administered through a nasogastric tube if the patient cannot tolerate oral medications. In addition, sodium iodide, 1 g in 500 ml of fluid, should be given daily to inhibit the release of stored hormone. Propranolol may be added for control of tachycardia and other sympathetic-like symptoms, if there is no evidence of cardiac failure. The initial propranolol dosage is 40 to 80 mg orally every 4 to 6 hours or 1 mg per minute intravenously for 2 to 10 minutes with concurrent maternal cardiac monitoring; the dose may be adjusted, depending on the patient's cardiac response. Dexamethasone, 1 mg orally or intramuscularly every 6 hours, or hydrocortisone, 100 mg intravenously every 8 hours, can further inhibit peripheral T_4-to-T_3 conversion. Oxygen, digitalis, fluid replacement, and acetaminophen (as an antipyretic) should be given as needed.

Thyroid Nodules and Cancer

Evaluation of thyroid nodules discovered during pregnancy should begin with ultrasound, needle biopsy, or aspiration. If malignant or suspicious cells are seen, surgery should be performed. If no suspicious cells are encountered, the nodule can be suppressed with levothyroxine.

There is no evidence that pregnancy affects the progression of thyroid cancer or that thyroid cancer affects the outcome of pregnancy. As a result, thyroid cancer or a history of it is not an absolute contraindication to pregnancy. Although pregnancy is not a contraindication to thyroid surgery, it is a contraindication to ^{131}I treatment.

Fetal Thyroid Function

The fetal thyroid gland is first capable of hormonal activity by the end of the first trimester, and there is normally a gradual increase in fetal T_4 concentrations during pregnancy. This increase represents fetal production rather than transplacental transfer, because both T_3 and T_4 cross the placenta only minimally. However, iodides, antithyroid medications, and TSIs cross the placenta easily.

Thyroid hormone deficiency during fetal development or during the first 2 years of life can cause irreversible brain damage, with the degree of disease related to the severity, duration, and gestational age at which the hypothyroidism occurs. Although neonatal hypothyroidism is not common (1 in 4000 live births in the United States), it is a potentially treatable cause of mental retardation and thus is now included in most newborn blood-screening programs.

At present, fetal hypothyroidism can be treated antenatally by direction hormone injection of the fetus via amniocentesis. Fetal hyperthyroidism can also be diagnosed before birth and may respond to prenatal treatment. Fetal or neonatal thyrotoxicosis occurs in 1 of 70 thyrotoxic mothers. It results from the transplacental transfer of TSIs and is a potentially serious disease with mortality rates of 10% to 16% due to prematurity and congestive heart failure. Hyperthyroid pregnant patients should be evaluated frequently for fetal tachycardia, and appropriate interval fetal growth should be confirmed. Fetal goiter may be identified on ultrasound examination, and fetal thyroid function can be assessed with fetal blood sampling. Because PTU and methimazole cross the placenta, maternal doses can be adjusted to correct the fetal hyperthyroidism; replacement T_4 can then be given to the mother, if necessary.

The diagnosis of neonatal thyrotoxicosis is usually clinically apparent, as the infant may have a goiter, exophthalmos, tachycardia, irritability, and growth restriction. The mother likely has a history of hyperthyroidism and may have had previous infants affected by this disease. Mild cases of neonatal thyrotoxicosis require no treatment; the symptoms resolve as maternal TSIs are cleared from the infant's system. Severely symptomatic babies are treated with propranolol and PTU.

Parathyroid Conditions

The parathyroid glands function to maintain maternal calcium and phosphate homeostasis. Total calcium levels decline in pregnancy because the binding protein albumin declines, but the level of ionized, biologically active calcium is unchanged. The fetus contains approximately 30 mg of calcium, which is actively transported across the placenta. Maternal calcium requirements increase from 0.5 mg per day to 1.5 mg per day at term. Serum parathyroid hormone (PTH) levels gradually increase during pregnancy, reflecting the increased calcium transfer to the fetus plus the increases in extracellular fluid volume and glomerular filtration rate.

Hyperparathyroidism

Hyperparathyroidism is a condition caused by excessive PTH production, often due to a clinically inapparent *parathyroid adenoma*. Hypercalcemia results and causes symptoms of fatigue, weakness, polyuria, polydipsia, nausea, anorexia, and constipation. During pregnancy, affected women may have

prolonged nausea and vomiting. Increased renal excretion of calcium may predispose to nephrocalcinosis, renal calculi, and symptomatic bony resorption. Although serum calcium measurements remain the best single diagnostic test, the physiologic changes of pregnancy may make the diagnosis of hyperparathyroidism difficult. A total calcium concentration of 10.5 mg/dl or greater in late pregnancy must be considered suspicious, and a total calcium concentration of 12.0 mg/dl or greater is definite evidence of hyperparathyroidism. Palpable parathyroid adenomas are extremely uncommon.

Hyperparathyroidism is associated with an increased incidence of perinatal morbidity and mortality; therapy is thus recommended. Up to 50% of infants of untreated mothers will develop hypocalcemia and tetany, which may be the first indicator of maternal disease. If the diagnosis is first established during pregnancy, surgical resection of the adenoma is generally indicated, although oral phosphate therapy (1 to 1.5 g daily in divided doses) may occasionally be attempted. Pregnancy termination need not be considered except in the rare case of advanced renal involvement.

Hypoparathyroidism

Hypoparathyroidism results from inadequate production of PTH and is characterized by weakness, fatigue, mental status changes, numbness and paresthesias of the extremities, muscular cramps, and tetany. It must be distinguished from pseudohypoparathyroidism, in which parathyroid function is normal but end organs do not respond to PTH. The signs and symptoms of hypoparathyroidism are the result of a decreased serum ionized calcium level and increased neuromuscular irritability. It occurs most commonly as the result of parathyroid gland injury or removal in association with thyroid surgery or irradiation, but it can be idiopathic. The increased calcium requirements of pregnancy may make patients with hypoparathyroidism more symptomatic. In addition, relative unavailability of calcium for the fetus may lead to secondary neonatal hyperparathyroidism. Symptomatic hypocalcemia can be prevented with calcitriol (1,25-dihydroxyvitamin D_3), dihydrotachysterol, large doses of vitamin D, and calcium gluconate or lactate. The patient should be on a low-phosphate diet and might benefit from consultation with an endocrinologist and a dietitian.

Adrenal Disease

In normal pregnancy, plasma concentrations of adrenal steroid hormones typically increase with advancing gestation. Because the amount of cortisol bound to nuclear receptors is actually slightly decreased (due to competition by progesterone), both total plasma cortisol and cortisol-binding globulin levels increase. Free cortisol levels are increased, and a diurnal variation is maintained. Aldosterone levels also rise, although the factor(s) responsible remain unclear; no consistent correlations exist with observed elevations in angiotensin II or progesterone. Adrenal function tests are un-

TABLE 12. *Causes of adrenal insufficiency*

Primary (Addison disease)
Autoimmune
Tuberculosis
Secondary
Exogenous glucocorticoids

altered. As with other endocrine disorders, abnormalities in adrenal function are usually associated with infertility. However, adrenal insufficiency and hyperfunction can complicate pregnancy.

Inadequate production of adrenal corticosteroids can be either chronic or acute. Although most cases of *adrenal insufficiency* are diagnosed outside of pregnancy, the disease may first occur during pregnancy and present a diagnostic challenge. The chronic form may present with numerous nonspecific signs and symptoms, whereas the acute form may present as vascular collapse.

The signs and symptoms of *chronic adrenocortical insufficiency* during pregnancy are identical to those in the nonpregnant state and include fatigue, hyperpigmentation, weakness, anorexia, nausea, vomiting, and weight loss. Because all of these problems may be encountered in the course of an otherwise normal gestation, the clinical diagnosis of adrenocortical insufficiency in pregnancy may be difficult. However, persistent weight loss or nausea and vomiting beyond the first trimester, particularly in association with any of the aforementioned signs or symptoms, should raise suspicions. The diagnosis and appropriate treatment of adrenocortical insufficiency during pregnancy are important because of the risks associated with the added stress of pregnancy and delivery and because of the increased likelihood of adrenal crisis, particularly during the puerperium.

Adrenal insufficiency can be primary (Addison disease), due to autoimmune adrenal destruction or tuberculosis, or secondary, due most often to exogenous glucocorticoids (Table 12). When *Addison disease* is suspected, a blood sample for plasma cortisol and ACTH levels should be obtained (Table 13). A cortisol less than 20 μg/dl is consistent with Addison disease. Treatment should be started promptly, consisting of intravenous hydrocortisone, 100 mg every 6 hours. When chronic adrenal insufficiency is suspected or confirmation of the diagnosis of acute adrenal insufficiency is needed, an ACTH challenge test can be performed and a 24-hour urinary free cortisol level determined. Chronic replacement thereafter consists of hydrocortisone, 12 to 15 mg/m^2 per day, and, if necessary (as guided by serum potassium), fludrocortisone acetate (Florinef Acetate), 100 g per day, for mineralocorticoid activity.

Additional cortisol replacement is recommended during periods of major stress, with criteria being fairly vague and liberal (e.g., injury, fever, surgery). In these instances, the dosage is increased to at least 200 mg per day until the stress has passed. For periods of minor stress (e.g., nausea, vomiting, low-grade fever), the routine daily dosage is doubled. Since glucocorticoids cross the placenta, transient suppression of the newborn hypothalamic–pituitary–adrenal axis may be observed, and the neonate may require cortisol replacement and treatment of hypoglycemia. Neonatal outcome is otherwise unaffected.

Cushing Syndrome (Hypercortisolism)

Elevated levels of glucocorticoids can result from bilateral adrenal hyperplasia, benign or malignant adrenal adenomas, or exogenous corticosteroid therapy. If adrenal hyperplasia occurs in response to an ACTH-producing pituitary tumor, the diagnosis is *Cushing disease.* Affected individuals are obese, hypertensive, and hirsute, with common complaints of weakness, easy bruising, and emotional lability. Classically described features of Cushing syndrome include round faces and full cheeks, together with increased centripetal fat distribution. Glucose intolerance, acne, and osteoporosis are also common in untreated patients.

The diagnosis of Cushing syndrome in pregnancy may be difficult because many of the previously mentioned signs and symptoms may also be seen in normal pregnancy. However, hirsutism and acne tend to be particularly prominent. These patients have elevated plasma cortisol levels, without diurnal variation, that do not suppress with dexamethasone (Table 14). Because of the possibility of adrenal carcinoma, any such patient must be carefully evaluated by appropriate laboratory and radiographic means. With Cushing symptomatology, adrenal cancers are typically very large (6 cm) and easily detectable on CT scan.

Cushing syndrome in pregnancy is associated with an increased incidence of miscarriage, premature labor, diabetes, hypertension, and stillbirth. Consequently, careful fetal surveillance is mandatory.

TABLE 13. *Laboratory diagnosis of adrenocortical insufficiency*

Test	Normal	Normal response	Addison disease
Corticotropin stimulation		> Doubling of cortisol at 1 h	< Doubling of cortisol at 1 h
Plasma adrenocorticotropic hormone	23 ± 5 pg/ml in first trimester 59 ± 16 pg/ml in last trimester	Increased during pregnancy	Increased with primary disease; decreased with secondary disease
Morning plasma cortisol	9 ± 3 μg/dl in first trimester 27 ± 11 μg/dl in last trimester	Increased during pregnancy	Decreased

TABLE 14. *Laboratory diagnosis of hypercortisolism*

Test	Normal	Normal response	Cushing syndrome
Morning plasma cortisol	9 ± 3 µg/dl in first trimester 27 ± 11 µg/dl in last trimester	Increased during pregnancy	Further increased with loss of dirunal variability
Evening plasma cortisol	4 ± 2 µg/dl in first trimester 15 ± 6 µg/dl in last trimester	—	—
24-h urinary free cortisol	30–100 µg/d in first trimester 90–140 µg/d in last trimester	Increased during pregnancy	Further increased
Plasma adrenocorticotropic hormone	23 ± 5 pg/ml in first trimester 59 ± 16 pg/ml in last trimester	Increased during pregnancy	Very low or undetectable

Congenital Adrenal Hyperplasia

Congenital adrenal hyperplasia (CAH) is the result of one of several enzyme defects in cortisol biosynthesis. The majority of patients have 21-hydroxylase deficiency, although 11β-hydroxylase deficiency or 18-hydroxysteroid dehydrogenase deficiency may rarely be encountered. Because these enzyme deficiencies are autosomal-recessive, the patient with this diagnosis has a negligible chance to have an affected child, unless she is related to the child's father.

Approximately 90% of patients with CAH during pregnancy have a partial or complete deficiency of the 21-hydroxylase enzyme. The resultant decrease in cortisol production leads to increased ACTH stimulation, which then results in both increased production of androgenic cortisol precursors (e.g., 17α-hydroxyprogesterone) and decreased production of aldosterone. Because these androgenic steroids readily cross the placenta, pregnancies complicated by significant maternal 21-hydroxylase deficiency are at increased risk for fetal virilization. Such virilization is most apparent in female infants, although male infants may also have somewhat enlarged external genitalia. The risk of fetal virilization is reduced if pregnant patients with CAH receive adequate basal glucocorticoid replacement, together with additional glucocorticoid in times of stress. Mineralocorticoid replacement should be continued as well.

Sometimes, the pregnant patient herself does not have CAH but has had a previous child with the disorder. The diagnosis of congenital adrenal hyperplasia in the fetus has historically been made on the basis of amniotic fluid measurement of 17α-hydroxyprogesterone. However, molecular genetic techniques are now available for evaluation of fetuses at risk by chorionic villus sampling (CVS) of chorionic villus cells or amniocytes. The affected fetus will produce high levels of androgenic steroids that can cause virilization. Fetal treatment consisting of maternal oral dexamethasone twice daily beginning at 6 to 7 weeks may prevent this. The treatment is discontinued if CVS or amniocyte analysis confirms that the fetus does not carry the enzymatic defect.

A newborn with ambiguous genitalia requires rapid diagnosis, treatment, and gender assignment. The karyotype, electrolytes, 17α-hydroxyprogesterone, and urinary 17-ketosteroids should be evaluated expeditiously. The clinical manifestations of cortisol and aldosterone deficiency can include hypoglycemia, hyperpigmentation, apneic episodes, seizures, emesis, hyperkalemia, dehydration, hypotension, vascular collapse, and shock. Resuscitation requires hydrocortisone administration and saline/glucose hydration. Elevated plasma renin activity indicates the need for mineralocorticoid replacement as well. Eventually, maintenance therapy with hydrocortisone (glucocorticoid) and fludrocortisone (mineralocorticoid) is guided by 17α-hydroxyprogesterone and plasma renin activity measurements, respectively. Undertreatment is accompanied by premature skeletal maturation, whereas overtreatment leads to slowing of skeletal maturation. It is hoped that using clinical variables such as height velocity and weight to guide replacement therapy will improve the mean adult height in patients with this disorder (i.e., 4th percentile for men and 25th percentile for women).

Pheochromocytoma

Pheochromocytoma is a rare but extremely serious complication of pregnancy, with increased maternal and perinatal morbidity and mortality rates. Hypertension is present in the majority of patients and may be either paroxysmal or sustained. Only a minority of patients have classic pheochromocytoma episodes, characterized by extreme hypertension, headache, diaphoresis, weakness, tremor, and palpitations. Such patients are often initially considered to have hyperthyroidism.

The diagnosis of pheochromocytoma is best made by measurement of 24-hour urinary catecholamines; normal values are unaffected by pregnancy. If the diagnosis is established by laboratory criteria, the tumor should be localized, using whatever combination of abdominal CT scan and selective venous sampling is clinically indicated. Eighty percent of these tumors are located in one adrenal, 10% to 15% are bilateral, and 10% are found in other locations, including the renal hilus, the organ of Zuckerkandl, and the periaortic sympathetic chain.

Because of the high morbidity and mortality associated with this condition, surgical removal during pregnancy is indicated when the diagnosis is established. The patient should be pretreated with alpha- and beta-blockers, usually phenoxybenzamine and propranolol, for 1 to 2 weeks before surgery to increase the likelihood of intraoperative symptomatic control. Multidisciplinary management is essential to maximize maternal and fetal outcomes.

◊ DERMATOLOGIC DISEASES

Physiologic Changes during Pregnancy

The systemic changes of pregnancy affect the skin in many ways; effects can be transient or permanent. Striae gravidarum, or stretch marks, develop in the majority of women, and although they may fade postpartum, they seldom disappear. Ninety percent of all pregnant women experience some degree of hyperpigmentation, the cause of which is unknown. It may involve melanocyte-stimulating hormone and estrogens, and/or other factors. Hyperpigmentation is more marked in darker-skinned women, more often permanent in lighter-skinned women, and involves the nipples, perineum, umbilicus, and the linea alba (nigra). Facial pigmentation, or melasma, is seen in at least 50% of pregnant women. It is melanin-related and aggravated by sunlight. Benign or melanocytic nevi commonly enlarge and darken and can be confused with malignant melanoma. Vascular changes are also prominent and may manifest as spider angiomas, palmar erythema, and venous varicosities. Finally, scalp hair growth is altered, with an increased proportion of growing hairs to resting hairs. This is reversed after delivery with the onset of telogen effluvium, an abrupt hair loss 1 to 4 months postpartum. By 6 to 12 months, normal hair growth is restored.

Pregnancy-specific Dermatologic Diseases

Intrahepatic Cholestasis of Pregnancy

Intrahepatic cholestasis of pregnancy is the second most common cause of jaundice in pregnant women (hepatitis is the most common cause) and can produce intense pruritus (Table 15). There may be a several-fold increase in maternal serum bile salts, alkaline phosphatase, aspartate aminotransferase (serum glutamic-oxaloacetic transaminase), alanine aminotransferase (serum glutamic-pyruvic transaminase), and bilirubin. Treatment is symptomatic but not always effective. Topical antipruritics, antihistamines, dexamethasone, cholestyramine, and ursodeoxycholic acid have been used with variable success. The pruritus and laboratory abnormalities typically resolve promptly after delivery, but half of patients will experience recurrence in subsequent pregnancies or with oral contraceptive use. Cholestasis is associated with an increased risk of adverse fetal outcome. Antepartum tests of fetal well-being and consideration of timely delivery are recommended.

Herpes Gestationis

Herpes gestationis, or pemphigoid gestationis, is a rare, serious, autoimmune dermatologic disease seen in pregnancy. The onset is typically in mid- to late pregnancy but occasionally occurs postpartum. It is characterized by severe pruritus, with urticarial papules, plaques, erythema, and vesicles and bullae involving the abdomen and extremities. It is occasionally generalized, and exacerbations and remissions are common. Treatment for these pruritic lesions typically includes antihistamines and topical steroids, with oral steroids considered in severe cases. Biopsy and histologic examination reveals subepidermal edema with inflammatory infiltrate, and immunofluorescent staining confirms complement and IgG deposition at the basement membrane. This complement-fixing IgG can cross the placenta and cause dermatologic manifestations in about 5% of newborns; these typically resolve within several weeks. Herpes gestationis has been associated with adverse fetal outcome, so fetal well-being testing is appropriate. Recurrence is seen in subsequent pregnancies, and it is often more severe and occurs earlier in gestation.

Pruritic Urticarial Papules and Plaques of Pregnancy

Pruritic urticarial papules and plaques of pregnancy (PUPPP) is the most common pruritic dermatosis of pregnancy. An intensely pruritic disorder, PUPPP appears late in pregnancy, with a frequency as high as 1%. It is more common in nulliparas and is not known to recur. The papules and plaques can be generalized or patchy, involving the abdomen, buttocks,

TABLE 15. *Dermatologic diseases in pregnancy*

Disorder	Frequency	Clinical characteristics	Perinatal outcome	Treatment
Intrahepatic cholestasis of pregnancy	Common	Jaundice; pruritus; increased liver function tests; 50% recurrence in subsequent pregnancy	Increased morbidity	Antipruritics; antihistamines; cholestyramine
Herpes gestationis	Rare	Severe pruritus; papules, plaques, bullae	Increased morbidity	Antipruritics; antihistamines; steroids
Pruritic urticarial papules and plaques of pregnancy	Common	Papules, plaques	Unaffected	Antipruritics; steroids
Impetigo herpetiformis	Rare	Pustules	Parallels severity of maternal disease	Antibiotics, supportive
Acne vulgaris	Common	—	Unaffected	Tretinoin, benzoyl Iperoxide
Malignant melanoma	Rare	Pigmented cutaneous lesions	Placental metastases reported	Surgery

thighs, and arms. On biopsy and immunofluorescent staining, the absence of antibody or complement deposition distinguishes PUPPP from herpes gestationis; instead, there is a nonspecific lymphocytic perivasculitis. Treatment consists of antipruritics and topical steroids. In severe cases, oral steroids may be considered. There is no associated increase in perinatal morbidity.

Impetigo Herpetiformis

Impetigo herpetiformis, which some consider to be pustular psoriasis, is a rare disease with an onset late in pregnancy. It initially involves intertriginous surfaces but can extend to involve the entire skin surface and mucous membranes. It classically appears as erythematous patches surrounded by sterile pustules that can become secondarily infected. Systemic symptoms and signs include fever, malaise, gastrointestinal distress, and hypocalcemia; maternal sepsis is not uncommon. Treatment is supportive, with maintenance of fluid and electrolyte balance, correction of hypocalcemia, and antibiotic therapy as needed. The utility of steroids is uncertain. Delivery is not necessarily accompanied with resolution. Perinatal morbidity and mortality parallel the severity of maternal disease; tests of fetal well-being are warranted in severe cases.

Non–Pregnancy-specific Dermatologic Diseases

Acne Vulgaris

Some, but not all, women will note that their acne vulgaris improves with pregnancy. Topical treatments, such as tretinoin (Retin-A) and benzoyl peroxide, as well as oral erythromycin, can be useful for the pregnant patient. Isotretinoin (Accutane), prescribed for severe cystic acne, and etretinate (Tegison), prescribed for psoriasis, are contraindicated, as they are teratogenic.

Malignant Melanoma

Malignant melanoma, a relatively common disease of women of childbearing age, should be considered if a skin lesion is enlarging and unusually colored, with bleeding and/or irregular borders. Diagnosis is by biopsy. Pregnancy is not thought to affect survival of stage I patients, and the disease does not usually affect pregnancy outcome, although placental metastases have been reported. Treatment is primarily surgical, with adjuvant chemo/immunotherapy. As the majority of recurrences manifest with 5 years, most experts recommend a delay in future pregnancies.

◊ SURGICAL DISEASES IN PREGNANCY

Excluding ectopic pregnancy, pregnancy does not increase the risk of surgical illness or malignancy and does not increase the risk of adverse outcome after an uncomplicated surgical procedure. Surgical diseases in the pregnant woman can be life-threatening, however, because the physiologic changes of pregnancy and the presence of a gravid uterus may delay accurate diagnosis and can make many surgical procedures more technically difficult. While nonemergent surgery should be postponed until after delivery if at all possible, a surgical emergency in a pregnant woman should prompt the same aggressive treatment that the nonpregnant individual would receive.

Appendicitis

Laparotomy is required during 1 in 500 to 1000 pregnancies; appendicitis is the most common diagnosis. Pregnancy does not increase the risk of appendicitis. It occurs with equal frequency in all three trimesters, and appendectomy can be performed safely throughout pregnancy. However, acute appendicitis has been associated with a maternal mortality rate as high as 5% and an increased risk of preterm labor and fetal loss. These complications most often result from a delay in diagnosis.

Intraabdominal pathology can be difficult to diagnose in the gravid woman. Bowel is progressively displaced upward and backward as the gravid uterus grows during pregnancy. Because bowel sounds are normally heard only in the upper abdomen, the absence of bowel sounds may not be appreciated. The appendix also assumes an increasingly more cephalad position, and associated inflammation and pain are therefore not localized to the right lower quadrant after the first trimester. Anorexia, nausea and vomiting, a change in bowel habits, and even epigastric or abdominal pain can be part of normal pregnancy and thus may not suggest pathology. Laboratory evaluation may not be helpful, as a mild leukocytosis is common in pregnancy. Nevertheless, it is in the patient's best interest to have a high index of suspicion because delayed diagnosis and therapy can be catastrophic. A ruptured appendix in pregnancy does not wall itself off well and is therefore very serious.

The patient typically presents with periumbilical or right flank pain that is increased by uterine manipulation. Placing the patient on her left side allows the uterus to fall away from the right flank, and may facilitate examination. Thirty percent of appendices are retrocecal in location; in this situation, the presenting complaint may be right flank or leg pain or pain on rectal examination, and the patient may have psoas or obturator muscle signs. Symptoms of anorexia, nausea, and vomiting are usually increased relative to normal pregnancy. The white blood cell count may be significantly elevated, and the patient may be febrile, especially if appendix rupture or generalized peritonitis is present. Sonographic examination can help rule out other diagnoses but generally cannot confirm appendicitis itself, as ultrasound penetrates gas-filled structures poorly. A plain x-ray film to identify air–fluid levels or free air in the abdomen can be very helpful and generally exposes the fetus to less than 300 mrad (0.0003 Gy) of radiation. Once appendicitis is suspected, laparotomy should be performed. A right paramedian vertical incision provides ideal visualization.

Intestinal Obstruction

The second most common nonobstetric indication for abdominal surgery is intestinal obstruction, which complicates 3 in 10,000 pregnancies. Risk factors include previous pelvic inflammatory disease and previous intraabdominal surgery. The incidence of abdominal obstruction increases as pregnancy advances because the enlarging uterus displaces the bowel upward and backward, placing preexisting adhesions on tension and increasing the risk of volvulus. As stated above, pregnancy makes assessment of bowel function difficult and may contribute to a delay in diagnosis. Maternal mortality as high as 10% to 20% has been reported, due primarily to maternal shock associated with nonrecognition of bowel infarction. As with appendicitis, once bowel obstruction unresponsive to conservative management has been diagnosed, surgical intervention should not be delayed.

Cholecystitis

Acute abdomen may also be due to cholecystitis. Cholecystitis occurs in 1 in 1000 to 1600 pregnancies; over 90% of cases are caused by cholelithiasis. Patients typically present with nausea, vomiting, and the acute onset of colicky midepigastric pain. Laboratory evaluation and ultrasound examination are helpful in making the diagnosis. The treatment is primarily medical, especially in the first and third trimesters. Surgery might be considered for the patient with repeated severe episodes of cholecystitis and unremitting pain, systemic toxicity, or persistent or recurring pancreatitis. The second trimester is preferable for elective surgery because the risks of surgery-associated fetal loss, preterm labor, or fetal compromise are lowest at this time and, although the pregnancy is well established, the uterus is still small enough to allow adequate visualization of the operative site without extensive uterine manipulation. Open laparoscopic second-trimester cholecystectomy has been reported with good results. Maternal mortality is minimal, and fetal mortality is usually less than 5%

Pancreatitis

Pancreatitis can also result in acute abdomen. In pregnancy, the most common etiology of pancreatitis is cholecystitis, with alcohol abuse, viral infection, and hyperlipidemia accounting for a small proportion of cases. Treatment is primarily medical, as outlined earlier, with surgery considered only if symptoms do not improve rapidly (1 to 2 days) or an abscess or pseudocyst develops. As with cholecystitis, ultrasound examination may be helpful in making the diagnosis and ruling out other entities. The patient should be followed closely with careful attention to fluid management. Fetal loss can occur in complicated cases as a result of acidosis, hypovolemia, and hypoxia.

Liver Disease

Abdominal pain, particularly right upper quadrant pain, may be due to liver disease. Most commonly, liver pathology in pregnancy is due to preeclampsia, hepatitis, or acute fatty liver. Very rarely, pregnancy is complicated by cirrhosis and/or portal hypertension. Because pregnancy increases the risk of bleeding from esophageal varices, such patients may require endoscopic sclerotherapy during pregnancy.

Peptic Ulcer Disease

Although peptic ulcer disease can cause symptoms of acute abdomen, it is rare in gravid women because the hormonal milieu and other physiologic changes of pregnancy confer a protective effect during pregnancy. Endoscopy can be performed to confirm the diagnosis. Management is primarily medical.

◊ MATERNAL TRAUMA

Physiologic Changes of Pregnancy

Accurate assessment of the pregnant trauma victim requires knowledge of the physiologic changes that normally occur during gestation. No organ system is unaffected, but the functions of the cardiovascular and respiratory systems are altered most dramatically. Plasma volume increases by 50%, while red cell mass increases by 25%, resulting in a physiologic anemia. Leukocytosis normally occurs, peaking in the third trimester with a white blood cell count of 12,000 to 18,000/mm^3 and 25,000/mm^3 in labor. Cardiac output increases by 4.5 to 6.0 l per minute (30% to 50%), primarily as a result of a gradual increase in stroke volume to 50% above nonpregnant levels. The majority of pregnant women have a widely split first heart sound, a third heart sound, and a systolic ejection murmur. Over 10% of cardiac output goes to the uterus at term, and veins in the pelvis and lower extremities are engorged. Renal blood flow increases by 30%, leading to a 30% to 50% increase in the glomerular filtration rate. As a result, the BUN and creatinine fall and should not be higher than 13 mg/dl and 0.8 mg/dl, respectively, during pregnancy. A hormonally mediated decrease in vascular resistance leads to a midtrimester decrease in both systolic and diastolic blood pressure. All these changes are affected by maternal position; in the supine position, the uterus compresses the vena cava, resulting in decreased venous return, decreased cardiac output, a drop in blood pressure, bradycardia, and syncope.

Hyperventilation begins as early as the first trimester, probably in response to increased progesterone levels. Because of gradual elevation of the diaphragm by the enlarging uterus, functional residual capacity, residual volume, and expiratory reserve volume all decrease, while inspiratory reserve volume increases. The normal gravida at term has a chronic respiratory alkalosis with a resting carbon dioxide tension below 30 mm Hg. Seventy-five percent of gravidas experience dyspnea in the third trimester. Although arterial oxygen tension generally rises toward term, a moderate hypoxemia can occur in the supine position. Thus, the midtrimester gravida lying in the emergency room on her back may be hypotensive, bradycardic, relatively hypoxemic, and anemic, all because of normal physiologic changes.

The ABCs

Taking into consideration the physiology of pregnancy, the pregnant trauma patient should initially be assessed as any trauma victim is assessed, according to the ABCs: airway, breathing, and circulation. In a rapid assessment of the patient's status, airway patency and adequacy of respirations should be established. Supplemental oxygen should be administered to all patients; the patient who is not breathing spontaneously should be intubated and mechanically ventilated. A wedge should be placed under the right hip to displace the uterus off the vena cava. Pregnancy significantly slows gastrointestinal motility; all pregnant women should be assumed to have a full stomach. The conscious patient should be given sodium citrate or a similar antacid, while the airway of the unconscious patient should be protected.

If cardiac function is adequate, attention should be turned to maintaining adequate circulating volume. One or two large-bore intravenous lines should be established and Ringer's lactate solution given; infusion of large volumes of sodium chloride should be avoided, as it can lead to hypoperchloremic acidosis that would exacerbate lactic acidosis caused by poor perfusion. If the patient is bleeding, packed red blood cells should be ordered and administered as soon as possible.

If cardiac arrest has occurred, full resuscitation should be initiated as for any other patient. Cardiopulmonary resuscitation (CPR) at most generates only 30% of the normal cardiac output; CPR of a pregnant woman in left lateral tilt will be even less effective. The patient must therefore remain supine, and someone must be assigned to manually elevate the uterus off the vena cava. It can be assumed that perfusion to the uterus will be negligible during CPR. The general consensus is that a fetus can survive total asphyxia for at most 4 to 6 minutes. If cardiac function has not been restored within 4 minutes of arrest and the fetus is still alive, an emergent, nonsterile, classical cesarean section should be performed without anesthesia at the bed side, and the uterus and abdominal incisions closed as rapidly as possible. If cardiac arrest has persisted for more than 6 minutes but fetal cardiac activity continues, delivery should still be performed; in addition to possibly saving the fetus, evacuation of the uterus will facilitate CPR by improving cardiovascular dynamics.

The American College of Obstetricians and Gynecologists recommends that any pregnant woman sustaining trauma beyond 22 to 24 weeks' gestation undergo fetal monitoring for a minimum of 4 hours. If more than four contractions per hour are observed, if rupture of membranes, bleeding, fetal arrhythmia, or fetal heart rate decelerations occur, or if the mother is seriously injured, the patient should be admitted with continuous fetal monitoring for at least 24 hours.

Abdominal Trauma

Blunt abdominal trauma commonly occurs during a motor vehicle accident, especially if the woman is unrestrained or is not wearing her lap belt as low as possible, under her uterus. Rupture of the liver or spleen occurs in up to 25% of cases of blunt trauma, and rupture of the uterus occurs in 10%. Bladder injury or rupture is more common after 20 weeks, when the bladder assumes an intraabdominal position and is no longer protected by the pelvis. Bladder injury may also result from pelvic fracture. The patient should be stabilized as above, with any signs of shock or peritoneal irritation raising the suspicion of major intraabdominal injury. Intraabdominal bleeding can be detected with intraperitoneal lavage, just as in the nonpregnant patient. Bladder injury is suspected when a Foley catheter cannot be successfully passed, fails to return urine, or returns grossly bloody fluid. Bowel injury is uncommon, except at points of fixation. The fetus is usually protected by amniotic fluid and the resilience of the uterus, although fetal skull fracture has been reported after pelvic trauma.

Placental abruption or uterine rupture can occur after fracture of the pelvis or a sudden deceleration injury. Abruption is associated with abdominal pain, uterine tenderness or irritability, and fetal heart rate decelerations. If the patient is otherwise stable and fetal viability is confirmed, emergent delivery should be considered. Uterine rupture usually results in vaginal bleeding, hypotension, absent fetal heart tones, and hematuria if the rupture involves the anterior uterine wall. The patient should be stabilized and a laparotomy performed as rapidly as possible. Counseling should be provided regarding the likelihood of hysterectomy, and multiple units of packed red blood cells should be made available.

If the patient is stable and a CT scan or other radiologic studies are necessary for diagnostic purposes, they should be performed. If at all possible, the patient should be positioned with a wedge under one hip to deflect the uterus off the vena cava. The amount of radiation exposure resulting from standard radiologic procedures is less than the minimum dose associated with fetal teratogenicity or growth effects. The fetus is most susceptible before 15 weeks' gestation, when radiation doses of 10 rad (0.1 Gy) or greater can cause mental retardation. At 16 to 25 weeks, the risk is considerably less, and radiologic procedures at greater than or equal to 25 weeks pose minimal to no risk. Most authorities recommend limiting fetal exposure to less than 5 rad (0.05 Gy). Most plain x-ray films entail doses of less than 1 rad (0.01 Gy); an abdominal CT scan exposes the fetus to 2 to 2.6 rad (0.02 to 0.026 Gy). MR imaging does not require ionizing radiation and thus does not entail risk at any gestational age. Medical and surgical care should not be compromised in any way just because the patient is pregnant. If the woman is Rh-negative and unsensitized, $Rh_0(D)$ immune globulin will protect her if there was fetal–maternal bleeding.

Penetrating Abdominal Trauma

Gunshot and knife wounds are responsible for most cases of penetrating abdominal trauma in pregnancy. As the uterus grows out of the pelvis, it becomes more likely that the uterus will be a site of injury. Penetration of the uterus results in fetal injury in 59% to 89% of cases, and fetal death in 41% to 71%. After penetrating abdominal trauma, the pregnant patient should be assessed as above and attempts made to determine the exact site(s) of injury and associated organ damage. The initial evaluation and subsequent surgical management should be the same as for the nonpregnant patient. If the uterus is the primary site of injury, exploratory laparotomy will likely be required. Bullet wounds must be explored surgically, because deflection of the bullet off intraabdominal structures can cause extensive damage and make it impossible to determine the projectile path. Knife wounds may also require exploration because the enlarged uterus compresses other intraabdominal organs and prevents structures underlying the stab wound from sliding away from the blade, as they would in the nonpregnant state. Ultrasound examination of the fetus to determine age and assess viability is essential.

Decisions about whether or not to empty the uterus should be individualized. If there is extensive intrauterine damage, if the pregnancy is near term, if there is a strong suspicion of fetal hemorrhage, or if uteroplacental insufficiency is present, the fetus should be delivered and the uterus thoroughly explored. If the uterus is uninjured or the injury can be repaired without entering the uterine cavity, if the fetus is previable or dead, and if uterine size does not preclude adequate exploration of the abdominal cavity, hysterotomy may be avoided as long as hemostasis is achieved.

Intraabdominal organs are compressed into the upper abdomen as pregnancy advances. Penetrating wounds in this area are especially traumatic because multiple organs are injured; in decreasing order of frequency, small bowel, liver, colon, and stomach are damaged most often. For this reason, many authorities recommend that upper abdominal wounds be explored by laparotomy in all pregnant patients. Broad-spectrum antibiotics should be administered, and tocolytic therapy can be used with caution in the postoperative period. β-Mimetics have maternal and fetal cardiovascular effects that may confuse postoperative assessment, while magnesium sulfate is associated with maternal nausea, vomiting, and dizziness. Maintenance of normal intravascular volume and close attention to fluid balance are crucial.

Head Trauma

The gravida with head trauma should be evaluated and treated in the same way as the nonpregnant patient. Assessment begins with the ABCs. The head and neck should be immobilized as a unit in case there is cervical spine injury. In the stable patient, gestational age and viability should be assessed. Unless precluded by vertebral fractures, the uterus should be rolled off the vena cava by placing a wedge under the backboard. Mannitol, steroids, and other medications should be given, if necessary. Because fluid restriction, osmotic diuresis, maternal hypotension, and hypothermia induced during neurosurgery may reduce uteroplacental blood flow, the viable fetus should be monitered and therapeutic adjustments made as required.

Burns

Burns are described as being partial- or full-thickness and quantitated according to the percentage surface area affected.

Extensive full-thickness burns result in severe thermal instability and dramatic fluid loss. Hypovolemic shock can occur, especially within the first 36 hours. Airway management and treatment of the burn itself should be the same for pregnant and nonpregnant patients. The pregnant burn victim, however, requires meticulous attention to fluid management, with consideration of the expanded intravascular volume and altered cardiovascular dynamics associated with pregnancy (see above). Fetal status is directly related to the adequacy of uteroplacental perfusion; poor outcome is associated with inadequate fluid resuscitation. If more than 50% of the patient's surface area is affected, immediate delivery of the viable fetus should be considered. However, in some cases, aggressive fluid resuscitation and close fetal monitoring may allow delivery to be deferred.

Thermal injury causes elevated prostaglandin levels and increased susceptibility to infection. These factors often contribute to preterm labor. Because complications typically associated with tocolytic therapy may not be tolerated by the gravid burn victim, tocolytics should be used cautiously if at all. Indomethacin (Indocin) may be the safest agent for use before 32 weeks. If fetal surveillance (greater than or equal to 24 weeks' gestation) indicates fetal compromise despite optimal maternal resuscitation, the fetus should be delivered.

Electrical Injury

There are very few reports of electrical injury during pregnancy. Because the uterus and amniotic fluid offer low resistance, current entering an upper extremity and exiting a lower extremity may traverse the uterus and fetus. Maternal cardiac and respiratory status should be assessed and treated as in any injured patient. Ultrasound examination and fetal monitoring should guide pregnancy management. Fetal survival without specific intervention has been reported, although immediate fetal death is also possible.

SUMMARY POINTS

◊ The obstetrician-gynecologist must be thoroughly familiar with the normal physiologic changes of pregnancy, as these changes affect the presentation of many diseases, as well as their management.

◊ Although many disease processes are unchanged by pregnancy, the course of some diseases is altered; this alteration often affects diagnosis and therapy.

◊ Necessary radiologic procedures can be performed during pregnancy.

◊ Very few medications need to be restricted in pregnancy.

◊ In general, a woman should not receive different care because she is pregnant, although fetal well-being must be kept in mind if the fetus is past the age of viability.

◊ RECOMMENDED READINGS

Hematologic Disease

American College of Obstetricians and Gynecologists. Hemoglobinopathies in pregnancy. *ACOG Techn Bull No. 220,* Feb 1996.

Burrows RF, Kelton JG. Incidentally detected thrombocytopenia in healthy mothers and their infants. *N Engl J Med* 1988;319:142–145.

Charache S, Terrin ML, Moore RD, et al. Effect of hydroxyurea on the frequency of painful crises in sickle cell anemia. *N Engl J Med* 1995;332:1317.

Cunningham FG, Pritchard JA, Mason R. Pregnancy and sickle cell hemoglobinopathies: results with and without prophylactic transfusions. *Obstet Gynecol* 1983;62:419.

Koshy M, Burd L, Wallace D, Moawad A, Baron J. Prophylactic red-cell transfusions in pregnant patients with sickle cell disease. *N Engl J Med* 1988;319:1447.

Rock GA, Shumak KH, Buskard NA, et al. Comparison of plasma exchange with plasma infusion in the treatment of thrombotic thrombocytopenic purpura. *N Engl J Med* 1991;325:393.

Romslo I, Haram K, Sagen N, Augen K. Iron requirements in normal pregnancy as assessed by serum ferritin, serum transferrin saturation, and erythrocyte protoporphyrin determinations. *Br J Obstet Gynaecol* 1983; 90:101.

Thompson MW, McInnes RR, Willard HF. The hemoglobinopathies: modes of molecular disease. In: *Thompson & Thompson genetics in medicine.* Philadelphia: WB Saunders, 1991:247.

Gastrointestinal Disease

Bohman VR, Steller W, Little BB, et al. Seroprevalence and risk factors for hepatitis C virus antibody in pregnant women. *Obstet Gynecol* 1992;80:609.

David A, Katz VL, Cox R. Gallbladder disease in pregnancy. *J Reprod Med* 1995;40:759.

Hanauer SB, Baert FJ. The management of ulcerative colitis. *Annu Rev Med* 1995;46:497.

Hod M, Orvieto R, Kaplan B, et al. Hyperemesis gravidarum: a review. *J Reprod Med* 1994;39:605.

Laifer SA, Guido RS. Reproductive function and outcome of pregnancy after liver transplantation. *Mayo Clin Proc* 1995;70:388.

Ramin KD, Ramin SM, Richey SD, Cunningham FG. Acute pancreatitis in pregnancy. *Am J Obstet Gynecol* 1995;173:187.

Rogers RG, Katz VL. Course of Crohn's disease during pregnancy and its effect on pregnancy outcome. *Am J Perinatol* 1995;12:262.

Sharp HT. Gastrointestinal surgical conditions during pregnancy. In: Pitkin RM, Scott JR, eds. *Clinical obstetrics and gynecology.* Philadelphia: JB Lippincott Co, 1994:306.

Wolf JL. Liver disease in pregnancy. *Med Clin North Am* 1996;80:1167.

Cardiovascular Disease

Bhagwat AR, Engel PJ. Heart disease and pregnancy. *Cardiol Clin* 1995;13:163.

Boughman JA, Berg KA, Astemborski JA, et al. Familial risks of congenital heart defect assessed in a population-based epidemiologic study. *Am J Med Genet* 1987;26:839.

Elkayam U, Gleicher N. *Cardiac problems in pregnancy: diagnosis and management of maternal and fetal disease,* 2nd ed. New York: Alan R. Liss, 1990.

Friederich PW, Sanson B, Simioni P, et al. Frequency of pregnancy-related venous thromboembolism in anticoagulant factor-deficient women: implications for prophylaxis. *Ann Intern Med* 1996;125:955.

Hankins GDV, Wendel GD, Leveno KJ, Stoneham J. Myocardial infarction during pregnancy: a review. *Obstet Gynecol* 1985;65:139.

Iturbe-Alessio I, del Carmen Fonseca M, Mutchinik O, Santos MA, Zajarias A, Salazar E. Risks of anticoagulant therapy in pregnant women with artificial heart valves. *N Engl J Med* 1986;315:1390.

Midei MG, De Ment SH, Feldman AM, Hutchins GM. Peripartum myocarditis and cardiomyopathy. *Circulation* 1990;81:922.

Perloff JK. Congenital heart disease and pregnancy. *Clin Cardiol* 1994;17:579.

Presbitero P, Somerville J, Stone S, Aruta E, Spiegelhalter D, Rabajoli F. Pregnancy in cyanotic congenital heart disease: outcome of mother and fetus. *Circulation* 1994;89:2673.

Sciscione AC, Callan NA. Pregnancy and contraception. *Cardiol Clin* 1993;11:701.

Szekely P, Turner R, Sraith L. Pregnancy and the changing pattern of rheumatic heart disease. *Br Heart J* 1973;35:1293.

Weiner CP. Diagnosis and management of thromboembolic disease during pregnancy. *Clin Obstet Gynecol* 1985;28:107.

Pulmonary Disease

Cunningham FG, Lucas MJ. Urinary tract infections complicating pregnancy. *Baillieres Clin Obstet Gynaecol* 1994;8:353.

Hilman BC, Aitken ML, Constantinescu M. Pregnancy in patients with cystic fibrosis. *Clin Obstet Gynecol* 1996;39:70.

Hou SH. Pregnancy in women on haemodialysis and peritoneal dialysis. *Baillieres Clin Obstet Gynaecol* 1994;8:481.

Houshiar AM, Ercole CJ. Urinary calculi during pregnancy: when are they cause for concern? *Postgrad Med* 1996;100:131.

Jones DC. Pregnancy complicated by chronic renal disease. *Clin Perinatol* 1997;24:483.

Katz VL, Kuller JA, McMahon MJ, Warren MA, Wells SR. Varicella during pregnancy: maternal and fetal effects. *West J Med* 1995;163:446.

Miller KS, Miller JM. Tuberculosis in pregnancy: interactions, diagnosis and management. *Clin Obstet Gynecol* 1996;39:120.

Renal Disease

Rigby FB, Pastorek JG. Pneumonia during pregnancy. *Clin Obstet Gynecol* 1996;1:107.

Schatz M, Zeiger RS. Asthma and allergy in pregnancy. *Clin Perinatol* 1997;24:407.

Wendel PJ, Ramin SM, Barnett-Hamm C, Rowe TF, Cunningham FG. Asthma treatment in pregnancy: a randomized controlled study. *Am J Obstet Gynecol* 1996;175:150.

Wong KM, Bailey RR, Lynn KL, et al. Pregnancy in renal transplant recipients: the Christchurch experience. *N Z Med J* 1995;108:190.

Neurologic Disease

Birk K, Ruddick R. Pregnancy and multiple sclerosis. *Arch Neurol* 1986;43:719.

Brown RH. Clinical aspects of myotonic dystrophy. *Neurogenet Adv* 1994;3:1.

Buehler BA, Delimont D, van Waes M, Finnell RH. Prenatal prediction of risk of the fetal hydantoin syndrome. *N Engl J Med* 1990;322:1567.

Dias MS. Neurovascular emergencies in pregnancy. In: Pitkin RM, Scott JR, eds. *Clinical obstetrics and gynecology.* Philadelphia: JB Lippincott Co, 1994:337.

Dias MS, Sekhar LN. Intracranial hemorrhage from aneurysms and arteriovenous malformations during pregnancy and the puerperium. *Neurosurgery* 1990;27:855.

Digre KB, Varner MW, Corbett JJ. Pseudotumor cerebri and pregnancy. *Neurology* 1984;34:721.

Gaily E, Granstrom ML, Hiilesmaa V, Bardy A. Minor anomalies in offspring of epileptic mothers. *J Pediatr* 1988;112:520.

Jaffe R, Mock M, Abramowicz J, et al. Myotonic dystrophy and pregnancy: a review. *Obstet Gynecol Surv* 1986;41:272.

Mitchell PJ, Bebbington M. Myasthenia gravis in pregnancy. *Obstet Gynecol* 1992;80:178.

Sadasivan B, Malik GM, Lee C, et al. Vascular malformations and pregnancy. *Surg Neurol* 1990;33:305.

Endocrine Disease

Kohlmeier L, Marcus R. Calcium disorders of pregnancy. *Endocrinol Metab Clin North Am* 1995;24:15.

Robertson GL. Diabetes insipidus. *Endocrinol Metab Clin North Am* 1995;24:549.

Rosen IB, Korman M, Walfish PG. Thyroid nodular disease in pregnancy: current diagnosis and management. *Clin Obstet Gynecol* 1997;40:81.

Sipes SL, Malee MP. Endocrine disorders in pregnancy. *Obstet Gynecol Clin North Am* 1992;19:655.

Yankowitz J, Weiner C. Medical fetal therapy. *Baillieres Clin Obstet Gynaecol* 1995;9:553.

Dermatologic Disease

Alsulyman OM, Ouzounian JG, Ames-Castro M, Goodwin TM. Intrahepatic cholestasis of pregnancy: perinatal outcome associated with expectant management. *Am J Obstet Gynecol* 1996;175:957.

Errickson CV, Matus NR. Skin disorders of pregnancy. *Am Fam Phys* 1994;49:605.

Uncu G, Ozan H, Tatlikazan S, et al. Gestational herpes: 3 cases. *J Obstet Gynecol* 1995;21:381.

Wong RC, Ellis CN. Physiologic skin changes in pregnancy. *J Am Acad Dermatol* 1984;10:929.

Surgical Disease

Epstein FB. Acute abdominal pain in pregnancy. *Emerg Med Clin North Am* 1994;12:151.

Kochhar R, Goenka MK, Mehta SK. Endoscopic sclerotherapy during pregnancy. *Am J Gastroenterol* 1990;85:1132.

Mazze RI, Kallen B. Appendectomy during pregnancy: a Swedish registry study of 778 cases. *Obstet Gynecol* 1991;77:835.

Mazze RI, Kallen B. Reproductive outcome after anesthesia and operation during pregnancy: a registry study of 5,405 cases. *Am J Obstet Gynecol* 1989;161:1178.

Munro A, Jones PF. Abdominal surgical emergencies in the puerperium. *BMJ* 1975;4:691.

Sharp HT. Gastrointestinal surgical conditions in pregnancy. *Clin Obstet Gynecol* 1994;37:306.

Maternal Trauma

Bocka J, Courtney J, Pearlman M, et al. Trauma in pregnancy. *Ann Emerg Med* 1988;17:829.

Hoff WS, D'Amelio LF, Tinkoff GH, et al. Maternal predictors of fetal demise in trauma during pregnancy. *Surg Gynecol Obstet* 1991;172:175.

Kissinger DP, Rozycki GS, Morris JA, et al. Trauma in pregnancy: predicting pregnancy outcome. *Arch Surg* 1991;126:1079.

Kuhlmann RS, Cruikshank DP. Maternal trauma in pregnancy. In: Pitkin RM, Scott JR, eds. *Clinical obstetrics and gynecology.* Philadelphia: JB Lippincott Co, 1994:274.

Nash P. Trauma in pregnancy. *BMJ* 1990;301:974.

Pearlman MD, Tintinalli JE, Lorenz RP. Blunt trauma during pregnancy. *N Engl J Med* 1990;323:1609.

Sakala EP, Kort DD. Management of stab wounds to the pregnant uterus: a case report and review of the literature. *Obstet Gynecol Surv* 1988; 43:319.

CHAPTER 24

Immunologic Disorders in Pregnancy

◇

James R. Scott
D. Ware Branch

◇ REPRODUCTIVE IMMUNOLOGY

The fascinating field of reproductive immunology has become important in the clinical practice of modern obstetrics. The obstetrician is in a unique position to observe the only natural grafting of living tissue from one person to another—pregnancy. It is still unclear how the fetus and its placenta survive in the immunocompetent maternal environment. Nevertheless, research on the maternal–fetal immunologic relation has contributed new information that has led to a better understanding and management of immunologic disorders in pregnancy.

Fundamental Immunobiology

The immune system is widely distributed and complex. Its primary function is to protect against foreign antigens and pathogens and to distinguish biological self from nonself. Immune responses are highly regulated and nonrandom processes. After exposure to a nonself antigen, a series of cellular and biochemical events occur, including antigen processing and presentation, recognition of the processed antigen by a specific T cell, clonal expansion of T cells and elaboration of lymphokines, and production of an antibody or cytotoxic immune response. Immune effector mechanisms are classified as either innate or adaptive, but these two systems interact extensively.

The innate immune system has many components, including physical and biochemical barriers to the entry of foreign material, primary effector cells such as mononuclear phagocytes, natural killer (NK) cells, and polymorphonuclear leukocytes, and circulating biochemical factors such as the complement system. After ingestion, phagocytes and NK cells enzymatically destroy antigens. Activation of these cells depends only on the foreign nature of the eliciting antigen. This nonspecific immune surveillance is continuous, but host resistance to a particular antigen is not enhanced by repeated exposure (Fig. 1).

The hallmark of adaptive immunity is the precise specificity of antigen recognition and memory, so that repeated exposures to a specific antigen elicit enhanced immune responsiveness. B cells are precursors of plasma cells that secrete specific antibodies and give rise to the humoral immune response. T cells control and regulate the cellular immune response. The histocompatibility system plays a central role in antigen recognition. Human leukocyte antigens (HLA) are products of a gene complex, the major histocompatibility complex (MHC), located in humans on the short arm of chromosome 6 (Fig. 2). Class I MHC antigens, expressed by nearly all nucleated cells, are essential cell surface recognition molecules identified by cytotoxic T cells. Class II MHC antigens have more restricted tissue expression (B cells, monocytes, macrophages, and activated T cells); they are cell surface recognition molecules important for presenting antigen to helper T cells. The class I MHC region is subdivided into individual loci termed HLA-A, -B, and -C; the class II region is subdivided into individual loci, including those that code for the HLA-DR, -DP, and -DQ antigens. Other molecules with immunobiological activities are also encoded within a MHC class III region.

Adaptive immune responses, such as allograft rejection, involve essential processes that occur in sequence in the lymphatic system (see Fig. 2). As proliferating T cells mature, they differentiate into an array of subtypes that have diverse functions. CD4+ helper cells help other cells proliferate and help B cells produce antibodies. CD4+ inducer cells control the subsequent development of other T cells. CD8+ cytotoxic cells lyse foreign or infected cells, and CD8+ suppressor cells prevent uncontrolled proliferation. These immune cells communicate through the production and release of cytokines (i.e., lymphokines). Interleukin (IL)-1 is largely macrophage- or monocyte-derived and promotes multiplication and activation of lymphocytes. Interleukin-2, produced in response to

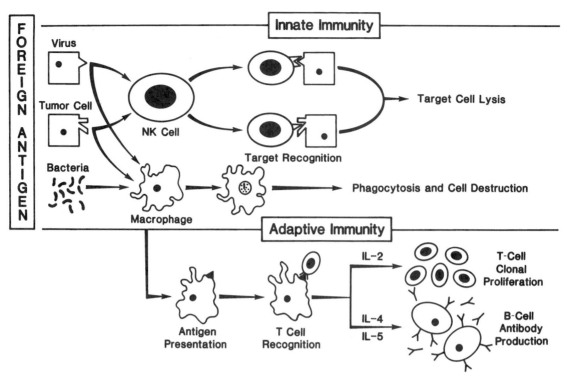

FIG. 1. Schematic view of innate and adaptive immune systems. Foreign antigen is recognized by phagocytic cells of the innate immune system. The foreign antigen can be a microbial pathogen, viral antigen, or tumor antigen. Innate immune responses result in direct cytotoxicity or destruction of the pathogen. Activation of the adaptive immune system depends on interaction with processed antigen provided by cells of the innate immune system. T-cell and B-cell activation results in T-cell clonal proliferation and B-cell antibody production, respectively. IL, interleukin; NK, natural killer. (From Dudley DJ. The immune system in health and disease. *Balliere's Clin Obstet Gynaecol* 1992;6:393.)

lymphocyte activation, is the major T-cell growth factor for the proliferation of activated T cells. Specifically committed lymphocyte subsets then migrate to the alien tissue or confront invading organisms. They destroy and remove these targets by direct binding and secretion of cytokines that recruit and activate macrophages.

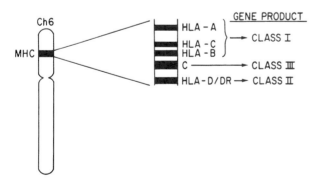

FIG. 2. Chromosomal location of the major histocompatibility complex (MHC). Within the complex are genes that encode as follows: for class I antigens (HLA-A, HLA-B, and HLA-C); for several components of the complement cascade, including complement components 2 and 4 and factor B, some of which are located at position C; and for class II antigens (HLA-D/DR). (From Scott JR, Rote NS, eds. *Immunology in obstetrics and gynecology.* Norwalk, CT: Appleton-Century-Crofts, 1985:35.)

B cells or plasma cells, on the other hand, produce specific antibody by gene rearrangement, a process that creates myriad possible immunoglobulin antigen-recognition sites. The antibody circulates through the bloodstream and destroys target cells, usually in concert with complement or antibody-dependent cellular cytotoxic cells. The primary antibody response to an antigen is IgM, which is soon superseded by a predominantly IgG response. Antibodies are heterogeneous proteins composed of several classes of immunoglobulins. Four subclasses of human IgG, each with slightly different properties, can be distinguished by differences in the highly specific allotypic markers of the heavy polypeptide chain of the Ig unit. Because antigens usually have multiple determinants, most humoral immune responses are polyclonal and contain a mixture of antibodies produced from multiple clones of lymphocytes.

Cells capable of recognizing self-antigens and producing an immune response are present in all normal people, but they are actively regulated and suppressed. Autoimmune diseases apparently result from a breakdown in this regulatory mechanism, leading to an inability to discriminate between self and nonself. Autoimmunity is characterized by persistent activation of immunologic effector mechanisms that affect the function and integrity of certain cells and organs. The process may be initiated by environmental agents, and it probably becomes sustained because of persistent T-cell activation that overrides normal tolerance of self-antigens. Because autoimmune diseases have a predilection for women in their reproductive years, associations with pregnancy are common.

Maternal–Fetal Immunology

Many reproductive immunologists regard the conceptus as a semi-allograft in that it bears paternal as well as maternal antigens, and initial interest in the maternal–fetal immunology derived from this orientation. It appears, however, that the immunologic interaction between the mother and conceptus may not fit into a traditional allogeneic immunology paradigm. Indeed, this interaction may be primarily healthy and growth-promoting, not destructive. In turn, there may be no need for a complex abrogation of the normal maternal immune response in order for pregnancy to survive, as many reproductive immunologists have suggested, and pregnancy is certainly not a state of generalized immune suppression.

After fertilization, the first immunologic recognition between genetically dissimilar cells, the developing semiallogeneic conceptus implants into the endometrium. From that point forward, differentiated fetal trophoblast cells are in direct and continuous contact with maternal uterine tissue and blood. Neither villous cytotrophoblast nor syncytiotrophoblast expresses classic HLA class I or class II MHC antigens, and hence, they resist lysis by cellular or antibody-mediated immunologic activity. As a result, the majority of trophoblastic cells in contact with maternal blood or tissues are immunologically inert from the viewpoint of allogeneic immune responses. Extravillous cytotrophoblastic cells also do not express class II MHC antigens, but they do express a nonclassic class I MHC antigen, known as HLA-G, with very limited polymorphic variation. HLA-G may be a specialized cellular recognitive molecule to limit lytic activity by activated NK cells or to regulate cytotrophoblast proliferation and invasion.

The presence of maternal serum factors that inhibit cell-mediated immune function has been suggested to explain the immunologic success of pregnancy. This hypothesis presumes that maternal cellular immune responses to the conceptus normally are blocked, and circulating blocking factors develop in all successful pregnancies. Theoretically, blocking antibodies are directed against maternal lymphocytes to prevent their reaction with receptors on fetoplacental tissues, or they block receptors on the fetoplacental semiallograft to prevent attack by maternal lymphocytes. They could also be antiidiotypic antibodies directed against the antigen-specific combining sites (idiotypes) on other antibodies. Similar idiotypes function as antigen receptors on the surface of T lymphocytes, so antiidiotypic antibodies might bind to antigen receptors to prevent maternal lymphocytes from interacting with the target cells of the conceptus.

Blocking antibodies and other alleged pregnancy-maintaining factors in maternal peripheral blood have never been well defined biochemically or immunologically. They usually are identified indirectly by *in vitro* tests such as the mixed lymphocyte reaction (MLR). There is, however, a wide variability in these assays among different patients and between the same couples tested at different times. No uniform method exists for reporting the results, and the results depend on equations used for calculating MLR data. Moreover, the actual relevance of circulating blocking antibodies in pregnancy is disputed. These antibodies frequently do not appear until late in the first or second trimester of the first pregnancy. Agammaglobulinemic women have normal pregnancies; animals rendered incapable of producing antibodies also have successful pregnancies.

Contemporary investigations have focused on local cellular events at the maternofetal tissue interface that are more likely to be of importance. The transformation of endometrial stromal cells into decidual cells and the unique properties of the invading trophoblast at the fetomaternal junction seem to play key roles in the successful implantation and development of the embryo. The decidua contains T lymphocytes and granulocytes. The lymphocytes are comprised of cells with either $\alpha\beta$ receptors or $\gamma\delta$ receptors. Of the $\alpha\beta$ T cells, a majority are of CD8+ phenotype and may have immunosuppressive activity. The $\gamma\delta$ T cells are enriched in early and late human decidua and, because they do not always require MHC restriction for cytotoxicity, may serve an antimicrobial role.

Large numbers of class II MHC-positive and non-B/non-T lymphoid cells similar to NK cells can be identified in luteal phase and early to midpregnancy decidua. These cells, called large granular lymphocytes, can kill standard NK cell targets but do not lyse trophoblast under normal circumstances. Abundant macrophages also are present in the decidua, and they are the predominant leukocyte in close proximity to the invading trophoblast. These cells may serve as antigen-processing or phagocytic cells.

Some cells may function as suppressor cells through the generation of soluble factors that impair IL-2-dependent lymphocyte responses. Other cytokines likely play important roles at the maternofetal interface. In addition to cytokines, hormones, enzymes, growth factors, and endometrial proteins within maternal decidual tissue have potent immunomodulatory properties. Although the significance of each is difficult to establish in isolation, this activity at the fetomaternal interface may be responsible for the favorable interaction between the conceptus and the mother.

The ontogeny of the immune system begins with the conceptus, but its development is not completed until after birth. During weeks 2 and 3 of gestation, pluripotential yolk sac stem cells form the precursors for all the blood cell series. The thymus develops in the human embryo at week 6 of gestation, and lymphocyte differentiation proceeds in the absence of foreign antigens. Small lymphocytes appear in the peripheral blood at week 7 and around lymphocyte plexuses by week 8. As early as 13 weeks of gestation, T cells that can respond to mitogens and recognize histoincompatible cells begin to appear. By 20 weeks of gestation, the human fetus responds to congenital infections by producing plasma cells and antibodies, and immunologic maturation continues in preparation for exposure to a highly contaminated world.

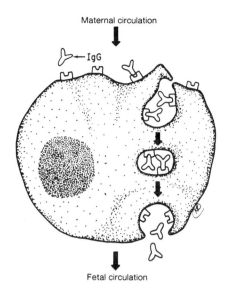

FIG. 3. The transport of maternal IgG across the trophoblast and into the fetal circulation is an active process. Maternal IgG binds to Fc receptors on the surface of the trophoblast and is internalized into vacuoles. These receptors are specific for the Fc portion of IgG and do not bind other classes of immunoglobulins. The interaction of IgG with the receptors probably protects the antibody from digestion during the transport of the vacuole across the cell. On the fetal side, IgG is released into the fetal circulation. (From Scott JR, Rote NS, eds. *Immunology in obstetrics and gynecology.* Norwalk, CT: Appleton-Century-Crofts, 1985:70.)

The presence of an intact trophoblastic cellular barrier prevents the movement of large numbers of immunocompetent cells into or out of the fetus during pregnancy. In contrast, maternal IgG, by virtue of its Fc fragment, is specifically selected for placental transfer (Fig. 3). Fetal IgG usually is about 10% of adult levels by the middle of the first trimester (Fig. 4). Adequate humoral immunity in the neonatal period depends on the circulating immunoglobulins that have crossed the placenta, and fetal blood levels of IgG reflect maternal levels. The specific antibody protection depends on the mother's own antigenic experience. Maternal antibodies, in addition to their primary role of protecting the neonate from infections, can result in disease syndromes that can be harmful to the infant.

♦ ERYTHROCYTE IMMUNIZATION

Rh Disease

Erythroblastosis fetalis (i.e., hemolytic disease of the newborn) is caused by an incompatibility between fetal and maternal blood. The Rh-negative mother becomes immunized by exposure to Rh-positive fetal erythrocytes during pregnancy or delivery, and antibodies formed by the mother pass through the placenta to the fetal circulation, where they react with the Rh-positive fetal erythrocytes, causing a hemolytic anemia.

Although the first description of erythroblastosis fetalis dates back to 1609, no rational treatment was possible until

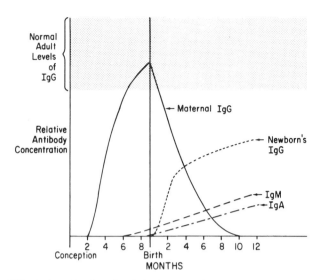

FIG. 4. Levels of antibody in the cord blood and neonatal circulation. Early in gestation, maternal IgG crosses the placenta and enters the fetal circulation. At the time of birth, the fetal circulation normally contains a near-adult level of IgG, which is almost exclusively maternal, and small amounts of fetal IgM and IgA. After delivery of the child, maternal IgG is rapidly catabolized, whereas neonatal IgG production increases. (From Scott JR, Rote NS, eds. *Immunology in obstetrics and gynecology.* Norwalk, CT: Appleton-Century-Crofts, 1985:69.)

this century, when the ABO blood groups and Rh factor were discovered. Advances in therapy have dramatically reduced perinatal mortality, and Rh immune globulin (RhIgG) is now available to prevent the condition. The incidence of erythroblastosis fetalis gradually has decreased since the introduction of RhIgG. Paradoxically, as the disorder becomes less frequent, physicians find it more difficult to keep abreast of new and sometimes controversial recommendations for prophylaxis and treatment.

Pathophysiology

Nomenclature

The Rh blood group was so named because rabbits immunized with rhesus monkey erythrocytes produced an antibody that agglutinated erythrocytes from 85% of Caucasians. Subsequently, the human blood group system was found to be extremely complex. The genetic locus for Rh antigens is located on the short arm of chromosome 1, but the number of genes controlling their synthesis is unclear. The final gene product on the erythrocyte is a small protein of 7000 to 10,000 molecular weight with multiple antigenic determinants. Rh antigens associated with membrane phospholipid are distributed in nonrandom clusters on the red blood cell surface, and the number of antigenic sites for a specific erythrocyte depends on the genotype.

Although several systems of terminology have been proposed, the Fischer-Race nomenclature is the most widely used in obstetrics and has been recommended by the World Health

Organization Expert Committee on Biological Standardization in the interest of simplicity and uniformity. The Fischer-Race system assumes the presence of three genetic loci, each with two possible alleles. Antigens produced by these alleles are identified by specific antisera and have been lettered *C, c, D, E,* and *e*. Because no antiserum specific for *d* has been found, *d* signifies the absence of a discernible allelic product. The following gene complexes have been identified: *CDe, cDE, cde, cDe, cdE, Cde,* and *CDE*. Genotypes are indicated as pairs of gene complexes, such as *CDe/cde*. For most clinical purposes, people are classified as Rh-positive or Rh-negative by testing their red blood cells with anti-*D* antiserum.

Several variations of *D* antigen expression form a heterogeneous group called Du variants (Fig. 5). Du phenotypes (the antigens expressed on the erythrocyte surface) that strongly express *D* antigen may react with sera that contain anti-*D;* other Du phenotypes are distinguished from *d* phenotypes only by sensitive assays. Most Du variant patients are considered to be Rh-positive because their erythrocytes can stimulate the production of anti-*D* antibodies, and they seldom produce anti-*D* antibodies themselves.

Fetomaternal Hemorrhage

Fetal blood often enters the maternal circulation during pregnancy and in the immediate postpartum period; fetal red blood cells have been detected in 6.7% of pregnant women during the first trimester, in 15.9% during the second trimester, and in 28.9% during the third trimester. The minimum number of Rh-positive fetal red blood cells necessary to cause immunization in the pregnant Rh-negative woman is unclear, but as little as 0.1 ml of Rh-positive blood has been shown to

TABLE 1. *Factors that influence whether a patient will become Rh immunized*

Conditions associated with increased risk of fetomaternal hemorrhage
Amniocentesis
Threatened abortion, placenta previa, placental abruption
Abdominal trauma
External version
Fetal death
Sinusoidal fetal heart tracing
Multiple pregnancy
Cesarean section
Anemic infant

Factors that influence Rh immunization
Incidence and size of fetomaternal hemorrhage
ABO compatibility between mother and fetus
Rh phenotype of fetal red cells
Gender of the baby
Genetic predisposition (responder)

sensitize Rh-negative volunteers. A fetomaternal hemorrhage sufficient to cause immunization is most common at the time of delivery. Factors that increase the risk of transplacental transfer of fetal red blood cells are listed in Table 1. Even though the quantity of fetal blood in the maternal circulation usually is small, larger transplacental bleeds can occur in an unpredictable manner.

Detection. The Kleihauer-Betke test was the first method described to detect fetal red blood cells. Fetal cells that contain stained fetal hemoglobin HbF can be distinguished microscopically from the adult erythrocyte ghost cells (Fig. 6). A

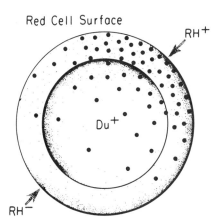

FIG. 5. Mechanism for the determination of D and Du positivity. One theory suggests that the density of the D antigen on the surface of the red cell determines the results of red cell typing. Patients with no antigen are typed Rh⁻, patients with low densities of the antigen are typed Du⁺, and patients with high densities of the antigen are typed Rh⁺. (From Kochenour NK, Scott JR. Rh isoimmunization in pregnancy. In: Scott JR, Rote NS, eds. *Immunology in obstetrics and gynecology.* Norwalk, CT: Appleton-Century-Crofts, 1984:143.)

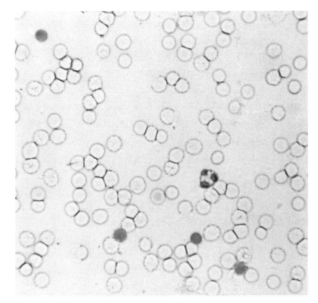

FIG. 6. Peripheral smear showing dark fetal red cells in contrast to light-colored maternal cells. The large, dark-staining cell near the middle is a maternal neutrophil. (From Scott JR, Warenski JC. Tests to detect and quantitate fetomaternal bleeding. *Clin Obstet Gynecol* 1982;25:277.)

count is made of fetal and adult cells on the smear, and the size of the fetomaternal bleed is determined according to the following formula:

$$\frac{\text{number of fetal erythrocytes}}{\text{number of maternal erythrocytes}} = \frac{x \text{ (ml of fetomaternal bleed)}}{\text{estimated maternal blood volume}}$$

A number of modifications of the original acid elution technique have been introduced, and rapid, simplified commercial tests are now available in kit form. An erythrocyte-rosetting test that specifically detects Rh-positive fetal red blood cells can also be used; because this test is qualitative, positive results should be followed by a quantitative acid elution test.

Immunology

Unlike the ABO system, in which patients produce antibodies against similar or identical antigens on bacteria or other substances, Rh-negative patients develop circulating titers of anti-D only when exposed to Rh-positive red blood cells. Moreover, about 30% of Rh-negative people are never sensitized (i.e., nonresponders), even when challenged with large volumes of Rh-positive blood. The maternal humoral immune system responds relatively slowly to Rh antigens, first by synthesizing low levels of IgM antibodies and later by producing IgG antibodies that usually are detectable within 6 weeks to 6 months. These antibodies are capable of crossing the placenta and can destroy fetal Rh-positive red blood cells. The heterogeneity of the IgG subclasses produced and the differences in transplacental transfer may be partially responsible for the variability of fetal involvement between patients.

The reaction of anti-D antibody with D antigens results in the eventual destruction of Rh-positive cells. This is not a complement-fixing reaction, and most IgG-coated red blood cells are hemolyzed extravascularly in the splenic reticuloendothelial system. Antibody-dependent cellular cytotoxicity mechanisms may also contribute; mononuclear phagocytes and some lymphoid cells have receptors that can interact with a portion of the antibody on the red blood cell surface to lyse the target cells, as has been shown *in vitro* with anti-D-coated erythrocytes.

Clinical Manifestations

In the fetus, red blood cell destruction leads to anemia and ultimately erythroblastosis fetalis, characterized by heart failure, edema, ascites, pericardial effusion, and extramedullary hematopoiesis. The severe anemia is associated with tissue hypoxia and acidosis, and extensive liver erythropoiesis results in replacement of normal hepatic parenchyma and architectural distortion. The consequences include a decrease in protein production, portal hypertension, ascites, and generalized anasarca.

In the neonate, the primary clinical problems are anemia and hyperbilirubinemia, but bleeding problems and difficul-

ties with heart failure can also occur. Although hemoglobin breakdown products (primarily bilirubin) are found in increased levels in amniotic fluid and cord blood, excessive amounts are readily cleared by the placenta and metabolized by the mother. Low levels of glucuronyl transferase in the neonate preclude the conjugation of large amounts of bilirubin and result in high levels of serum bilirubin, which lead to kernicterus by the deposition of the bilirubin complexes in the basal ganglia of the central nervous system.

Prevention

Mechanisms

Immunization to the D antigen can be prevented by the administration of RhIgG either before or shortly after exposure to Rh-positive cells. There are three potential mechanisms of action from an immunologic standpoint: antigen blocking (i.e., competitive inhibition), clearance and antigen deviation, and central inhibition.

Antigen Blocking–Competitive Inhibition. This classic explanation assumes that passively administered antibodies produce suppression by attaching to or covering antigenic sites on the Rh-positive red blood cells, rendering them unavailable to the receptors on the maternal lymphoid cells that are necessary to initiate the immune response. Evidence against this theory is the fact that a ratio of 20 µg of exogenous antibody per milliliter of red blood cells prevents the synthesis of endogenous anti-D antibody even though only a small percentage of the antigenic sites are bound.

Clearance and Antigen Deviation. This theory is based on the concept that the antigen is directed away from the reticuloendothelial system, preventing the formation of antibodies. Presumably, ABO incompatibility protects against Rh immunization in this manner. Because other antigens, such as C and E, present on the carrier molecule also are directed away from the immune system, the use of RhIgG should prevent the formation of antibodies to C and E in addition to D. Evidence for this type of nonspecificity suggests that antigen deviation may in some way be involved in antigen-mediated immune suppression for the Rh system.

Central Inhibition. Immune responses are modulated much like a thermostat by effector lymphocytes that are responsible for augmenting (i.e., helping) or abrogating (i.e., suppressing) the response. Suppressor cells have membrane receptors for the altered Fc portion of IgG and can be stimulated by IgG-containing immune complexes. This suggests that the immune response to the D antigen can be prevented by the generation of antigen-specific suppressor cells near the time of exposure to Rh-positive erythrocytes. RhIgG, in the presence of fetal Rh-positive erythrocytes, may generate the immune complexes responsible for the induction of these cells (Fig. 7). This hypothesis is consistent with the observation that antibody-mediated immune suppression appears to prevent only a primary response and has no effect on the secondary response in Rh-sensitized patients.

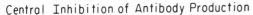

Central Inhibition of Antibody Production

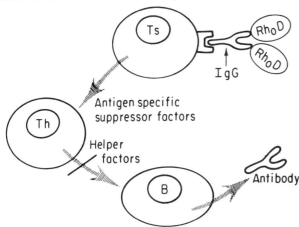

FIG. 7. The theoretical mechanism that best explains the known facts about Rh prophylaxis is central inhibition of antibody production. The immune response to the Rh antigen is modulated by effector lymphocytes that augment (helper cells; Th) or suppress (suppressor cells; Ts). Suppressor cells can be stimulated by the Fc portion of IgG in immune complexes with Rh antigen to produce soluble substances that suppress the stimulating effect of helper lymphocytes. This blocks the production of endogenous antibody against the Rh antigen. (From Kochenour NK, Scott JR. Rh isoimmunization in pregnancy. In: Scott JR, Rote NS, eds. *Immunology in obstetrics and gynecology.* Norwalk, CT: Appleton-Century-Crofts, 1984:145.)

Clinical Use of RhIgG

Rh immune globulin, first released for general use in 1968, has been remarkably successful in the prevention of sensitization to the Rh antigen. Concern about the possibility of transmitting human immunodeficiency virus [HIV; acquired immunodeficiency syndrome (AIDS)] through RhIgG prompted an investigation by the Food and Drug Administration, which revealed that all viruses are inactivated by the manufacturing process. More than 350,000 women in the United States receive RhIgG annually, and there is no evidence to implicate this product as a source of HIV infection or to change recommendations for its use.

One vial of RhIgG (i.e., 300 µg of anti-*D*) can suppress immunity to about 30 ml of whole Rh-positive blood or 15 ml of packed Rh-positive red blood cells. To reduce the morbidity and mortality of Rh erythroblastosis fetalis to the minimum, it is imperative that all women at risk be identified and treated. RhIgG is 100% effective immunologically if given before sensitization. Potential reasons for postabortal and postpartum clinical failures include the following:

◊ Failure to type the patient's blood at the first prenatal visit or to order RhIgG when indicated;
◊ Error in transmitting the proper blood type to the mother's chart and to the physician;
◊ Error in typing the mother's, father's, or baby's blood;
◊ Failure to administer RhIgG when ordered;
◊ Unrecognized fetomaternal hemorrhage during pregnancy;

◊ Inadequate RhIgG dosage for the volume of fetomaternal hemorrhage;
◊ Patient refusal.

In each pregnancy, a woman should have her blood and Rh type determined and an antibody screen performed as early as practical so that she can be managed appropriately (Table 2). If the father is homozygous for *D*, then all his offspring will be *D*-positive. On the other hand, if he is heterozygous, there is a 50% chance that any given child of his will be Rh-negative and unaffected by Rh hemolytic disease caused by *D*. Sixty percent of white, Rh-positive men are heterozygous, and 40% are homozygous, for the *D* antigen.

First-Trimester Abortion. The *D* antigen has been identified on the fetal red blood cell as early as day 38 of gestation, and the risk of sensitization in both induced and spontaneous abortions is 3% to 5.5% but varies with length of gestation. The embryo has a circulation by 4 weeks postconception, and transplacental passage of erythrocytes could theoretically occur by 6 to 8 weeks of gestation. How early and often this actually happens has not been well documented, and the necessity for prophylaxis after menstrual extractions or spontaneous abortions with blighted ova before 6 weeks has never been satisfactorily resolved. Nevertheless, until the minimum amount of Rh-positive blood necessary to immunize is more firmly established, and because the fetal blood type usually is not known, all Rh-negative women with any type of abortion episode should be protected with RhIgG when the pregnancy is terminated. Commercially available 50-µg RhIgG preparations (i.e., Mini-Gamulin Rh, MicRhoGam) protect against 5 ml of whole fetal blood or 2.5 ml of packed red blood cells and are sufficient prophylaxis against all fetomaternal hemorrhages that occur during the first trimester.

A similar potential for sensitization exists with ectopic pregnancy, but whether RhIgG is necessary after a hydatidiform mole is uncertain. Histologic analysis of hydatidiform moles reveals no nucleated fetal red blood cells or fetal vessels in the

TABLE 2. *Evaluation and management of an unsensitized Rh-negative, Du-negative pregnant patient*

Time in gestation	Management
First prenatal visit	Determine ABO blood group and Rh, including Du
	Antibody screen (indirect Coombs' test)
28 weeks	Antibody screen negative: administer 300 µg RhIgG
	Antibody screen positive: check Rh of baby's father and manage as Rh-sensitized
35 weeks (optional)	Antibody screen negative (<1 : 4): observe
	Antibody screen positive: manage as Rh sensitized
Postpartum	Antibody screen negative: administer 300 µg RhIgG if infant is Rh-positive of Du-positive
	Antibody screen positive: manage next pregnancy as Rh-sensitized

villi, and most investigators have found that trophoblastic cells do not contain Rh antigens. In the only reported case of Rh immunization associated with a hydatidiform mole, it is likely that antepartum sensitization during the next pregnancy was actually the cause.

Amniocentesis. Amniocentesis for intrauterine diagnosis of genetic disease carries a risk of fetomaternal hemorrhage and sensitization in Rh-negative patients even when performed under ultrasound direction. Therefore, until further data show a more selective protocol to be safe, it is recommended that all Rh-negative patients who undergo midtrimester amniocentesis receive 300 µg of RhIgG. One theoretical risk of RhIgG used in this way is the phenomenon of enhancement. This term refers to facilitation of an immune response in the presence of a low antibody level at the time of antigen exposure. Because the half-life of RhIgG is about 25 days, augmentation could take place in the third trimester as fetal red blood cells gain access to the maternal circulation. Although immunologic enhancement has not been clearly proved in this situation, it is one reason to avoid the lower, 50-µg dose of RhIgG with amniocentesis and to make sure that the patient receives an additional 300-µg dose at 28 weeks of gestation.

Even in the third trimester, the use of ultrasound for amniocentesis and the absence of macroscopic blood in the amniotic fluid are not adequate guarantees against the appearance of fetal red blood cells in the maternal circulation. If delivery is to be accomplished within 72 hours, it is reasonable to withhold RhIgG at the time of amniocentesis and to administer it immediately after delivery if the infant is Rh-positive.

Antepartum Bleeding. Although the risk of sensitization with threatened abortion is not known, fetomaternal bleeding may be more common in this setting. One way to manage the situation is to test for fetal red blood cells in maternal blood and to administer RhIgG if they are present. If this course is followed, RhIgG should be repeated again at 28 weeks of gestation if the pregnancy continues; if the pregnancy proceeds to abortion, it is unlikely that more RhIgG is necessary.

It may also be worthwhile to look for fetal red blood cells in the maternal circulation during certain other obstetric complications known to increase the risk of fetomaternal hemorrhage. They include antepartum bleeding from placenta previa or placental abruption, abdominal trauma, fetal hydrops, sinusoidal fetal heart rate patterns, and unexplained fetal demise.

Antepartum Prophylaxis. It has become apparent that the standard postpartum RhIgG regimen fails to protect 1% to 2% of Rh-negative women who deliver an Rh-positive infant. Most often this is because of occult transplacental transfer of a sufficient number of fetal red blood cells during the pregnancy. Antepartum prophylaxis was first suggested in 1967, and trials of antepartum administration of RhIgG were started in Canada in 1968. Sensitization occurred in only two of 1799 Rh-negative women who delivered Rh-positive infants, representing a failure rate of 0.11% as compared with the expected failure rate of 1.6%. The beginning of the third trimester and a 300-µg dose were chosen because most sensitizations occur

after this time and adequate levels of RhIgG are still present at the end of pregnancy.

A protocol for the antepartum administration of RhIgG is shown in Fig. 8. Whether an anti-*D* titer is necessary at 35 weeks of gestation to detect the rare patient who might become sensitized despite antepartum RhIgG is unresolved at this time. This did not occur in 1357 pregnancies when the indirect Coombs test at 28 weeks was negative before giving RhIgG, and it is extremely unlikely that such a case would require active intervention before delivery.

It is important to realize that the patient has recently received RhIgG if blood is crossmatched at delivery and to remember that the infant may have a weakly positive direct Coombs test. Each patient should be thoroughly informed and given a card showing that she has received antepartum RhIgG in case she is seen later by a different physician or delivers at another hospital. Otherwise, postpartum RhIgG might be withheld because of a mistaken diagnosis of Rh immunization based on a positive indirect Coombs test from the circulating anti-*D* antibody.

Postpartum Use. The most common cause of Rh immunization is delivery of an Rh-positive or Du-positive child by an Rh-negative woman. Ordinarily, 300 µg of RhIgG injected intramuscularly within 72 hours of delivery prevents sensitization. There is evidence that RhIgG is effective even when given later than this arbitrarily chosen time limit. Therefore, RhIgG should be administered as soon as possible after delivery, but it is still indicated after 72 hours if an error is recognized. Postpartum administration of RhIgG protects the mother against sensitization by the just-completed pregnancy only. It is necessary to test and treat the mother as needed after delivery of each subsequent Rh-positive or Du-positive child.

Even when appropriately timed, about 0.4% of patients have a fetomaternal hemorrhage large enough that 300 µg of RhIgG is not sufficient prophylaxis. Ideally, the volume of the fetomaternal bleed could be determined by using one of

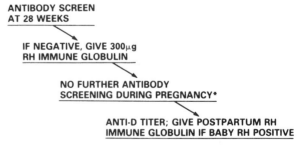

ANTEPARTUM RH IMMUNE GLOBULIN

ANTIBODY SCREEN
AT 28 WEEKS

IF NEGATIVE, GIVE 300µg
RH IMMUNE GLOBULIN

NO FURTHER ANTIBODY
SCREENING DURING PREGNANCY*

ANTI-D TITER; GIVE POSTPARTUM RH
IMMUNE GLOBULIN IF BABY RH POSITIVE

FIG. 8. Two-dose (antepartum–postpartum) regimen for unimmunized Rh-negative patients. (Some authorities recommend obtaining an anti-*D* antibody titer at 35 weeks of gestation because a titer of 1:4 or higher represents active immunization. Lower levels of antibody can be detected because of the circulating RhIgG.)

the acid elution tests; however, because the incidence of patients not protected by 300 μg is so low, it is probably not cost-effective to screen every Rh-negative woman for fetal red blood cells at the time of delivery. If a large fetomaternal hemorrhage is found either on routine screening or because clinical suspicion led to the test, additional RhIgG at a dose of 300 μg for each 15 ml of fetal red blood cells is indicated.

One confusing scenario is the pregnant woman who is reported to be Rh-negative, Du-positive late in pregnancy or after delivery. This can mean either that the patient is actually Du-positive (and does not require RhIgG) or that she is Rh-negative but has a large number of Rh-positive fetal cells in her circulation (and therefore is a candidate for RhIgG). In this case, it is helpful to have prior information about the patient's blood type either when she was not pregnant or early in pregnancy. If there is any question, it is best to check for the presence of Rh-positive fetal cells in the maternal circulation before deciding against giving RhIgG.

Management

Once a pregnant patient is identified as being Rh-immunized, the goal is to time the delivery so that morbidity and mortality risks to the infant are minimized. With this in mind, patients are grouped into one of three categories:

1. Mildly affected fetuses, who can be allowed to remain *in utero* until they have achieved pulmonary maturation.
2. Moderately affected fetuses, who may need to be delivered before pulmonary maturity but who do not need active fetal treatment of the condition.
3. Severely affected fetuses, who require active intervention to reach a gestational age at which the risks of delivery and neonatal intensive care are less than the risks of *in utero* therapy.

Because there are clinical variations among patients with Rh-immunized pregnancies, protocols for fetal assessment and treatment must be individualized. The severity of previously affected pregnancies, the possibility of an Rh-negative fetus, and the results of testing in the current pregnancy are important factors in formulating a management plan for fetal evaluation, treatment, and delivery.

Maternal Antibody Titers

In a first sensitized gestation, the risk of fetal involvement is low. Thus, women in their first immunized pregnancy and those without a history of an affected infant can be evaluated with monthly anti-*D* titers. As long as the titer remains low, there is little risk of fetal anemia, and the pregnancy usually can be allowed to continue to near term without other testing or intervention. After the first affected pregnancy, maternal anti-*D* titers are poorly predictive of fetal status, and closer evaluation is required. Although each laboratory has its own critical titer, anti-*D* titers of 1:16 or greater in most centers

demand amniocentesis and analysis of amniotic fluid bilirubin concentration.

Unlike first immunized pregnancies, in which the incidence of fetal anemia and hydrops is less than 10%, the pattern of fetal involvement in successive pregnancies is one of equal or greater severity. If hydrops occurred in one pregnancy, the next Rh-incompatible fetus has an 80% to 90% chance of becoming hydropic.

Amniocentesis and Amniotic Fluid Analysis

Although not excreted in large amounts by the fetal kidneys, bilirubin diffuses into the amniotic fluid across such fetal membranes as the skin and umbilical cord. The reliability of spectrophotometric analysis of amniotic fluid bilirubin concentration has been questioned, but it remains a clinically useful method for evaluating fetal status. The timing of the initial amniocentesis requires judgment as to when the risk of intrauterine morbidity becomes appreciable. Factors involved in the decision include severity of involvement in previous pregnancies and changes in or absolute value of antibody titers. The amniocentesis is done under ultrasound guidance, and the aspirated amniotic fluid is sent for determination of the optical density at Δ450 μm (Fig. 9). Using the Liley graph, the ΔOD[450] is then plotted on a semilogarithmic

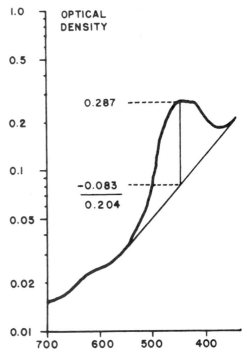

FIG. 9. Spectrophotometric scan of amniotic fluid containing bilirubin. An arbitrary line *(thick line)* has been drawn to show where the scan would have been traced if there had been no increase in bilirubin. The peak absorption of bilirubin occurs at 450 μm. The difference between the peak and the arbitrary line equals 0.204.

scale versus gestational age (Fig. 10). To understand the Liley curve, it is important to remember that the concentration of bilirubin pigments in the amniotic fluid gradually declines during a normal pregnancy. A significant hemolytic process results in a higher ΔOD^{450} level that is constant or rising. The absolute value as well as the trend plotted against gestational age determine the plan of management. When the bilirubin concentration is in the lower zone (i.e., zone I), the fetus usually is Rh-negative or relatively mildly affected. When it is in zone II, most fetuses are moderately affected; values in zone III indicate that the fetus is in danger of dying *in utero.*

The fetal Rh antigen status can be determined from amniotic cells using polymerase chain reaction. Therefore, the first amniocentesis can now be used to determine whether the fetus is Rh-negative or Rh-positive. This procedure greatly simplifies the management of pregnancies in which the fetus is Rh-negative.

Fetal Blood Analysis

The degree of fetal anemia can be determined by fetal blood sampling by way of ultrasound-guided umbilical cord puncture. This technique is useful to evaluate the fetus at risk for severe hemolytic disease. Transplacental needle passage is associated with some degree of fetomaternal hemorrhage in more than 50% of cases, and other morbidity and fetal deaths occasionally occur.

Ultrasound

Serial ultrasound examinations are also helpful to evaluate fetal status in Rh immunization. Because there is not complete correlation between amniotic fluid ΔOD^{450} values and ultrasound findings, they should be used together (Fig. 11). Ascites and soft tissue edema are definite signs of severe fetal involvement with erythroblastosis fetalis. Once hydrops has

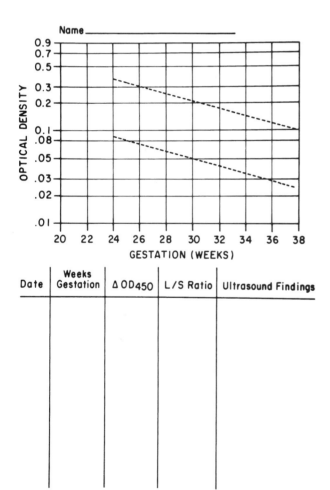

Date	Weeks Gestation	Δ OD₄₅₀	L/S Ratio	Ultrasound Findings

FIG. 10. This form is used to record serial data on each Rh-immunized patient. The modified Liley graph is divided into three zones to predict the outcome of the pregnancy in terms of umbilical cord blood hemoglobin, intrauterine deaths, or unaffected fetuses.

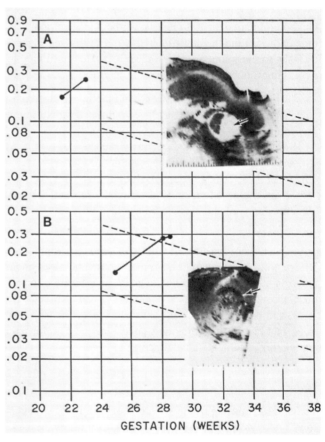

FIG. 11. Ultrasound findings in two patients with severe Rh immunization. **(A)** Marked fetal ascites *(broken line)* is already demonstrated by sonogram at 23 weeks of gestation, even though the amniotic fluid ΔOD^{450} value has not yet reached the upper zone on the Liley graph. **(B)** The amniotic fluid ΔOD^{450} value is in the upper zone by 30 weeks of gestation, with no ultrasound evidence of fetal hydrops *(broken line).* (From Kochenour NK, Scott JR. Rh isoimmunization in pregnancy. In: Scott JR, Rote NS, eds. *Immunology in obstetrics and gynecology.* Norwalk, CT: Appleton-Century-Crofts, 1984:153.)

developed, the fetus is severely anemic, with a hemoglobin level less than 5 g/dl. On the other hand, a patient with high ΔOD^{450} values and no sonographic evidence of hydrops fetalis may have a less severely involved fetus than would be expected from the amniotic fluid analysis alone.

Doppler ultrasound–determined blood velocity waveforms have been investigated as noninvasive predictors of fetal anemia. Doppler indices are of limited clinical usefulness for predicting those fetuses that require transfusion, and properly designed prospective studies are needed before this technique can be recommended in the management of Rh immunization.

Fetal Monitoring

Although antepartum fetal heart rate monitoring has been reported to be helpful, its exact role in Rh immunization is unclear. Important management decisions often are made late in the second and early in the third trimesters, when these tests are of less value. The severely compromised fetus moves less frequently than a normal fetus, and lack of fetal movement, either as visualized by ultrasound or as perceived by the mother, has been used as a sign of worsening fetal condition. There are few data to indicate whether serial nonstress tests or contraction stress tests are useful in this situation. The appearance of a sinusoidal pattern suggests anemia and a worsening fetal condition, and as with any high-risk pregnancy, intrapartum electronic monitoring is recommended.

Fetal Management

Mildly to Moderately Involved Fetus

A sonogram for gestational age is obtained at 14 to 16 weeks to avoid errors in dating. Unless the maternal antibody titer is low, amniotic fluid analysis and serial sonograms are used to follow the fetus' status. If the current pregnancy is the first sensitized pregnancy, or if the preceding infant was only mildly involved, the first amniocentesis should be performed at about 26 to 28 weeks of gestation. The timing of each subsequent amniocentesis as well as the optimal time of delivery depend on the results of the previous amniotic fluid analyses and ultrasound findings.

The use of the amniotic fluid lecithin–sphingomyelin ratio level is extremely beneficial in management decisions in these patients. If the ΔOD^{450} value is in zone II and falling, delivery should be accomplished as soon as the fetus is mature. If the ΔOD^{450} level is in zone II and rising, or there is sonographic evidence of hydrops, it may be appropriate to deliver the fetus before maturity. In many instances, however, the ΔOD^{450} value is in zone I, and delivery should be undertaken between 38 and 40 weeks, as soon as the cervix is favorable for induction.

One of the most common errors in the management of the Rh-sensitized patient is to underestimate the severity of the condition. When a fetus has attained pulmonary maturity, there is little reason not to deliver because the condition will continue to worsen *in utero*. Even when the OD^{450} is low, in-

dicating that the infant may be Rh-negative, the patient should be delivered by 40 weeks in an institution with the personnel and facilities to treat the infant with unexpected hyperbilirubinemia with exchange transfusions.

Severely Involved Fetus

For the potentially severely involved fetus, an ultrasound should be obtained at 14 to 16 weeks of gestation and repeated every 1 to 2 weeks to detect fetal ascites and edema and to direct the timing of the first amniocentesis. The relatively poor correlation between Liley graph values and fetal hematocrit in the second trimester of pregnancy has modified the evaluation and therapy of severely affected fetuses before 27 weeks of gestation. When bilirubin levels plotted on the Liley graph or the presence of hydrops indicates severe anemia, percutaneous umbilical blood sampling is performed. Provisions are made at the same time for an *in utero* blood transfusion. Hydropic changes already present on the ultrasound mean that the fetal hematocrit is less than 15%. In general, fetuses whose hematocrits are less than 25% should be transfused, but the need for transfusion is individualized according to the hematocrit and gestational age.

At the University of Utah, fetuses that reach 34 to 36 weeks usually are delivered. This policy is based on an infant survival rate greater than 95% at 32 weeks of gestation in the university's neonatal intensive care unit and concern about the occasional patient with an unexplained fetal death after an uncomplicated intrauterine transfusion. Because the procedure has become technically easier, continuing intrauterine transfusions until nearer term may be in order to avoid the problems of prematurity.

Intrauterine Transfusions

Intraperitoneal Approach. Placing blood in the fetal peritoneal cavity reverses fetal anemia by uptake of erythrocytes into the subdiaphragmatic lymphatics.

Under sedation and with sterile technique, the patient is first scanned with either static or real-time ultrasound to assess fetal position, placental location, and the presence of fetal ascites or peripheral edema. The orientation of the fetal spine facilitates the transfusion if it is either to the side or posterior. The transfusion site and the necessary depth of the needle insertion are then calculated. Under local anesthesia, and with the bladder used as a landmark, a large-gauge needle is guided into the fetal abdominal cavity with real-time ultrasound. Type O-negative, irradiated, leukocyte-poor, high-hematocrit packed red blood cells that have been maternally crossmatched and deglycerized are then infused at a rate of 5 to 10 ml/min. The formula for the amount of blood transfused is as follows: (number of weeks of gestation − 20) × 10 ml. If fetal ascites is present, some of the fluid should be removed before the transfusion to avoid excessive intraabdominal pressure. Depending on fetal position, the infused blood is almost always visualized in the peritoneal cavity of the fetus by real-time ultrasound. During the transfusion, it is important to monitor the fetal heart rate. This can be done with either real-time ultrasound or a hand-held Doppler. An increase in fetal heart rate usually is associated with a good outcome, whereas bradycardia is ominous. Fetal heart tones are again carefully monitored after completion of the procedure. If the number of weeks of gestation is less than 24, the heart tones are checked every 4 hours, and the mother is discharged in 12 to 24 hours. If the number of weeks is more than 24, the patient is transferred to the labor and delivery suite, where continuous electronic fetal monitoring is performed; if signs of fetal distress (e.g., persistent bradycardia) occur, then delivery is accomplished.

Intravascular Approach. Preparation of the patient is the same as for fetal intraperitoneal transfusion. The tip of a 20- or 22-gauge needle is followed and guided to the umbilical cord by using continuous real-time ultrasound. When the placenta is anterior, a transplacental approach is used to enter the umbilical vein (Fig. 12). Otherwise, the vessel is entered by traversing the amniotic fluid and puncturing the cord near its insertion into the placenta. When vascular access is attained, a small amount of blood is withdrawn for immediate hematocrit determination. The volume of blood to be transfused can then be determined according to the method described by Nicolaides. The goal is to achieve a posttransfusion hematocrit of 40% to 45%. The blood is infused at a rate of about 10 ml/min, and a posttransfusion sample is drawn for measurement of the hematocrit. Posttransfusion fetal surveillance is the same as for the intraperitoneal approach, and subsequent transfusions are timed to keep the fetal hematocrit above 25%.

Once the infant has been transfused by either method, frequent ultrasound examinations are used for timing the next intrauterine transfusion. Specifically, ultrasound evidence of increasing or decreasing fetal peritoneal fluid accumulation can be used to determine whether transfusion intervals should be decreased or increased. If transfusion is unsuccessful, or if severe fetal hydrops does not improve with transfusion, preterm delivery may be required. Because the cervix usually is unfavorable for vaginal delivery at this stage of pregnancy, cesarean section often is necessary. Even if the transfusion is successful, severely involved fetuses usually have been delivered soon after 34 weeks of gestation.

Intravascular transfusions have become popular, but direct comparison of the results reported with intraperitoneal transfusions is difficult because of differences in indications, techniques, experience of the operator, and the quality of neonatal intensive care facilities at each institution. All these factors play an important role in fetal survival. Specifically, no prospective, randomized trials have been conducted to com-

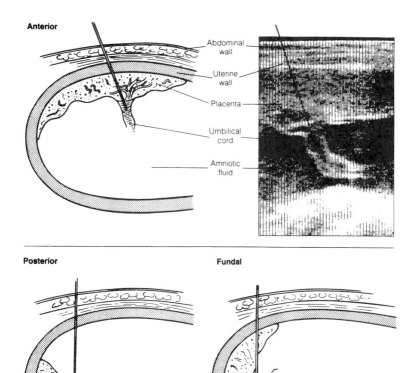

FIG. 12. Technique for intravascular fetal transfusion.

pare the results of each route in a similar population. Intraperitoneal transfusions potentially allow a larger red blood cell volume to be administered so that the interval between transfusions can be increased, and they may be technically easier to administer, particularly later in gestation. However, blood is erratically absorbed from the fetal peritoneal cavity in hydropic infants. Advantages of intravascular transfusions include the ability to check the fetus' antigenic status and actual hematocrit and directly infuse red blood cells into the fetal circulation early in gestation. A disadvantage of this technique is an increased risk of fetomaternal bleeding and the potential for increasing the severity of maternal sensitization during the current and future pregnancies. Both procedures are associated with a fetal loss rate of about 1% to 2% per transfusion.

It is clear that intravascular transfusion is more effective in treating hydropic infants and often is lifesaving. It is not clear whether the intravascular route is superior in the fetus that is not hydropic or in the fetus that has resolved hydrops and is receiving a subsequent transfusion. Fetal survival rates are excellent and comparable by either technique (Table 3). It is likely that indications for combining intraperitoneal and intravascular transfusions eventually will be better defined and may become the optimum treatment.

Aggressive and early use of new diagnostic techniques and advances in fetal therapy, proper timing of delivery, and modern changes in neonatal care have all contributed to the improved perinatal outcome for severely Rh-immunized patients. It is doubtful that measures advocated in the past are justified today. There is little convincing evidence that plasmapheresis; treatment with immunosuppressive agents such as promethazine, corticosteroids, and azathioprine; or oral desensitization regimens significantly improve the outcome in severely Rh-sensitized patients, and each poses some risk to the mother and infant.

Neonatal Care

One of the most important facets of the overall management of the Rh-affected baby is the close cooperation necessary between the obstetric and pediatric teams and the blood bank. The successful management of markedly premature erythroblastotic infants requires all the resources of a tertiary intensive care nursery, including respiratory assistance, correction of acidosis, and exchange transfusion.

Intravascular transfusion in particular suppresses fetal erythropoiesis, and many infants so treated have no fetal cells apparent in the circulation at delivery. They commonly require few or no neonatal exchange transfusions. Reticulocytes may not appear for 3 to 4 months, however, and many of these infants need several transfusions after discharge. Studies of long-term follow-up indicate that most children who have required intrauterine transfusions for severe erythroblastosis fetalis grow and develop normally.

Atypical Antibodies

Because of the decreasing frequency of erythroblastosis fetalis from antibodies to the *D* antigen, an increased proportion of autoantibodies and alloantibodies are now directed against other red blood cell antigens. Differences in the frequencies of these antibodies and whether they cause hemolytic disease depend on the following variables:

◊ Size and frequency of the antigenic stimulus,
◊ Relative potency of the antigen,
◊ Capacity of the fetus to respond to the antigenic stimulus,
◊ Alteration of the antigen when it combines with Rh-positive cells,
◊ Type of antibody response (IgG or IgM),
◊ When the antigen appears on fetal red blood cells.

TABLE 3. *Neonatal survival of infants with severe Rh immunization treated with intrauterine transfusions*

	Nonhydrophic		Hydrophic		Overall	
	Number of patients	(%)	Number of patients	(%)	Number of patients	(%)
Intraperitoneal						
Bowman and Manning, 1982	16/16	(100)	6/8	(75)	22/24	(92)
Scott et al., 1984	12/14	(86)	4/6	(67)	16/20	(80)
Watts et al., 1988	26/26	(100)	4/9	(44)	30/35	(86)
Harman et al., 1990	19/23	(83)	10/21	(48)	29/44	(66)
Total	73/79	(92)	24/44	(55)	97/123	(79)
Intravascular						
Nicolaides et al., 1986	8/8	(100)	9/10	(90)	17/18	(94)
Berkowitz et al., 1988	13/16	(81)	0/1	(0)	13/17	(76)
Grannum et al., 1988	5/6	(83)	16/20	(80)	21/26	(81)
Poissonier et al., 1989	55/60	(92)	29/47	(62)	84/107	(79)
Harman et al., 1990	22/23	(96)	18/21	(86)	40/44	(91)
Weiner et al., 1991	35/35	(100)	11/13	(85)	46/48	(92)
Total	138/148	(93)	83/112	(74)	221/260	(85)

TABLE 4. *Hemolytic disease resulting from irregular antibodies*

Blood group system	Antigen	Severity of hemolytic disease	Proposed management	Blood group system	Antigen	Severity of hemolytic disease	Proposed management
Rh subtype	C	+ to +++	AF ΔOD450	Lutheran	Lua	+	Expectant
	Cw	+ to +++	AF ΔOD450		Lub	+	Expectant
	c	+ to +++	AF ΔOD450	Diego	Dia	+ to +++	AF ΔOD450
	E	+ to +++	AF ΔOD450		Dib	+ to +++	AF ΔOF450
	e	+ to +++	AF ΔOD450	P	P	−	None
Lewis	Lea	−	None		PPIPk (Tja)	+ to +++	AF ΔOD450
	Leb	−	None				
I	I	−	None	Xg	Xga	+	Expectant
Kell	K	+ to +++	AF ΔOD450	Public antigens	Yta	+ to +++	AF ΔOD450
	k	+	Expectant		Ytb	+	Expectant
	Ko	+	Expectant		Lap	+	Expectant
	Kpa	+	Expectant		Ena	+ to ++	AF ΔOD450
	Kpb	+	Expectant		Ge	+	Expectant
	Jsa	+	Expectant		Jra	+	Expectant
	Jsb	+	Expectant		Coa	+ to +++	AF ΔOD450
Duffy	Fya	+ to +++	AF ΔOD450		Coab	+	Expectant
	Fyb	−	None	Private antigens	Batty	+	Expectant
	Fy3	+	Expectant		Becker	+	Expectant
Kidd	Jka	+ to +++	AF ΔOD450		Berrens	+	Expectant
	Jkb	+ to +++	AF ΔOD450		Biles	+ to ++	AF ΔOD450
	Jk3	+	Expectant		Evans	+	Expectant
MNSs	M	+ to +++	AF ΔOD450		Gonzales	+	Expectant
	N	−	None		Good	+ to +++	AF ΔOD450
	S	+ to +++	AF ΔOD450		Heibel	+ to ++	AF ΔOD450
	s	+ to +++	AF ΔOD450		Hunt	+	Expectant
	U	+ to +++	AF ΔOD450		Jobbins	+	Expectant
	Mia	++	AF ΔOD450		Radin	+ to ++	AF ΔOD450
	Mta	++	AF ΔOD450		Rm	+	Expectant
	Vw	+	Expectant		Ven	+	Expectant
	Mur	+	Expectant		Wrighta	+ to +++	AF ΔOD450
	Hil	+	Expectant		Wrightb	+	Expectant
	Hut	+	Expectant		Zd	+ to ++	AF ΔOD450

−, not a proven cause of hemolytic disease of the newborn; +, mild; ++, moderate; +++, severe; expectant, no further diagnostic testing or intervention is necessary until delivery; AF ΔOD450, amniocentesis with amniotic bilirubin studies may be necessary.

(Adapted from Weinstein L. Irregular antibodies causing hemolytic disease of the newborn: a continuing problem. *Clin Obstet Gynecol* 1982;25:321.)

For a red blood cell alloantibody to cause erythroblastosis, the antigen must be present on the fetal red blood cell and absent in the mother. The minor antigens that cause hemolytic disease are listed in Table 4.

Because both Rh-positive and Rh-negative mothers can produce these antibodies, pregnant women who have previously received blood products or are multiparas are candidates for an antibody screen as part of their initial prenatal testing. If the antibody screen is positive, it should be serially titrated and the patient managed as shown in Fig. 13.

Anti-Kell, usually produced in response to previous blood transfusion, is the single most important non-Rh cause of fetal hemolytic disease. When the mother is found to have anti-Kell antibody, paternal Kell genotyping should be carried out. Ninety percent of fathers and their fetuses are Kell-negative, and no further diagnosis or treatment is required as long as paternity is certain. Because anti-Kell titers and amniotic fluid ΔOD450 values are of less predictive value than in

Rh disease, aggressive fetal surveillance and, in some cases, cordocentesis are necessary when the infant is Kell-positive.

Women with autoimmune hemolytic anemia produce antibodies that can cause similar effects in the fetus. Although maternal anemia may be severe during pregnancy, it is more often mild in both mother and fetus and requires no active treatment. No correlation exists between maternal autoantibody titer and severity of hemolysis in the neonate, and management is similar to that for alloantibodies.

ABO Incompatibility

A comparison of Rh and ABO incompatibility is important because they are the most frequent causes of immune hemolytic disease in the neonatal period. In about 20% to 25% of pregnancies, ABO incompatibility exists between mother and infant, but a clinically recognizable hemolytic process in the

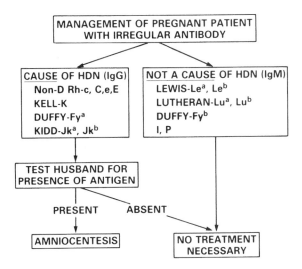

FIG. 13. Flow sheet for the management of a pregnant patient with irregular antibodies. It is important to determine that the husband is the father of the baby before deciding against amniocentesis.

infant occurs in only 10%. ABO hemolytic disease affects the firstborn child in about 50% of cases, and it is not uncommon for multiple siblings to be affected with comparable severity.

The pathophysiology involves the transplacental passage of maternal antibody and its interaction with fetal or neonatal red blood cell antigens, yielding erythrocyte destruction, variable anemia, and hyperbilirubinemia. Clinically, ABO hemolytic problems are confined almost exclusively to the A (specifically A_1 rather than A_2) or B infants of group O mothers. Anti-A and anti-B "natural" antibodies produced early in life by group A or B individuals are predominantly IgM. In contrast, group O individuals produce anti-A or anti-B that is predominantly IgG and capable of crossing the placenta. Yet, for reasons not completely understood, these antibodies seldom cause harm during pregnancy. There is no relationship between the antibody titer and the severity of hemolytic disease. The discordance between the high frequency of ABO-incompatible pregnancies and the low frequency of hemolytic disease as well as the broad spectrum of the severity has been attributed to such factors as immature, weak, nonspecific, or altered antigens on the fetal red blood cell; absorption of the antibodies by ABO antigens present in all body tissues; and the presence of soluble blood group substances in fetal plasma and tissue fluids that can neutralize maternal antibody. No single test exists that can forewarn the physician of impending ABO hemolytic disease. Because this problem does not occur until after birth, amniocentesis and preterm induction of labor are not justified. The most common manifestations of ABO incompatibility in the neonate are early-onset jaundice (i.e., within 24 hours) and a variable elevation of the indirect bilirubin fraction. In contrast to Rh disease, kernicterus and anemia are rare. The cornerstones of management of ABO incompatibility are bilirubin surveillance, phototherapy (required in about 10% of infants), and, occasionally, exchange transfusion.

◊ IMMUNE THROMBOCYTOPENIA

Immunologic thrombocytopenia can be viewed as two diseases with similar potential fetal but very different maternal consequences: autoimmune (formerly idiopathic thrombocytopenic purpura) and alloimmune (formerly isoimmune thrombocytopenic purpura). Perinatal morbidity and mortality are associated with both disorders, but maternal and neonatal thrombocytopenia can also be asymptomatic or result from other complications of pregnancy.

In many cases of maternal thrombocytopenia, the low platelet count is first noted on a complete blood count as part of routine automated prenatal screening tests. Normal values for platelet counts usually do not change during pregnancy, and the mean antepartum platelet count for healthy pregnant women is 246,000/mm^3. Platelet counts that are less than 150,000/mm^3 occur in up to 7.6% of pregnant women; counts less than 100,000/mm^3 occur in fewer than 1%. The single most common etiology of maternal thrombocytopenia is the benign condition known as incidental thrombocytopenia of pregnancy. It occurs in asymptomatic women without a history of bleeding diathesis, and, in most cases, the platelet count is above 100,000/mm^3. A small proportion of cases present with platelet counts less than 100,000/mm^3, and other causes of thrombocytopenia must be excluded. There are no serious maternal or fetal consequences of incidental thrombocytopenia of pregnancy.

The most serious condition commonly confused with autoimmune thrombocytopenia late in pregnancy is atypical preeclampsia or HELLP syndrome (hemolysis, elevated liver enzymes, and low platelet count). A low platelet count can also be the first sign of AIDS, systemic lupus erythematosus (SLE), antiphospholipid syndrome, sepsis, cocaine abuse, thrombotic thrombocytopenic purpura, transfusion reaction, or blood dyscrasias, or it may be caused by medications. Low neonatal platelet counts also are seen with prematurity and infections and, occasionally, in infants born to women who are preeclamptic or Rh-sensitized.

Pseudothrombocytopenia can result from laboratory artifacts such as platelet clumping induced by ethylenediaminetetraacetic acid (EDTA) in the collection tube, blood clotting related to techniques of blood withdrawal, and an inadequate amount of anticoagulant. These factors can be confirmed by examining a stained peripheral maternal blood smear. A fingerstick blood sample can be obtained by using an ammonium oxalate Unopette (Becton-Dickinson, Rutherford, NJ), and the blood cells counted by phase microscopy. Another method involves analysis of a venous blood sample from one test tube anticoagulated with EDTA and another with 3.8% sodium citrate. Once the diagnosis of pseudothrombocytopenia is established, no further treatment is needed for mother or infant.

Autoimmune Thrombocytopenia

Autoimmune thrombocytopenia (ATP) is the most common autoimmune bleeding disorder encountered during pregnancy. The coexistence of ATP and pregnancy is relatively frequent because the disease usually presents in the second to third decade of life and has a female preponderance of 3:1. Autoimmune thrombocytopenia is characterized by the production of IgG antibodies directed against both maternal and fetal platelets. The spleen is a major site of antiplatelet antibody production, and the thrombocytopenia occurs from increased platelet destruction. An IgG antibody binds to the platelets, rendering them more susceptible to sequestration and premature destruction in the reticuloendothelial system. The rate of destruction exceeds the compensatory ability of the bone marrow to produce new platelets.

The course of ATP is not substantially influenced by pregnancy. However, pregnancy may be adversely affected by ATP, and abnormal bleeding in the peripartum period can be hazardous for the mother. Because the placenta selectively transports maternal IgG antiplatelet antibodies into the fetal circulation, fetal thrombocytopenia may also occur and result in hemorrhagic consequences.

Diagnosis

Most women with ATP have a history of easy bruising, petechiae, ecchymoses, menorrhagia, or other bleeding problems. The diagnosis is based on a maternal platelet count repeatedly less than 100,000/mm^3, with or without megathrombocytes on the peripheral blood smear; a bone marrow aspirate with a normal or increased number of megakaryocytes; exclusion of other diseases or drugs associated with thrombocytopenia; and the absence of splenomegaly.

Both direct and indirect assays of antiplatelet antibodies are now available clinically. About 90% of patients with ATP have increased levels of bound immunoglobulins, primarily IgG, on platelet surfaces. This platelet-associated IgG (PAIgG) correlates with the severity of thrombocytopenia in the mother but not the fetus. Increased levels of unbound circulating antiplatelet antibody are unreliable predictors of thrombocytopenia in the mother or the fetus.

Treatment

Treatment of the mother should aim to prevent bleeding by maintaining a platelet count greater than 20,000/mm^3 in the antepartum period and over 50,000/mm^3 for delivery.

Glucocorticoids

Glucocorticoid drugs are the cornerstone of therapy in pregnancy. Prednisone, 1 to 2 mg/kg per day in divided doses, is the standard regimen used for 2 to 3 weeks. A rise in platelet count to more than 50,000/mm^3 accompanied by a decrease in clinical bleeding typically is achieved within 21 days. Platelet response of some degree is seen in more than 70% of patients, and a complete remission in up to 25%. The prednisone dose is then tapered by 10% to 20% decrements at 2-week intervals to a dose that maintains the platelet count above 50,000/mm^3. Glucocorticoids appear to function ther-

apeutically by decreasing antiplatelet antibody production by the reticuloendothelial system; reducing platelet-bound IgG by interfering with the interaction of antiplatelet antibody at the platelet surface; increasing platelet survival by decreasing the clearance of antibody-coated platelets by macrophages in the spleen and liver; and improving abnormal capillary fragility. Dexamethasone and betamethasone, which readily cross the placenta, do not ensure a normal fetal platelet count. The side effects of glucocorticoids in pregnancy include steroid-induced moon facies, diabetes mellitus, psychosis, adrenocortical insufficiency, osteoporosis, and aseptic necrosis.

Immunoglobulin

High doses of immune globulin (i.e., 400 mg/kg per day for 5 days) given intravenously (IVIG) usually induce a peak platelet count within 7 to 9 days. More than 80% of patients treated with this regimen have a peak platelet count greater than 50,000/mm^3, and the response lasts for more than 30 days in 30% of patients. The exact mechanism of action of IVIG is not clear, but it appears to depress antiplatelet antibody production, interfere with antibody attachment to platelets, inhibit macrophage receptor-mediated immune complex clearance, or interfere with platelet receptor mechanisms in the reticuloendothelial system. In responders, only 2 to 3 days of IVIG therapy may be needed, and doses greater than 800 mg or 1 g/kg may suffice as a single or double infusion. Although expensive, IVIgG therapy initiated 1 to 2 weeks before delivery or surgery is useful in obstetric patients who must undergo operative procedures or who develop bleeding problems and require emergency treatment. The IgG is selectively transported across the placenta, and the amount transferred increases with gestational age and dose. Thus, maternally infused IgG may also have a beneficial fetal effect after 32 weeks of gestation. It does not guarantee a normal platelet count in the fetus, however, because thrombocytopenia has occurred in infants after IVIG administration to the mother. No cases of HIV transmission have been reported with the use of IVIG, but adverse effects include thrombosis, alopecia, liver function disturbances, transient neutropenia, chills, nausea, flushing, tightness of the chest, wheezing, and anaphylactic reactions in patients with IgA antibodies.

Splenectomy

Splenectomy, which removes the site of destruction of damaged platelets as well as the major source of antibody production, is used only in pregnant patients with ATP who are refractory to or cannot tolerate glucocorticoids and IVIG. A complete remission is obtained in 80% of patients. The postsplenectomy platelet count increases rapidly and often is normal within 1 to 2 weeks. The surgery is associated with a modest risk of spontaneous abortion or preterm labor and technically more difficult late in gestation. If splenectomy is unavoidable, it is best performed in the second trimester; it has also been combined safely with cesarean section at term. Splenectomy does not always protect the fetus from thrombocytopenia because antibodies to platelets also are produced in other lymphoid tissues.

Platelet Transfusions

Platelet transfusions are used only as a temporary measure to control life-threatening hemorrhage or to prepare a patient for splenectomy or cesarean section. The survival of transfused platelets is decreased in patients with ATP because antiplatelet antibodies also bind to donor platelets. The usual elevation in the platelet count of about 10,000/mm³/m² per unit of platelet concentrate is not achieved in ATP patients, but 6 to 10 units is useful during the perioperative period to temporarily control hemostasis.

Other Therapies

The use of other agents has been reserved for patients who are refractory to glucocorticoids and splenectomy. Those most commonly used, such as azathioprine, cyclophosphamide, vinca alkaloids, and danazol, are to be avoided in pregnancy because of their toxicity and potential adverse effects on the fetus. Plasmapheresis has also been tried, but the results of this treatment are variable.

Obstetric Management

No maternal deaths from ATP in pregnancy have been recorded since the early 1980s, but peripartum bleeding associated with vaginal or cesarean delivery remains a major risk.

Because the placenta is permeable to circulating maternal antiplatelet antibody, fetal thrombocytopenia may occur. This infrequently results in clinical bleeding such as purpura, ecchymoses, hematuria, melena, or intracranial hemorrhage. These hemorrhagic complications are extremely unlikely if the infant's platelet count remains greater than 50,000/mm³. Most cases of perinatal intracranial hemorrhage have been reported in infants born vaginally. Although it is not clear that vaginal delivery is the causative factor in intracranial bleeding, many consider it prudent to avoid labor and vaginal delivery if the fetus is markedly thrombocytopenic. The optimal obstetrical management, however, remains controversial because (1) the fetal platelet count is greater than 50,000/mm³ in 80% of cases, (2) it is difficult to predict which infants will be thrombocytopenic, and (3) the overall frequency of serious neonatal morbidity or mortality from ATP is quite small. Even when the maternal platelet count is less than 100,000/mm³, many of the infants have normal platelet counts (Fig. 14). The fetal platelet count does not correlate closely enough with maternal PAIgG, circulating antiplatelet antibody levels, or previous treatment regimens to determine the safest route of delivery for an individual patient (Figs. 15 and 16). The futility of using a maternal factor as a predictor of fetal involve-

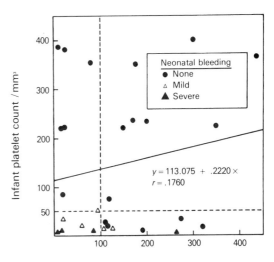

FIG. 14. Relation of maternal and infant platelet counts in pregnant patients with immunologic thrombocytopenic purpura from a series of patients managed at the University of Utah Medical Center and the University of Iowa Hospitals.

ment is illustrated by patients with twins in which one infant has a normal platelet count and the other is thrombocytopenic.

The use of fetal scalp blood sampling for platelet determinations early in labor or at the time of elective induction has been suggested as one way for obstetricians to ascertain the safety of vaginal delivery. This method, which uses a widely available pediatric Unopette system, identifies the 80% of infants of ATP mothers with a platelet count sufficient to safely deliver vaginally. As with scalp blood sampling performed

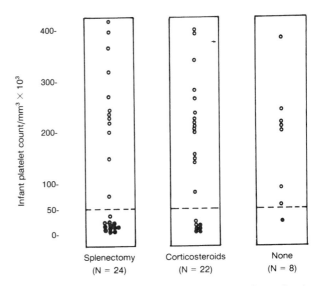

FIG. 15. Relation of maternal treatment to infant platelet counts. Eight mothers had previously had a splenectomy and were also receiving corticosteroids. The *solid dots* represent infants who had purpura, petechiae, or symptomatic bleeding. (From Scott JR, Rote NS, Cruikshank DP. Antiplatelet antibodies and platelet counts in pregnancies complicated by autoimmune thrombocytopenic purpura. *Am J Obstet Gynecol* 1983;145:932.)

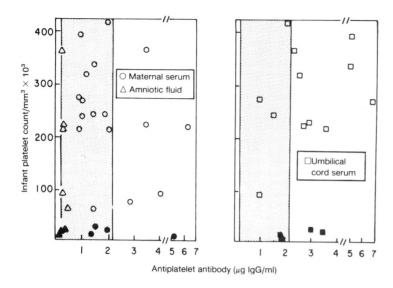

FIG. 16. Relation of maternal serum, amniotic fluid, and umbilical cord serum antiplatelet antibody concentrations to infant platelet counts. Normal values are indicated by the shaded areas; the solid symbols represent infants who had purpura, petechiae, or symptomatic bleeding. (From Scott JR, Rote NS, Cruikshank DP. Anti-platelet antibodies and platelet counts in pregnancies complicated by autoimmune thrombocytopenic purpura. *Am J Obstet Gynecol* 1983;145:932.)

for any reason, technical problems can occur with limited cervical dilation, a high presenting part, or inaccurate platelet counts if the blood clots in the sample collected. Percutaneous umbilical cord sampling (PUBS) has also been proposed to determine the fetal platelet count. However, most authorities feel that PUBS, as well as fetal scalp platelet counts, need not be performed because of the overall low frequency of fetal bleeding in ATP.

Vaginal delivery usually is indicated unless a markedly thrombocytopenic infant is identified. External fetal monitoring rather than scalp electrodes should be used in these patients in early labor until the fetal platelet count is known. Injectable anesthetics and forceps manipulations should be avoided, and careful attention should be given to the repair of lacerations or the episiotomy.

Delivery is best accomplished in a setting in which platelets, fresh frozen plasma, and immune globulin are available for the mother. A neonatologist or pediatrician familiar with the disorder should be present to promptly treat hemorrhagic complications in the neonate. The platelet counts of affected neonates usually fall after delivery, and the lowest counts may not be reached for several days. Although most infants are asymptomatic and the thrombocytopenia is self-limited, daily platelet counts should be obtained. For the seriously thrombocytopenic infant, treatment with high-dose immune globulin, glucocorticoids, or platelet or exchange transfusions is effective in raising the platelet count. Early in the puerperium, breast-feeding may theoretically induce neonatal thrombocytopenia because of the passage of antiplatelet antibodies in the colostrum, but it is considered to be a safe and reasonable option.

Alloimmune Thrombocytopenia

Alloimmune thrombocytopenia should be suspected when a thrombocytopenic infant is delivered by a mother with a normal platelet count and whenever a severely thrombocyto-

penic infant is delivered. The disorder is the result of maternal alloimmunization by platelet antigens that are lacking on her own platelets, analogous to neonatal hemolytic anemia caused by fetomaternal erythrocyte incompatibility. Fetomaternal incompatibility for the platelet-specific alloantigen HPA-1a (formerly called PL^A1) is responsible for most of the serologically proven cases of neonatal alloimmune thrombocytopenia. The antigen is inherited as a codominant trait; 69% of people are homozygous HPA-1a-positive, and 28% are heterozygous. Other platelet-specific alloantigens, including HPA-1b (PL^A2), HPA-2a and b (Ko), HPA-3a and b (BAK), HPA-4a and b (Pen), and HPA-5a and b (Br) as well as class I HLA antigens, can also be involved. Two percent of mothers are HPA-1a-negative, and 98% are married to HPA-1a-positive men. Yet alloimmune thrombocytopenia occurs in only one to two per 10,000 neonates, indicating that unknown factors prevent sensitization from occurring more frequently. In some cases, the disorder may remain subclinical because the maternal anti-HPA-1a antibodies are of insufficient levels to induce thrombocytopenia in the infant. The more frequent development of HPA-1a antibodies in association with a certain maternal HLA phenotype seems to be another reason. A woman who possesses the DR3 antigen is 76.5 times more likely to form anti-HPA-1a antibodies than a woman who is DR3-negative. In contrast to Rh immunization, alloimmune thrombocytopenia occurs in many infants of primiparas not previously exposed to a sensitizing stimulus or blood transfusions, and the diagnosis usually is not made until after delivery. Future siblings of an infant with alloimmune thrombocytopenia have about a 75% chance of also having the disorder, depending on the alloantigen and paternal zygosity.

Obstetric Management

Although less common than ATP, alloimmune thrombocytopenia often has more serious consequences for the infant. Neurologic abnormalities from intracranial bleeding occur in about 25% of infants, and neonatal mortality rates of 10% to 15% have been reported. Intracranial hemorrhages have been detected in about 10% of affected infants by sonography in utero. Therefore, serial ultrasound examinations to detect this complication have been advocated. Antepartum maternal administration of IVIgG is accepted to elevate the fetal platelet count in 75% of cases and is the current treatment of choice. Direct intravascular fetal transfusions of IVIgG have been unsuccessful in raising the fetal platelet count in some cases. Serial fetal transfusion of HPA-1a-negative platelets has also been recommended, but this treatment is not universally accepted because of the potential risks involved with repeated cordocenteses. Intracranial hemorrhage has occurred as early as the end of the first trimester, when intrauterine platelet transfusion is not yet possible. Fetal platelet transfusions may have merit in severely thrombocytopenic fetuses during the third trimester to minimize the risk of fetal intracranial bleeding and in preparation for delivery.

Although the obstetric management of alloimmune thrombocytopenia is similar to that for ATP, a stronger case can be made for antepartum fetal blood sampling and delivery by cesarean section near term for significant fetal thrombocytopenia. Whenever a PUBS is being done for suspected alloimmune thrombocytopenia, HPA-1a-negative, crossmatched platelet concentrates should be available for immediate transfusion of the thrombocytopenic neonate. These can be obtained by plasmapheresis from the mother or known antigen-negative donors and can be stored for up to 5 days. Before infusion, the platelets must be washed to remove maternal antibody. Once the maternal antiplatelet antibody has been cleared from the infant's circulation, the disorder is self-limiting.

◊ SYSTEMIC LUPUS ERYTHEMATOSUS

A chronic, multisystem inflammatory disease, SLE is one of the most frequent serious disorders that affect women of childbearing age. Despite the general impression that the disease is rare, more than 250,000 persons are known to have SLE, and about 50,000 new cases are diagnosed each year. Although the cause remains unknown, it has been established that the development of antibody to autologous DNA and other cell components leads to the deposition of antigen–antibody complexes and to resultant inflammatory responses in target tissues. The frequency of SLE among identical twins and familial aggregations as well as abnormal distributions of HLA antigens in these patients also strongly implicate genetic factors. With an increased awareness of the disease, more sophisticated diagnostic methods, and improved drug therapy, the outlook for these patients has greatly improved. The 10-year survival rate for SLE now appears to exceed 90%.

Diagnosis

The disease is easily overlooked initially because it may begin with mild and vague symptoms such as fatigue and is characterized by periods of exacerbation and remission. The presence of autoantibodies, characteristically against nuclear components, is a hallmark of the disorder.

The American Rheumatism Association has set criteria for the diagnosis of SLE that incorporate immunologic abnormalities and improve disease classification for purposes of clinical studies (Table 5). The most common clinical manifestations include arthralgia or arthritis (90%), dermatologic involvement (70% to 80%), renal disease (46%), hematologic abnormalities (50%), and cardiovascular disease (30% to 50%). The most frequent laboratory findings are thrombocytopenia, leukopenia, and the presence of autoantibodies.

Lupus should be suspected when a woman in her reproductive years presents with glomerulonephritis, nephrotic syndrome, hemolytic anemia, leukopenia, or thrombocytopenia. A positive antinuclear antibody test occurs in virtually all (98%) patients; in its absence, the diagnosis must be critically reevaluated. High titers of antibodies to double-stranded DNA and antibodies to the Smith (Sm) antigen are also specific for SLE.

Systemic Lupus Erythematosus and Pregnancy

The cause of flares and remissions remains unknown, and in general, the clinical course of the disease is not adversely influenced by pregnancy. In the past, most maternal deaths occurred during the puerperium, but more recent studies show little or no increase in disease activity postpartum. Maternal complications correlate most closely with the activity of the disease and with cardiac or renal involvement. Diffuse proliferative lupus glomerulonephritis carries a risk of renal failure, hypertension, and superimposed preeclampsia. In fact, sometimes superimposed preeclampsia is difficult to differentiate clinically from a lupus flare.

TABLE 5. *Diagnostic criteria for systemic lupus erythematosus[a]*

Finding	Frequency
Malar rash (fixed erythema over malar eminences)	85%
Discoid rash (erythematous, raised patches with scaling)	15%
Photosensitivity	Common
Oral or pharyngeal ulcers	50%
Arthritis (nonerosive, involving two or more joints)	90%
Pleuritis or pericarditis	25% to 46%
Proteinuria, 0.5 g/day, or cellular casts	50%
Seizures or psychosis	20%
Anemia, leukopenia, thrombocytopenia	>95%
Positive antinuclear antibody titer	>95%
Positive lupus erythematosus preparation, anti-DNA, anti-Sm, or false-positive test results for syphilis	>95%

[a]The presence of any four criteria, serially or simultaneously, in any given period of observation is sufficient to make the diagnosis of systemic lupus erythematosus.

Spontaneous abortion, preterm delivery, fetal growth retardation, and stillbirths are more frequent in SLE patients. About 20% to 30% of patients develop preeclampsia, and premature birth occurs in 30% to 50%. Most fetal losses are predicted by the presence of antiphospholipid antibodies (aPL), lupus anticoagulant (LA), or anticardiolipin (aCL; see Antiphospholipid Syndrome). Fetal loss is also related to disease activity and poor renal status. In contrast, SLE patients with mild to moderate renal disease who are in remission before conception have a successful live birth rate of 80% to 90%.

Pregnancy Management

Most patients should be counseled to postpone conception until at least 1 to 2 years after the diagnosis of SLE, when the disease is in good control with low doses of corticosteroids. Diaphragm, condom, and sterilization are the preferred methods of fertility regulation. Although elective termination of pregnancy should be an option, induced abortions exert little, if any, positive influence on the subsequent clinical course. There is little evidence that therapeutic abortion alone is therapeutic in a flare.

The mainstay of therapy for active SLE is corticosteroids. An initial regimen of prednisone (60 to 100 mg/day) induces remission in most patients. With a satisfactory response, the dosage usually can be tapered over several weeks to 10 to 15 mg/day. Intravenous hydrocortisone, 100 mg every 8 hours during labor and delivery, and continuation of adequate corticosteroid treatment during the first 2 months postpartum are recommended to limit the chances of exacerbation. Dialysis, plasmapheresis, or azathioprine therapy may be needed in seriously ill patients, but cyclophosphamide should be avoided because of its significant teratogenicity in the human. In contrast, adverse fetal effects from maternal corticosteroid administration are rare. The relation between corticosteroids (and other immunosuppressive drugs) and infection should be appreciated because infection is now a leading cause of death among SLE patients.

Clinical precautions in pregnancies associated with SLE are similar to those required for other high-risk pregnancies. Recommended laboratory studies in addition to routine prenatal tests are listed in Table 6. There is no uniform definition for SLE flare, and it may be difficult to distinguish from preeclampsia. Proteinuria may reflect prior damage rather than active nephritis or preeclampsia. Immunologic signs of activity (i.e., high anti-DNA antibody and low complement) are of uncertain importance for pregnancy if not associated with clinical illness.

The gestational age should be firmly established early in pregnancy. Serial ultrasonography and antepartum and intrapartum fetal heart rate monitoring are useful to diagnose fetal growth retardation and prevent stillbirths. The route of delivery should be based on appropriate obstetric indications; SLE *per se* is not an indication for cesarean delivery.

TABLE 6. *Management of systemic lupus erythematosus during pregnancy*

Testing parameter[a]	First trimester	Second trimester	Third trimester
Blood count with platelets	×	×	×
Microscopic urinalysis	×	×	×
24-hr urine for protein, creatinine clearance	×	×	×
Urine culture	×		
Lupus anticoagulant	×		
Anticardiolipin	×		
Anti-Ro and anti-LA antibodies	×		
SMA	×		
Clinic visits	Biweekly	Biweekly	Weekly
Sonographic examination	Once	Monthly	Monthly
Fetal heart rate testing			Weekly

[a] × denotes that the test should be performed in the trimester indicated.

Neonatal Lupus Erythematosus

Neonatal lupus erythematosus (NLE), a rare condition caused by placental transfer of maternal autoantibodies, is characterized by specific dermatologic, hematologic, or cardiac manifestations. About 50% of mothers who deliver infants with NLE have SLE or another autoimmune condition. Many other women who deliver infants with NLE develop SLE or a related autoimmune condition months or years later.

The typical infant skin lesions are erythematous and scaly, usually involving the face or scalp. They appear within the first several weeks after delivery and disappear by 12 months of age. Hematologic abnormalities include hemolytic anemia, leukopenia, thrombocytopenia, and hepatosplenomegaly.

The NLE cardiac lesions are congenital complete heart block (CCHB) and endocardial fibroelastosis, which are associated with maternal anti-Ro (SSA) or anti-La (SSB) antibodies. Most mothers with these autoantibodies, however, have normal infants, and the overall risk of CCHB is probably less than 5%. If CCHB occurs, recurrence risk in a subsequent pregnancy is probably about 20% to 30%. Screening mothers with SLE for anti-Ro and anti-La alerts the physician to the possibility of disease in the fetus. Furthermore, the recognition of CCHB may avoid a needless cesarean section for "fetal distress." The usual presentation is a fixed fetal bradycardia ranging from 60 to 80 beats per minute detected between weeks 16 and 25 of gestation. Ultrasonographic examination of the fetal heart shows a structurally normal heart with atrioventricular dissociation. The histologic lesion is one of fibrosis and interruption of the conduction system, particularly in the region of the atrioventricular node. Most fetuses tolerate CCHB throughout pregnancy and labor, but hydrops fetalis can develop *in utero.*

If CCHB is diagnosed *in utero,* most authorities recommend treating the fetus via maternally administered glucocorticoids that cross the placenta (e.g., dexamethasone, 4 mg per day) in the hope of preventing further autoantibody-mediated damage to the fetal heart. Biophysical assessment with ultrasound examinations to detect pericardial and pleural effusions is the best way to monitor the fetus. The goal is to achieve fetal maturity, but delivery is indicated if the fetal condition is deteriorating. Vaginal delivery usually is possible and may be achieved by continuous fetal heart rate monitoring and fetal scalp blood sampling in labor. A registry of CCHB cases is maintain by J.P. Buyon, M.D. at the Hospital for Joint Diseases in New York City (212-598-6283).

◊ ANTIPHOSPHOLIPID SYNDROME

Antiphospholipid syndrome (APS) is an autoimmune disorder characterized by the production of moderate to high levels of antiphospholipid antibodies (aPL) and specific clinical features. The most frequent clinical manifestations are thrombotic episodes, thrombocytopenia, and pregnancy loss. When APS occurs in patients with other autoimmune diseases, such as SLE, it is classified as secondary APS. Primary APS, encountered more frequently in obstetrics, is diagnosed when the syndrome occurs in women with no recognizable autoimmune disease. To be classified as APS, a patient must have at least one clinical feature of the syndrome along with moderate to high levels of aPL (Table 7).

Laboratory Determination and Interpretation

There are three aPL with well-established assays: the biological false-positive test for syphilis (BF-STS), lupus anticoagulant (LA), and anticardiolipin (aCL). All three autoantibodies bind moieties on negatively charged phospholipids, and it has been suggested that aCL binding depends on a circulating gly-coprotein, β_2-glycoprotein-I. Both BF-STS and aCL are detected by conventional immunoassay methods. The assay for aCL is standardized, using sera obtainable from the Antiphospholipid Standardization Laboratory (Atlanta, GA). Results calibrated against these standards are measured as GPL (IgG aCL) or MPL (IgM aCL) units and should be reported and interpreted in semiquantitative terms as negative, low positive, medium positive, or high positive. Low-positive and isolated IgM aCL results (i.e., IgM positive, LA and IgG aCL negative) are of questionable clinical significance and should be carefully interpreted in the light of the clinical situation.

The LA is detected in plasma using phospholipid-dependent clotting assays, such as activated partial thromboplastin time, dilute Russell viper venom time, and kaolin clotting time. Because LA binds to the phospholipid portion of the clotting tests, the clotting time is prolonged, even though the patients have a thrombotic, not a bleeding, tendency. The prolongation of the clotting time is not specific for LA, and further tests typically are performed to exclude factor deficiencies and other antibody inhibitors of clotting. The clinician need only know whether or not the laboratory detected LA. The sensitivity of the various clotting assays for LA varies considerably, and a laboratory known to perform reliable and sensitive LA testing should be used.

Whether LA and aCL are distinct or are the same immunoglobulin being detected by different laboratory methods remains controversial. Both LA and aCL seem to be members of the same family of autoantibodies and are associated with the same set of clinical problems. Most patients with APS have both LA and IgG aCL, but some patients have only LA or aCL. Both tests should be obtained when the diagnosis of APS is considered. The use of other aPL (e.g., antiphosphatidylserine, antiethanolamine) is controversial.

TABLE 7. *Clinical and laboratory criteria for antiphospholipid syndrome*[a]

Clinical features
  Pregnancy loss
    Recurrent pregnancy loss
    Fetal death
  Thrombosis
    Venous
    Arterial, including stroke
  Autoimmune thrombocytopenia
  Other
    Coombs'-positive hemolytic anemia
    Livedo reticularis
Laboratory features
  Lupus anticoagulant
  Anticardiolipin antibodies
    IgG, medium- or high-positive
    IgM, medium- or high-positive and lupus anticoagulant

[a]Patients with antiphospholipid syndrome should have at least one clinical and one laboratory feature at some time in the course of their disease. Laboratory test results should be positive on at least two occasions more than 8 weeks apart.

Prevalence

During pregnancy, aPL antibody levels do not differ significantly from nonpregnant levels. Fewer than 2% of normal pregnant women have IgG aCL, and fewer than 4% have IgM aCL. More than 80% of these positive results are in the low-positive range, with only 0.2% of IgG and 0.7% of IgM results in the clinically significant medium- or high-positive range. Other studies have confirmed the relatively small proportion of positive results in unselected obstetric patients. For this reason, aPL testing in the general population as a screening test for pregnancy complications is not cost-effective and not recommended. In contrast, testing for aPL in patients with recurrent pregnancy loss or fetal deaths is more productive because the prevalence of positive results is 5% to 10%.

The prevalence of aPL antibodies in patients with SLE is about 30% to 40%. The fetal loss rate in SLE patients with aPL is 73%, compared with 19% in SLE patients without aPL. However, well over 50% of women with APS who present with obstetric problems have no underlying autoimmune disease. The risk of fetal loss in patients without SLE but with

LA or aCL is also high, with a wide variation in the reported prevalence. Differences in the methodology and sensitivity of LA and aCL assays among laboratories, fluctuations of aPL during the course of disease, and patient selection probably explain these discrepancies. The firm relationship between fetal loss and aPL is apparent only in patients with a prior history of thrombosis, fetal loss, SLE, or other autoimmune manifestations.

Clinical Manifestations

It is now recognized that a small subset of patients with pregnancy loss have significantly positive tests for aPL as the only explanation (or marker). A history of midtrimester fetal death (i.e., loss of pregnancy after the detection of fetal heart tones) appears to be a specific clue for APS because 90% of patients with aPL as the cause of their pregnancy loss have at least one midtrimester fetal death. The more consecutive pregnancy losses, the worse the prognosis for future pregnancies. Women with aPL are also at risk for a variety of serious medical problems, including thromboembolic disease, stroke, and thrombocytopenia. Thirty percent to 50% of women with APS have a history of thrombotic episodes, and more than 80% of the thrombotic events occur while the patient is pregnant or taking oral contraceptives.

Pathogenesis

The mechanism of aPL-related pregnancy loss and thrombotic events has not been resolved. Decidual vasculopathy is a prominent feature in patients with APS, and decidual vessel thromboses, small placentas, and placental infarctions have all been reported. These lesions are nonspecific, however, and the degree of placental pathology is not always sufficient to explain the fetal death. The original hypothesis proposed an imbalance of local prostacyclin and thromboxane production leading to vasoconstriction, platelet aggregation, and intravascular thrombosis, but subsequent studies have not confirmed this. A recent study indicates that aPL leads to a diminution of annexin V on trophoblastic cells. Other proposals for the thrombotic tendency include decreased activation of protein C, inhibition of fibrinolysis, platelet activation, and decreased functional antithrombin III. Although animal studies strongly suggest a pathogenic role for aPL, it is not certain whether these antibodies are the cause of fetal loss or simply represent epiphenomena reflecting other mechanisms of thrombosis.

Pregnancy Management

A positive result of a test for aPL does not invariably indicate a poor prognosis, and some patients with APS have achieved successful pregnancies without specific medical therapy. A well-documented history of previous unexplained fetal deaths or the presence of underlying autoimmune disease (i.e., SLE, APS) should be established before therapy is considered.

Many reports suggest that women with APS and previous pregnancy loss can be treated during their next pregnancy to improve their chance of delivering a live infant.

Prednisone, 40 to 60 mg/day, and low-dose aspirin (i.e., 80 mg/day) were used initially in pregnant patients with LA and eventually in patients with aCL. Direct comparison of various reports is virtually impossible because of the nature of the patients (e.g., SLE vs. no SLE and differences in numbers of previous fetal deaths) and their diagnoses (LA and aCL vs. LA alone or aCL alone). Although no controlled trials have been published, the pregnancy outcome was improved in all series but one. Treatment with glucocorticoids has been complicated by numerous adverse effects, including gestational diabetes, hypertension, oropharyngeal candidiasis, facial acne, facial abscess, postpartum adrenal insufficiency, pneumonia, mycobacterial infection, osteoporosis leading to vertebral collapse, and osteonecrosis of the hip.

Today, most authorities favor the use of subcutaneous heparin treatment, with or without low-dose aspirin, to treat APS pregnancy because the results seem comparable to or better than those achieved with glucocorticoids (Table 8) and there are fewer side effects. Within the last 3 years, two well-designed studies indicate a better fetal outcome for women with antiphospholipid antibodies and recurrent pregnancy loss who were treated with heparin and low-dose aspirin compared to aspirin alone. The treatment regimen at the University of Utah includes one baby aspirin taken daily (i.e., 80 mg/day) throughout pregnancy in an attempt to prevent or ameliorate preeclampsia. Subcutaneous heparin (15,000 units daily in divided doses) is begun after first-trimester documentation of a live fetus, and the dose is changed to approximately 20,000 units daily in the second and third trimesters. The most significant risks are bleeding from trauma, heparin-induced osteoporosis, and idiosyncratic thrombocytopenia. The latter is uncommon in pregnancy. To avoid osteoporosis, it may be helpful for women treated with either glucocorticoids or heparin to take at least 1 g of calcium daily and exercise regularly. The concomitant use of glucocorticoids and heparin should be avoided because this combination has not been shown to be better than either alone in achieving a live birth. Moreover, severe osteoporosis with fractures has been reported in several women with APS who were treated with a combination regimen.

The use of low-dose aspirin (i.e., 80 mg/day) alone has also been suggested, particularly for women not previously pregnant or considered to be at low risk for fetal loss. Other therapeutic approaches that have been tried include intravenous immunoglobulin, plasma exchange, and azathioprine, but none appears to be superior to the usual regimens.

Even with treatment, patients with true APS have complicated pregnancies, and careful antepartum management, including serial monitoring for fetal growth and well-being, is essential. Fetal loss may occur despite treatment, and complications include maternal thrombocytopenia, chorea gravidarum, severe early-onset preeclampsia, fetal growth retardation, fetal distress, and thrombotic episodes. The high rate

TABLE 8. *Outcome of antiphospholipid syndrome—treated pregnancies*

	Total number	Spontaneous abortions (%)	Fetal deaths (%)	Live births (%)
Prednisone and low-dose aspirin				
Lubbe and Liggins 1988	18	NA[a]	NA	15 (78)
Gatenby et al., 1989	27	NA	NA	17 (63)
Ordi et al., 1989	9	0	2 (22)	7 (78)
Lockshin et al., 1989	11	3 (27)	6 (55)	2 (18)
Cowchock 1991	19	NA	NA	13 (68)
Reece et al., 1990	18	3 (17)	1 (5)	14 (78)
Branch et al., 1992	39	8 (21)	8 (21)	23 (59)
Total	141			91 (68)
Heparin or heparin and low-dose aspirin				
Rosove et al., 1987	15	NA	NA	14 (93)
Cowchock 1991	8	NA	NA	6 (75)
Branch et al., 1992	19	1 (5)	2 (11)	16 (84)
Total	42			36 (84)

[a]NA, not applicable.

of preeclampsia in patients with APS has prompted a search to determine whether APS may present or manifest itself as preeclampsia. In a series of patients with severe early-onset preeclampsia, 16% had significant levels of aPL. Three of these women suffered serious peripartum or postpartum sequelae, including cerebral infarction, amaurosis fugax, transient global amnesia, deep venous thrombosis, pulmonary embolus, and autoimmune flare. Moreover, treatment of APS patients during pregnancy does not appear to markedly diminish the risk or severity of preeclampsia, which often is an important contributor to preterm delivery. The typical sequence of fetal compromise develops as limitation of fetal growth followed by abnormalities of the fetal heart rate tracing indicative of hypoxemia and decreased amniotic fluid volume. With any of these findings, twice-weekly fetal cardiotocography and weekly ultrasonic measurements of the amniotic fluid volume have been recommended as soon as delivery for fetal distress would be considered.

Although close fetal monitoring is a key to successful pregnancy, the relative contribution of fetal surveillance versus pharmacologic treatment is yet to be determined. Even careful fetal surveillance cannot prevent fetal or neonatal death before 22 to 24 weeks of gestation. Although preterm delivery is common because of obstetric complications, infants born to women treated for APS during pregnancy follow a course similar to the offspring born of normal women at the same gestational age.

Several women with APS have developed features suspicious for an autoimmune flare in the postpartum period, consisting of unexplained fever, pleurisy, pulmonary infiltrates, pleural effusion, thromboses, and cardiomyopathy. Perhaps the most dangerous feature is thrombosis, but the pleuropulmonary disease is also life-threatening. After infection was thoroughly excluded, these women with unexplained fever and pleuropulmonary disease were successfully treated with glucocorticoids and supportive care. Finally, the role of long-term prophylactic aspirin or anticoagulation in nonpregnant

patients with APS is unresolved. Certainly, this therapy should be considered for all patients who have already suffered a life-threatening thrombotic episode.

Subclinical Autoimmunity

Although other autoantibodies have also been suggested as the cause of reproductive disorders, this entity is less well defined and more controversial. The idea that a subclinical autoimmune condition or polyclonal B lymphocyte abnormality may in some way cause other reproductive problems arose primarily from the observation that many patients with recurrent pregnancy loss have detectable levels of other autoantibodies. This has stimulated further interest in the role of these autoantibodies in infertility, endometriosis, preeclampsia, and fetal death. The conclusions in this area are complicated by differences in autoantibody measurements and types of assays. Most published reports have focused on antinuclear antibodies, but other autoantibodies or autoimmune aberrations have also been implicated. Given the available data, it is difficult to support the routine performance of autoantibody profiles in the evaluation of patients with these disorders. The statistical chance of obtaining false-positive test results in normal patients increases with the number of tests performed, and no reasonable recommendation is available regarding the management of patients with positive results.

◊ RHEUMATOID ARTHRITIS

Rheumatoid arthritis is a chronic inflammatory process that can affect several organ systems but primarily involves synovia-lined joints, which become swollen and painful. The following criteria must be met to establish the diagnosis of rheumatoid arthritis (i.e., seven criteria for classic rheumatoid arthritis, five criteria for definite rheumatoid arthritis, three criteria for probable rheumatoid arthritis, two criteria for possible rheumatoid arthritis):

◊ Morning stiffness,
◊ Pain and tenderness in at least one joint,
◊ Swelling of at least one joint,
◊ Swelling of at least one other joint,
◊ Symmetric joint swelling,
◊ Subcutaneous nodules,
◊ X-ray changes typical of rheumatoid arthritis,
◊ Positive test result for rheumatoid factor,
◊ Poor mucin precipitate of synovial fluid,
◊ Characteristic histologic changes of synovium,
◊ Characteristic histologic changes of nodules.

Most cases are mild and require little or no medical treatment; in others, however, the disease is characterized by an intermittent course with ultimate progression over many years to typical joint deformities and the findings already listed.

The signs and symptoms improve in at least 50% of pregnant patients, a phenomenon that may be related to elevated blood levels of free cortisol or to enhanced phagocytosis of immune complexes. The rheumatoid factors (i.e., IgM antibodies against autologous IgG) do not cross the placenta, and there is no fetal or neonatal involvement.

Because half or more of women with rheumatoid arthritis have spontaneous remission during pregnancy, treatment must be directed along lines that will do no harm to mother or fetus. Management includes an appropriate balance of rest and exercise, heat, and physical therapy. The basic reliance on large doses of salicylates, nonsteroidal antiinflammatory drugs, and analgesics should be modified during pregnancy. Low-dose steroids (e.g., prednisone, 5 mg/day) and lower doses of aspirin are recommended. Gold compounds cross the placenta, but no fetal adverse effects or teratogenicity have been reported; it appears that gold therapy can be continued in selected pregnant patients whose rheumatoid arthritis is of such severity as to warrant it. Other nonsteroidal antiinflammatory agents, penicillamine, and antimalarials are not recommended because of potential detrimental effects on the fetus.

Because rheumatoid arthritis appears to have little adverse effect on pregnancy outcome, fetal surveillance is necessary only for specific obstetric indications. Special problems with delivery usually can be anticipated. Mechanical problems are rare but may occur if there is significant hip involvement. For the actual delivery, special stirrups or no stirrups may be necessary. The need for cesarean section and the type of anesthesia, whether general or regional, are determined by the obstetric indications or special problems such as atlantoaxial subluxation.

Other Rheumatic (Collagen Vascular) Diseases

Most disorders of undetermined cause characterized by inflammation of various tissues have been termed systemic rheumatic or collagen vascular diseases. More recently, many have been classified as autoimmune disorders because of their association with the production of autoantibodies and other immunologic aberrations. This group includes mixed connective tissue disorder, Sjögren syndrome, polyarteritis nodosa, dermatomyositis, and scleroderma. The risk of both maternal and perinatal death is particularly high in patients with polyarteritis nodosa. For scleroderma, the maternal and fetal risks are of concern in that nearly 10% of women had their disease worsen during pregnancy, and nearly 5% have serious complications. Scleroderma with renal or pulmonary involvement may represent a particularly high-risk state.

◊ AUTOIMMUNE THYROID DISEASE

Although disorders of thyroid function are covered more completely in Chapter 23, it should be mentioned here that autoimmune thyroid diseases in pregnancy are of biological importance to the mother and fetus. The clinical spectrum is broad, and the key issue is the level of thyroid hormone secretion. Affected women may have hyperthyroidism or hypothyroidism, or they may be euthyroid, with or without ophthalmopathy or goiter. The major forms of autoimmune thyroid disease are Graves' disease and chronic autoimmune (Hashimoto) thyroiditis. Both have familial associations, and many patients have demonstrable antibodies to various thyroid antigens. Graves' disease is characterized by thyroid hypersecretion and cellular hyperplasia caused by thyroid-stimulating autoantibodies that bind to and activate the thyroid-stimulating hormone (TSH) receptors on thyroid follicular cells. Hypothyroidism in chronic autoimmune thyroiditis is caused by immune destruction of the thyroid gland and by autoantibodies that block the binding of TSH to its receptors without activating the receptors.

The transplacental transport of thyroid-stimulating antibodies can have a significant impact on the fetus. Mothers with Graves' disease may give birth to children with neonatal hyperthyroidism. The likelihood of thyrotoxicosis in the infant usually can be predicted by antepartum observation of the fetal heart rate for tachycardia and monitoring maternal thyroid-stimulating antibody activity during pregnancy. Marked differences in thyroid function are seen between mother and child. This may relate to different populations of autoantibodies (i.e., thyroid-stimulating antibodies vs. thyrotropin-binding inhibitory immunoglobulins) and facilitated transfer across the placenta. Serum T_4 and TSH levels from cord blood immediately after delivery and on day 2 of life are used to follow infants for evidence of thyrotoxicosis. The neonate with this condition is jittery and underweight with tachycardia, tachypnea, goiter, and diarrhea. The duration of the neonatal disease is almost always less than 3 months, and most affected infants recover without incident.

◊ MYASTHENIA GRAVIS

Myasthenia gravis is a chronic neuromuscular autoimmune disease characterized by fatigue and weakness, typically of the extraocular, facial, pharyngeal, and respiratory muscles.

It is worsened by exertion and relieved by rest and anticholinesterase drugs. Antibodies to human acetylcholine receptors (AChR) are detectable in up to 90% of patients with myasthenia. The anti-AChR antibodies are involved in complement-dependent destruction of the postsynaptic membrane of the myoneural junction, resulting in decreased nerve impulse transmission. The disorder often is accompanied by a thymoma, thymic hyperplasia, or other autoimmune diseases. The functional abnormalities associated with the disease are similar to those induced by curare. The course during pregnancy is variable, although there is a tendency for relapse during the puerperium.

The cholinesterase inhibitors and their equivalent doses most commonly used to alleviate symptoms are 0.5 mg of intravenous neostigmine, 1.5 mg of subcutaneous neostigmine, 15 mg of oral neostigmine, 60 mg of oral pyridostigmine, and 5 mg of oral ambenonium. Drugs are adjusted to the dose at which the patient's muscle strength is optimal with a minimum of cholinergic adverse effects. Oral pyridostigmine or a sustained-release preparation of pyridostigmine are the most commonly used medications. Excessive cholinergic medication results in unpleasant effects such as abdominal cramps, flatulence, diarrhea, nausea, vomiting, and excessive secretion of saliva and tears. Advanced effects include muscle weakness and respiratory failure, which can mimic myasthenic crises and may be fatal. Treatment with high-dose corticosteroids has also been used successfully in some patients. Regular rest periods with limited physical activity should be prescribed for the pregnant patient with myasthenia gravis, and aggressive treatment of any infections is indicated because infections appear to exacerbate the disorder. Some antibiotics, such as the aminoglycosides, may produce a myasthenic crisis and should be avoided.

Careful plans should be made for drug therapy during pregnancy, labor, delivery, and the postpartum period. Labor typically progresses normally or even more rapidly than usual because smooth muscle is unaffected. Vaginal delivery is the rule; cesarean section is reserved for obstetric reasons. Assisted ventilation should be available in the event of respiratory difficulty. During labor, the patient's oral dose of anticholinesterase should be discontinued and replaced with an intramuscular equivalent. Many patients with myasthenia are sensitive to sedatives, analgesics, tranquilizers, and especially narcotics. Muscle relaxants should be avoided, if possible; local or regional anesthetics are preferable. Magnesium sulfate is contraindicated because the drug diminishes the acetylcholine effect and has been known to induce a myasthenic crisis.

About 12% to 20% of infants born to women with myasthenia exhibit neonatal myasthenia, which lasts from a few hours to several days. The manifestations are caused by the transplacental transfer of acetylcholine-blocking factor. Interestingly, neonatal myasthenia may not occur in all infants born to the same patient with myasthenia. The classic features of neonatal myasthenia gravis differ from those seen in the adult form. The symptoms usually do not develop until day 1 or 2 of life, probably because of some protection to the infant from the maternal blood levels of anticholinesterase agents. It is clinically important to recognize this phenomenon because an infant who appears healthy at birth may later develop respiratory failure with asphyxia. The involved infant shows generalized muscle weakness and hypotonic limbs and is limp and motionless. The Moro reflex often is weak or absent, and there may be a feeble cry, inability to suck, and associated difficulty in swallowing and breathing. Arthrogryposis (i.e., joint contractures), which may develop as a result of reduced intrauterine movement, has been reported in several infants of mothers with myasthenia.

◊ TRANSPLANTATION

Organ transplantation has evolved from a fledgling clinical experiment into an effective treatment that restores many patients to near-normal lifestyles. The number of young women with organ allografts is dramatically increasing, and many now become pregnant (Fig. 17). Most pregnancies have resulted in live births, but concerns include potential adverse effects of immunosuppressive drugs and other medications on the fetus, an increased chance for pregnancy complications, and the heightened psychological stress of being a transplant recipient and an expectant mother. Although the prognosis for a successful pregnancy generally is good, it is apparent that these are high-risk pregnancies that require expert obstetric care.

Kidney Transplantation

The experience with pregnancy is greatest in patients who have received living-donor or cadaver kidney transplants. About one in 50 women of childbearing age with a functioning renal allograft becomes pregnant, and more than 3000 pregnancies have now occurred. Some women have successfully delivered twins and triplets, and many others have undergone more than one pregnancy. One patient has had five live births and one spontaneous abortion with no deleterious effect on the kidney evident 16 years after transplantation (see Fig. 1).

Although the transplanted kidney usually functions satisfactorily during gestation, few patients have the increased glomerular filtration rate (GFR) seen in normal pregnant women. Rather, GFR characteristically decreases during the third trimester, although this deficit has been reversible after delivery except in a few cases. Deterioration of renal function, rejection, and even maternal death have occurred during gestation. Urinary tract infections are particularly common, and the incidence of pyelonephritis increases as much as twofold. Other reported infections attributed to immunosuppression include endometritis, wound infection after cesarean section, skin abscess, HIV and cytomegalovirus infections, sepsis, and pneumonia with unusual organisms such as *Aspergillis, Pneumocystis, Mycobacterium tuberculosis,* and *Listeria.* Hypertension and preeclampsia (30%) are also

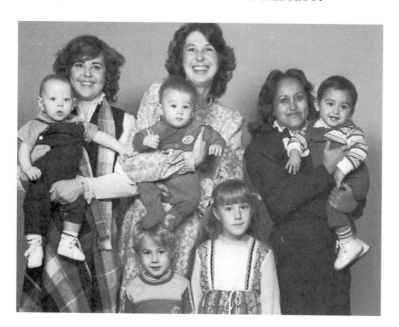

FIG. 17. Three women who have had successful pregnancies after kidney transplantation are pictured with their children. The patient in the middle now has four children. (From Scott JR, Rote NS, eds. *Immunology in obstetrics and gynecology.* Norwalk, CT: Appleton-Century-Crofts, 1985:203.)

prominent complications in these pregnancies and contribute to the increase in preterm births (45%), fetal growth retardation (20%), and, occasionally, fetal death.

Other Organ Transplantation

Although fewer patients with other organ allografts have had pregnancies, maternal complications and perinatal outcome appear to parallel those of kidney transplant recipients. Since the early 1980s, women of childbearing age with malignant and nonmalignant hematologic disorders have been treated with bone marrow transplantation. Ovarian failure from pretransplant cyclophosphamide and irradiation reduces fertility in some patients, but at least 11 normal children have been born to women after bone marrow transplantation. Preeclampsia occurred in one woman, but the others had relatively uncomplicated pregnancies and deliveries. Twentynine pregnancies have been reported in liver transplant recipients. Maternal complications have included elevated liver function tests, rejection, recurrent hepatitis, decreased renal function, urinary tract infection, adrenal insufficiency, and endometritis. The rates of fetal growth retardation, preeclampsia, preterm births, and neonatal infections were also increased. Five cases of pregnancy after combined pancreas and kidney transplantation have been reported in addition to one successful pregnancy at the University of Utah. The patients remained normoglycemic, but preeclampsia and fetal growth retardation resulted in preterm birth in two cases. Thirty pregnancies are known to have occurred in heart ($n = 27$) and heart and lung ($n = 3$) allograft recipients. Cardiac function remained normal in all patients; five episodes of rejection requiring treatment and three late maternal deaths occurred. Frequent pregnancy complications included hypertension (48%), preeclampsia (24%), and preterm labor (28%). Of the 27 births, there were two sets of twins, 10 premature births, five infants who were small for gestational age, and four infants with neonatal complications.

Immunosuppressive Drugs

The most commonly used maintenance regimens for immunosuppression in transplant patients consist of combinations of daily prednisone, azathioprine, and cyclosporine. Prednisone is an antiinflammatory glucocorticoid that decreases both humoral and cell-mediated immune responses. Potential adverse steroidal effects on the mother include glucose intolerance, peptic ulcer, osteoporosis, fluid retention, infections, impaired wound healing, and mood changes. Azathioprine is a purine analog whose principal action is to decrease delayed hypersensitivity and cellular cytotoxicity while leaving antibody-mediated responses relatively intact. The primary maternal hazards of azathioprine administration are an increased risk of infection and neoplasia. Sometimes bone marrow depression and liver toxicity occur but usually resolve with a decrease in dose. Cyclosporine, a relatively new immunosuppressive agent, is used in transplant patients. It is a fungal metabolite whose major inhibitory effect is on specific T-lymphocyte subsets, particularly the cells that mediate allograft rejection. Although infection and bone marrow depression are less frequent, hepatotoxicity and nephrotoxicity are problems. Other adverse effects include hirsutism, tremor, gingival hyperplasia, and the development of lymphomas.

All these immunosuppressive drugs cross the placenta to some degree. The reason for the increased incidence of fetal growth retardation is unclear but has been attributed to both the drugs and the underlying maternal disease. Despite studies in animals that show anomalies in offspring secondary to ingestion of glucocorticoids, azathioprine, and cyclosporine, no statistical increase in the rate of congenital anomalies has been noted in humans.

Prepregnancy Evaluation

Preconception counseling is desirable for all transplant patients. A woman who is contemplating pregnancy after transplantation should be in good health and show no evidence of graft rejection. Medical problems such as diabetes mellitus, recurrent infections, and serious effects from the immunosuppressive drugs make pregnancy inadvisable. The ideal timing of pregnancy appears to be between 2 and 5 years after transplantation, when allograft function has stabilized and immunosuppressive medication has been reduced to moderate doses. The rate of spontaneous abortion is not increased above that in the general population, but both the physician and the patient should be aware that bacterial, viral, and fungal infections secondary to immunosuppression are common in pregnancy. Rejection or permanent impairment of organ function can occur, but it is probably unrelated to pregnancy because the incidence is similar to that in the transplant population at large. Finally, an assessment of the patient's psychological status and family support as well as a tactful but honest discussion of the potential pregnancy problems are important. Because long-term organ allograft survival rates are not 100%, not all transplant recipients will live to raise their children to adulthood. All female recipients should be offered effective contraception and permanent sterilization when they have completed their families.

Prenatal Care

Early diagnosis of pregnancy is important so that meticulous antepartum care can be given. An early ultrasound examination is invaluable in establishing an accurate date of delivery. Possible fetal growth retardation should be monitored by serial ultrasound examinations. Antepartum management requires serial assessment of organ allograft function, diagnosis and treatment of rejection, blood pressure control, treatment of infection, and careful evaluation of fetal well-being.

The incidence of intraepithelial and invasive cancer of the genital tract in patients taking immunosuppressive drugs is increased, and regular Papanicolaou tests and surveillance for cancer are vital components of clinical care. Some patients have become Rh-sensitized from the allograft, and others have acquired herpes genitalis, human papillovirus, HIV, or hepatitis. Because of the high incidence of hypertension in transplant patients, prophylactic low-dose aspirin seems reasonable to attempt to decrease the incidence of preeclampsia. Pregnancy may alter the pharmacokinetics of cyclosporine metabolism, and adjustment or conversion to divided doses is necessary in some patients. Most of the commonly used antihypertensive agents can be continued during pregnancy with little risk to the fetus. Angiotensin-converting enzyme inhibitors should be discontinued, however, because of potential adverse effects on the fetus, such as oligohydramnios, pulmonary hypoplasia, and long-lasting neonatal anuria.

In general, the management of obstetric complications does not differ from that in nontransplant patients. The risk of infection, however, warrants a more aggressive approach to prolonged ruptured membranes and avoidance of invasive procedures when possible. The isolated onset or worsening of proteinuria has been observed in some kidney transplant patients near term, but this usually resolves postpartum and, in the absence of other signs of preeclampsia, requires no specific management.

Labor and Delivery

The timing of delivery frequently is dictated by an untoward event, such as premature labor, premature ruptured membranes, or severe preeclampsia. The renal allograft is placed extraperitoneally in the iliac fossa and usually does not interfere with vaginal delivery. Rare cases of obstructed labor from soft tissue dystocia caused by the graft or pelvic osteodystrophy have been reported. If the fetal head is not engaged in the pelvis during labor, dystocia can be assessed by ultrasound and computed tomographic scan pelvimetry. There are no particular contraindications to induction, labor, or vaginal delivery in other organ graft recipients. Because of the concern with their increased susceptibility to infection, vaginal examination should be kept to a minimum and artificial rupture of membranes and internal monitoring performed only when specifically indicated. Cultures and antibiotics are warranted with the earliest sign of infection.

The decision to deliver by cesarean section is based on accepted obstetric indications. Operative deliveries in these patients usually are managed with prophylactic antibiotics and additional glucocorticoids and require strict asepsis, careful attention to hemostasis, and good surgical technique. A lower midline vertical incision provides the greatest exposure and avoids the region of the transplanted kidney. A low transverse uterine incision usually is possible, but the surgeon should be aware of the anatomic alterations associated with the transplanted kidney so that no damage is inadvertently done to the blood supply or urinary drainage.

Neonatal Problems

Despite the high-risk status of pregnancy in the transplant population, most of their offspring have had an uncomplicated neonatal course. Of those neonates who have experienced complications, the following problems have been noted: respiratory distress syndrome, increased susceptibility to infection, congenital infection (especially cytomegalovirus, hepatitis, and HIV), hypoglycemia, hypocalcemia, adrenal insufficiency, thymic atrophy, bone marrow hypoplasia, transient leukopenia, transient chromosomal abnormalities, reduced levels of IgM and IgG, and transiently elevated serum creatinine levels. We have advised mothers against breast-feeding, because immunosuppressive drugs have been detected in breast milk. Because the incidence of infections and neoplasms is increased in association with primary immunologic deficiencies and the administration of immunosuppressive drugs, it is important that a child exposed to these agents *in utero* have a careful evaluation of the immune system and long-term follow-up. From all reports to date, the children progress normally through infancy and childhood.

Maternal Neoplasms and the Fetus

Immunologic competence is greatest during young adulthood, when neoplasms are uncommon; as immunologic competence decreases with age, the incidence of cancer increases. The incidence of cancer in the 25- to 35-year age group is about 0.06%, and this is not altered by pregnancy. Gestation does not change the 5-year survival rates of women with leukemia, Hodgkin disease, and various solid tumors, even when the cancer is one that typically is affected by the endocrine milieu, such as carcinoma of the breast.

Relatively little attention has been focused on the possibility of fetoplacental metastasis in pregnant women with common types of cancers because it has never become a clinical problem. For example, carcinoma of the cervix occurs once in every 2000 to 6000 pregnancies, but no cases of placental or fetal invasion by this tumor have been verified. Although leukemia and Hodgkin disease are not uncommon in women of reproductive age, and as many as one in every 35 patients with carcinoma of the breast is pregnant, transmission of these cancers to the fetus is also exceedingly rare. This is particularly surprising in the case of hematologic cancers, in which relatively large numbers of malignant stem cells are in the maternal bloodstream. There is a possibility that diseases such as leukemia are oncogenic viral diseases and that the virus occasionally is transmitted early in fetal life.

Although the spread of cancer to the placenta is unusual, it can occur, as shown by cases listed in Table 9, in which the placenta and fetus were studied in detail. It is apparent that the representation of melanoma is out of proportion to its incidence, but the reason for this phenomenon is unknown. Careful histologic observation in pregnant women with can-

cer has shown that tumor cells may be present in the intervillous spaces, but only seldom is there invasion of the villi. Moreover, in the extremely unusual instances of congenital neoplasia, such as neuroblastoma, melanoma, and leukemia, the tumor does not spread from the fetus to the mother. The placental villus thus appears to be an effective barrier to the spread of tumor cells from the maternal to the fetal circulation as well as in the opposite direction. Once malignant tumor cells enter the fetal bloodstream, they can be disseminated throughout the entire fetus and usually are sequestered in the liver.

Because fetal and maternal tissues are genetically dissimilar, maternal–fetal metastasis can logically be considered an allograft or the transplantation of foreign cells. The rare cases of fetal dissemination of maternal malignant disease may be isolated examples of acquired tolerance in which fetuses were exposed to maternal antigen before the development of immunologic competency and, as a result, did not recognize the maternal tumor cells as foreign. Conversely, those cases in which maternal malignant melanoma has widely metastasized to the fetus and then regressed spontaneously after birth are probably examples of true allograft rejection. This phenomenon could also explain what may be underdiagnosed cases of placental transmission of other maternal malignant diseases, particularly during the latter half of pregnancy, after the establishment of fetal immunocompetence.

◊ RECOMMENDED READINGS

Reproductive Immunology

Dudley D, Daynes R. The immune system in health and disease. *Baillieres Clin Obstet Gynaecol* 1992;6(3):393.

Kovats S, Main EK, Librach C, et al. A class I antigen, HLA-G, expressed in human trophoblast. *Science* 1990;248:220.

Mori T, Takakura K, Narimoto K, et al. Endocrine and immune implications of human endometrial decidualization in implantation. *Ann NY Acad Sci* 1992;626:321.

Silver RM, Branch DW. The immunology of pregnancy. In: Creasy R, Resnik R, eds. *Maternal fetal medicine, 3rd ed.* Philadelphia: WB Saunders, 1998:115.

Erythrocyte Alloimmunization

American College of Obstetricians and Gynecologists. *Prevention of D isoimmunization. Technical bulletin no. 147.* October 1990.

American College of Obstetricians and Gynecologists. *Management of isoimmunization in pregnancy. Technical bulletin no. 227.* August 1996.

Bennet PR, Van Kim CL, Colin Y, et al. Prenatal determination of fetal RhD type by DNA amplification. *N Engl J Med* 1993;329:607.

Harman CR, Bowman JM, Manning FA, Menticoglou SM. Intrauterine transfusion—intraperitoneal versus intravascular approach: a case control comparison. *Am J Obstet Gynecol* 1990;162:1053.

Jackson GM, Branch DW. Isoimmunization in pregnancy. In: Gabbe S, Niebyl J, Simpson JL, eds. *Obstetrics: Normal and problem pregnancies, 3rd ed.* New York: Churchill Livingstone, 1997.

Nicolini U, Kochenour NK, Greco P, et al. Consequences of fetomaternal hemorrhage after intrauterine transfusion. *Br Med J* 1988;297:1379.

Olofsson P, Stangenberg M, Seibing A, et al. Fetal heart rate responses to anemia in Rh isoimmunization. *J Perinat Med* 1990;18:187.

Poissonier MH, Brossard Y, Demedairos N, et al. Two hundred intrauterine exchange transfusions in severe blood incompatibilities. *Am J Obstet Gynecol* 1989;159:1497.

TABLE 9. *Reported cases of metastasis of neoplastic disease to placenta or fetus*

Malignancy	Total number of patients	Placental metastasis	Fetal metastasis
Malignant melanoma	16	10	6
Hepatic carcinoma	2	1	1
Sarcoma	2	1	1
Leukemia	7	5	2
Hodgkin disease	1	0	1
Bronchial carcinoma	4	4	0
Breast carcinoma	6	6	0
Gastric carcinoma	2	2	0
Pancreatic carcinoma	1	1	0
Ethmoid carcinoma	1	1	0
Adrenal carcinoma	1	1	0
Ovarian carcinoma	1	1	0
Total	42	33	11

Polesky HF. Detection of fetomaternal hemorrhage: how, when, and why. *Transfusion* 1991;31:288.

Spinnato JA. Hemolytic disease of the fetus: a plea for restraint. *Obstet Gynecol* 1992;80:873.

Weiner CP, Williamson RA, Wenstrom KD, et al. Management of fetal hemolytic disease by cordocentesis. II. Outcome of treatment. *Am J Obstet Gynecol* 1991;165:1302.

Immunologic Thrombocytopenia

Burrows RF, Kelton JG. Low fetal risks in pregnancies associated with idiopathic thrombocytopenia purpura. *Am J Obstet Gynecol* 1990;163: 1147–1150.

Burrows RF, Kelton JG. Pregnancy in patients with idiopathic thrombocytopenic purpura: Assessing the risks for the infant at delivery. *Obstet Gynecol Surv* 1993;48:781–788.

Bussel JB, Berkowitz RL, Lynch L, et al. Antenatal management of alloimmune thrombocytopenia with intravenous gamma globulin: A randomized trial of the addition of low dose steroid to intravenous gamma globulin. *Am J Obstet Gynecol* 1996;174:1414–1423.

Bussel JB, Zabusky MR, Berkowitz RL, McFarland JG. Fetal alloimmune thrombocytopenia. *N Engl J Med* 1997;337:22–26.

Nicolini U, Tanniranadorn Y, Gonzales P, et al. Continuing controversy in alloimmune thrombocytopenia: fetal hyperimmunoglobulinemia fails to prevent thrombocytopenia. *Am J Obstet Gynecol* 1990;163:1144.

Silver RM, Branch DW, Scott JR. Maternal thrombocytopenia in pregnancy: Time for a reassessment. *Am J Obstet Gynecol* 1995;173:479.

The American Society of Hematology ITP Practice Guideline Panel. Diagnosis and treatment of idiopathic thrombocytopenic purpura: recommendations of the American Society of Hematology. *Ann Intern Med* 1997; 126:319–326.

Systemic Lupus Erythematosus

Condemi JJ. The autoimmune diseases. *JAMA* 1992;268:2882.

Gimovsky ML, Montoro M. Systemic lupus erythematosus and other connective tissue diseases in pregnancy. *Clin Obstet Gynecol* 1991; 34:35.

Lockshin MD. Pregnancy associated with systemic lupus erythematosus. *Semin Perinatol* 1990;14:130.

Olah KS, Gee H. Fetal heart block associated with maternal anti-Ro (SS-A) antibody—current management. A review. *Br J Obstet Gynaecol* 1991; 98:751.

Risto K, Julkunen H, Ammala P, et al. Congenital heart block: successful prophylactic treatment with intravenous gamma globulin and corticosteroid therapy. *Am J Obstet Gynecol* 1991;165:1333.

Silver RM, Branch DW. Autoimmune disease in pregnancy. Systemic lupus erythematosus and antiphospholipid syndrome. *Clin Perinatol* 1997; 24:291.

Antiphospholipid Syndrome

Branch DW, Andres R, Digre KB, Scott JR. The association of antiphospholipid antibodies with severe preeclampsia. *Obstet Gynecol* 1989;73:541.

Branch DW, Silver RM, Blackwell JL, et al. Outcome of treated pregnancies in women with antiphospholipid syndrome: an update of the Utah experience. *Obstet Gynecol* 1992;80:614.

Branch DW, Silver RM, Pierangeli SS, van Leeuwen I, Harris EN. Antiphospholipid antibodies in women with recurrent pregnancy loss, fertile controls, and antiphospholipid syndrome. *Obstet Gynecol* 1997;89:549–555.

Harris EN, Exner T, Hughes RV, Asherson RA, eds. *Phospholipid-binding antibodies.* Boca Raton: CRC Press, 1991.

Kochenour NK, Branch DW, Rote NS, Scott JR. A new postpartum syndrome associated with antiphospholipid antibodies. *Obstet Gynecol* 1987; 69:460.

Kutteh WH. Antiphospholipid antibody-associated recurrent pregnancy loss: Treatment with heparin and low-dose aspirin is superior to low-dose aspirin alone. *Am J Obstet Gynecol* 1996;174:1584.

Pollard JK, Scott JR, Branch DW. Growth and development of children from women treated during pregnancy for the antiphospholipid syndrome. *Obstet Gynecol* 1992;80:365.

Rai R, Cohen H, Dave M, Regan L. Randomised controlled trial of aspirin and aspirin plus heparin in pregnant women with recurrent miscarriage associated with phospholipid antibodies (or antiphospholipid antibodies). *Br Med J* 1997;314:253.

Rai RS, Regan L, Clifford K, et al. Antiphospholipid antibodies and B2-glycoprotein-I in 500 women with recurrent miscarriage: results of a comprehensive screening approach. *Hum Reprod* 1995;10:2001–2005.

Rand JH, Wu X-X, Andree HAM, et al. Pregnancy loss in the antiphospholipid syndrome: a possible thrombogenic mechanism. *N Engl J Med* 1997; 337:154–160.

Rheumatoid Arthritis

Klipple GL, Cecere FA. Rheumatoid arthritis and pregnancy. *Rheum Dis Clin North Am* 1989;15:213.

Other Rheumatic (Collagen Vascular) Diseases

Goplerud CP. Scleroderma. *Clin Obstet Gynecol* 1983;26:587.

Olah K, Redman CWG. Overlap syndrome and its implications in pregnancy. *Br J Obstet Gynaecol* 1991;98:728.

Autoimmune Thyroid Disease

Davidson KM, Richards DS, Schatz DA, Fisher DA. Successful *in utero* treatment of fetal goiter and hypothyroidism. *N Engl J Med* 1991;324: 543.

Lowe TW, Cunningham FG. Pregnancy and thyroid disease. *Clin Obstet Gynecol* 1991;34:72.

Peterson CM. Autoimmune thyroid disease in pregnancy. In: Coulam CB, Faulk WP, McIntyre JA, eds. *Immunological obstetrics.* New York: WW Norton, 1992:645.

Myasthenia Gravis

Mitchell PJ, Bebbington M. Myasthenia gravis in pregnancy. *Obstet Gynecol* 1992;80:178.

Plauche WC. Myasthenia gravis in mothers and their newborns. *Clin Obstet Gynecol* 1991;34:82.

Varner MW, Digre KB. Myasthenia gravis. In: Coulam CB, Faulk WP, McIntyre JA, eds. *Immunological obstetrics.* New York: WW Norton, 1992:666.

Transplantation

Bumgardner GL, Matas AJ. Transplantation and pregnancy. *Transplant Rev* 1992;6:139.

Hill NCW, Morris NH, Shaw RW, et al. Pregnancy after orthotopic liver transplantation. *Br J Obstet Gynaecol* 1991;98:719.

Norton P, Scott JR. Gynecologic and obstetric problems in renal allograft recipients. In: Buchsbaum HJ, Schmidt J, eds. *Gynecologic and obstetric urology, 3rd ed.* Philadelphia: WB Saunders, 1993:657.

Scott JR, Wagoner LE, Olsen SL, et al. Pregnancy in heart transplant recipients: management and outcomes. *Obstet Gynecol* 1993;82:324.

Sims CJ. Organ transplantation and immunosuppressive drugs in pregnancy. *Clin Obstet Gynecol* 1991;34:100.

Maternal Neoplasms and the Fetus

Anderson JF, Kent S, Machin GA. Maternal malignant melanoma with placental metastasis: a case report with literature review. *Pediatr Pathol* 1989;9:35.

CHAPTER 25

Human Immunodeficiency Virus and Other Perinatal Infections

— ◊ —

Howard L. Minkoff

◊ HUMAN IMMUNODEFICIENCY VIRUS

In the 17 years since acquired immunodeficiency syndrome (AIDS) was first reported, the public perception of human immunodeficiency virus (HIV) disease has evolved from that of a mysterious, untreatable, invariably lethal illness affecting gay men to a disease increasingly infecting women—and increasingly responsive to an array of new therapies. As these treatments become available, particularly those capable of reducing mother-to-child transmission of HIV, it becomes ever more important for obstetricians to stay abreast of rapid developments in the field.

Microbiology

HIV is one of five known human retroviruses: single-stranded RNA-enveloped viruses that have the ability to become incorporated into cellular DNA. HIV-1, which used to be called human T-cell lymphotrophic virus III (HTLV-III), has a diameter of about 100 nm. Other retroviruses, all of which are significantly less common than HTLV-III, are HTLV-I, which causes adult T-cell leukemia/lymphoma and tropical spastic paraparesis; HTLV-II, which causes hairy cell leukemia; HTLV-IV (also called HIV-2), which causes AIDS; and HTLV-V, which causes cutaneous T-cell lymphoma/leukemia. As a retrovirus (RNA virus), HIV can be reverse-transcribed into DNA and incorporated into the host genome. It is composed of core proteins (p18, p24, and p27), surface proteins (gp120 and gp41), genomic RNA, and the reverse transcriptase enzyme, surrounded by a lipid bilayer envelope. Recently, gp120 has been studied as a potential predictor of infectivity and an important focus for vaccine research. The virion contains three structural genes (*gag, pol,* and *env*) and a complex set of regulatory genes, including *tat, vif, nef, vpu,* and *ref,* that control the rate of virion production. It preferentially infects cells with the CD4+ antigen, particularly helper lymphocytes, but also macrophages, cells of the central nervous system (CNS), and, according to some evidence, cells of the placenta.[1] Recent research has shown that at least two other cell surface molecules help HIV enter cells. These coreceptors for HIV, called CXCR4 and CCR5, are receptors for chemokines.[2] Recently, it has also been been discovered that individuals who are homozygous for a deletion at the CCR5 gene are less likely to acquire HIV, while deletion heterozygotes progress less rapidly, if infected.[3]

Epidemiology

By the end of 1995, 71,818 cases of AIDS occurring among adolescent and adult women had been reported to the Centers for Disease Control and Prevention (CDC); 13,764 of these cases were reported in 1995.[4] It is estimated that 107,000 to 150,000 women in the United States are currently infected with HIV. Although the annual HIV incidence among women and minorities is remaining relatively constant,[5] trends vary across the country. In New York state, for example, there is some evidence that the number of pregnancies in infected women is declining, while in some parts of the South numbers continue to rise. The women at greatest risk in the United States are women of color, women in relationships with users of injectable drugs, and women of younger ages. Women accounted for 19% of AIDS cases reported in 1995,[4] an increase from 6.5% (534 of 8153) of AIDS cases reported in 1984.

The rate of increase in AIDS cases among women between 1990 and 1994 (89%) was more than three times the increase reported among men (29%), and the male-to-female ratio of AIDS incidence decreased from 7.5 to 1 in 1990 to 5.1 to 1 in 1994.[5] By 1995, HIV infection had become the third leading cause of death in the United States among all women aged 25 to 44 years and the leading cause of death among African-American women of this age group and among all reproductive-age women in some urban centers.[6]

The "face" of the HIV epidemic is evolving. Between 1990 and 1994, AIDS incidence among African-American women doubled, with 1994 rates twofold higher than those of Hispanic/Latina women and 17 times those among white women.[7] By 1995, the racial/ethnic distribution of reported AIDS cases was 22.6% among white women, 55.8% among black women, and 20.7% among Hispanic women. AIDS incidence rates per 100,000 women in 1995 were 3.8 among white women, 59.2 among black women, and 61.9 among Hispanic women.[4] The majority of new cases of AIDS in women are reported among those 20 to 29 years of age, indicating that their HIV infection was probably acquired in late adolescence or earlier.

Increasingly, women are acquiring HIV heterosexually, with cases attributable to heterosexual contact growing in 1994 by 146%, compared to a 59% AIDS incidence growth among women who themselves use injectable drugs.[5] The risk-group assignation of women diagnosed with AIDS in 1995, which would reflect HIV acquisition in the mid-1980s and beyond, was 36% users of injectable drugs and 47% heterosexual contact with either a drug user or a bisexual man. Fifteen percent of women either did not report or could not identify their exposure category.

United States 1991 data on HIV seroprevalence among pregnant women, based on anonymous infant heel stick data, revealed an HIV seroprevalence rate of 1.5 per 1000 childbearing women. The highest rates were seen among women delivering in the Northeast, and the lowest rates were noted in the Midwest.[8,9] Based on combined metropolitan national data surveys from 1992 and back-calculation data, HIV seroprevalence rates among all women in the United States were estimated to 1.1 to 1.4 per 1000 women.[8]

The vast majority of cases of pediatric AIDS are secondary to vertical transmission of HIV from mother to fetus (Fig. 1).

HIV infection is now among the 10 leading causes of death among children aged 1 to 4 years. As of 1990, estimates of the number of children with HIV infection in the United States ranged from 5000 to 10,000. The World Health Organization estimates 30% excess infant and child mortality in major United States, Western European, and sub-Saharan African cities, where AIDS has become the leading cause of death for women aged 20 to 40 years.

Pathophysiology

HIV infection leads to progressive debilitation of the immune system, rendering individuals susceptible to opportunistic infections (e.g., *Pneumocystis carinii* pneumonia [PCP] and CNS toxoplasmosis) and neoplasia (e.g., Kaposi's sarcoma) that rarely afflict patients with intact immune systems. An HIV-infected patient with one of several specific opportunistic infections, neoplasia, dementia encephalopathy, or wasting syndrome is diagnosed as having AIDS. The diagnosis of AIDS can also be made in the absence of laboratory evidence of infection if a patient has no other known cause of immune deficiency and has the definitive diagnosis of one of a number of indicator diseases.[3] In 1993, the CDC changed the case definition to include all individuals with HIV infection whose CD4+ cell count drops below 200/mm^3, as well as HIV-infected individuals with advanced cervical cancer, pulmonary tuberculosis, or recurrent pneumonia.[10] At the time of initial infection, an individual may be asymptomatic or may experience an acute mononucleosis-like syndrome that can be accompanied by aseptic meningitis. Recent studies have shown an immediate viremia of substantive proportions (up to 10 billion viral particles turned over per day) and an equally impressive immune responsive with similar levels of T-cell turnover.[11] Antibodies can be detected in almost all individ-

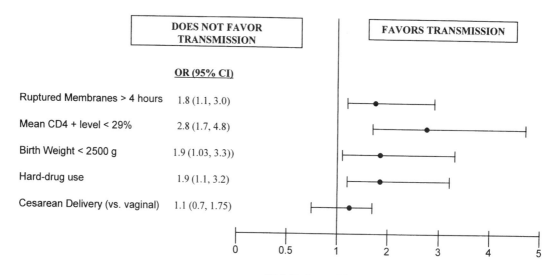

	DOES NOT FAVOR TRANSMISSION	FAVORS TRANSMISSION
	OR (95% CI)	
Ruptured Membranes > 4 hours	1.8 (1.1, 3.0)	
Mean CD4 + level < 29%	2.8 (1.7, 4.8)	
Birth Weight < 2500 g	1.9 (1.03, 3.3))	
Hard-drug use	1.9 (1.1, 3.2)	
Cesarean Delivery (vs. vaginal)	1.1 (0.7, 1.75)	

Risk Ratios and 95% Confidence Intervals

FIG. 1. Obstetric factors associated with vertical transmission of HIV-1 from mother to child. (Adapted from ref. 29.)

uals 6 to 12 weeks after exposure, but in rare circumstances this latent period (the so-called window phase) can be longer. After seroconversion has occurred, an asymptomatic period of variable length usually follows. The median clinical latency is estimated at approximately 11 years.[12] Very few infected persons (fewer than 5%) develop AIDS within 3 years.[13] Evidence of immune dysfunction may be followed by clinical conditions ranging from fever, weight loss, malaise, lymphadenopathy, and CNS dysfunction to infections such as herpes simplex virus or oral candidiasis. These nonspecific conditions are usually progressive and are a prelude to an opportunistic infection that is diagnostic of AIDS. Studies of infected individuals have noted that 5 years after infection was confirmed, up to 35% had progressed to AIDS.[14,15] A study of subjects with hemophilia demonstrated that the incidence rate of AIDS after seroconversion was 2.67 per 100 person-years and was directly related to age (AIDS developed in younger individuals at a slower rate).[16] It should be noted that all these statistics antedate the use of new, more powerful antiretroviral agents that have already been shown to have a significant effect on surrogate markers of disease progression. The level of virus in the plasma can provide an estimate of the probability that AIDS will develop in an individual within 5 years.

Once AIDS is diagnosed, the short-term prognosis is improving (e.g., surviving an initial episode of PCP), although the long-term prognosis remains poor. The effect that the newest antiretrovirals, including protease inhibitors, will have on survival cannot be clearly gauged yet, but there is reason for cautious optimism. Most data on the natural history of HIV disease predate the newer therapies and are based on studies of men. The cumulative probability of survival in men has been estimated at 49% at 1 year after diagnosis and only 15% after 5 years.[17] In one study of 4323 patients, the median reported survival time after diagnosis was 12.5 months, with a 5-year survival rate of 3.4%.[18] The time of initial diagnosis, patient age, and use of zidovudine (ZDV; Retrovir; formerly azidothymidine [AZT]) were significant predictors of survival. Those with PCP survived longer than those with

Kaposi's sarcoma. Viral load and CD4+ counts can be used to predict the likelihood that AIDS will develop in an individual during a given follow-up period. At present, there is no convincing evidence that the natural history of HIV infection is influenced by sex or pregnancy (Fig. 2).[19]

Management

The guiding principle in the care of HIV-infected pregnant women is rigorous adherence to the standards of care that apply to all other HIV-infected individuals. The first step is to monitor the immune status with CD4+ counts and viral load determinations. These should be performed at regular intervals because they predict the course of disease and allow rational decisions to be made regarding therapeutic interventions. If the CD4+ count remains greater than 500/mm^3 and the viral load less than 5000 copies/ml, the obstetrician can anticipate an unremarkable course. ZDV will be required as part of a regimen to prevent transmission of HIV, but additional therapy can be deferred (Fig. 3). If these viral load and CD4+ conditions are not met, multidrug antiretroviral therapy should be instituted. Although protocols for antiretroviral therapy are not uniformly agreed on, several references are available to guide clinicians in the management of HIV-infected pregnant women.[20]

It must be understood that new agents will shortly appear on the market, and more information on risks may also be discerned. Obstetricians must stay abreast of an evolving literature if they are to provide optimal care to their patients. Pending the publication of additional information supporting early intervention with antiretroviral agents, most women with CD4+ counts greater than 500/mm^3 and low viral loads who are *not* pregnant will not receive antiretroviral therapy. Therefore, the current focus of therapy in pregnant women with high CD4+ counts is the prevention of mother-to-child transmission of HIV. This is the circumstance that most closely matches that of the multisite study that demonstrated that ZDV could reduce the rate of mother-to-child transmission of HIV; it is also the situation for which the most empiric information

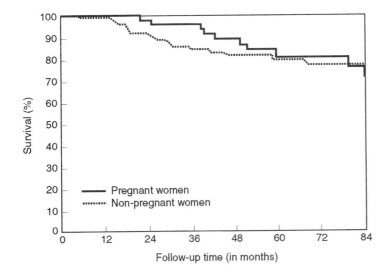

FIG. 2. Probability of survival in pregnant and non-pregnant human immunodeficiency virus–seropositive women. (Adapted from ref. 19.)

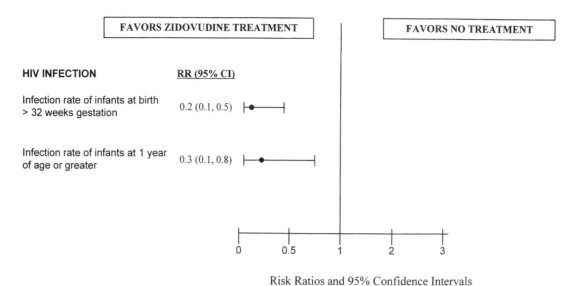

FIG. 3. Reduction of maternal–infant transmission of HIV-1 with antepartum and intrapartum zidovudine. (Adapted from ref. 28.)

exists regarding efficacy for prevention of perinatal transmission. Accordingly, recommendations for the use of ZDV in pregnancy, as promulgated by a public health task force, are most directive for this group. The specific regimen recommended by the task force should be prescribed in the antepartum, intrapartum, and neonatal periods.[21] It should be noted, however, that data showing reduced efficacy of many treatment regimens among patients previously treated with ZDV (compared to ZDV naive) raise concerns, even in this group, regarding the use of monotherapy during the antepartum period.

For pregnant women whose CD4+ count falls below 500/mm³, as for nonpregnant individuals with similar counts, consideration should be given to the use of combination therapy. If monotherapy has limited clinical or virologic effects and hastens the development of resistance, it would be inappropriate to continue such substandard care solely because a woman is pregnant. Whichever regimen is eventually shown to be optimal should be considered for use in pregnancy as well. Only in rare circumstances should considerations related to pregnancy lead clinicians to choose one approach over another. One such consideration could be differences in reported side effects. For example, while ritonavir (Norvir) is associated with gastrointestinal upset, which may be particularly problematic in early gestation, indinavir (Crixivan) is associated with hyperbilirubinemia and nephrolithiasis, potentially more serious pregnancy events. Thus, in pregnancy, ritonavir or nelfinavir (Viracept) might be a more appropriate first choice among protease inhibitors. Although definitive evidence of the safety of the newer antiretroviral agents when used during pregnancy is lacking, no greater reassurance regarding the safety of ZDV was available when clinicians first used it in pregnancy.

If the regimen chosen to treat HIV disease does not include ZDV, it would seem judicious to continue its use anyway, according to the regimen recommended by the public health

panel, if the patient is pregnant. Alternative agents may eventually be shown to have efficacy in preventing mother-to-child transmission, but until that effect is demonstrated, it would be imprudent to use them. The recommendation to use ZDV, as opposed to other antiretroviral agents, for the prevention of mother-to-child transmission of HIV is based on two considerations. First, empiric data strongly support its use for this purpose; no other agent has been similarly studied. Second, pharmacokinetic studies demonstrate that high levels of drug are available in the fetal compartment.[22] Similar information is unavailable for most other agents.

The importance of placental passage of drug is not certain. If viral load thresholds are truly central to transmission risk, then viral dynamics on the maternal side of the placenta might be as important as placental passage of drug. Several recent publications suggest that a correlation exists between maternal viral load and rates of mother-to-child HIV transmission and further hint at the existence of a clinically relevant threshold (Fig. 4).[23,24] Other researchers disagree.[25,26] Differences in study populations and techniques for storing and assaying samples may explain some of the conflicting results. If appropriately designed studies confirm the initial reports of a threshold, it may have bearing on the choice of therapeutic regimen for use by pregnant women. If, for example, viral load remains above the threshold for transmission despite initial therapy, clinicians may consider the addition of other antiretroviral agents that might reduce the load. That possibility, however, remains conjectural. For the present, viral load should be used to monitor and modify therapy directed toward maternal well-being, not to adjust treatments in pursuit of lower mother-to-child HIV transmission rates.

Currently, there are insufficient data to justify the substitution of any agent for ZDV in most circumstances. Even if there is evidence of ZDV resistance, which might make ther-

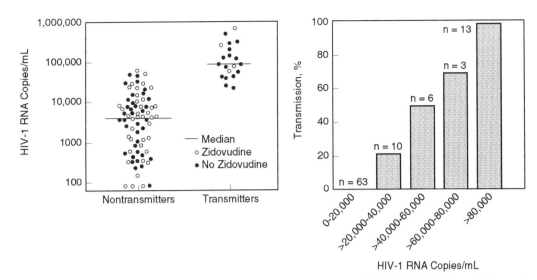

FIG. 4. Left: Maternal plasma human immunodeficiency virus type 1 (HIV-1) RNA levels at delivery in infected nontransmitting and transmitting mothers. Mothers who received zidovudine (ZDV) during gestation and/or labor and delivery are indicated by *open circles;* mothers who did not receive ZDV during gestation, labor, or delivery are indicated by *darkened circles. Horizontal bars* indicate the median for each of the measured variables. **Right:** Perinatal transmission rate according to HIV-1 RNA levels at delivery. (Adapted from ref. 24.)

apy for the prevention of mother-to-child transmission seem futile, ZDV might still have a role. The demonstration of transmission of escape mutants from mother to child[27] suggests that an individual ZDV-susceptible virus might be transmitted, even if the predominant strain or strains in the mother are not susceptible. Further research is needed to see whether or not there is advantage to combination therapy as part of a strategy to prevent transmission of resistant strains. If the mother is intolerant of ZDV, it is reasonable to consider using an alternative agent, which could potentially reduce viral load during the antepartum period, and then adding ZDV for the intrapartum (depending on the type of toxicity experienced by the mother) and neonatal periods.

In summary, pregnant women should be the beneficiaries of any clinical advantage offered by new regimens and should not be restricted to single-drug therapy. However, the continued use of the public health service panel's recommended ZDV regimen as part of any therapeutic strategy should be assured.

In regard to prophylaxis for opportunistic infections, if the CD4+ count drops below 200/mm,[3] PCP prophylaxis should be instituted; if it falls below 50/mm,[3] prophylaxis for *Mycobacterium avium-intracellulare* complex should be given and an ophthalmology consult obtained. The specific details of management of the myriad infections to which these women are prone is beyond the scope of this chapter.

Preventing Perinatal Transmission

In 1994, the results of AIDS Clinical Trial Group (ACTG) protocol 076 were released, demonstrating that a regimen of ZDV given during pregnancy and labor and to the newborn for 6 weeks was able to remarkably reduce the risk of perinatal

HIV-1 transmission. Almost a 70% reduction in transmission risk was observed, from 25% in the placebo group to 8% in the ZDV group.[28] More recently, ACTG protocol 185 demonstrated that similar results could be seen even among women who had previous exposure to AZT or who had CD4+ counts less than 200/mm[3]. The ZDV regimen from ACTG protocol 076 has begun to be successfully integrated into clinical practice in the United States and Europe and has been accompanied by dramatic declines in perinatal transmission rates. The protocol 076 regimen consists of ZDV, 100 mg orally five times a day or 200 mg orally 3 times a day, in the antepartum period (beginning after 14 weeks). In the intrapartum period, intravenous therapy is used, with a loading dose of 2 mg/kg over the first hour followed by a maintenance dose of 1 mg/kg per hour thereafter. In the neonatal period, infants receive a ZDV syrup, 2 mg/kg every 6 hours for 6 weeks. Preliminary data regarding the safety of this regimen have been reassuring. Almost 1000 children have been tracked for 4 years, and they have shown no increase in risks of neurodevelopmental delay or carcinogenesis. Some concern has been raised, however, as a result of mouse data reported from the National Cancer Institute (NCI). That report suggested that mice exposed to high dose rates of ZDV in the third trimester bore pups who were subsequently found to have high rates of liver, lung, skin, and genitourinary tumors in midlife. Although other investigators have not reported similar findings, the NCI data should chasten those who would dismiss all concerns regarding these therapies, and should reinforce the need for thorough counseling and long-term follow-up. In regard to monitoring of mothers on ZDV, only a blood count and measures of liver function are required on a monthly basis. The only abnormality that occurs with any frequency is anemia.

The vast majority of perinatal HIV-1 infection occurs in the developing world. Unfortunately, the ACTG protocol 076 ZDV regimen is too costly and logistically complex for many nonindustrialized countries to implement on a wide scale, and its efficacy in a breast-feeding population (where postpartum transmission remains a real concern) is unknown. An ideal preventive intervention would be cheap, nontoxic to mother and fetus, easy to administer, be given once or for a limited period of time, and have utility in preventing postpartum transmission. The results of ACTG protocol 076 have spurred a worldwide evaluation of many other modalities for reducing transmission.

Potential interventions to reduce transmission have focused on (1) reduction of maternal viral load, (2) enhancement of maternal and infant HIV-1-specific immune response, (3) prophylaxis of the newborn, and (4) attempts to reduce peripartum and postpartum exposure to the virus. Reduction of intrapartum exposure could include attempts to minimize the duration of ruptured membranes, which has been related to the rate of mother-to-child transmission of HIV (Fig. 5).[29] At the moment, only ZDV has been proven to significantly reduce the rate of mother-to-child transmission of HIV. Recently recommendations have been made that HIV infected women be offered cesearean section as a way to further reduce mother-to-child transmission of HIV. The future challenge for researchers is to utilize the increasing understanding of the pathogenesis of perinatal HIV-1 transmission to design preventive regimens that will be applicable on a global basis.

◊ TOXOPLASMOSIS

Primary maternal toxoplasmosis during pregnancy occurs in approximately 1 of every 900 pregnancies in the United States.[30] This estimate is based on a prospective study of sera from 23,000 pregnant women done in early and late gestation.[31] The study, conducted by the National Institutes of Health, showed that 38% of the women tested had antibody to *Toxoplasma gondii*, indicating previous infection with the organism. The presence of antibody correlated with increasing patient age and was twice as frequent among blacks as among whites. None of the mothers tested had evidence of significant clinical disease. It has been estimated that 3000 babies are born each year with congenital *T. gondii* infection.

Microbiology: Transmission

Cats

The definitive host for *T. gondii* is the cat. About one-half of cats tested in the United States have antibodies to *T. gondii*. It is thought that cats become infected by eating infected wild rodents and birds. A week after infection, they begin to shed oocysts in their feces. Shedding of oocysts persists for about 2 weeks before spontaneous recover occurs. These animals are susceptible to reinfection and may also shed *Toxoplasma* oocysts when infected with other organisms.

Cat feces are extremely infectious. The fecal oocysts are spread through the air and, when inhaled, are likely to cause infection. Sporulation of the organism occurs after 1 to 5 days in the litter and may be prevented by changing the litter daily. Care must be taken in disposing of cat liter.

Meat

In Europe, where the use of refrigeration is more limited and meat is usually not frozen, ingestion of infected meat is an important cause of toxoplasmosis. In contrast, in the United States much of the meat is frozen at some point during storage or transport. Freezing is probably one of the factors responsible for the difference in incidence of toxoplasmosis here and in Europe. Worldwide, about 1% of cattle, 20% of hogs, and 30% of sheep have toxoplasmosis, according to estimates based on isolation of the organism from animal muscle tissue. To avoid contagion from meat, it should be cooked thoroughly at adequate temperatures.

Epidemiology

T. gondii has a worldwide distribution and has been reported wherever cats are found. It is somewhat more common in tropical and coastal regions and are less common in regions

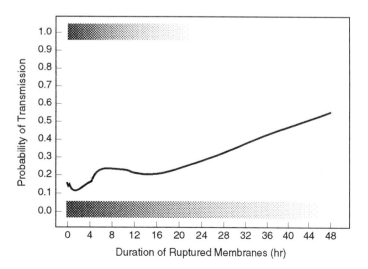

FIG. 5. Probability of HIV-1 transmission in relation to the duration of ruptured membranes. The *dots* at the top represent women who transmitted HIV-1 to their infants, and those at the bottom women who did not transmit HIV-1. Data on women whose membranes were ruptured for more than 48 hours are shown at the 48-hour mark. (Adapted from ref. 29.)

that are either cold, warm and arid, or at high elevation. The infection rate in the United States is significantly lower than that in France. Within the United States, seroprevalence rates are lower in the West Central and Mountain states and higher in the East Atlantic and East Central states.

Pathophysiology

T. gondii exists in three forms: trophozoite or proliferative form, tissue cyst, and oocyte. The organism undergoes a substantial portion of its life cycle in the cat, and then between 5 and 8 days of infection, the cat has peak oocyst production. As many as 10 million oocysts per day can be shed in feces for periods varying between 7 and 20 days. These oocytes sporulate within 1 to 3 days and can remain infectious for several months in moist soil. At that point, they may be carried from point of deposition by other animals (e.g., flies) and deposited in food. It has also been suggested that they can become airborne from a dried-out litter box and lead to human infection. Humans most commonly become infected by eating undercooked or raw meat that contains tissue cysts. In humans, the trophozoite form of *T. gondii* is seen in the acute phase of infection, during which host cells are invaded. Thereafter, the organism multiplies every 4 to 6 hours until the cytoplasm becomes so filled with trophozoites that cells rupture, releasing organisms to invade other cells.

In Utero Transmission

Newborns with congenital toxoplasmosis become infected *in utero* by transplacental passage of the parasite when the mother has acute infection. Chronic infections (those whose onset precedes pregnancy) do not lead to congenital infection, except in the rare circumstance of an immunocompromised host (e.g., HIV disease, those taking steroids for systemic lupus erythematosus).[32] In general, the likelihood of fetal infection increases with each trimester of pregnancy, being approximately 15%, 25%, and 60% in the first, second, and third trimester, respectively.[33] The severity of damage associated with congenital toxoplasmosis is also related to the timing of maternal infection, but the risks decrease toward term.[33] Severe fetal disease or fetal death occurs in about 10% of cases when infection occurs in the first trimester, and is extremely rare with infection in the third trimester. Mild damage is more frequent in the second and third trimesters (about 5%). Subclinical infections increase from about 2% with first-trimester infections to 50% with third-trimester infections.

The results of a case–control study of women with poor pregnancy outcomes suggested that acute infection can also be associated with preterm delivery and stillbirth, but not with spontaneous abortion. Chronic infections were not associated with any untoward outcomes.[34]

Diagnosis in Pregnancy

Mother

Maternal infection with *T. gondii* is usually asymptomatic, although 10% to 20% of infected mothers present with lymphadenopathy. Posterior cervical lymphadenopathy is the most frequent finding associated with acute maternal toxoplasmosis. The infection can also result in a mononucleosis-like syndrome with fatigue, lassitude, and, rarely, encephalitis. Acute toxoplasmosis should be considered in any pregnant women who presents with lymphadenopathy, particularly involving the posterior cervical chain, and/or mononucleosis-like symptoms. However, the vast majority of those acutely infected with *T. gondii* are asymptomatic.

The diagnosis of primary infection with *T. gondii* during pregnancy requires either (1) demonstration of a seroconversion, (2) a significant rise in antibody titer obtained from maternal serum taken at two different times, or (3) detection of *Toxoplasma*-specific IgM antibody. Adults with primary infection rapidly develop IgG and IgM antibodies to *Toxoplasma*. *Toxoplasma*-specific IgG antibody develops within 2 weeks after infection, peaks in 6 to 8 weeks, declines over the subsequent several months, and then persists for life. *Toxoplasma*-specific IgM develops within 10 days after infection and remains elevated for 6 months to more than 6 years.[35]

Since IgM antibody remains elevated for many months, this test may not provide useful information to document recent primary infection in pregnant women. The enzyme-linked immunosorbent assay (ELISA) test for IgM frequently shows the development of high titers of antibody that persist for many years. Indirect immunofluorescence antibody (IFA) tests for *Toxoplasma*-specific IgM usually show high titers for only about 6 months after infection, after which the titer rapidly delines. Thus, the IFA test is more useful than ELISA in differentiating remote from recent primary infection in pregnant women.

Approximately 50% of placentas of congenitally infected infants will show *T. gondii* cysts on histologic examination, supporting the diagnosis of acute maternal infection during pregnancy. The organism has also been isolated from placental tissue of acutely infected mothers in 2% to 25% of cases.[36] Recovery was more frequent when infection occurred later in pregnancy. Isolation of organisms from tissue specimens, buffy coat heparinized blood, and body fluids can also be used for diagnosis. These specimens produce the organism after inoculation into tissue culture or the intraperitoneal cavities of mice.

Prenatal Diagnosis

Antenatal diagnosis of fetal toxoplasmosis has relied on culture of amniotic fluid (15 to 20 ml) or fetal blood (1.5 to 3 ml) obtained at the time of diagnostic amniocentesis or cordocentesis, respectively. The specimen is commonly cultured in mice or fibroblast cells. The main difficulties with culture techniques have been that some assays may take up to several weeks to get complete results, and very few laboratories are able to perform the assay.

Toxoplasma-specific IgM, when present in fetal blood from cordocentesis, has also been used to diagnose fetal infection prenatally. Unfortunately, fetal-specific IgM antibody frequently does not develop until after 21 to 24 weeks' gestation and is only positive in about 50% of infected cases.

Identification of *T. gondii* by polymerase chain reaction (PCR) is useful in the detection of fetal infections *in utero*.[37,38] In one large series that evaluated 339 fetuses, of which 34 were found to be infected by conventional methods, PCR performed better than conventional tests (sensitivity, 97.4% vs. 89.5%; negative predictive value, 99.7% vs. 98.7%).[39] More recently, it has been shown that detection of *Toxoplasma*-specific IgA may be a reliable method for the diagnosis of toxoplasmosis in the newborn.[40]

Child

Most congenitally infected newborns are asymptomatic at birth. A number of these asymptomatic, untreated infants will later exhibit delayed and potentially serious manifestations. The 20% of infected infants with clinically obvious symptoms at birth present with multiple findings. The most frequent findings are chorioretinitis, jaundice, fever, and hepatosplenomegaly. Hydrocephaly or microcephaly and cerebral calcifications may also be seen in severe cases. Demonstration of *Toxoplasma*-specific IgM may be diagnostic, although approximately 20% of newborn infections are not detectable by *Toxoplasma*-specific IgM at birth.

Treatment and Prevention

In adults, the treatment of acute toxoplasmosis is primarily supportive. The prognosis following acute infection is good, except in the setting of profound immunosuppression.

Pregnant women with acute infection should be treated with a combination of pyrimethamine, folinic acid, and a sulfonamide. Although not certain, treatment with this regimen may prevent maternal-to-fetal transmission of the infection or improve the outcome among infected fetuses. In one study from France, 163 mothers diagnosed with toxoplasmosis prior to 28 weeks were treated with spiramycin (23 also received pyrimethamine and sulfadiazine). Three fetuses died *in utero*, and 27 were diagnosed with congenital toxoplasmosis. All 27 were free from symptoms and had normal neurologic development at 15 to 71 months.[41]

The standard regimen is pyrimethamine, 25 mg orally daily, and sulfadiazine, 1 g orally four times daily for 1 year. Pyrimethamine is a folic acid antagonist and therefore may have teratogenic effects when given in the first trimester. Whenever possible, treatment with pyrimethamine in the first trimester should be weighed against the potential risk of drug teratogenicity to the infant. Folinic acid, 6 mg intramuscu-

larly or orally every other day, should be used to correct the depletion of folic acid induced by pyrimethamine.

Spiramycin, another agent used in the treatment of acute toxoplasmosis, can be obtained in the United States through the CDC; it is more commonly used in Europe. There are no good controlled studies of its efficacy in this country. It has not been found to be teratogenic in humans or animals to date. Serosusceptible pregnant women should be counseled to avoid eating raw or undercooked meats that may contain *T. gondii* cysts and to avoid close contact with cat feces, such as changing cat litter. Other important preventive measures for pregnant women at risk include routinely boiling water for consumption, vigorously washing fruits and vegetables, and consuming meats that have been either cooked to at least 159°F, smoked, or cured.

In countries with extremely high seroprevalence rates, such as France, programs of routine seroscreening have proven successful in diagnosing recent seroconverters and allowing for prenatal diagnosis of fetal status and either termination of pregnancy or prenatal therapy.[42] Currently, there is no consensus for routine screening in the United States.

Most recently, programs have been undertaken that focus on screening of newborns and the institution of treatment in the neonatal period to minimize the morbidity that would otherwise accrue to congenitally infected children. Many infected children can be detected with IgM assays who would otherwise be missed on routine clinical examination. Treatment of these infants has been shown to be associated with very low rates of subsequent neurologic or retinal disease.[43]

CYTOMEGALOVIRUS

Cytomegalovirus (CMV), a member of the herpesvirus family, is the most common congenital viral infection, affecting approximately 1% of all live births; about 35,000 infants are born infected with CMV annually in the United States.[44,45] Congenital CMV infections are acquired by the fetus *in utero* when the mother is infected while pregnant or experiences reactivation of a prior infection. Although reactivated disease in pregnant women accounts for more than 50% of congenital infections, primary maternal CMV infection is much more likely to result in a severely affected and symptomatic infant.[46] Passive *in utero* transfer of maternally derived CMV-specific IgG antibody appears to provide some protection to the fetus when CMV is reactivated during pregnancy.[47]

The great majority of infants (90%) with congenital CMV infection are asymptomatic, but some (10%) have evidence of disease in the newborn period. About 10% of symptomatic infants present with full-blown cytomegalic inclusion disease. An additional 10% of infected infants who are asymptomatic at birth later present with symptoms related to CMV infection. The most common late-onset symptoms in these cases are mental retardation and deafness.[48] These infants usually shed high titers of virus in the urine and saliva for a number of months.

CMV infections can be acquired by infants during the post-partum period through (1) exposure to infectious maternal body fluids such as cervical secretions, urine, saliva, and breast milk,[49,50] (2) following blood transfusion or tissue transplantation from an infected donor,[51] or, most frequently, (3) through contact with infected individuals, such as in the newborn nursery, in day care centers, or in the family household. These cases are called acquired CMV infections, in contrast to congenital infections.

Microbiology

CMV, a herpesvirus, has a diameter of about 180 nm and is encapsulated by an icosahedral capsid containing 162 capsomeres. Within the capsid is double-stranded DNA of about 240 kilobases that is enclosed by a lipid bilayer envelope. The diagnosis of CMV infection requires laboratory confirmation and cannot be made on clinical grounds alone. Seroconversion, monoclonal antibody to CMV, and PCR are among the tools currently available for diagnosis. Antibody response, whether maternal or fetal, may play a less important role in transmission and subsequently in the development of symptomatic disease than other viral factors such as the amount of maternal viremia or the time in pregnancy when infection and subsequent maternal-to-fetal transmission occur.

Epidemiology

Seroprevalence to CMV among adult populations shows significant geographic variability. Rates range from 40% to 100%, depending on the region surveyed.[52,53] Countries or regions with low socioeconomic status usually demonstrate very high seroprevalence rates.[53] The risk of seroconversion for a pregnant seronegative woman is approximately 2% during pregnancy.[54] There are two periods in life when infection rates are particularly high: perinatal (related to mother-to-child, breast-feeding, and child-to-child transmission) and reproductive age (putatively related to sexual transmission). Pregnant women acquire CMV infection either through exposure to infected children[55] (who shed virus in urine, saliva, and nasopharyngeal secretions and are infectious for a prolonged time)[56] or through sexual contact.

Pathophysiology

Mother

The vast majority of pregnant women with primary CMV infection are asymptomatic. Symptomatic disease, if present, usually appears as a mononucleosis-like syndrome, including some lymphadenopathy, lassitude, malaise, pharyngitis, and fever. CMV-specific antibody (IgM) develops within a few days following infection and remains detectable for a few months. CMV-specific IgG develops rapidly and persists for life.

Following primary infection, the virus goes into a latent phase. Intermittent periods of reactivation frequently occur, and virus is again excreted in the nasopharynx, cervix, urine, saliva, and breast milk. Maternal shedding of the virus increases throughout pregnancy, and neonatal infection becomes increasingly likely as cervical shedding rates increase toward term.[57]

Infant

Acquisition of disease by neonates at the time of birth is much more common then congenital infection but much less devastating. After primary infection, the congenital infection rate has been reported to be as high as 55%.[47] Severe cases of congenitally acquired symptomatic infection result from primary rather than recurrent infection in pregnant women and from infections occurring early in pregnancy. The most common findings in these cases include hepatosplenomegaly, jaundice, a generalized petechial rash, and microcephaly. Less common findings include chorioretinitis (with or without optic atrophy), pneumonitis, cerebral calcifications, microphthalmia, seizures, and cerebral and cerebellar atrophy. The mortality of newborns with symptomatic disease is approximately 30%. Approximately 10% of infants who are asymptomatic at birth will later exhibit symptoms related to CMV infection. The most common findings include mental retardation and hearing loss.

Diagnosis

Mother

About one-third to two-thirds of all pregnant women have IgG antibody to CMV, indicating previous infection. Detection of CMV-specific IgM in the acute phase of infection is useful for making the diagnosis of CMV infection, but only 80% of women with primary infection demonstrate this antibody.[58] In addition, more than a one-third of mothers with recurrent CMV from latent infection will be positive for CMV-specific IgM. CMV-specific IgM antibody may persist for 4 to 9 months, and some test methods may give false-positive results because of cross-reactions with other herpesviruses, antinuclear antibody, or rheumatoid factor.[35] Even though CMV is hepatotropic, elevations in liver enzymes are rarely seen in primary or recurrent infections. Virus culture is the gold standard for the diagnosis of CMV infection but does not distinguish between primary and recurrent infection. Virus is usually detected in the cervix, nasopharynx, and urine of infected individuals.

Prenatal

Sonography may be useful for identifying some abnormalities in the fetus that may be related to CMV infection. Nonspecific sonographic findings including fetal hydrops, intrauterine growth retardation, polyhydramnios, fetal ascites, and specific CNS anomalies (e.g., ventriculomegaly, periventricular calcifications) suggest an intrauterine infection, possibly CMV, and should be evaluated further with amniocentesis or cord blood sampling. Lynch et al.[59] reported the successful prenatal diagnosis of fetal infection by a combination of amniotic fluid culture and measurement of total and CMV-specific IgM and τ-glutamyl transpeptidase (τ-glutamyltransferase) in fetal blood samples. Further studies are needed defining the sensitivity and specificity of these methods of identifying infected infants prior to birth.

Management

Mother

Susceptible pregnant women have a 2% risk of seroconverting primary infection while pregnant. Because this is a relatively low risk, because there is a somewhat low rate of possible damage to the fetus, and because no effective therapy is available for infected infants, routine serologic testing of pregnant women is not recommended.

Probably, the single most important method of preventing primary infection during pregnancy is minimizing exposure in high-risk areas, such as nurseries, day care centers, and other places that have a high concentration of young children. Careful handwashing techniques, as well as proper handling of potentially infectious body fluids, should be instituted to minimize spread of the infection.

No protocols currently exist for the use of antiviral agents—acyclovir (Zovirax) and ganciclovir sodium (Cytovene)—during pregnancy to decrease the risk of mother-to-child transmission of CMV.

Infants

Clinically evident infection in newborns and infants is treated with supportive measures. In the most severe cases of neonatal infection, antiviral agents such as acyclovir and ganciclovir have been used to suppress the infection, but discontinuation of the medication results in reappearance of the infection. Foscarnet sodium (Foscavir) has also been used in primary symptomatic neonatal disease and has been effective in reducing viral shedding.

◊ HERPES SIMPLEX VIRUS

Herpes simplex virus (HSV) is an extremely common sexually transmitted pathogen with potentially devastating consequences for perinatally infected neonates. Management of HSV infection in pregnancy has undergone substantive evolution over the last several years, aimed at reducing reliance on operative delivery.

Microbiology

HSV is an encapsulated, double-stranded DNA virus that infects susceptible mucosal surfaces. There is an approximately 50% concordance in the DNA sequences of HSV-1 and HSV-2, the latter being predominantly genital and the former predominantly oral. Either virus can cause serious illness in neonates. Immunity to one type of HSV may lead to an attenuated presentation if an individual becomes infected with the other.

Epidemiology

Whereas only approximately 5% of the reproductive-age population gives a history of clinical herpes infections, serologic surveys suggest that up to 20% of the sexually active population has had genital herpes. The discordance may be related to the presence of antibody to HSV-1 that offers sufficient protection from HSV-2 to mute any symptoms. The infection is transmitted both from symptomatic and asymptomatic individuals. There is little evidence to suggest that pregnancy in itself increases either the frequency or the severity of genital HSV infections. In one study of an unselected patient population, HSV shedding occurred in only 0.1% to 0.4% of all deliveries.[60] In other studies of pregnant women with histories of HSV infection, positive cultures were found in 0.2% to 7.4% of asymptomatic women.[61] It has been estimated that if PCR is used in lieu of cultures, shedding would be detected about eight times as frequently.[62] The rate of shedding at term is no higher than at other times in pregnancy. Unfortunately, from the therapeutic perspective, most women who shed virus are not aware that they infected with HSV.

Pathophysiology

HSV has an incubation period of 2 to 10 days followed by a primary infection characterized by focal vesicle formation and a pronounced cellular immune response. The infection enters a latent phase, with the virus ascending peripheral sensory nerves and coming to rest in nerve root ganglia. Recurrent exacerbations occur intermittently, stimulated by poorly understood mechanisms. Infection may be primary (2- to 3-week course of treatment), recurrent (5- to 10-day course of treatment), or asymptomatic. Primary infection poses the greatest risk to both mothers and infants. Clinically, it is extremely difficult to distinguish primary from recurrent disease.[63] One-half of infants born vaginally to mothers with a primary infection will themselves have HSV infection, compared with only 4% of those born to mothers with recurrent infection.[64] Primary infection may also be associated with abortion, low birthweight, preterm birth, and, rarely, congenital infection.[65] Virus shedding occurs for a significantly longer time with primary infection (1 to 2 weeks) than with recurrent infection (3 to 6 days).

Antibodies appear approximately 7 days following the onset of primary infection, reaching a peak in 2 to 3 weeks, and generally remain detectable for life. Titers do not rise significantly with recurrent infections. The significant difference in infection rates in neonates born to mothers with primary infections (50%) versus those born to women with recurrent infections (4%) suggests that maternal antibodies provide some protection. With recurrent infection, the infection rate has been estimated to range from 0% to 8% when virus is present at the time of vaginal delivery.

Fortunately, disseminated primary HSV infections in pregnant women are rare. When HSV infection becomes disseminated during pregnancy, mortality is high for both mothers and fetuses, and systemic antiviral therapy is recommended.

Although HSV shedding occurs in approximately 0.1% to 0.4% of deliveries,[60] neonatal infection occurs much less frequently, encountered in approximately 0.01% to 0.4% of deliveries. The reason for this 10-fold difference in infection between mothers and newborns is unknown but is probably related to both a protective benefit of maternal antibodies and the size of viral inoculum to which the fetus is exposed during birth. The viral inoculum associated with asymptomatic shedding is several log less than that associated with primary infection.

Neonatal infection may result from either HSV-1 or HSV-2. The majority of cases of neonatal HSV infections, however, are caused by HSV-2, with only 25% of isolates being HSV-1.[66] It is estimated that approximately 90% of cases of neonatal HSV infections can be traced to a maternal source of infection[66] and are secondary to either ascending infection with ruptured membranes or colonization during the actual birth process.

As noted, approximately 50% of mothers with a primary genital HSV infection delivering vaginally will give birth to an infant with HSV infection.[61] Of these infected neonates, 60% will die in the neonatal period. Of equal concern is that approximately 50% of the survivors will have significant sequelae such as microcephaly, mental retardation, seizures, microphthalmia, retinal dysplasia, chorioretinitis, meningitis, encephalitis, hypertonicity, apnea, and coma. Less commonly, neonates may also acquire infection from exposure during the neonatal period to either or both parents or other infected family members,[67] other infected infants,[68] or infected health care workers.[67]

Although there have been isolated reports of "congenitally infected" fetuses with malformations,[69] other investigators have found no such associations.[60]

Diagnosis

The diagnosis of primary HSV infection is relatively easy to make from a clinical standpoint, whereas recurrent infections may be more difficult to diagnose solely on clinical grounds. However, other ulcerative lesions (e.g., syphilis, chancroid) may also occur. Virus isolation by tissue culture remains the most accurate method of confirming the diagnosis of HSV infection. Cytologic tests such as Pap smear and Tzanck preparations tend to be less sensitive and accurate. Rapid, accurate tests for HSV, such as PCR, have been demonstrated to have utility in research settings and will undoubtedly eventually have a role in clinical medicine.

Management

Antepartum

It is important to remember the HSV infection is a sexually transmitted disease (STD), and women diagnosed with it during pregnancy should be screened for other STDs. In regard to preventing mother-to-child transmission of HSV, management has greatly changed over the last decade. It was previously recommended that pregnant women who were suspected of having a genital HSV infection, had a history of prior HSV infection, or had sexual partners with HSV infections be monitored closely with third-trimester cultures for recurrent infection or asymptomatic HSV shedding. Women who had a positive culture near term were scheduled for elective cesarean section to avoid contact between the neonate and the virus during delivery.

This protocol has had little impact on the overall incidence of neonatal HSV infection for several reasons. Most women who deliver infants with neonatal HSV infection have no history of infection and no lesions at the time of delivery,[70] and thus would not have met the criteria for monitoring in the first place. It was calculated that a weekly screening strategy would cost approximately $1.8 million for each case of neonatal HSV infection averted.[71] It is not clear whether the neonatal morbidity and mortality actually prevented by such a protocol would outweigh the maternal mortality that would result from complications of cesarean delivery. Moreover, cesarean delivery, even with intact membranes, will not prevent all cases of neonatal HSV infection secondary to maternal genital HSV infection. In a recent multicenter study, it was found that 12% of the reported cases of neonatal HSV infection occurred in spite of delivery by cesarean section with intact membranes.[72]

Current recommendations for pregnant women with HSV infections include the following:

◊ Cultures should be done when a women has active HSV lesions during pregnancy to confirm the diagnosis. If there are no visible lesions at the onset of labor, vaginal delivery is acceptable.
◊ Weekly surveillance cultures of pregnant women with a history of HSV infection, but no visible lesions, are not necessary, and vaginal delivery is acceptable.
◊ Amniocentesis in an attempt to rule out intrauterine infection is not recommended for mothers with HSV infection at any stage of gestation.

Recently, it has been suggested that oral acyclovir prophylaxis might have a role in the prevention of recurrence and thereby could reduce the need for cesarean section.[21] Cost savings with that strategy have been suggested, based on decision analysis. Although acyclovir is a nucleoside drug that incorporates into DNA, registries have not, to date, revealed an untoward rate of adverse outcomes among exposed infants. Preliminary trials with acyclovir in pregnancy have found that the need for cesarean section was reduced with no increase in morbidity for exposed neonates.[73]

Intrapartum

Currently, it is recommended that term patients who have visible HSV lesions and are in labor or have ruptured membranes undergo cesarean delivery. The duration of ruptured membranes should not influence the decision to perform cesarean delivery, because some infants born to mothers with HSV lesions and ruptured membranes for 24 hours or longer remain uninfected.

Recently, some authorities have questioned the policy of cesarean delivery for women with recurrent HSV lesions, primarily because the presence of HSV antibody in such women may render the mother-to-child HSV transmission rate quite low. However, until official American College of Obstetricians and Gynecologists recommendations change, most clinicians in the United States will opt for cesarean delivery in women with recurrent HSV lesions.

For patients with active HSV infections and premature rupture of membranes remote from term, there are not enough data to recommend a management protocol that would apply in all clinical situations. The risk of extreme prematurity must be weighed against the risk of neonatal HSV infection. There have been several case reports of infants born without sequelae after prolonged periods of conservative management.

Although the use of scalp electrodes has been implicated as a rare etiology of neonatal infection,[71] monitoring by fetal scalp electrode is not contraindicated if needed to adequately assess fetal condition in women with a history of HSV infection but without lesions or symptoms.

It has been suggested that cultures be obtained at delivery in women with a history of HSV infection to aid in assessing the need for therapy in the newborn.

Treatment

There is presently no known cure for HSV infection. The purine analog acyclovir has been used both to treat primary HSV infections and to prevent recurrent HSV infections in nonpregnant women.

Prevention

Although it is not necessary to isolate an infant from an infected mother, the infected parturient should be counseled regarding handwashing and good hygiene to prevent infection of the infant. Every effort should be made to avoid direct contract of the newborn with herpetic lesions.

SUMMARY POINTS

◊ All pregnant women should have HIV testing recommended to them.

◊ HIV-infected pregnant women should have regular monitoring of their CD4+ count and viral load.

◊ All HIV-infected women should receive ZDV per the ACTG 076 protocol.

◊ Standards of care for HIV infection should be upheld during the prenatal period.

◊ During the intrapartum period, the duration of ruptured membranes among women with HIV infection should be minimized.

◊ All pregnant women should be counseled regarding ways in which to minimize the risk of acquiring infection with *T. gondii.*

◊ Pregnant women who acquire *T. gondii* infections should have studies performed to ascertain the status of the fetus.

◊ If congenital infection with *T. gondii* is diagnosed and the patient continues the pregnancy, antiparasitic therapy should be instituted.

◊ CMV is the most common congenital infection in the United States.

◊ Although patients with CMV antibody may have reactivation resulting in infected newborns, these children are less frequently and less severely infected than those whose mothers have primary infection.

◊ Primary first-episode genital HSV infection increases the risk of untoward perinatal events, including preterm birth, low birthweight, and congenital infection.

◊ HSV-infected women with active lesions who are in labor or have ruptured membranes at term should be delivered by cesarean section.

◊ Nucleoside analogs may be used to reduce the frequency of HSV viral shedding and thereby the need for cesarean section.

◊ REFERENCES

1. Maury W, Potts BJ, Rabson AB. HIV-1 infection of the first-trimester and term human placental tissue: a possible mode of maternal-fetal transmission. *J Infect Dis* 1989;160:583–588.
2. Levy JA. Infection by human immunodeficiency virus—CD4 is not enough. *N Engl J Med* 1996;335:1528–1530.
3. Liu R, Paxton WA, Choe S, et al. Hoozygous defect in HIV-1 co-receptor accounts for resistance for some multiply-exposed individuals to HIV-1 infection. *Cell* 1996;86:367–377.
4. Rosenberg PS. Scope of the AIDS epidemic in the United States. *Science* 1995;270:1372–1375.
5. Ward JW, Karon J, Fleming P, Gayle H. Trends in AIDS incidence in the United States, 1990–1994. Presented at the XIth international conference on AIDS, Vancouver, British Columbia, July 7–12, 1996 (abst Mo.C.332, p 36).
6. Centers for Disease Control and Prevention. Morbidity and mortality weekly report. Update: mortality attributable to HIV infection among persons aged 25–44 years—United States, 1994. *MMWR* 1996;45(6): 121–125.
7. Rosenberg PS. Scope of the AIDS epidemic in the United States. *Science* 1995;270:1372–1375.
8. Gwinn M, Pappaioanou M, George JR, et al. Prevalence of HIV infection in childbearing women in the United States: surveillance using newborn blood samples. *JAMA* 1991;265:1704–1708.
9. Chin J. Current and future dimensions of the HIV/AIDS pandemic in women and children. *Lancet* 1990;336(8709):221–224.
10. Centers for Disease Control. 1993 Revised classification system for HIV infection and expanded surveillance case definition for AIDS among adolescents and adults. *MMWR* 1992;41(RR-17):1–19.

11. Ho DD, Neumann AU, Perelson AS, Chen W, Leonard JM, Markowitz M. Rapid turnover of plasma virons and CD4 lymphocytes in HIV-1 infection. *Nature* 1995;373:123–126.
12. Lemp GF, Payne SF, Rutherford GW, et al. Projections of AIDS morbidity and mortality in San Francisco. *JAMA* 1990;263:1497–1501.
13. Hessol NA, Lifson AR, O'Malley PM, Doll LS, Jaffe HW, Rutherford GW. Prevalence, incidence, and progression of human immunodeficiency virus infection in homosexual and bisexual men in hepatitis B vaccine trials, 1978–1988. *Am J Epidemiol* 1989;130:1167–1175.
14. Goedert JJ, Biggar RJ, Weiss SH, et al. Three-year incidence of AIDS in five cohorts of HTLV-III-infected risk group members. *Science* 1986;231:992–995.
15. Lifson AR, Rutherford GW, Jaffe HW. The natural history of human immunodeficiency virus infection. *J Infect Dis* 1988;158:1360–1367.
16. Goedert JJ, Kessler CM, Aledort LM, et al. A prospective study of human immunodeficiency virus type 1 infection and the development of AIDS in subjects with hemophilia. *N Engl J Med* 1989;321:1141–1148.
17. Rothenburg R, Woelfel M, Stoneburner R, Milberg J, Parker R, Truman B. Survival with the acquired immunodeficiency syndrome: experience with 5833 cases in New York City. *N Engl J Med* 1987; 317:1297–1302.
18. Lemp GF, Payne SF, Neal D, Temelso T, Rutherford GW. Survival trends for patients with AIDS. *JAMA* 1990;263:402–406.
19. Hocke C, Morlat P, Chene G, Dequae L, Dabis F. Prospective cohort study of the effect of pregnancy on the progression of human immunodeficiency virus infection. *Obstet Gynecol* 1995;86:886–891.
20. Minkoff H, Augenbraun M. Antiretroviral therapy of the pregnant women. *Am J Obstet Gynecol* 1997;176:478–489.
21. Randolph AG, Hartshorn RM, Washington AE. Acyclovir prophylaxis in late pregnancy to prevent neonatal herpes: a cost-effectiveness analysis. *Obstet Gynecol* 1996;88:603–610.
22. O'Sullivan MJ, Boyer PJJ, Scott GB, et al. The pharmacokinetics and safety of zidovudine in the third trimester of pregnancy for women infected with human immunodeficiency virus and their infants: phase I ACTG study (protocol 082). *Am J Obstet Gynecol* 1993;168:1510–1516.
23. Fang G, Burger H, Grimson R, et al. Maternal plasma human immunodeficiency virus type 1 RNA level: a determinant and projected threshold for mother-to-child transmission. *Proc Natl Acad Sci U S A* 1995; 92:12100–12104.
24. Dickover RE, Garratty EM, Herman SA, et al. Identification of levels of maternal HIV-1 RNA associated with risk of perinatal transmission. *JAMA* 1996;275:599–605.
25. Landesman S, Burns D. Quantifying HIV. *JAMA* 1996;275:640–641.
26. Misrahi M, Teglas JP, N'Go N, et al. CCR5 chemokine receptor variant in HIV-1 mother-to-child transmission and disease progression in children. *JAMA* 1998;279:277–280.
27. Wolinsky SM, Wike CM, Korber BT, et al. Selective transmission of human immunodeficiency virus type-1 variants from mothers to infants. *Science* 1992;255:1134–1137.
28. Connor EM, Sperling RS, Gelber R, et al. Reduction of maternal-infant transmission of human immunodeficiency virus type 1 with zidovudine treatment. *N Engl J Med* 1994;331:1173–1180.
29. Landesman S, Kalish L, Burns D, et al. The relationship of obstetrical factors to the mother-to-child transmission of HIV-1. *N Engl J Med* 1996;334:1617–1623.
30. Sever JL, Sison AV. Toxoplasmosis in pregnancy. In: Queenan JT, ed. *Management of high-risk pregnancy*. Boston: Blackwell Science, 1994;32:302–307.
31. Sever JL. Perinatal infections affecting the developing fetus and newborn. In: *The prevention of mental retardation through the control of infectious diseases*. Washington DC: U.S. Public Health Service, 1968. Publication no. 1692.
32. Minkoff H, Remington J, Holman S, Ramirez R, Goodwin S, Landesman S. Vertical transmission of toxoplasma by HIV-infected women. *Am J Obstet Gynecol* 1997;176:555–559.
33. Sever JL, Larsen JW, Grossman JH. Toxoplasmosis. In: *Handbook of perinatal infections,* 2nd ed. Boston: Little Brown, and Company, 1989:160.
34. Djurkovic-Djakovic O. *Toxoplasma* infection and pathologic outcome of pregnancy. *Gynecol Obstet Invest* 1995;40:36–41.
35. Fung JC, Tilton RC. TORCH serologies and specific IgM antibody determination in acquired and congenital infections. *Ann Clin Lab Sci* 1985;15:204–211.
36. Desmonts G, Couvreur J. Toxoplasmosis in pregnancy and its transmission to the fetus. *Bull N Y Acad Med* 1974;50:146–159.
37. Burg JL, Grover CM, Pouletty P, et al. Direct and sensitive detection of a pathogenic protozoan, *Toxoplasma gondii*, by polymerase chain reaction. *J Clin Microbiol* 1989;27:1787–1792.
38. Grover CM, Thulliez R, Remington JS, et al. Rapid prenatal diagnosis of cogenital toxoplasma infection by using polymerase chain reaction and amniotic fluid. *J Clin Microbiol* 1990;28:2297–2301.
39. Hohfeld P, Daffos F, Costa JM, Thulliez P, Forestier F, Vidaud M. Prenatal diagnosis of congenital toxoplasmosis with a polymerase-chain-reaction test on amniotic fluid. *N Engl J Med* 1994;331:695–699.
40. Stepick-Biek P, Thulliez P, Araujo FG, et al. IgA antibodies for diagnosis of acute congenital and acquired toxoplasmosis. *J Infect Dis* 1990;162:270–273.
41. Berrebi A, Kobuch WE, Bessieres MH, et al. Termination of pregnancy for maternal toxoplasmosis. *Lancet* 1994;344:36–39.
42. Daffos F, Forestier F, Capella-Pavlovsky, et al. Prenatal management of 746 pregnancies at risk of congenital toxoplasmosis. *N Engl J Med* 1988;318:271–275.
43. Guerina NG, Hsu HW, Meissner HC, et al. Neonatal serologic screening and early treatment for congenital *Toxoplasma gondii* infection: the New England Regional Working Group. *N Engl J Med* 1994;330: 1858–1863.
44. Sison AV, Sever JL. Cytomegalovirus infections in pregnancy and the neonate. In: Queenan JT, ed. *Management of high-risk pregnancy*. Boston: Blackwell Science, 1994;34:315–321.
45. Alford CA, Stagno S, Pass RF, et al. Congenital and perinatal cytomegalovirus infections. *Rev Infect Dis* 1990;12 Suppl 7:S745–S753.
46. Stagno S, Cloud G, Pass RF, et al. Primary cytomegalovirus infections in pregnancy: incidence, transmission to fetus, and clinical outcome. *JAMA* 1986;256:1904–1908.
47. Stagno S, Pass RF, Dworsky ME, et al. Congenital cytomegalovirus infection: the relative importance of primary and recurrent maternal infection. *N Engl J Med* 1982;306:945–949.
48. Stagno S, Pass RF, Dworsky ME, et al. Congenital and perinatal cytomegalovirus infection. *Semin Perinatol* 1983;7:31–42.
49. Reynolds DW, Stagno S, Hosty TS, et al. Maternal cytomegalovirus excretion and perinatal infection. *N Engl J Med* 1973;289:1–5.
50. Stagno S, Reynolds DW, Pass RF, et al. Breast milk and the risk of cytomegalovirus infection. *N Engl J Med* 1980;302:1073–1076.
51. Yeager AS, Grument FC, Hafleigh EB, et al. Prevention of transfusion acquired cytomegalovirus infections in newborn infants. *J Pediatr* 1981;90:281–287.
52. Krech U, Jung M, Jung F, eds. *Cytomegalovirus infections of man.* New York: S Karger, 1971.
53. Krech U. Complement-fixing antibodies against cytomegalovirus in different parts of the world. *Bull World Health Organ* 1973;49:103–106.
54. Griffiths PD, Campbell-Benzie A, Heath RB. A prospective study of primary cytomegalovirus infection in pregnant women. *Br J Obstet Gynaecol* 1980;87:308–314.
55. Pass RF, Little EA, Stagno S, et al. Young children as a probable source of maternal and congenital cytomegalovirus infection. *N Engl J Med* 1987;316:1366–1370.
56. Murph JR, Bale JF. The natural history of acquired cytomegalovirus infection: cytomegalovirus infection among children in group day-care. *Am J Dis Child* 1988;142:843–846.
57. Stagno S, Reynolds D, Tsiantos A, et al. Cervical cytomegalovirus excretion in pregnant and non-pregnant women: suppression in early gestation. *J Infect Dis* 1975;131:522–527.
58. Stagno S, Tinker MK, Irod C, et al. Immunoglobulin M antibodies detected by enzyme-linked immunosorbent assay and radioimmunoassay in the diagnosis of cytomegalovirus infections in pregnant women and newborn infants. *J Clin Microbiol* 1985;21:930–935.
59. Lynch L, Daffos F, Emanuel D, et al. Prenatal diagnosis of fetal cytomegalovirus infection. *Am J Obstet Gynecol* 1991;165:714–718.
60. Brown ZA, Vontver LA, Benedetti J, et al. Genital herpes in pregnancy: risk factors associated with recurrences and asymptomatic viral shedding. *Am J Obstet Gynecol* 1985;153:24–30.
61. Stagno S, Whitley RJ. Herpesvirus infections of pregnancy. Part II: herpes simplex virus and varicella zoster virus infections. *N Engl J Med* 1985;313:1327–1330.
62. Cone RW, Hobson AC, Brown Z, et al. Frequent detection of genital herpes simplex virus DNA by polymerase chain reaction among pregant women. *JAMA* 1994;272:792–796.
63. Hensleigh PA, Andrews WW, Brown Z, Greenspoon J, Yasuka L, Prober C. Genital herpes during pregnancy: inability to distinguish primary and recurrent infections clinically. *Obstet Gynecol* 1997;89:891–895.

64. Brown ZA, Vontver LA, Benedetti J, et al. Effects on infants of a first episode of genital herpes during pregnancy. *N Engl J Med* 1987;317:1246–1251.

65. Brown ZA, Benedetti J, Selke S, Ashley R, Watts DH, Corey L. Asymptomatic shedding of herpes simplex virus at the onset of labor: relationship to preterm labor. *Obstet Gynecol* 1996;87:483–488.

66. American Academy of Pediatrics, Committee on Fetus and Newborn, Committee on Infectious Diseases. Perinatal herpes simplex virus infections. *Pediatrics* 1980;66:147–149.

67. Yeager AS, Ashley RL, Corey L. Transmission of herpes simplex virus from father to neonate. *J Pediatr* 1983;103:905–907.

68. Linnerman CC Jr, Buchman TG, Light IJ, et al. Transmission of herpes-simplex virus type 1 in a nursery for the newborn: identification of viral isolates by DNA "fingerprinting." *Lancet* 1978;1(807):964–966.

69. South MA, Tompkins WA, Morris CR, et al. Congenital malformation of the central nervous system associated with genital type (type 2) herpes virus. *J Pediatr* 1969;75:13–18.

70. Prober CG, Hensleigh PA, Boucher FD, Yasukawa LL, Au DS, Arvin AM. Use of routine viral cultures to identify neonates exposed to herpes simplex virus. *N Engl J Med* 1988;318:887–891.

71. Binkin NJ, Koplan JP, Cates W Jr. Preventing neonatal herpes: the value of weekly viral cultrues in pregnant women with recurrent genital herpes. *JAMA* 1984;251:2816–2821.

72. Stone KM, Brooks CA, Guinan ME, et al. Neonatal herpes—results of one year's surveillance. In: *Abstracts of the 25th interscience conference on antimicrobial agents and chemotherapy*. Washington DC: American Society for Microbiology, 1985:185(abst 515).

73. Scott LL, Sanchez PJ, Jackson GL, Zeray F, Wendel GD Jr. Acyclovir suppression to prevent cesarean delivery after first-episode genital herpes. *Obstet Gyecol* 1996;87:69–73.

CHAPTER 26

Placenta Previa and Abruption

◇

James R. Scott

Bleeding during the latter half of gestation occurs in 3% to 4% of all pregnancies. It can be inconsequential or signal a serious condition, but all vaginal bleeding is alarming to pregnant women and warrants immediate evaluation. Although lesions of the vagina and cervix are rarely the cause of significant bleeding late in pregnancy, polyps, friable condyloma acuminata, and other lesions occasionally bleed from minor trauma. Invasive cervical carcinoma must also be considered, but cervical cytology obtained during a prenatal examination usually excludes this diagnosis. In some cases, no specific reason for the bleeding can be found.

The most common causes of serious bleeding during the latter half of pregnancy are placenta previa and placental abruption, which are potentially fatal to the mother and fetus. The condition of the fetus and mother requires prompt assessment. However, rectal or vaginal examinations should be delayed until preparations have been made to deal with potential consequences, such as severe hemorrhage.

◇ SECOND-TRIMESTER BLEEDING

Vaginal bleeding during the second trimester of pregnancy is seldom discussed in the obstetric literature. Nevertheless, it has important implications regarding the management of repeated episodes of bleeding and fetal salvage. Midtrimester bleeding is more common than generally appreciated, and the perinatal mortality rate of 23% to 32% is higher than that associated with third-trimester bleeding.[1,2] The etiology of bleeding at this stage of gestation falls into five general categories: placenta previa, premature placental separation, hydatidiform mole, cervical or vaginal lesions, and undetermined causes. The prognosis becomes progressively more grave with greater amounts of blood loss, a higher number of bleeding episodes, and uterine contractions. These three signs often indicate placental abruption.

Proper evaluation involves techniques similar to those used later in pregnancy, including hospitalization, stabiliza-tion of the maternal condition if necessary, placental localization by sonography, and assessment of the fetal status by electronic fetal heart rate (FHR) monitoring. Speculum examination is generally less dangerous than in third-trimester bleeding. Except with hydatidiform mole or when the fetus is in jeopardy, conservative management is almost always indicated initially in an attempt to achieve fetal maturity. Pregnancies maintained into the third trimester have a much lower perinatal mortality rate than those in which delivery occurs during the second trimester. If premature labor ensues or delivery becomes necessary in the late second trimester because of continued bleeding or fetal distress, the route of delivery is determined by obstetric indications. Because infant morbidity and mortality are primarily related to hypoxia and the high incidence of prematurity, it is desirable to have expert perinatal and neonatal care available for these very high-risk patients at the time of delivery.

◇ PLACENTA PREVIA

Placenta previa is defined as implantation of the placenta in the lower uterine segment, with the placenta either overlying or reaching the cervix, usually in advance of the fetal presenting part. Traditionally, placenta previa has been categorized into three types (Fig. 1):

1. Total previa: the internal os is entirely covered by the placenta.
2. Partial previa: the os is partially covered, expressed as the percentage covered at the time the diagnosis is made.
3. Marginal previa: the placental edge reaches the internal os and may extend into the os as the cervix dilates. The low-lying placenta implanted in the lower uterine segment but not reaching the cervical os has similar clinical manifestations.

However, these terms are of limited prognostic value and do not necessarily predict different antepartum courses. All

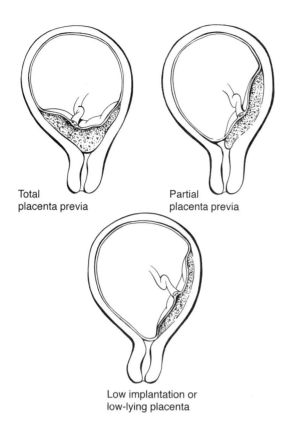

Total placenta previa

Partial placenta previa

Low implantation or low-lying placenta

FIG. 1. Variations of placenta previa.

are associated with potential life-threatening hemorrhage during labor, and classifications have become less important as cesarean section has become the preferred method of delivery for most patients with any degree of placenta previa.

Incidence

Placenta previa occurs in approximately 1 in 200 births. It is much more common in parous women, occurring in only one in 1500 nulliparas and in up to 1 in 20 grand multiparas. The incidence seems to be decreasing in the United States, perhaps as the result of a decline in the number of women of high parity and an increase in the number of primigravidae. This is most likely related to more readily available means of contraception and more liberal attitudes toward surgical sterilization.

Etiology

The specific cause of placenta previa is unknown, but a number of factors may affect the location of implantation in any pregnancy. These include abnormalities of endometrial vascularization, delayed ovulation, and prior trauma to the endometrium or myometrium. It is likely that more than chance controls the site of implantation. Multiple pregnancy predisposes to placenta previa because of the increased surface area of placenta or placentas. In patients who have in-

trauterine synechiae or a scar from a uterine incision after such operations as cesarean section, hysterotomy, myomectomy, or metroplasty, it is quite common to find that subsequent placental sites include the area of the scar. There is a sixfold increase in the incidence of placenta previa in patients who have had a delivery by low cervical cesarean, regardless of whether the uterine incision was vertical or transverse. These risk factors suggest that extensive endometrial scarring promotes either trophoblast nidation or subsequent migration of the trophoblast into the relatively unscarred lower uterine segment. Presumably, previous gestations permanently damage the endometrium underlying the placental site. The change in size and contour of the uterine cavity after any pregnancy may also be related to the development of placenta previa in multiparas. These factors suggest a need for increased placental surface area to compensate for reduced uteroplacental oxygen delivery or increased fetal nutritional requirements that promote previa formation.

Clinical Course

Classically, placenta previa presents as painless vaginal bleeding in the third trimester, but it can occur as early as 20 weeks of gestation. Uterine activity is sometimes evident.

During late pregnancy, the lower uterine segment thins, and the softening cervix begins to efface and dilate. If the placenta is implanted in the lower pole, the size and margins of the implantation site become altered by these uterine changes. Various degrees of detachment of the placenta result, and maternal bleeding occurs from the intervillous space. The earlier in pregnancy the lower uterine segment begins to form, and the lower the placenta, the earlier the first episode of bleeding occurs. Blood loss associated with the first episode ranges from slight to heavy, but it is rarely fatal. Unless major uterine sinuses have been opened, the initial bleeding tends to stop as clots form, but it often recurs with renewed intensity as further cervical changes occur. The bleeding can be precipitated by pelvic examination, intercourse, or labor. It often begins without any inciting cause; the patient may simply awaken in the middle of the night in a pool of bright red blood.

The mean gestational age at diagnosis is 32.5 weeks of gestation, with about one-third of patients presenting before 30 weeks of gestation and an additional one-third after 36 weeks of gestation. Asymptomatic placenta previa may be found by sonography, occasionally at the time of repeat cesarean, or rarely, the patient may bleed for the first time after labor is well established.

The baby is usually not adversely affected unless placental exchange is compromised by major placental detachment or maternal hypovolemia from blood loss. However, placenta previa is associated with an increased incidence of congenital abnormalities[3] and fetal growth retardation.[4] Preterm delivery is the greatest threat to the infant, and the stage of pregnancy during which the first bleeding occurs is an important factor in perinatal outcome.

Diagnosis

Painless vaginal bleeding in the second half of pregnancy means placenta previa until proved otherwise, particularly if associated with multiparity, a soft uterus, an abnormal presentation, or a floating presenting part. A careful abdominal examination can raise or lower the suspicion.

Because fewer than one-half of patients who experience painless vaginal bleeding have placenta previa, it is of major importance to confirm it or rule it out to avoid unnecessary, prolonged observation in the hospital. Transabdominal ultrasonography is currently the initial diagnostic technique of choice because of its safety and availability (Fig. 2).[5] If sonography is available in the labor–delivery area, the placenta can be localized quickly in all patients with third-trimester bleeding unless the hemorrhage is extreme and immediate delivery by cesarean is necessary because of the mother's unstable condition.

Although transabdominal ultrasonography represents an important advance in diagnostic accuracy, it has limitations. Patient obesity may cause poor imaging of the placenta. Posteriorly and laterally situated placentas are not always well imaged. When it presents by the vertex, the fetal head may cast an acoustic shadow over the internal os and the placenta. An overdistended bladder may push the lower uterine segment into the horizontal position and lead to a false diagnosis of placenta previa.[6] Postvoid views may be needed for confirmation, but this is inconvenient and time consuming. Moreover, an empty bladder makes the examination more difficult because there is no acoustic window. Magnetic resonance imaging can overcome some of these technical difficulties, but its lack of portability, relatively lengthy examination time, and expense limit its value, particularly in emergency situations.[7]

Placental migration confounds the traditional classification of placenta previa and results in inaccurate sonographic diagnosis. The earlier in pregnancy that sonography is performed, the more frequently the placenta appears to cover the cervix. Therefore, the diagnosis of placenta previa, when made by ultrasound in the second trimester, must be interpreted cautiously. A low-lying placenta has been reported in up to 45% of pregnant women with second-trimester bleeding, and approximately 5% of all pregnant women display sonographic evidence of a complete, partial, or marginal placenta previa in midgestation. However, 95% of these patients will experience no symptoms, will have a sonographically normal placental location by 28 weeks of gestation, and will have no previa at term.

It has been suggested that transvaginal ultrasonography is more instructive than conventional transabdominal examination for the diagnosis of placenta previa.[8] Potential advantages include closer apposition of the probe to the target area without the interposition of other structures, and it allows the use of a transducer with a higher frequency, which gives superior resolution, and the woman does not need a full bladder. Advocates of transvaginal ultrasound caution that the probe should be inserted no more than 3 cm into the vagina and should not come into contact with the cervix or lower segment and that the improved images outweigh the theoretical disadvantages of provoking bleeding. This technique seems to be relatively safe, well tolerated, and more accurate than transabdominal ultrasonography.[6,8]

The definitive antepartum diagnosis of placenta previa is made by palpation of the placenta on vaginal examination. This examination, in itself, can provoke hemorrhage sufficient to endanger the mother's life. It should be performed only after preparations for immediate cesarean delivery have been made (i.e., double-setup examination) and only if expectant management is not appropriate. Some have questioned the need to confirm the ultrasound diagnosis of placenta previa by vaginal examination. However, even with optimal technique, ultrasound is not infallible. Accuracy of transabdominal ultrasound ranges from 93% to 97%;[5–8] false-negative and false-positive results have been reported. Conversely, little is gained by double-setup examination in the face of active hemorrhage mandating immediate delivery or fetal malposition precluding vaginal delivery.

Management

All patients with significant bleeding should be admitted to the hospital and be placed at bed rest in an area of high-intensity care such as the labor–delivery suite. An intravenous catheter should be inserted, blood drawn for type and screen, intravenous fluids started, and serial vital signs and hematocrit levels checked. The systemic manifestations of hemorrhage depend on the amount of blood lost. Bleeding episodes usually occur during late pregnancy, when the circulating blood vol-

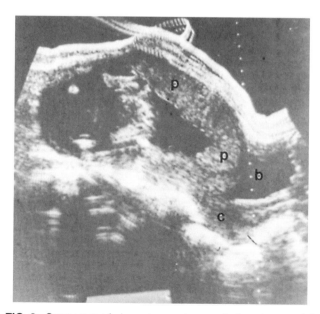

FIG. 2. Sonogram of placenta previa reveals the placenta (p) in the lower uterine area, covering the internal os of the cervix (c), which is situated posterior to the junction of the base and posterior walls of the bladder (b).

ume is increased by 20% to 40%, so there may be deceptively minor changes in pulse and blood pressure. Evidence of hypovolemia indicates that hemorrhage has been severe.

The details of the episode, history of previous bleeding, and past obstetric and medical history should be obtained. The time spent completing the history depends on the patient's clinical and hemodynamic status, and she should be rapidly assessed for manifestations of hypovolemic shock. If her condition is stable, the physical examination should also be a complete one with the exception of a vaginal or rectal examination. Inspection of the lower extremities and perineum usually reveals blood. On examination of the abdomen, the uterus is most often soft, normal in tone, and nontender. A high presenting part with a breech, oblique, or transverse lie is characteristic. The status of the fetus should be quickly evaluated by means of continuous electronic FHR monitoring. Fetal distress or fetal death is unusual in the absence of significant placental detachment or maternal hemorrhagic shock.

Once the diagnosis of placenta previa is confirmed by physical examination and sonography, management decisions depend on the gestational age of the fetus, the amount of bleeding, and the condition of the mother and fetus. The two major factors responsible for improved perinatal outcome have been expectant management and the liberal use of cesarean section (Fig. 3).[3,9–12] In the patient who is remote from term, expectant management is the treatment of choice. The goal is to extend the period of gestation long enough to allow for fetal maturity without compromising maternal health. Maternal blood loss should be replaced to maintain her hematocrit above 30%, and the use of autologous blood transfusions is sometimes feasible. Up to 20% of patients de-

velop uterine contractions, but it is difficult to diagnose preterm labor when vaginal examinations are contraindicated. Tocolytics have been used safely in selected patients with placenta previa having preterm labor, but this is controversial. No studies have proved their efficacy in this situation.[9,13] Maternal hemodynamic stability is necessary before these drugs are considered. β-Mimetics produce tachycardia and hypotension, making the evaluation of maternal blood volume status difficult. Therefore, magnesium sulfate may be a better choice in these patients if tocolysis is used.[13] Because nearly one-third of patients fail expectant management, the use of antenatal steroids to reduce the incidence of respiratory distress syndrome is reasonable in patients presenting between 26 and 32 weeks of gestation. Cervical cerclage has been proposed as a temporizing measure for treatment of patients with placenta previa,[14] but this procedure introduces its own risks and has not become common clinical practice.

If the mother responds to conservative management, the safest course is to continue bed rest with bathroom privileges in the hospital setting. Fetal surveillance with ultrasound examinations every 2 to 3 weeks is indicated to evaluate fetal growth, amniotic fluid volume, and placental localization. The current costs of prolonged hospitalization and the psychological toll in some women have recently led to attempts at outpatient management. Home care can realistically be considered only under ideal circumstances. It requires a highly motivated patient who understands the risks involved, can maintain strict bed rest, lives near the hospital, and has 24-hour transportation availability. The data on whether hospitalization or outpatient management at home is more cost effective than bed rest at home are conflicting.[15–17]

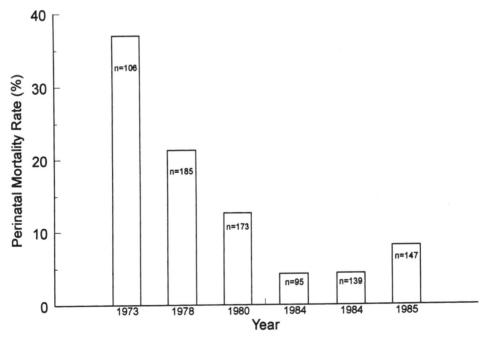

FIG. 3. Perinatal mortality rates in patients with placenta previa have decreased over the years. (Data from references 3, 10, and 11.)

Delivery

Repetitive bleeding and transfusions may require emergency cesarean delivery at any time. More ideal is a well-planned elective delivery at approximately 36 to 37 weeks of gestation. Amniocentesis studies to determine fetal maturity are helpful in deciding on the optimal time for delivery. Waiting longer than necessary invites further episodes of hemorrhage that endanger the mother and the fetus.

Cesarean delivery has replaced vaginal delivery for all but a small number of patients with minor degrees of placenta previa. Unusual circumstances under which the vaginal approach might be considered include:

◊ A dead fetus,
◊ Major fetal malformations,
◊ A clearly previable fetus,
◊ Active labor with engagement of the fetal head,
◊ Uncertainty about the degree of placenta previa.

Prolonged attempts at vaginal delivery are unwise from the standpoint of blood loss even in these circumstances. Moreover, a posterior placenta previa is likely to obstruct engagement of the presenting part and represents a relative contraindication. Therefore, with a living, viable fetus, cesarean delivery is usually the method of choice. The advantage in terms of perinatal survival is striking, and this advantage applies equally to marginal and partial placenta previa and to total placenta previa.

If a sonogram performed within several days of the delivery date demonstrates only a low-lying placenta or is inconclusive, a double-setup examination is reasonable. The patient should be prepped and draped for cesarean delivery. A vein must be kept open with a large-bore catheter, intravenous fluids should be running, and blood for transfusion should be available in the room. An anesthesiologist should be present, the operating room ready, and the pediatric staff and nursery notified to expect a high-risk infant. A careful sterile speculum examination is performed first to visualize any placental tissue in the cervical os. If the diagnosis is not apparent on speculum examination, the obstetrician examines the vaginal fornices for fullness suggesting the presence of placenta extending to the cervix. Next, one examining finger is carefully introduced into the cervical canal. If placental tissue covers the os, there is a gritty feel to the tissue palpated. When only a portion of the internal os is covered, the placental edge can be felt. The examination should be stopped at that point in either case because even a gentle examination may precipitate severe hemorrhage. If no placental tissue is palpated over the os or at its margin, a finger is placed carefully into the cervix to palpate gently 360° around the internal os. If placental tissue is palpated during this maneuver, a diagnosis of a low-lying placenta is made. Because this examination may cause heavy bleeding, it should not be undertaken unless immediate diagnosis is essential or prompt delivery is planned.

At the time of double-setup examination, if the cervix is dilated 3 cm or more and the placenta does not cover any of the internal os, rupture of the membranes permits the presenting part to advance against the placenta and tamponade it against the bleeding maternal sinuses. If this does not control the bleeding, and labor does not ensue and progress normally, cesarean delivery is indicated.

Opinions differ regarding the type of cesarean that should be performed in patients with placenta previa. The location of the placenta and the fetal presentation as revealed by sonogram and prominence of lower uterine segment blood vessels help the physician to make the decision. If the placenta is implanted on the posterior uterine wall and there is a polar lie, either a transverse or a vertical incision in the lower segment will avoid the placental tissue and permit easy delivery. If the placenta is anterior, or there is a transverse lie, a vertical incision is the best choice. The baby is delivered by the obstetrician passing a hand around the margin of the placenta or incising the placenta. It may be easier for the obstetrician to bring down one of the baby's feet and perform breech extraction than to try to deliver a very high head past a placenta that occupies the uterine incision. Incising the placenta may involve additional blood loss, and prolonged delay in delivery can lead to fetal exsanguination. In either case, the baby should be delivered promptly, the cord clamped, and the pediatrician advised to check the infant's hemoglobin or hematocrit level.

Complications

Morbidity may result from the placenta previa, but the maternal mortality rate is now less than 1%, and perinatal mortality has been reduced to less than 5% with modern treatment. Conditions associated with placenta previa are placenta accreta, placenta percreta, and placenta increta, occurring in up to 15% of cases. Because of an underdeveloped or absent decidua basalis layer, the placenta invades myometrium and forms an abnormally firm attachment to the uterine wall. In the lower uterine segment, where muscle content is diminished, interlacing muscle bundles contracting around open vessels may be less effective. Severe postpartum bleeding can occur with attempts at placenta removal because there is no distinct plane of separation; uterine compression and oxytocic drugs are often ineffective. If uterine preservation is important, bilateral hypogastric artery ligation may be useful. In many cases, cesarean hysterectomy is necessary and may be lifesaving.

◊ RUPTURED VASA PREVIA

Ruptured vasa previa is a rare cause of bleeding in late pregnancy or during labor and is often associated with placenta previa or multiple gestation. When there is a velamentous insertion of the umbilical cord, the abnormal portion of the membranes is located in the lower uterine segment. The umbilical vessels course through the membranes, unsupported, in advance of the fetal presenting part, extending across the cervical os. The vessels are commonly torn at the time of spontaneous or artificial rupture of the membranes, but tearing can occur before that time. Fetal exsanguination can follow rapidly, and the fetal mortality rate is at least 50%. Antenatal diagnosis of vasa previa requires a high index of suspicion, but color-flow Doppler imaging is a promising modality for future diagnosis.[18] New-onset vaginal bleeding at the time of membrane rupture should alert the physician to this possibility. Tests for nucleated red blood cells or fetal hemoglobin in the expelled blood, palpation of the vessels, and sonographic or direct visualization of the bleeding vessel through a lighted vaginal cone used for fetal scalp blood sampling have all been used to confirm the diagnosis. However, these tests are not always readily available when the emergency arises, and none are completely reliable. Significant vaginal bleeding and fetal distress, particularly fetal tachycardia, a sinusoidal FHR tracing, or variable decelerations, coinciding with membrane rupture require immediate delivery by cesarean to save the infant.

◊ **PLACENTAL ABRUPTION**

Abruptio placenta refers to premature separation of the normally implanted placenta before birth of the fetus. This most often takes place in the third trimester, but it can happen at any time after 20 weeks of gestation. Complicating approximately 1% of pregnancies, placental abruption is the most common cause of intrapartum fetal death and accounts for nearly 15% of perinatal mortality. Frequently, the placental separation is an acute process that increases in severity over a few hours. At other times, it has a variable presentation. It may be self-limited, or it may become quiescent and then recur. Permanent neurologic impairment occurs in up to 14% of surviving infants.[19] The placental separation may be complete, may be partial, or may involve only the placental margin (Fig. 4). The latter is commonly referred to clinically as marginal sinus rupture or marginal sinus bleeding, an entity that has been difficult to demonstrate pathologically. Minor degrees of abruption, involving less than a few centimeters of the placenta, are usually trivial, whereas complete detachment can be fatal to the mother and fetus. Approximately 48% of abruptions are designated as mild (grade I), 27% as moderate (grade II), and 24% as severe (grade III).

Pathophysiology

Separation of the placenta is initiated by bleeding into the decidua basalis. The bleeding usually originates from the small vessels in the basal layer of decidua, but it may be from fetoplacental vessels. The bleeding splits the decidua and spreads beneath the placenta, shearing it off. As a hematoma forms, it causes additional separation of the placenta from the uterine wall with destruction and compression of adjacent placental tissue. Occasionally, blood will extravasate into and through the myometrium to the peritoneal surfaces, resulting in the Couvelaire uterus. An organized clot lying within a depression on the maternal surface of the placenta can often be

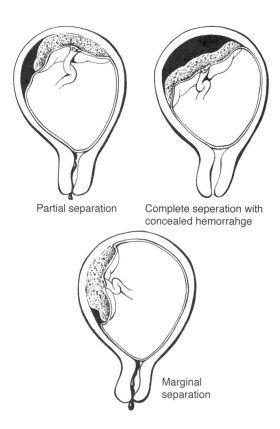

Partial separation   Complete seperation with concealed hemorrahge

Marginal separation

FIG. 4. Various degrees of separation of a normally implanted placenta.

defined at delivery. The effects on the fetus depend mainly on the degree of disruption at the uteroplacental interface. Marginal separation may have no apparent effect, and intermediate degrees produce variable effects. In cases of complete or near-complete abruption, fetal death from anoxia is virtually certain.

A number of etiologic factors, such as maternal smoking, a short umbilical cord, uterine anomalies, advanced maternal age, physical work, and poor nutrition, have been associated with some cases, but the cause is obscure in most patients.[20] Maternal hypertension is the most consistently identified predisposing factor (Fig. 5). This relationship is true for all degrees of placental abruption but is most strongly associated with severe cases, in which nearly one-half of patients are hypertensive.[21–23] A direct blow to the uterus, forceful external version, placental site bleeding from a needle puncture at amniocentesis, and sudden decompression of the overdistended uterus with rupture of membranes are all rare but have been implicated. Physical trauma now complicates approximately 1 in every 12 pregnancies, and a direct blow to the uterus as a result of violence or an automobile accident represents an increasingly important cause. Finally, obstetricians are now aware that abruption is also associated with cocaine-induced transient hypertension.[24] In most cases, the symptoms of headache, lower back pain or contractions, and vaginal bleeding occur soon after the cocaine use.

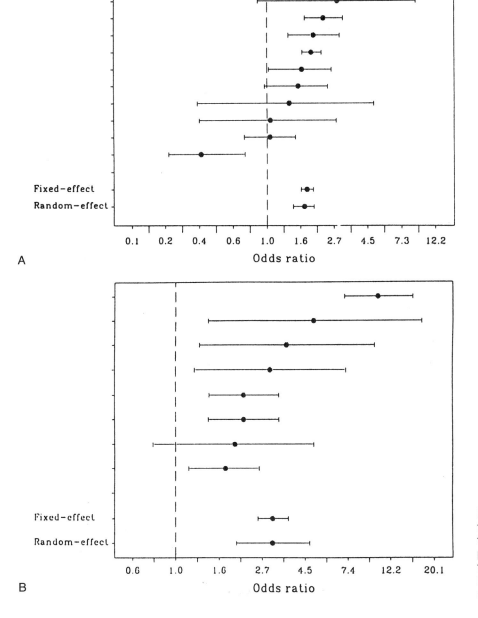

FIG. 5. (A) Association between placental abruption and preeclampsia derived from 12 studies. **(B)** Association between placental abruption and chronic hypertension derived from eight studies. Odds ratios with 95% confidence intervals. (Modified from ref. 21.)

A history of placental abruption increases the risk of recurrence in a subsequent pregnancy by at least 10-fold,[21,22,25] and the perinatal mortality in repeat abruption is as high as 15%. A woman who has twice suffered placental abruption has a 25% chance of developing an abruption in her next pregnancy, frequently in a more severe form. Presently, there is no proven management regimen to reduce this risk.

Signs and Symptoms

The diagnosis of placental abruption is essentially a clinical one because no pathognomonic laboratory tests are available. The classic findings are vaginal bleeding, abdominal pain,

uterine contractions, and uterine tenderness (Fig. 6). Uterine contractions are characteristically of high frequency and low amplitude, with elevated baseline uterine tonus (Fig. 7). However, the signs and symptoms vary considerably. In 80% of patients, the abruption presents as vaginal bleeding. In 20%, the blood remains trapped or concealed. It may extravasate into the amniotic sac, causing port wine staining of the amniotic fluid. Combinations are also seen, with the external bleeding representing only a portion of the actual maternal blood loss.

The clinical manifestations vary greatly depending on the degree of detachment, and the diagnosis requires a high degree of suspicion. It is now apparent that a number of patients

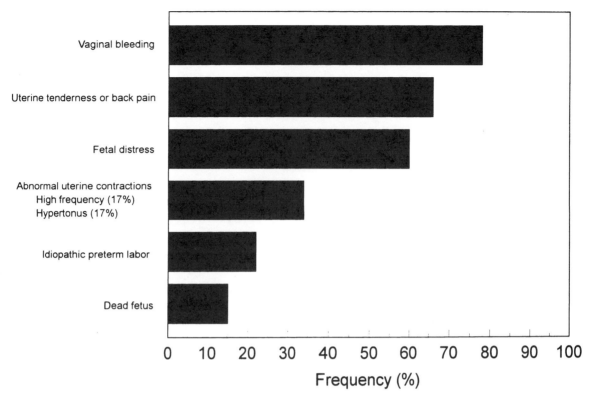

FIG. 6. Prevalence of signs and symptoms of placental abruption. (From ref. 26, with permission.)

do not develop the classic picture and that symptoms may be deceptively minimal, particularly if the placenta is implanted posteriorly. A concealed abruption should be considered when a patient presents with premature labor, and she should be monitored carefully. Differential diagnoses include pla-

centa previa, "bloody show" of term labor, uterine rupture, severe preeclampsia, and intraabdominal pain of nonuterine origin (Table 1). Ultrasonography is useful in excluding placenta previa, but it is much less reliable for establishing the diagnosis of abruption and appears to have little impact on the

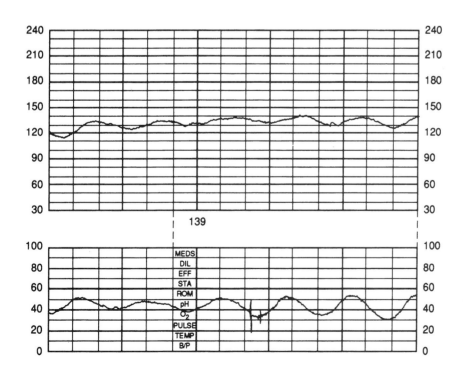

FIG. 7. Fetal heart rate tracing from a patient with placental abruption illustrates increased baseline intrauterine pressure and hypertonic uterus with frequent contractions.

TABLE 1. *Differential diagnosis of bleeding late in pregnancy*

Signs and symptoms	Placenta previa	Marginal separation	Moderate abruption	Severe abruption	Antepartum rupture of scarred uterus
External bleeding	Mild to severe	Mild	None to moderate	None to severe	None to mild
Pain	None to mild	None to mild	None to moderate	None to severe	None to severe
Myometrial tone	Normal	Normal	Increased	Hypertonic	Normal to increased
Uterine tenderness	None	Usually none	Marked, usually diffuse	Marked and diffuse	None to moderate
Fetal status at first examination	Alive	Alive	Frequently alive; in jeopardy	Dead or in jeopardy	Dead or in jeopardy
Presentation	High incidence of breech, oblique, transverse	Normal distribution	Normal distribution	Normal distribution	Normal distribution if not extruded
Station of presenting part	High	Variable	Variable	Variable	High
Shock	Uncommon	None	Frequent	Usual	Frequent
Coagulopathy	None	None	Occasional	Frequent	Rare
Association with hypertension	Normal distribution	Normal distribution	Increased	Increased	Normal distribution

course of management.[26,27] In 20% to 25% of cases, the diagnosis is strengthened by sonographic demonstration of a retroplacental mass, but negative findings do not exclude life-threatening placental abruption. Valuable time should not be lost performing an ultrasound when there is obvious fetal distress or when the maternal condition is unstable.

In marginal and mild degrees of premature separation of the placenta, scant to moderate dark vaginal bleeding may occur. The uterus is often irritable, and the patient may have vague lower abdominal or back discomfort. There may be contractions of relatively normal frequency, duration, and intensity. The fetus is rarely affected, and maternal vital signs are unchanged. Although these patients usually require no immediate intervention, careful monitoring is indicated because these findings may herald a more severe degree of separation. Approximately 30% of patients with mild abruption have few or no signs or symptoms, and the diagnosis is often made retrospectively after delivery of a placenta with a small retroplacental clot.

In the case of moderate abruption, the clinical findings are more classic, but the fetus is still alive. Usually, more than one-fourth but less than one-half of the placental surface has separated. The onset of symptoms may be gradual or abrupt and may consist of continuous abdominal (uterine) pain followed promptly by vaginal bleeding. The uterus is tender, contracting, and fails to relax completely between contractions. Fetal distress is common. The patient's fibrinogen level is usually mildly reduced to 150 to 250 mg/dl. Although external bleeding is typically moderate in amount, the total blood loss may be much more. Cold, clammy skin, tachycardia, hypotension, and oliguria indicate shock.

With severe abruption, more than one-half of the placenta separates from the uterus. The onset is characteristically abrupt, with brief or absent premonitory signs. The uterine pain is agonizing, often described as tearing, knife-like, and unremitting. The uterus is continuously board-like and ten-

der. In most patients, external bleeding is moderate to severe, but it may be concealed. The fetus is almost always stillborn. Nearly one-half have died by the time the mother is admitted.[28] Fibrinogen levels are often reduced, and shock ensues with astonishing speed.

Coagulopathy

The most common cause of consumptive coagulopathy in pregnancy is placental abruption.[23] Overt hypofibrinogenemia (<150 mg/dl), elevated levels of fibrinogen–fibrin degradation products, and variable decreases in other coagulation factors can be demonstrated in about 30% of women with a placental abruption severe enough to kill the fetus. These coagulation defects are less common in cases in which the fetus survives. The major mechanisms are disseminated intravascular coagulation (DIC) and, to a lesser degree, retroplacental bleeding.

Renal Failure

Acute renal failure is rare with lesser degrees of placental abruption, but it is seen in the severe forms when there is delayed or incomplete treatment of hypovolemia. Although renal failure from cortical necrosis is seen in fatal cases, acute tubular necrosis is more commonly encountered. The precise cause of renal damage is unclear. Major factors include seriously impaired renal perfusion from reduced cardiac output and intrarenal vasospasm as a consequence of massive hemorrhage and, at times, coexisting acute or chronic hypertensive disorders.

Management

When abruption is suspected, management depends on the stage of gestation and the condition of the mother and infant.

With even a mild abruption, the patient should be observed closely, with continuous external FHR monitoring in the labor–delivery area for at least 4 to 6 hours or until signs and symptoms have subsided. Abruption mistaken for false labor or premature labor may have disastrous consequences if the patient is sent home. The severity of placental separation can progress, particularly after abdominal trauma. In such cases, there may be sudden fetal distress or loss of fetal heart tones requiring immediate cesarean section.[29,30] Placental abruption is rare in trauma patients who have no uterine contractions or who have contractions at a frequency of less than one every 10 minutes after 4 hours of monitoring. Of those women who have uterine contractions with greater frequency, almost 20% have placental abruption.

Although the incidence of fetomaternal hemorrhage in patients with abruption is low, it is fivefold higher in women who have experienced trauma.[31] The mean estimated fetal to maternal bleed is usually less than 15 ml, and 300 µg of Rh immune globulin (i.e., one ampule) will protect nearly all D-negative patients from D immunization.[31,39] Fetal and neonatal anemia, fetal cardiac arrhythmias, and fetal death have all been reported, but it is doubtful that the routine use of the Kleihauer–Betke assay or similar testing can help prevent adverse outcomes.

If external bleeding stops and there are no signs of further separation, the patient should remain in the hospital for a longer period of observation before a final decision is made on the safety of conservative management. Monitoring should be continued and further evaluation carried out if uterine contractions, a worrisome FHR pattern, vaginal bleeding, or significant uterine tenderness or irritability is present. Blood loss is typically underestimated, and serial vital signs should be followed. A rational goal of therapy is to achieve a urine output of at least 30 ml/hr and a hematocrit of greater than 30% with the liberal use of intravenous fluids and blood products. With any signs of maternal or fetal compromise, or if the patient is past 37 weeks of gestation, it is usually best to prepare for delivery after performing a double-setup examination. Once the absence of placenta previa is confirmed, the membranes can be ruptured. An oxytocin infusion is started if labor is desultory or incoordinate, and continuous electronic monitoring of the fetus should be maintained. Continued bleeding, failure of the uterus to relax between contractions, and fetal distress are indications for cesarean delivery.

With greater degrees of abruption, a more aggressive approach and prompt delivery will most often be the treatment of choice. The immediate objectives of treatment are to restore blood loss, maintain constant surveillance of the fetus, and anticipate and treat clotting defects. In the case of actual or impending shock, the following should be done rapidly:

1. At least 3 U of blood should be screened or matched. A vein should be kept open with a large-bore catheter and infusion of Ringer lactate or a crystalloid solution. Blood should be drawn for hemoglobin, hematocrit, and coagulation studies (e.g., fibrinogen, platelet count, fibrin degradation products, prothrombin time, and partial thromboplastin time). These should be repeated at frequent intervals until the patient is out of danger. While waiting for the initial results of the laboratory tests, the physician can perform a rapid clot test. Blood is placed in a red-topped tube. If a clot does not form within 6 minutes or forms and lyses within 30 minutes, a coagulation defect is probably present, and the fibrinogen level is less than 150 mg/dl. The management of shock and the correction of DIC associated with abruption are outlined in Chapter 32.

2. In all cases of moderate abruption, the fetus is at high risk, and fetal distress will develop in as many as 60% of patients. Continuous electronic fetal heart monitoring is essential if abnormalities are to be detected in time for the obstetrician to deal with them.

3. A vaginal examination should be carried out, and the membranes ruptured. Many patients with placental abruption will be in spontaneous labor. If labor does not ensue promptly, an oxytocin infusion should be started at a rate of 1 mU/min and increased at appropriate intervals until effective labor occurs. With careful electronic FHR monitoring, up to 48% of these patients may be delivered vaginally.[23] The mother should be observed closely for the amount of bleeding, vital signs, urinary output, and coagulation defects. Cesarean section is performed if there is evidence of fetal distress, maternal bleeding becomes excessive, effective labor is not established, or delivery cannot be anticipated within a reasonable period of time.

The appropriate method of delivery is somewhat controversial, but cesarean section is now used much more liberally. Vaginal delivery is possible in patients with mild and moderate abruption if there is no evidence of fetal distress and bleeding is not excessive. However, sudden changes in FHR patterns and fetal death can occur in labor, and increased fetal survival in patients who have been delivered by cesarean has been reported.[28]

If severe separation has caused fetal death, vaginal delivery is preferred unless brisk hemorrhage cannot be successfully managed with vigorous blood replacement or because of other obstetric complications. The patient's clotting status should be determined and corrected along with hypovolemia and hypotension (see Chapter 30). Coagulation defects present serious bleeding problems with cesarean delivery.

Complications

Maternal complications associated with moderate and severe placental separation may result from either the disease or the treatment. Hypofibrinogenemia and thrombocytopenia are the coagulation abnormalities most prominently associated with severe abruption. Uncontrolled bleeding from DIC is treated with lactated Ringer solution, blood replacement, cryoprecipitate-containing fibrinogen, and platelet packs. Postpartum hemorrhage should be anticipated, especially with severe separation. Although the uterus may feel firm, its contractile efficiency and ability to close off bleeding sinuses may be greatly impaired by extravasation of blood between the muscle fibers throughout the myometrium, as in the Couvelaire uterus. The problem may be compounded by the persistence of a clotting defect. If conservative measures, such as correction of the coagulopathy, bimanual compression of the uterus, and administration of oxytocic drugs, fail, the ultimate means of controlling the bleeding is by ligation of the hypogastric arteries or by hysterectomy. However, the usual course for the coagulopathy is gradual improvement after delivery. Therefore, surgical procedures should be avoided if possible because difficulties with hemostasis often lead to even more problems with hematomas and increased bleeding.

Prevention of renal failure consists mainly of early detection and treatment of shock, meticulous replacement of blood loss, and proper treatment of any infection that may be present or anticipated. Monitoring the response of the central venous or pulmonary wedge pressure and urinary output to a provocative test may allow early detection of renal difficulty and prevent renal failure (see Chapter 30).

Pituitary necrosis (i.e., Sheehan syndrome), which may follow ischemia, results from the same changes that precipitate renal failure. Lactation at the proper time in the puerperium suggests that the pituitary gland has escaped serious damage. Thyrotropic, adrenotropic, and gonadotropic pituitary function may be destroyed singly or in combination. Return of menses is adequate evidence of gonadotropic activity. Tests of thyroid and adrenal function 4 to 6 months after delivery are appropriate follow-up for patients who have suffered severe abruptio placenta.

◊ CIRCUMVALLATE PLACENTA

An uncommon variation of placental abruption is circumvallate placenta (see Chapter 4), which can also cause bleeding in the second or third trimester of pregnancy. In addition to antepartum hemorrhage, prematurity, and perinatal death, fetal malformations are increased in patients with this condition.[32] The bleeding is bright red, moderate, and nearly always painless. When bleeding occurs before fetal maturity, the patient may be treated expectantly. Ultrasonic placental localization usually rules out placenta previa. If bleeding is persistent or heavy, if the patient is in labor, and if placenta previa cannot be ruled out, double-setup examination is indicated. In most cases, the treatment is induction of labor unless there is another indication for cesarean. At times, this complication is responsible for the spontaneous onset of preterm labor; as a result, there is an increased perinatal mortality rate. The definitive diagnosis is made by inspection of the placenta after delivery.

◊ RUPTURE OF THE UTERUS

Either spontaneous or traumatic rupture of the uterus may occur before or during labor (see Chapter 29). It is a serious hazard to the mother, and the fetus usually dies if it is ex-truded into the peritoneal cavity or if the maternal hypovolemia is so profound that fetal oxygenation becomes inadequate. The major causes of rupture of the uterus are weakness of the uterine wall because of incision (e.g., for a previous cesarean, hysterotomy, myomectomy, metroplasty) and difficult operative delivery (e.g., breech extraction or difficult forceps delivery, especially version and extraction). Injuries such as gunshot wounds and seat belt injuries account for a small percentage of cases. This is not to suggest that pregnant women should abandon seat belts; uterine rupture is less serious than possible death if this protection is not used. Improperly monitored or inappropriate use of oxytocic agents, especially in parous women, has been associated with a significant number of cases. The use of constant-infusion pumps allows for safer administration, and the continuous monitoring of the frequency, duration, and strength of uterine contractions is mandatory to avoid uterine tetany. Lower uterine segment rupture because of neglected obstructed labor now occurs rarely in developed countries.

As with any ruptured viscus, pain usually, but not always, precedes the definitive tear. Pain and shock follow, but the pain may lessen after the rupture occurs. Depending on the location of the rupture, bleeding may be scant or heavy, and some of the blood may escape vaginally. The therapeutic surgical procedure must be tailored to the findings at laparotomy. If the tear is clean and amenable to repair, the edges may be freshened and the defect sutured. If repair is not reasonable, the uterus should be removed. In a patient whose condition is compromised, a supracervical hysterectomy may solve the immediate emergency more quickly and easily than a total hysterectomy.

◊ SUMMARY

The most serious causes of antepartum hemorrhage are placenta previa and placental abruption. The basic principles of immediate care of these women include assessment of the fetus and prompt maternal resuscitation if required. Ultrasonography has become important to establish or rule out the diagnosis of placenta previa. Expectant management for both complications is appropriate if the mother's condition is stable and the infant is premature. Early delivery is necessary with repeated or severe bleeding and with fetal distress if the baby is sufficiently mature to be capable of survival.

◊ REFERENCES

1. Scott JR. Vaginal bleeding in the midtrimester of pregnancy. *Am J Obstet Gynecol* 1972;113:329.
2. Nielson EC, Varner MW, Scott JR. The outcome of pregnancies complicated by bleeding during the second trimester. *Surg Obstet Gynecol* 1991;173:371.
3. McShane PM, Heyl PS, Epstein MF. Maternal and perinatal morbidity resulting from placenta previa. *Obstet Gynecol* 1985;65:176.
4. Brar HS, Platt LD, DeVore GR, et al. Fetal umbilical velocimetry for the surveillance of pregnancies complicated by placenta previa. *J Reprod Med* 1988;33:741.
5. Oppenheimer LW, Farine D, Knox Ritchie JW. The classification of placenta praevia—time for a change? *Fetal Matern Med Rev* 1992;4:73.

6. Thorp JM, Councell RB, Sandridge DA, Wiest HH. Antepartum diagnosis of placenta previa percreta by magnetic resonance imaging. *Obstet Gynecol* 1992;80:506.
7. Boive J, Rochester D, Cadkin A, et al. Accuracy of placental localization by ultrasound. *Radiology* 1978; 128:177.
8. Tan NH, Abu M, Woo JLS, Tabir HM. The role of transvaginal ultrasonography in the diagnosis of placenta previa. *Aust NZ J Obstet Gynecol* 1995;35:42.
9. Cotton D, Ead J, Paul R, Quilligan EJ. The conservative aggressive management of placenta previa. *Am J Obstet Gynecol* 1980;17:687.
10. Silver R, Depp R, Sabbaga RE, et al. Placenta previa: aggressive expectant management. *Am J Obstet Gynecol* 1984;150:15.
11. Newton ER, Barss V, Cetrulo CL. The epidemiology and clinical history of asymptomatic midtrimester placenta previa. *Am J Obstet Gynecol* 1984;148:743.
12. Lavery JP. Placenta previa. *Clin Obstet Gynecol* 1990;33:414.
13. Watson WJ, Cefalo RC. Magnesium sulfate tocolysis in selected patients with symptomatic placenta previa. *Am J Perinatol* 1990;7:251.
14. Arias F. Cervical cerclage for the temporary treatment of patients with placenta previa. *Obstet Gynecol* 1988;71:545.
15. D'Angelo LJ, Irwin LF. Conservative management of placenta previa: a cost-benefit analysis. *Am J Obstet Gynecol* 1984;149:320.
16. Love CD, Wallace EM. Pregnancies complicated by placenta previa: what is appropriate management? *Br J Obstet Gynaecol* 1996;103:864.
17. Wing DA, Paul RH, Miller LK. Management of symptomatic placenta previa: a randomized, controlled trial of inpatient versus outpatient expectant management. *Am J Obstet Gynecol* 1996;175:806.
18. Harding JA, Lewis DF, Major CA, et al. Color flow Doppler—a useful instrument in the diagnosis of vasa previa. *Am J Obstet Gynecol* 1990;163:1566.
19. Abdella TN, Sibai BM, Harp JM, et al. Perinatal outcome in abruptio placentae. *Obstet Gynecol* 1984;63:365.
20. Kramer MS, Usher RH, Pollack R, et al. Etiologic determinants of abruptio placentae. *Obstet Gynecol* 1997;89:221.
21. Anath CV, Savitz DA, Williams MA. Placental abruption and its association with hypertension and prolonged rupture of membranes: a methodologic review and meta-analysis. *Obstet Gynecol* 1996;88:309.
22. Pritchard JA, Cunningham FG, Pritchard SA, Mason RA. On reducing the frequency of severe abruptio placentae. *Am J Obstet Gynecol* 1990;33:406.
23. Lowe TW, Cunningham FG. Placental abruption. *Clin Obstet Gynecol* 1990;33:406.
24. Chasnoff IJ, Burns WJ, Schnoll SH, et al. Cocaine use in pregnancy. *N Engl J Med* 1985;313:666.
25. Karegard M, Gennser G. Incidence and recurrence rate of abruptio placentae in Sweden. *Obstet Gynecol* 1986;67:1986.
26. Hurd WW, Miodovnik M, Hertzberg V, Lavin JP. Selective management of abruptio placentae: a prospective study. *Obstet Gynecol* 1983;61:467.
27. Sholl JS. Abruptio placentae. Clinical management in nonacute cases. *Am J Obstet Gynecol* 1987;156:40.
28. Knab DR. Abruptio placentae. An assessment of the time and method of delivery. *Obstet Gynecol* 1978;52:625.
29. Kettel ML, Branch DW, Scott JR. Occult placental abruption following maternal trauma. *Obstet Gynecol* 1988;71:449.
30. Pearlman MD, Tintinalli JE, Lorenz RP. A prospective controlled study of outcome after trauma during pregnancy. *Am J Obstet Gynecol* 1990;162:665.
31. Goodwin TM, Breen M, Kelly JV. Pregnancy outcome and fetomaternal hemorrhage after non-catastrophic trauma. *Am J Obstet Gynecol* 1990;126:665.
32. Bey M, Dott A, Miller JM. The sonographic diagnosis of circumvallate placenta. *Obstet Gynecol* 1991;78:515.

CHAPTER 27

Malpresentations and Umbilical Cord Complications

$$\Diamond$$

Dwight P. Cruikshank

◊ BREECH PRESENTATION

Breech presentation, the most common obstetric malpresentation, complicates approximately 4% of deliveries.

Definitions

Breech presentation is a polar alignment of the fetus in which the fetal buttocks present at the maternal pelvic inlet. Three types are recognized: frank, incomplete, and complete. In frank breech presentation, the fetal hips are flexed and the knees extended, so that the thighs are apposed to the abdomen and the lower legs to the chest (Fig. 1). The buttocks are the most dependent part of the fetus, and the presenting part fills the pelvis and presents a good dilating wedge to the cervix. Overall, frank breech presentation accounts for 60% to 65% of breech presentations; it is more common at term.

In the incomplete breech presentation, the fetus has one or both hips incompletely flexed so that some part of the fetal lower extremity, rather than the buttocks, is the most dependent part (hence the terms single footling or double footling). The presenting part does not fill the pelvis well and is a poor dilating wedge. This presentation accounts for 25% to 35% of breech presentations and is more common among premature fetuses.

Complete breech presentation is the least common type, accounting for about 5% of breech presentations. In this situation, the fetal hips and knees are both flexed so that the thighs are apposed to the abdomen and the legs lie on the thighs. The buttocks are the most dependent part, providing the advantages described above for the frank breech presentation. However, some of these fetuses convert to incomplete breech presentations as labor progresses.

The position of the breech fetus is described with the fetal sacrum as the reference point; thus, it is right sacrum anterior, left sacrum posterior, left sacrum transverse, and so forth.

A spontaneous breech delivery is one in which the entire infant delivers vaginally without manual aid. The recommended form of vaginal delivery is the assisted breech delivery, also known as partial breech extraction. In this delivery the fetus is allowed to deliver by the forces of uterine contractions and maternal bearing-down efforts until the fetal umbilicus has passed over the mother's perineum. After this, delivery of the legs, trunk, and arms is assisted manually; the head may be delivered manually or with forceps. A complete breech extraction, in which manual assistance is applied by traction in the groins or on the lower extremities before complete delivery of the buttocks, is rarely, if ever, indicated in singleton breech presentations.

Incidence

Breech presentation is associated closely with birthweight. Breech presentation accounts for 4% of births overall but occurs in 15% of deliveries of low-birthweight (<2500 g) infants. Furthermore, the smaller the infant, the higher is the incidence of breech presentation, which rises to 30% among infants weighing 1000 g to 1499 g and to 40% among those weighing less than 1000 g.

Viewed from another perspective, the association between breech presentation and low birthweight is even more striking. Only 70% of infants who present as breeches weigh more than 2500 g; 30% weigh less than 2500 g (compared with 5% to 6% of infants who are in vertex presentation), and 12% are of very low birthweight, weighing less than 1500 g.

Cause

Factors that predispose to breech presentation are listed in Table 1. The importance of fetal anomalies cannot be overemphasized (Table 2). Malformations of the central nervous system complicate 1.5% to 2.0% of breech births: the incidence

419

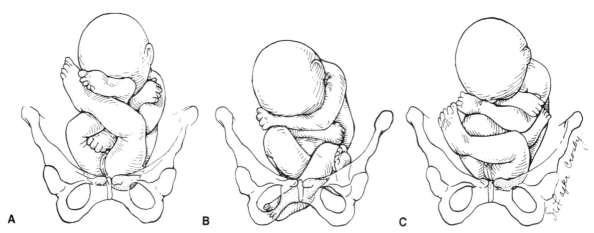

FIG. 1. Fetal attitude in **(A)** frank, **(B)** incomplete, and **(C)** complete breech presentations.

of hydrocephalus is 10-fold greater, and that of anencephaly twofold to fivefold greater, than among infants presenting as vertex. Up to 1% of infants in breech presentation have a significant chromosomal anomaly: one in 200 has Down syndrome, and the incidence of other autosomal trisomies is also increased. Of those infants presenting as breeches, the incidence of major congenital anomalies overall is 17% among premature infants, 9% among term infants, and 50% among term infants who die in the perinatal period. It is prudent to keep these numbers in mind when deciding on a method of delivery for a fetus in breech presentation.

An association between cerebral palsy and breech presentation (although not with vaginal breech delivery) has been recognized for many years. The realization that most fetal insults leading to cerebral palsy occur before delivery suggests that neurologic dysfunction may be a cause of breech presentation.

In more than 50% of cases, no causative factor for breech presentation can be identified.

TABLE 1. *Factors predisposing to breech presentation*

Fetal anomalies
Head anomalies
Anencephaly
Hydrocephalus
Chromosomal anomalies
Autosomal trisomies
Multiple anomaly syndromes
Uterine anomalies
Septate
Bicornuate
Unicornuate
Uterine overdistension
Polyhydramnios
Multiple gestation
High parity with lax abdominal
and uterine musculature
Pelvic obstruction
Placenta previa
Myomata
Other pelvic tumors

Diagnosis

On abdominal examination, Leopold's first maneuver demonstrates the fetal head in the fundus. The third maneuver reveals the softer breech over the pelvic inlet. It is useful to remember that the head narrows down to the neck before attaching to the body, whereas there is no such tapering between the breech and body. Auscultation of fetal heart tones with a stethoscope usually reveals them to be loudest in the upper quadrants of the uterus when the fetus is in a breech presentation.

The diagnosis is often made by vaginal examination when the cervix is open. In frank or complete breech presentation, the anal orifice may be felt, with the bony prominences of the ischial tuberosities directly lateral to it. Face presentation may be difficult to distinguish from frank breech presentation, with the fetal mouth being mistaken for the anus. It is helpful to remember that the mouth is surrounded by bone, whereas the anus is not. In incomplete breech presentations, palpation of the feet on vaginal examination is diagnostic. During labor, any presentation that is not clearly vertex by vaginal examination should be confirmed by ultrasound.

Perinatal Mortality

Perinatal mortality is much higher in breech presentation than in vertex, being fourfold greater among term infants and

TABLE 2. *Congenital malformations among term infants in breech presentation*[a]

Type of malformation	Incidence (%)
Central nervous system	1.7
Hydrocephalus	0.6
Anencephaly	0.4
Trisomy 21	0.5
Cardiovascular	0.6
Gastrointestinal	0.5
Genitourinary	0.1
Overall	9.0
Overall among term infants who die	50.0

[a]From ref. 15, with permission.

twofold to threefold greater among premature infants. Much of this excess mortality is not preventable; according to Kaupilla,[15] 64% of deaths among term infants in breech presentation are caused by malformations or infection. Among premature infants, malformations, infection, maternal disease, and intrauterine death before labor account for 56% of perinatal mortality, and complications of prematurity unrelated to the method of delivery account for another 11%. Thus, only about one-third of perinatal deaths among infants who present as breeches are related to potentially preventable factors. These factors basically fall into two groups: trauma and asphyxia.

Trauma to the head is a significant risk in both term and premature breech infants regardless of the route of delivery. Unlike the situation in vertex presentation, in which the fetal head is in the maternal pelvis for hours or days, during which molding can occur, the aftercoming head of the breech fetus must come through the pelvis as is—there is no time for molding. Thus, minor variations in maternal pelvic architecture, which would be insignificant in vertex presentation, may become major risks. This problem is compounded for the premature infant, in whom the head is the largest part. In these circumstances the fetal body may deliver through an incompletely dilated cervix, which then entraps the head. Performance of a cesarean does not ensure atraumatic delivery of the aftercoming head. An inadequate incision or suboptimal uterine relaxation may result in head entrapment as serious as that which can occur with vaginal delivery.

Damage to fetal muscles, soft tissue, and viscera may occur with both vaginal and cesarean delivery if the fetus is grasped by the operator in places other than its bony pelvis. Likewise, either type of delivery may be associated with nerve injury if the arms are not delivered properly, especially if there are nuchal arms. Finally, trauma to the cervical spinal cord may occur with vaginal delivery of a breech fetus with hyperextension of the neck.

Asphyxia may be caused by prolapse of the umbilical cord. The incidence of cord prolapse in term fetuses in frank breech presentation is 0.4%. In complete breech presentation, the incidence is 5% to 6%, and with incomplete breech presentation, the incidence may be as high as 10%. Cord prolapse in incomplete breech presentation, although an indication for prompt cesarean delivery, is often not the devastating event that it is in vertex or frank breech presentation. Because the cord is prolapsed between the fetal legs, it often is not markedly compressed during subsequent contractions.

Not all of the excess asphyxia among fetuses in breech presentation is caused by overt cord prolapse. Abnormalities of the fetal heart rate pattern are four to eight times more common in fetuses in a breech presentation than in fetuses in vertex. An unknown percentage of this is undoubtedly a result of occult cord prolapse and other forms of cord compression.

Antepartum Management

Breech presentation diagnosed before 32 of weeks gestation should be managed expectantly. The fetuses of approximately two-thirds of multiparas and one-third of primigravidas who are diagnosed as being in breech presentation before 32 weeks of gestation will convert to vertex presentation spontaneously before labor. Breech presentation that persists into the late third trimester should be evaluated by an ultrasound examination for congenital anomalies. Pelvimetry and other radiographic evaluations are best delayed until the onset of labor for two reasons: (1) the fetus may convert to vertex presentation before labor, making exposure of the mother and fetus to radiation unnecessary, and (2) radiographs early in labor give essential information about the attitude of the fetal head, neck, and arms and the relationship of the fetus to the maternal pelvis—information that is needed to determine the route of delivery.

When a breech presentation persists beyond 32 weeks of gestation, some obstetricians recommend attempts at converting the presentation to vertex by external cephalic version. Ranney reported his experience with 860 patients managed by external version.[24] Attempts were made to turn the fetus to vertex whenever breech presentation was found in the third trimester, and some patients had repeated versions performed. Ranney was able to lower the incidence of breech presentation at term to 0.6%, about one-sixth the expected number, and encountered no fetal trauma or death and no increase in the incidence of placental abruptions.

The results of Kasule and co-workers[14] are less optimistic. All patients with fetuses in breech presentation after 30 weeks of gestation were prospectively randomized to either an external version group (310 patients) or a control group (330 patients). The subjects in the external version group had the procedure performed between 33 and 36 weeks of gestation. If the first attempt failed, or if the fetus reverted to breech presentation, the procedure was repeated up to three times in subsequent weekly visits. No attempts at external version were made after 36 weeks of gestation. Although their immediate success rate was 80%, 46% of fetuses spontaneously reverted to breech presentation. There were three perinatal deaths attributed to the procedure: two from abruptio placentae and one from premature labor and delivery. Most importantly, the incidence of breech presentation at delivery was 52% in the external version group and 51% in the control group, with 49% of fetuses in the control group converting to vertex presentation spontaneously before delivery. The authors surmised that many, if not all, of their successful external versions may have been in patients whose fetuses would have converted spontaneously had nothing been done. This hypothesis, coupled with the three perinatal deaths, led them to conclude that "there is no place for external cephalic version before 36 weeks gestation."

This view is supported by the data of Westgren and associates,[27] who investigated the incidence of spontaneous conversion of breech presentation to vertex in the last trimester. Of all fetuses identified at 32 weeks of gestation to be in breech presentation, 57% spontaneously converted to vertex by term, whereas 43% persisted as breech. Factors that reduced the likelihood of spontaneous conversion included nulliparity, previous breech delivery, and extended fetal legs. The data of Westgren and associates[27] are presented in Table 3. These data, combined with those of Kasule,[14] seem to indicate that the most opportune time to attempt external cephalic version is at 36 weeks of gestation in the nullipara and 38 weeks in the multipara.

If external version is to be attempted, monitoring of the fetal position and heart rate by real-time ultrasound is prudent. In the past, the consensus has been that no anesthesia should be used, and pain is considered a reason to discontinue the attempt. Recently, however, those who believe that vaginal breech birth is not an option and that the delivery must be by cesarean unless the external version is successful have proposed a different approach. This involves waiting until the pregnancy has progressed at least to 37 weeks of gestation, at which time epidural anesthesia is instituted. External version is attempted, and, if this is successful, the patient has an immediate induction of labor; if unsuccessful, the patient is delivered by cesarean. In either case, the epidural used for the external version attempt is used for the delivery as well. This approach seems to have merit provided one is careful not to be overly aggressive with attempts at external version in an anesthetized patient. Some physicians also recommend tocolysis with subcutaneous terbutaline during attempts at external version, although in many cases this does not seem to be necessary.

Lau and associates[18] reported a prospective case-controlled study of external version. They reported an overall success rate of 57% in nulligravidas and 84% in multiparous. They also found a rate of reversion to breech presentation of 4%. Complications included a 3.3% incidence of transient fetal bradycardia and a 0.4% rate (one case) of what the authors called placental abruption. This particular patient had a 3-minute episode of fetal bradycardia and some vaginal spotting, although nothing suggesting abruption was found at the time of emergency cesarean. These same investigators[19] have recently reported another series of 243 women who underwent attempts at external version. Regression analysis identified three independent predictors of failed version: (1) engaged presenting part, (2) difficulty palpating the fetal head, and (3) nulliparity. The chance of success was 0% if all three

TABLE 3. *Spontaneous conversion of breech to vertex presentation[a]*

Gestational week	Probability of spontaneous conversion	
	Multipara (%)	Nullipara (%)
32	78	46
33	75	35
34	70	30
35	65	22
36	53	15
37	35	10
38	22	2
39	7	1

[a]Adapted from ref. 27, with permission.

variables were present, less than 20% if any two were present, 30% to 60% if only one was present, and 94% if none were present. Interestingly, placental location, position of the fetal spine, attitude of the fetal legs, and maternal obesity were not significant variables for predicting successful version when the other variables were controlled.

It should be noted that successful external version does not necessarily reduce the cesarean rate to that found in other vertex presentations. Lau and colleagues[18] reported a 32% cesarean rate in nulliparous patients after successful external version to vertex presentation; the rate in multiparous patients was 11%. Likewise, Laros and colleagues[17] reported a 30% cesarean rate after successful external version compared to a 15% rate in all other term singleton vertex pregnancies.

Active labor and ruptured membranes are absolute contraindications to the procedure. Relative contraindications include an engaged presenting part and an estimated fetal weight of 4000 g or more. Whether a previous cesarean contraindicates attempts at external version is uncertain, although a recent series of 56 such patients reported a success rate of 82%, with no serious maternal or fetal complications. That success rate seems high, however. Most recent studies of external version in patients without previous cesarean report overall success rates of 50% to 70%.

Management of Labor and Delivery

Term Breech Presentation

Cheng and Hannah[6] published a critical review of the literature on singleton term breech pregnancies, reviewing all articles in the English language literature between 1966 and 1992. They found that there were only 24 studies that presented results according to the intended mode of delivery and that presented outcome data in sufficient detail to be analyzable. Of these 24 reports, only two were randomized trials; eight were prospective cohort studies, and 14 were retrospective cohort studies. Twenty-two of these studies, including both prospective trials, did not demonstrate a statistically significant difference in corrected perinatal mortality between those patients for whom a vaginal delivery was planned and those for whom a cesarean was planned. Two series did show significantly worse outcomes among those for whom vaginal delivery was planned. Furthermore, when the authors combined all of the data, they produced a "typical odds ratio" of 3.86, for the 95% CI of 2.22 to 6.69. Their data on low 5-minute Apgar scores and traumatic neonatal morbidity were similar to the data on perinatal mortality in that the overwhelming majority of individual studies did not find a difference between those for whom vaginal birth was planned and those for whom cesarean was planned. However, when the studies were combined, the planned vaginal delivery group faired worse in both categories. The authors of this review carefully point out all of the flaws in the papers they reviewed and conclude that most of these studies were too poorly done to allow definitive conclusions. They conclude their paper by stating "the only way to obtain more definitive information regarding the effectiveness of a policy of elective cesarean vs. that of a trial of labor in women with breech presentation at term is to mount an appropriately sized, randomized control trial. In the absence of such a trial, a policy of elective cesarean delivery appears to be a reasonable option for the woman with breech presentation at term."

The enthusiasm for universal cesarean delivery for term fetuses in breech presentation must be tempered by the data of Green and colleagues[13] from the Royal Victoria Hospital in Montreal. During the years 1963 through 1973, they delivered 595 term infants in breech presentation, 22% by cesarean. From 1978 through 1979, they delivered 175 term infants in breech presentation, 94% by cesarean. Despite a greater than fourfold increase in the rate to nearly universal cesarean delivery, there was no difference between the two time periods in the incidences of intrapartum fetal death, neonatal death, fetal/neonatal trauma, asphyxia neonatorum, or neonatal central nervous system abnormality. The most recent update of the register of clinical trials maintained by the Cochrane Pregnancy and Childbirth Group (Fig. 2) concludes that the policy of planned cesarean section was associated with significantly more actual cesarean sections (odds ratio 6.44, 95% confidence interval 3.93 to 10.53); increased maternal morbidity (1.63, 1.03 to 2.57); a nonsignificant trend toward fewer brachial plexus injuries and 5-minute Apgar scores below 7; and in one study reduced short-term neonatal morbidity. *The studies were too small to address the question of perinatal morbidity adequately* (emphasis added). It must be pointed out, however, that the Cochrane review could identify only three randomized controlled trials regarding delivery method for term breeches, and only 20 cited cases met the predefined inclusion criteria. The "evidence-based" approach to this problem, therefore, is hampered by the paucity of "evidence."

As noted, there are only two randomized controlled trials regarding term breech presentation. Collea and associates[8] performed a randomized, prospective study of term fetuses in frank breech presentation. Of the 208 patients enrolled in the study, 93 were randomized to the group to be delivered by cesarean; five had vaginal deliveries before the cesarean could be done. One hundred fifteen women were randomized to the trial of labor category; these women then had radiographic pelvimetry performed, and the criteria for pelvic nor-

malcy were so rigid that 52 were deemed to have pelves inadequate for vaginal breech delivery. Of the patients with radiologically adequate pelves, 49 had vaginal deliveries. Thus, 43% of patients (49 of 115) originally randomized to the trial-of-labor category had vaginal deliveries. As expected, maternal outcomes in terms of febrile morbidity, need for blood transfusions, and the length of hospital stay were much better in the group whose infants were delivered vaginally. The perinatal mortality was zero in both groups. There was one significant fetal injury among the patients who delivered vaginally, but this occurred in a patient whose delivery was in violation of the protocol. These authors concluded that the properly selected term fetus in frank breech presentation can be delivered vaginally with safety.

Gimovsky and associates[11] performed a similar randomized prospective study of patients with term, nonfrank (complete and incomplete) breech presentations, except that two patients were randomized to the trial-of-labor category for each one randomized to cesarean delivery. Once again, rigid criteria for pelvic adequacy led to 33% of patients originally randomized to the trial-of-labor group being excluded after radiographic pelvimetry. Overall, 44% of those allowed a trial of labor had vaginal deliveries. The vaginal delivery rate was 56% for complete and 34% for incomplete breech presentations. Maternal morbidity was much better in the group who had vaginal deliveries. Neonatal morbidity, as reflected by cord blood gas analyses, Apgar scores, birth injury, and hospital stay, was not different between the two groups. One infant in each group died of congenital malformations. A third infant delivered vaginally without difficulty died because of "inadequate resuscitation." The conclusion of this study was that a trial of labor under carefully selected conditions is a reasonable alternative to cesarean delivery for the term fetus in a nonfrank breech presentation.

Schiff and colleagues[25] published a retrospective review of 846 term breeches managed by protocol at a single institution. They evaluated their data based on intention to treat, with 613 patients being in the trial of labor group and 233 in the planned cesarean group. They found an excess perinatal mortality in the trial-of-labor group of two infants, an incidence of one in 300. They reported that one of these deaths was from group B streptococcal infection and not preventable by the method of delivery. The other death was a result of trauma. They concluded that, in the 1990s, excess mortality

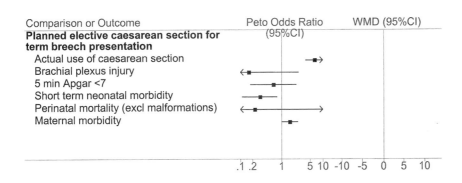

Comparison or Outcome	Peto Odds Ratio (95%CI)	WMD (95%CI)
Planned elective caesarean section for term breech presentation		
Actual use of caesarean section		
Brachial plexus injury		
5 min Apgar <7		
Short term neonatal morbidity		
Perinatal mortality (excl malformations)		
Maternal morbidity		

FIG. 2. Planned cesarean section for term breech. From the Cochrane Database of Systematic Reviews.

for a trial of labor in term breech presentation is approximately one in 300, and "probably is not significant."

Brown and co-workers[5] published a retrospective observational study of breeches born between 1980 and 1987. There was not a standard protocol for management of these cases. Interestingly, the authors did correct for cesareans done for the indication of fetal distress, feeling that including cesareans done for that indication could tend to make the outcomes in the cesarean group worse. They found no differences between the vaginally and cesarean-delivered groups in any perinatal outcome, including mortality, Apgar scores, and neonatal morbidity.

Bingham and colleagues[3] reported a retrospective review of 313 term singleton term breech deliveries delivered at one institution over a 3-year period. They found that there was no difference in any neonatal outcome parameter between those delivered vaginally and those delivered by cesarean. However, they did report a failed trial-of-labor rate of 40%, which is higher than that reported by Collea[8] or Gimovsky.[11] Many of their failures were in the second stage of labor and may have been related to the large number of patients who had epidural anesthesia. Nonetheless, they correctly point out that a high failed trial-of-labor rate makes a trial of labor less desirable because cesareans done after a failed trial of labor, or done on an emergency basis, carry more risk than those done electively.

The series of Crougham-Minihane et al.[9] and Kiely[16] are further reviews of the effect of route of delivery on neonatal morbidity and mortality.

Premature Breech Presentation

No randomized prospective data are published regarding delivery of the premature infant in breech presentation. Penn and co-workers[23] attempted a multicenter randomized controlled trial in 26 hospitals in England in an effort to determine the optimal mode of delivery for breech infants at gestational ages between 26 and 32 weeks. After 17 months of attempting to enroll patients, the study was abandoned because only 13 women from six hospitals had been recruited. The authors stated that the "low accrual rate was due to clinicians' reluctance to randomize eligible women." Therefore, management decisions must be made based on retrospective data, which suffer from serious shortcomings.

In 1977, Goldenberg and Nelson[12] advocated cesarean delivery for all infants in a breech position who weigh less than 2500 g. Their data showed an advantage for cesarean-delivered infants weighing 500 g to 1499 g in perinatal mortality and with low 5-minute Apgar scores. However, for infants weighing 1500 g or more, no such advantage could be demonstrated. Woods[28] found a 63% neonatal mortality rate for vaginally delivered breech infants weighing 1000 g to 1499 g, compared with 25% for those delivered by cesarean—a statistically significant difference. Among breech infants weighing 1500 g to 2500 g, there was no significant difference in neonatal mortality between the vaginal and cesarean groups. Most importantly, Woods' study in-

cluded long-term follow-up of the survivors and could not demonstrate an advantage for the cesarean group in terms of morbidity. Mann and Gallant[20] found a 47% neonatal mortality rate among vaginally delivered breech infants weighing 1000 g to 1499 g, compared with 30% in those delivered by cesarean, but could find no advantage to cesarean delivery for those weighing 1500 to 2500 g. The available retrospective data, therefore, suggest that breech presentation infants who weigh less than 1500 g are best delivered by cesarean.

Incomplete Breech Presentation

Because of the 10% incidence of cord prolapse, most obstetricians have advocated cesarean delivery for all infants in incomplete breech presentation. There are occasions, however, when exceptions to this rule should be made. For example, a multiparous patient or one near complete dilation with an incomplete breech that is well down in the pelvis probably may be delivered vaginally if she meets the other criteria for a vaginal birth.

The Primigravida

To separate primigravidas whose fetuses are in breech presentation as a group needing cesarean delivery is fallacious for two reasons. First, there are no data to suggest that primigravidas are at more risk than parous women for fetal injury, cord prolapse, difficult vaginal delivery, or perinatal death. Second, this philosophy implies that the parous woman in labor with a fetus in breech presentation is not at very high risk. Because this fetus may be larger than her previous infants, and because her pelvis may be adequate for vertex presentation but not for the unmolded head of a breech fetus, the parous woman is at no less risk. All women in labor with fetuses in breech presentations, whether parous or not, need to be evaluated and managed according to the same rigid criteria.

Extension of the Fetal Neck

Ballas and Toaff[2] demonstrated that when the fetal neck is hyperextended to an angle greater than 90° (Fig. 3), vaginal delivery is associated with a 70% incidence of fetal spinal cord transections. In their study, lesser degrees of extension (Fig. 4) were not associated with this complication; however, prudence dictates that extension of the fetal neck beyond the straight vertical is best managed by cesarean delivery because further extension may occur when the head enters the pelvis. However, the military attitude, in which the neck is neither flexed nor extended (Fig. 5), is not an indication for cesarean delivery.

Therefore, radiographic or ultrasound evaluation of the attitude of the fetal neck is mandatory if the physician is contemplating a trial of labor. Because extension of the neck is an intrinsic fetal condition caused by increased extensor muscle tone, and because the condition waxes and wanes, this evaluation should be performed early in labor rather than before.

A fetus with a normally flexed head but with the arms extended over the head is shown in Fig. 6. The potential for

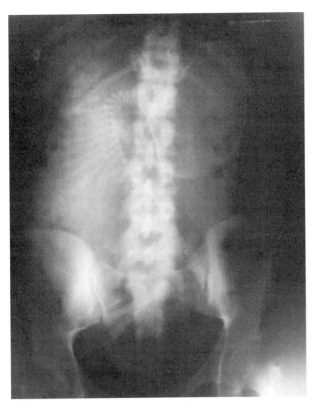

FIG. 3. Hyperextension of the fetal neck.

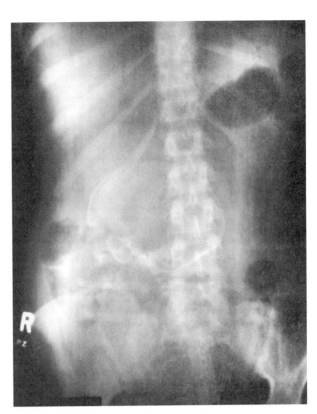

FIG. 5. The military attitude of the fetal head and neck: neither well flexed nor extended.

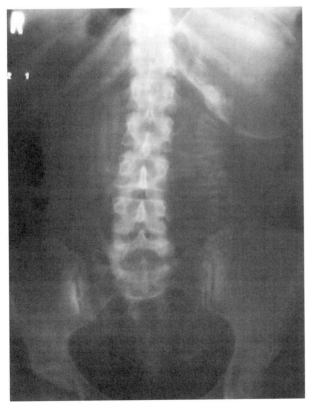

FIG. 4. Extension of the fetal neck.

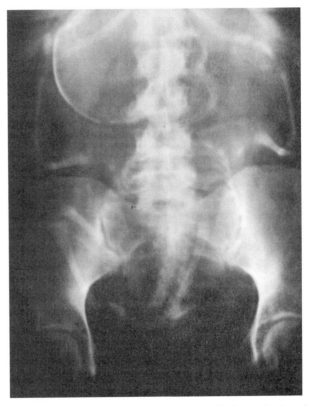

FIG. 6. Breech fetus with both arms extended over the head.

brachial plexus and arm injury is great in this circumstance. The patient should be delivered by cesarean with a generous uterine incision, and special care must be taken to deliver the arms atraumatically.

Patient Selection for Trial of Labor

The patient who arrives in labor with a fetus in breech presentation must be promptly evaluated to ascertain whether she is a candidate for a trial of labor. If she had previous cesarean, I believe she should undergo a repeat cesarean delivery, although there are insufficient data to either support or refute this recommendation.

The next deciding factor is the estimated fetal weight (EFW). If the EFW is less than 1500 g, most physicians would recommend a cesarian delivery based on the retrospective data presented above. Equally important is the other end of the spectrum, because the large fetus is at risk for entrapment of the unmolded head in the mother's bony pelvis. If the EFW is more than 3800 g (8.5 lb), cesarean delivery is indicated, even if in the past the woman was delivered of large infants vaginally from vertex presentation.

If the best estimate of fetal weight is between 1500 g and 3800 g, the next step is radiographic evaluation of the maternal pelvis. This must reveal the maternal pelvis to be gyne- coid in shape and the dimensions of the inlet and midpelvis to be of average size or greater. Guidelines for pelvic adequacy are 11 cm for the anteroposterior diameter of the inlet, 12 cm for the transverse diameter of the inlet and the anterior–posterior diameter of the midpelvis, and 9.5 cm for the transverse of the midpelvis (i.e., interspinous distance).

While the pelvimetry is being obtained, a radiograph of the maternal abdomen that includes the fetal body and head should be performed. The purpose of this film is twofold: to be certain the fetal neck is not extended and to search for fetal anomalies that would contraindicate cesarean delivery (e.g., anencephaly, massive hydrocephalus, thanatophoric dwarfism). This evaluation should be obtained before delivery, even if one is committed to cesarean delivery for all infants in breech presentation, to prevent the delivery of nonviable infants by this route. However, a thorough ultrasound is an adequate substitute for radiographs if cesarean delivery is planned.

The ideal method of radiographic pelvimetry is computed tomography (CT) scan. The chief advantage is that the radiation exposure to the fetus (2.3 mGy or 0.23 rad) is 80% lower than that with conventional x-ray pelvimetry (13 mGy or 1.3 rad). An additional advantage is that much better images are obtained in less time. Typically, three views are obtained, a lateral digital scout view (Fig. 7), an anteroposterior digital scout view (Fig. 8), and one axial section through the foveae of the femoral heads (Fig. 9). The lateral view is used to measure the anteroposterior diameters of the inlet and midpelvis, and the anteroposterior view to measure the transverse di-

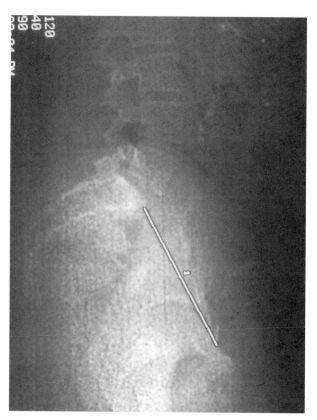

FIG. 7. Computed tomographic pelvimetry. Lateral digital scout view is used to measure the anteroposterior diameters of the inlet and midpelvis.

ameter of the inlet. It is stated in the radiologic literature that the ischial spines are difficult to identify on the anteroposterior digital scout view, although I have not found that to be the case. Nevertheless, the interfoveal distance on axial scan has been taken to represent the interspinous distance, a potentially se-

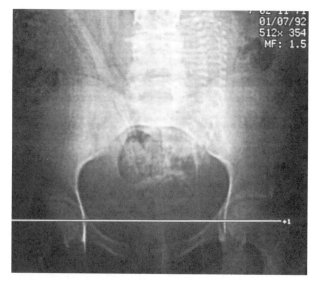

FIG. 8. Computed tomographic pelvimetry, anteroposterior digital scout view, is used to measure the transverse diameter of the inlet and the interspinous distance.

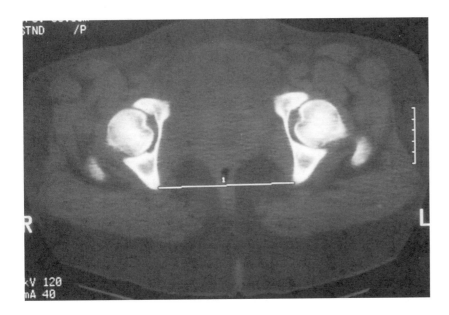

FIG. 9. Computed tomographic pelvimetry, axial section through the foveas of the femoral heads, is used to measure the intrafoveal distance. This method can result in overestimation of the interspinous diameter.

rious error. Aronson and Kier[1] recently have shown that in at least 65% of women, the ischial spines are below the level of the foveae, and that using the interfoveal measurement overestimates the interspinous distance by an average of 1.0 cm. Therefore, the obsterician should either personally measure the interspinous from the anteroposterior digital scout film or, if the interfoveal measurement is used, consider the minimal acceptable interspinous distance for vaginal delivery of a term breech to be 10.5 cm rather than 9.5 cm.

Management of Labor

Management of the fetal membranes must be individualized. Certainly a significant cord prolapse will not occur as long as the membranes are intact, and intact membranes against the cervix are a good dilating wedge. Therefore, a case can be made for leaving them intact as long as possible. This must be balanced against the need for effective monitoring of contractions and the fetal heart rate. If a good external tracing can be obtained, the physician should leave the membranes intact. If membranes have ruptured spontaneously, the wisest course is to apply the internal monitors. If the membranes are intact but the external monitor is either showing signs of heart rate abnormality or not obtaining a satisfactory tracing, a decision must be made concerning amniotomy. This can be done safely in frank or complete breech presentations if the breech is in the maternal pelvis and well applied to the cervix.

Careful attention to the course of labor is essential in breech presentation. Once the active phase of labor is entered, the nullipara's cervix should dilate at the rate of at least 1 cm/hr, and the parous woman's at 1.5 cm/hr. Furthermore, descent of the presenting part must occur simultaneously with dilation. The patient whose fetus remains above the ischial spines at complete or near-complete dilation is best managed by cesarean delivery. Likewise, arrest of dilation in the active

phase is an indication for cesarean delivery. If labor is dysfunctional and progress ceases, cesarean delivery is usually preferable to oxytocin stimulation of labor. Dysfunctional labor may be a symptom of fetopelvic disproportion, and stimulation with oxytocin in such circumstances runs the risk of forcing the fetal body through the maternal pelvis and subsequently entrapping the head.

The definition of what is a normal duration of the second stage of labor is modified with breech presentation. A prolonged second stage may be another symptom of fetopelvic disproportion. As a general rule, if a nullipara cannot push the breech fetus out in 1 hour, or the parous woman in 30 minutes, cesarean delivery is indicated. This may need to be individualized somewhat, depending on the anesthetic management of the patient.

Once the patient is in the active phase of labor, epidural anesthesia is excellent in breech presentation. The main advantage of epidural anesthesia is prevention of undue maternal expulsive efforts before the cervix is completely dilated. However, profound epidural anesthesia may interfere with maternal expulsive efforts after complete dilation, leading to prolongation of the second stage. Bingham and Lilford[3] summarized six studies that demonstrated prolongation of the second stage of labor with epidural anesthesia in breech presentation, although there were no increases in the rates of breech extraction or cesarean delivery. In such circumstances, continuous monitoring of the fetal heart is essential. Epidural anesthesia is not mandatory in term breech presentation if the patient is cooperative and able to refrain from pushing until the cervix is completely dilated.

Management of Vaginal Delivery

Vaginal delivery of a fetus in breech presentation requires the attendance of at least an obstetrician and an anesthesiologist. It is preferable to have a pediatrician in attendance as well.

The fetal monitor should be taken to the delivery room, and monitoring should be continued until one is committed to a vaginal delivery. Such a commitment occurs when the fetal umbilicus passes over the mother's perineum, at which time the fetal head is in the maternal pelvis. Traction on the fetus before that point constitutes a total breech extraction and should be avoided. If immediate delivery becomes necessary before that point (e.g., cord prolapse at complete dilation), cesarean delivery is indicated.

Once the fetal umbilicus passes over the maternal perineum, a loop of cord 4 to 6 inches in length should be brought down to prevent subsequent excessive traction on the cord. The legs may then be delivered by flexing the knees and sweeping the legs out from in front of the fetus. A towel is placed around the fetal pelvis, which is then grasped, and downward traction is applied until the fetal scapulae pass under the maternal symphysis. Then the fetal body is rotated so that the shoulders are in an anteroposterior position, and the anterior arm is flexed and swept out under the symphysis. The fetus is then rotated 180 degrees in the direction that will keep the fetal back toward the maternal symphysis, and the other arm is swept out in a similar manner. It is important during delivery of a breech that the fetus not be allowed to assume a position with the fetal face or abdomen toward the maternal symphysis.

Delivery of the fetal head often is best accomplished with Piper forceps. Milner[21] has shown that at any given birthweight, neonatal mortality is better among those delivered with forceps to the aftercoming head than among those delivered without. This is probably in part because this produces a more controlled, less explosive delivery of the head. It is also probably true that those obstetricians using forceps in Milner's[21] series were more skilled in all aspects of management of breech labor and delivery. An assistant must support the fetal body during application of these forceps (Fig. 10). The temptation to elevate the fetal body to provide better visualization must be resisted because this maneuver hyperextends the neck. Rather, the fetal body should be supported parallel to the floor, and the operator should drop to

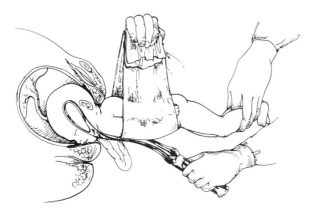

FIG. 10. Breech delivery is accomplished with Piper forceps applied to the aftercoming head. Note that the infant's body is being supported parallel to the floor.

his or her knee for application of the forceps. The application is pelvic rather than cephalic, with the forceps being applied to the lateral aspects of the maternal pelvis, not wandered around from the posterior using landmarks on the fetal head, as one would do in vertex presentation. Controlled delivery of the fetal head is then accomplished, with suctioning of the fetal airway as soon as the mouth passes over the perineum.

A generous episiotomy is necessary for any vaginal breech birth. For the term-sized infant, a mediolateral episiotomy may be appropriate.

An anesthesiologist capable of a rapid induction of general anesthesia should be present throughout the delivery because it may be necessary to perform an immediate cesarean at any time up until delivery of the fetal umbilicus.

The patient who arrives at the hospital ready to deliver, with the breech fetus on the perineum, presents special problems because there is no time for much of the evaluation outlined above. In such circumstances, three things need to be done quickly: abdominal examination for estimation of fetal weight, pelvic examination to be certain the cervix is completely dilated, and the ultrasound examination to be certain the fetal neck is not extended and the fetus is alive. If the EFW is more than 3800 g or the fetal neck is extended, rapid induction of general anesthesia should be performed, followed by cesarean delivery.

Management of Cesarean Delivery

Abdominal delivery does not guarantee atraumatic birth of the fetus in breech presentation. Just as in vaginal delivery, it is important to grasp the fetal bony pelvis rather than soft tissue during extraction. The most serious complication is head entrapment by the uterus contracting down around the neck after delivery of the body. Some physicians have advocated a vertical uterine incision so that it may be extended should this occur. This may be the best choice for the premature fetus accompanied by a poorly developed lower uterine segment. Because such an incision compromises future childbearing, the obstetrician should perform a low transverse cervical incision for the term fetus or the premature fetus when labor has resulted in a well-developed lower segment. Such an incision can be extended in a J-shaped (rather than a T-shaped) manner if necessary. A technique that may obviate the need for this in the face of head entrapment is general anesthesia with an agent that rapidly relaxes the uterus. The anesthesiologist should be alerted that this may become necessary, even if the cesarean is begun under regional anesthesia.

After any breech delivery, whether vaginal or cesarean, an umbilical arterial blood pH should be obtained from a clamped segment of the umbilical cord. Apgar scores do not always reflect the true condition of the newborn, and the cord blood pH can be most useful in the immediate management of the infant. Christian and Brady[7] have demonstrated that term breeches delivered vaginally without complications and with good Apgar scores have a slightly lower umbilical arterial pH (mean 7.23) and a slightly higher umbilical arterial P_{CO_2} (mean 51.2 mm Hg), than uncomplicated vaginally born vertex infants, although the values were still quite normal. Umbilical arterial P_{O_2} and base deficit and all umbilical venous parameters were the same in vaginally born breech and vertex infants.

Practical Considerations

Management of labor and delivery in a patient with breech presentation requires considerable judgment and skill acquired through supervised experience. Unfortunately, in the past, many residency training programs stopped teaching vaginal breech delivery. Although this trend is now being reversed, there is a group of obstetricians with very limited breech experience. These physicians' patients whose fetuses are in breech presentation are best served by cesarean delivery.

◊ FACE PRESENTATION

In face presentation, the fetal neck is hyperextended so that the occiput touches the back. The presenting part is that part of the fetal face between the orbital ridges and the chin (Fig. 11). The incidence is approximately one in 550 births.

Cause

Proposed causative factors include anencephaly, high parity, contracted pelvis, large infant, small infant, and nuchal cord. It is interesting to note that, in the majority of studies, one of the larger categories is that in which no causative factor can be identified; this varies from 2% to 97%, with an average frequency of 38%.

Anencephalic fetuses frequently present by the face if the fetal presentation is cephalic. However, because the course and mechanism of labor, management of delivery, and perinatal outcome are entirely different in this situation, these cases should be excluded from consideration of face presentation. The association between face presentation and anencephaly is important to remember, however, because when face presentation is suspected clinically, ultrasound studies are indicated to rule out this anomaly.

Most series demonstrate an association between high parity and face presentation; whether this relationship is causal is not clear. The average reported incidence of contracted pelves in series of face presentations is 15%. In reality, the incidence is probably much lower because in most series only those patients with arrested labor were studied radiographically. Contracted pelvis or cephalopelvic disproportion is probably diagnosed clinically with excessive frequency in face presentation because the extended head feels larger on abdominal palpation and because the head is often floating at the onset of labor. However, if large series of radiographically diagnosed pelvic contractions are examined, it is rare to find a case of face presentation, none being reported in three series of radiographically diagnosed pelvic contractions totaling more than 700 patients. The weight of evidence seems to indicate that pelvic contraction is not of causative significance in face presentation.

Many authors associate face presentation with large infants, on the assumption that cephalopelvic disproportion may result from excessive fetal size in spite of a normal pelvis. The argument that large infants cause cephalopelvic disproportion, and thus face presentation, is weakened by the high proportion of vaginal deliveries in most series of face presentations. Furthermore, the average incidence of large infant (variously defined) in series of face presentations is 12%, not significantly different from that in the general obstetric population.

Many series have demonstrated an increased proportion of low-birthweight infants among face presentations and ascribed causative significance to prematurity, although other studies have found no excess of low-birthweight infants. Part of the discrepancy results from the inclusion of anencephalic fetuses in many series—fetuses that usually are small for gestational age. Although the average incidence of low birthweight is 15%, it is 11% in those series in which it is possible to exclude anencephalics; this is not significantly different from the incidence of low birthweight in the general population. Thus, it is difficult to conclude that low birthweight or prematurity is a causative factor in face presentation.

Nuchal cord occurs in approximately 25% of cephalic deliveries, and cases have been reported in which as many as eight loops have been associated with normally flexed necks. The average incidence of nuchal cord in face presentation is 10%. Nuchal cord is not a cause of face presentation.

Of all the proposed causative factors in face presentation, there is no unanimity of opinion regarding their significance, and as reported by Cruikshank and Cruikshank,[10] none can withstand careful scrutiny. There does seem to be an association between face presentation and high parity, but 34% of face presentations occur in primigravidas. All of the postulated causes presume that face presentation develops after the onset of labor. Cases of face presentation that occur before labor are called primary and are thought to result from

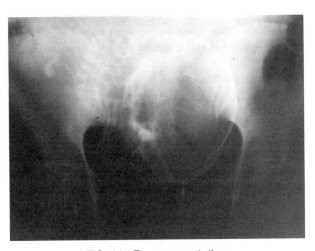

FIG. 11. Face presentation.

increased tone in the extensor muscles of the fetal neck. The usual attitude of the fetal head is flexion caused by greater tone in the flexor muscles, but occasionally infants are seen in whom the extensors predominate. In addition to face presentation, hyperextension of the neck occurs in transverse lie (i.e., "flying fetus") and in breech presentation; in fact, up to 5% of breech fetuses have hyperextended necks.

To ascertain the true incidence of primary face presentation, it is necessary to examine large series of x-ray films obtained before labor. In three such series, seven primary face presentations were found among 1762 patients, an incidence of one face presentation in 251 cases, which is more than twice the reported incidence of face presentation at delivery. These data, coupled with the uncertainties surrounding the proposed causative factors, make it most likely that all face presentations are primary and intrinsic to the fetus and that there are no significant causative factors. The preponderance of multiparas in series of face presentation is compatible with this theory. Increased extensor muscle tone cannot cause extension of the neck if the head is fixed in the pelvis; thus, face presentation is less likely to occur during the last 1 to 2 weeks of pregnancy in a primigravida with an engaged presenting part than in a multipara in whom the head often is not engaged until after the onset of labor.

Diagnosis

Traditional obstetric wisdom states that face presentation is diagnosed by Leopold's maneuvers, with palpation of the cephalic prominence on the same side as the fetal back and with a deep groove between them. In reality, the diagnosis usually is made by vaginal examination during labor followed by ultrasound studies. Only 3% of cases are diagnosed antepartum, with 35% of cases being diagnosed in the first stage of labor, 27% in the second stage, and 35% at the time of delivery.

At the time of diagnosis, 60% of face presentations are mentum (chin) anterior (MA), 15% are mentum transverse (MT), and 25% are mentum posterior (MP).

Mechanism and Course of Labor

The best study of the mechanism of labor in face presentation is that of Borell and Fernstrom,[4] who studied seven patients with two to six sets of x-ray pelvimetry during labor. This study concluded that, in face presentation, the presenting diameter is the tracheloparietal (trachelobregmatic), which is 0.7 cm longer than the presenting diameter in vertex presentation (the suboccipitobregmatic).

They also demonstrated that internal rotation in face presentation occurs between the ischial spines and the ischial tuberosities, lower than in vertex presentation. After internal rotation has placed the fetal chin under the maternal symphysis, delivery occurs by flexion of the fetal neck. It is important to remember that in face presentation, the distance from the leading edge to the largest presenting diameter is greater than

that in vertex presentation. Thus, engagement of the presenting part probably has not occurred until the face is at a +2 station.

Safe vaginal delivery of a term-sized persistent MP is impossible for two reasons: the short fetal neck cannot span the full length of the maternal sacrum, so the fetal head and shoulders must enter the maternal pelvis at the same time, and even if this should occur, the persistent MP would have to deliver under the symphysis by extension, but the neck is already maximally extended. Many MPs will spontaneously rotate and convert to MA; the average reported rate being 35%. This may be an artificially low value because, as pointed out above, rotation does not occur until the head is well down in the pelvis. Surgical intervention before that point would make the incidence of spontaneous rotation seem lower. In fact, some series report spontaneous rotation rates of 50% to 65%. When the face is MT at the time of diagnosis, spontaneous rotation to MA usually occurs.

Most patients with face presentations have durations of the first stage of labor similar to those of patients with vertex presentations, although there may be some prolongation in MP presentations. Likewise, the length of the second stage is similar to or only slightly longer than that in vertex presentation.

Management

The average reported incidence of spontaneous or elective low forceps delivery in face presentation is 72% (range 40% to 90%). The average rate of cesarean delivery is 15%, and in only two series was it greater than 29%. In older series, up to 12% of face presentations were delivered by various operative vaginal procedures, including midforceps rotation, version and extraction, and manual conversion of face to vertex (Thom maneuver). These procedures are associated with high perinatal mortality and maternal morbidity; although they are advocated by the authors of several older series, there is no place for them in the modern management of face presentation.

Face presentation alone is not a contraindication to oxytocin stimulation of labor, and it can be done for the same reasons and with the same precautions as in vertex presentation. Likewise, outlet forceps delivery in MA presentation can be accomplished using the same criteria one would use in vertex presentation, but midforceps delivery in face presentation should be abandoned. Because of the altered diameters of the presenting part, if the face is not bulging the perineum, any forceps delivery is probably a midforceps operation and should not be attempted.

The old adage "if a face is progressing, leave it alone" is still valid. This applies to MT and MP presentations as well as to MA because of the likelihood that these presentations will convert to MA. Rotation may not occur, however, until the presenting part is on the pelvic floor. In any face presentation, as in vertex presentation, if progress in dilation and descent ceases despite adequate contractions, delivery should be accomplished by cesarean. Conversely, as long as dilation and descent continue, management should be expectant.

The only series using fetal monitoring extensively in the management of face presentation, reported variable decelerations in 59% of 29 infants, severe variables in 29%, and late decelerations in 24%. Only 14% of patients in the study (4 of 29) had no fetal heart rate abnormality. It seems plausible that the increased incidence of fetal heart rate abnormalities results in part from abnormal pressure on the extended head, neck, or eyes, similar to the mechanism of heart rate abnormalities described in occiput-posterior presentations. Face presentation is an indication for electronic fetal monitoring. Decisions regarding fetal distress will need to be made on the basis of electronic monitoring alone, because fetal blood sampling for pH determination is contraindicated.

◊ BROW PRESENTATION

In brow presentation, the fetal head is midway between flexion and hyperextension; the presenting part is that portion of the head between the orbital ridges and the anterior fontanelle. Brow presentation is less common than face presentation; the reported incidence is approximately one in 1400 births.

Cause

As in face presentation, numerous factors have been proposed as causative in brow presentation. Most series report a few cases of brow presentation associated with placenta previa, polyhydramnios, uterine anomalies, and fetal malformations, but these are no longer seriously proposed as causes of brow presentation. Likewise, the reported incidence of nuchal cord in brow presentation is lower than that in the general obstetric population, and nuchal cord seems to be related to brow presentation only by coincidence. The average incidence of low birthweight among brow presentations is only 13%. This does not seem to be etiologically significant. Most data suggest that cephalopelvic disproportion is more commonly associated with brow presentation than with face presentation.

There are those who believe that brow presentation, like face presentation, is nearly always primary (i.e., caused solely by factors intrinsic to the fetus). Others believe that brow is an unstable or transitional presentation, representing a head in the process of converting from vertex to face presentation or vice versa. If this is true, and if, as proposed above, all face presentations are primary, then all brow presentations must likewise be primary. If so, how can the apparent association between brow presentation and cephalopelvic disproportion be explained? Two factors seem germane: (1) "relative" cephalopelvic disproportion is more likely to occur in brow presentation because the presenting diameters of the fetal head are greater than in face or vertex presentation (see Mechanism and Course of Labor), and (2) persistent brow presentation probably selects for patients with smaller pelves because, in patients with larger pelves, the brow converts to face or to vertex before being recognized.

Diagnosis

Theoretically, brow presentation may be diagnosed by abdominal examination, with both fetal chin and occiput being palpable. In reality, the diagnosis is nearly always made by vaginal examination or sonographic studies, or both. Most cases are diagnosed in labor, with approximately one-half diagnosed during the second stage. If labor is progressing, the diagnosis is often missed until late in the second stage of labor.

Mechanism and Course of Labor

When the fetal head engages as a brow presentation, there are three possible mechanisms of labor, depending on whether the brow converts to a face, converts to a vertex, or persists as a brow. Spontaneous conversion to face or vertex occurs in approximately 50% of cases, with 30% converting to face and 20% to vertex. However, in those series in which the brow presentation was diagnosed early in labor, spontaneous conversion rates of 67% to 75% are reported. In fact, presentations probably enter the pelvis as brows but are never diagnosed as such.

Regardless of the eventual outcome, the brow usually engages transversely at the pelvic brim. Borell and Fernstrom[4] have demonstrated radiographically that the engaging diameter is the mentoparietal. The mentoparietal diameter is about 1.5 cm longer than the engaging diameter in vertex presentation and 0.8 cm longer than that in face presentation.

Most would agree that there is no mechanism of labor for a term-sized persistent brow under most circumstances, and therefore, vaginal delivery is impossible. Vaginal delivery can occur if the fetus is quite small or the pelvis very large, however.

Most series report a definite prolongation of labor with brow presentation, but the duration of labor in those patients who eventually convert to face or vertex is no different from the duration of labor with vertex presentation. It appears that those cases destined to convert to face or vertex and deliver spontaneously have normal to slightly prolonged labor, whereas those destined to persist as brows often have very prolonged labors unless timely intervention is undertaken.

Management

The best recommendation for management of brow presentations is the same as that for face presentations. If dilation and descent are progressing normally, expectant management is best. If progress ceases, delivery should be by cesarean. The association of cephalopelvic disproportion with brow presentation seems to contraindicate the use of oxytocin to stimulate labor. Forceps deliveries are acceptable if the brow converts to MA face or vertex. Persistent brow presentations, once progress in labor has ceased, require delivery by cesarean, and all forceps operations are contraindicated.

In assessing whether progress in labor has stopped, it is important to remember that if the fetus becomes arrested at the pelvic brim, tremendous caput succedaneum may form over the brow, giving a false impression of descent of the head.

◊ SHOULDER PRESENTATION (TRANSVERSE LIE)

When the long axis of the fetus lies perpendicular to that of the mother, the condition is termed a shoulder presentation or transverse lie. This malpresentation complicates one in 300 births.

Definitions

In transverse lie, the fetal head lies in one maternal iliac fossa and the breech in the other. A better term for this would be transverse presentation, but this term is avoided because it is often confused with transverse position of vertex presentation. Because the fetal shoulder usually lies over the pelvic inlet, the formal term is shoulder presentation, which should be considered synonymous with transverse lie. The fetal position is described with the fetal acromion used as a reference point and is termed left or right acromion, according to the side of the mother to which the fetal shoulder is directed. Because the fetal back may be directed anteriorly, posteriorly, superiorly, or inferiorly, the additional qualifying terms dorsum superior, dorsum anterior, and so on are used as well. Thus, a fetus with its head on the mother's left and its back toward the mother's head would be described as left acromion dorsum superior.

If one fetal pole lies in a maternal iliac fossa and the other pole lies in the opposite upper quadrant of the uterus, the lie is said to be oblique or unstable.

Cause

The most common causative factors are high parity with lax abdominal wall and uterine musculature as well as conditions in which the fetus is small in relation to the volume of the uterus (i.e., prematurity and polyhydramnios). Shoulder presentation may also be caused by anything that prevents descent of a fetal pole into the maternal pelvis, such as pelvic contraction, placenta previa, lower uterine segment myoma, or an ovarian tumor in the cul-de-sac. These conditions should be kept in mind for any patient who presents with a transverse lie, but especially in the patient of low parity who has this malpresentation at or near term.

Diagnosis

The diagnosis usually can be made by physical examination of the maternal abdomen, with the fetal head and buttocks palpable in the iliac fossae and no fetal pole at the pelvic inlet. A very high or unreachable presenting part on vaginal examination suggests transverse lie. All such findings on physical examination should be confirmed by ultrasound, which also should be used in such circumstances to search for placenta previa and pelvic masses.

Mechanism of Labor

The tiny fetus in transverse lie may deliver by the mechanism of conduplicato corpore, in which the fetal body doubles up on itself and the fetal head and buttocks enter the maternal pelvis simultaneously. This is often associated with rupture of fetal abdominal viscera.

If the fetal weight is greater than about 800 to 1000 g, there is no mechanism of labor. Uterine contractions will wedge the fetal shoulder into the pelvis, and eventually the membranes will rupture and the fetal arm will prolapse into the vagina. Such a condition is termed a neglected transverse lie. If labor is permitted to continue, there will be progressive thinning of the lower uterine segment, a Bandl retraction ring will form, the uterus will rupture, and eventually both the fetus and the mother will die.

Management

Shoulder presentations diagnosed before term should be managed expectantly because most will convert to polar presentations before labor. If the patient is not at term but the cervix is significantly dilated (>3 cm), hospitalization at bed rest should be considered because the incidence of cord prolapse in such a patient is 10% to 15% if rupture of membranes occurs.

If the patient is at term (38 completed weeks of gestation or more), external version may be attempted with the same techniques and precautions as described for breech presentation. If the version is successful, and the cervix favorable, induction of labor may be undertaken immediately. External version may also be attempted in early labor, provided the membranes are intact and no fetal part has entered the pelvis. Before any version attempt, ultrasound must be used to rule out placenta previa and pelvic masses.

If the patient is in active labor or has ruptured membranes, and the fetus is of a gestational age to be considered potentially viable, delivery must be by cesarean. Because of exceedingly high morbidity and mortality for both mother and fetus, there is no role for internal version and extraction in the management of transverse lie. Because the lower uterine segment may be poorly developed, vertical uterine incisions are often necessary. If, however, the fetus can be manipulated to a polar presentation after opening the abdomen but before entering the uterus, a low transverse incision may be performed. This usually is possible only if the membranes are still intact and is easiest if general anesthesia with a uterine relaxing agent is used.

The patient with a neglected transverse lie is an obstetric emergency. Usually she is septic, and often the fetus is dead. If the uterus is still intact, it is exceedingly thin. Many patients are completely dilated on arrival at the hospital, but the temptation to try vaginal maneuvers such as internal version must be resisted because this will often result in uterine rupture and may lead to maternal death. Such patients should have basic laboratory studies, coagulation indices, and blood cultures obtained. Rapid intravenous hydration and antibiotic therapy should be instituted, type-specific blood should be available, and the patient should be taken promptly to the operating room for cesarean delivery. Cesarean hysterectomy is often the best procedure for such patients, especially if the uterus has ruptured or is grossly infected. In the past, various vaginal fetal destructive procedures were described for treating the neglected transverse lie with a dead fetus. Because few obstetricians today have any training in such procedures, and few hospitals have the appropriate instruments, such procedures should be abandoned in favor of cesarean delivery, even in the event of a dead fetus.

◊ COMPOUND PRESENTATIONS

A compound presentation occurs whenever some part of a fetal extremity is prolapsed alongside the presenting part. By far the most common type is vertex/hand or vertex/arm, in which some part of the upper extremity is alongside the head. Much less common types are breech/arm and vertex/foot. The reported incidences ranges between one in 400 and one in 1200 births.

Cause

Situations in which the presenting part poorly fills the pelvis predispose to compound presentation. The most obvious of these is prematurity, which is associated with most compound presentations. In fact, the incidence of this complication among infants who weigh more than 1500 g is only one in 1600 births.

Diagnosis

The diagnosis almost invariably is made by vaginal examination and generally is made late in labor. At least 50% of these malpresentations are diagnosed in the second stage of labor. Whenever a fetal hand or arm is palpated on vaginal examination, the examiner must be certain that the fetal head is in the pelvis as well before concluding that the presentation is compound. If the head is not easily palpated in the pelvis in such circumstanes, most likely the diagnosis is shoulder presentation with a prolapsed arm, a much more serious and urgent obstetric condition.

Management

Management of vertex/arm and vertex/hand presentations should be expectant. One of three outcomes will occur: (1) the prolapsed part will withdraw back up into the uterus as labor progresses, (2) the baby will deliver with the arm or hand alongside the head, or (3) progress in labor will cease, in which case cesarean delivery is indicated.

The reported incidence of cord prolapse in compound presentation is 10% to 20%, but many of these are related to attempts to replace the prolapsed arm into the uterus, which often necessitates upward displacement of the fetal head. For this reason, attempts at replacement of the prolapsed part in any compound presentation should be avoided.

Because of the increased incidence of cord prolapse, electronic fetal monitoring should be used in these situations. Vertex/arm and vertex/hand presentations are not indications for cesarean delivery in and of themselves. Indications for cesarean delivery in such circumstances include failure to progress in labor, cord prolapse, and fetal distress.

Cases of breech/arm presentation should be managed as any other breech presentation would be managed. Cases of vertex/foot presentation are rare, but those few reported cases have a perinatal mortality two to three times that of other compound presentations and are best managed by cesarean delivery. In essence, these are variants of shoulder presentation.

There is no role for version and extraction in the modern management of compound presentation, although this was commonly done in years past.

◊ UMBILICAL CORD COMPLICATIONS

The mean length of the umbilical cord at term is 55 to 60 cm, and the normal range (fifth to 95th percentile) is 35 to 80 cm. The longest umbilical cord reported in the literature measured 129 cm. The length of the cord is related to fetal activity in the first two trimesters; there is little change in the length of the cord after 28 weeks of gestation. At term, mean cord length is slightly (1.6 cm) but significantly longer in male than in female fetuses and is 4.5 cm greater in vertex infants compared with breech. There is no correlation between cord length and either fetal or placental weight.

Cord Prolapse

The reported incidence of prolapse of the umbilical cord varies between 0.2% and 0.6% of births. Cord prolapse almost never occurs with cords shorter than 35 cm; the incidence is 0.4% with normal-length cords (35 to 80 cm) and 4% to 6% with cords longer than 80 cm. Other than excessive cord length, causative factors include malpresentation in approximately 50% of cases, low birthweight (less than 2500 g) in 30% to 50% of cases, grand multiparity (more than five pregnancies) cases, multiple gestation in 10%, and obstetric manipulation including artificial rupture of membranes in 10% to 15%. Table 4 shows the association between cord prolapse and malpresentation, especially with nonfrank breech, compound, and shoulder presentations. Nearly 50% of cord prolapses occur during the second stage of labor.

The diagnosis of cord prolapse should be suspected in any patient who develops fetal heart rate abnormalities after rupture of the membranes, either spontaneous or artificial. The heart rate abnormalities usually observed are sustained bradycardia and, less frequently, profound variable decelerations (Fig. 12). All such patients should be promptly examined or

TABLE 4. *Incidence of cord prolapse*

Presentation	Incidence (%)
Vertex	0.14
Breech	2.5–3.0
Frank	0.4
Complete	5.0
Incomplete	10.0
Shoulder (transverse lie)	5.0–10.0
Compound	10.0–20.0
Face–brow	Rare

reexamined, and the diagnosis confirmed by palpation of the cord alongside the presenting part or in the cervix or vagina.

When cord prolapse is diagnosed, every effort should be made to prevent compression of the cord by the presenting part. The patient should be placed in steep Trendelenburg or the knee–chest position, and the presenting part should be manually elevated as far out of the pelvis as possible and held there until delivery is accomplished. Once the diagnosis is made, further palpation of the cord must be avoided because this causes spasm of the umbilical arteries and may further compromise the fetus. Confirmation of fetal cardiac activity should be by ultrasound rather than by cord palpation. In fact, ultrasound is the only certain way to confirm fetal viability. There are at least two reported cases in which nonpulsatile cords were palpated, no fetal heart tones were heard with Doppler or stethoscope, but ultrasound revealed fetal heart rates of 50 to 80. In both cases, prompt delivery resulted in surviving infants.

Cesarean delivery is the treatment of choice in almost all cases if there is fetal cardiac activity. Even at complete dilation, the perinatal outcome is better with cesarean delivery than with such maneuvers as breech extraction or high forceps. If no fetal cardiac activity is present by ultrasound, and the fetal lie is polar, the mother usually is better served by allowing continued labor and vaginal delivery.

In most series of cord prolapse, perinatal mortality is approximately 15%. Among term infants and among all infants delivered by cesarean within 10 minutes of cord prolapse, mortality is less than 5%. Murphy and MacKenzie[22] reported a retrospective study of 132 consecutive cases of cord prolapse in a single hospital. The overall perinatal mortality was 9% (12 of 132 infants). However, all but one death was from either extreme prematurity or congenital malformations; the perinatal mortality rate attributable to asphyxia was 0.8% (one case). Of the 120 survivors they reported, only one infant had a major neurologic handicap.

True Knots

The reported incidence of true knots in the cord is 0.3% to 2.1% of births, the mean being about 1.0%. As is true of all cord accidents, true knots are more common if the cord is abnormally long. Ten percent of true knots occur in cords more than 80 cm in length, and 3% of cords longer than 80 cm have true knots. However, many true knots must form early in pregnancy, for the incidence in aborted fetuses is 0.9%. True knots can be diagnosed only after delivery in the vast majority of cases because, unless the knot is pulled tight, there is no reduction of flow or increase in perfusion pressure and, thus, no abnormality of the fetal heart rate or Doppler velocimetry. The patient with a tight knot will demonstrate a typical cord pattern of variable decelerations (Fig. 13) and will, of necessity, be managed like any other patient with fetal heart rate abnormalities.

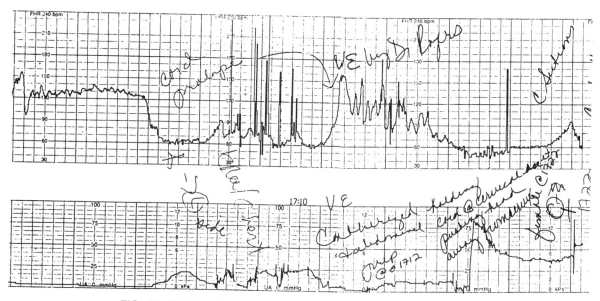

FIG. 12. Fetal monitor tracing associated with umbilical cord prolapse.

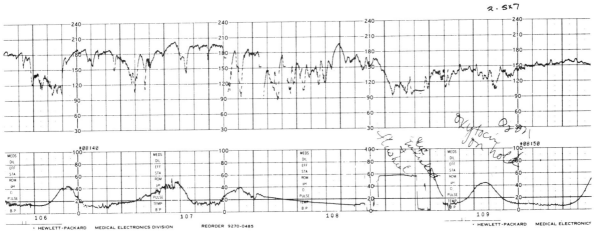

FIG. 13. Monitor tracing of a fetus subsequenty found to have a tight true knot in the umbilical cord.

The Collaborative Study of Cerebral Palsy[26] found no difference in 5-minute Apgar scores or neurologic abnormalities at age 1 year between controls and infants born with true knots in the cord. There is an association between true knots and antepartum stillbirths, however. About 4% to 5% of stillborns have true knots in the cord, compared with 1% of liveborn infants.

Nuchal Cord

The incidence of loops of umbilical cord around the fetal neck is 24.6% of liveborn infants, with 21% having one loop around the neck and 3.5% having two or more. In fact, 0.1% of fetuses have four or more loops of nuchal cord; the maximum reported number is nine. The incidence is 14% with short cords (<35 cm), 23% with normal-length cords, and 53% with cords longer than 80 cm. There is no evidence that nuchal cords cause fetal death or significant degrees of fetal distress. The Collaborative Study of Cerebral Palsy found no increase in the incidence of depressed 5-minute Apgar scores, perinatal mortality, or abnormal neonatal development among infants with nuchal cords. It did demonstrate reduced 1-minute Apgar scores in these infants, however. Although nuchal cords are at times diagnosed by ultrasound, the excellent outcome of these infants demonstrates that no alteration in management is indicated unless the fetus develops bona fide distress during labor.

Body Coils of Cord

The incidence of coils of umbilical cord around various parts of the fetal body other than the neck is 0.5% to 2.0% and is greater with long cords. As with nuchal cords, body coils are not associated with any increase in low Apgar scores, perinatal mortality, or neonatal morbidity.

SUMMARY POINTS

1. Most studies regarding the optimal route of delivery for the term breech are too poorly done to allow definitive conclusions. The only two randomized prospective trials concluded that vaginal delivery is safe in selected patients.

2. There are no randomized prospective data regarding optimal route of delivery for the premature breech. The available retrospective data suggest that those less than 1500 g and/or 32 weeks of gestation are best delivered by cesarean.

3. Fetal anomalies and chromosome abnormalities are an important cause of breech presentation. Likewise, fetuses that have sustained neurologic insults leading to cerebral palsy often present as breeches.

4. Nearly all cases of mentum anterior face presentation and compound presentation should be managed expectantly, and vaginal delivery anticipated. Persistent mentum posterior face, persistent brow, and essentially all cases of shoulder presentation should be delivered by cesarean.

5. External cephalic version is appropriate for most patients with breech presentation late in the third trimester. The ideal time to attempt the meneuver is 36 weeks of gestation in primigravidas and 37 to 38 weeks in parous women.

◊ REFERENCES

1. Aronson D, Kier R. CT Pelvimetry: the foveae are not an accurate landmark for the level of the ischial spines. *Am J Roentgenol* 1991;156:527.
2. Ballas S, Toaf R. Hyperextension of the fetal head in breech presentation: radiological evaluation and significance. *Br J Obstet Gynaecol* 1976;83:201.
3. Bingham P, Hird V, Lilford RJ. Management of the mature selected breech presentation: an analysis based on the intended method of delivery. *Br J Obstet Gynaecol* 1987;94:746.

4. Borell V, Fernstrom I. The mechanism of labour in face and brow presentation: a radiologic study. *Acta Obstet Gynecol Scand* 1960; 39:626.

5. Brown L, Karrison T, Cibils LA. Mode of delivery and perinatol results in breech presentation. *Am J Obstet Gynecol* 1994;171:28.

6. Cheng M, Hannah M. Breech delivery at term: a critical review of the literature. *Obstet Gynecol* 1993;82:605.

7. Christian SS, Brady K, Read JA, Kopelman JN. Vaginal breech delivery. A five-year prospective evaluation of a protocol using computed tomographic pelvimetry. *Am J Obstet Gynecol* 1990;163:848.

8. Collea JV, Chein C, Quilligan EJ. The randomized mangement of term frank breech: a study of 208 cases. *Am J Obstet Gynecol* 1980;137:235.

9. Croughan-Minihane MS, Peitti DB, Gordis L, Golditch I. Morbidity among breech infants according to method of delivery. *Obstet Gynecol* 1990;75:821.

10. Cruikshank DP, Cruikshank JE. Face and brow presentation: a review. *Clin Obstet Gynecol* 1981;24:333.

11. Gimovsky ML, Wallace RL, Schifrin BS, Paul RH. Randomized management of the nonfrank breech presnetation at term: a preliminary report. *Am J Obstet Gynecol* 1983;146:34.

12. Goldenberg RL, Nelson KG. The premature breech. *Am J Obstet Gynecol* 1977;127:240.

13. Green JE, McLean F, Smith LP, Usher R. Has an increased cesarean section rate for term breech delivery reduced the incidence of birth asphyxia, trauma, and death? *Am J Obstet Gynecol* 1982;142:643.

14. Kasule J, Chimbira THK, Brown IM. Controlled trial of external cephalic version. *Br J Obstet Gynaecol* 1985;92:14.

15. Kaupilla O. The perinatal mortality in breech deliveries and observations on affecting factors: a retrospective study of 2227 cases. *Acta Obstet Gynecol Scand* 1975;39(Suppl):1.

16. Kiely JL. Mode of delivery and neonatal death in 17587 infants presenting by the breech. *Br J Obstet Gynaecol* 1991;98:898.

17. Laros RK, Flanagan TA, Kilpatrick SJ. Management of term breech presentation: a protocol of external cephalic version and selective trial of labor. *Am J Obstet Gynecol* 1995;172:1916.

18. Lau TK, Lo KWK, Rogers M. Pregnancy outcome after successful external cephalic version for breech presentation at term. *Am J Obstet Gynecol* 1979;176:218.

19. Lau TK, Lo KWK, Wan D, Rogers MS. Predictors of successful external cephalic version at term: a prospective study. *Br J Obstet Gynaecol* 1997;104:798.

20. Mann LI, Gallant JM. Modern management of the breech delivery. *Am J Obstet Gynecol* 1979;134:611.

21. Milner RDG. Neonatal mortality of breech deliveries with and without forceps to the aftercoming head. *Br J Obstet Gynaecol* 1975;82:783.

22. Murphy DJ, Mackenzie IZ. The mortality and morbidity associated with umbilical cord prolapse. *Br J Obstet Gynaecol* 1995;102:826.

23. Penn ZJ, Steer PJ, Grant A. A multicentre randomised controlled trial comparing elective and selective caesarean section for the delivery of the preterm breech infant. *Br J Obstet Gynaecol* 1996;103:684.

24. Ranney B. The gentle art of external cephalic version. *Am J Obstet Gynecol* 1973;116:239.

25. Schiff E, Friedman SA, Mashiach S, et al. Maternal and neonatal outcome of 846 term singleton breech deliveries: seven-year experience at a single center. *Am J Obstet Gynecol* 1926;175:18.

26. Spellacy WN, Gravem H, Fisch RO. The umbilical cord complications of true knots, nuchal coils and cords around the body. Report from the Collaborative Study of Cerebral Palsy. *Am J Obstet Gynecol* 1966;94:1136.

27. Westgren M, Edvall H, Nordstrom L, et al. Spontaneous cephalic version of breech presnetation in the last trimester. *Br J Obstet Gynaecol* 1985;92:19.

28. Woods JA. Effects of low birth weight breech delivery on neonatal mortality. *Obstet Gynecol* 1979;53:735.

CHAPTER 28

Complications of Labor

—————— ◊ ——————

Donald J. Dudley

From 1970 to 1990, the cesarean delivery rate in the United States increased from 5% to 25%. The four primary indications for cesarean delivery include dystocia, repeat procedure, fetal distress, and abnormal fetal presentation. *Dystocia,* translated, means "difficult birth" and includes all of the labor abnormalities that may occur in women during labor. Although the incidence of cesarean delivery has recently equilibrated at between 20% and 25%, it is generally accepted that this number of abdominal deliveries remains excessively high. Perhaps one reason for the continued high rate of cesarean delivery is a poor understanding of the labor process and the lack of an organized approach to the management of labor. This fundamental lack of understanding often leads to unnecessary induction of labor, which has an *a priori* risk of cesarean delivery of at least 25%, and to inadequate medical treatment, or augmentation, of abnormal labor. With fewer inductions of labor and better augmentation of labor, one can expect a decline in the cesarean delivery rate.

Efforts at reducing the cesarean delivery rate have more recently focused on the categories of dystocia and repeat cesarean section. Obviously, the best method to decrease the incidence of repeat cesarean deliveries is not to do one initially. Hence, new efforts are being directed at the diagnosis and management of labor abnormalities in term pregnancies. The purpose of this chapter is to review these labor abnormalities and management options. A thorough examination of the management of labor and delivery is available in a recently published comprehensive text.[2]

◊ KEYS TO THE MANAGEMENT OF NORMAL LABOR

The normal labor process is reviewed in Chapter 7. There are several key points in the management of labor (Table 1). First is that normal labor progresses in a predictable fashion after the diagnosis of labor is made. However, determining the start of labor is one of the most difficult diagnoses. If the diagnosis of labor is made in error, all subsequent actions are incorrect, as one is essentially doing an induction of labor, and different management is required. Labor is defined as cervical change effected by regular, painful uterine contractions. In nulliparous women in their first labor, cervical change is usually manifest by cervical effacement, or thinning, followed by cervical dilation (Fig. 1). Cervical effacement is often associated with a "bloody show," or the passage of blood-tinged mucus per vagina. Conversely, in the multiparous patient, the initial stage of labor is often characterized by cervical dilation followed by effacement. The amniotic membranes may or may not be intact.

The normal labor curve as defined by Friedman is shown in Fig. 2. This curve was developed by Emanuel Friedman based on the observation of several thousand laboring women. The first stage of labor is divided into the acceleration phase, active phase, and deceleration phase. The acceleration phase occurs when the active phase of labor starts. At this time, concerted uterine activity overcomes some of the basic resistances of the lower uterine segment and cervix. The cervix is usually effaced and less than 4 cm dilated. In the active phase, one can anticipate approximately 1 cm of dilation per hour (Table 2). The deceleration phase may or may not occur. In the second stage of labor, from complete dilation until delivery, again one can anticipate the laboring woman gaining at least 1 cm of station of the fetal head in relation to the maternal pelvis per hour. Cervical examinations should be performed periodically to confirm that progress is being made. Students should be encouraged and allowed to perform examinations hourly so that full educational opportunities are gained. More experienced obstetricians often will perform examinations every 2 to 3 hours, depending on the presentation of the patient. After each examination, the progress in labor should documented on the specific patient's labor curve, and a plan formulated with regard to future examinations and potential interventions.

Nulliparous women and multiparous women behave fundamentally differently in labor. Figure 3 is the labor curve used on Labor and Delivery at the University of Utah Hospitals, and

TABLE 1. *Keys to the management of labor*

Labor progress is predictable
Diagnosis of labor is critical
Labor in nulliparas is different from labor in multiparas
Labor progress should be graphically followed
Cardinal movements of labor should occur
Prompt intervention is needed if labor does not progress
   appropriately
Medical therapy with oxytocin is effective
Clinical judgment must be made regarding the role
   of cesarean delivery

this curve reflects two different labor patterns for nulliparous and multiparous women. Labor, in its simplest terms, is the force of uterine contractions overcoming resistance of the female reproductive tract including the lower uterine segment, cervix, vagina, and perineum. In nulliparous women, more uterine force is required to overcome resistance in the reproductive tract, and the uterus tends to be less effective in maintaining effective uterine contractions. In multiparous women, less uterine force is required, and the tissues of the reproductive outlet, having been stretched by the previous delivery, have less resistance. Additionally, the uterus usually maintains more effective contractile activity. Thus, nulliparous women are more likely to develop labor abnormalities that require intervention. Multiparous women usually labor quickly and meet all expected milestones without the need for significant intervention.

In addition to following the changes in the cervical examination, the practitioner should pay special attention to the cardinal movements of labor (Table 3). This term refers to the changes that occur in the flexion and position of the fetal head throughout the labor process. The cardinal movements of labor usually occur in the following sequence: engagement of

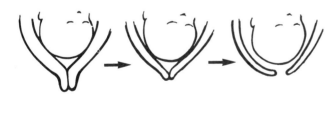

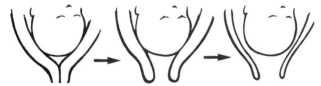

FIG. 1. Cervical effacement and dilation: nulliparas versus multiparas. The upper portion of the figure depicts the cervical changes in early labor of the nulliparous woman. Note that cervical effacement precedes significant dilation. The lower portion depicts the cervical changes of the multiparous woman in early labor. Significant cervical dilation may precede achievement of complete cervical effacement.

the fetal head, descent of the fetal head, flexion of the fetal head, internal rotation (assuming an occiput-transverse position), extension (as the fetal head progresses through the birth canal and crowns at the perineum), external rotation (or restitution to the transverse position), and then shoulder rotation after the head has delivered. Abnormalities in the normal progress of labor as manifest in these cardinal movements may be reflected by abnormal fetal position and other specific abnormalities discussed below.

If labor is progressing appropriately, then a noninterventional approach is indicated, providing for maternal comfort and encouragement. However, if these landmarks are not achieved by the patient, then prompt intervention is recommended. Thus, the next important key in the management of labor is prompt intervention when labor progress is inadequate. Ineffective uterine contractions lead to increased tissue acid content in myometrium, which further contributes to poor contractility.[17] The longer labor continues in a dysfunctional pattern, the less likely it becomes that one can correct the underlying problem with medical therapy. Prompt medical therapy for desultory labor is, therefore, another important key to success in the management of labor.

A schematic employing these key components of labor management is shown in Fig. 4. Normal labor is characterized by coordinated uterine contractions, cervical dilation, gain in station of the fetal head, and normal progress in the cardinal movements of labor. With careful attention to achieving these milestones of normal labor, a successful vaginal delivery is likely. However, should the parturient not achieve these milestones, prompt intervention is more likely to increase the chances for vaginal delivery. Although an aggressive approach with regard to diagnosing labor abnormalities may enhance maternal and fetal outcome, the last important key to the successful management of labor is to develop clinical judgment on when to abandon medical therapy in favor of surgical management. Obviously, obstetricians strive for healthy mothers having healthy babies. If the judgment is made that continuing medical therapy may compromise either mother or fetus, then prompt surgical delivery (cesarean or operative vaginal delivery) should be considered.

◊ INCIDENCE OF DYSTOCIA

The precise incidence of dystocia is difficult to determine and varies with different populations and different labor and delivery units based on local practice patterns. Dystocia is far more common in nulliparous women than in multiparous women and is more common in the first stage of labor than in the second stage of labor. Labor abnormalities occur in approximately 25% of nulliparous women and 10% to 15% of multiparous women. Dystocia occurs in the second stage of labor in about 5% to 10% of nulliparous women and is relatively rare in multiparas (<2%).

Labor problems are a common indication for cesarean delivery. In the United States in 1996, 20.6% of pregnancies were delivered by cesarean (National Center of Health Sta-

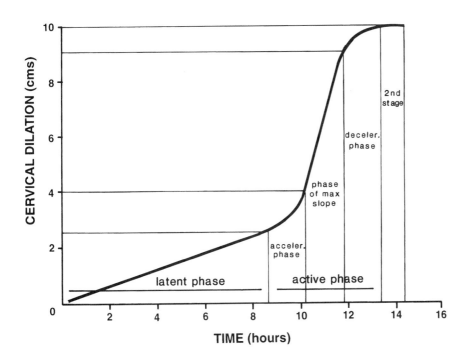

FIG. 2. The Friedman labor curve. This figure depicts the normal labor curve developed by Friedman. Note the different phases of the first stage of labor, including the latent phase, acceleration phase, active phase, and deceleration phase. (Adapted from ref. 2, with permission.)

tistics), down from the highest incidence of 25% in 1988. In 1990, the overall rate was 23.6%, with 7.1% for the indication of "failure to progress" or dystocia and 8.5% for a repeat procedure.[15] Other indications included abnormal presentation (2.6%), fetal distress (2.3%), and other problems (3.2%). Improved management of labor with a decrease in the number of cesarean deliveries for dystocia (and then having less need for repeat procedures) should be an emphasis of every Labor and Delivery unit in the United States. Most authorities believe that a cesarean delivery rate of less than 15% is both optimal and achievable.

◊ ETIOLOGY OF DYSTOCIA

Traditionally, the causes of slow progress in labor have been attributed to the "powers" (uterine contractility), the "passage" (maternal pelvimetry), and/or the "passenger" (position and size of the fetus). In more scientific terms, these represent a primary dysfunctional labor, cephalopelvic or fetopelvic disproportion, abnormal fetal head position, and asynclitism.

TABLE 2. *Expected length of different phases of labor*[9]

Phase of labor	Average duration (hr)	Maximum slope (cm/hr)	Upper limit of normal
Nulliparous labor			
Latent phase	8.6		>20 hr
Active phase	4.9	1.2 or less	
Second stage	0.95	1.0 or less	None[a]
Multiparous labor			
Latent phase	5.3		>14 hr
Active phase	2.2	1.5 or less	
Second stage	0.24	2.0 or less	None[a]

[a]There is no limit to the length of the second stage so long as progress is being made and there is no fetal distress.

This section evaluates each of these potential causes of dystocia. The generic term "failure to progress" is often used as a diagnosis to justify cesarean delivery. This term is more appropriately used as a sign of an underlying problem and does not represent a diagnosis. Hence, the term "failure to progress" is not sufficient to describe the labor problem and should not be used.

Primary Dysfunctional Labor

Primary dysfunctional labor refers to inadequate uterine contractility to maintain appropriate progress in labor. In general, an adequate uterine contraction pattern is one in which there are four contractions every 10 minutes (Fig. 5). However, some women contract less frequently and continue to progress adequately in labor such that no intervention or treatment is required. The uterus has no defined nervous system for the conduction of electric signals to stimulate muscle contrac-

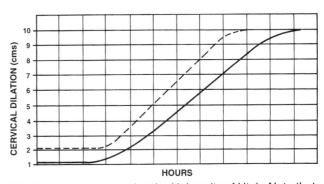

FIG. 3. Labor curve used at the University of Utah. Note that different labor slopes are expected between nulliparous *(solid line)* and multiparous women *(dotted line)*.

TABLE 3. *The cardinal movements of labor*

Engagement
Descent
Flexion
Internal rotation
Extension
External rotation
Shoulder rotation

tions, as can be found in cardiac contractility. The readiness of the uterus for labor is heralded by the occurrence and widespread distribution of gap junctions throughout the myometrium. Gap junctions allow for the rapid transmission of calcium fluxes through the uterine musculature and, hence,

the occurrence of global uterine contractions. The uterus commonly has focal contractions during pregnancy (Braxton Hicks contractions), which are not of sufficient strength or duration to effect cervical change and therefore do not constitute labor.

Smooth muscle cells of the uterus are not randomly distributed but are arranged in a specific fashion such that maximal force can be generated to effect vaginal delivery. In women with uterine embryologic abnormalities such as uterus didelphys and bicornuate uterus, labor is not often successful in achieving vaginal delivery, as global, concerted uterine contractions cannot occur because of the abnormal arrangement of uterine smooth muscle cells. Similar problems may be noted in women exposed to diethylstilbestrol (DES) *in utero* with uterine anomalies characteristic of this

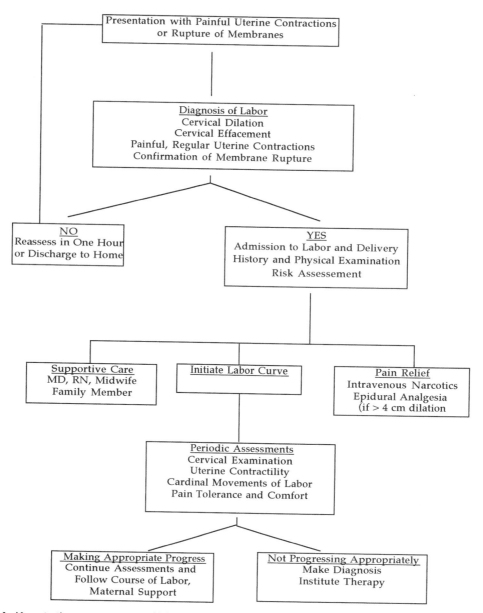

FIG. 4. Keys to the management of labor. This schematic drawing depicts how the keys to the management of labor can be used to help ensure good maternal and fetal outcomes.

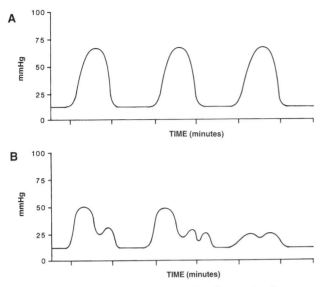

FIG. 5. Uterine contractions patterns. Uterine contractions can be depicted using tocodynometry (external monitoring) or direct uterine pressures (using intrauterine pressure catheters). A shows the contraction pattern of a normal labor. Significant pressure is obtained with contractions every 2 to 3 minutes. B shows uterine contraction patterns typical of primary dysfunctional labor. Contractions achieve varying degrees of pressure and are often combined (coupling).

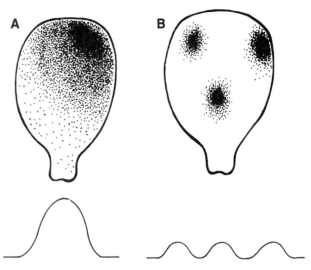

FIG. 6. Uterine pacemakers and contractions. A shows the normal uterine contraction pattern associated with a single dominant pacemaker focus. B depicts a uterus with three separate pacemakers, all firing sequentially. Note that the uterine pressures achieved in this situation is less than that shown with a single dominant pacemaker.

teratogen (e.g., T-shaped uterus). In the structurally normal uterus, contractions begin to occur in a less random timing days to weeks before the initiation of labor. Moreover, there is a distinct diurnal variation of uterine contractility such that, in most women, uterine contractions occur more frequently and labor most often commences at night.[13] These rhythmic variations may be the result of hormonal patterns in which specific and predictable changes in different hormones (e.g., corticotropin-releasing hormone, progesterone, estradiol) allow for more frequent and stronger uterine contractions until the final signal for labor. The precise nature of this signal to the maternal uterus in women is not known.

As the normal uterus approaches term and the start of labor begins, different foci for the initiation of a uterine contraction may be present (Fig. 6). This phenomenon often leads to the clinical scenario in which some contractions are quite hard and lengthy whereas other contractions are mild and of short duration. Women will have mild contractions interspersed with firmer, more painful contractions because of the lack of a dominant pacemaker in the uterine musculature. Eventually, as labor progresses, one of these foci of uterine contractility predominates over other foci, resulting in more concerted, painful uterine contractions. As this occurs, true labor commences with effacement and dilation, and this change is reflected in the uterine tocodynometry patterns (Fig. 5). In a primary dysfunctional labor, uterine activity shifts from the concerted global contractions to more focal and less efficient contractions by allowing the reemergence of other pacemaker foci (Fig. 6). Medical therapy with oxytocin is effective at

correcting the underlying pathophysiology and restoring the pattern of global and concerted uterine contractions.

Although usually quite effective, oxytocin therapy may be of little benefit if the woman has intrauterine infection complicating labor. Should the parturient have clinical signs of intrauterine infection (also known as chorioamnionitis), then labor progress is often desultory and not accelerated with oxytocin augmentation.[4] Clinical signs of intrauterine infection include maternal fever (>38°C), fetal tachycardia (baseline fetal heart rate of >160 beats per minute), elevated maternal white cell count, uterine tenderness when the uterus is relaxed, and foul-smelling vaginal discharge. With the diagnosis of intrauterine infection, broad-spectrum antimicrobial agents should be administered and uterine activity stimulated with oxytocin if labor is not progressing adequately. Because oxytocin often does not work well in this scenario, the obstetrician should be prepared to move to cesarean delivery promptly if dystocia occurs and oxytocin is ineffective to avoid excessive neonatal infectious morbidity.

Cephalopelvic Disproportion

True cephalopelvic disproportion (CPD) (or fetopelvic disproportion) is likely a rare occurrence on the labor and delivery suite. Some authorities believe that CPD occurs in no more than one in 250 pregnancies.[16] Cephalopelvic disproportion happens when the fetal birthweight or the fetal head is of sufficient size or orientation to preclude entry into the maternal pelvic inlet. This diagnosis if often made in retrospect after the birthweight is known and the positioning of the fetal head has been determined at the time of cesarean delivery. However, in the United States, the term CPD is used to describe almost any unsuccessful attempt at vaginal delivery. Further, the diagnosis of CPD is often used when labor progress is not sufficient and medical therapy is not successful. These cases often reflect inadequate use of oxytocin and are not problems with large fetal size or a small maternal pelvis. Cephalopelvic disproportion is an important diagnosis because it has prognostic information for subsequent pregnancies when vaginal birth after cesarean (VBAC) is considered. In women with a prior diagnosis of CPD, success rates of VBAC vary from 50% to 70%. Additionally, they should be managed differently during the VBAC with prompt repeat cesarean if labor does not progress appropriately.

Another important contribution to the fetopelvic relationship is the size of the fetus. Pregnancies with macrosomic fetuses (>4000 g birthweight) have a greater risk of cesarean delivery for dystocia as a result of true CPD. In a study by Turner et al.,[26] fetal macrosomia was associated with longer first and second stages of labor, greater need for oxytocin therapy, and a greater risk for cesarean delivery for CPD refractory to oxytocin. In their patient population, they had an overall incidence of cesarean delivery of 5.2%, but if birthweight was 4000 to 4500 g, the incidence of cesarean delivery was 13.8%. Also, forceps delivery was employed in 31.8% of infants with a birthweight of 4000 to 4500 grams, whereas forceps were used in 13.6% of deliveries overall. Unfortunately, there are no good predictors of fetal weight to guide management. Sonographic estimates of fetal weight at term are notoriously spurious and can miscalculate birthweight by 500 g or more. The obstetrician employing Leopold's maneuvers to estimate fetal weight by palpation of the maternal abdomen can only estimate small, average, or large fetal size. Hence, it is not advisable to induce labor or perform a cesarean delivery for presumed macrosomia, unless the obstetrician judges a dangerous situation exists for vaginal delivery (e.g., high risk of shoulder dystocia).

If the obstetrician suspects that the patient may have CPD because of small pelvic dimensions on clinical pelvimetry at the initial prenatal visit, then this finding should be noted in the prenatal chart, but the patient should not be told she might be "too small for the baby." First, informing the patient at this early stage of pregnancy that she may be at risk for CPD establishes in the patient the expectation of cesarean delivery. Second, the maternal pelvis is a dynamic structure, and pelvimetry will change as the patient approaches term and the pelvic ligaments soften and expand under the hormonal influences of pregnancy. Third, perhaps the best measure of the maternal pelvis is made by the fetal head at the time of labor. Obviously, if the obstetrician truly believes that CPD is inevitable and labor is contraindicated based on examination of clinical pelvimetry and assessment of fetal size, then cesarean delivery should be planned. However, this problem is exceptionally rare.

When the diagnosis of a labor abnormality is made, clinical pelvimetry should be performed to assess the dimensions of the maternal pelvis (Fig. 7). Only in the rare cases in which the maternal pelvis is markedly small should ce-

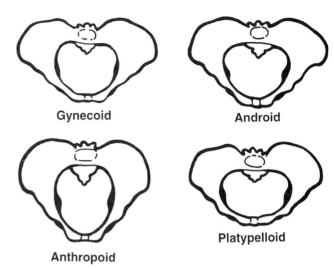

FIG. 7. Pelvic types. There are four primary pelvic types: gynecoid, android, anthropoid, and platypelloid. Women may have a mixed pelvic type with features suggestive of different pelvic types and do not fit conveniently into one of these four types.

sarean delivery be performed without the prior use of oxytocin. For example, labor through a platypelloid pelvis with a normal term-sized fetus is rarely successful because of the markedly shortened anterior–posterior diameter that characterizes this pelvic structure. After assessment of the pelvic type, approximations of the fetal size should be undertaken. Unless the fetus appears to be markedly macrosomic (greater than 4500 g), medical therapy with oxytocin should be instituted. Only in those cases of small pelvic fit or obvious excessive fetal size should oxytocin be foregone and cesarean delivery performed.

More precise measurements of the maternal pelvis can be made with x-ray, computed tomography, or magnetic resonance imaging (x-ray, CT, and MRI pelvimetry, respectively). Direct measurements of the maternal pelvic structures (inlet, midpelvis, and outlet) can be made with any of these modalities. However, these determinations have proved to be of little use in the normal laboring patient at term with a cephalic presentation. Currently, radiographic imaging of the maternal pelvis is reserved for pelvic measurements when vaginal delivery is considered for a fetus with a breech presentation. In some cases, pelvimetry has been used to predict outcome in women considering VBAC. Recently, the concept of the fetopelvic index[25] has been advanced to help select those women who are more likely to have successful VBAC. To determine the fetopelvic index, the fetal head diameter is measured by sonography, and the maternal pelvis is measured with x-ray pelvimetry. If the index is positive (indicating fetal head dimensions larger than maternal pelvic dimensions), then the likelihood of cesarean delivery is high, with a sensitivity of 80%, specificity of 98%, and a positive predictive value of 97%. This test has not gained widespread acceptance, perhaps because of maternal radiation exposure.

Abnormal Position of the Fetal Head

Abnormal positions of the fetal head include occiput posterior (OP), deep transverse arrest, and deflexion abnormalities such as face and brow presentations. Different positions of the fetal head are depicted in Figure 8. An OP position is unfavorable for successful vaginal delivery, particularly if the parturient has an android pelvic structure, as the long diameter of the fetal head negotiates the maternal pelvis at a relatively high station, leading to poor descent. Additionally, the fetal heart tracing may have some unusual decelerations that are difficult to interpret, leading to more advanced testing of the fetal acid–base status (e.g. fetal scalp pH determinations). The OP position is a relatively rare cause of dystocia, accounting for about 1 in 250 cesarean deliveries,[16] but can be corrected with medical therapy. Operative vaginal delivery, either via a Scanzoni maneuver or via a straight OP pull, is another option for delivery. A Scanzoni maneuver involves rotating the OP fetus to an OA position with forceps and then completing the delivery. A Scanzoni maneuver is associated with a higher incidence of maternal trauma (third- and fourth-degree lacerations of the perineum and sulcus tears of the vagina) and fetal trauma (spinal cord transection). Hence, these deliveries should be performed only by obstetricians skilled in these techniques. Moreover, delivery of the OP fetus via forceps should probably be attempted only if the fetal head has attained at least at -1 to -2 station. At higher stations, cesarean delivery is the more prudent alternative.

A deep transverse arrest is an abnormality of the cardinal movements of labor in the second stage in which the fetus maintains an OT position at a low pelvic station. Deep transverse arrests are often associated with abnormal maternal pelvic architecture and may not be easily delivered via forceps. The ideal forceps to use for a deep transverse arrest are Keilland forceps. If the fetal position cannot be accurately assessed, and operative assistance is being considered, then vacuum extraction may be a reasonable option. However, excessive traction of the fetus with a deep transverse arrest can result in birth trauma, and cesarean delivery is a prudent option if the fetal station is not sufficiently low for operative vaginal delivery or if excessive traction is required to effect delivery. Operative vaginal delivery for a deep transverse arrest should be performed only by obstetricians skilled in the use of forceps for this problem.

Deflexion abnormalities also cause dystocia. Deflexion refers to an abnormality in the cardinal movements of labor in which flexion of the fetal head does not occur as expected. The classic forms of deflexion abnormalities include brow and face presentations. Typically, a brow presentation is characterized by the long axis of the fetal head negotiating the short axis of the midpelvis, precluding vaginal delivery. Whereas fetuses with a brow presentation rarely deliver vaginally (except in women with generously sized midpelvic dimensions with a small fetus), face presentations often will deliver vaginally if the mentum, or chin, is positioned anteriorly (mentum anterior). Although these extreme flexion abnormalities are usually easily diagnosed (albeit relatively rare), other mild flexion abnormalities may not be so readily evident. Flexion abnormalities may be suspected in a prolonged or protracted labor unresponsive to oxytocin. Unfortunately, there is no safe and accepted means to correct the flexion of the fetal head.

Often, abnormal fetal position may occur as the result of the maternal pelvic type (Fig. 7). For example, android pelvic types often lead to deep transverse arrest or occiput posterior position because of the progressive narrowing of the pelvis. Women with an anthropoid pelvis tend to have fetal positions persistently occiput anterior or posterior, thus interfering with the normal cardinal movements of labor. Finally, women with a true platypelloid pelvis have transverse arrests, assuming the fetal head negotiates the shortened pelvic inlet. Because many women have mixed pelvic types, careful clinical pelvimetry may provide valuable information in the management of dystocia.

Epidural Analgesia and Asynclitism

The impact of epidural analgesia on the occurrence of dystocia and the cesarean delivery rate has been controversial. Epidural analgesia is an excellent form of pain relief for the laboring woman, and in some labor and delivery units the majority of laboring women opt for this therapy. This anesthetic approach involves the introduction of thin-gauged plastic catheter into the maternal epidural space and is thoroughly discussed in Chapter 8. At the time of epidural placement, some anesthetic agents may be injected directly into the spinal canal, and most epidurals involve injection of a local anesthetic into the epidural space. In this respect, epidural analgesia is a vital part of the obstetrician's and anesthesiologist's armament to provide pain relief during labor. However, epidural analgesia may have contributed significantly to the cesarean delivery epidemic of the past two decades. A metaanalysis of epidural use in the laboring woman cites an increase risk of 10% for cesarean delivery.[14]

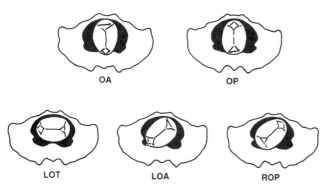

FIG. 8. Position of the fetal head. The sutures of the fetal head should be palpated, and the fetal head position should be recorded to ensure that the normal cardinal movements of labor are being followed. The fetal occiput, with the maternal position, are the reference points. Hence, OA refers to the occiput anterior position; OP, occiput posterior; LOT, left occiput transverse; LOA, left occiput anterior; ROP, right occiput posterior. Any fetal position can occur and should be noted on the labor curve.

An important concept in the management of laboring women with epidural analgesia involves assessment of the attitude, or lie, of the fetal head. When applied too early in labor (less than 4 or 5 centimeters dilation), epidural analgesia can adversely affect the progress of labor. While ineffective uterine activity can be corrected with oxytocin administration, epidural analgesia may alter the attitude of the fetal head as it traverses the maternal mid-pelvis with paralysis of the pelvic musculature. Asynclitism of the fetal head is the result (Fig. 9). When asynclitism of the fetal head occurs, the sagittal suture of the head is either deviated posteriorly or anteriorly in relation to the maternal outlet. As with other abnormal positioning of the fetal head, a larger diameter of the fetal head is expected to negotiate the bony pelvis of the mother. Thus, the second stage of labor in women with epidural analgesics is often prolonged, and operative vaginal delivery is more commonly needed to accomplish delivery. An important aspect of performing operative vaginal delivery involves correction of the asynclitism of the fetal head. This correction can often be accomplished with forceps that have a sliding lock or via vacuum extraction of the fetus, where the precise attitude and positioning of the fetus is of less importance.

Fetal Abnormalities

Specific fetal abnormalities may contribute to the etiology of dystocia. Fetuses with neuromuscular disease, and particu-

larly those who have suffered an *in utero* demise, may have flexion abnormalities. Also, fetal conditions such as hydrocephalus, hydrops fetalis, and tumors of the head or sacrum can lead to mechanical obstruction of the birth canal and hence cause dystocia, which is usually not remedied except by cesarean delivery.

◊ DIAGNOSIS OF LABOR ABNORMALITIES

Only if the progress of labor is closely monitored can labor abnormalities be diagnosed. Moreover, the timely diagnosis of these labor abnormalities, with prompt medical therapy, should improve the chances of achieving a vaginal delivery. These labor abnormalities can be classified as either arrest disorders (Fig. 10) or protraction disorders (Fig. 11). Table 2 provides parameters for abnormal labor.

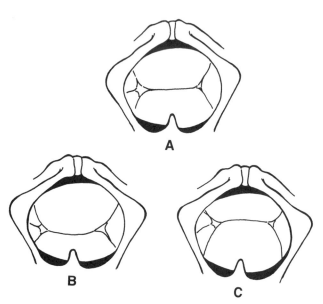

FIG. 9. Synclitism. The term synclitism refers to the relative orientation of the fetal sagittal suture with the maternal bony pelvis. **A** depicts a normal synclitism of a fetus in LOT position, with the sagittal suture equidistant between the anterior and posterior segments of the maternal pelvis. **B** shows a posterior asynclitism, where the sagittal suture is closer to the posterior bony pelvis, and more of the right parietal bone is palpated. **C** depicts an anterior asynclitism in which the sagittal suture is more anteriorly located, and the left parietal bone is more readily evident.

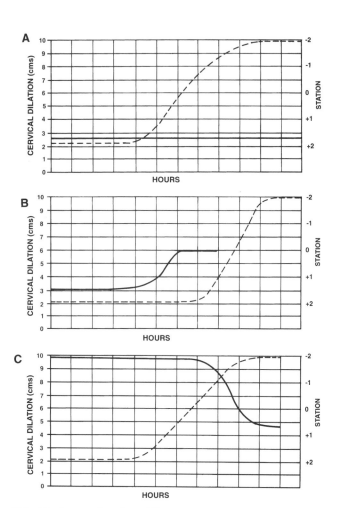

FIG. 10. Arrest disorders. These figures depict examples of different arrest disorders. **A** shows a prolonged latent phase. Although one might say that a prolonged latent phase is not strictly an arrest disorder, it reflects an abnormality in the normal progress of labor in which the change into the active phase is arrested. **B** depicts an arrest of dilation, in which the cervix achieves 6 cm of dilation but then does not change for 2 hours. **C** is an example of an arrest of descent. The fetal head moves from a −2 station to a 0 to −1 station but then makes no further progress.

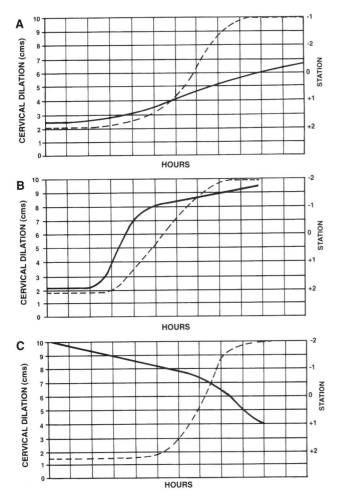

FIG. 11. Protraction disorders. These examples of protraction disorders are exaggerated to depict each abnormality. In each case, these abnormalities should be detected early, and appropriate therapy instituted. **A** depicts a protracted active phase. Note that the average slope is much less than 1.5 cm/hr. **B** is an example of a prolonged deceleration phase. Although somewhat rare, this type of labor pattern is associated with a need for cesarean delivery. **C** depicts a prolonged and neglected second stage. Intervention should occur sooner than indicated on this partogram.

Prolonged Latent Phase

A prolonged latent phase (Fig. 10A) occurs when regular painful uterine contractions are present for an extended period of time without entering the active phase of labor. Although a prolonged latent phase is not generally classified as an arrest disorder, one can make the case that the normal progress into normal labor is being arrested by abnormalities in the normal labor process. In nulliparous women, the definition of a prolonged latent phase is a period of uterine activity without cervical change for more than 20 hours, and in multiparas this time period is 14 hours. The cervix is often up to 4 cm dilated and completely effaced. The precise etiology is not clear but likely reflects ineffective uterine contractions without a dominant myometrial pacemaker.

The management of a prolonged latent phase is controversial, and there are two possible approaches. Some authorities believe that a prolonged latent phase of labor reflects an underlying labor abnormality that should be managed aggressively, whereas others recommend a more conservative course. One approach is to manage a prolonged latent phase aggressively with amniotomy and oxytocin. The other approach is to provide supportive measures including intravenous hydration and narcotic pain relief. Studies comparing these approaches have not shown either to be a clearly superior choice, so either treatment plan is acceptable as long as the patient understands the plan and risks. The more aggressive approach runs the risk of performing an induction of labor with the attendant higher risk of cesarean delivery, whereas the more conservative approach runs of the risk of prolonging a potentially dysfunctional labor. Either option is acceptable, and deciding which course to take requires obstetric judgment and a motivated, informed patient.

Arrest of Dilation

An arrest of dilation occurs when there is no cervical change after 2 hours in the active phase of labor despite uterine activity (Fig. 10B). In most cases, arrest of dilation occurs as a result of ineffective uterine contractions. Uterine contractions may be noted to couple (Fig. 5), an example of the loss of a dominant myometrial pacemaker with the expression of two pacemakers firing independently and without coordinated uterine contractions. Sometimes multiple pacemakers may be evident. In any case, prompt medical therapy with oxytocin usually corrects the underlying problem.

Arrest of Descent

After complete dilation is achieved, the primary goal of the second stage of labor is to gain station of the fetal head through the maternal pelvis with eventual delivery. At this time the patient often has an uncontrollable urge to push (because of Ferguson's reflex, in which the signal to push is given when the fetal head stretches the maternal pelvic floor). If the patient has an epidural catheter and is unable to generate effective pushing efforts, then she may be asked to rest and descend and allow the uterus to gain station until the urge to push occurs as the epidural analgesic wanes. If the patient does not gain station of 1 cm after an hour of adequate pushing efforts, an arrest of descent is diagnosed (Fig. 10C). The cause of this arrest disorder may be one or a combination of several underlying abnormalities, including inadequate uterine contractions, CPD, abnormal fetal position, and asynclitism. If an arrest of descent is diagnosed, the obstetrician has several options including the use of oxytocin, operative vaginal delivery, or cesarean delivery. The choices for therapy should be guided by the fetal status, station of the fetal head, and maternal status.

Protracted Active Phase

When cervical change continues with adequate uterine contractions in the active phase of labor, but over a longer time period than anticipated, then a prolonged active phase is the diagnosis (Fig. 11A). In nulliparous patients, cervical change is less than 1.2 cm/hr, whereas in multiparous patients cervical change is occurring at less than 1.5 cm/hr. A prolonged active phase may be the result of inadequate uterine contractility, but often both the timing and strength of uterine contractions appear to be normal, and the cervix continues to change slowly despite oxytocin therapy. The underlying problem may be true cephalopelvic disproportion or an undiagnosed flexion abnormality. Oxytocin therapy often is not successful in accelerating labor, and an arrest of dilation or descent may be inevitable regardless of the therapies employed. Should a protracted active phase lead to an arrest of labor despite oxytocin therapy, cesarean delivery is the best therapeutic course.

Prolonged Deceleration Phase

Some authorities argue that there is no deceleration phase of active labor, but prolonged time in achieving complete dilation after a previously normal labor is an ominous sign (Fig. 11B). Typically, the parturient progresses normally through labor and then slows progress after 8 cm. The uterine contraction pattern often will become dysfunctional and not be corrected with oxytocin. The cervix becomes swollen and edematous and seems to lose effacement. When a prolonged deceleration phase is diagnosed, cesarean delivery is often required, as the underlying problem is an abnormal fetal position (e.g., OA or OP at high station such that the long diameter of the fetal head is negotiating the shortest diameter of the fetal pelvis) or true CPD. One should not succumb to the temptation of pushing the cervix over the fetal head while having the mother push through a contraction in hopes of reducing the cervix and obtaining complete dilation, as the resultant tissue trauma often merely exacerbates cervical edema. This maneuver often leads one to believe that the cervix is completely dilated when, in fact, the fetal head has not descended into the maternal pelvis and the cervix is not truly completely dilated. Pushing efforts in this circumstance can lead to significant trauma to the cervix and prolongs the inevitable. Cesarean delivery for a prolonged deceleration phase after an adequate trial of oxytocin is recommended.

Prolonged Second Stage

An exaggerated example of a prolonged second stage is shown in Fig. 11C. A prolonged second stage is diagnosed when the fetal head descends less than 1 cm per hour. In the recent past, a second stage lasting longer than 2 hours was considered abnormal and an indication for operative vaginal delivery or cesarean delivery. Currently, as long as the fetus is tolerating the stresses of the second stage well, and some gain in station is being made, there is no indication for terminating the second stage early regardless of the cumulative time of pushing efforts. Because epidural analgesia may increase the length of the second stage, there is no reason for intervention on the obstetrician's part if the fetal heart rate tracing is acceptable and the mother is comfortable. However, maternal exhaustion will often occur with the need for operative intervention. As with the other labor abnormalities, an attentive obstetrician with a plan of management for any contingency should improve both maternal and fetal outcome in abnormal second stages of labor.

In summary, several specific labor abnormalities may occur and can easily be diagnosed. With a rational plan of management, the need for cesarean delivery can be avoided and salutary maternal and fetal outcomes accomplished. The term "failure to progress" thus is not sufficient for a diagnosis. For example, a woman may have "arrest of dilation" followed by treatment with oxytocin. Should this be unsuccessful, then she may require cesarean delivery for "arrest of dilation refractory to oxytocin therapy." Addressing labor abnormalities in more specific terms enables more rational treatment strategies to be utilized in the current and future pregnancies, regardless of the outcome.

◊ OPTIONS FOR THE MANAGEMENT OF DYSTOCIA

Once dystocia is diagnosed with a specific abnormality, the obstetrician has a number of therapeutic options that can lead to vaginal delivery rather than immediate resort to cesarean delivery. Oxytocin should be administered first unless there is a clear contraindication to this medication, as this is an effective and safe therapy in experienced hands and can correct most labor abnormalities. A schematic showing how to manage abnormal labor is depicted in Fig. 12.

Mapping the Progress of Labor

A key adjunct to the management of labor is the use of some form of a labor curve, such as a Friedman curve. The use of a labor curve has improved maternal and fetal outcomes while lowering the cesarean delivery rates, including sites in underdeveloped countries.[5] Many labor and delivery units utilized the concept of "alert" and "action" lines (Fig. 13).[18] In this type of partogram, crossing an alert line merely means that labor progress is slowing, while crossing the action line indicates that a specific action must be taken. Mapping labor progress allows for the timely diagnosis of dysfunctional labor and the prompt application of medical therapy. Therefore, most contemporary labor and delivery suites have incorporated the use of labor curves into the routine management of laboring women.

Amniotomy

Artificial rupture of membranes has been used in the management of slow or desultory labor for decades (Fig. 14). This intervention has been deplored by some obstetricians as

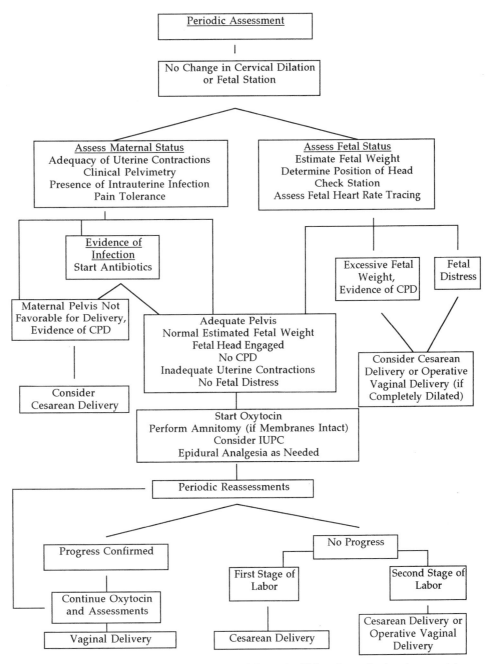

FIG. 12. Therapeutic options in the management of dystocia. This schematic drawing provides one algorithm for the management of dystocia. The primary goal is to effect vaginal delivery with good maternal and neonatal outcomes.

needless intervention and recommended by others as a useful adjunct. Retrospective studies with relatively small sample sizes suggested that amniotomy could speed normal labor and stimulate abnormal labor to again meet normal milestones. However, recent large-scale prospective randomized studies[8,27] do not support the routine use of amniotomy in the management of dystocia (Fig. 15). Although normal labor is accelerated modestly, particularly in multiparous women, patients in whom amniotomy was routinely used did not have lower rates of cesarean delivery. Additionally, there is a mod-

est increase in the rate of intrauterine infection in women who underwent amniotomy early in the course of labor (e.g., less than 4 cm dilation). Rupture of the membranes is also associated with variable decelerations of the fetal heart rate as a result of umbilical cord constriction. This problem can in some cases be remedied via amnioinfusion, or infusion of warm saline into the uterine cavity via an intrauterine pressure catheter (IUPC). However, the measure undertaken to improve outcome (amniotomy) leads to further interventions that otherwise could have been avoided.

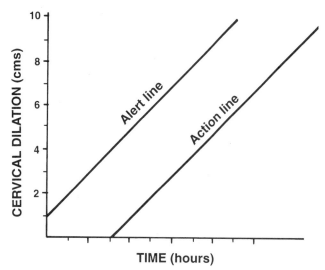

FIG. 13. Action and alert lines in the management of labor. This figure depicts the alert and action lines graphically. This type of labor curve has been used successfully to manage labor in many different settings. With this curve, slowing of the labor curve is first marked by an alert that labor is not progressing normally. Then, with further lack of progress, the action line is crossed, mandating that some form of action (medical or surgical therapy) be instituted. (Adapted from ref. 18, with permission.)

Conversely, there are reasonable indications for amniotomy. Amniotomy is an excellent method for labor induction if the cervix is favorable and the fetal head well applied to the cervix. The judicious use of amniotomy after 5 cm does accelerate labor in the multiparous woman, but less so in the nullipara. Also, oxytocin tends to work more efficiently if the membranes have been ruptured. Disruption of the membranes is required for internal monitoring of the fetal heart rate tracing or of uterine activity. Rupturing of the membranes will detect meconium staining of the amniotic fluid and alert the obstetrician and pediatrician to be prepared for a potentially

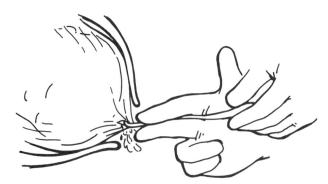

FIG. 14. Performing an amniotomy. The first and middle digits of one hand are placed in the cervical os, and then a plastic hook or clamp is inserted with the free hand to rupture the membranes. The fetal head should be well applied to the cervix with no obvious umbilical cord preceding the head (i.e., funic presentation).

high-risk circumstance regarding care of the newborn and the prevention of meconium aspiration.

Thus, amniotomy can be a useful adjunct in the management of labor, but only if used wisely and in appropriate circumstances. As long as the parturient is making adequate progress in labor and the fetal heart rate tracing is normal, there is no indication for amniotomy. Spontaneous rupture of the membranes usually occurs at between 7 and 9 cm dilation. Elective amniotomy should not be performed at only 4 or 5 cm of cervical dilation or before the patient is shown to be in active labor. Cervical examinations should be minimized after the membranes have been ruptured to decrease the chance of infection because the number of cervical examinations correlates well with the risk of intrauterine infection. When possible, amniotomy is useful in women being treated with oxytocin for abnormal labor. If there are concerns regarding the fetal heart tracing, the membranes should be ruptured and an internal fetal scalp lead placed. Similarly, amniotomy should be done before placement of an IUPC.

Intrauterine Pressure Catheters

An intrauterine pressure catheter is often introduced into the amniotic cavity to help determine the adequacy of uterine contractions (Fig. 16). The catheter is a thin, soft plastic device that is slipped past the fetal presenting part into the uterus. Application of the catheter usually requires that the fetal membranes are ruptured, either through spontaneous or artificial rupture of the membranes. Older devices required a pressure transducer at the bedside, which required calibration, in the hopes of obtaining reliable pressure measurements. More recent devices have the pressure transducer in the tip of the catheter, yielding more reliable pressure measurements.

Many different quantitative approaches to uterine contractility have been proposed using IUPC technology. For example, the Montevideo unit, introduced in the late 1950s, is equal to the average intensity of the uterine contractions multiplied by the number of contractions over a 10-minute period (expressed as mm Hg/10 min). A total of 200 Montevideo units indicated that there was adequate uterine contractility to effect labor progress. If this level of uterine activity was achieved and no labor progress resulted, then one could state that an adequate trial of labor had been completed and justify cesarean delivery. In another approach, computer-generated estimates of uterine contractility have been calculated and oxytocin administration then calibrated according to total area of uterine contractions.[7] Although these approaches provide a mathematical solution to attempt to optimize uterine action, they do not decrease the incidence of cesarean delivery. Because the use of IUPCs in the management of labor has not been shown conclusively to improve labor outcome, there is no compelling reason to use them. Perhaps their best application is in assisting nursing personnel with the use of oxytocin so that the precise timing of uterine contractions can be determined.

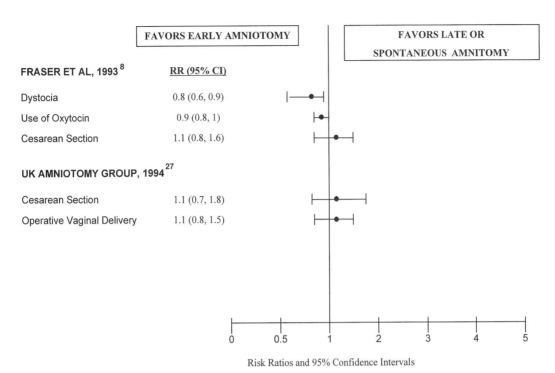

		FAVORS EARLY AMNIOTOMY	FAVORS LATE OR SPONTANEOUS AMNITOMY

FRASER ET AL, 1993 [8]

RR (95% CI)

Dystocia	0.8 (0.6, 0.9)
Use of Oxytocin	0.9 (0.8, 1)
Cesarean Section	1.1 (0.8, 1.6)

UK AMNIOTOMY GROUP, 1994 [27]

Cesarean Section	1.1 (0.7, 1.8)
Operative Vaginal Delivery	1.1 (0.8, 1.5)

Risk Ratios and 95% Confidence Intervals

FIG. 15. Odds ratio of the effect of amniotomy on labor dystocia. Amniotomy has little effect on the course of labor, the incidence of dystocia, or the incidence of cesarean delivery.

Epidural Analgesia

Although application of epidural analgesia early in labor may in some cases be detrimental to outcome, epidural pain relief can be of great benefit with regard to labor progress when used appropriately. Women with excessive labor pain may have greater anxiety, which in some cases may lead to poor labor progress. Thus, one potential adjunct to the management of labor is the use of epidural analgesia. With adequate pain re-lief, many women will progress more rapidly in labor. Additionally, oxytocin administration is associated with more painful uterine contractions, and adequate pain relief can aid in the appropriate dosing of oxytocin. The initial infusion of oxytocin should not be delayed while waiting for epidural placement; epidural placement usually takes less than 30 minutes, and oxytocin infusion should be commenced as soon as dystocia is diagnosed, as or before the epidural catheter is being placed. Delaying oxytocin for an excessive period of time may contribute to a poor uterine response.

Oxytocin

In 1953, du Vigneaud and co-workers sequenced the oxytocin peptide.[6] Oxytocin is a nine-amino-acid peptide (Fig. 17) normally produced in the hypothalamus and secreted by the posterior pituitary in a spurting or pulsatile fashion. During normal pregnancy, serum oxytocin concentrations remain essentially unchanged throughout gestation, and there is little increase in total serum concentrations before labor. However, with labor, plasma levels increase and then peak in the

FIG. 16. Placement of an intrauterine pressure catheter (IUPC). The first and middle digits of one hand are inserted into the cervical os, and then the IUPC is placed alongside the fetal head into the uterine cavity with the free hand. The fetal membranes usually require amniotomy if not previously ruptured.

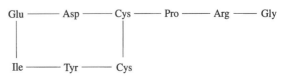

FIG. 17. The amino acid structure of oxytocin. Oxytocin is a nine-amino-acid peptide with two disulfide bonds.

second stage. Receptors for oxytocin increase in decidua in the weeks preceding the onset of labor and increase sharply just before labor. Oxytocin receptors are expressed primarily in decidua, myometrium, and breast tissue. Myometrial sensitivity to oxytocin parallels expression of oxytocin receptors such that responsiveness begins at about 20 weeks of gestation and then dramatically increases at about 30 weeks of gestation. Oxytocin is cleared from peripheral blood by the liver and kidney and is also significantly metabolized by oxytocinase, an enzyme produced in abundant quantities by the placenta and gestational tissues.

When oxytocin is administered intravenously, there is a concentration-dependent increase in its serum levels, but there is wide variation in responsiveness to oxytocin.[1] Intravenous administration of oxytocin has effects only on tissues expressing receptors, and as a result, oxytocin has an excellent therapeutic index. Oxytocin administration not only results in an increase in the frequency of uterine activity but also increases the total force generated by each contraction and the duration of each contraction. The myometrial response to oxytocin is highly variable, and uterine hyperstimulation may occur at any dose of administered oxytocin, depending on the individual patient. Uterine hyperstimulation necessitating discontinuation of the drug or a decrease in the dose being used is the most common side effect of the medication. The only known side effects of oxytocin not related to uterine activity include disturbances in water homeostasis and electrolytes. Oxytocin has approximately 1% the antidiuretic effect of vasopressin, and these side effects are usually seen only at high concentrations of oxytocin infusion (e.g., 40 to 50 units administered total). Also, intravenous boluses of oxytocin can lead to hypotension and tachycardia as a result of a paradoxical relaxation of vascular smooth muscle.

From the first clinically described use of oxytocin in the 1940s, there has been controversy as to the best and most appropriate regimen for oxytocin use. Table 4 summarizes some different acceptable oxytocin protocols currently used. Historically, early regimens of oxytocin administration were highly individualized by physician preference, ranging from relatively low doses to extremely high doses. In the 1980s, Seitchik and co-workers published studies in which carefully administered low-dose protocols resulted in salutary outcomes. In their first study, Seitchik and Castillo[22] found that the most important determinant of the maximum oxytocin dose and the frequency of hyperstimulation was dose incrementation interval. Those patients who received lower dose

increments (every 30 to 40 minutes) by 1.0 mU/min had lower oxytocin doses and less hyperstimulation with good outcomes. In a nonrandomized study comparing two different oxytocin regimens, Seitchik et al.[23] found that a more aggressive oxytocin regimen (starting at 5 mU/min and increasing according to uterine response) did not improve outcomes over the low-dose regimen.

However, recent studies have shown that low-dose protocols may result in higher cesarean delivery rates when compared to high-dose protocols. Satin et al.[20] utilized two different methods of oxytocin administration. In one 5-month period, they used a low-dose regimen in 1251 women where the starting dose of 1 mU/min was increased by 1 mU/min every 20 minutes until 8 mU/min was reached, and then the incremental increase was by 2 mU/min every 20 minutes up to a maximum of 20 mU/min. For the next 5-month period (1537 women), they studied the high-dose regimen advocated by O'Driscoll et al.[16] in which the starting dose of 6 mU/min was increased by 6 mU/min every 20 minutes up to a maximum of 42 mU/min. Among those patients being augmented, the average maximum oxytocin dose was greater in the high-dose protocol (14.7 mU/min vs. 6.6 mU/min), as was the incidence of uterine hyperstimulation (52% vs. 39%). Notably, there was a significant decrease in the cesarean section rate for dystocia (9% vs. 12%), the use of forceps (12% vs. 16%), rates of neonatal sepsis (8% vs. 12%), and a shorter time from admission to delivery (10.1 hours vs. 13.4 hours).

In a following study, Satin et al.[21] compared two incremental dosing intervals of high-dose oxytocin, comparing a 20-minute dosing interval versus a 40-minute dosing interval. In those women receiving oxytocin for labor augmentation, 603 were in the 20-minute interval group and 564 in the 40-minute interval group. The results of this study showed that the maximum oxytocin dose, the time from admission to delivery, and the incidence of uterine hyperstimulation were similar in each group. However, women receiving incremental increases in oxytocin at 20-minute intervals had a significantly lower cesarean section rate for dystocia (8% vs. 12%).

Finally, in a randomized study by Xenakis et al.,[28] the low-dose protocol was compared to a higher-dose protocol in which oxytocin was commenced at 4 mU/min and increased by 4 mU/min every 15 minutes. They found a significantly greater number of cesarean deliveries in women receiving the lower-dose regimen (10.4% vs. 25.7%). There were no differences in maternal or neonatal outcome or in the incidence of hyperstimulation. The average maximal dose of oxytocin

TABLE 4. *Acceptable oxytocin protocols*

Starting oxytocin dose	Incremental dose increase	Timing of incremental dose increase	Source
1 mU/min	1 mU/min	40 min	Seitchik and Castillo[22]
1 to 2 mU/min	1 to 2 mU/min	30 min	University of Utah
3 mU/min	3 mU/min	20 min	Author's preference
4 mU/min	4 mU/min	15 to 20 min	Houston, Texas
6 mU/min	6 mU/min	15 to 20 min	AMOL protocol[16]

in the high-dose regimen was only 9 mU/min, suggesting that achieving a more rapid response with higher doses does not require excessive amounts of oxytocin and that prompt correction of the labor abnormality is critical for success.

These studies suggest that a higher dose of oxytocin will stimulate a higher proportion of patients earlier, resulting in more timely correction of dysfunctional labor and in a lower risk for cesarean delivery (Fig. 18). There are numerous factors that can account for the wide variation in responsiveness to oxytocin infusions, including differences in oxytocin receptor expression, differences in oxytocin plasma concentrations, and differences in oxytocinase concentrations and activity.

Regardless of the choice of protocols, clinical judgment should be used when oxytocin therapy is prescribed.[3] There should be no evidence of fetopelvic disproportion based on clinical pelvimetry and estimated fetal weight. If the pelvis is not adequate, or the fetus is large, then the dysfunctional labor may be a sign that vaginal delivery is not possible, and cesarean delivery would be the more appropriate therapy. Additionally, oxytocin should not be used in women with prior classical cesarean section scars (Fig. 19) because the risk of uterine rupture is high. Care should be utilized when women with prior low transverse cesarean sections are being augmented with oxytocin. Although the studies regarding the use of oxytocin and the risk of scar dehiscence are mixed, one should know the total dose given and follow the course of labor carefully. Vaginal birth after cesarean section is addressed more fully in Chapter 27. Oxytocin is an extremely effective drug when used appropriately but can be dangerous for mother and fetus if used inappropriately. Therefore, clin-

ical judgment is required whenever oxytocin is utilized in the management of dystocia.

Operative Vaginal Delivery

The rules for performing successful operative vaginal delivery include complete cervical dilation, engagement of the fetal head filling the hollow of the sacrum, and known position of the fetal head. Forceps- or vacuum-assisted vaginal delivery should be performed only on behalf of the mother or fetus and not for the convenience of the obstetrician. In the context of dystocia, the primary reason for moving to assisted vaginal delivery is an arrest of descent of the fetal head. This arrest may be due to inadequate uterine contractions, insufficient maternal pushing efforts, abnormal position of the fetal head (OP or deep transverse arrest), or asynclitism of the fetal head. In these situations, the mother often has pushed for 2 hours or more and may be unable to continue with effective pushing efforts because of exhaustion. However, maternal exhaustion should not be listed as the sole indication for moving to forceps or the vacuum extractor. A precise diagnosis should be provided, such as "arrest of descent."

Use of the appropriate forceps or the indications for vacuum extraction are dependent on the experience of the obstetrician. Experienced obstetricians skilled in the use of forceps have the judgment to use the appropriate instruments and traction for a successful and safe vaginal delivery. Less experienced providers may find vacuum extraction more successful but still require judgment and skill to execute a safe vacuum-assisted delivery. Even with vacuum extraction, pru-

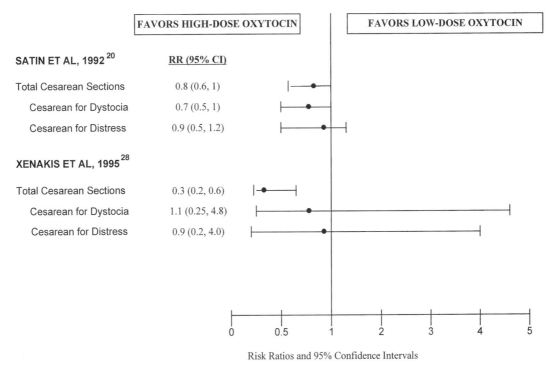

FIG. 18. Odds ratio of low-dose oxytocin versus high-dose oxytocin. High-dose oxytocin results in lower overall cesarean delivery rates.

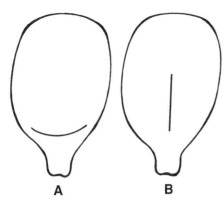

FIG. 19. Low transverse versus classical cesarean delivery. **A** depicts the uterine scar of a low transverse cesarean section; **B** shows the uterine scar after a classical cesarean delivery. Classical cesarean section scars are inherently weaker than scars from a low transverse cesarean section and have a higher risk of rupture with labor.

dent use in specific situations will decrease the incidence of maternal and fetal complications. An all too common occurrence is the inappropriate use of operative vaginal delivery with adverse obstetric and neonatal outcome. In experienced hands, there are no differences in neonatal outcome in infants delivered by normal vaginal delivery or by outlet forceps.

Cesarean Delivery

If all the above measures are not successful, then cesarean delivery is likely needed to obtain a good maternal and neonatal outcome. Although one should not move to cesarean delivery before all options are entertained, similarly one should not hesitate to operate if a successful vaginal delivery is not possible without potential serious risk or harm to the fetus and neonate. Delay in moving to cesarean delivery when indicated can potentially lead to adverse maternal and neonatal outcomes, such as postpartum hemorrhage, uterine rupture, and birth injury. Cesarean section is discussed in detail in Chapter 29.

◊ ACTIVE MANAGEMENT OF LABOR

Since the mid-1960s, an organized approach to the active management of labor (AMOL) has been developed and advocated by the obstetric staff at the National Maternity Hospital in Dublin, Ireland. Initially developed by Kieran O'Driscoll,[16] this approach has been modified over the years. The advocates of AMOL cite a continuing low cesarean delivery rate (less than 10%) with excellent outcomes for mother and infant. The primary goal of AMOL is to prevent prolonged labor. Women are guaranteed that they will either be delivered, or close to delivery, within 12 hours of admission to Labor and Delivery. The style and content of this labor management have generated much controversy and misunderstanding in the United States. For example, many obstetricians believe

that the active part of AMOL is aggressive intervention in the laboring women, but in fact it refers to the fact that an obstetrician (usually the head of the department) reviews the labor progress of each patient to ensure that optimal outcomes are achieved.

Basic Concepts of AMOL

Table 5 lists the primary components of the active management of labor. Perhaps the hallmark feature of AMOL is that no patients are admitted to Labor and Delivery unless the diagnosis of labor has been made. The diagnosis of labor is defined as painful, regular uterine contractions with complete cervical effacement, regardless of cervical dilation. The average dilation of the cervix at the time of admission is 2 to 3 cm. AMOL applies only to the nulliparous patient, as multiparous women who have had previous vaginal delivery usually deliver vaginally with little intervention and without prolonged labor. After the diagnosis of labor has been made, amniotomy is performed at the time of admission regardless of cervical dilation. The diagnosis of labor is key because, if this is incorrect, an induction of labor is being initiated with increased risk for cesarean delivery.

On admission, a nurse-midwife or student midwife is assigned to the patient, and she stays with only that patient for her entire labor. There are no provisions for change of nursing shifts. One aspect of AMOL is that the parturient is guaranteed delivery (or being near delivery) within 12 hours of admission. Also, these women receive detailed instructions on expectations during labor in prenatal birthing classes. One-on-one nursing care, with a clear vision of the ensuing labor, alleviates maternal anxiety and is perhaps the most distinguishing feature of AMOL over other styles of labor management as practiced in the United States. Cervical examinations to corroborate labor progress are performed by the midwives every 1 to 2 hours.

If the patient does not make adequate progress in labor, oxytocin administration is promptly initiated at 6 mU/min and increased by 6 mU/min every 15 minutes until seven to eight contractions occur every 15 minutes (Table 4). During labor, the patient is never left unattended by the midwife

TABLE 5. *Key concepts of active management of labor*

Comprehensive prenatal education
Admission only after labor is diagnosed
Strict criteria for the diagnosis of labor
Delivery with 12 hr of admission
One-on-one nursing care
Immediate amniotomy at admission (if membranes still intact)
Frequent cervical examinations to ensure progress in labor
Prompt intervention if labor progress not confirmed
High-dose oxytocin protocols
Epidural analgesia is available
Midpelvic and rotational forceps not used
Continuous internal audit
"Active" involvement of attending obstetrician

assigned to her care, and uterine activity is directly palpated by the midwife. The midwife assigned to the parturient will then perform the delivery with the head midwife in attendance. The attending obstetrician is asked to intervene only when there is need for an obstetric operation, such as episiotomy, forceps delivery, or cesarean delivery. Midforceps delivery and rotational forceps are not performed because of concerns of birth trauma.

With AMOL as it is done at the National Maternity Hospital, cesarean delivery rates for dystocia are less than 10%. Oxytocin is used in 50% to 60% of nulliparas and only 10% to 15% of multiparas (who are not managed with this program). Delivery occurs in less than 12 hours in 98% of women. Cerebral palsy rates approximate that of the United States, or about 2 per 1000 births. Birth trauma is a rare occurrence. The occurrence of abnormal fetal position (OP) is about 1 in 250 births. Epidural analgesia is allowed and does not impact significantly on the cesarean delivery rate. Clearly, AMOL suits the population served at the NMH well.

Lessons from AMOL

There have been three prospective randomized trials of AMOL in the United States (Table 6). Lopez-Zeno et al.[12] found a significant decrease in the cesarean delivery rate in nulliparous patients in the AMOL arm of the studies, from 14.1% to 10.5%. Frigoletto et al.[10] randomized over 1200 to AMOL or traditional management and found no decrease in the cesarean delivery rate but were able to show a modest decrease in the duration of labor in the AMOL arm. In the third study, Rogers et al.[19] also found no significant decrease in cesarean delivery rate but confirmed a decrease in the length of labor. These discrepancies may be because AMOL may not significantly reduce the cesarean delivery rate if the baseline rate is 11% or less. In other nonrandomized studies, AMOL has been shown to decrease the primary cesarean delivery rate by 25% to 50%, and a recent metaanalysis showed that the risk of cesarean delivery for dystocia was decreased on average by 34%.[11] In an analysis of these three randomized trials, AMOL resulted in a lower risk for cesarean delivery (Table 6, Fig. 20) and a greater incidence of delivery within 12 hours of delivery (Fig. 21).

Although critics of AMOL cite perceived excessive intervention (based on the use and doses of oxytocin), proponents of AMOL counter that a cesarean delivery rate of 20% to 25% versus less than 10% is the greater intervention. Many lessons can be derived from the protocol of AMOL. First, AMOL is a regimented approach to the management of labor in all nulliparous women admitted to the hospital. In many ways, this philosophy runs counter to the concept of individualizing patient care according to her specific situation. However, application of protocols in some situations (so-called "clinical practice guidelines") leads to more standardized application of appropriate therapies with concomitant improved outcomes. Whereas much has been made of the use of early amniotomy and the relatively high doses of oxytocin employed in AMOL protocols, a recent detailed analysis indicates that the most important component of AMOL in achieving a low cesarean birth rate is one-on-one nursing.[24] And perhaps the most important aspect of nursing care in this setting is the alleviation of maternal anxiety and the prompt diagnosis and treatment of dystocia. The precise oxytocin regimen is likely among the least important aspects of AMOL in the management of dystocia.

Active management of labor is an excellent example of how an organized approach to labor management can lead to better outcomes. Although AMOL cannot be adopted in its entirety in all labor and delivery units in the United States, the principles of AMOL can be adapted in many situations. First, normal women at term with uterine contractions should be admitted when they are in active labor. Obviously, there are exceptions to this concept, but premature admission with interventions usually implies that an induction of labor is being performed for no clear indication. Second, dysfunctional labor should be diagnosed and treated with appropriate medical therapy promptly. Third, efforts to alleviate maternal anxiety through prenatal education and attentive sympathetic caregivers should be maximized. Unfortunately, labor and delivery units in the United States would find it impossible to provide one-on-one nursing care throughout labor with the current staffing policies of most units. However, more personal interactions with all caregivers, from nurses to obstetricians, should be encouraged. And last, there is little delay in making the decision to move to cesarean delivery, improving both maternal and neonatal outcomes.

TABLE 6. *Cesarean delivery incidence in randomized studies of active management of labor*

Study	Total number of patients	Traditional n	Traditional n (%) CS	AMOL n	AMOL n (%) CS	p
Lopez-Zeno et al.[12]	705	354	50 (14.1)	351	37 (10.5)	<0.05
Frigoletto et al.[10]	1263[a]	585	66 (11.3)	678	62 (9.2)	ns[b]
Rogers et al.[19]	405	205	24 (11.7)	200	15 (7.5)	0.36
Total	2373	1144	140 (12.2)	1229	114 (9.3)	0.02[c]

[a]This value includes only those women eligible for the study protocol.
[b]Nonsignificant.
[c]Simple chi-square analysis.

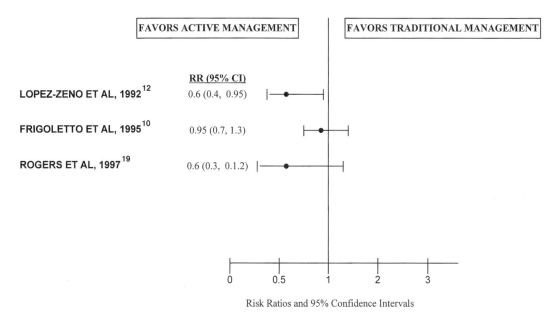

FIG. 20. Odds ratio of the effect of active management of labor on cesarean delivery rate. AMOL is associated with a lower risk of cesarean delivery in one study but with equivocal results in two studies.

◊ CONCLUSION AND SUMMARY POINTS

Key points regarding the management of dystocia, from the perspective of evidence-based medicine, include the following:

1. Dystocia is common, particularly in the nulliparous patient, and is a common indication for cesarean delivery.
2. Early amniotomy does not improve labor outcomes. However, amniotomy after 5 cm of dilation can shorten the time of labor, but at the expense of a modest increase in infectious morbidity.

3. Early application of epidural analgesia can contribute to labor abnormalities, particularly in the second stage, and lead to an increased need for operative vaginal delivery.
4. Active management of labor protocols can decrease the cesarean delivery rate in some populations.
5. Oxytocin protocols using higher doses (3 to 6 mU/min and increasing concentrations every 15 to 20 minutes) decrease the need for cesarean delivery for dystocia with adequate safety for mother and fetus.

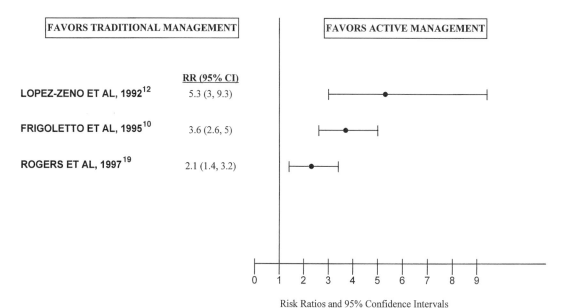

FIG. 21. Odds ratio of the effect of active management of labor on delivery within 12 hours. AMOL is associated with delivery within 12 hours of presentation to the labor and delivery units in each study depicted.

All authorities agree that the primary goal in managing women in labor is to obtain healthy babies with minimal maternal morbidity. However, the methods used to achieve these goals elicit a great deal of controversy among obstetricians. Nevertheless, following the principles of labor management as outlined in this chapter should ensure good maternal and fetal outcomes.

◊ **REFERENCES**

1. Amico JA, Seitchik H, Robinson AG. Studies of oxytocin in plasma of women during hypocontractile labor. *J Clin Endocrinol Metab* 1984;58:274–279.
2. Creasy RK (ed). *Management of labor and delivery.* Maulden, MA: Blackwell Science, 1997.
3. Dudley DJ. Oxytocin: use and abuse, science and art. *Clin Obstet Gynecol* 1997;40:516–524.
4. Duff P, Sanders R, Gibbs RS. The course of labor in term patients with chorioamnionitis. *Am J Obstet Gynecol* 1983:147:391–395.
5. Dujardin B, De Schampheleire I, Sene H, Ndiaye F. Value of the alert and action lines on the partogram. *Lancet* 1992;339:1336–1338.
6. du Vigneaud V, Ressler C, Trippett S. The sequence of amino acids in oxytocin, with a proposal for the structure of oxytocin. *J Biol Chem* 1953;205:949–957.
7. Fairlie FM, Philips GF, Andrews BJ, Calder AA. An analysis of uterine activity in spontaneous labor using a microcomputer. *Br J Obstet Gynecol* 1988;95:57–64.
8. Fraser WD, Marcoux S, Moutquin JM, et al. Effect of early amniotomy on the risk of dystocia in nulliparous women. *N Engl J Med* 1993;328:1145–1149.
9. Friedman EA. *Labor: Clinical evaluation and management, 2nd ed.* New York: Appleton, 1978.
10. Frigoletto RD, Leiberman E, Lang JM, et al. A clinical trial of active management of labor. *N Engl J Med* 1995;333:495–490.
11. Glantz JC, McNanley TJ. Active management of labor: a meta-analysis of cesarean delivery rates for dystocia in nulliparas. *Obstet Gynecol Surv* 1997;52:497–505.
12. Lopez-Zeno J, Peaceman AM, Adashek JA, Socol ML. A controlled trial of a program for the active management of labor. *N Engl J Med* 1992;326:450–454.
13. Moore TM, Iams JD, Creasy RK, Burau KD, Davidson AL. Diurnal and gestational patterns of uterine activity in normal human pregnancy. *Obstet Gynecol* 1994;83:517–523.
14. Morton SC, Williams MS, Keeler EB, Gambone JC, Kahn KL. Effect of epidural analgesia for labor on the cesarean delivery rate. *Obstet Gynecol* 1994;83:1045–1052.
15. Notzon FC, Cnattingius S, Bergsjo P, Cole S, Taffel S, Irgens L, Daltveit AK. Cesarean section delivery in the 1980s: international comparison by indication. *Am J Obstet Gynecol* 1994;170:495–504.
16. O'Driscoll K, Meagher D, Boylan P. *Active management of labor: the Dublin experience, 3rd ed.* London: Mosby-Yearbook, 1993.
17. Parratt J, Taggart M, Wray S. Abolition of contractions in the myometrium by acidification *in vitro. Lancet* 1994;344:717–718.
18. Philpott RH, Castle WM. Cervicographs in the management of labor in primigravidae: II. The action line and treatment of abnormal labor. *J Obstet Gynecol Br Commonw* 1972;79:599–602.
19. Rogers R, Gibson GJ, Miller AC, Izquierdo LE, Curet LB, Qualls CR. Active management of labor: does it make a difference? *Am J Obstet Gynecol* 1997;177:599–605.
20. Satin AJ, Leveno KJ, Sherman ML, Brewster DS, Cunningham FG. High- versus low-dose oxytocin for labor stimulation. *Obstet Gynecol* 1992;80:111–116.
21. Satin AJ, Leveno KJ, Sherman ML, McIntire D. High-dose oxytocin: 20- versus 40-minute dosage interval. *Obstet Gynecol* 1994;83:234–238.
22. Seitchik J, Castillo M. Oxytocin augmentation of dysfunctional labor. I. Clinical data. *Am J Obstet Gynecol* 1982;144:899–905.
23. Seitchik J, Castillo M. Oxytocin augmentation of dysfunctional labor. V. An alternative oxytocin regimen. *Am J Obstet Gynecol* 1985;151:757–761.
24. Thorton JG, Lilford RJ. Active management of labor: current knowledge and research issues. *Br Med J* 1994;309:366–369.
25. Thurnau GR, Hales KA, Morgan MA. Evaluation of the fetal–pelvic relationship. *Clin Obstet Gynecol* 1992;35:570–581.
26. Turner MJ, Rasmussen MJ, Turner JE, Boylan PC, MacDonald D, Stronge JM. The influence of birthweight on labor in nulliparas. *Obstet Gynecol* 1990;76:159–163.
27. U.K Amniotomy Group. A multicenter randomized trial of amniotomy in spontaneous first labor at term. *Br J Obstet Gynecol* 1994;101:307–309.
28. Xenakis EMJ, Langer O, Piper JM, Conway D, Berkus MD. Low-dose versus high-dose oxytocin augmentation of labor—a randomized trial. *Am J Obstet Gynecol* 1995;173:1874–18.

CHAPTER 29

Cesarean Delivery

───── ◇ ─────

James R. Scott

Cesarean section is a term commonly used in obstetrics to describe the delivery of a viable fetus through an incision in the abdominal wall (laparotomy) and the uterus (hysterotomy). However, the words cesarean and section used together are actually redundant because both imply incision. Cesarean birth and cesarean delivery are preferable terms and are used interchangeably in this chapter.

Cesarean delivery has played a major role in lowering both maternal and perinatal morbidity and mortality rates during the past century. The initial purpose was to preserve the life of the mother with obstructed labor, but indications have expanded over the years to include delivery for a variety of more subtle dangers to the mother or the fetus.[1,2] Contributing to its more frequent use is its increased safety, which is largely a result of better surgical technique, improved anesthesia, effective antibiotics, and availability of blood transfusions. Nevertheless, there has been increasing concern over what is considered by many to be an excessive cesarean rate in contemporary obstetrics.

The percentage of women in the United States delivered by cesarean dramatically increased from less than 5% in 1965 to 25% in 1990. It is now the most common operative procedure performed in many hospitals in this country. The reasons for this striking increase are multiple. During the 1970s and 1980s, it was assumed that cesarean delivery would be the solution to numerous obstetric problems. Facing increasing medical-legal pressures, obstetricians gradually abandoned most vaginal breech and forceps deliveries, broadened the definition of intrapartum fetal distress, and liberalized the diagnosis of dystocia. Also, a greater number of older women and primigravidae, whose primary cesarean rate is higher, were having children. Finally, the escalation in primary cesareans increased the overall cesarean rate because until recently most women were delivered by repeat cesarean birth in subsequent pregnancies.

Although perinatal outcome in the United States improved during the time when the cesarean rate increased, it has also improved in other countries where cesarean rates remained low. Moreover, the incidence of cerebral palsy has not declined during the past 20 years because perinatal morbidity and mortality are more often a function of antepartum events, abnormal fetal growth, congenital anomalies, and premature birth.[3] Delivery by cesarean is usually associated with an increased cost for the health-care system when compared to vaginal birth. These factors have led to efforts to reduce the rate of cesarean birth. Most emphasis has been placed on decreasing the number of repeat cesareans. Periodic review of all cesarean deliveries has also been encouraged as useful and desirable. A number of studies show that a critique of the indications for cesarean birth can identify and alter a too-liberal or too-restricted use of the procedure.[4]

◇ INDICATIONS

Cesarean birth is necessary whenever labor is unsafe for either mother or fetus, when labor cannot be induced, when dystocia or fetal problems present significant risks with vaginal delivery, and when an emergency mandates immediate delivery. It is not practical to list all potential indications for cesarean delivery or to discuss the numerous changes in obstetric management that have influenced these over the years (Table 1). Many indications are well accepted, a number are subjective or selectively applied in individual patients, and others are more controversial.[1,2] The majority of cesareans are performed for fetal indications, a few are solely for maternal reasons, and some benefit both fetus and mother. Repeat cesarean accounts for approximately 30% of cesarean births in the United States, dystocia is the indication for up to 30%, and fetal distress, breech, and other conditions are responsible for the remaining cases.

Labor Contraindicated

Uterine contractions can be hazardous to the mother under certain circumstances. These include central placenta previa,

457

TABLE 1. *Common indications for cesarean delivery*

Accepted
Failed induction
Cephalopelvic disproportion
Failure to progress in labor
Proven fetal distress
Placental abruption
Placenta previa
Umbilical cord prolapse
Obstructive benign and malignant tumors
Active genital herpes infection
Abdominal cerclage
Conjoined twins

Controversial (or selective)
Breech presentation
Repeat cesarean
Immune thrombocytopenia
Severe Rh immunization
Congenital fetal anomalies, major
Cervical carcinoma
Prior vaginal colporrhaphy
Large vulvar condylomata

previous classical uterine incision, myomectomy transecting the uterine wall, or uterine reconstruction. In these situations, labor and vaginal delivery may result in uterine rupture and hemorrhage, endangering the life or future health of the mother. Conditions in which labor is dangerous to the fetus include placenta previa, velamentous insertion of the cord or other forms of vasa previa, and cord presentation. More recent indications include treatable fetal anomalies such as meningomyelocele and certain degrees of hydrocephaly.

Failed Induction

Conditions such as isoimmunization, diabetes mellitus, intrauterine growth retardation, and hypertensive disorders constitute a threat to the mother or fetus and often require delivery when the cervix is unfavorable for induction. If attempts to induce labor are inappropriate or unsuccessful, cesarean birth is the only alternative. More effective methods of softening the cervix before inducing labor preterm are reducing the need for cesarean.

Dystocia

Mechanical problems of the uterus, fetus, or birth canal or ineffective uterine contractions that result in unsuccessful progress of labor and vaginal delivery are collectively referred to as dystocia. This term encompasses a variety of commonly used clinical terms, such as failure to progress, cephalopelvic disproportion (CPD), and dysfunctional labor (see Chapter 28). It is also a relative term. For example, fetal macrosomia sometimes causes CPD, but most cesarean births for abnormal labor involve a normal-sized infant. Dystocia occasionally is caused by soft tissue tumors and abnormal fetal presentations (see Chapter 28).

Fetal Distress

Electronic fetal monitoring improves the chance of detecting fetal distress, but its inaccuracy (false-positive rate) has also contributed to the increased number of cesarean births. Nonreassuring fetal heart rate (FHR) patterns and the diagnosis of fetal distress are discussed in Chapter 15. Many clinicians have replaced vaginal breech deliveries with cesarean delivery to avoid the risk of intrapartum asphyxia or delivery-related trauma from head entrapment and umbilical cord prolapse (see Chapter 28).

Maternal or Fetal Emergency

Certain maternal or fetal conditions require immediate delivery of the baby because vaginal delivery is either impossible or inappropriate. Such circumstances include severe placental abruption, hemorrhage from placenta previa, prolapse of the umbilical cord, active genital herpes, and impending maternal death.

◊ COMPLICATIONS

Cesarean section is not an innocuous procedure.[5] A variety of postpartum complications—including unexplained fever, endometritis, wound infection, hemorrhage, aspiration, atelectasis, urinary tract infection, thrombophlebitis, and pulmonary embolism—occur in up to 25% of patients. The frequency of maternal death related to cesarean section varies with the institution and with the condition necessitating the procedure. Maternal mortality rates are fewer than one per 1000 operations, and many deaths are related to the underlying maternal illness or anesthetic complications.

Late maternal complications of cesarean delivery include intestinal obstruction from adhesions and dehiscence of the uterine incision in subsequent pregnancies. Both of these complications are more common with the classic incision than a lower uterine segment incision. A rare complication not generally appreciated is the combination of uterine infection and classic incision. Invasion of the incision by the infecting organism may lead to dehiscence, allowing the uterine infection to drain freely into the peritoneal cavity. Prompt surgical intervention and vigorous antibiotic therapy are indicated, and hysterectomy may be required. The incidence of abnormal myometrial invasion by the placenta (accreta/increta/percreta) is also increased with each cesarean and can cause severe and intractable hemorrhage at repeat cesarean.

◊ TYPES OF CESAREAN OPERATIONS

Almost all contemporary cesareans are performed by using a transperitoneal approach to reach the uterine wall. An extraperitoneal technique was sometimes used in the past in patients with an infected uterus in an attempt to reduce the chance of peritonitis. More effective antibiotics have now made this approach unnecessary.

The two major types of cesarean operations are classified by the location and direction of the uterine incision. The first are those incisions made in the upper segment of the uterus (Fig. 1). The vertical incision usually made in the anterior fundus is referred to as a classical incision. It is used primarily when it is difficult to deliver the infant through a low uterine segment incision. The second type is characterized by incisions made in the lower portion of the uterus after the bladder has been displaced downward (Fig. 2). The preferred and most frequently used is the low transverse incision. A vertical incision may also be made in this area, but it usually involves the upper uterine segment unless the lower segment is quite elongated by labor.

Occasionally, variations are used because of unanticipated difficulty (Fig. 3). These incisions are best avoided by careful assessment and planning. A J-shaped incision is made when the obstetrician begins a transverse lower uterine segment incision and finds the lower uterine segment to be too narrow. It is often not realized that the incision is inadequate until delivery is attempted. A vertical extension from one end is necessary to avoid extension into the broad ligament. The T-shaped incision is made for similar reasons.

◊ ANESTHESIA

The choice of anesthetic technique and agents is dictated by a number of factors, as discussed in Chapter 8. Patients with fetal distress, hemorrhage, shock, previous injury or surgery to the spine, or skin infections of the lower back are not usually candidates for spinal or epidural anesthetic techniques. Conversely, a patient with active pulmonary disease such as pneumonia or tuberculosis or one who will be difficult to intubate is not a good candidate for inhalation anesthesia.

In most cases, there is no clear-cut indication or contraindication, so the technique utilized depends primarily on such factors as urgency of delivery, patient choice, and skill of the anesthesiologist. The choice between regional block and inhalation anesthesia is made after a discussion among the patient, anesthesiologist, and obstetrician.

Maternal and fetal hemodynamics are markedly affected by maternal position. In the dorsal recumbent position, the

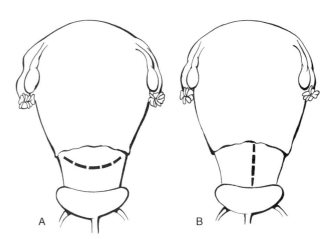

FIG. 2. Incisions in lower uterine segment. **(A)** Low transverse incision. **(B)** Low vertical incision.

gravid uterus compresses the inferior vena cava. Decreased venous return and maternal cardiac output result in hypotension and reduced uterine perfusion, referred to as the inferior vena cava syndrome. The weight of the pregnant uterus also progressively compresses the aorta as the mean arterial pressure falls, thus reducing blood flow to the pelvis. Hypotension produced by regional anesthetic techniques compounds this problem. Devices attached to the operating table, inflatable wedges or towels placed under the patient, or tilting the table, can be used to displace the uterus to the patient's left in preparation for cesarean section. Rapid intravenous infusion of physiological solution containing sodium immediately before the initiation of regional anesthesia also reduces the incidence of hypotension.

The status of the fetus worsens as the time of exposure to anesthesia lengthens. Progressive fetal depression as induction-to-delivery time is prolonged makes it important to avoid unnecessary delay before and during surgery. The abdomen should be fully prepped, draped, and ready for the incision before general anesthesia is induced. On the other hand, reckless

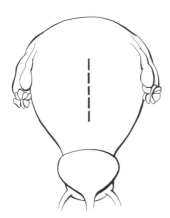

FIG. 1. Classic incision in the upper segment of the uterus.

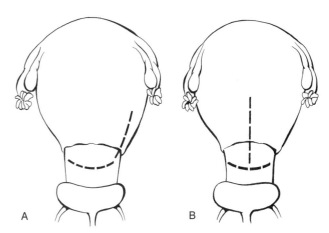

FIG. 3. Undesirable variations of uterine incisions. **(A)** J-shaped incision. **(B)** T-shaped incision.

surgical techniques for rapid delivery of the fetus are unwise. An induction-to-delivery time of 5 to 15 minutes is reasonable if maternal oxygenation, blood pressure, and displacement of the uterus are monitored and maintained.

◊ OPERATIVE PROCEDURE

Cesarean delivery requires the same preoperative care as for any major surgery and additional consideration for the status of the fetus. A patient who is dehydrated from prolonged labor needs correction with intravenous fluids. Because anemia is relatively common in pregnancy, a hemoglobin or hematocrit should be checked preoperatively. Blood is typed and screened to be available for immediate transfusion. Routine preparation of autologous blood is not cost effective for most cesarean patients because few patients are transfused. However, autologous blood can be prepared during the antepartum period if the patient is at high risk for hemorrhage as with placenta previa or accreta. Because the bladder will be in the operative field, it is necessary to place an indwelling catheter before beginning surgery. The patient and her partner should be given an explanation of the details of the operation, the risks involved, and the reason it is necessary. Informed written permission for the procedure, anesthetic, administration of blood, and possible hysterectomy if necessary is then signed by the patient.

With elective cesarean delivery, it is the obligation of the physician to obtain evidence of fetal maturity.[6] Documentation by noninvasive techniques is outlined in Table 2. These criteria are not intended to preclude the use of menstrual dating. If the criteria confirm gestational age assessment on the basis of menstrual dates in a patient with normal menstrual cycles and no immediately antecedent use of oral contraceptives, delivery can be scheduled at greater than 39 weeks by menstrual dates. Ultrasound is considered confirmatory of menstrual dates if there is gestational age agreement within 1 week by crown–rump measurement obtained at 6 to 11 weeks, or within 10 days by the average of multiple measurements obtained at 12 to 20 weeks. When the fetal gestational age is uncertain, amniocentesis for amniotic fluid studies should by used to ensure fetal maturity. Awaiting the onset of spontaneous labor is another option.

Preparation

Preparation of the abdomen includes scrubbing the skin with soap and an antiseptic agent such as nonorganic iodide. The abdomen is then draped, leaving the area for the incision exposed.

Aspiration of the acidic contents of the stomach is a known risk when general anesthesia is used in pregnant women. The resulting pneumonitis is called Mendelson syndrome. Pretreatment with any of several medications reduces the risk of aspiration (see Chapter 8).

Prophylactic antibiotics are used in appropriate patients to reduce the incidence of postpartum infection.[7] The risk of postpartum endometritis is increased by duration of labor, prolonged rupture of the membranes, and number of cervical examinations. A single dose of a broad-spectrum antibiotic, such as 1 g of a cephalosporin, is usually given at delivery after the umbilical cord has been clamped. With a clinically apparent intrapartum infection, therapeutic antibiotics started before surgery are continued into the postoperative period.

A pediatrician, neonatologist, or other physician should also be available in the operating room if there is indication that the infant will need rescusitation.

Surgical Technique

A lower abdominal midline vertical incision and the transverse Pfannenstiel incision are the two most commonly used skin incisions. Speed of entry through the low vertical incision is facilitated by diastasis of the rectus muscles during pregnancy, which permits rapid access to the lower uterine segment in emergencies. This incision minimizes blood loss and allows extension for examination of the upper abdomen if necessary. However, the transverse Pfannenstiel incision is used more frequently in modern obstetrics because of the cosmetic result preferred by most women. Moreover, entry through this incision is relatively rapid in the hands of an experienced surgeon, visualization of the pelvis is adequate, and there is less risk of subsequent herniation.

The abdomen is opened in layers, and any large bleeding vessels encountered are clamped, but meticulous hemostasis is not attempted at this time if it will unduly delay delivery of the fetus. The abdominal cavity is briefly inspected, and the direction and degree of rotation of the uterus are noted. Retractors are placed in the abdominal incision and pulled laterally to expose the anterior surface of the uterus and the bladder covering the lower uterine segment.

The fold of peritoneum between the serosa of the uterus and the serosa of the bladder is identified (Fig. 4A). This loose peritoneum is elevated in the midline with forceps and incised, allowing entry into the space between the bladder and the lower uterine segment (Fig. 4B). The peritoneum is incised in a lateral direction, further separating the bladder from the overlying peritoneum, avoiding underlying veins in the broad

TABLE 2. *Fetal maturity assessment before elective repeat cesarean delivery*[a]

Fetal heart tones documented for 20 weeks by non-electronic fetoscope or for 30 weeks by Doppler

36 weeks since a positive serum or urine human chorionic gonadotropin pregnancy test was performed by a reliable laboratory

An ultrasound measurement of the crown–rump length, obtained at 5 to 11 weeks that supports a gestational age of >39 weeks

An ultrasound obtained at 12 to 20 weeks that confirms the gestational age of >39 weeks determined by clinical history and physical examination

[a]Adapted from ACOG Committee Opinion No. 98. September 1991.

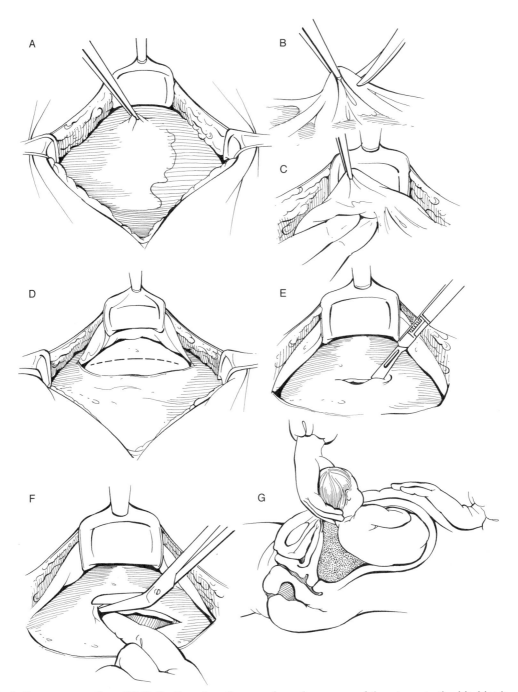

FIG. 4. Cesarean section. **(A)** Reflection of peritoneum from the serosa of the uterus to the bladder is identified. **(B)** Peritoneal reflection between the uterus and bladder is elevated and incised. **(C)** The bladder is displaced away from the lower uterine segment. **(D)** The bladder is retracted, and the incision is planned to be 2 to 3 cm below the peritoneal incision. **(E)** A small incision is made through the uterine wall to the fetal membranes. **(F)** A uterine incision is made in a curvilinear shape, using bandage scissors. **(G)** The fetal head is elevated through the uterine incision by the operator's hand.

and cardinal ligaments. The operator then reflects the bladder from the lower uterine segment (Fig. 4C,D).

The operator is now looking directly at the fascia covering the lower uterine segment. A few centimeters below the peritoneal incision, a small transverse incision is made in the midline with a scalpel (Fig. 4E). If care is taken, the fetal

membranes will bulge into the incision without being ruptured. The operator then inserts a finger between the fetal membranes and the wall of the uterus. Using this finger as a guide, the operator inserts the lower blade of bandage scissors to extend the incision laterally in a gentle upward curve (Fig. 4F). The assistant retracts the abdominal wall firmly on the side the operator is dissecting. Under direct vision, this half of the incision is extended as far laterally as possible without entering the broad ligament. The procedure is repeated on the opposite side. Once it is completed, a crescent-shaped or curvilinear incision is present in the lower uterine segment, and the fetal membranes are bulging into the incision.

An alternative method of opening the uterus is to make a shallow curvilinear incision through the pubocervical fascia. In a small area in the center, the incision is extended through to the fetal membranes. Inserting both index fingers into the opening, the operator pulls laterally, bluntly opening the uterus. This method works best in a patient with a thin lower uterus segment.

The operator now ruptures the membranes and inserts one hand beneath the lower edge of the uterine incision and over the fetal membranes to feel the presenting fetal part. With a vertex presentation, the occiput is identified, and the fetal head is flexed. The hand is gradually inserted between the uterine wall and the fetal head, and the head is brought into the uterine incision (Fig. 4G). The assistant or operator exerts fundal pressure on the fetal buttocks to gently deliver the fetal head through the incision. Once the head is delivered, the assistant suctions the mouth and the nares with a bulb syringe while the operator completes the delivery. If meconium is present in the amniotic fluid, a catheter and suction should be immediately available for complete suctioning of nasopharynx and oropharynx. The fetal shoulders are delivered with gentle traction on the fetal head in a manner similar to a vaginal delivery. Specially designed forceps or a vectis can also be used instead of the operator's hand in delivering the head through the uterine incision.

After delivery, the umbilical cord is clamped and divided, and the fetus is handed to an assistant outside the operative field. The placenta is delivered spontaneously if possible. If manual removal is necessary, it is delivered by separating it bluntly from the uterine wall with the fingers held extended in a rigid manner and the back of the hand facing the uterine wall. The uterine cavity is inspected for any structural abnormality, and any retained placental tissue or adherent membranes are removed. Dilation of the endocervical canal from above is unnecessary unless an unusual circumstance suggests nonpatency of the canal. Oxytocin is added to the patient's intravenous infusion to stimulate uterine contractions and reduce the amount of bleeding.

The cut edges of the uterine wall are now grasped with ring forceps or other noncrushing clamps for traction and to compress bleeding venous sinuses. With a two-layer closure, the first layer (Fig. 5A) is a continuous locked or unlocked absorbable suture anchored securely at the angle of the incision. The second layer of closure (Fig. 5B) imbricates the first with the use of absorbable sutures placed as interrupted figures-of-eight, Lembert, or continuous sutures to completely cover the first layer. Any persistent bleeding in the incision line is controlled with interrupted figure-of-eight sutures. When the low transverse uterine segment is thin, a one-layer closure is satisfactory and is commonly used.[8] The peritoneum can either

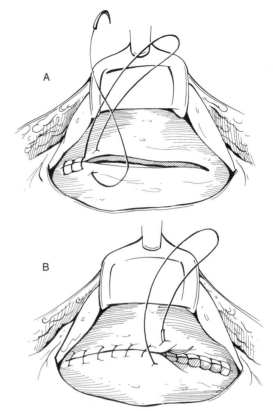

FIG. 5. Wound closure. **(A)** First layer of closure. **(B)** Second layer of closure. **(C)** Closure of visceral peritoneum.

be left open or reapproximated with a continuous layer of absorbable suture (Fig. 5C).

Any packs in the abdominal cavity are removed, and residual blood or amniotic fluid is removed by suction. If meconium soilage or exposure to infected amniotic fluid has occurred, the pelvic cavity should be copiously lavaged with normal saline solution. The ovaries, tubes, and other organs are inspected, and the abdomen is then closed in layers. The use of a mass ligature closure such as the Smead-Jones technique for vertical incisions should be considered for patients at high risk of disruption. A delayed absorbable synthetic suture is most commonly used on fascia, but nonabsorbable suture is also acceptable.

Postoperative management is similar to that of any patient who has had major surgery. Because the postpartum patient who has undergone cesarean delivery is at risk for thrombophlebitis and thromboembolism, spontaneous leg movement and early ambulation are encouraged. The urinary catheter may be removed on the first postoperative day, and the patient is soon able to tolerate oral feedings. Currently, discharge from the hospital is often dictated by economic and insurance factors rather than medical condition. If there is a contraindication to early discharge, the physician should insist on continued inpatient management and document the reason in the patient's record. With early discharge, adequate support and professional care at home must be an integral part of management.

Closure of the Classic Incision

The thickness of the upper uterine wall may require a three-layer closure to and including the serosa. Continuous suture techniques may be used, but interrupted sutures frequently give a more exact closure. The first layer should include about half the thickness of the wall and can be simple or figures-of-eight. The second layer is placed to avoid leaving a space between the layers. The third layer should close the serosa in a manner that minimizes the raw surface exposed to the abdominal cavity. This absorbable suture is continuous and not locked. Each bite with the needle should begin on the raw surface of the wound and exit through the serosa a few millimeters from the cut edge. With this technique, the cut edge is infolded, and the serosal surfaces are brought over to cover. Sometimes this is referred to as a baseball stitch.

Variations

After prolonged obstructed labor, the fetal head can be deeply impacted in the midpelvis with a greatly elongated and thinned lower uterine segment. Under these circumstances, it may be necessary for an assistant to dislodge the fetal head with a hand inserted into the vagina either immediately before or during the cesarean. Manipulation of the fetal head necessary for the delivery combined with the thin lower uterine segment risks lateral extension of a transverse incision and laceration of uterine vessels.

Occasionally, in the presence of a posterior placenta previa, footling breech presentation, or preterm delivery, the lower uterine segment is too narrow for an adequate transverse incision. Under these circumstances, a vertical incision in the lower segment is usually necessary, even if it extends into the upper segment of the uterus. Other breech presentations after labor can usually be safely managed through a transverse low cervical incision, but the incision should be as wide as possible to deliver the head.

A transverse lie with the fetal back down or shoulder presentation is one indication for a classic incision in the uterus. Attempts to deliver the fetus through a transverse lower segment incision may result in extension of the uterine incision into the uterine vessels. A transverse lie with the fetal back up ("umbrella" position) usually does not need a classic incision for delivery.

When the maternal surface of the placenta is encountered as the uterus is opened, considerable hemorrhage can result. Suction must be available so the operative field can be kept reasonably clear for visualization, and the operator should quickly enlarge the incision for delivery of the fetus. The placenta should not be cut or fractured because disruption of the vessels on the chorionic plate may result in fetal hemorrhage. Instead, the placenta should be separated from the uterine wall to allow access to the fetal membranes. The membranes are then punctured, and the fetus is delivered through this opening and through the uterine incision. It may be possible to deliver the fetus by the vertex in this situation, but the op-erator may find it necessary to grasp the feet and deliver the fetus by internal podalic version and breech extraction instead. A rare occurrence is the inadvertent displacement of the vertex into the fundus during the initial attempt to deliver the fetus. In most instances, the feet can be grasped and the fetus extracted as in a breech delivery.

◊ SURGICAL STERILIZATION

Tubal ligation adds little time or morbidity to cesarean delivery and does not significantly prolong postpartum recovery. The Pomeroy method (Chapter 35) is the simplest sterilization technique and gives satisfactory results. Other methods may result in fewer failures but also are associated with higher morbidity.

◊ POSTMORTEM CESAREAN SECTION

Events that lead to cesarean birth after death of the mother are fortunately so rare that most obstetricians never perform such an operation. The principles are relatively simple. The certainty of maternal death must be quickly established, on clinical grounds if necessary, but preferably by electrocardiographic or electroencephalographic findings if the patient is being monitored. Aseptic precautions are ignored, and the abdomen and uterus are opened rapidly with vertical and classical incisions. The fetus is quickly delivered, given immediate resuscitation, and moved to an intensive care nursery as soon as possible. The placenta is removed, and the uterus and abdomen are closed. Efforts to document fetal heartbeat before deciding on cesarean section may give erroneous information because the time from apparent fetal death to actual fetal death or serious damage is unknown. The prognostic factors of importance are length of gestation, cardiovascular status of the mother before death, and interval between maternal death and delivery. Unfortunately, the prognosis for the fetus is usually ominous.[9] The infant may survive if delivery is accomplished within 10 minutes of maternal death, but the presence and severity of brain damage from cerebral hypoxia are difficult to predict. With modern life-support systems, the outlook for the fetus is improved if the cesarean section can be done before the mother's actual death. A significant ethical dilemma occurs when a parturient with a lethal disease may succumb before birth of the fetus but opposes intervention. A position against court-ordered intervention has been expressed by the American College of Obstetricians and Gynecologists.

◊ VAGINAL BIRTH AFTER PREVIOUS CESAREAN

The rising number of women delivered by repeat cesarean has been one of the principal reasons for the steady increase in the cesarean delivery rate in the United States during the last 20 years. However, it is no longer assumed that all women who have had a cesarean need to be delivered by repeat cesarean. There is now a general consensus that a trial of labor (TOL) is desirable and outweighs the risk in most cases. Consequently, the number of repeat cesareans is decreasing, and more women with previous cesarean sections are being delivered vaginally.

Following the wave of enthusiasm for vaginal birth after cesarean (VBAC), some third-party payers and managed care organizations have mandated that all women who have had previous cesarean deliveries must undergo TOL. However, it is becoming increasingly recognized that there are potential risks to VBAC and that some repeat cesareans are clinically indicated.[10,11] Common sense and clinical judgment are important factors in deciding whether TOL or repeat cesarean is best in each specific case.

Acceptance of VBAC varies greatly among patients and is also related to the way it is presented by the physician. It is certainly reasonable to encourage women to undertake TOL in a safe setting, but possible complications should be honestly discussed. Approximately 40% to 50% of women eligible for TOL refuse it in favor of a repeat cesarean.[11] This is most common when the labor preceding the prior cesarean was long and painful, and the patient fears a similar scenario.

Safety

Numerous reports on the benefits and safety of VBAC can be found.[1,2,12–14] However, recent studies suggest that a more selective and cautious approach to VBAC may be indicated.[11] The most recent series show that major complications are more likely for women undergoing TOL than for those who elected repeat cesarean[15] (Fig. 6). The increased incidence of infection and morbidity in women who fail a TOL has received relatively little attention until lately (Fig. 7). Infants born by repeat cesarean after failed TOL also have increased rates of infections.[16]

Prelabor Considerations

Most studies of vaginal birth after cesarean delivery have been conducted in university or tertiary level centers under ideal conditions with staff coverage and in-house anesthesia.[17]

However, the majority of obstetric patients in this country are delivered where manpower may be limited. A recent national survey on obstetric anesthesia found that anesthesiologists are available in house on nights and weekends in 77% of hospitals with more than 1500 births per year, in 26% of hospitals with 500 to 1499 births per year, and in only 3% of hospitals with fewer than 500 births per year.[18] There have been too few studies with sufficient numbers of patients to determine the results of VBAC in rural hospitals. Nevertheless, it is incumbent on the physician to provide a safe setting if VBAC is to be undertaken.

Although patients were carefully selected in initial studies, there has been a tendency to expand the list of obstetric conditions for which VBAC is recommended. These conditions include multiple previous cesareans, unknown uterine scar, breech presentation, twins, postterm pregnancy, and suspected macrosomia.[1,2,11,17] Although success has been re-

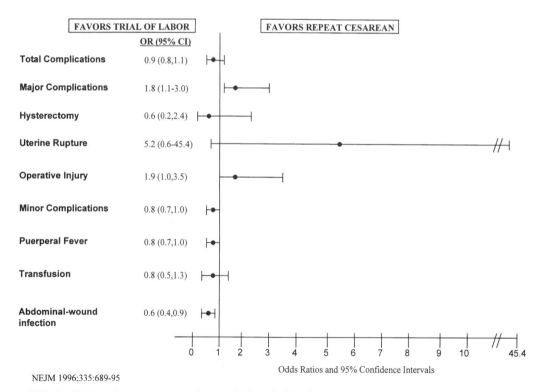

NEJM 1996;335:689-95

FIG. 6. Odds ratio graph comparing morbidity of trial of labor versus elective repeat cesarean.

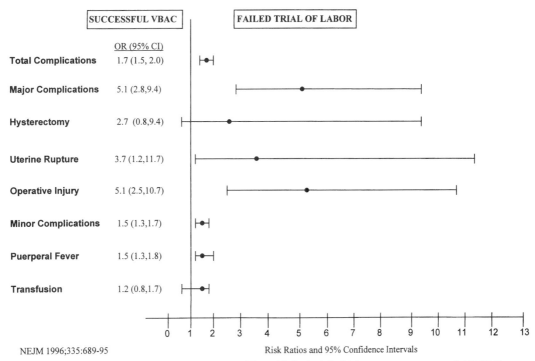

NEJM 1996;335:689-95

FIG. 7. Odds ratio graph comparing morbidity of failed trial of labor versus successful VBAC.

ported in small series, careful and individualized analysis of the risk of adverse outcome is necessary before VBAC is attempted in these settings.

Preparation

Reports of uterine ruptures resulting in perinatal deaths and neurologically impaired infants validate a judicious approach with careful patient selection and counseling regarding the risks and possible sequelae of TOL. Thorough, impartial, and factual counseling beginning early in pregnancy is desirable to prepare for TOL after a previous cesarean. If the type of previous incision is in doubt, medical records should be obtained (Table 3). It is generally agreed that contraindications to TOL include a classical scar, a low vertical scar that extends into the upper segment of the uterus, and a T-shaped scar. The patient also should be aware that problems could

TABLE 3. *Risk of uterine rupture depending on scar location*

Previous uterine incision	Incidence of uterine rupture (%)
Low segment transverse	0.2–2.3
Classic	4.3–8.8
T-shaped incision[a]	4.3–8.8
Low vertical[b]	0.5–6.5

[a]Estimate based on clinical impression.

[b]Estimate. If scar is truly lower segment, rate is closer to that of the low segment transverse. If scar extends into the upper segment, rate probably approaches that for prior classic incision.

arise during the prenatal course that could necessitate repeat cesarean delivery. After appropriate evaluation, the potential success and safety of labor should be discussed with the patient and documented in the prenatal record. When the decision to attempt VBAC is made, patient support and encouragement are in order. Global mandates for TOL after previous cesarean are inappropriate because individual risk factors are not considered.

Success of Labor

Most published series indicate that approximately 60% to 80% of TOL after a previous cesarean delivery result in successful vaginal births.[1,2,11–14,19] However, these success rates usually represent a selected population. Patients judged inappropriate for TOL have often been excluded, and the exact percentage of women undergoing TOL is not always stated.

For women whose first cesarean was done for a nonrecurring indication, the rate of successful vaginal delivery is similar to the overall incidence of vaginal delivery in laboring patients who have not undergone previous cesarean. A woman who has delivered vaginally at least once before or after her previous cesarean also is more likely to have successful TOL than the woman who has yet to deliver vaginally.[19]

Many patients with a previous diagnosis of dystocia are able to deliver vaginally, but the percentage is consistently lower (50% to 70%) than those with nonrecurring indications.[11,12,19] The lower rate is undoubtedly related to the stringency and accuracy of the original indication (Table 4). Although scoring systems may be helpful, no totally reliable

TABLE 4. *Incidence of vaginal birth after previous cesarean delivery* [a]

Indication for prior cesarean	Successful vaginal delivery (%)
Fetal distress	71–75
Twins	72
Breech	84–88
Failure to progress or dystocia	
Overall	65–68
Latent-phase diagnosis	79
Active-phase diagnosis	61

[a]Adapted from ref. 19.

way to predict whether a TOL will be successful has been identified.[20,21] Radiographic pelvimetry alone has not been predictive, and a proposed fetopelvic index using x-ray pelvimetry and ultrasound has not been widely adopted.[22]

Candidates for Vaginal Birth After Cesarean

Selection

The following criteria are clinically useful to identify candidates and conditions most predictive of a safe and successful TOL:

1. One or two prior low-segment transverse cesareans.
2. Clinically adequate pelvis in relation to fetal size.
3. No other uterine scars, anomalies, or previous rupture.
4. Patient consent.
5. Physician available throughout labor capable of monitoring labor and performing a cesarean.
6. Availability of anesthesia and personnel for emergency cesarean.

Potential Contraindications

There are other circumstances in which the risk of adverse outcome may outweigh the advantages of TOL:

1. Prior classical or T-shaped incision or other transmural uterine surgery. Whether TOL should be encouraged after a low vertical incision is controversial.
2. Contracted pelvis, macrosomia, or both.
3. Medical or obstetric complication that precludes vaginal delivery.
4. Patient refusal.
5. Inability to immediately perform emergency cesarean because of unavailable surgeon, anesthesia, inadequate staff or facility.

Management of Labor

Despite an extensive literature on VBAC, there is relatively little information on how labor should be conducted. Labor and delivery of these patients is safest in facilities where anesthesia, obstetric, and blood bank personnel are immediately available at all times. Each hospital should develop a

protocol for management of VBAC (Fig. 8). A reasonable regimen includes the following measures:

◊ Intravenous access on admission.
◊ Blood count, type, and screen.
◊ Nothing by mouth.
◊ Continuous electronic fetal monitoring.
◊ Alert anesthesia, obstetric, and neonatal personnel.

Analgesia

There are few contraindications to epidural anesthesia, and adequate pain relief may encourage a greater percentage of women to choose TOL.[2,11] Epidural analgesia rarely masks the signs and symptoms of uterine rupture, and success rates for VBAC are similar to those experienced by women who receive other types of pain relief.

Intrapartum Management

Spontaneous labor may be preferable in a woman who has previously undergone cesarean delivery.[23] Once labor has

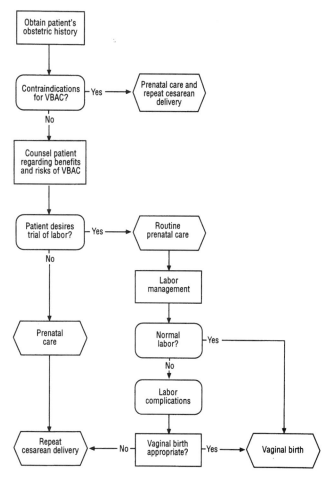

FIG. 8. Flow sheet showing one management scheme for VBAC. (Reproduced from ref. 14 with permission from the American College of Obstetricians and Gynecologists.)

begun, she should be promptly evaluated and monitored. Most authorities recommend continuous electronic monitoring for these patients.

Personnel should be present who are familiar with the potential complications of VBAC and to watch closely for fetal distress and inadequate progress of labor. If the patient was originally delivered by cesarean for fetal distress, fetal distress may occur again. Because 20% to 50% will have an unsuccessful TOL, these women should be considered at high risk for labor problems. When the previous cesarean was for dystocia, prompt diagnosis of a subsequent labor disorder is especially important to avoid the added risk of obstructed labor. In general, the progress of labor should be evaluated by standard criteria used for nulliparas if there have been no previous vaginal births and by criteria for multiparas if prior babies have been delivered vaginally.

Oxytocin

Oxytocin is often suspected as a factor responsible for uterine rupture. Although a metaanalysis found no relationship between the use of oxytocin and rupture of the uterine scar,[12] several more recent studies indicate that high infusion rates of oxytocin place women at greater risk.[24,25] Therefore, oxytocin to induce or augment labor should be used cautiously to avoid hyperstimulation.

Delivery

There is nothing unique about delivery of the infant after TOL. The need to routinely explore the uterus after successful vaginal delivery is controversial. Scar separation can be difficult to palpate, rarely results in significant bleeding, and usually causes no major clinical problem. Most asymptomatic dehiscences heal well, and there are no data to suggest that future pregnancy outcome is better if the dehiscence is surgically repaired. Nor has the safety of a trial of labor in a subsequent pregnancy after a known dehiscence been established. Obviously, excessive vaginal bleeding or signs of hypovolemia at delivery require complete assessment of the previous scar and the entire genital tract.

Uterine Rupture

Rupture of the uterine scar is the most serious complication of VBAC. It can be life-threatening for both mother and baby.[17]

The best predictor of the safety of labor after previous cesarean is the location of the previous uterine scar (Table 3).

Scar dehiscence is defined as an opening of the previous scar with intact overlying visceral peritoneum and no expulsion of intrauterine contents (also termed a "window"). This type of scar separation rarely produces hemorrhage or causes a major clinical problem. Incomplete or partial rupture refers to an opening of the previous scar but not the overlying peritoneum, and the extraperitoneal extrusion of intrauterine contents, often into the broad ligament. A complete rupture is a separation of the previous scar and overlying peritoneum with extrusion of intrauterine contents into the abdominal cavity.

Spontaneous ruptures before labor are most commonly associated with classic incisions. Intrapartum uterine ruptures requiring emergency treatment occur in approximately 0.5% of patients with a transverse low-segment scar.[11,17] The rupture usually involves the previous scar and lower uterine segment, but it may be stellate and extend intraperitoneally or retroperitoneally. Contributing factors include hyperstimulation with oxytocin, dysfunctional labor, more than one cesarean delivery, high parity, and even previous perforation of the nonpregnant uterus at curettage, hysteroscopy, metroplasty, and myomectomy. The rate of rupture has not been shown to be increased with previous intrapartum or postpartum infection or to be related to the method or number of layers of closure.

In most cases, the reason uterine rupture occurs in a particular VBAC patient is unknown. Unfortunately, poor outcomes have occurred even in appropriate candidates. To date, there is no way to detect the individual patient who is at high risk for rupture of the uterine scar. Imaging techniques are being investigated as a way to identify those patients, but the reliability has not been established.[26]

Diagnosis

Because uterine rupture may be difficult to diagnose, close surveillance and a high index of suspicion is necessary. A constellation of signs and symptoms may initially be subtle, but they usually gradually or rapidly progress to a clearer clinical picture. The most common sign of uterine rupture is fetal distress.[17,27,28] A fetal heart rate (FHR) pattern with variable decelerations often rapidly evolves into late decelerations, bradycardia, and undetectable fetal heart tones (Fig. 9). Because FHR abnormalities occur in 50% to 70% of uterine ruptures, all FHR changes in patients undergoing TOL should be evaluated thoroughly.

Uterine or abdominal pain most commonly occurs in the area of the previous incision, but it may range from mild to "tearing" in nature. Uterine contractions often diminish in intensity and frequency. Vaginal or intraabdominal bleeding is associated with anxiety, restlessness, weakness, dizziness, gross hematuria, shoulder pain, and shock. This clinical picture can be mistakenly attributed to abruption. Loss of station of the presenting part is diagnostic.[17]

Management

Any of these findings warrant an immediate exploratory laparotomy. The condition of the infant is dependent on the severity of the rupture as well as its relationship to the placenta and umbilical cord. When the umbilical cord is compressed or the placenta is detached, low Apgar scores, hypoxia, or fetal death can occur.

In the majority of patients, repair of the uterus is possible. The tear can be repaired if the patient wants to retain fertility, if her condition is not jeopardized by continued hemorrhage,

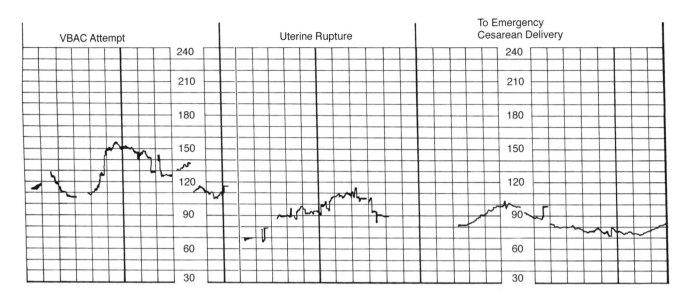

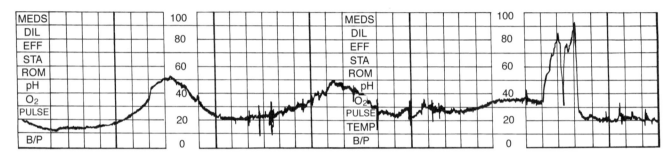

FIG. 9. Fetal heart rate (FHR) tracing shows changes in FHR pattern during uterine rupture.

and if repair is technically feasible. The wound edge should be debrided before the edges are reapproximated, and suturing techniques are similar to those used for cesarean repair. Extension of the rupture into the broad ligament vessels, extensive damage to the uterine myometrium, or associated placenta accreta may require hysterectomy.

Future Pregnancies After Uterine Rupture

If the site of the ruptured scar is confined to the lower segment, the rate of repeat rupture or dehiscence in labor is 6%.

If the scar includes the upper segment of the uterus, the repeat rupture rate is 32%.[29,30] Therefore, women with a prior uterine rupture are best delivered by repeat cesarean as soon as the fetus is mature or at 36 to 37 weeks of gestation before the onset of labor.

Conclusions and Recommendations

There are no randomized trials comparing VBAC with elective repeat cesarean section to definitively prove that outcomes are better with a trial of labor. There is strong sentiment in favor of VBAC, but overall outcomes from TOL and elective repeat cesarean delivery appear medically equiva-

lent.[31,32] When VBAC is successful, it is associated with less morbidity than repeat cesarean. With careful patient selection and close attention during labor, the majority of women previously delivered by cesarean can safely and more economically deliver vaginally. Most problems occur when the patient is not under direct observation or when the diagnosis of uterine rupture is delayed.

◊ CESAREAN HYSTERECTOMY

Indications

Occasionally, hysterectomy must be performed immediately after cesarean section or vaginal delivery. A useful classification is based on emergency indications (e.g., uterine rupture, uncontrollable uterine hemorrhage, placenta accreta, uterine infection) and nonemergency indications (e.g., for significant uterine pathology such as carcinoma *in situ* or uterine leiomyomas).

Emergency Indications

Uncontrollable uterine hemorrhage may result from uterine rupture, uterine atony, placenta accreta, placental site sinusoids after placenta previa, or a coagulation defect. When surgery is indicated to control hemorrhage of uterine origin, the patient's desire to preserve childbearing capacity and the current danger are assessed. Nonsurgical management is indicated in such circumstances as uterine atony and coagulation defect.

Bimanual uterine massage, oxytocin, prostaglandin administration, and blood replacement should be used before surgical intervention is considered. Hemorrhage from sinusoids in the lower uterine segment associated with placenta previa can sometimes be controlled with mattress or figure-of-eight 2-0 to 0 absorbable sutures. With uterine atony, surgical interruption of the arterial flow to the uterus may be tried as the first measure of control. The operator may proceed to bilateral ligation of the hypogastric or the uterine arteries. If this is not efficacious, hysterectomy may be necessary.[1]

Hysterectomy can also be lifesaving as treatment of severe uterine infection. The patient who has experienced a second-trimester septic abortion with septic shock, peritonitis, or uterine perforation may be saved by prompt hysterectomy. Clostridial infection, dehiscence of a classic incision with uterine infection, or a severe uterine infection unresponsive to antibiotics should also be treated by hysterectomy.

Nonemergency Indications

The risks and benefits of hysterectomy for nonemergency indications are much less certain than for emergency conditions. Hysterectomy performed at term is associated with hemorrhage, infection, thromboembolism, and injury to contiguous organs.[33] The declining use of hysterectomy despite an increase in the incidence of cesarean section reflects a generally accepted conservative approach in most situations. Tubal ligation is a safer operation at term than hysterectomy. When carcinoma *in situ* must be treated, removal of the cervix at the time of hysterectomy is much more certain and technically less complicated in the nonpregnant state. The decision to perform a nonemergency hysterectomy requires good judgment, which is based on existing skills, facilities, and the needs of the individual patient.

Procedure

The technique for hysterectomy is described in Chapter 45, but some points are especially pertinent to its performance immediately after cesarean section or vaginal delivery.[1] In general, blood is conserved if the uterine wound for cesarean section is rapidly closed before beginning the hysterectomy. Normal ovaries should be preserved, and the operator should be aware that the relative shortening of the uteroovarian ligament at term necessitates extra care in the placement of clamps and sutures in this area. The increased vascularity of the pregnant uterus requires considerable care in the correct placement of clamps and sutures.

In the uterus at term, it can be difficult to determine by palpation the location of the portio of the cervix when performing a hysterectomy. Because of this difficulty, sometimes portions of the cervix are inadvertently left behind. Clips or clamps placed vaginally on the cervix preoperatively can be more easily palpated, or a vertical incision can be made in the lower uterine segment and extended caudad until the limits of the cervix can be identified. Drainage of the pelvic cavity may be necessary, depending on the adequacy of hemostasis. In emergent situations or when the patient is unstable, a supracervical hysterectomy is simpler and quicker and may be preferable to total hysterectomy.

◊ SUMMARY

Cesarean delivery has contributed greatly to the low maternal and infant morbidity and mortality rates in modern obstetrics. However, ways to eliminate inappropriate indications and lower what is perceived as an excessive cesarean rate in the United States have been emphasized recently. Vaginal birth after cesarean (VBAC) is successful in many women. Although rare, uterine rupture is the most serious complication associated with VBAC. Proper selection and close monitoring of the mother and infant during the trial of labor are warranted in all VBAC patients.

◊ REFERENCES

1. Phelan JR, Clark SL, eds. *Cesarean delivery.* New York: Elsevier Science, 1988.
2. Flamm BL, Quilligan EJ. *Cesarean section. Guidelines for appropriate utilization.* New York: Springer-Verlag, 1995
3. Scheller JM, Nelson KB. Does cesarean delivery prevent cerebral palsy or other neurologic problems of childhood? *Obstet Gynecol* 1994;83:623.
4. Lagrew DC, Morgan MA. Decreasing the cesarean section rate in a private hospital: success without mandated clinical changes. *Am J Obstet Gynecol* 1996;174:184.
5. Chazotte C, Cohen WR. Catastrophic complications of previous cesarean section. *Am J Obstet Gynecol* 1990;163:738.
6. American College of Obstetrics and Gynecology. Assessment of fetal lung maturity. *ACOG Educ Bull* 1996;230:1.
7. Duff P. Prophylactic antibiotics for cesarean delivery: a simple cost-effective strategy for prevention of postoperative morbidity. *Am J Obstet Gynecol* 1987;157:794.
8. Hauth JC, Owen J, Davis RO. Transverse uterine incision closure: one versus two layers. *Am J Obstet Gynecol* 1992;167:1108.
9. Katz VL, Dotters DJ, Droegemueller W. Perimortem cesarean delivery. *Obstet Gynecol* 1986;68:571.
10. Gregory KD, Henry OA, Gellons AJ, et al. Repeat cesareans: How many are elective? *Obstet Gynecol* 1994;84:574.
11. Scott JR. Avoiding labor problems during vaginal birth after cesarean delivery. *Clin Obstet Gynecol* 1997;40:533.
12. Rosen MG, Dickinson JC, Westhoff CL. Vaginal birth after cesarean section: a meta-analysis of morbidity and mortality. *Obstet Gynecol* 1991;77:465.
13. Flamm BL, Goings JR, Liu Y, et al. Elective repeat cesarean versus trial of labor: a prospective multicenter study. *Obstet Gynecol* 1994;83:927.
14. American College of Obstetricians and Gynecologists. *Vaginal delivery after previous cesarean birth. ACOG practice patterns.* Washington: American College of Obstetricians and Gynecologists, 1995:1.
15. McMahon MJ, Luther ER, Bowes WA, Olshan AF. Comparison of a trial of labor with an elective second cesarean section. *N Engl J Med* 1996;335:689.
16. Hook B, Kiwi B, Amini SB, et al. Neonatal morbidity after elective repeat cesarean section and trial of labor. *Pediatrics* 1997;100:348.
17. Scott JR. Mandatory trial of labor after cesarean delivery: an alternative viewpoint. *Obstet Gynecol* 1991;77:811.

18. Hawkins JL, Gibbs CP, Orleans M, et al. Obstetric anesthesia work force survey, 1981 versus 1992. *Anesthesiology* 1997;87:135.

19. Pridjian G. Labor after prior cesarean section. *Clin Obstet Gynecol* 1992;35:445.

20. Pickhardt MG, Martin JN, Meydrech EF, et al. Vaginal birth after cesarean delivery: are there useful and valid predictors of success or failure? *Am J Obstet Gynecol* 1991;165:353.

21. Flamm BL, Geiger AM. Vaginal birth after cesarean delivery: an admission scoring system. *Obstet Gynecol* 1997;90:907.

22. Thurnau GR, Scates DH, Morgan MA. The fetal–pelvic index: a method of identifying fetal–pelvic disproportion in women attempting vaginal birth after previous cesarean delivery. *Am J Obstet Gynecol* 1991; 165:353.

23. Wing DA, Lovett K, Paul RH. Disruption of prior uterine incision following misoprostol for labor induction in women with previous cesarean delivery. *Obstet Gynecol* 1998;91:828.

24. Jones RO, Nagashima AW, Hartnett-Goodman MM, et al. Rupture of low transverse cesarean scars during trial of labor. *Obstet Gynecol* 1991;77:811.

25. Grubb DK, Kjos SL, Paul R. Latent labor with an unknown uterine scar. *Obstet Gynecol* 1996;88:351.

26. Rozenberg P, Goffinet F, Phillipe HJ, et al. Ultrasonographic measurement of lower uterine segment to assess risk of defects of scarred uterus. *Lancet* 1996;347:281.

27. Arulkumarun S, Chua S, Ratnam SS. Symptoms and signs with scar rupture: value of uterine activity measurement. *Aust NZ Obstet Gynecol* 1992;3:208.

28. Cowan RK, Kinch RAH, Ellis B, et al. Trial of labor following cesarean delivery. *Obstet Gynecol* 1994;83:933.

29. Reyes-Ceja L, Cabrera R, Insfran E, et al. Pregnancy following previous uterine rupture. *Obstet Gynecol* 1969;34:387.

30. Ritchie EH. Pregnancy after uterine rupture of the pregnant uterus. *J Obstet Gynaecol Br Commonw* 1971;78:642.

31. Hadley CB, Mennuti MT, Gabbe SG. An evaluation of the relative risks of a trial of labor versus elective repeat cesarean section. *Am J Perinatol* 1986;3:107.

32. Roberts RG, Wall EM, Hess GH, et al. Trial of labor versus elective repeat cesarean section for the woman with a previous cesarean section: Task Force on Clinical Policies for Patient Care. *Am Acad Fam Practice* 1995:1–29.

33. Plauche WC, Gruich FG, Bourgeois MO. Hysterectomy at the time of cesarean section: analysis of 108 cases. *Obstet Gynecol* 1981;58:459.

CHAPTER 30

Critical Care Obstetrics

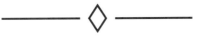

Steven L. Clark

The critically ill obstetric patient presents unique challenges to the clinician. Pregnancy alters the function of virtually every organ system; thus, both the baseline state and the patient response to physiological aberrations are different in the pregnant patient compared with her nonpregnant counterpart. In addition, fetal considerations often are important in designing a diagnostic and therapeutic approach to the critically ill gravida; numerous situations may be encountered in which the physiological demands of mother and fetus may be opposite. Many of the principles that apply to the critically ill nongravid patient apply in pregnancy as well. This chapter explores a number of conditions in critical care medicine that are unique to pregnancy.

◇ SHOCK IN PREGNANCY

Shock encompasses various pathophysiological aberrations that lead to inadequate tissue perfusion and impaired cellular metabolism. Although hypotension often is the most obvious clinical sign in shock of any cause, such blood pressure changes are the final common manifestation of a number of distinct pathologic processes. The successful clinical management of patients in shock depends on the proper definition of the underlying pathophysiology as well as an understanding of the unique effects of pregnancy on such conditions.

Several types of shock have been defined. This chapter focuses on the pathophysiology, diagnosis, and treatment of hypovolemic and septic shock, the types most commonly encountered in the pregnant patient.

In the nonpregnant patient, hypotension is defined as a systolic blood pressure less than 90 mm Hg or a mean arterial pressure less than 60 mm Hg. During pregnancy, this definition has less value because blood pressures as low as 80/50 mm Hg commonly are seen in healthy pregnant women. Further, although a mean arterial pressure of 60 mm Hg may be adequate for perfusion of the adult heart and brain in a nonpregnant adult, the effects of a given blood pressure on uteroplacental perfusion cannot easily be generalized but are related to gestational age and placental condition. Whereas a blood pressure of 80/50 mm Hg may be adequate in one pregnant woman, another woman with pregnancy-induced hypertension and uteroplacental insufficiency may suffer inadequate placental perfusion and fetal distress with a diastolic blood pressure of 90 mm Hg. During pregnancy, shock is more reliably diagnosed on the basis of the overall clinical picture, including heart rate, mental status, urine output, and fetal condition, than on the basis of an absolute arterial pressure.[1]

◇ HYPOVOLEMIC SHOCK

Despite the availability of modern blood-banking techniques, hemorrhage remains a major cause of maternal mortality.[2] Pertinent physiological changes that affect a woman's response to hemorrhage during pregnancy include a 50% increase in plasma volume with slightly lesser increases in circulating red blood cell mass. These changes as well as an increase in resting heart rate of 10 beats per minute result in about a 50% increase in resting cardiac output in the term gravida compared with her nonpregnant counterpart.[3] Such changes are accompanied by a decrease in systemic vascular resistance resulting in a net decrease in mean arterial pressure during the second trimester.[4] At term, an average of 500 ml of blood is lost with vaginal delivery compared with a mean blood loss of 1000 ml with cesarean section.[3] Such losses usually are well tolerated by the pregnant woman because of the physiological hypervolemia.

Early in the course of massive hemorrhage, there are decreases in mean arterial pressure, cardiac output, central venous pressure and pulmonary capillary wedge pressure (PCWP), stroke volumes, and oxygen consumption and increases in arterial venous oxygen content difference.[1] These changes are accompanied by compensatory increases in heart rate, systemic and pulmonary vascular resistance, and myocardial contractility.[1] In addition, the redistribution of cardiac output and blood volume result in diminished perfusion to the kidneys, gastrointestinal tract, skin, and uterus with relative maintenance of blood flow to the heart and brain. In the pregnant patient, such redistribution may result in fetal hypoxia and distress even in the absence of an overt maternal hypotension. To some extent, the fetus acts like a miner's canary: regardless of absolute maternal blood pressure, significant maternal shock is virtually never seen in the presence of a reassuring fetal heart rate pattern.[1] During this initial phase, initial oxygen extraction by the maternal tissues is increased. Further maldistribution of blood flow results in local tissue hypoxia and metabolic acidemia. If not promptly corrected, such shunting of blood from the renal and splanchnic beds may result in acute tubular necrosis and may contribute to pulmonary capillary endothelial damage resulting in the adult respiratory distress syndrome (ARDS) even if resuscitation eventually is successful.[5,6,7]

As the blood volume deficit exceeds 25%, the compensatory mechanisms become inadequate to maintain cardiac output and blood pressure. At this point, small additional losses of blood result in rapid clinical deterioration that produces a cycle of cellular death and vasoconstriction leading to organ ischemia, loss of capillary membrane integrity, and additional loss of intravascular fluid volume to the extravascular spaces. Thus, time is of the essence in restoring hemodynamic and oxygenation parameters to normal if survival is to be optimized.[8]

The management of the patient in hemorrhagic hypovolemic shock is directed toward two goals: restoring circulating blood volume and eliminating the source of hemorrhage. The management of the most common causes of obstetric hemorrhage (e.g., lacerations, retained placenta, uterine atony) is described in detail elsewhere. The therapeutic restoration of circulating blood volume begins with a rapid infusion of crystalloid solution and packed red blood cells. These maneuvers form the cornerstone of therapy for hemorrhagic shock. Patients with normally functioning hearts may respond better to hypovolemic shock with blood volume replacements that are 500 to 1000 ml in excess of their predicted norm.[8] Such expansion dilates the constricted capillary networks that persist from the initial hypotensive phase and assist in resolving acidosis at the cellular level.

Continued replacement of blood loss with crystalloid solutions and packed red blood cells alone results in eventual depletion of labile clotting factors and platelets and may result in a dilutional coagulopathy, which itself may contribute to further bleeding. A fibrinogen level below 100 mg/dl or prolongation of the prothrombin and active partial thromboplastin times in a bleeding patient are indications for fresh frozen plasma infusion. Platelet transfusion should be guided by platelet counts. One unit of platelets raises the platelet count by 8000 to 10,000/mm^3 and should be considered in a bleeding patient with a platelet count below 50,000/mm^3.

◊ SEPTIC SHOCK

The incidence of septic shock appears to be increasing.[10] Septic shock accompanies up to 50% of bacteremias caused by gram-negative organisms and 5% of those caused by gram-positive organisms. In the overall hospital population, the mortality rate once clinical shock is evident is 40% to 50%.[11] Pregnancy classically is thought to be a factor that predisposes a patient to septic shock. In obstetrics, septic abortion, chorioamnionitis, pyelonephritis, and endometritis are the most common conditions associated with septic shock.[11] Although it may be presumed that with a younger population, the mortality with septic shock is somewhat less than in the overall population, this condition continues to account for a significant percentage of maternal mortality.[2,11]

Septic shock in obstetrics most commonly is associated with infection caused by endotoxin-releasing gram-negative aerobic coliform organisms. Endotoxin, a complex cell wall–associated lipopolysaccharide, is released into the circulation at the time of bacterial death, resulting in multiple hemodynamic effects. The subsequent activation of lymphocytic T cells and mast cells results in histamine and kinin activation as well as the activation of kallikrein and a decrease in kallikreinigen and kallikrein inhibitor.[12] These changes result in the release of bradykinin, a potent arterial dilator. Some studies also suggest a role for complement activation as well as arachidonic acid metabolites, nitric oxide, and β-endorphins in the pathophysiology of septic shock.[12–15] This generalized inflammatory response, similar to that seen with other conditions such as anaphylaxis, is responsible for much of the pathophysiology seen with these conditions and has been termed the systemic inflammatory response syndrome (SIRS).[16]

Early septic shock is a classic example of distributive shock, related to a systemic maldistribution of relatively normal or even increased cardiac output. Clinical findings include hypotension, fever, and chills. Initial hemodynamic findings include decreased systemic vascular resistance and high normal or elevated cardiac output.[1,14] The continued maldistribution of cardiac output leads to local tissue hypoxia and the development of lactic acidosis and end-organ dysfunction. This decrease in systemic vascular resistance is caused by the release of vasoactive substances as well as by vascular endothelial cell injury, which promotes capillary plugging secondary to complement-induced leukocyte aggregation. These factors lead to increased arteriovenous shunting.[14]

The treatment of septic shock in this early phase involves optimizing preload by restoring relative intravascular volume with crystalloid infusion as well as aggressively treating the underlying infection.[1] Although some authorities advocate the use of colloid solutions for volume replacement, there is no convincing evidence that the use of such solutions decreases the incidence of pulmonary edema or ARDS.[17] If the offending organism is known, single-agent antibiotic therapy may be used. More commonly in obstetrics, the infection is polymicrobial, and broad-spectrum coverage for gram-negative and gram-positive aerobic and anaerobic organisms is most appropriate. If an abscess is involved, prompt surgical drainage after initial resuscitation is mandatory.

If the process continues, the patient may enter a second hemodynamic phase of septic shock. Of primary importance in this late phase is the development and progression of myocardial dysfunction leading to ventricular failure.[18,19,20] Although commonly viewed as a late finding, studies assessing stroke work index and ventricular ejection fraction have demonstrated depressed intrinsic ventricular function even in the early stages of septic shock, when increases in heart rate are compensatory and associated with a normal or high cardiac output.[18–21] This myocardial depression is a direct effect of myocardial depressant substance in the sera of patients with septic shock.[19] When ventricular function has deteriorated to the point where cardiac index is frankly depressed (i.e., less than 3 to 4 liters/min/m² in pregnancy) in the presence of adequate preload, the prognosis is extremely grave.[21] Pulmonary hypertension, another important hemodynamic alteration often associated with septic shock, may have additional profound hemodynamic consequences.[22]

For most pregnant patients in septic shock, maximum ventricular function is obtained by means of Starling's law with a PCWP of about 16 mm Hg.[13] Patients who remain hypotensive after such preload manipulation should be treated with dopamine hydrochloride. This agent, in doses of less than 5 µg/kg/min, improves renal blood flow by way of dopaminergic mesenteric vasodilation; in doses of 5 to 30 µg/kg/min, a positive inotropic effect also is seen. In doses that exceed 30 µg/kg/min, the favorable effect on blood pressure is principally one of α-adrenergic vasoconstriction. Additional inotropic or vasoconstrictive agents may need to be administered in refractory septic shock.[12] The hemodynamic manipulation of patients whose hypotension fails to respond rapidly to volume infusion may be assisted by pulmonary artery catheterization, allowing the clinician to achieve optimal preload before the institution of inotropic or vasoconstrictive therapy.

Patients who recover from the initial hemodynamic instability of septic shock may suffer prolonged morbidity secondary to endotoxin-mediated pulmonary capillary injury and noncardiogenic pulmonary edema (i.e., ARDS). Such lung failure is a major cause of death in patients with septic shock.[12] Similarly, pregnant patients whose hypotension was prolonged may experience acute tubular necrosis. Endotoxin-mediated endothelial cell injury and associated thromboplastin-like activity as well as prolonged shock from any cause may also lead to activation of the coagulation cascade and to a clinical picture of disseminated intravascular coagulation (DIC). Although the use of high-dose corticosteroids has been advocated in the acute management of septic shock, reports have failed to demonstrate a benefit from such therapy.[23,24] Naloxone, an endorphin-receptor blocker, is under investigation in the treatment of hypotension associated with septic shock.[25]

◊ FETAL RESPONSE TO MATERNAL HEMODYNAMIC INSTABILITY

Fetal well-being depends principally on the maintenance of maternal oxygenation and uterine blood flow. During severe fetal hypoxia, cardiac output decreases, and pulmonary vasoconstriction occurs, with redistribution of the fetal circulation favoring blood flow to the brain, heart, and adrenals at the expense of splanchnic and even placental blood flow. Although Starling's law is operative in the fetus, ventricular stroke work varies over a much smaller range of end-diastolic pressures. Changes in cardiac output manifest themselves primarily by changes in fetal heart rate alone. As maternal arterial PO_2 falls, there appears to be no corresponding fall in fetal PO_2 as long as the maternal PO_2 exceeds 60 mm Hg. Because the fetus operates on the steep portion of the oxygen dissociation curve (i.e., normal fetal PO_2 range, 10 to 33 mm Hg), further falls in maternal and fetal PO_2 result in dramatic decreases in fetal oxygen saturation and fetal hypoxia.[1] The administration of oxygen to the mother produces only a minor increase in fetal PO_2. However, such changes in fetal PO_2 may produce significant increases in fetal oxygen saturation and, thus, may benefit the marginally hypoxic fetus, especially if maternal hyperoxia is achieved (Fig. 1).[26]

Near term, uterine blood flow approaches 500 ml/min and accounts for about 10% of total maternal cardiac output. The uterine arteries show little capacity for autoregulation; thus, uterine and placental blood flow fall in direct proportion to maternal systemic arterial pressure. In the hypotensive mother, compensatory maternal vasoconstriction aimed at maintaining circulation to the heart and brain decreases uterine blood flow even further. Thus, maternal hypotension, whether caused by supine venacaval compression, conduction anesthetic, or even amniotic fluid embolism (AFE), may be first heralded by fetal bradycardia. Because maternal compensatory mechanisms maintain systemic arterial pressure at the expense of uterine blood flow, such abnormal patterns may be seen even in the absence of overt maternal hypotension.[1] Thus, during the critical course of a gravely ill mother, careful monitoring of fetal well-being is essential. Even in a medical or surgical intensive care setting, continuous electronic fetal heart rate monitoring

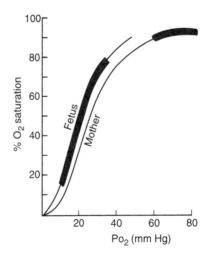

FIG. 1. Oxygen dissociation curves for human maternal and fetal blood, indicating the physiological range of PO_2 and O^2 saturation for mother and fetus. (Adapted from *Clark SL, Phelan JP. Critical care obstetrics, 2nd ed.* Boston: Blackwell Scientific, 1990:343.)

is often an important part of the care of the critically ill and unstable pregnant patient.

◊ INVASIVE HEMODYNAMIC MONITORING

Since its introduction into clinical medicine in the early 1970s, the pulmonary artery catheter has come to play an important role in the management of critically ill patients with hemodynamic instability. Several prospective trials demonstrate the benefits of this technique in select, critically ill patients, including a reduction in morbidity and mortality in some subsets.[21,27–32] On the other hand, the risk–benefit ratio of invasive monitoring in the general population of seriously ill patients has been questioned.[33] When obstetric patients require such monitoring, optimal patient outcome is predicated on the clinician's understanding of the hemodynamic changes associated with pregnancy as well as a working knowledge of indications for invasive hemodynamic monitoring.[22]

The pulmonary artery catheter is a multilumen catheter with a thermistor located near the distal end (Fig. 2). When saline solution at a known temperature is injected through the proximal port, the detection of resultant temperature changes by the distal thermistor allows the calculation of cardiac output with the assistance of a cardiac output computer. Catheter placement most commonly occurs through the internal jugular or subclavian vein. As the catheter is advanced through the great vessels and heart, its location can be precisely determined by observing characteristic pressures and waveforms (Fig. 3). When the catheter is correctly placed, the lumens terminate in the pulmonary artery and the superior vena cava or right atrium and allow direct assessment of central venous pressure, PCWP, pulmonary artery pressure, and cardiac output. These pressures may be combined with mean arterial pressure and body surface area and heart rate to calculate additional important hemodynamic indices, such as systemic vascular resistance and left ventricular stroke work index (Table 1). In critically ill obstetric patients, discrepancies are often seen between measurements of PCWP and central venous pressure. In such circumstances, clinical use of the central venous pressure measurement alone would be misleading and possibly deleterious. With rare exceptions, the complications seen with pulmonary artery catheterization are associated with obtaining central venous access and are similar whether a central venous pressure line or pulmonary artery catheter is used. For these reasons, in a modern perinatal intensive care unit, central venous pressure monitoring alone seldom is indicated.

Determinants of Cardiac Output

In addition to heart rate, important determinants of cardiac output are preload, afterload, and an assessment of myocardial contractility.

Preload

Preload represents the volume or pressure generated within the ventricles at end-diastole. According to Starling's law, ventricular output is directly proportional to ventricular preload. Clinically, right ventricular preload is measured as central venous pressure, and left ventricular preload as PCWP. Because the left side of the heart perfuses the myocardium, brain, and uteroplacental unit, PCWP is the preload measurement of interest in clinical practice. When central venous pressures are used, it is done with the tacit assumption that the preloads of the right and left sides of the heart are equivalent. In a critically ill patient, this often is not the case, thus further limiting the usefulness of central venous pressure in the hemodynamically unstable obstetric patient.

Afterload

Afterload describes the resistance to the flow of blood during ventricular systole. It is not measured directly; rather, after the measurement of cardiac output, central venous pressure, and mean arterial pressure, afterload is calculated as systemic vascular resistance. Cardiac output fluctuates inversely with systemic vascular resistance. Septic shock and preeclampsia are examples of frequently encountered conditions in obstetrics that may markedly influence systemic vascular resistance.[11]

Ventricular Stroke Work Index

Ventricular stroke work is also a calculated parameter (see Table 1). The assessment of ventricular stroke work on a

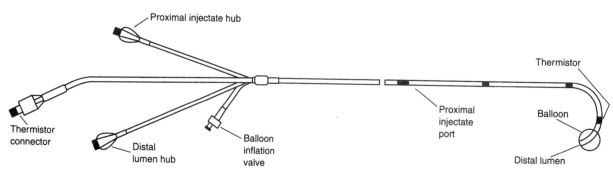

FIG. 2. Pulmonary artery catheter. (Adapted from Clark SL, Phelan JP. *Critical care obstetrics, 2nd ed.* Boston: Blackwell Scientific, 1990:63.)

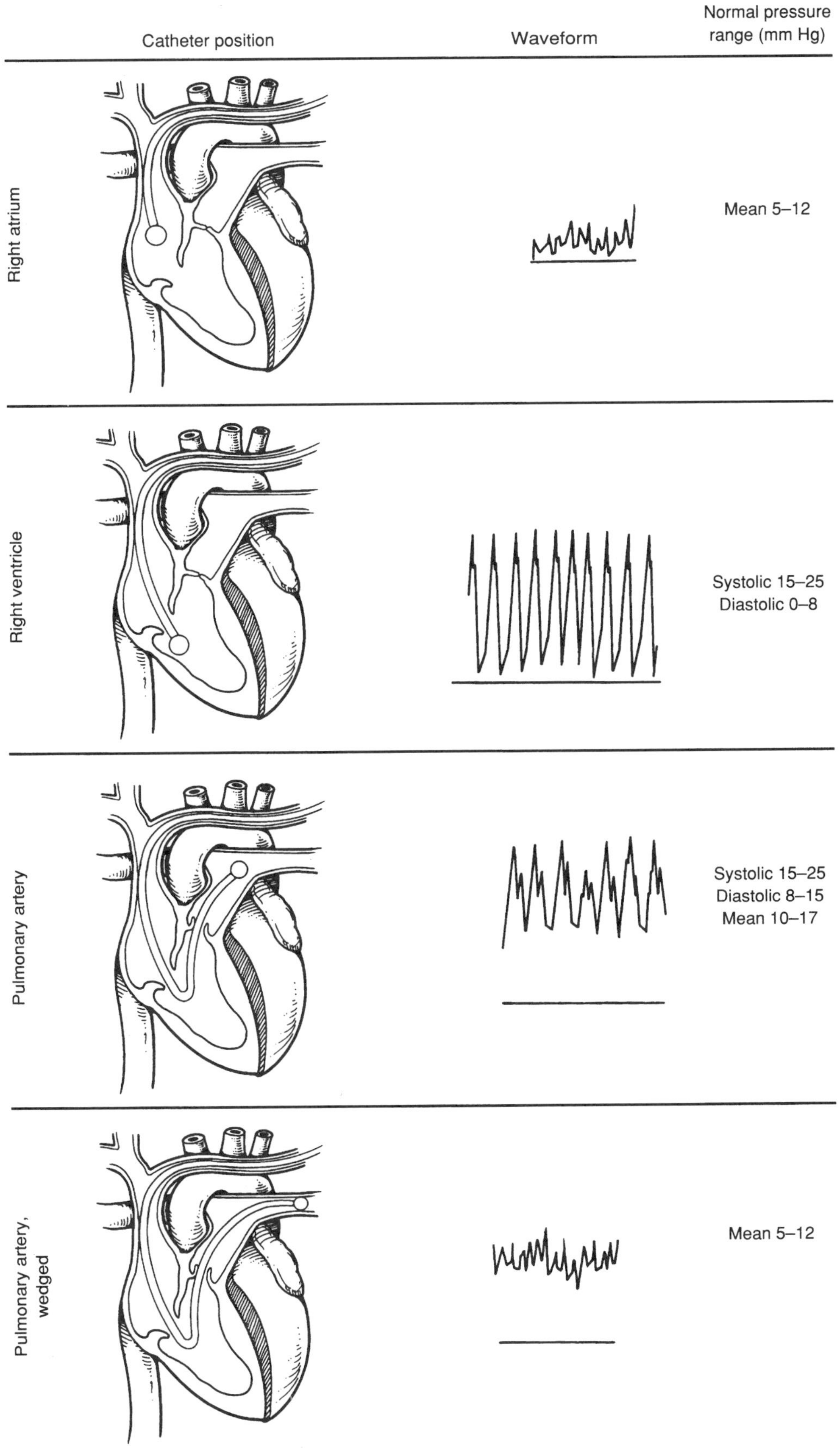

Catheter position	Waveform	Normal pressure range (mm Hg)

Right atrium — Mean 5–12

Right ventricle — Systolic 15–25, Diastolic 0–8

Pulmonary artery — Systolic 15–25, Diastolic 8–15, Mean 10–17

Pulmonary artery, wedged — Mean 5–12

FIG. 3. Pulmonary artery catheter placement. Catheter position, corresponding waveforms, and pressures are shown. (Adapted from Clark SL, Phelan JP. *Critical care obstetrics, 2nd ed.* Boston: Blackwell Scientific, 1990:67.)

TABLE 1. *Derived hemodynamic parameters*

Parameter	Derivation[a]	Normal nonpregnant range
Stroke volume index	$\dfrac{CO}{(HR)(BSA)}$	34–45 ml/beat per m²
Mean arterial pressure	$\dfrac{(Systolic) + 2\,(diastolic)}{3}$	85–95 mm Hg
Systemic vascular resistance	$\dfrac{(MAP - CVP)}{CO} \times 79.9$	900–1200 dynes-sec-cm⁻⁵
Pulmonary vascular resistance	$\dfrac{MPAP - PCWP}{CO} \times 79.9$	150–250 dynes-sec-cm⁻⁵
Left ventricular stroke work index	$SVI \times (MAP - PCWP) \times 0.0136$	51–61 g-m-m⁻²

[a]CO, cardiac output; BSA, body surface area; CVP, central venous pressure; HR, heart rate; MAP, mean arterial pressure; MPAP, mean pulmonary artery pressure; PCWP, pulmonary capillary wedge pressure; SVI, stroke volume index.

modified Starling curve (Fig. 4) allows the clinician to directly assess the intrinsic contractility of the left ventricle and to classify myocardial function as normal, hyperdynamic, or hypodynamic. After preload has been optimized, ventricular function may be further affected by the administration of inotropic agents such as dopamine. The use of such agents may shift the intrinsic contractility of the ventricle from the hypodynamic to the normal range, resulting in improved cardiac performance (Fig. 5).

Indications

The indications for pulmonary artery catheterization in pregnancy include many of the conditions common to all critical care medicine. These include patients with severe cardiac disease during labor and delivery, patients with septic shock, and hemodynamically unstable patients in whom volume status is uncertain. Select patients with complicated severe preeclampsia form a subset unique to pregnancy.[27–30] It has been suggested that patients with severe hypertension unresponsive to conventional antihypertensive medication, those with pulmonary edema of unknown cause, and those with persistent oliguria may benefit from invasive hemodynamic monitoring.[28] In contrast, hemodynamic monitoring seldom is indicated in cases of hypovolemia associated with obstetric hemorrhage. Normal values for invasively obtained hemodynamic indices have been described and are valuable in managing the critically ill obstetric patient (Table 2).[4,34] Techniques to avoid several catheter-related complications have been recently reviewed.

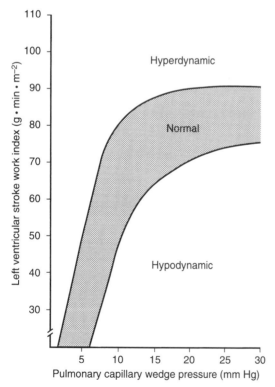

FIG. 4. Pulmonary capillary wedge pressure versus left ventricular stroke work index. Normal relationship is represented by the *shaded area*. (Adapted from Clark SL, Phelan JP. *Critical care obstetrics, 2nd ed.* Boston: Blackwell Scientific, 1990:399.)

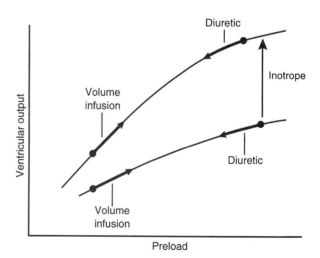

FIG. 5. Effect of volume manipulation and inotrope administration on ventricular output in two patients with septic shock. (Adapted from Clark SL, Phelan JP. *Critical care obstetrics, 2nd ed.* Boston: Blackwell Scientific, 1990:181.)

TABLE 2. *Central hemodynamic changes*[a]

Parameter	Nonpregnant	Pregnant
Cardiac output (liters/min)	4.3 ± 0.9	6.2 ± 1.0
Heart rate (beats/min)	71 ± 10.0	83 ± 10.0
Systemic vascular resistance (dyne-cm-sec⁻⁵)	1530 ± 520	1210 ± 266
Pulmonary vascular resistance (dyne-cm-sec⁻⁵)	119 ± 47.0	78 ± 22
Colloid oncotic pressure (mm Hg)	20.8 ± 1.0	18.0 ± 1.5
Colloid oncotic pressure– pulmonary capillary wedge pressure (mm Hg)	14.5 ± 2.5	10.5 ± 2.7
Mean arterial pressure (mm Hg)	86.4 ± 7.5	90.3 ± 5.8
Pulmonary capillary wedge pressure (mm Hg)	6.3 ± 2.1	7.5 ± 1.8
Central venous pressure (mm Hg)	3.7 ± 2.6	3.6 ± 2.5
Left ventricular stroke work index (g-m-m⁻²)	41 ± 8	48 ± 6

[a]From Clark SL, Cotton DB, Lee W, et al. Central hemodynamic assessment of normal term pregnancy. *Am J Obstet Gynecol* 1989; 161:1439.

◇ DISSEMINATED INTRAVASCULAR COAGULOPATHY ASSOCIATED WITH PREGNANCY

Disseminated intravascular coagulopathy is not a distinct clinical entity; rather, it represents a manifestation of various disease processes that have in common activation of intravascular clotting and fibrinolysis, resulting in excess consumption of soluble coagulation components. In obstetrics, secondary fibrinogenolysis commonly dominates the clotting aberration and results in the circulation of fibrin and fibrinolytic split products, which further accentuate the clinical presentation of hemorrhage. In addition, sometimes a dilutional coagulopathy is encountered in pregnancy. This condition obtains when massive hemorrhage is replaced only by red blood cells and crystalloid solution, resulting in a dilutional depletion of platelets and soluble clotting factors. From both a clinical and a laboratory standpoint, dilutional coagulopathy may be confused with a more classic process of intravascular consumption and fibrinolysis. In practice, the hemorrhage associated with dilutional coagulopathy often results in hypotension and shock. The tissue hypoxia that accompanies shock of any cause is well known to potentially activate the coagulation–fibrinolysis cycle associated with DIC. Thus, it is not always possible to draw a clear distinction between dilutional and consumptive coagulopathy.

Pathophysiology

A number of conditions in obstetrics may trigger the intravascular coagulation–fibrinolysis sequence. All have in common some form of endothelial disruption or release of tissue thromboplastins into the central circulation. Thus, clotting may occur by either the intrinsic or the extrinsic coagulation pathways. After activation of the clotting cascade, fibrin monomer polymerizes, forming insoluble fibrin.[37,38]

Serum plasminogen simultaneously begins the degradation of fibrin. The breakdown products of fibrin and fibrinogen (i.e., fibrinolytic split products) then bind the soluble fibrin monomer to prevent further polymerization. In addition, plasmin inactivates factors V, VIII, IX, and XIII and inhibits the platelet-mediated primary phase of coagulation. The fibrin monomer that does polymerize is filtered within the microvasculature, resulting in fibrin plugs. Such plugging reduces blood flow, which causes tissue hypoxia and organ ischemia. The subsequent endothelial damage further enhances the clotting cascade. Thrombocytopenia results from both consumption and destruction secondary to fibrinolytic split products in the microvasculature, a process that also results in microangiopathic hemolytic anemia. The release of thromboplastic material from damaged red blood cells and complement activation further propagate the vicious cycle of intravascular coagulation–fibrinolysis (see Fig. 5).

Diagnosis

Disseminated intravascular coagulation is clinically suggested by excess bleeding from surgical incision sites or the postpartum uterus. In severe cases, spontaneous bleeding from intravenous sites and other mucous membranes may also be seen. Table 3 lists some laboratory abnormalities that may be present in DIC. The prothrombin and partial thromboplastin times are relatively insensitive indicators of clotting status because these tests are not prolonged until 40% to 50% of the clotting factors have been consumed. Although levels of fibrinolytic split products and paracoagulation tests are thought to be sensitive indicators of DIC, they may be normal in 10% to 15% of patients with acute DIC.

Causes

Numerous causes of DIC may be encountered in obstetrics (Fig. 6). The most common are placental abruption and dead fetus syndrome. Amniotic fluid embolism (AFE), a rare obstetric catastrophe, is often associated with DIC.[39] Rarely, severe preeclampsia may be associated with frank intravascular

TABLE 3. *Laboratory abnormalities in disseminated intravascular coagulation*[a]

Antithrombin III consumption
Elevated fibrinopeptide A
Abnormal prothrombin time
Abnormal partial thromboplastin time
Abnormal platelet count
Elevated fibrinogen–fibrin split products
Schistocytosis
Leukocytosis
Positive protamine sulfate test
Abnormal clot retraction

[a] From Clark SL, Cotton DB, Hankins GDV, Phelan JP, eds. *Critical care obstetrics,* 2nd ed. Boston: Blackwell Scientific, 1991:184.

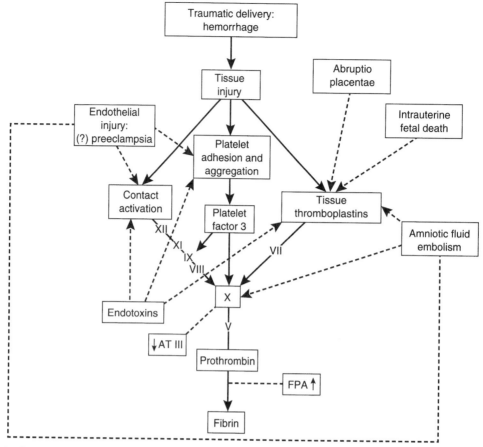

FIG. 6. Obstetric disorders that initiate disseminated intravascular coagulation. (Adapted from Clark SL, Phelan JP. *Critical care obstetrics, 2nd ed.* Boston: Blackwell Scientific, 1990:182.)

coagulation; more commonly, isolated thrombocytopenia is seen with normal tests of intravascular clotting.[40] Other conditions not unique to obstetrics, such as septic shock and transfusion disorders, may also be associated with DIC in obstetrics. The management of acute DIC in obstetrics principally involves resolution of the underlying pathophysiological process. Although possibly severe, the DIC associated with abruption, dead fetus syndrome, or AFE usually is self-limiting, and its resolution may begin with delivery of the fetus and placenta. In most cases, the replacement of soluble clotting factors or platelets is effective in preventing clinical hemorrhage for the short term while delivery is accomplished; little evidence exists to support the use of heparin or fibrinolytic agents in obstetric DIC syndromes. One exception may be dead fetus syndrome, in which low-dose heparin therapy (5000 U subcutaneously twice daily) may correct moderate coagulation abnormalities during delivery. In the presence of bleeding or surgery, platelet transfusion should be considered for patients with a platelet count less than 30,000/mm³, and fibrinogen replacement with fresh frozen plasma is appropriate for the bleeding patient with a fibrinogen level less than 100 mg/dl or elevated clotting tests such as prothrombin and partial thromboplastin times. In the nonsurgical patient without clinical hemorrhage, clotting abnormalities associated with a mild to moderate intravascular coagulopathy may simply be observed while delivery is accomplished.

◊ BLOOD TRANSFUSION

Indications for blood or component transfusion include restoration of circulating volume, improvement in oxygen transport, and correction of coagulation disorders.[41–52] The third indication has been addressed in the preceding paragraphs. This section addresses blood and component transfusion considerations in the patient with massive blood loss.[50]

The incidence of blood transfusion in patients undergoing vaginal delivery is less than 1%, whereas from 2% to 12% of patients undergoing cesarean delivery receive blood.[41] To anticipate the potential for peripartum blood loss, blood often is sent for type and screen and, occasionally, type and cross match. To type and screen blood, first the ABO group and Rh(D) type of the patient's cells are determined. Her serum is then mixed with reagent red blood cells that contain the antigens with which most clinically significant antibodies will react. An antibody-enhancing solution, such as bovine serum albumin, may be added at this point to enhance the detection of nonagglutinating antibodies. After incubation and washing, the appearance of an agglutination indicates the presence in the recipient serum of antibodies to one or more antigens in the reagent blood cells.[49]

Type and cross match procedures are similar to those described for typing and screening except that potential donor red blood cells are used rather than standard reagent erythrocytes. If blood that has been screened but not cross matched is used, a transfusion reaction might take place if the recipient serum contains an antibody to an antigen present on the donor cells that was not present on the reagent red blood cells. Because only 0.03% to 0.07% of patients who were determined not to have antibodies on type and screening are subsequently found to have preexisting antibodies determined by cross match, the type-and-screen approach has been about 99% effective in preventing incompatible transfusions.[57] Type-and-screen testing is much less costly than typing and cross matching blood and allows blood to be made available for more than one potential recipient, thus decreasing the wastage of banked blood. Therefore, this method is appropriate for both vaginal delivery and most cases of cesarean section and, under these circumstances, is preferred to typing and cross matching.[43,44]

Whole Blood

A unit of whole blood contains about 450 ml of blood. One unit of whole blood can raise the recipient's hematocrit by 3% to 4%. When stored for longer than 24 hours, whole blood retains few functioning granulocytes or platelets. Clotting factors are maintained in adequate concentration for the life of the unit, but levels of factors V and VIII may be reduced. Because whole blood is not readily available, whole blood transfusion is uncommon in modern obstetric practice; red blood cells plus component replacement is preferred.

Red Blood Cells

Packed red blood cells are prepared from whole blood by separating the cells from plasma by centrifugation or sedimentation.[52] They have a hematocrit of about 70% to 75%. A unit of packed cells contains the same number of erythrocytes as a unit of whole blood; thus, it can raise the recipient's hematocrit by 3% to 4%. Packed red blood cells provide the same oxygen-carrying capacity as whole blood in about half the volume.

Platelets

Platelets are prepared from whole blood by centrifugation and then are resuspended in 50 to 70 ml of plasma. Unlike red blood cells, they cannot tolerate prolonged storage; under special circumstances, however, they may be stored for up to 5 days.[52] The donor plasma in which the platelets are suspended must be ABO-compatible with the recipient's red blood cells. A unit of random donor platelets should raise the platelet count by 8000 to 10,000/mm³. Platelets are available in packs of 8 or 10 units. No consensus has been reached regarding minimal platelet levels that indicate the need for transfusion. In the nonbleeding or nonsurgical patient, platelet transfusion seldom is indicated with a platelet count that exceeds 10,000/mm³ because antibody formation and platelet destruction are rapid. In the bleeding or surgical patient, the platelet count should be maintained above 30,000/mm³ to prevent further hemorrhage.

Fresh Frozen Plasma

Fresh frozen plasma contains all soluble clotting factors, similar to whole blood. In addition, it contains significant amounts of factors V and VIII. The plasma is first separated from whole blood and then frozen. The volume of an unit is about 250 ml.[52] Fresh frozen plasma is indicated for patients with a consumptive or dilutional coagulopathy in whom replacement of soluble clotting factors, including fibrinogen, is indicated. In the bleeding patient, a fibrinogen level less than 100 mg/dl associated with prolongation of prothrombin and partial thromboplastin times is an indication for fresh frozen plasma infusion. One unit will raise the serum fibrinogen level by approximately 25 mg/dl.

Cryoprecipitate

A unit of cryoprecipitate is prepared by thawing a unit of fresh frozen plasma, removing the supernatant plasma, and then refreezing the precipitate.[52] Cryoprecipitate contains factors VIII, VIIIc, and XIII; von Willebrand factor; fibrinogen; and fibronectin. The sole advantage of cryoprecipitate over fresh frozen plasma is the ability to infuse relatively large amounts of factors in a small volume. In practice, volume restriction seldom is desirable for the hemorrhaging patient; thus, fresh frozen plasma is nearly always preferable to cryoprecipitate in the management of obstetric hemorrhage associated with consumptive or dilutional coagulopathy.

In cases of dilutional coagulopathy, bleeding is more likely to be secondary to thrombocytopenia than to factor deficiency.[58] All the blood and clotting factors contained in cryoprecipitate and fresh frozen plasma carry with them the risk of blood-borne disease transmission, although such a risk is minimal in properly screened and donated blood.

Transfusion Reactions

Acute transfusion reactions are seen in about 5% of blood recipients, and delayed transfusion reactions in up to 7% of recipients.[41] Nonhemolytic febrile reactions may accompany 1% of all transfused units.[49] Most nonhemolytic febrile and allergic reactions are unavoidable. Most hemolytic reactions may be prevented by proper attention to cross-matching procedures.

Hemolytic transfusion reactions may be acute or delayed. Acute intravascular hemolysis most commonly results from the transfusion of ABO-incompatible blood. Such errors are the most frequent cause of fatalities resulting from blood transfusion and usually are related to technical errors in blood specimen labeling and in patient identification.[49] Such hemolysis is complement-mediated. Signs and symptoms of acute hemolytic reaction include lumbar pain, facial flushing, chest pain that may be accompanied by fever, tachycardia, hypotension, and shock.[49] In severe cases, DIC associated with oliguria and pulmonary edema may be seen. Acute tubular necrosis or ARDS may be encountered in patients who survive the acute episode. The key laboratory findings in the diagnosis of intravascular hemolytic transfusion reaction are a decrease in the plasma haptoglobin level with an increase in free serum hemoglobin. These findings typically are accompanied by hemoglobinuria if plasma levels exceed 25 mg/dl.[49]

Acute extravascular hemolytic reactions are not mediated by complement but by the development of IgG antibodies to antigens such as D or Kell. Clinical findings are less severe and often manifest by simply a fever and hemolytic anemia.[50] Severe clinical symptoms are infrequent.

Delayed hemolytic reactions occur within 3 to 7 days of a blood transfusion. These reactions are caused by a serum antibody that is present in low, undetectable levels at the time of transfusion. The clinical parameters are similar to those seen with acute extravascular hemolysis but are not as severe.

Management of Hemolytic Transfusion Reactions

The goals of therapy in managing a severe hemolytic transfusion reaction are to maintain the blood pressure and avoid respiratory failure or acute tubular necrosis associated with oliguria.[49] When hemolytic transfusion reaction is suspected, the transfusion should be stopped immediately. An intravenous line should be maintained with normal saline solution. Crystalloid solution and pressor agents, if necessary, should be infused rapidly to maintain blood pressure. Oxygen should be administered; assisted ventilation may also be necessary. Urine output should be maintained to prevent the development of renal shutdown and acute tubular necrosis. Mannitol (20 to 25 mg intravenously over 5 minutes) should be administered and may be repeated up to four times within 24 hours. Specimens of the transfused blood as well as the recipient's blood should be sent to the blood bank for analysis. The recipient's plasma should also be checked for hemolysis. Plasma and urine samples should be checked for hemoglobin, and direct antiglobulin tests should be performed on the postreaction blood sample.

◊ ACUTE RESPIRATORY DISTRESS SYNDROME

Acute respiratory distress syndrome is a complex pathophysiological process resulting from either primary lung epithelial injury by way of the airways or capillary endothelial injuries initiated by way of the pulmonary vasculature. Such injury results in increased pulmonary capillary permeability, loss of lung volume, and shunting with resultant arterial hypoxemia.[53] The physiological criteria required for the diagnosis of ARDS are listed in Table 4. In pregnancy, sepsis,

TABLE 4. *Physiological criteria for adult respiratory distress syndrome[a]*

$P_{O_2} < 50$ with $F_{I}O_2 > 0.6$
Pulmonary capillary wedge ≤ 12 mm Hg
Total respiratory compliance < 50 ml/cm (usually 20–30 ml/cm)
Functional residual capacity reduced
Shunt $(Q_s/Q_t) > 30\%$
Dead space $(V_D/V_T) > 60\%$
Alveolar–arterial gradient on 100% oxygen ≥ 350 mm Hg

[a]$F_{I}O_2$, fraction of inspired oxygen; P_{O_2}, partial pressure of oxygen; Q_s, blood flow to nonventilated areas; Q_t, total blood flow to both ventilated and nonventilated areas; V_D, dead space volume; V_T, tidal volume. (From Clark SL, Cotton DB, Hankins GDV, Phelan JB, eds. *Critical care obstetrics, 3rd ed.* Boston: Blackwell Scientific, 1997.)

viral pneumonic processes, hypovolemic shock, and aspiration pneumonia are the most common causes of ARDS.[53,54]

ARDS represents a final common pathway of a cascade of events initiated by the alveolar, epithelial, or endothelial injury (Fig. 7).[53] After the initial injury to alveolar epithelial cells or vascular endothelial cells, the complement system, leukocytes, macrophages, and platelets may all play important roles in perpetuating the injury. During the initial lung injury, phospholipids are released from red blood cell membranes, resulting in a secondary mechanism of injury. Free arachidonic acids serve as a substrate for the synthesis of both prostaglandins and thromboxanes by way of the cyclooxygenase system and, possibly, leukotrienes by way of the lipoxygenase system. All of these arachidonic acid metabolites have been implicated in perpetuating the injury of ARDS.

Clinically, the course of ARDS can be divided into four phases.[53] Each is distinguishable by histologic changes in the lungs and reflected in various physiological parameters in the patient. In phase I, hyperventilation is the only physiological aberration seen, and arterial oxygenation remains adequate. During phase II (i.e., the latent period), there may be minor auscultatory and radiographic evidence of pulmonary disease. Mild decreases in lung compliance and increases in intrapulmonary shunting of blood are common. Histologically, these stages are characterized by progressive alveolar and interstitial edema formation and the movement of inflammatory cells into the interstitium. Damage to type I alveolar cells occurs, and hyaline membrane formation begins. Phase III is characterized by acute respiratory failure with severe dyspnea, tachypnea, and arterial hypoxemia. During this phase, lung volume is lost, resulting in the deterioration of pulmonary compliance and an increase in intrapulmonary shunting. Chest x-ray films taken during this stage demonstrate marked abnormalities, including bilateral lung opacification. During phase III, intubation and assisted ventilation are required. Histologically, phase III is characterized by thickening of the alveolar septum and marked infiltration by leukocytes, plasma cells, and macrophages. Hyaline membranes begin to form and organize during this phase, and the

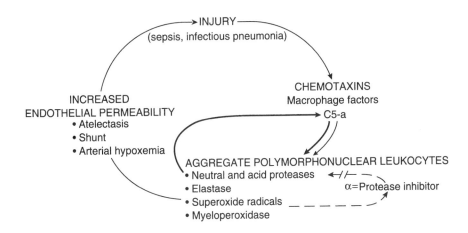

FIG. 7. Schematic diagram of the proposed mechanism of lung injury. After the cycle is established, loop 1 feeds back on itself to perpetuate the injury. Amplification of the first loop is provided by the neutral and acid proteases *(bold line)*; disruption of the amplification loop is prevented by myeloperoxidases *(dashed line)*. PMNS, polymorphonuclear leukocytes. (Adapted from Clark SL, Phelan JP. *Critical care obstetrics, 2nd ed.* Boston: Blackwell Scientific, 1990:343.)

proliferation of fibroblasts and type II alveolar cells is prominent. In phase IV, interpulmonary shunting in excess of 25% results in hypoxemia refractory to all measures. Dead space during this period may exceed 60% of tidal volume. Metabolic and respiratory acidemia may be found and may result in increased myocardial excitability, which often leads to terminal dysrhythmia. Intraalveolar fibrosis is severe, and pathologic and physiological derangements are irreversible.

Clinical Management

Four considerations are essential in understanding the clinical management of the pregnant patient with ARDS. These are oxygen delivery and tissue extraction, pulmonary compliance, interpulmonary shunt fraction, and eradication of the underlying cause.[53–63]

Oxygen delivery is directly proportional to cardiac output; it is also influenced by the oxygen-carrying capacity of the blood. Thus, oxygen delivery can be optimized by maintaining cardiac output and correcting anemia. In the presence of suboptimal cardiac output or significant anemia, marked increases in the inspired concentration of oxygen have little effect on actual oxygen delivery. However, high inspired concentrations of oxygen are toxic to the lung.[58] The goals in caring for a patient with severe ARDS are first to optimize cardiac output and hematocrit and then to maintain a PO_2 of 60 to 70 mm Hg. Because increased body temperature and metabolic acidosis produce a rightward shift in the oxyhemoglobin dissociation curve, these conditions may favorably affect peripheral oxygen delivery. Thus, the patient should not be chilled either in the operating room or through the administration of large volumes of intravenous fluids or blood that is below body temperature. Further, respiratory alkalosis should be corrected. Indeed, a mild metabolic acidemia may result in better tissue oxygen delivery than would be obtained with complete correction of the patient's acid–base status.

Arterial–venous oxygen content difference may be used to assess the adequacy of oxygen delivery. During pregnancy, the arterial–venous gradient narrows.

In the critically ill patient who is receiving assisted ventilation, pulmonary compliance can be calculated by using parameters obtainable from the ventilator. With severe ARDS, pulmonary compliance may fall from a normal value of about 75 ml/cm H_2O to as low as 20 ml/cm H_2O. Serial calculation of compliance may be useful in evaluating the effects of various therapeutic maneuvers, including positive end-expiratory pressure (PEEP). Longitudinal evaluation of pulmonary compliance may serve as a useful method of following the resolution or progression of ARDS.

The normal shunt in the healthy gravida is 2% to 5% of cardiac output. Mild pulmonary dysfunction may result in shunting of 10% to 15%.[68] A shunt that exceeds 25% suggests and, in the absence of other causes, may be diagnostic of ARDS.[60] The shunt may be estimated either by analyzing an arterial blood sample alone or by analyzing simultaneously obtained arterial and pulmonary artery blood samples. In the former method, the greatest accuracy is obtained by having the woman breathe 100% oxygen. In a patient who is intubated and receiving 100% inspired oxygen, the arterial oxygen pressure should exceed 500 mm Hg; values below 300 mm Hg suggest severe shunting.

During initial treatment of the pregnant gravida with ARDS, the physician should simultaneously conduct an aggressive search for and attempt to eliminate the underlying cause of the lung injury. Early intubation is essential for the patient in incipient respiratory failure (Table 5).[60] Mechanical ventilation requires a volume-cycled ventilator. Appropriate initial settings may include a rate of 12 breaths per minute, a tidal volume of about 15 mm/kg body weight with a sigh volume of 200 to 400 ml above tidal volume, a PEEP of 5 cm H_2O, and 100% inspired oxygen. Fifteen to 30 minutes after the initial therapy, an arterial blood sample is analyzed, and the ventilator settings are adjusted to obtain a P_aO_2 of 60 to 70 mm Hg with a PCO_2 of 35 to 45 mm Hg. The level of PEEP often must be increased to optimize PO_2 and oxygen saturation. The use of high levels of PEEP is preferable to the continued use of toxic concentrations of oxygen. If possible, the F_1O_2 should be reduced to less than 60% to minimize the potential for long-term oxygen toxicity. The criteria for using higher levels of

TABLE 5. *Guidelines for instituting ventilator therapy[a]*

	Normal	Intubate
Respiratory rate	12–20	>35
Vital capacity (ml/kg)	65–75	<15
FEV_1 (ml/kg)	50–60	<10
Inspiratory force (cm H_2O)	75–100	<25
P_aO_2 (mm Hg)	100–75 air	<70 mask 0.4
		<300 F_1O_2
P_aCO_2 (mm Hg)	35–45	>55
V_D/V_t	0.25–0.40	>0.6

[a]FEV_1, forced expiratory volume in 1 sec; F_1O_2, forced inspiratory oxygen concentration; P_aCO_2, arterial carbon dioxide pressure; P_aO_2, arterial oxygen pressure; V_D/V_t, ratio of dead space volume to tidal volume. (From Clark SL, Cotton DB, Hankins GDV, Phelan JP, eds. *Critical care obstetrics, 2nd ed.* Boston: Blackwell Scientific, 1991:357.)

TABLE 6. *Signs and symptoms noted in patients with amniotic fluid embolism[a]*

Sign or symptom	No. of patients	%
Hypotension	43	100
Fetal distress	30	100
Pulmonary edema or adult respiratory distress syndrome	28	93
Cardiopulmonary arrest	40	87
Cyanosis	38	83
Coagulopathy	38	83
Dyspnea	22	49
Seizure	22	48
Atony	11	23
Bronchospasm	7	15
Transient hypertension	5	11
Cough	3	7
Headache	3	7
Chest pain	1	2

[a]From ref. 48.

PEEP include a static compliance less than 40 ml/cm H_2O, a shunt fraction exceeding 20%, or an alveolar–arterial oxygen gradient on 100% oxygen exceeding 400 mm Hg.[53] At high levels of PEEP (>20 cm H_2O), cardiac output may fall; thus, invasive hemodynamic monitoring often is useful in assessing the cardiac output response to high levels of PEEP. Fluid therapy in patients with ARDS may also be facilitated by the use of invasive hemodynamic monitoring, and the PCWP should be maintained as low as is consistent with adequate cardiac and urine output.

The management of the patient with ARDS often is a long-term process. Ventilation and circulation may be supported by using some of the techniques outlined in this section. After the underlying cause of ARDS has been eliminated, therapy involves support of respiration and circulation while allowing the lungs time to heal. Despite aggressive and optimal management, the mortality rate for adults with ARDS exceeds 50%, and in many instances, such patients may expire despite optimal therapy. Recently, surfactant replacement as well as nitric oxide therapy have shown promise in the treatment of severe ARDS; however, at present, the use of these agents remains investigational.[64–66]

◊ AMNIOTIC FLUID EMBOLISM

Amniotic fluid embolism is an uncommon obstetric catastrophe with a mortality as high as 80%.[39] It is a biphasic process that is triggered by the sudden embolization of amniotic fluid or debris of fetal origin into the maternal venous circulation. The initial physiological disturbances involve profound alterations in hemodynamics and oxygenation, often followed by the development of a consumptive coagulopathy. Either of these phases may predominate, and occasionally, bleeding may be the presenting manifestation. The most common presentation is that of sudden dyspnea and hypotension commonly followed within minutes by cardiorespiratory arrest. In up to 50% of these cases, these initial events may be accompanied by seizure activity. Common signs and symptoms of AFE are presented in Table 6.[67] One-half of all patients

with AFE die within 1 hour after the onset of symptoms; in survivors, neurologic damage or brain death secondary to the initial severe hypoxia is not uncommon. Data from the National AFE Registry suggested an overall mortality rate of 61%; only half of those who survive do so without significant neurologic sequelae.[67] Women with AFE generally exhibit left ventricular dysfunction or failure accompanied by elevated PCWP and, in most cases, depressed left ventricular stroke work index.[67,68] Systemic vascular resistance is decreased. Elevations of pulmonary artery pressure and pulmonary vascular resistance often are in the range attributable to left ventricular failure. The existence of an initial but transient phase of pulmonary hypertension and elevated right ventricular pressure is supported by some animal and clinical data. A component of noncardiogenic pulmonary edema (i.e., ARDS) often is present and may become the predominant clinical problem in survivors.

A hemorrhagic phase is reported in at least 50% of patients with AFE. This problem commonly is compounded by the simultaneous occurrence of uterine atony, perhaps as a direct result of a myometrial depressant effect of amniotic fluid.[67] Although AFE has been reported under many conditions, most cases have occurred during labor.[67] In the past, a pattern of vigorous labor or hypertonic uterine contractions associated with oxytocin infusion had often been implicated in the pathogenesis of this condition. Evidence of this association was anecdotal and is clearly invalid.[67,69] Placental abruption is present in up to 50% of cases, with fetal death reported in some cases before the acute clinical presentation.

Early studies suggested that meconium or particulate matter in amniotic fluid is the pathologic agent, but more recent data suggest that a humoral substance, rather than particulate matter, is responsible for the observed hemodynamic changes.[67] It is also clear the infusion of clear amniotic fluid, *per se,* is innocuous, both in the human and in animal models.[67] Further,

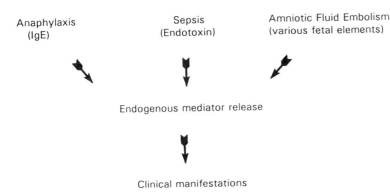

FIG. 8. Proposed pathophysiological relationship among amniotic fluid embolism, septic shock, and anaphylactic shock. Each syndrome may also have direct physiological effects (e.g., fever in endotoxin-mediated sepsis). (From ref. 48, with permission.)

the marked similarities between the clinical manifestations of AFE and both septic and anaphylactic shock suggest the involvement of endogenous mediators in the pathophysiology of this condition.[67] Azagami demonstrated that in an animal model of AFE, pretreatment with an inhibitor of leukotriene synthesis prevents the development of AFE syndrome and death.[70,71] Thus, it has been suggested that the term *amniotic fluid embolism* is a misnomer because the syndrome is not caused by amniotic fluid *per se,* nor are clinical manifestations those commonly seen with embolic events. Clark and coworkers proposed the term *anaphylactoid syndrome of pregnancy* to describe this condition (Fig. 8).[67]

Classically, the definitive diagnosis of AFE has been made at autopsy with the demonstration of fetal squamous cells, mucin, hair, or vernix in the pulmonary artery vasculature. More recently, it has been demonstrated that squamous cells and other debris of presumed fetal origin may be demonstrated in blood aspirated from the central venous or pulmonary artery circulation of living patients with AFE.[72] Studies of pregnant women undergoing pulmonary artery catheterization for various medical indications have suggested that the detection of squamous cells in the maternal pulmonary artery circulation is a common phenomenon that may in part be attributable to contamination with adult squamous epithelium from the site of central venous access.[72] Further, such debris is detected in only 50% to 75% of patients with clinical AFE, even when examined with special stains and techniques.[67] Thus, the detection of squamous cells in the maternal pulmonary artery circulation during life is neither sensitive nor specific for the diagnosis of AFE. Such a diagnosis must be made principally on the basis of clinical presentation. The differential diagnosis of AFE includes septic shock, aspiration pneumonitis, acute myocardial infarction, pulmonary thromboembolism, and, in cases in which coagulopathy is a dominant feature, placental abruption.

Treatment revolves around three goals: oxygenation, maintenance of cardiac output and blood pressure, and resolution of what usually is a self-limiting, albeit severe, coagulopathy. When sudden intrapartum hypotension and dyspnea suggest AFE, the following steps should be taken.[73] First, administer oxygen if the patient is conscious. Intubate and ventilate with 100% F_IO_2 if the patient is in respiratory failure.

Monitor the fetal heart rate carefully if gestational age is sufficient to consider intervention for fetal distress. Hypotension usually is on the basis of cardiogenic shock; treatment involves initial optimization of cardiac preload by rapid crystalloid administration followed by dopamine infusion if the patient remains hypotensive. A flow-directed pulmonary artery catheter may be helpful in guiding later hemodynamic management. After resolution of hypotension, fluid therapy should be restricted to maintenance levels to minimize pulmonary edema caused by developing ARDS. Administer component therapy to treat bleeding secondary to DIC. Packed red blood cells and fresh frozen plasma are the mainstay of such therapy.

In patients who survive AFE, recurrence during subsequent vaginal or cesarean delivery has not been reported.[73]

◊ REFERENCES

1. Clark SL. Shock in the pregnant patient. *Semin Perinatol* 1990;14(1):52.
2. Rochat RW, Kooniu LM, Atrash HK, et al. Maternal mortality in the United States. *Obstet Gynecol* 1988;72:91.
3. Pritchard JA. Changes in blood volume during pregnancy and delivery. *Anesthesiology* 1965;26:393.
4. Clark SL, Cotton DB, Lee W, et al. Central hemodynamic assessment of normal term pregnancy. *Am J Obstet Gynecol* 1989;161:1439.
5. Shoemaker WC. Pathophysiologic basis of therapy for shock and trauma syndromes. *Seminars in Drug Treatment* 1973;3:211.
6. Slater G, Vladeck BA, Bassin R, et al. Sequential changes in the distribution of cardiac output in various stages of experimental hemorrhage shock. *Surgery* 1973;73:714.
7. Clark SL; Hypovolemic Shock. In: Clark SL, Cotton DB, Hankins GDV, Phelan JP, eds. *Critical care obstetrics. 3rd ed.* Boston: Blackwell Scientific, 1997:191.
8. Shoemaker WC, Montgomery ES, Kaplan E, et al. Physiologic patterns in surviving and non-surviving shock patients. *Arch Surg* 1973;106:630.
9. American Association of Blood Banks. Circular of information for the use of human blood and blood components. *American Red Cross*, May 1986;25.
10. Duff P. Pathophysiology and management of septic shock. *J Reprod Med* 1980;24:109.
11. Lee W, Clark SL, Cotton DB, et al. Septic shock during pregnancy. *Am J Obstet Gynecol* 1988;159:410.
12. Mason JW, Kleeberg U, Dolan P, et al. Plasma kallikrein and Hageman factor in gram negative bacteremia. *Ann Intern Med* 1970;73:545.
13. Parker MM, Parillo JE. Septic shock, hemodynamics and pathogenesis. *JAMA* 1983;250:3324.
14. Parillo JE. Septic shock in humans. In: Shoemaker WC, Ayers SM, Grenvik A, et al, eds. *Textbook of critical care. 2nd ed.* Philadelphia: WB Saunders, 1989:1018.

15. Bernton EW, Long JB, Holoday JW. Opioids and neuropeptides: mechanisms in circulatory shock. *Federal Proceedings* 1985;44:290.

16. Dinerman JL, Lowenstein CJ, Snyder SH. Molecular mechanisms of nitric oxide regulation: Potential relevance to cardiovascular disease. *Circ Res* 1993;73:217.

17. Holcroft JW, Trunky DD. Extravascular lung water following hemorrhage shock in the baboon: comparison between resuscitation with Ringer's lactate and Plasmanate. *Ann Surg* 1974;180:408.

18. Parker MM, Shelhamer JH, Bacharach SL, et al. Severe reversible myocardial depression in septic shock. *Crit Care Med* 1983;11:229.

19. Parillo JE, Buuch C, Shelhamer JH, et al. A circulatory myocardial depressant substance in humans with septic shock. *J Clin Invest* 1985;76:1539.

20. Weil MH, Nishijima H. Cardiac output in bacterial shock. *Am J Med* 1978;64:920.

21. Mimoz O, Rauss A, Rekik N, et al. Pulmonary artery catheterization in critically ill patients: a prospective analysis of outcome changes associated with catheter-prompted changes in therapy. *Crit Care Med* 1994;22:573.

22. Sibbald WJ, Paterson NAM, Holliday RL, et al. Pulmonary hypertension in sepsis. *Chest* 1978;73:583.

23. Bone RG, Fisher CJ, Clemarer TP, et al. A controlled trial of high dose methylprednisolone in the treatment of severe sepsis and septic shock. *N Engl J Med* 1987;317:653.

24. Veterans Administration, Systemic Sepsis Cooperative Study Group. Effects of high-dose glucosteroid therapy on mortality in patients with clinical signs of sepsis. *N Engl J Med* 1987;317:659.

25. Rock P, Silverman A, Pluys D, et al. Efficacy and safety of naloxone in septic shock. *Crit Care Med* 1985;13:28.

26. Behrmann RE, Lees MH, Peterson EM, et al. Distribution of the circulation in the normal and asphyxiated fetal primate. *Am J Obstet Gynecol* 1970;108:956.

27. Cotton DB, Gonik B, Dorman K, et al. Cardiovascular alterations in severe pregnancy induced hypertension: relationship of central venous pressure to pulmonary capillary wedge pressure. *Am J Obstet Gynecol* 1985;151:762.

28. Clark SL, Cotton CB. Clinical indications for pulmonary artery catheterization in severe pregnancy induced hypertension. *Am J Obstet Gynecol* 1988;158:453.

29. Clark SL, Phelan JP. Pre-eclampsia/eclampsia: hemodynamic and neurologic correlations. *Obstet Gynecol* 1985;66:337.

30. Hankins GDV, Wendel GD Jr, Cunningham FG, Leveno KJ. Longitudinal evaluation of hemodynamic changes in eclampsia. *Am J Obstet Gynecol* 1984;150:506.

31. Sola JE, Bender JS. Use of the pulmonary artery catheter to reduce operative complications. *Surg Clin North Am* 1993;73:253.

32. Coles NA, Hibberd M, Russell M, et al. Potential impact of pulmonary artery catheter placement on short term management decisions in the medical intensive care unit. *Am Heart J* 1993;126:815.

33. Connors AF, Speroff T Jr, Dawson NV, et al. The effectiveness of right heart catheterization in the initial care of critically ill patients. *JAMA* 1996;276(11):889–897.

34. Clark SL, Cotton DB, Pivarnik JM, et al. Position change and central hemodynamic profile during normal third trimester pregnancy and postpartum. *Am J Obstet Gynecol* 1991;164:883.

35. US Food and Drug Administration. Precautions necessary with central venous catheters. *FDA Drug Bull* 1989;July:15.

36. Wadas TM. Pulmonary artery catheter removal. *Crit Care Nurs* 1994;14:63.

37. Bick RL. Disseminated intravascular coagulation and related syndromes: etiology, pathophysiology, diagnosis, and management. *Am J Hematol* 1978;5:265.

38. Kopec M, Wegrzynourczy Z, Budzynski A, et al. Interaction of fibrinogen degradation products with platelets. *Exp Biol Med* 1968;3:73.

39. Clark SL. New concepts of amniotic fluid embolism. *Obstet Gynecol Surv* 1990;45:360.

40. Pritchard JA. Cunningham FG, Mason FA. Coagulation changes in eclampsia. Their frequency and pathogenesis. *Am J Obstet Gynecol* 1976;124:855.

41. Sacks DA. Blood and component therapy in obstetrics. In: Clark SL, Cotton DB, Hankins GDV, Phelan JP, eds. *Critical care obstetrics. 3rd ed.* Boston: Blackwell Scientific, 1997:191.

42. Penney GC, Moores HM, Boulton FE. Development of a rational blood-ordering policy for obstetrics and gynaecology. *Br J Obstet Gynaecol* 1982;89:100.

43. Kamani AA, McMorland CH, Wadsworth LD. Utilization of red blood cell transfusion in an obstetric setting. *Am J Obstet Gynecol* 1988;159:1177.

44. Chestnut DH. Blood replacement for repeat cesarean section: "type and screen" preferable to cross matching. *N C Med J* 1985;46:139.

45. Friedman BA. An analysis of surgical blood use in United States hospitals with application to the maximum surgical blood order schedule. *Transfusion* 1979;19:268.

46. Boral LI, Hill SS, Apollon CJ, Folland A. The type and antibody screen, revisited. *Am J Clin Pathol* 1979;71:578.

47. Heisto H. Pretransfusion blood group serology. *Transfusion* 1979;19:761.

48. Hardy NM, Bolen FH, Shatney CH. Maximum surgical blood order schedule reduces hospital costs. *Am Surg* 1987;53:223.

49. Committee on Standards. *Standards for blood banks and transfusion services. 13th ed.* Arlington, VA: American Association of Blood Banks, 1989.

50. Murphy S, Kahn RA, Holme S, et al. Improved storage of platelets for transfusion in a new container. *Blood* 1982;60:194.

51. Kruskall MS, Mintz PD, Bergin JJ, et al. Transfusion therapy in emergency medicine. *Ann Emerg Med* 1988;17:327.

52. Snyder EL, ed. *Blood transfusion therapy. 2nd ed.* Arlington, VA: American Association of Blood Banks, 1987.

53. Hankins GDV. Acute pulmonary injury and respiratory failure during pregnancy. In: Clark SL, Cotton DB, Hankins GDV, Phelan JP, eds. *Critical care obstetrics. 3rd ed.* Boston: Blackwell Scientific, 1997:347.

54. Eriksen NL, Parisi VM. Adult respiratory distress syndrome and pregnancy. *Semin Perinatol* 1990;14:68.

55. Petty TL. Adult respiratory distress syndrome. *Semin Respir Med* 1982;3:219.

56. Orell SR. Lung pathology in respiratory distress following shock in the adult. *Acta Pathol Microbiol Scand* 1971;79:65.

57. Bachoten M, Weibel ER. Alterations of the gas exchange apparatus in adult respiratory insufficiency associated with septicemia. *Am Rev Respir Dis* 1977;116:589.

58. Clark JM. The toxicity of oxygen. *Am Rev Respir Dis* 1974;110:40.

59. Pontoppidan H, Geffin B, Lowenstein E. Acute respiratory failure in the adult. *N Engl J Med* 1972;287:743.

60. Weisman IM, Rinaldo JE, Rogers RM. Positive endexpiratory pressure in adult respiratory failure. *N Engl J Med* 1982;307:1381.

61. Temmesfeld-Wollbruck B, Walmrath D, Grimminger F, et al. Prevention and therapy of the adult respiratory distress syndrome. *Lung* 1995;173:139.

62. Marinelli WA, Ingbar DH. Diagnosis and management of acute lung injury. *Clin Chest Med* 1994;15:517.

63. Bernard GR, Artigas A, Brigham KL, et al. The American–European Consensus Conference on ARDS. Definitions, mechanisms, relevant outcomes, and clinical trial coordinations. *Am J Respir Crit Care Med* 1994;149:818.

64. Pontoppidan H, Geffin B, Lowenstein E. Acute respiratory failure in the adult. *N Engl J Med* 1972;287:743.

65. Haslam PL, Hughes DA, Mac Naughton PD, et al. Surfactant replacement therapy in late-stage adult respiratory distress syndrome. *Lancet* 1994;343:1009.

66. Rossaint R, Gerlach H, Falke KJ. Inhalation of nitric oxide—a new approach in severe ARDS. *Eur J Anaesthesiol* 1994;11:43.

67. Clark SL, Hankins GDV, Dudley DA, et al. Amniotic fluid embolism: analysis of the national registry. *Am J Obstet Gynecol* 1995;172:1158–1169.

68. Clark SL, Cotton DB, Gonik B, et al. Central hemodynamic alterations in amniotic fluid embolism. *Am J Obstet Gynecol* 1988;158:1124.

69. Morgan M. Amniotic fluid embolism. *Anaesthesia* 1979;34:29.

70. Clark SL. Arachidonic acid metabolites and the pathophysiology of amniotic fluid embolism. *Semin Reprod Endocrinol* 1985;3:253.

71. Azegami M, Mori N. Amniotic fluid embolism and leukotrienes. *Am J Obstet Gynecol* 1986;155:1119.

72. Clark SL, Pavlova A, Horenstein J, et al. Squamous cells in the maternal pulmonary circulation. *Am J Obstet Gynecol* 1986;154:104.

73. Clark SL. Pregnancy following amniotic fluid embolism. *Am J Obstet Gynecol* 1992;167:551.

CHAPTER 31

Primary Care in Gynecology

———— ◇ ————

Thomas E. Nolan

Health care reform is changing both the training of physicians and the practice of medicine. The major emphasis of the medical care system in this century has primarily been the acute care of disease. Over the past decade, the model of primary and preventive care has been suggested as a better alternative. In many cases, evidence suggests that certain preventive strategies are cost effective and lower morbidity and mortality risks. An example of preventive care is immunizations, which have either reduced or eliminated human scourges such as smallpox, measles, mumps, polio, rubella, hepatitis, and chickenpox. Other strategies, such as cancer screening and prevention by early recognition and precursor treatment of cancer, are reducing premature death.

Another aspect of health care reform is the behavior of physicians in a cost-conscious fiscal environment. Since the 1970s, the number of medical students has skyrocketed, leading to an excess of physicians in several geographic areas. In the 1960s, the concept of subspecialists began to emerge, with various medical specialty boards recognizing the need to regulate and grant special status to those individuals with advanced training. In the 1970s and 1980s, subspecialties proliferated, with fewer American-trained physicians entering primary care as generalists. Despite the addition of family practice as a recognized specialty, many physicians in the United States opted to do advanced training beyond the initial board certification. This has not been the case in obstetrics and gynecology. More than 90% remain in a general practice, even though obstetricians and gynecologists perform specialty-related surgical procedures. The surgical nature of the specialty has led to difficulties in obtaining primary care status. Subspecialists and individuals in procedure-oriented specialties were reimbursed at much higher levels than their colleagues in the so-called "cognitive specialties." The cost of caring for many common diseases was greater when a subspecialist managed the patient, with little demonstrable change in patient outcome.

At the same time, the American people have demanded that a physician provide a wider range of services. Fortunately, most American women are comfortable with their obstetrician and gynecologist and, in many cases, wish to remain with that physician. In the recent past, the ability of the "specialist" obstetrician/gynecologist to provide services outside the scope of the reproductive tract has been limited. Training programs are changing and reflect primarily the drop in surgical volume because of better medical therapies and changes in reimbursement policies. The services that most health maintenance organizations desire include preventive care, nutrition and fitness counseling, and management of anemia, depression, thyroid dysfunction, hypercholesterolism, low back pain, hypertension, diabetes, and chest pain.[1] The purpose of this chapter is to better define and broaden the scope of primary care for women.

◇ WELLNESS

The concept of "wellness" is to live in such a way as to minimize destructive behaviors (e.g., tobacco abuse, obesity) and enhance behavior that maximizes health and longevity (e.g., exercise and wearing seat belts). Accident prevention, immunization, and lifestyle adjustments such as smoking cessation and moderation in alcohol consumption are examples of beneficial behaviors. Weight control, a problem of increasing concern in the United States, can help prevent such diseases as diabetes.[2] Limiting saturated fat ingestion may reduce weight and, in susceptible individuals, reduce the risk of heart disease. The role of physical activity and health is the sole focus of a recent report issued by the Office of the Surgeon General.[3] Exercise programs have a positive impact on weight control, diabetes, constipation, and blood lipids. Other aspects of screening and maintaining a healthy lifestyle include recognition and control of common chronic diseases, including hypertension, hyperlipidemia, diabetes, and depression. Because many of these diseases have a higher prevalence in the older age groups, the gynecologist needs to be more knowledgeable about the treatment of these diseases.

Immunizations, which have a direct impact on disease prevention, are sometimes overlooked. Current adult recommendations are shown in Table 1.

Nutritional counseling is rarely requested for health reasons alone; most often it is sought because of obesity. The rate of obesity has progressively increased in the past 20 years. The recent introduction of new pharmaceutical agents for weight control, albeit with significant side effects, is evidence of the problem. In the United States, 35% of nonpregnant women are classified as overweight.[4] At the other extreme, and most often encountered in more affluent younger populations, are eating disorders such as bulimia and anorexia nervosa. Individuals with severe eating disorders usually require intense specialty counseling outside the realm of the generalist. Vegetarians represent yet another area of

TABLE 1. *Routine immunizations for adults*[a]

- Tetanus–diphtheria booster. Should be administered every 10 years, or a single midlife (at age 50 years) booster for individuals who have had the full series.
- Influenza vaccine. Annually beginning at age ≥65 and for high-risk groups including health care workers and individuals with chronic disease. Should be offered to young adults.
- Pneumococcal vaccine. Given at age ≥65 and repeated at 6 years. Before age 65, high-risk groups include those with cardiopulmonary disease or asplenic individuals as a result of trauma or autolysis from hemoglobinopathies. Currently, it is unknown if this vaccine is safe in pregnancy.[b]
- Mumps, measles, rubella. For adults born after 1956. Additional criteria: women of childbearing age lacking evidence of immunity should receive a rubella vaccine. If possible, this vaccine should be given before pregnancy in nonimmune women. A second measles immunization, preferably as MMR (measles, mumps, and rubella vaccine), should be given to all women unable to show proof of immunity. Mumps vaccine should not be given during pregnancy.
- Hepatitis B. Sexually active young adults and high-risk individuals include health care workers, intravenous drug users, current recipients of blood products, persons in health-related jobs with exposure to blood or blood products, household and sexual contacts with HBV carriers, and individuals with recently acquired sexually transmitted diseases.

Recent vaccines (1995)

- Hepatitis A. For high-risk groups such as health care, sanitation workers, and international travelers (military) in areas with poor sanitation.
- Varicella. Individuals at high risk such as health care workers without evidence of immunologic conversion are candidates.

[a]Modified from The American College of Physicians. *Guide for adult immunization.* Philadelphia: American College of Physicians, 1994:2.

[b]Centers for Disease Control and Prevention. Recommendation of the Immunization Practices Advisory Committee (ACP): Pneumococcal vaccine. *MMWR* 1989; 64–68, 73–76.

nutritional concern, though many are well informed on the nutritional aspects of their lifestyle. In contrast, food faddism and certain more extreme groups (vegans) may require close assessment and occasional monitoring (i.e., total protein and albumin levels). Certain ethnic groups (such as Mexican-American and African-American women) are at higher risk for malnutrition. Depending on the population served, questions concerning sufficient money to buy food and ability to refrigerate and prepare food should be asked.

Diet has assumed greater importance in the past decade as information has emerged regarding the relationship between various foods and cardiovascular disease, diabetes, and osteoporosis. In the past, most medical aspects of nutritional assessment focused on avoiding chronic deficiencies and disease states. Vitamin deficiencies are rarely encountered today. However, because many food preparations are supplemented, there is a current fascination with vitamin supplements, but physicians should recognize that the American diet remains higher in fats and lower in fiber than optimal recommendations. Also, relative protein deficiencies may present as iron deficiency anemia, and an expanded workup (primarily for gastrointestinal cancers) may be warranted. Nutritional assessment in the outpatient environment should consist of screening, counseling, diagnosis, and management. Any program implemented must be sensitive to local and ethnic cultures. If a family cannot afford or is unwilling to eat certain foods, no aspect of counseling will help. Recommended daily allowances (RDAs) change periodically and are currently being adjusted for age and gender. Nutritional counseling should reinforce appropriate eating practices, identifying and changing inappropriate practices, correct misinformation, and identifying disease or deficiency states. Risk factors for poor nutrition include adolescence and old age, low income, cigarette or substance abuse, pica, frequent dieting, skipping of meals, and vegan diets. Medical and psychiatric conditions that contribute to poor nutrition include mental illness (psychosis or major depression), muscle weakness involving the muscles of mastication, and certain medications.

A practical approach to assessing nutritional intake is the 24-hour diet recall history or a diary. Information provided by the patient should include type and quantity of food intake, meals eaten, and meals skipped. Recent weight changes should be documented, and consumption of alcohol, candy, soft drinks, and vitamin and mineral supplements obtained. A simple questionnaire may be obtained from a registered dietitian or hospital nutritionist and filled in by the patient in advance.

Counseling

Counseling in the office environment is an art form and requires sensitivity, empathy, and insight on the part of the examining physician. One role that all physicians should be comfortable with is counseling patients on effects of tobacco abuse (Table 2).

TABLE 2. *Principles of counseling to prevent tobacco abuse[a]*

- Direct face-to-face advice and suggestions. A brief, direct, unambiguous, and informative statement should be used. Content should include short- and long-term benefits of cessations including health, economic, and social aspects.
- Reinforcement. Support visits or telephone calls in the first 2 weeks when relapse is the highest.
- Office reminders. Label the chart to remind the patient on each visit to give an antitobacco message.
- Self-help materials. May be obtained from volunter organizations.
- Community programs should be utilized if available.
- Drug therapy. Various techniques and patches are available and should be used on weaning individuals away from nicotine. Remember to reinforce that they should be used solely instead of and not with tobacco products.

[a]U.S. Preventative Services Task Force. *Guide to Clinical Preventive Services, 2nd ed.* Alexandria. VA: International Medical Publishing, 1996: 597–609.

Ideally, counseling should result in a therapeutic response. Ten steps recommended for effective counseling by the United States Preventive Task Forces are[5]:

1. Develop a therapeutic alliance.
2. Counsel all patients.
3. Ensure that patients understand the relationship between behavior and health.
4. Work with patients to assess barriers to behavior change.
5. Gain commitment from patients to change.
6. Involve patients in identifying risk factors.
7. Use a combination of strategies.
8. Design a behavior modification protocol.
9. Monitor progress through follow-up contract.
10. Involve office staff.

Sufficient time for free discussion is a necessity. If time is limited, ask the patient to return when more time is available. Often the individual has made some attempt at correcting her problem. Depending on the circumstances, the initial assessment should include:

◊ Evaluating suicide risk, including any previous attempts,
◊ Learning about prior counseling, diagnosis, and medication use,
◊ Documenting steps the patient has taken in resolving the problem,
◊ Determining what efforts have helped or hindered in the process (many self-described "solutions" become part of the problem),
◊ Enhancing communication, particularly important in sexual and family dysfunction,
◊ Discussing behavioral modification or the use of certain medications such as the serotonin-selective reuptake inhibitors (SSRI),

◊ Considering referral, depending on physician comfort level, of patients likely to represent a high suicide risk or psychosis.

Principles of Screening

Screening is the assessment of the risk of a disorder occurring in individuals or a population with no evidence of disease.

Screening begins not with a laboratory test but with a reliable history and physical examination performed during the initial visit. In performing the history and physical examination, the practitioner should selectively utilize available resources and testing for the individual rather than the "all or nothing" approach. Screening also can be used to stratify the risk of a disease in patients. Testing should be focused on risk factors or risk assessment. For instance, cholesterol therapy now weights various risk factors and the serum cholesterol levels before initiating therapeutic interventions. As a consequence:

◊ Screening may identify individuals who are free of disease or at low risk for the development of a disease. An obvious example is the use of screening mammography.
◊ Screening may identify individuals who are susceptible to the development of a disease. Cervical cancer is more common in individuals with AIDS. Therefore, screening of AIDS patients with Pap smears every 6 months may identify precursors of cervical cancer such as cervical intraepithelial neoplasia.
◊ Screening may identify a patient with a precursor of a disease. Individuals treated with radiation or chemotherapy are at higher risk of associated carcinomas, such as thyroid cancer following neck irradiation for Hodgkin's disease or certain leukemias following chemotherapy.
◊ Screening may identify individuals with a disease or condition before it becomes clinically manifest. Screening mammography before detection of a palpable breast cancer or development of lymph node metastasis is an example.
◊ Screening may identify individuals who have a disease or condition that poses a risk to others. Tuberculosis and syphilis testing in individuals with HIV/AIDS is an example.

The benefit of screening is based on the *prevalence* of the disorder (i.e., the proportion of individuals with the disease) and the *sensitivity* and *specificity* of a test (i.e., how good is the test at identifying or excluding disease).

Screening tests should also be evaluated for their clinical usefulness and limitations in terms of accuracy and reproducibility, risks, and cost. The physician should use such information in order to assess what can be expected from the test. A mathematical determination can be used to define these issues in the following terms:

Sensitivity. The ability of a test or procedure to identify individuals with the disease.

Specificity. The ability of a test or procedure to identify persons without the disease.

Positive predictive value. The likelihood that a positive test result will identify persons with the disease.

Negative predictive value. The likelihood that a negative test result will identify persons without the disease.

◊ CARDIOVASCULAR DISEASE

Cardiovascular disease kills more women than all female cancers combined. Most cardiovascular disease has four major components: family history, hypertension, tobacco abuse, and hyperlipidemias. Diabetes may be a contributing factor in some cases.

Hypertension

Hypertension is the most prevalent factor in cardiovascular disease and usually coexists with obesity and hyperlipidemias. The overall average blood pressure in United States populations has declined in the past several decades.[6] Body weight and fat distribution are important factors in risk stratification.[7] Hypertension contributes significantly to other causes of disease in women, primarily cerebrovascular and renal disease. Many factors in the etiology of hypertension are multifactoral with no clear genetic predisposition. Ethnic background also has an influence. African-Americans are considered a high-risk group, whereas native Africans are a low-risk group. Physical labor or exercise often is involved in the daily life of the native African, and the diet is high in complex carbohydrates, vegetable protein, and potassium.[8] In turn, these environmental influences are directly related to obesity, the most important predictor of hypertension.[9]

A classification of hypertension is found in Table 3. Men and women whose blood pressure is controlled below 140/90 experience normal survival over a 10- to 20-year follow-up. Hypertension is defined in most studies as a blood pressure greater than 140/90 taken on two separate occasions ("sustained") using Korotkoff V (disappearance, not muffled) sounds. Measurement of blood pressure should be standardized and performed properly.

The patient should be allowed to rest for 5 minutes in a seated position, and the right arm is used for all measurements unless there is a medical contraindication such as a vascular access shunt. Cuff placement on the arm and the cuff size are important variables. Attention to detail eliminates high and low readings. A common problem is to place too small a cuff on an obese patient, resulting in so-called "cuff hypertension." The cuff should be applied 20 mm above the bend of the elbow with the arm parallel to the floor. Once the cuff is applied, it should be inflated to 30 torr above the disappearance of the brachial pulse or to 220 mm Hg. The cuff should be deflated slowly at a rate no more than 2 mm Hg/sec. Failure to follow these guidelines may result in falsely high or low readings of the systolic and diastolic blood pressure.

TABLE 3. *Classification of blood pressure for adults aged 18 years and older* [a,b]

Category	Systolic (mm Hg)	Diastolic (mm Hg)
Normal	<130	<85
High normal	130–139	85–89
Hypertension[c]		
Stage 1 (mild)	140–159	90–99
Stage 2 (moderate)	160–179	100–109
Stage 3 (severe)	180–209	110–119
Stage 4 (very severe)	≥210	≥120

[a]All measurements are in patients who are healthy and on no medications. If measurements fall into two different categories, then the higher category should be used for classification purposes. Additionally, if other diseases are present, such as diabetes, then it should be noted in parathesis.

[b]Modified from: The fifth report of the Joint National Committee on the Detection, Evaluation, and Treatment of High Blood Pressure. *Arch Intern Med* 1993; 153:154–183.

[c]Requires the performance of two additional measures after initial reading.

In 20% to 30% of women with initially elevated blood pressure in the office, the blood pressure will decrease into the normal range after a period of rest. The elevation induced by the stress of seeing a physician is labeled "white coat" hypertension, a well-known clinical syndrome. Some studies suggest that this phenomenon is more prevalent in women.[10]

Baseline laboratory evaluations are recommended in the initial evaluation to rule out secondary or reversible causes of hypertension. Young patients with severe and very severe levels of hypertension should be considered for referral to rule out secondary causes of hypertension. The initial battery of tests consist of:

◊ Dipstick urinalysis for protein and glucose (microscopic is indicated if any abnormalities appear);

◊ Hemoglobin or hematocrit;

◊ Creatinine or blood urea nitrogen (BUN), potassium, fasting glucose level;

◊ Total cholesterol, HDL-cholesterol, and fasting triglycerides;

◊ Electrocardiogram (to evaluate for hypertensive changes such as left ventricular hypertrophy or previous evidence of myocardial infarction);

◊ Optional: Chest radiographs (hypertensive cardiomyopathy, coarctation of the aorta).

Management

Once the diagnosis of hypertension is made, various therapeutic interventions should be considered (Fig. 1). For most patients, the physician should assess overall risk and then attempt to modify the lifestyle. Nonpharmacologic interventions should be used only for initial therapy when the diastolic blood pressure is persistently >110 mm Hg. If the blood pressure

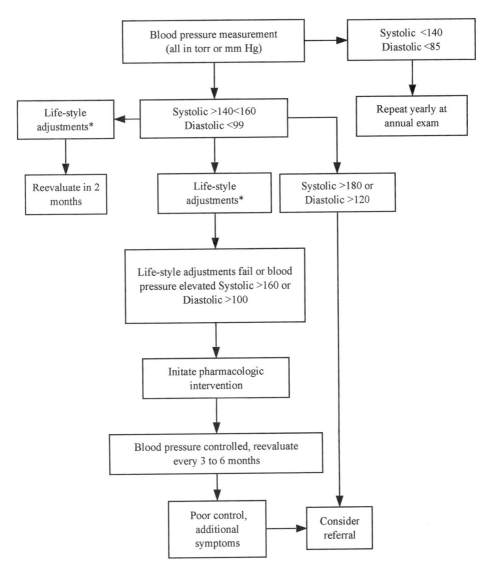

*Excercise, dietary changes, weight and alcohol reduction.

FIG. 1. Algorithm for the management of essential hypertension. (From Nolan TE. *Primary care for the obstetrician and gynecologist.* New York: Wiley-Liss, 1995,82; with permission.)

does not respond after 3 to 6 months of nonpharmacologic intervention, medical therapy should be initiated. With persistent blood pressures above 180 systolic and 110 diastolic, medical interventions should be initiated earlier. Therapeutic schemes have changed over the past 15 years because of the multitude of excellent medications currently available. The goal of therapy is to lower blood pressure into the "normal range" or achieve a systolic <140 mm Hg and a diastolic of <85 mm Hg.

Although medical therapies for hypertension are outside the scope of this chapter, the following brief guidelines should be considered:

◊ Diuretics are inexpensive and most effective in African-Americans. Current dosages have lessened concerns over potassium depletion. Side effects of glucose intolerance and an increase in total cholesterol and LDL-cholesterol raise theoretical concerns on the impact on atherosclerosis.

◊ β-Blockers are also inexpensive but have side effects that may impact on overall cardiovascular disease such as raising total cholesterol and LDL-cholesterol while decreasing HDL-cholesterol. Other side effects are desirable, specifically the ability to calm certain patients and decrease the frequency of migraine headaches. β-Blockers are poorly tolerated in individuals with asthma, chronic obstructive pulmonary disease, and diabetes.

◊ Calcium channel blockers work well for moderate to severe hypertension and are especially effective in the elderly and in African-Americans. Concern about an increased rate of myocardial infarctions relates to the use of the short-acting formulations and primarily in individuals with compromised left ventricular function. Since these medications have become generic, the long-acting forms are more affordable for a larger group of patients.

◊ Angiotensin-converting enzyme inhibitors (ACE inhibitors) have become widely used as a first-level therapy because of less-frequent dosing and relatively safe use with other medications and medical conditions. The second-generation formulations have fewer side effects. As a group, they are less effective in African-Americans unless used in combination with a diuretic agent.

◊ α_1-Adrenergic drugs are popular because of potency issues in men and an increase in HDL-cholesterol. Unfortunately, in women, they may cause stress urinary incontinence.

◊ Central blockers (methyldopa and clonidine) have become less popular because of anticholinergic side effects. Clonidine, however, is a potent antihypertensive and is relatively inexpensive.

◊ Smooth muscle relaxants such as minoxidil and hydralazine have side effects that limit their usefulness. In extreme cases, clinicians may use minoxidil because of potency, but excessive hair growth is a problem in women.

Blood pressure monitoring is initiated once therapy is started. Individuals with nonpharmacologically controlled hypertension or mild hypertension should have their blood pressure measured monthly. Those who use home devices should perform their measurements at least twice a week and at the same time of day. The interval of reassessment varies with the compliance of the individual and blood pressure control. In stable patients, once every 3 to 6 months is adequate.

If pharmacologic therapy is necessary, a return appointment should be scheduled in 2 to 4 weeks to assess effectiveness of the medication and to review side effects. Once the blood pressure is stable, then office visits for review of blood pressures every three months are appropriate. If side effects are intolerable, then a different class of medication should be initiated, or a second medication added after lowering the dose of the primary medication. Patients with multiple medical problems or who fail to respond with two agents should be referred.

Cholesterol

Hypercholesterolemia is a risk factor for atherosclerosis and cardiovascular events (myocardial infarction and stroke). Cholesterol-testing guidelines vary by organization.[11,12] The testing of women without risk factors such as tobacco abuse, diabetes mellitus, hypertension, or a family history of cardiovascular disease is of unproven efficacy. The second United States Preventative Services Task Force (1996) recommended testing every 5 years between the ages of 45 and 65,[10]

whereas the American College of Physicians recommended testing once between ages 45 and 55.[11] The American College of Obstetricians and Gynecologists uses the first United States Preventative Services Task Force (USPSTF) guidelines published in 1988, which state that total cholesterol testing should be initiated at age 20 and performed every 5 years. Patients with a family history of cardiovascular disease (history of premature coronary artery problems and strokes before age 55) should be considered for lipid testing in their 20s.

Metabolism

Cholesterol metabolism is divided into two pathways: the *exogenous* pathway, derived from dietary sources, and the *endogenous* pathway, which is the posthepatic or the lipid transport pathway. Individual variations in the ability to metabolize cholesterol exist, which may explain why dietary interventions in some individuals have minimal impact. Individuals are classified as normals, hyporesponders (diet has little impact), and hyperresponders (exaggerated response to diet).[13] Hyporesponders, despite cholesterol-laden diets, show no effect on serum cholesterol measurements. Normal individuals will have fluctuation reflecting dietary intake, whereas hyperresponders have a high serum cholesterol regardless of dietary intake.

Multiple variables may influence lipid levels, including exercise before testing, laboratory standards, recent diet intake, tobacco use, and intake of exogenous hormones. Many management and risk stratifications require knowledge of levels of LDL-cholesterol and HDL-cholesterol, and standard collection techniques are necessary. The following are recommended: (1) sit quietly for 15 minutes before sampling; (2) maintain normal diet for several days before sampling with a 12-hour fast; (3) avoid exercise during the fasting period; (4) continue alcohol, tobacco, and caffeine intake at current levels; (5) keep tourniquet time less than 2 minutes and preserve samples in EDTA tubes.

Management

Current recommendations for the treatment of hypercholesterolemia by the National Cholesterol Education Program are diet, weight loss for the obese, and medications if the individual is unresponsive to diet.[14] Risk factors for cardiovascular disease should be assessed and modified if possible. Two diets are recommended. The step I diet limits dietary fats to 30% of daily intake with less than 10% consisting of saturated fats and less than 300 mg of cholesterol. If, after 3 months, lipids levels are still elevated above recommended levels, then the step II diet should be initiated (saturated fats are reduced to less than 7%, and dietary cholesterol to less than 200 mg). A management algorithm is shown in Fig. 2.

Currently, there are three lines of medical therapy: bile acid-binding resins, nicotinic acid, and the "statin" drugs (lovastatin, simvastatin, and pravastatin). The use of bile acid

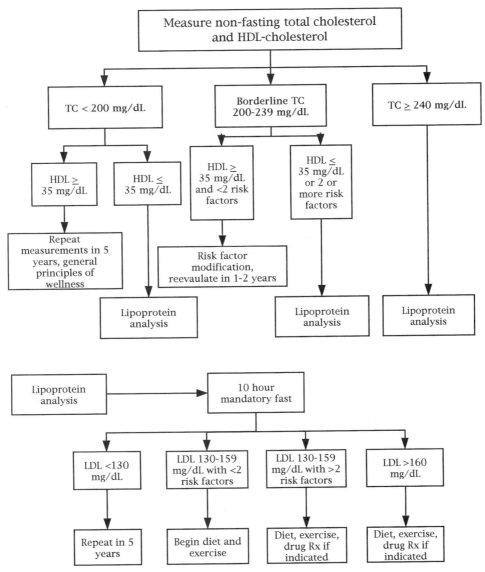

FIG. 2. Management scheme for measurement and therapy of increased levels of cholesterol. TC, total cholesterol; LDL, LDL-cholesterol. (Adapted from ref. 14.)

resins is limited by side effects such as abdominal bloating and gas.[15] Nicotinic acid use is associated with facial flushing; however, longer-acting preparations have decreased this problem. Aspirin, 325 mg given before dosing may help control flushing and may have additional therapeutic benefit by decreasing platelet aggregation. The "statin" drugs have had a major impact on therapy because of their profound ability to decrease total cholesterol and LDL-cholesterol. Side effects are uncommon but significant (elevated liver function tests, myonecrosis in combination with other medications).

◊ DIABETES MELLITUS

Diabetes mellitus (DM) is a chronic metabolic disorder characterized not only by altered glucose and insulin metabolism but also by abnormalities in carbohydrate, protein, and fat metabolism. The linkage between hyperglycemia and macrovascular disease such as coronary artery disease is becoming better defined. Recently the American Diabetes Association redefined standards from the original 1979 criteria and changed the definitions and diagnostic criteria for the classification of diabetes.[16] The terms insulin-dependent diabetes mellitus (IDDM) and non-insulin-dependent diabetes (NIDDM) are no longer used. The terms type 1 and type 2 are now the accepted standard and represent the continuum of hyperglycemic states.

Type 1 diabetes is characterized by beta cell destruction leading to absolute insulin deficiency. Two forms are now recognized: immune-mediated diabetes mellitus (more common) and idiopathic diabetes mellitus. Immune-mediated diabetes mellitus is the result of widespread autoimmune destruction of pancreatic beta cells and hence a total lack of insulin, which results in ketoacidosis. Idiopathic type 1 refers to other forms of the disease without a known etiology.

Type 2 diabetes occurs in individuals with insulin resistance and relative insulin deficiency. Over many years, these individuals may have progressive loss of beta cells and become insulin-requiring. Type 2 diabetics may range from predominantly insulin resistant with relative insulin deficiency to absolute deficiency in insulin secretion with insulin resistance. Associated risk factors include obesity, hypertension, and a sedentary lifestyle.

In the new classification, individuals with a fasting glucose of ≥110 mg/dl but <126 mg/dl are defined as having "impaired fasting glucose" (IFG). The classification "impaired glucose tolerance" (IGT) is defined as an oral glucose tolerance test value of ≥140 mg/dl but <200 mg/dl at 2 hours (Table 4). Both of these stages of glucose intolerance are intermediate metabolic stages between normal glucose homeostasis and diabetes. These are not clinical entities in the own right but are recognized as risk factors for cardiovascular disease and future diabetes. Evidence suggests that retinopathy may occur at mean glucose levels of 126 mg/dl and progressively worsen with increasing levels. Additionally, there are data to suggest that microvascular disease begins many years before the clinical diagnosis of diabetes, and by lowering the threshold for diagnosis, therapy may be started sooner and complications lessened.

Gestational diabetes mellitus is retained in the new classification system, but universal screening is not recommended. Criteria for screening include age >25 years, obesity, a family member with a history of diabetes, and a high-risk ethnic background (Hispanic, African-American, Native American, or Asian). Criteria for the diagnosis remain the same with a 1-hour glucose threshold of 140 mg/dl after a 50-g glucose load. The criteria for a 3-hour oral glucose tolerance test remain unchanged. Figures 3 and 4 show algorithms for the diagnosis of diabetes.

Only 50% of the estimated 14 million Americans with diabetes are aware they have the disease. Micro- and macrovascular changes are late manifestations, and the course of vascular disease may be modified by early diagnosis and glucose control. To be effective in disease modification, screening programs must be implemented, but it is unknown if these programs are cost effective. Suggested criteria for testing asymptomatic patients are found in Table 5.

Proper metabolic control ("tight glucose control") is widely recognized to minimize though not eliminate complications of type 1 diabetes. An important aspect of disease management is the recognition that diabetic ketoacidosis usually results from infections of the genitourinary tract, including pelvic inflammatory disease. Chronic monilial infections may be an early diagnostic clue for diabetes. Treatment of these infections is made difficult by poor glucose control. Because patients with type 1 disease are followed primarily by internists, the remaining text is limited to type 2 diabetes.

Type 2 diabetes is a heterogeneous form of diabetes that commonly occurs in age groups 55 years of age or older. In many cases, there is a first-degree family member with the disease. Of interest, concordance in identical twins for type 2 diabetes is 90% to 95% versus 25% to 50% in type 1 diabetes. The metabolic defect in type 2 diabetes is reduced insulin secretion and/or relative insulin resistance. In most cases, these individuals will survive long periods without insulin, in comparison to the type 1 diabetics. Obesity alone may cause some degree of insulin resistance, even if increased fat distribution is limited to the abdomen. Impaired glucose uptake in target tissues may result in a compensatory (but inadequate) increase in insulin secretion. Therefore, in early stages of the disease, there are higher than normal circulating levels of insulin. Other associated conditions common to the type 2 diabetic are hypertension and hyperlipidemia. Obesity is found in 85% of affected patients. Patients with the familiar triad of obesity, hypertension, and diabetes should have aggressive control of each disease entity. Additionally, lipid screening should be performed more frequently, and abnormalities treated. In the early stages of therapy, diet, weight control, and oral preparations are useful for glucose control.

The later stages of type 2 diabetes mellitus differ from the early stages because of exhausted insulin stores in the pancreas. When this stage is reached, insulin injections are

TABLE 4. *Metabolites and apoproteins in cholesterol metabolism*

- Lipoprotein particle. Made from three major components: central core of nonpolar lipids (triglycerides and cholesterol esters), a surface coat of phospholipids consisting of apoproteins, and structural proteins. As lipoprotein particles are metabolized, lipids are removed for energy production and become more dense. Apoproteins are modified as cholesterol moves from the so-called "exogenous pathway" (dietary) to the "endogenous pathway" (postabsorption and metabolized by the liver).
- Apoprotein. A specific recognition protein exposed at the surface of a lipoprotein particle. Apoproteins are associated with specific types of cholesterol. Abnormalities in apoprotein structure have been associated with premature cardiovascular disease.

Prehepatic metabolites
- Chylomicrons and remnants. Large particles consisting of dietary cholesterol and triglycerides.

Posthepatic metabolites
- VLDL (very low-density lipoprotein). Transient remnants found after initial liver metabolism. They represent only 10% to 15% of cholesterol particles.
- IDL (intermediate-density lipoprotein). Posthepatic remnants derived from dietary sources.
- LDL-Cholesterol. Approximately 60% to 70% of total measured cholesterol. Structurally abnormal B-100 apoproteins (part of the whole lipoprotein) have been associated with premature atherosclerosis and heart disease in some families.
- HDL-Cholesterol. About 20% to 30% of total cholesterol. High levels of HDL-cholesterol are associated with longevity. The ability of estrogen to raise HDL-cholesterol is considered a primary influence in lowering coronary artery disease in women.

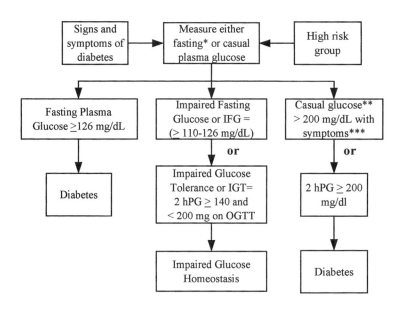

*Fasting glucose defined as no caloric intake for at least 8 hours
** Casual glucose defined as glucose drawn at anytime regardless of last meal.
***Symptoms are polyuria, polydipsia, unexplained weight loss.

FIG. 3. Diagnostic criteria for diabetes mellitus.

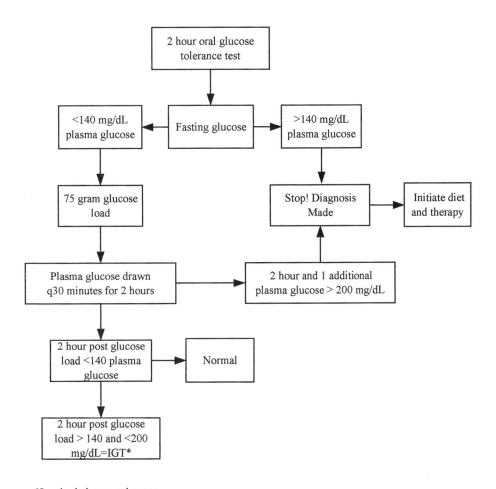

*Inpaired glucose tolerance

FIG. 4. Oral glucose tolerance test.

TABLE 5. *Screening criteria for diabetes in asymptomatic, undiagnosed individuals*

1. Consideration should be given to all individuals 45 years or older, and if normal repeated every 3 years.
2. Testing should be considered earlier if the following clinical conditions obtain:
   - Obesity (≥120% desirable body weight or a BMI ≥27 kg/m²)
   - High-risk ethnic group
   - First-degree relative with diabetes
   - Diagnosis of gestational diabetes in pregnancy or delivered an infant >9 lb
   - Hypertensive
   - On lipid profile have a triglyceride level of ≥250 mg/dl or HDL-cholesterol ≤35 mg/dl
   - Previous diagnosis of impaired glucose tolerance or elevated fasting glucose

necessary for glycemic control. These diabetics are insulin-requiring type 2 diabetics as opposed to insulin-dependent diabetics, type 1. Insulin is necessary to move glucose across cell membranes and allow it to enter various metabolic pathways. In complete absence of insulin, ketoacidosis (DKA) will result. Type 2 diabetics, primarily with infections or severe stresses such as surgery, may develop DKA. After the infection and stress have resolved, they no longer require insulin and can return to diet or oral medications. The more common metabolic decompensation for type 2 diabetes is a *hyperglycemic hyperosmolar nonketotic state* (HHNS) more commonly seen in the elderly. These patients usually present with altered mental states and plasma glucose levels as high as 800 mg/dl or greater. Once the blood sugar is lowered, the individual usually becomes responsive.

The current screening criteria in Table 5 are from a specialty group and are not outcome generated. The number of patients affected with diabetes is estimated as 16 million in the united States, with up to 50% undiagnosed.[16] Despite the availability of laboratory testing for common autoantibodies resulting in type 1 diabetes, accurate cutoff values and costs limit the usefulness of these tests. The benefit of widespread testing is probably minimal because the incidence of type 1 diabetes is less than 0.5%. If an autoantibody is found, there is currently no effective therapy to prevent beta cell destruction.

The effect of lowering plasma glucose to prevent complications of diabetes has been proven in type 1 diabetes. Data to support this concept in type 2 have not been collected, but most experts agree that the same problems exist regardless of disease type. Screening for type 2 diabetes may be effective in reducing cardiovascular disease, including stroke, coronary artery disease, and peripheral vascular disease.

Because of individual variation in response to glucose loading, most experts suggest that the fasting plasma determination is superior to glucose challenge testing. Because the fasting state represents a known physiological state, whereas glucose loading is artificial, the results are thought to better represent the individual's normal glucose state. Cost considerations associated with stress testing, including time spent by the patient in testing, are also important. For these reasons,

the most effective screening paradigm is to rely on fasting tests. The role of the oral glucose tolerance test is to assist in borderline cases. However, there can be as many as 10% false positives (guidelines of glucose levels are met, but the disease is not clinically evident). The patient with borderline values should be started on lifestyle adjustments rather than medications. Individuals with IGT or IFT should be considered for annual testing.

Treatment

The following are guidelines for general care of diabetes regardless of type to decrease long-term complications:

◊ Establish the diagnosis of diabetes mellitus (DM) and classify it. It is important that the diagnosis is well documented because of life and medical insurance issues.
◊ Initiate diabetes education classes and enlist the patient as a coparticipant. The signs and symptoms of hypo- and hyperglycemia should be stressed. Discuss complications, specifically infections (urinary tract are very common), blood glucose monitoring, medications, complications, and how to contact the physician.
◊ Place the patient on an ADA diet with appropriate caloric intake, sodium, and lipid restrictions.
◊ Establish cardiac risk factors and aggressively treat hypertension and lipidemias. Tobacco use in DM forms a lethal combination.
◊ Establish the baseline kidney function with a serum creatinine and 24-hour urine collection for albumin. Evaluate initially and annually for presence of nephropathy (e.g., 1+ albumin on dip stick, presence of difficult-to-control hypertension, serum creatinine >1.5 mg/dl). If there is evidence of renal disease, consultation or transfer of care to nephrologist should be considered.
◊ Establish the extent of any funduscopic lesion and refer to an ophthalmologist for baseline evaluation.
◊ Stress foot care and inspect feet and toenails at each visit.
◊ Use the fingerstick blood glucose for diabetic monitoring. Urine should be checked for ketones when establishing a medication regimen to avoid ketosis (but do not use the first morning void!).
◊ Follow chronic glycemic control by HgbA$_{1c}$ every 2 to 3 months (every 6 months in the elderly) in the office. Remember that HgbA$_{1c}$ is not a diagnostic test and reflects the status of glucose control in the bone marrow when red cells are made, 90 days before.

A general health evaluation should be performed at least annually. The following laboratory tests should be used in the initial evaluation: CBC with differential, chemistry profile, lipid profile, urinalysis, thyroid function tests, and baseline ECG. Annual assessment of renal function and lipid status is indicated.

Diet is the most important component of management in type 2 diabetes and unfortunately is the hardest to achieve. The approach to overweight diabetics consists of three major strategies: weight loss, a low-fat diet (≤30% kcal from fat), and exercise. Obese patients should be advised to reduce to their ideal body weight if possible, but any weight loss will improve glucose control. Other advantages of weight reduction and exercise are lower triglycerides, total cholesterol, and LDL-cholesterol with increased HDL-cholesterol and improved glucose control. Exercise improves weight loss and insulin sensitivity as well as the lipid profile, especially for those at high risk for cardiovascular and microvascular diseases. General guidelines in management are:

◊ Place the patient on the ADA-prescribed reducing diet (50% CHO, 30% fat, 20% protein, high fiber) with three meals a day to achieve and maintain ideal body weight or to reduce weight by 5% to 15% in 3 months (if >130% above ideal body weight).
◊ Encourage risk factor modification (tobacco cessation, exercise, reduce fat intake, etc.).
◊ After dieting for 2 to 3 weeks, check the fasting blood glucose (FBG) daily for 2 months. If the FBG declines during this period, no other therapy is necessary. If FBG does not decline or increases, consider use of oral hypoglycemic agents (OHA). Criteria for oral medications include (1) diabetic less than 10 years, (2) fasting blood sugar <250 mg/dl, (3) no severe hepatic or renal disease, and (4) no allergy to sulfonylurea.
◊ After starting OHAs, check FBS and the 2-hour postprandial glucose every 2 months (in conjunction with daily home glucose monitoring [HGM]). If the postprandial glucose is <200 mg/dl, diet alone is sufficient. If FBG is consistently >200 mg/dl, insulin therapy should be initiated.
◊ If insulin is necessary, a dosage of 0.5 to 1 unit/kg of actual body weight should be used.
◊ If the total daily insulin requirement is less than 30 U/day, the entire dose may be given as NPH or lente before a major meal. Goals for glucose control are FBS <140 mg/dl and the 2-hour postprandial glucose <200, with no blood sugar <60 mg/dl.
◊ If a single insulin injection does not achieve control, a mixture of regular and NPH (50:50) in split doses 30 minutes before breakfast and dinner may be given.
◊ Very obese type 2 diabetics may require more insulin per kilogram body weight, with more regular insulin than long-acting agents.
◊ In well-motivated patients, consider a regimen of regular insulin injections before each meal with a bedtime injection of NPH or lente insulin.

Oral Hypoglycemic Agents

Blood sugar may be lowered pharmacologically at different physiological steps of glucose metabolism. Oral hypoglycemic agents (OHA) are recommended for many type 2 patients but should never be used in type 1 patients. Currently, there are four classes of agents (sulfonylureas, biguanides, thiazolidinediones, and α-glucosidase inhibitors) available for glucose control, but only two are approved by the FDA. Most patients successfully controlled on oral agents have mild to moderate increases in plasma glucose. Higher levels of glucose (>250 mg/dl) are less successfully treated without the addition of insulin.

Sulfonylureas' mode of action is by two different mechanisms. They primarily enhance insulin secretion from the beta cells of the pancreas and also increase the number of receptors in target tissues to enhance insulin binding. Second-generation agents, glipizide and glyburide, have fewer hepatic side effects but differ little in effectiveness. The lowest possible dose should be initiated and increased after 2 to 4 weeks if necessary. Side effects of these agents include hypoglycemia (less frequent than with insulin but more severe) and weight gain.

Dimethylbiguanide (metformin) has recently been approved for use in the United States. The mechanism of action is to increase insulin sensitivity in the liver (reduce hepatic glucose production) and increase glucose intake in skeletal muscles. Because there are fewer effects on pancreatic secretion, hypoglycemia is rare. Because weight gain is less often a side effect, it may be a better choice in obese patients. These drugs may be added to the sulfonylureas because of the different mode of action. A beneficial effect is noted on serum lipid profiles, with mild decreases in triglycerides and LDL-cholesterol and mild increases in HDL-cholesterol. Gastrointestinal upset has been noted in some patients and may be lessened by taking medication with meals.

α-Glucosidase inhibitors are useful in postprandial hyperglycemia and may be used with sulfonylureas. The mode of action is to slow the digestion of sucrose, maltose, and complex carbohydrates. The limiting factors in these drugs are gastrointestinal side effects (pain, flatulence, and diarrhea).

The OHAs have no effect in the absence of endogenous insulin. If a question arises about the adequacy of beta cell actions, measure the insulin C-peptide. Annually, 3% to 5% of patients need to be switched to insulin because of pancreas failure. Patients who refuse home glucose monitoring should have blood glucose measured every 2 months to avoid loss of sugar control.

Insulin Therapy in Type 2 Diabetes

In some patients, a combination of NPH or combined NPH–regular at supper or bedtime, followed by a morning dose of OHA, is effective in the control of hyperglycemia. This method is controversial and probably outside the usual scope of a primary care physician. The newly available fixed combinations of NPH and regular insulin (70/30; 50/50) may be an alternative in patients with fasting hyperglycemia or poor control on oral agents.

Assessment of Glucose Control

The only acceptable method for assessment of glucose control is by blood glucose determination. The cost of glucose meters has dropped substantially in the past decade, and the role of test strips is probably of historical interest. Remember that the results are whole-blood determinations, not serum. The only role for urine testing is to determine whether caloric intake is adequate by testing for ketones. Urine determinations for ketones should be done if blood sugars are elevated. When blood sugars are >300 mg/dl, then medical advice should be sought by the patient. Infection remains the most common cause of loss of glycemic control in the compliant patient.

Glycohemoglobin

Unreliable patients are difficult to manage in any clinical situation, and diabetics can be the most vexing. Some diabetics are notorious for not reporting accurate glucose values. In some situations, chronic glycemic assessments are necessary. Glycohemoglobin is a product of a ketoamine reaction between glucose in the blood and N-terminal amino acids of the beta chains of hemoglobin. Hemoglobin A has three subtypes: A_{1a}, A_{1b}, and A_{1c}. The glycohemoglobin level reflects the glycemic state over the previous 12 weeks (the approximate half-life of a red cell). The normal level of $HgbA_{1c}$ is between 4% and 6%, depending on the laboratory method used. Most diabetologists consider values below 7% as excellent control, and values over 10% are considered poor control.

Individual patients who do not respond to diet and OHAs are best referred because of the difficulty in managing these patients and the associated vascular complications. These patients are obese, hypertensive, and often have other diseases better managed by an internist. Patients with vascular disease, other medical disorders, or insulin resistance (defined as >200 U insulin/day) should be referred.

◊ THYROID DISEASE

The incidence of thyroid disorders in women is approximately 10 times greater than that in men.[17] A familial tendency has been noted, but the exact pattern of inheritance has not been determined. Thyroid dysfunction affects up to 1% of a young population and progressively increases with age to 2% to 3% of the elderly population. The diagnosis of thyroid disease may be elusive, especially in the early stage of presentation. The diagnosis may be difficult in reproductive-aged women. Pregnancy and exogenous hormones affect thyroid-binding globulins, which makes the interpretation of thyroid function difficult. Inexpensive and sensitive thyroid-stimulating hormone (TSH) assays have eliminated the need to consider the effect of hormonal alterations when screening. However, knowledge of the hormonal effects of thyroid physiology in women is vital for obstetricians and gynecologists (Table 6).

Thyroid hormones act in target tissues by binding to cellular nuclear receptors. Thyroxine (T_4) is the main hormone released by the thyroid gland and provides a stable reservoir for extrathyroidal conversion to the more active hormone, triiodothyronine (T_3). T_3 has a higher affinity for the nuclear

TABLE 6. *Common abbreviations in thyroid physiology*[a]

TRH Thyroid-releasing hormone. Hypothalamic regulatory hormone.

TSH Thyroid-stimulating hormone. Pituitary regulatory hormone, stimulated by TRH and with negative feedback by peripheral hormones

T_3 Triiodothyronine. Active thyroid hormone, primarily by peripheral conversion of thyroxine (T_4).

T_4 Thyroxine. Primary hormone released from thyroid gland, requires peripheral conversion to T_3 to become activated. Commonly given for replacement therapy.

TBG Thyroid-binding globulin. Synthesized in the liver, specific carrier protein for thyroxine. Affected by hormones such as estrogen and testosterone.

TSI Thyroid-stimulating immunoglobin. An IgG antibody that stimulates pituitary to produce inappropriate high levels of TSH. May pass placenta causing neonatal hyperthyroidism.

[a]From Nolan TE. *Primary care for the obstetrician and gynecologist.* New York: Wiley-Liss, 1995, with permission.

receptor and affects cellular function at that level. Thyrotropin-releasing hormone (TRH) is released from the hypothalamus and affects pituitary TSH by classic negative feedback mechanisms. Pituitary TSH regulates thyroid gland growth and hormone production. Thyroid-stimulating immunoglobulin (TSI), formerly referred to as long-acting thyroid stimulator (LATS), binds to the TSH receptor and is one cause of Graves' disease.

Approximately 99% of circulating T_4 and T_3 is bound by plasma proteins, primarily thyroxine-binding globulin (TBG). The levels of active or free thyroid hormone in circulating serum proteins remain constant despite physiological alterations such as changes in sex hormones or glucocorticoid levels. Changes in total serum protein levels have no effect on the patient's clinical status. Estrogenic compounds, regardless of source, increase TBG plasma concentration by decreasing hepatic clearance of TBG. Androgens, especially testosterone, and corticosteroids have the opposite effect: hepatic clearance of TBG increases, decreasing circulation levels. Therefore, elevated thyroid hormone levels may be the result of increased protein binding from altered albumin and estrogen states and/or decreased peripheral conversion of T_4 to T_3.

Thyroid function test results may also be misleading in individuals taking certain medications (e.g., propranolol and amiodarone) or who have systemic illnesses (e.g., malignancy, sepsis, multiple organ failure, and acute renal failure). Hyperemesis gravidarum may cause very low TSH and T_4 levels, which makes the diagnosis of thyroid disorders in this condition difficult. Life transitions from puberty through menopause may change TBG levels but do not alter free thyroid hormone concentrations.

Screening

The neck should be palpated during routine physical examinations. Approaching the patient from behind and asking her to swallow is the best method to palpate the gland. Patients exposed to even low doses of radiation are at increased risk of thyroid carcinoma and should be closely screened. Ultrasound is limited because of the high number of asymptomatic nodules detected—up to 30% in some series—and should not be used for routine screening.[18]

Only in neonates has laboratory testing been found to be cost effective.[19] Recent data suggest that screening every 5 years in women 35 or older is cost effective.[20] Early treatment of thyroid disease does modify the course of the disease but may impact on other medical problems such as coronary artery disease, congestive heart failure, and lipid disorders. Elderly patients frequently have thyroid dysfunction with minimal symptoms, which makes the diagnosis difficult. Elderly patients with new-onset psychiatric prob-

lems or exacerbation of medical disorders may also have thyroid disease.

Periodic screening is justified in first-degree relatives of patients with thyroid disease, but there are no set guidelines or recommendations for periodic screening.[21] Reasonable criteria include patients with familial tendencies for thyroid dysfunction, autoimmune diseases, and unfavorable lipid profiles. These individuals should probably be screened every 5 years from age 20 to 30 and then every 3 years after age 35. Women after 65 should be screened biannually, especially if psychiatric disease is present.[22]

The TSH assay is the primary test used in screening because of the lack of hormonal influence. An algorithm for interpretation and management of abnormal TSH levels and goiters is shown in Fig. 5.

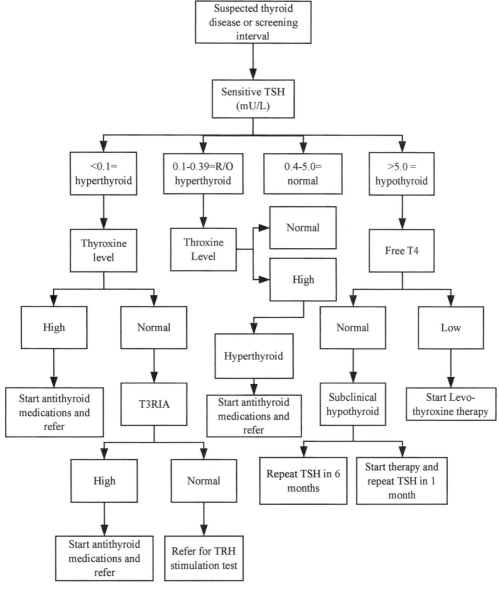

FIG. 5. Algorithm for the management of thyroid disorders. (From Nolan TE. *Primary care for the obstetrician and gynecologist.* New York: Wiley-Liss, 1995: 22; with permission.)

Diagnosis

The clinical diagnosis of hypothyroidism includes signs and symptoms of fatigue, lethargy, cold intolerance, nightmares, dry skin, hair loss, constipation, myalgias, carpal tunnel syndrome, and weight gain. Menstrual dysfunction is common but not always present. Menorrhagia is the most frequent complaint, but amenorrhea may also be the presenting symptom. Anovulatory women with normal thyroid function do not benefit from thyroid replacement therapy. Neuropsychiatric symptoms associated with thyroid dysfunction include depression, irritability, and impaired memory; dementia is the most common presentation in the elderly. Women with amenorrhea, galactorrhea, and hyperprolactinemia should undergo TSH testing to distinguish hypothalamic and pituitary hypothyroidism from prolactin-secreting pituitary adenomas.

Hyperthyroid patients present with signs of symptoms of fatigue, diarrhea, heat intolerance, palpitations, dyspnea, sleep disorders, nervousness, and weight loss. Paradoxically, young patients may gain weight as a result of increased appetite. Tachycardia, lid lag, tremor, proximal muscle weakness, and warm moist skin are the most common physical signs. Ophthalmologic changes include lid retraction, periorbital edema, and proptosis, but these changes are uncommon and occur in fewer than one-third of affected women. Elderly patients may present with unexplained weight loss, atrial fibrillation, or new-onset angina pectoris. Hyperthyroid women usually have regular menses but with lighter flow, and anovulation is common. Goiter is commonly noted in younger women, but it may be absent in the elderly. A toxic nodular goiter ("hot nodule") is associated with nonhomogeneous glandular enlargement, but subacute thyroiditis should be suspected if the thyroid gland is enlarged, hard, and very tender to palpation.

Treatment

The treatment of choice for hypothyroidism is thyroid replacement with L-thyroxine (T_4). The mode of action of exogenously absorbed T_4 is identical to that of endogenous thyroid production—conversion to T_3 in peripheral tissues. A parenteral formulation is available but rarely necessary because oral preparations have a half-life of 7 days. The average patient undergoing surgery or delivery can safely miss several days of medication. Aluminum hydroxide, cholestyramine, ferrous sulfate, or sucralfate may decrease absorption of oral preparations. The replacement dose of T_4 is related to patient weight (approximately 1.6 μg/kg) but is less in the elderly. Formulations are available to start at 0.025 mg and increase in increments of 0.025 to 0.050 mg. The normal daily dose in most healthy individuals is 0.1 to 0.15 mg, but the final dosage should be adjusted to maintain the serum TSH within the normal range. In pregnant women, the T_4 dose requirement may be increased by 25% to 100%, but the final dosage should be adjusted by monitoring serum TSH. Thyroid status should be assessed at 20 to 24 weeks of gestation and adjusted as necessary. If the replacement dose is modified in pregnancy, the prepregnancy dosage can be resumed immediately postpartum.

Thyroid testing after initiation of replacement therapy should be obtained 3 weeks later or after dosage changes because of the medication's long half-life. The goal of therapy is to keep TSH levels in the normal range. A mild increase of T_4 has been associated with cortical bone loss and osteoporosis. Individuals with coronary artery disease should be treated with low doses of L-thyroxine (0.025 mg) because a sudden increase in the basal metabolic rate could precipitate a myocardial infarct or worsen angina. Elderly patients (>65 years of age) should also be started on lower doses to prevent cardiac problems.

The hyperthyroid patient is usually best served by referral unless she is pregnant, but the gynecologist may initiate therapy. Initial therapy includes β-adrenergic blocking drugs to control sympathomimetic symptoms by blocking peripheral conversion of T_4 to T_3. The mainstay of therapy for hyperthyroidism is propylthiouracil (PTU), 50 to 300 mg every 6 to 8 hours, or methimazole (Tapazole), 10 to 30 mg per day. Both antithyroid drugs block thyroid hormone biosynthesis, but there are major differences: PTU partially inhibits extrathyroidal T_4-to-T_3 conversion, whereas methimazole has the advantage of a longer half-life and therefore can be administered in a single daily dose.

Antithyroid medications have minor side effects of fever, rash, and arthralgias in approximately 5% of cases. Major drug toxicity occurs in <1% of patients and is manifested as hepatitis, vasculitis, and agranulocytosis. Agranulocytosis usually presents as sore throat, usually from group B streptococcal organisms. Any patient who complains of orophagia should be promptly evaluated and treated with antibiotics.

Individuals treated medically for hyperthyroidism require lifelong follow-up because of the high relapse rate. In younger patients, relapses commonly occur in the postpartum period. With medical therapy, the euthyroid state is typically restored within 3 to 10 weeks. Fifty percent of individuals treated by medication alone will have a relapse and/or possible thyroid storm (usually presentation is fever, tachycardia, and abdominal pain). Treatment should be continued for 6 to 24 months unless total ablation by radioiodine or surgery is performed. Thyroid ablation by radioiodine results in permanent hypothyroidism in most cases. Surgery has become less common because of potential complications such as inadvertent parathyroid removal, which commits the patient to lifelong calcium therapy.

Ablation of the thyroid gland with 131-iodine results in a permanent cure rate of 70% to 80%. The principal drawback to radioactive iodine therapy is a high rate of postablative hypothyroidism. Most medical endocrinologists assume hypothyroidism will develop and recommend that patients receive lifetime thyroid replacement therapy.

Thyroid storm is a rare but potentially lethal problem in untreated hyperthyroidism. Therapy includes high doses of PTU, β-blocking agents, high doses of glucocorticoids (60 to

80 mg of methylprednisolone or equivalent every 6 to 8 hours), and high-dose iodine preparations (potassium iodide or 1 g of intravenous sodium iodide). Admission to an intensive care unit is advisable, but therapy should be initiated quickly.

Thyroid Nodules

Thyroid nodules can be palpated in an estimated 5% of patients during routine examination. Most symptomatic nodules are benign, but malignancy and hyperthyroidism must be excluded. An important risk factor for thyroid cancer is previous radiation exposure, even in low doses.[23] Virtually all nodules require evaluation by tissue examination. Most surgical biopsies have been replaced by fine needle aspiration and biopsy (FNAB) techniques. An algorithm for the workup of a thyroid nodule is found in Fig. 6. Before FNAB is performed, thyroid function tests should be obtained. If evidence of thyroid dysfunction is detected, appropriate therapy may eliminate the nodule. Biopsy should be performed if the individual is euthyroid or the nodules persist after therapy. Most nodules are "cold" on scanning or imaging. Direct tissue sampling by FNAB is cost effective and successful in approximately 95%

of cases. In 5% of cases that are indeterminate, open surgical biopsy is required.

Seventy-five percent of malignancies are papillary carcinoma, but cure rates are >90% even in the presence of cervical lymph node metastases. Good prognosis is associated with patients less than 50 years of age and with a primary tumor less than 4 cm. Radioiodine therapy and surgical ablation are the most common methods of therapy for all thyroid tumors.

The approach to the pregnant woman with a suspicious thyroid nodule is FNAB followed by thyroxine suppression therapy. If malignancy is strongly suspected, surgical exploration should be undertaken in the second trimester. If the nodule is not suspicious for cancer, the FNAB may be delayed until the postpartum period.

◊ UPPER RESPIRATORY AND PULMONARY DISORDERS

The most common reason for patients to seek medical attention in a primary care practice is upper respiratory disease. Fevers, myalgias, cough with or without sputum production,

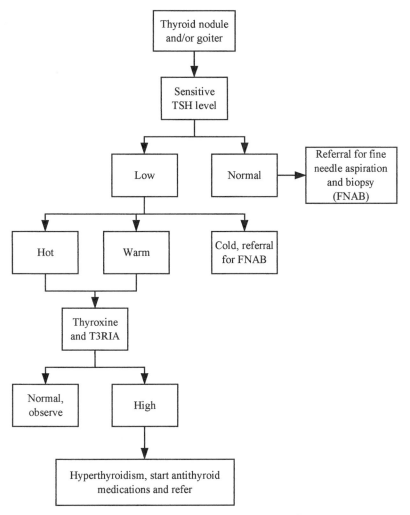

FIG. 6. Algorithm for the management of thyroid nodule. (From Nolan TE. *Primary care for the obstetrician and gynecologist.* New York: Wiley-Liss, 1995: 128; with permission.)

dyspnea, and chest and head pain are the common symptoms that result in practitioner visits. Most infections are viral and spread by coughing, sneezing, or just talking. Because of increasingly virulent and resistant organisms, one of the most important aspects of caring for upper respiratory infections is to resist the temptation to overtreat with antibiotics.[24] For instance, bacterial sinusitis is estimated to occur in only 0.5% of cases, and otitis media may occur in 2% of otherwise uncomplicated colds. However, the clinician is under patient pressure to "do something" and give antibiotics.

Common Cold

The common cold may be caused by any of five different viral groups with hundreds of antigenic variations. Despite progress in viral culturing to identify infectious organisms, many "colds" continue to defy identification. Most infections occur between early fall and spring. In most cases, patients are correct in their diagnosis based on the common symptoms of a runny nose, scratchy sore throat, mild myalgias, and low-grade fever (usually <100.4°F). The physical exam should be targeted toward identifying bacterial infections. The woman with a severely injected pharynx and exudate should be cultured for group A β-hemolytic streptococcal infection. The need to treat adults immediately for presumed streptococcal pharyngitis should be tempered by the knowledge that rheumatic fever and acute glomerular nephritis are unlikely in patient's older than 21. The ears should be examined to rule out bacterial otitis media with erythema and inflammation, which benefit from antibiotics.[25,26] Serous otitis is common and results in fluid behind the tympanic membrane. In many cases, fluid bubbles are seen, and antihistamines give symptomatic relief.

Sinusitis

A common problem in clinical practice is the patient with self-diagnosed "sinus problems." A wide range of other medical conditions such as headaches, postnasal drainage, halitosis, and dyspepsia may be caused by sinus inflammation.[27] Even though the entire respiratory system may be infected by a particular virus or pathogen (a global term for this is the sinobronchial syndrome), one anatomic area usually produces the most symptoms. During the evaluation for sinusitis, other systemic infections or conditions should be considered.

The mucosa of the nose and sinus may be irritated or inflamed by multiple agents including infectious, chemical, nervous, physical, emotional, and hormonal stimuli. Poor health, systemic diseases, nutritional deficiencies, work environment, geographic location (cold, wet, and/or humid weather) may contribute to chronic sinus inflammation. Sinus disease may be the result of other common stimuli such as atmospheric pollutants, tobacco smoke, dental disease, anatomic deformities (septal defects and misalignments), and neoplasms.

The primary infection is usually viral and located in the nose and nasopharynx. In most cases, bacterial infections follow viral infection (the normal sinus is sterile). Normal ciliary function in the sinus is compromised by a viral infection, which causes inflammatory exudates and edema formation. Common bacterial agents associated with sinusitis are *Streptococcus pneumoniae, Haemophilus influenzae, Staphylococcus aureus, Streptococcus pyogenes,* and α *Streptococcus* species. The maxillary and frontal sinuses are commonly affected in adults. The diagnosis of bacterial sinusitis is clinical and rarely made by culture.[28] Symptoms of bacterial sinus infection include fever, malaise, a feeling of "fullness" in the face, pain on sudden motion, vague headache, and referred dental pain (usually to the maxillary teeth). On physical exam, pain is elicited by direct pressure or percussion over the affected sinus. Nose and throat inspection will usually reveal purulent exudates in the middle meatus or in the nasopharynx. Imaging is rarely necessary but, if done, will reveal thickened mucosa in early infections or air–fluid levels in advanced infections. Broad-spectrum antibiotic coverage is necessary to cover common aerobic and anaerobic organisms. These include amoxicillin/clavulanate, erythromycin with sulfonamide, cefaclor, clarithromycin, and doxycycline. Hot packs, analgesics, decongestant drops such as phenylephrine, and systemic medications such as pseudoephedrine should be limited to the first few days of therapy. Symptoms should improve within 2 days, and complete resolution is usual by 10 days. A delay in improvement may be secondary to antibiotic resistance or abscess formation.

In primary care, the most important aspect in treatment of sinus conditions is to recognize complications. Untreated sinus infections may lead to orbital cellulitis and abscess formation, subperiosteal abscess formation, and cavernous sinus thrombosis. Parenteral antibiotics and surgical drainage are the usual therapy. Acute meningitis may be the result of bacterial spread either by local extension of primary infections or through venous channels. Dural abscess and brain abscess are rare but usually are secondary to direct bacterial spread. Symptoms include persistent dull headache, fatigue, weight loss, and vomiting.[29] The diagnosis is usually made by either CT or MRI scan followed by abscess drainage.

Bronchitis

Acute bronchitis is defined as inflammation of the tracheobronchial tree associated with a generalized respiratory infection. It is most common during the winter at the peak of upper respiratory viral infections. The common cold viruses (rhinovirus and coronavirus), adenovirus, influenza virus, and a nonviral pathogen, *Mycoplasma pneumoniae,* are the usual etiologic agents. Persistent cough, hoarseness, and fever are presenting symptoms. Three to four days after the initial acute infection resolves, a persistent cough begins, which may last as long as 4 weeks.[30] Sputum production is present in up to 50% of patients.

Physical examination should be directed toward ruling out pneumonia. On auscultation, rhonchi and coarse rales are usually noted, but signs of consolidation and alveolar involve-

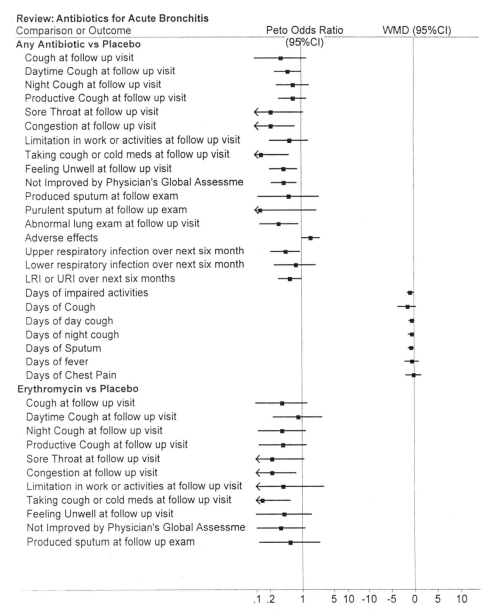

FIG. 7. Antiobiotics for acute bronchitis. (From Becker L, Glazier R, McIsaac W, Smucny J. The Cochrane Library, 1997.)

ment are absent. If there is a question of pneumonia (fine rales, decreased breath sounds in specific lung segments), a chest radiograph should be obtained. As the initial viral syndrome subsides, sputum may become more purulent. Sputum culture is rarely helpful because of contamination with normal oral flora. Treatment should be directed at symptomatic relief such as cough suppressants. However, antibiotics appear to have a modest beneficial effect in the treatment of acute bronchitis with a corresponding small risk of adverse effects (Fig. 7). Erythromycin or a macrolide derivative (azithromycin) is the drug of choice in patients with *M. pneumoniae.*

Chronic bronchitis is defined as a productive cough for at least 3 months of the year for two consecutive years and a form of chronic obstructive pulmonary disease (COPD). The usual etiology is tobacco abuse but may include chronic in-

fections and/or the inhalation of environmental pathogens found in dust. Incessant productive cough, especially on arising, is the cardinal manifestation of disease, and affected individuals have other associated pulmonary diseases. Because of the chronic nature of these diseases, referral to a general internist or pulmonologist is recommended.

Asthma: Reversible Obstructive Airway Disease

Asthma is a clinical syndrome of recurrent reversible airway obstruction that resolves either spontaneously or with bronchodilator therapy. The etiology remains unknown, but it is currently thought to be an inflammatory response. Bronchoconstriction is the *sine qua non* of asthma and is associated with hyperresponsiveness of the airways to physical and/or chemical irritants.[31]

Stimuli commonly associated with bronchoconstriction include viral infections, oxidant air pollutants (such as nitrogen dioxide or sulfur dioxide), allergies, pharmacologic stimuli (such as aspirin and nonsteroidal antiinflammatory drugs), exercise, occupational factors, and emotional stress. The disease usually presents before age 25, but it may appear at any age.

The clinical hallmarks of asthma are wheezing and dyspnea. Spirometry findings are normal except during episodes of bronchospasm. Symptoms are variable and range from a chronic cough to life-threatening episodes of hypoxia.

The pathophysiology of asthma consists of (1) airway smooth muscle constriction, (2) thickening of airway epithelium (which results in increased resistance), and (3) inflammatory secretions in the airway lumen. The release of bioactive mediators (histamine, acetylcholine, kinins, adenosine, leukotrienes, etc.) and neurotransmitters causes airway constriction. During the acute attack, airway resistance increases, which results in airway obstruction and decreased gas flow rates. The impact on pulmonary air flow is during the expiratory rather than the inspiratory phase.

An acute attack causes progressive shortness of breath, cough, wheezing, and anxiety. Physical examination reveals tachypnea of 25 to 40 breaths per minute and a hyperinflated chest with a prolonged expiratory phase. Accessory muscles of the neck are often used. Marked wheezing and rhonchi are heard on auscultation, usually in all lung fields. Decreasing wheezing may be the initial sign of resolution or, paradoxically, of impending respiratory arrest.

Multiple spirometric variations have been described, but they are essentially useless in the acute setting. A useful diagnostic measurement is the peak expiratory forced rate (PEFR). The measuring device is simple cylinder with a calibrated piston that measures expiratory effort. The PEFR maybe used during the acute phase of an attack or chronically (daily, before and after inhalation therapy) to assess medical treatment. During the resolution of an acute attack, the PEFR will normalize. Chest radiographs should not be routinely obtained unless there is a strong suspicion of an associated pneumonia (fever, chills, and productive cough). Pulse oximetry may be helpful in evaluating oxygen saturation and trends in the clinical course, but arterial blood gases are not used unless the attack is severe.

The "usual" asthma attack begins with tachpnea and respiratory alkalosis with a P_aCO_2 between 25 and 35 mm Hg and a P_aO_2 on room air between 55 and 75 mm Hg. If the attack worsens, pH may begin to normalize as a result of respiratory acidosis. A "normal P_aCO_2" signals impending pulmonary failure with inability to remove CO_2 because of severe air trapping. Before the onset of respiratory arrest ("status asthmatica"), a sharp rise in P_aCO_2 is noted, with a profound drop in pH from physical tiring. Emergent intubation and intensive care transfer are mandatory.

β-Adrenergic inhalation agents cause smooth muscle relaxation of the bronchioles and have been the mainstay of therapy. These drugs are absorbed topically and may be given via aerosol, which lessens (but does not eliminate) many systemic side effects. The onset of action is within minutes, and the bronchodilation effect lasts from 3 to 6 hours. Older systemic and inhalation agents, such as epinephrine and isoproterenol, stimulate both β₁ (causing tachycardia and anxiety) and β₂ receptors. β₂-Selective drugs common in clinical use are metaproterenol, albuterol, and salmeterol. Ipratropium bromide, an atropine-like compound, blocks parasympathetic stimulation associated with bronchospasm. Side effects are minimal, but bronchodilation is less than with the β-adrenergics. Ipratropium is usually added to the β-adrenergics.

Theophylline was the mainstay of therapy for many years, but its use has declined because of problems with toxicity and the wide variation of metabolism. Cigarette smoking, patient age, and various medications, including many antibiotics and antihypertensive agents, influence drug levels and hence toxicity.

Corticosteroids are commonly used in patients who are more labile and difficult to control by less toxic agents. The mechanism of action is unknown, but they are thought to prevent down-regulation of β-adrenergic receptor sites or to decrease inflammatory effects of mast cells in the tracheobronchial tree. Corticosteroids may be given by inhalation, orally, or intravenously, depending on the clinical situation. Intravenous corticosteroids are given in acute situations when β-adrenergics have failed or in patients with steroid-dependent asthma. In the acute situation, 20 to 80 mg of methylprednisolone every 6 hours is given, followed by 40 to 60 mg daily. The prednisone dosage is then decreased 5 mg daily until the course is finished or a baseline daily dosage is reached. Commercially available packs are useful for tapering oral dosages.

Pneumonia

Pneumonia is defined as inflammation of the distal lung including terminal airways, alveolar spaces, and the interstitium. The clinical classification of pneumonia as either community acquired or nosocomial is helpful in determining the most likely organism, prognosis, and therapy. Pneumonia remains a common cause of death. Risk factors for mortality include advanced age (>65 years of age),[32] chronic cardiopulmonary diseases, alcoholism, diabetes, renal failure, malignancy, and general poor nutrition. Clinical features associated with poor outcome include more than two-lobe involvement, respiratory rate greater than 30 breaths/min on presentation, severe hypoxemia, malnutrition with associated hypoalbuminemia, and septicemia.[33] Adult respiratory distress syndrome (ARDS) complicating pneumonia has a 50% to 70% mortality rate.

Signs and symptoms of pneumonia vary depending on the patient's immune status and the infecting organism. Viral pneumonia is usually caused by influenza virus types A or B, respiratory syncytial virus, or parainfluenza virus. Viral respiratory infections typically are acute in onset and spontaneously resolve after 1 to 2 weeks. Patients with viral pneumonia appear sicker than those individuals with typical upper respiratory tract infections. Influenza viruses are classified as types A, B, or C. Types A and B typically are associated with febrile illness and are spread primarily by aerosolization from coughing, sneezing, or talking. The incubation period is typically 1 to 3 days, followed by the acute onset of fever, chills, headache, myalgia, pain, and fatigue. Once the fever resolves, symptoms of cough, rhinorrhea, and pharyngitis may persist. Only 1% of the influenza cases evolve into pneumonia. However, mortality rates as high as 30% are reported. Elderly patients are more likely to develop secondary bacterial pneumonia, which increases the risk.

The best prevention for influenza is annual vaccination with a trivalent vaccine in high-risk groups such as the elderly, individuals with chronic cardiopulmonary disease (especially COPD), malignancy, diabetes, renal disease-and collagen vascular disease. If an unvaccinated individual is suspected to have viral pneumonia, the antiviral agent amantadine may be prescribed. Treatment for viral pneumonia is primarily supportive, but secondary bacterial infections should be treated with appropriate broad-spectrum antibiotics.

Typical (versus atypical) bacterial pneumonia usually presents with a high fever, productive cough, chills, and pleuritic chest pain. Common etiologic agents causing bacterial pneumonia include *Streptococcus pneumoniae* ("pneumococcal pneumonia"), *Haemophilus influenzae, Kelbsiella pneumoniae,* and other gram-negative and anaerobic bacteria. Atypical pneumonias are insidious in onset (the so-called walking pneumonia) and have a moderate fever, but without chills or rigors. Other symptoms include a nonproductive cough, headache, myalgias, and mild leukocytosis. Chest roentgenogram of typical pneumonia usually shows a discrete infiltrate, whereas atypical pneumonias reveal a more diffuse interstitial pattern or bronchopneumonia. Common etiologic agents of atypical pneumonia include viruses, *Mycoplasma pneumoniae, Legionella pneumophila,* and *Chlamydia pneumoniae.* In HIV infections, *Pneumoccystis carinii* is the most common organism, and *Mycobacterium tuberculosis* and fungal infections should also be considered in immunocompromised hosts.

Elderly (>65 years of age) and immune-impaired patients may have a more subtle presentation, lacking the high fever and chills usually found with "typical agents." In the elderly, confusion or exacerbation of other underlying illnesses may be the only clinical clue because elderly individuals may be unable to mount a fever, and an increased respiratory rate of greater than 25/min is the most reliable sign of pneumonia.

Chest x-ray should be performed if the chest examination reveals rales and decreased breath sounds, the oral temperature is >37.8°C, and the pulse rate is >100 beats/min.[34] Other tests useful in confirming the diagnosis of community-acquired pneumonia are the sputum Gram stain, sputum culture, and blood cultures. Before culturing, the sputum specimen should have >25 neutrophils with <10 epithelial cells per low-powered field on microscopic examination. *Legionella pneumoniae* requires special techniques such as direct fluorescent antibody staining of sputum or indirect serologic tests utilizing enzyme-linked immunosorbent assays (ELISA). *Mycoplasma pneumoniae* is suspected when the appropriate clinical syndrome exists with positive cold agglutinins.

Streptococcal pneumonia usually presents with a sudden onset of fever and chills and rusty sputum with gram-positive cocci on Gram stain. Bacteremia is present in approximately 25% of cases, and occasionally the diagnosis is confirmed by blood culture before sputum culture. Penicillin was classically the drug of choice. However, resistance is now reported in 4% to 5% of *S. pneumoniae* isolates.[35] Suggested treatment regimens for the various pneumonias are found in Table 7.

◊ GASTROINTESTINAL DISORDERS

Gastroesophageal Reflux

Gastric acid is essential to the breakdown and digestion of complex foodstuffs. The stomach possesses protective mechanisms against the erosive effects of acid, but damage may occur when defense barriers are compromised. Two pertinent examples of acid damage are (1) gastroesophageal reflux disease (GERD) or "heartburn," in which esophageal tissues are irritated by stomach acids, and (2) peptic ulcer disease (PUD), when the mucosa of the stomach and duodenum are damaged by peptic acid.

TABLE 7. *Treatment regimens for bacterial pneumonia*[a]

Bacterium	Antibiotic[b]	Dose
Streptococcus pneumoniae	Cefuroxime	750 mg q12h
	Ceprozil	500 mg q12h
	Erythromycin	1 g q6h
Staphylococcus pyogenes	Erythromycin	1 g q6h
Legionella	Erythromycin	1 g q6h
	Ciprofloxacin	400 mg q12h
	Rifampin	600 mg q12h
Mycoplasma pneumoniae	Erythromycin	500 mg q6h
	Tetracycline	500 mg q6h
	Doxycycline	100 mg q12h
Chlamydia pneumoniae	Erythromycin	500 mg q6h
	Tetracycline	500 mg q6h
	Doxycycline	100 mg q12h
Haemophilus influenzae	Third-generation cephalosporin	
Klebsiella	Second- and third-generation cephalosporin	
Staphylococcus aureus	Nafcillin	500–1,000 mg q4h
	Oxacillin	500–1,000 mg q4h
	Vancomycin[c]	1 g q12h

[a]From Nolan TE. In: *Precis VI.* Washington, DC: American College of Obstetricians and Gynecologists:97.
[b]Macrolides such as azithromycin and clarithromycin may be substituted for erythromycin.
[c]Consider infectious disease consult because of emerging resistance of nosocomial organisms to vancomycin (not necessarily *Staphylococcus* species).

GERD is caused by the reflux of gastric acid to sensitive esophageal tissues and usually results in substernal chest pain, which can radiate to the neck and be confused with cardiac chest pain. Certain myocardial infarctions (inferior wall) may be associated with "severe heartburn" and be misdiagnosed as GERD. Any chest pain syndrome that is atypical or consistent with the pattern and distribution of cardiac symptoms requires immediate evaluation and referral.

Heartburn is the cardinal manifestation of GERD and is the result of retrograde movement of acid from the stomach to the columnar-lined, sensitive esophagus. This usually occurs because of decreased tone and pressure in the lower esophageal sphincter (LES). Common causes of GERD are found in Table 8.

Symptoms occur after consumption of a large meal, eating certain foods, and after lying down. Prolonged esophageal exposure to acid may lead to stricture formation and dysphagia. Fortunately, strictures are rare, but affected patients experience prolonged periods of chest pain and may require esophageal dilation. Erosive esophagitis from chronic GERD may cause subclinical mucosal bleeding and eventually iron deficiency anemia. Nocturnal aspiration is usually silent, causing laryngitis and, in extreme cases, wheezing that may be mistaken for asthma.

Because of the recent release of over-the-counter H_2 blockers, patients may present with more advanced disease. Patients with anemia, excessive weight loss, symptoms consistent with pulmonary aspiration (sudden awakening with cough, choking, wheezing, or laryngospasm), and dysphagia should undergo further evaluation. Initial diagnostic studies consist of either an air-contrast barium study or upper gastrointestinal endoscopy. The air-contrast barium study is less sensitive than endoscopy, and with the decreasing cost of endoscopy, direct visualization may be preferable. These studies can be used to eliminate other potential causes of GERD, including esophageal motility disorders ("nutcracker esophagus"), erosive esophagitis, and peptic ulcer disease (gastric or duodenal).

Treatment should include lifestyle adjustments as well as medication. Cigarette smoking should be eliminated because it lowers LES pressure and delays esophageal acid clearance, increasing acid exposure to the esophageal mucosa. Patients should avoid recumbency for 2 to 3 hours after consuming a large meal. Foods with high acid content, such as citrus juices, should be eliminated from the diet, as well as fatty foods and chocolate, which decrease LES pressure and delay

TABLE 8. *Common causes of gastrointestinal reflux (GERD)*

Obesity and pregnancy
Girdles, abdominal binders
Foods: fatty foods, chocolate, high-acid content (citric juice)
Carminative substances: onion, garlic, peppermint
Cigarette smoking
Calcium channel blockers
Nonsteriodal antiinflammatory agents
Progestins in high doses

gastric emptying. Carminatives are naturally occurring substances found in onions, garlic, peppermint, and certain after-dinner liquors and cause increased gas, belching, and lower LES pressure.

H_2 antagonists interfere with gastric acid production and are the first-line treatment of GERD. Cimetidine (200 mg), ranitidine (150 mg), and famotidine (20 mg) are available over the counter and have become widely popular for the treatment of heartburn and GERD. Patients who are resistant to H_2 antagonists should be referred for more extensive workup. Omeprazole is a new medication that inhibits the gastric hydrogen–potassium pump, neutralizing stomach acid, and may be used in resistant cases. Other etiologies of abdominal pain should also be considered, such as pancreatitis and gallbladder disease.

Peptic Ulcer Disease

Peptic ulcer disease (PUD) is caused by acid and pepsin damage to the mucosa of the stomach and duodenum because of disruption of normal host factors. Activity of *H. pylori* is currently considered a primary etiologic factor for PUD. Peptic ulcer disease may also be the result of an increase in acid and pepsin production or a breakdown of host defenses. Alteration of peptic acid secretion and treatment of *H. pylori* infection form the cornerstone of therapy for PUD. Secretion of peptic acid is controlled by three endogenous chemicals: (1) acetylcholine, which is released by vagus nerve stimulation, (2) gastrin, which is released by protein in food, and (3) histamine, which is secreted by mast-like cells via a paracrine mechanism.[36]

To counter the effect of these destructive chemicals, three levels of defense are postulated to protect gastric and duodenal mucosa:

1. Secretion of mucus and bicarbonate by surface epithelial cells, creating a mucosal protective barrier.
2. A neutral pH at the mucosal level despite an acid environment in the lumen of the stomach or intestine.
3. Extensive blood flow in the gastrointestinal tract that rapidly removes acid from the mucosal epithelium.

The gut also has a rapid cell renewal process that replaces damaged and sloughed cells. Endogenous prostaglandins (PGE_1, PGE_2) enhance cellular renewal and increase mucus production, bicarbonate production, and blood flow. Disruption of prostaglandin production may contribute to the genesis of peptic ulcer disease.

Breakdown of the mucosal barrier is the single most important factor in the evolution of peptic ulcer disease. Definite factors associated with the disruption of the mucosal barrier include (1) infection with *Helicobacter pylori*, (2) cigarette smoking, and (3) use of NSAIDs including aspirin. *Helicobacter pylori* is associated with inflammation and disruption of the mucosal barrier, which allows further disruption by acid and pepsin.[37]

Symptoms of PUD are dyspepsia, upper abdominal pain, nausea, vomiting, anorexia, fullness, and bloating. Pain may be described as cramping, gnawing, or burning anywhere in the upper abdomen, or it may be elusive and of short duration. Response to meals is variable, and the correlation between symptoms and demonstrated ulcers is poor. Physical examination is rarely helpful except when serious complications such as gastric or duodenal perforation or obstruction result in an acute abdomen.

Because radiographic studies miss up to 20% of ulcers, endoscopy has become the procedure of choice. Direct visualization of ulcers and erosions is possible, and if carcinoma is suspected, direct biopsies may be performed. In some cases, neither diagnostic test identifies an ulcer despite the presence of classic symptoms such as pain disappearing with food or antacids. This condition is referred to as nonulcer dyspepsia, and a trial of therapy is warranted.

In many cases, empirical therapy for *H. pylori* infections is begun using one of the regimens found in Table 9. Several other therapies are also effective. Ulcers usually require a minimum of 12 weeks of treatment to heal. Antacids, because of the need for frequent dosing and side effects, are used less often then previously. Side effects include diarrhea with magnesium hydroxide and constipation with aluminum hydroxide. If antacids are used, a low-sodium formulation should be considered. Anticholinergic drugs were also used in the past, but the troublesome side effects of blurred vision and dry mouth limit their usefulness. Antisecretory agents, including H_2-receptor antagonists (cimetidine, ranitidine, and famotidine), are still commonly used in the treatment of ulcer disease with infrequent side effects and a high degree of patient compliance.[38]

Prostaglandin analogs such as misoprostol are most effective in the treatment of NSAID-related ulcers but also cause diarrhea. Because of associated uterine contractions, they should not be used in women of childbearing age. Sucralfate is an aluminum hydroxide salt of sucrose octasulfate, a large molecule that acts as a coating agent. The coating protects the mucosal barrier and is most successful in duodenal ulcer treatment. Omeprazole, a proton pump inhibitor that counteracts the hydrogen–potassium pump in the stomach, enhances healing by limiting acid production. This class of medications has been very successful, and they are replacing the H_2-receptor antagonists as therapy for PUD.

Cholecystitis may be mistaken for PUD, and an ultrasound of the gallbladder should be performed in the initial workup. Blood in the stool or melena should raise suspicion of gastrointestinal cancer in older patients. Individuals over the age of 40 should undergo diagnostic studies of the lower gastrointestinal system with either a barium enema and flexible sigmoidscopy or colonoscopy if the cause of pain is unclear. Depending on the experience of the physician, referral or consultation should be considered in the evaluation of these patients.

Gallbladder Disease

Gallbladder disease affects 2 million people annually in the United States, resulting in an estimated one-half million surgical procedures. The incidence of gallbladder disease is three times greater in women than in men, so an awareness of its presentations and treatment modalities is essential for the primary care physician.

Although gallbladder disease can occur at any age, 70% of patients are over the age of 40. Other factors such as high-estrogen states and pregnancy may predispose patients to cholelithiasis. Estrogen (both natural and pharmacologic) affects the solubility of bile constituents and contributes to the formation of gallstones. Obesity is also a commonly recognized risk factor. Women 15 to 20 lb overweight have a twofold increase, and with an excess of 50 to 75 lb, the risk increases sixfold.[39] Interestingly, rapid weight loss also increases the risk of cholelithiasis, probably by altering the steady-state solubility of bile salts and cholesterol esters. Other conditions that increase risk of stone formation include cirrhosis, diabetes, Crohn's disease, and a family history of cholelithiasis in siblings or children. Finally, American Indians (especially Pima Indians) and Mexican-Americans are at greater risk of developing disease.

An altered cholesterol-to-bile acid ratio increases the risk of cholelithiasis. Cholesterol stone formation may also occur as bilirubin concentrations increases in conditions such as hemolytic anemia. Biliary stasis further increases the risk of cholesterol precipitation for reasons such as mechanical changes in the biliary tree, dietary changes, or hormonal factors. A small stone may become a nidus and acquire further layers of cholesterol, mucin, and bilirubin salts. Eventually, the stone reaches a critical size and obstructs biliary outflow.

The clinical progression of cholelithiasis is variable. Four percent of patients with gallstones remain asymptomatic, but 50% of asymptomatic patients eventually develop symptoms, and 20% eventually experience severe complications. Common clinical symptoms include dyspepsia, fatty food intolerance, nausea and vomiting, biliary colic, and, rarely, jaundice. Biliary colic is the result of intermittent obstruction of

---

TABLE 9. *Therapy for* H. pylori *infections*

Dual therapy (Rx for 2 weeks)
   Omeprazole, 20 mg. bid
   Clarithromycin, 250 mg bid

Triple therapy (2 weeks)
   Omeprazole, 20 mg. bid or H_2-receptor antagonist
   Bismuth subsalicylate, 2 tabs qid
   Metronidazole, 250 tid
   Either tetracycline, 500 mg tid, or amoxicillin, 500 mg qid

"New triple therapy" (1 week)
   Omeprazole, 20 mg. bid
   Either clarithromycin, 250 mg bid, and metronidazole, 500 mg bid
   or Clarithromycin, 500 mg bid, and amoxicillin, 1 g bid

Alternative therapy
   Ranitidine bismuth citrate, 400 mg bid, for 4 weeks
   Clarithromycin, 500 mg tid, for first 2 weeks

the biliary tree and may present with various sites of pain, including right upper quadrant, midepigastric, or subscapular pain. Fever may be a sign of ascending cholangitis, a medical-surgical emergency that requires rapid diagnosis and therapy. Jaundice may be confused with hepatitis and occurs when the common duct is obstructed.

The most common complication of gallbladder disease is acute cholecystitis, which presents with severe pain, nausea, and vomiting. Anatomically, obstructions usually occur in the neck of the gallbladder or the cystic bile duct. If left untreated, obstructions may result in ischemia followed by gangrene of the gallbladder. Vomiting is present in 75% of patients and may resolve in 12 to 18 hours if the obstruction is transient. Symptoms are often mistaken for indigestion by both the patient and the clinician. Acute cholecystitis may lead to chronic cholecystitis, with repeated attacks. Cholangitis, inflammation in the bile-collecting system, is usually caused by an enteric organism and associated with colicky pain, fever, and jaundice. Untreated, an infected gallbladder can cause significant morbidity and mortality, especially in the elderly.

Two other associated conditions of gallbladder disease are worth noting. Pancreatitis is probably the most serious complication of gallstone disease. Cholelithiasis should be strongly considered as the etiology of acute pancreatitis. Approximately 50% of cases of pancreatitis are secondary to biliary tract disease. Cancer of the gallbladder is a rare complication of cholelithiasis, occurring in 0.2% to 5% of affected patients. Unfortunately, this cancer is insidious in onset and usually presents in an advanced stage as painless jaundice. An elevated serum bilirubin level may be useful in diagnosing ductal obstruction, and an elevated serum amylase value suggests pancreatitis. Elevated serum transaminase values (SGOT or SGPT) may indicate hepatic damage from obstruction.

The best test to diagnose cholelithiasis is the abdominal ultrasound, which is 96% accurate in diagnosing sludge or a stone. Ultrasonography has replaced oral cholecystography because of the rate of false negatives. Only 20% of stones have sufficient calcium (most stones are cholesterol in origin) for accurate imaging with abdominal flat-plate roentgenography. Nucleotide imaging (HIDA scans) may be useful for the diagnosis of acute cholelithiasis, but it is unable to detect stones in asymptomatic patients.

Controversy exists over the need for surgical treatment of gallstones that are asymptomatic or rarely symptomatic. However, complications of cholelithiasis markedly increase the risk of emergency surgery, resulting in a dramatic increase in the risk of morbidity and mortality. Therefore, management of cholelithiasis depends on a number of factors, including patient and physician preference. Variables in selecting therapy include the severity and character of symptoms, stone composition and size, and availability of various treatment modalities. In some patients, dietary modification aimed at reducing cholesterol and fatty food intake may decrease the frequency and severity of recurrences. However, expectant management usually does not alter the progression of symptoms over time because spontaneous reabsorption of existing gallstones is rare.

Surgery remains the definitive therapy for gallstones. It is indicated with recurrent symptoms, pancreatitis, and stones greater than 2 cm in size. Cholecystectomy ranks second only to diagnostic endoscopy in the frequency of digestive system surgery. Surgical complications are relatively common, with 0.7% to 1.2% mortality in asymptomatic patients, rising to almost 5% in cases complicated by acute cholangitis or pancreatitis. The risk of surgery also increases with age and is greater when common duct exploration is necessary.

Laparoscopic cholecystectomy has significantly decreased the number of "open" surgeries. Two large trocars are positioned (one umbilical and one midline midway between the umbilicus and subxiphoid), followed by two or three abdominal punctures in the right subcostal area to allow dissection with laser, cautery, and clips. Complications occur in about 5% of cases done with laparoscopy and include bleeding from the cystic artery or liver bed, bile leakage, or damage to the common duct. A 5% conversion from laparoscopy to conventional surgery results from unexpected findings or problems. Arguments for laparoscopy are similar to those in gynecology with reduction in cost, operating time, hospital stay, and postoperative morbidity.[40]

Lithotripsy has been used to mechanically disrupt gallstones but has no effect on resorption. Lithotripsy has been combined with oral medications (chenodesoxycholic acid and ursodeoxycholic acid) to hasten absorption and decrease the possibility of small fragments becoming a nidus for further stone growth. Success with this combined approach has been good, but recurrence rates within 2 years of therapy are 10% to 15%.

Irritable Bowel Syndrome, Diarrhea, and Constipation

Irritable bowel syndrome (IBS) is the most common gastrointestinal disorder encountered in a general medical practice. Additionally, IBS is often overlooked as a cause of chronic pelvic pain in young patients.[41] It occurs twice as often in women as in men, and most patients are young to middle-aged. The pathophysiology of IBS is unclear, but affected patients have altered motor reactivity to various stimuli such as psychological stress and meals. This hyperactivity is related to bowel wall neural control mechanisms and may cause spasm and pain. Transit time of the fecal stream gut is modified, resulting in pain, constipation, and diarrhea.

Functional gastrointestinal symptoms affect from 15% to 50% of patients, and there are three common clinical variants:

1. Spastic colitis, characterized by constipation and chronic abdominal pain.
2. An intermittent diarrhea-type syndrome, usually multiple small, usually painless stools.
3. The classically described combination of alternating diarrhea and constipation.

Patients with IBS often exhibit behavioral patterns similar to those linked with chronic pelvic pain—hysteria, depression, somatization, and bipolar personality disorders. Because

IBS has a significant emotional factor, the history is more important than physical examination. The patient–physician relationship is probably the most important component of treatment. Inquiries concerning bowel function in relationship to situations as well as symptoms are important. Irritable bowel syndrome is ultimately a diagnosis of exclusion after other disease states are eliminated.

The workup of IBS is similar to that for chronic pelvic pain. Older patients with sudden onset of symptoms are more likely to have organic disease. A rectal examination should be performed, and a guaiac test performed if the patient is over 40 years of age. In the presence of bloody stools, colonoscopy should be performed to rule out pathologic changes. Ulcerative colitis and Crohn's disease should be considered with symptoms such as weight loss and bloody stools. In the older patient, gastrointestinal cancers should be ruled out. However, most affected patients have no anatomic pathology, and diagnostic studies may be counterproductive in reinforcing to the patient that something is wrong or "has been missed."

Treatment of IBS is complicated by psychological problems and chronicity of the disorder.[42] After organic pathology has been excluded, psychological support should be given. The practitioner should emphasize the chronic nature of the disorder and that control of symptoms is important for longterm success.[43] Most therapy is aimed at regulation of bowel function by using bulk agents with increased dietary fiber. Patients should avoid situations that induce stress and trigger symptoms, and mild sedation with benzodiazepine-type medications may afford some relief.

Many patients respond poorly to treatment and tend to doctor shop, sometimes in search of antianxiety medications. Regardless of therapy, individuals do poorly unless they acquire insight into their disease process and accompanying coping skills. Resistant cases should be referred to a gastroenterologist.

Diarrhea

Diarrhea is the second most common illness after respiratory diseases in the United States. It is the most common affliction in developing parts of the world because of poor food-processing facilities and water sanitation. Acute diarrhea lasts less than 7 to 14 days, is usually self-limited, and commonly results from an infectious process. Chronic diarrhea lasts beyond 2 to 3 weeks, and the etiology may be either psychological or pathologic. Acute diarrhea can be further subdivided based on the presence or absence of blood in the stool and/or the presence of systemic illness. Chronic diarrhea syndromes are more commonly related to systemic diseases (Crohn's disease, ulcerative colitis, and celiac disease) and should be referred to a gastroenterologist.

In more affluent nations (high fat content with less fiber in the diet), diarrhea is defined as an increase in daily stool weight over 200 g. Strict adherence to this criterion is necessary to differentiate those individuals with IBS who may have up to 10 to 12 bowel movements daily. Stool consistency has been difficult to quantify because of a lack of standardization in liquid measurement, but normal stool should not contain blood, white blood cells, parasites, fat, or muscle fibers.

History is the most important tool in the initial evaluation of diarrhea. Most patients with acute diarrhea seek care within 48 hours of the onset of symptoms. Appendicitis, pelvic inflammatory disease, and adnexal torsion should be considered in evaluating acute diarrhea. Certain infectious agents may cause right lower-quadrant pain and mimic appendicitis. Diagnostic laparoscopy should be considered in questionable cases with peritoneal signs or high clinical suspicion of gynecologic etiologies.

The complaint of "diarrhea" should be confirmed and not accepted purely as a patient compliant. The number of normal bowel movements and the consistency should be determined. With a long history of IBS or "colitis," a complete history of the size and frequency of bowel movements should be obtained. Occasionally, fecal incontinence or incomplete evacuation is mistaken for diarrhea, especially in the elderly.

The initial evaluation should focus on:

◊ The acuteness or chronicity of the diarrhea. Individuals with diarrhea for >14 days without obvious IBS should be considered for consultation. Referral is indicated when weight loss and chronicity are discovered.

◊ The presence of blood. In younger patients with bloody diarrhea, the usual etiology is an infectious agent, especially if associated with recent travel. In older patients (>50 to 55 years old), diarrhea may be the first sign of colorectal cancer. A history of anorectal disorders (i.e., internal and external hemorrhoids, rectal fissures) can disclose important diagnostic possibilities and should be fully evaluated. In elderly individuals, diarrhea should be assumed to be cancer until proven otherwise.

◊ The presence of systemic disease. Symptoms such as anorexia, weight loss, fever, fatigue, and chills suggest an inflammatory or neoplastic disease.

Nonbloody diarrhea in the absence of systematic symptoms is usually secondary to food poisoning, irritable bowel syndrome, lactose intolerance, or any of various drugs (antibiotics, osmotic agents in the diet). Diarrhea from contaminated food is reported in clusters. Certain foods commonly implicated are eggs, chicken products, and shellfish. In most outbreaks, affected groups become ill within 24 to 36 hours of exposure. Other causes of acute nonbloody diarrhea are antibiotics and magnesium-containing antacids (surreptitious cathartic use is common in chronic laxative abusers with self-treated "constipation"). Sorbitol, found in sugarless chewing gum, and fructose in diet drinks may be responsible and often overlooked. Lactose intolerance may be familial, is common in African-Americans and Asians, and should be strongly considered if diarrhea follows the consumption of diary products.

Drinking of contaminated water sources, especially from fresh streams in western mountain areas, should raise suspicion for giardiasis. Adults in contact with children, especially in a child care environment, may become infected with viral agents that cause diarrhea.

Bloody diarrhea, in the absence of systemic illness, should raise suspicion of colorectal carcinoma. Rectal bleeding may be the first sign of diverticulosis, ulcerative colitis, or proctitis. Ulcerative colitis is associated with systemic illness, fatigue, and weight loss. If a scant amount of blood appears on toilet paper, hemorrhoids may be the cause. Recurrent blood in the stool or on toilet tissue warrants more extensive evaluation.

Common bacterial agents associated with bloody diarrhea include *Shigella, Salmonella, Campylobacter,* and *Yersinia* species. Additionally, pathologic forms of *E. coli* have caused outbreaks in the United States and have raised concerns about domestic meat-processing factories. Pseudomembranous colitis is associated with recent antibiotic use but is rare with long-term antibiotic therapy.

In acute outbreaks, history alone usually confirms the diagnosis and the etiology. Routine culturing for bacterial agents is rarely helpful but may be required to diagnose causes of bloody diarrhea that persists. If evidence of systemic illness is present, or colorectal carcinoma is suspected, a diagnostic workup (including either a barium enema with flexible sigmoidoscopy or colonoscopy) is indicated.

Most cases of diarrhea are self-limited and should be treated with hydration and observation. "Traveler's diarrhea" has become more common because of cheaper airfares to regional and international designations. The use of broad-spectrum antibiotics is discouraged to minimize evolving bacterial resistance. A nonantibiotic regimen should be prescribed before travel. If giardiasis is suspected (on the basis of mobile trophozoites identified in a stool sample by wet preparation), a 1-week course of metronidazole (250 mg three times daily) is indicated.

Constipation

"Constipation" means many things to different people, including infrequent stools, difficult bowel movements, bloating, or incomplete evacuation. Constipation is more common with aging, especially in individuals over 65. However, it is not limited to the elderly and is often underdiagnosed in young women. Laxative use increases in elderly individuals, and many so-called "normal" stool frequencies may be medically induced.

Constipation, by strict definition, is fewer than three bowel movements weekly. Strict adherence to this criteria should be avoided, and individual variation should be taken into consideration. The most important aspect of evaluating constipation is not the frequency of stooling but rather the associated symptoms of bloating or painful defecation. Decrease in bowel frequency, especially in the elderly, may result from pelvic floor dysfunction and decreased motility in the anorectal region. This condition, termed dyschezia, is failure of the puborectalis of the pelvic diaphragm to relax during defecation attempts.

Multiple drugs are associated with altered bowel function, and an expanded history of medication and diet should be obtained. Antacids containing aluminum hydrazide and calcium carbonate are commonly ingested drugs that cause constipation. Anticholinergic medications and antidepressants (especially tricyclics) are frequently implicated in bowel dysfunction. The calcium channel blocking agent verapamil is a well-known cause of severe constipation. Iron, in therapeutic doses, contributes to hard stools. Narcotic agents, nonsteroidal antiinflammatory drugs, and sympathomimetics (pseudoephedrine commonly added to combat sedation in combination cold preparations) may result in difficult bowel movements.

Hypothyroidism is a common cause of constipation, and a screening TSH is useful in evaluation. Other causes of constipation include long-standing insulin-dependent diabetes (especially with gastroparesis), neuropathy of any etiology, scleroderma, Parkinson's disease, and hypercalcemia from malignancy.

Patient age and the rapidity of onset of symptoms are important factors in determining the etiology. Sudden changes in stooling such as change in caliber of stool, intermittent diarrhea, or bloody stools should be evaluated for carcinoma of the colon. Colorectal cancer usually is detected in patients over the age of 50, but a distinct number of patients may present as early as their teens.[44]

Hirschsprung's disease, a condition limited to the colon, can cause constipation and is often is diagnosed in children, but it may occur at any age. Other conditions that may result in severe constipation include idiopathic megarectum and megacolon. These conditions are associated with a dilated rectum without distal narrowed colonic segments. Presentation is usually severe constipation accompanied by intermittent abdominal pain associated with distention.

Physical examination yields little information in most cases except when associated with tympanitic bowel sounds or with large masses secondary to retained stool or tumor mass. Digital examination of the rectum may differentiate between rectal diseases (masses, large quantities of hard stool) and colonic diseases (minimal stool in the vault). Often it is necessary to document abnormal gut motility by assessing stool transient times. Twenty radiopaque markers (made by cutting up a nasogastric tube) are ingested daily for 3 days. On days 4 and 7, plain abdominal films are obtained. The number of markers in the right and left colon and rectosigmoid are counted and multiplied by 1.2 to determine the transient time in hours for each colonic segment. The normal range is from 35 to 72 hours.[45]

A lateral radiograph revealing a rectal diameter of more than 6.5 cm at the pelvic brim is necessary to establish the diagnosis of megacolon and megarectum. If the suspected cause of megarectum or megacolon is cancer, water-soluble rather than lipid-soluble dyes should be used in imaging to prevent barium impactions. Anorectal physiology studies to measure muscle contractions should be considered if the individual does not respond to dietary changes and other simple maneuvers. If laxative abuse is suspected, flexible sigmoidoscopy may reveal pigment changes in colonic mucosa, referred to as melanosis coli. This unique discoloration is confirmatory of anthraquinone class (cascar and senna) laxative abuse.

Bowel training is important in patients of all ages once organic disease or dietary causes are eliminated. Patients should be instructed to attempt a bowel movement daily, either in the morning or in the evening. Timing is important because the gastrocolic reflex is most common at these times of day. The gastrocolic reflex is critical in elderly patients because of a natural decline in the defecation reflex. Attempts at defecation should be no less than 10 undistracted minutes, usually in the morning. Regular exercise, especially in the elderly, may help relieve constipation. Physical exercise stimulates the gastrointestinal tract and increases fluid intake. An exercise program, tailored to limitations such as visual problems to prevent falls and fractures, should be recommended. Fast walking may be all that is necessary to stimulate normal bowel function.

Increased consumption of fiber is advocated for good health in general and may reverse constipation. Dietary fiber may be purchased as a pill supplement in health food stores. Increased fiber intake may worsen some problems, primarily bloating and gas. Fluid intake should be increased, and if fiber pills are used, one glass of water should be consumed with each pill.

If lifestyle changes do not alter the frequency of bowel movements, laxatives may become necessary. All medications should be reviewed, and, if possible, known contributors to constipation replaced or eliminated. If laxatives are used, the effectiveness of the particular agent should be documented before therapy is initiated. Laxatives are divided into five major categories either by their mechanisms of action or by chemical grouping. A general classification of agents includes bulk agents, saline, hyperosmotics, stimulants, and emollients.

Bulk agents include bran, wheat husk, methylcellulose, and psyllium derivatives. The ease of administration and availability as over-the-counter agents contribute to their popularity. Most agents in this class are hydrophilic and increase stool mass while softening the stool. Flatulence and abdominal distention are distressing side effects but eventually resolve.

Commonly used hyperosmolar agents include saline laxatives, milk of magnesia, magnesium citrate, and sodium phosphate enemas. Use of these compounds results in active fluid secretion from the colonic wall into the gut lumen. Saline laxatives are often used as preprocedural bowel preparations. These agents are not suitable for long-term use but rather should be reserved for episodic use when bulk and other agents have proven unsuccessful. Lactulose is a semisynthetic disaccharide agent that has been actively promoted for patients with constipation. Because of frequent dosage intervals (three or four times daily) and quantities (30 ml/dose) necessary to be consumed, this medication never became popular.

Emollients or stool softeners such as dioctyl sodium sulfosuccinate (Colace) and mineral oil are bulk agents useful in elderly individuals. They act by incorporating water into the stool mass, which softens fecal material. Additionally, after metabolism by the enterhepatic circulation, bulk agents stimulate the colon. Glycerin suppositories lubricate the anorectal area and stimulate the defecation reflex when inserted.

Stimulant laxatives directly stimulate the myenteric plexus of the colon. There are two representative classes: anthroquinone derivatives (aloe, senna, and cascara) and polypenolic derivatives. These agents should be used only episodically because of potential permanent damage to the myenteric plexuses that results in refractory constipation. Unfortunately, this class of medications is abused regularly, resulting in a vicious cycle of increasing doses, which may progress to permanent damage. Castor oil inhibits glucose and sodium absorption while stimulating water and electrolyte secretion. When used in large quantities, it may lead to serious fluid and electrolyte disturbances. Bisacodyl (Dulcolax) remains within the lumen of the gut and has a direct stimulatory affect on the myenteric plexus. If large doses are used, diarrhea with hypokalemia and salt overload may result. Stimulative laxatives should be used only as a last resort rather than as a primary mode of therapy.

The presence of recurrent and resistant constipation or obstipation requires a workup for colorectal carcinoma. Megacolon or megarectum is a difficult problem to manage and should be referred to a gastroenterologist. If constipation is unresponsive to simple maneuvers such as diet or addition of bulk agents and emollients, long-term management by a gastroenterologist should be considered.

Colorectal Cancer

Colorectal cancer is the second most common cancer in the United States, with an estimated 160,000 new cases occurring annually. Most individuals are over age 50, with an annual mortality of 60,000. The primary sites of origin have changed over the past several decades from the rectum to equal distribution between the rectum and the proximal descending colon. Genetic predispositions are reported to be associated with the colorectal cancer. Large-bowel cancers may be related to environmental factors such as high socioeconomic level, urban environments, high level of dietary fat and meat protein intake, hypercholesterolemia, and coronary artery disease.[46] In contrast, Seventh Day Adventists, who are vegetarians, have a lower incidence of colorectal cancer than do other Americans.

Two theories (transit time and bacterial content) have been presented to link dietary influences to the occurrence of colorectal carcinoma. Stools of individuals in areas with a high prevalence of colorectal cancer have been cultured and found to be high in anaerobic flora. These microorganisms are thought to convert bile salts to carcinogens. High-fiber diets, which are common in Africa, are associated with a reduced occurrence of bowel cancers. High-fiber diets contribute to decreased stool transit times, which limits bowel wall contact with potential carcinogens found in fecal material. Because there are other confounding cultural considerations, these theories continue to be speculative.

The symptoms of bowel cancer are nonspecific and do not correlate with either the stage of disease or prognosis. Therefore, screening becomes an important issue in identifying early lesions, which are more easily cured.

Colorectal carcinomas have been associated with multiple syndromes and high-risk groups (anatomic locations in parentheses are where carcinomas are known to occur):

◊ Gardner's syndrome (small and large intestine),
◊ Familiar colonic polyposis (large intestine),
◊ Turcot's syndrome (large intestine),
◊ Nonpolyposis syndrome (large intestine),
◊ Cancer family syndrome (large intestine, ovary, endometrium),
◊ Ulcerative colitis (large intestine),
◊ Family history of cancers:
  ◊ Gynecologic: cervix, endometrium, ovary, and breast,
  ◊ Head and neck cancer,
  ◊ Lymphomas,
  ◊ Previous colorectal cancers,
◊ *Streptococcus bovis* on blood culture (reason unknown).

These patients should be considered at very high risk for the development of carcinoma at an early age. Intense surveillance should be initiated, and referral for continuity of follow-up should be considered.

Initial screening is done in two steps: (1) rectal examination or rectovaginal examination for masses, and (2) fecal occult blood testing (FOBT). The value of the rectovaginal exam is argued in younger patients, but it should be performed in all patients >50 years of age. FOBT, although inexpensive to perform, remains controversial. In a normal population, the rate of false-positive results ranges from 1% to 4%.[48] False-negative results may be as high as 50% because of the intermittent nature of bleeding in some lesions. The dilemma posed by false-positive test results and the resultant uncertainty about whether a more extensive workup is indicated has yet to be resolved. A recent large prospective study has proven that FOBT will reduce the mortality rate of colorectal cancer, but issues relating to cost-effectiveness remain. Despite objections over the utility of FOBT, no better screening test is currently available.

At the time of pelvic examination, a stool sample should be obtained. Because false-positive results can be caused by the trauma to the cervix during the performance of the Pap test, the examining glove should be changed if cervical bleeding is evident. Another option is to give the patient FOBT cards and have three to six samples obtained and returned to the office for development. The samples should be rehydrated before developer is applied to decrease the number of false negatives. Because ingestion of red meat may result in false-positive results, a red-meat-free diet should be consumed 3 to 5 days before testing. Any positive test result is an indication for invasive diagnostic testing.

For years, The American Gastrointestinal Society and the American Cancer Society (ACS) recommended that all patients over the age of 50 undergo sigmoidscopy at 3- to 5-year intervals. The newly released United States Preventive Services Task Force (1996) suggests that screening occur every 10 years. Ongoing assessments of outcomes under way in managed-care environments may provide answers to questions regarding the benefit and cost-effectiveness of flexible sigmoidoscopy versus colonoscopy and the interval between tests.

Rectal bleeding may be the first sign of bowel cancer. Unfortunately, bleeding is not always associated with early lesions. Low rectal carcinomas are associated with hematochezia, tenesmus, and narrowing of stool. Suggestive symptoms of cancer are abdominal pain, bloating, constipation, and diarrhea. Bright red bleeding is classically associated with left-sided colonic lesions, whereas occult bleeding from the mixing of blood with stool occurs with right-sided lesions. The characteristic of blood in the stool, either dark or clotted, has no clinical significance to location of the lesion or prognosis.

Associated medical conditions are anemia, new onset of angina, increasing frequency of angina, heart failure, or general malaise and fatigue. Any postmenopausal patient who has iron deficiency anemia should be considered at high risk for carcinoma of the gastrointestinal tract. Barium studies of the upper gastrointestinal system or upper endoscopy to investigate possible esophageal and gastric lesions, in addition to an assessment of the lower gastrointestinal tract, should be performed.

If a barium enema is chosen, a flexible sigmoidoscopy should be performed to examine the first 25 cm of the rectum and sigmoid colon. Two radiographic techniques of barium enema are available: (1) a single stream of barium, which is the easiest to perform and most comfortable for the patient; and (2) the air contrast technique, which has greater sensitivity (95% vs. 90%) but is time-consuming and uncomfortable for the patient. If a lesion is discovered, colonoscopy is performed to inspect the entire colon, with biopsy of any suspicious lesions. For cost-containment purposes, colonoscopy is probably preferable to performing both a barium enema and a flexible sigmoidoscopy examination. Carcinoembryonic antigen (CEA) is neither a screening nor a diagnostic test but is useful only to monitor known disease activity.

The primary goal in colorectal cancer treatment is early detection and removal of lesions. Prognosis of colorectal carcinoma is directly related to size and penetration of lesions into underlying mucosa and distal tissues. The Dukes classification is the most commonly used system:

A. Cancer limited to mucosa and submucosa
B. Cancer extending into muscularis or serosa of bowel wall
C. Regional lymph node involvement
D. Distant metastases (commonly lung, brain, liver, and supraclavicular lymph nodes)

Staging is performed during surgical resection, and lymph node findings are considered in the Dukes classification. Mortality rates are directly related to the stage of disease at discovery. With the exception of lower rectal lesions, the only effective therapy for colon cancer is surgery. Recent evidence suggests that some chemotherapeutic regimens may prolonged disease-free intervals. Lower rectal lesions differ from colonic lesions and respond to radiation. Anal carcinomas respond to both chemotherapy and radiation. Unfortunately, individuals with either advanced or recurrent disease respond poorly to adjunctive and salvage chemotherapies.

Patients who are at high risk of colorectal cancer should be evaluated periodically by a gastroenterologist. Patients with ulcerative colitis usually undergo yearly colonoscopy examination with Pap tests of lesions. When significant dysplasia arises in colonic lesions, total colectomy is recommended. Patients who have ulcerative colitis are at high risk for malignant transformation after 15 years, especially if they have pancolitis at a young age.

◊ DEPRESSION

Depression is a common psychiatric disorder that is probably underrecognized by most practitioners. The incidence of depression in the population has increased every decade since 1900. Many researchers think this represents the increasing societal pressures and influences placed on women. Women have a lifetime risk of 15% to 25%, twice that of men. This increased risk may be misleading because women are more likely than men to seek care.[49] Despite the high frequency of depression in our culture, fewer than 25% of patients receive treatment.[50] Many individuals feel that depression is a sign of either weakness or an inability to control their lives. Physicians may contribute to this by seeing symptoms as "normal" or expected reactions to family or workplace stress. Physical symptoms are more acceptable to most patients than emotional symptoms. In gynecology, many patients with chronic pelvic pain have an underlying depressive disorder. The dynamics and view of depression as a "weakness" may be changing. The stigma of depression seems to be lessening, and with more effective medication, more individuals are seeking help.

The etiology of depression is not well established. Depression has been viewed by many researchers as an underlying endogenous biochemical problem. The results of these studies have demonstrated regulation abnormalities of norepinephrine and decreased serotonin activity. Pharmaceutical research and the development of newer and more effective medications such as selective serotonin reuptake inhibitors (SSRI) support this view. Behaviorists believe that psychological factors, such as unexpressed anger, unresolved grief, and learned helplessness, are operative and are finally expressed as depression.

Depression is considered to have an endogenous component, but external pressures may precipitate a major depressive disorder. Even though these episodes are thought to be "situational" disruptions, they may herald the beginning of major depressive episode. Women specifically have unique conditions that may initiate an episode: (1) early childhood loss or prolonged illness of a parent; (2) physical or sexual abuse and domestic violence; (3) genetic predisposition; (4) socioeconomic deprivation; and (5) lifestyle stress, especially that of multiple roles (worker, mother, and spouse).[25]

Women are more susceptible to depression during certain defined periods of their lives. The physician should be aware of these events and the accompanying risk of depression. Perinatal loss has been underrecognized as a time of grief, anger, and, in many cases, depression. Counseling and support should be provided to the patient and her family at 6-week, 3-month, and 6-month intervals. Infertility is a well-recognized cause of depression in reproductive-age women, and group therapy may be useful. Postpartum depression is well known as a life event for major depression. Many patients with postpartum depression have a history of previous depression and should be closely monitored for suicide risk. Aging and the menopause are times of physiological and psychological changes, which may contribute to relapses or primary depression. However, the concept of involutional melancholia should be discarded, and specific etiologies in the social and psychological context should be pursued rather than dismissed as the "change in life."[51]

The most common time for an initial episode of depression in women is between the ages of 20 and 45. Once an individual has experienced a major depressive episode, additional episodes are more likely. Therefore, if a patient has a history of depression, then further history should be obtained on characteristics and courses of previous episodes. The practitioner needs to obtain information on pervious psychotic behavior and suicidal ideation, gestures, and attempts. Previous treatments for depression, including medication, duration of therapy, and episodes, should be documented. Patients with a history of previous severe episodes should be referred for long-term therapy, including hospitalization and intensive pharmacologic and psychological support.

If patterns of depression in the past have been episodic and of short duration, simple office counseling and follow-up in many cases will suffice. Any history of manic episodes is important and requires early referral. Mania has been described in up to 30% of patients with bipolar depression. Historically, these patients have a history of higher activity levels, overestimation of their abilities, increased energy levels, pressured speech, and decreased need for sleep. A history of hypomania (similar to mania, but without the psychotic episodes or fugue states) may also be obtained.

A history of substance abuse, which may represent a method of self-medication, is more common in depression. Patients with a long history of depression who present with acute relapse may be noncompliant with their medication. These individuals commonly explain that the "don't like drugs" and can "handle it themselves."

Diagnosis

Depressive symptoms may be normal for short periods in response to loss, disappointment, or change. True depression extends beyond feelings of sadness and becomes a dominant affect or mood disorder. In addition to a change in mood, there are thinking, behavioral, and biological alterations. The most common are listed below.

◊ Mood (emotional tone): Lack of motivation for normal life events, apathy, sadness, tearfulness, unhappiness, discouragement, and, in some cases, hostility. The first clue to an underlying depressive episode may be anhedonia, or the loss of capacity to feel happiness.
◊ Negative thinking: Self-blame, worthlessness, guilt, and a generalized feeling that things cannot get better. Recurrent thoughts of dying, suicidal ideation, or suicide attempts are specific warning signs and require intervention.
◊ Cognitive disorders: Slow thinking, difficulty remembering, indecisiveness, and inability to concentrate.
◊ Behavior changes: Passiveness, dependency, helplessness, a lack of direction. Commonly these symptoms may be evident in marital discord, alienation of friends, problems at work, and self-destructive behavior (e.g., accident proneness).
◊ Biological functions: Sleep disturbance or eating disorders including weight gain or loss. Many patients have trouble falling and staying asleep, whereas some will sleep too much. "Energy levels" are self-described as "decreased." Examples of other historical or physical complaints include weakness, fatigue, dizziness, and constipation.

Depression has been classified into different clinical types to assist in research, communication, and evaluation of medical and physiological therapies. The standard for classification is in the current *Diagnostic and Statistical Manual of Mental Disorders* (fourth edition) or *DSM-IV*. The *DSM* is updated on a regular basis and is the standard in psychiatric diseases.[52] Following are important categories in the classification of mood disorders that may be seen in primary care:

◊ Major change of mood: The loss of ability to experience pleasure.
◊ Major depression characterized by an endogenous, melancholic, or vegetative state.
◊ Major depression with psychosis: These patient may have delusions, loss of reality testing, and hallucinations.
◊ Dysthymia: A chronic, low-grade depressive episode that lasts for at least 2 years.
◊ Bipolar personality disorder, previously called the manic–depressive disorder.
◊ Seasonal affective disorder (SAD): Light-related; increased incidence in fall/winter when days are shorter.

Despite the prevalence of first episodes of depression occurring in the reproductive age group, depression may begin at any age. The recurrence rate of depression after one single major depressive episode increases the risk of a second episode to 50% to 60%. There is a 15% chance of suicide associated with any major depressive episode. Therefore, the usual patient will have several recurrences of depression, and in most cases, each recurrence lasts longer and is more severe. Bipolar depression recurs twice as often as unipolar depression. In 50% of patients with acute depression, symptoms remit spontaneously without intervention. In the remaining patients, symptoms improve with prolonged therapy in 35%, but 15% of patients remain ill for prolonged periods.

Depression may affect the results of some laboratory tests listed below. Some researchers have advocated that these changes support the organic nature of depression.

◊ Dexamethasone suppression test. As many as 50% of depressed patients will fail to suppress endogenous cortisol after the single-dose dexamethasone suppression test (1 mg of dexamethasone at bedtime followed by an 8 a.m. serum cortisol).
◊ Thyrotropin-releasing hormone (TRH) stimulation test. One-third of patients will have a blunted rise in thyroid-stimulating hormone levels after a 500 μmicrogram injection of TRH.
◊ Sleep electroencephalogram (EEG) has shown 80% of patients with depression to have decreased rapid eye movement (REM).

Depression may be the manifestation of other underlying diseases.[53] The following illnesses or diseases should be considered:

◊ Viral infections, specifically hepatitis and mononucleosis,
◊ Cancer, especially pancreatic cancer in the elderly,
◊ Collagen vascular diseases,
◊ Endocrine disorders, including hypothyroidism, hypo-adrenalism (Addison's disease), and panhypopituitarism,
◊ Stroke in the elderly, especially if coexisting hypertension and peripheral vascular disease are present,
◊ Organic brain disease including dementia and Alzheimer's disease.

Eating disorders and substance abuse may be causes or symptoms of major depression.[54] Certain gynecologic conditions are commonly associated with unrecognized depression. These ailments are among the most challenging conditions to diagnose and treat in gynecology and include chronic pelvic pain, idiopathic vulvodynia, vaginal pain and burning, poorly characterized dyspareunia, and incapacitating and severe premenstrual symptoms. Exaggerated or prolonged depression can also be associated with any major surgery that may alter or impact on femininity such as a hysterectomy, infertility, mastectomy, and menopause.

Commonly prescribed medications may produce depression, which may be dose or type specific. Agents that may produce these side effects include:

◊ Oral contraceptives, usually the progesterone component,
◊ Propranolol (lipid-soluble β-blockers more commonly than water-soluble agents),

◊ Cimetidine, usually in the elderly,

◊ Digitalis,

◊ Phenytoin,

◊ Spironolactone,

◊ Reserpine,

◊ Withdrawal syndromes with amphetamine, cocaine, and sedatives/tranquilizers,

◊ Alcohol.

As newer formulations are introduced to the market, the clinician will need to stay current. Additionally, as more medications become readily available (H_2 blockers), patients will be more prone to self-medication and will not recognize the relationship between the medications and symptoms.

Treatment

Treatment should focus on identifying immediate problems such as suicide risk and severity of disease. Physician comfort should also be an element in caring for these patients. Once these issues are resolved, then options for medication and counseling should be initiated. Most individuals who ultimately commit suicide visit their primary care physician shortly before death. Early in the initial assessment of the depressed patient, questioning should be directed to evaluate suicidal thoughts and ideation. If these feelings are present, the possibility and immediacy of a suicide attempt or gesture should be considered and documented. Most gynecologists develop a sixth sense about patients and should act on it. Clues that may be present are an overburdened individual, poor eye contact, and shutting out of all suggestion. If the risk of suicide is high, immediate transfer and hospitalization should be implemented.

Psychotherapy appears to be as effective as pharmacotherapy in the treatment of mild to moderate depression.[29] Principles of psychotherapy require an open discussion of problems. Resolution of problems is gained through insight, emotional support, and understanding from the patient–therapist relationship. Many psychologists feel that depression in women is linked with a negative viewpoint of themselves with expanded roles in the workplace, home, and society.[27] Psychotherapy should be directed at positive thinking and a realistic appraisal of self-worth with enhancement of independence and autonomy. Psychotherapy requires certain time commitments, which may limit this approach in a busy gynecologic practice.

New classes of medications for depression have revolutionized treatment and patient expectations. Until the release of the selective serotonin reuptake inhibitors (SSRIs), medical therapy was considered only for patients with severe depression. In current practice, however, with medications with fewer side effects, mild to moderate depression is commonly treated with the SSRIs. The major classes of medications for treatment of depression are tricyclics, heterocyclics, selective serotonin reuptake inhibitors (SSRIs), and monoamine oxidase (MAO) inhibitors. Monamine oxidase inhibitors are not

reviewed because of their multiple serious side effects; they remain outside the scope of most gynecologic practices.

Tricyclics were the original and only antidepressant medications available for a number of years. Major formulations in this class of medications include amitriptyline, doxepin, desipramine, imipramine, and nortriptyline. Common side effects for the class are related to their anticholinergic actions such as dry mouth, blurred vision, urinary hesitancy, and constipation. Imipramine is more commonly used for its side effect of increasing urethral tone and relaxing the detrusor, as a result of its α-adrenergic-stimulating properties, than as an antidepressant. Many patients using tricyclics feel drowsy or "hung-over." Less common but sometimes distressing side effects include orthostatic hypotension, cardiac arrhythmias, and, occasionally, weight gain. Because of the long half-lives and renal excretion of these medications, dosages should be closely monitored in the elderly. These drugs are usually given in a single evening dose and require a minimum of 3 weeks for therapeutic efficacy. These drugs may be lethal in combination with MAO inhibitors. The side effects in many cases have led to compliance problems.

Common tricyclic agents available and dosage ranges are noted below.

◊ Amitriptyline (Elavil, Endep), 75 to 300 mg hs,

◊ Doxepin (Adapin, Sinequan), 75 to 300 mg hs,

◊ Imipramine (Janimine, Tofranil), 75 to 300 mg hs,

◊ Nortriptyline (Aventyl, Pamelor), 40 to 200 mg hs,

◊ Desipramine (Norpramin, Pertofrane), 75 to 300 mg hs.

The heterocyclics were the next class of medications introduced for the treatment of depression. Major advantages for heterocyclics over the tricyclics were a reduction in anticholinergic side effects, orthostatic hypotension, and cardiac arrhythmias. Drowsiness was still present but decreased in most patients. Amoxapine, bupropion, maprotiline, and trazodone are common examples of formulations of this class of medications. As a group, they require a single daily dose. They also may be lethal when used in combination with MAO inhibitors. The antidepressant response is delayed and may require up to 4 to 6 weeks for a noticeable clinical response.

Common agents and dosages are:

◊ Amoxapine (Asendin), 10 to 40 mg hs,

◊ Bupropion (Wellbutrin), 225 to 450 mg hs,

◊ Maprotiline (Ludiomil), 100 to 225 mg hs,

◊ Trazodone (Desyrel), 150 to 600 mg hs.

The newest agents available for treatment of depression are the SSRIs. The widespread use of these medications has been no less than dramatic for the past decade. Medications representative of this class are fluoxetine, paroxetine, venlafaxine, and sertraline. These medications produce virtually no anticholinergic side effects or drowsiness, which has been instrumental in their popularity. Most serious cardiovascular side effects found with other agents have been eliminated. Gastrointestinal distress, though, in contrast to the other agents, is more prevalent. Because of the absence of significant side effects (most of which were CNS), these medications have changed perceptions about depression. Therapeutic effects may not be noted for 4 to 8 weeks, but most patients note a change within 2 weeks. These medications require single daily dosing and may be raised after 4 to 6 weeks. As with the other medications, their use with MAO inhibitors may cause fatal side effects. The widespread use of SSRIs has raised many questions about their appropriateness. Additionally, some managed care organizations have suggested that they be used for first-line therapy rather than psychotherapy.

Common agents and dosages are:

◊ Fluoxetine (Prozac), 10 to 40 mg hs,
◊ Paroxetine (Paxil), 20 to 50 mg hs,
◊ Sertraline (Zoloft), 50 to 150 mg hs,
◊ Venlafaxine (Effexor), 75 to 225 mg bid or tid.

These medications increase appetite and decrease weight loss, increase energy, decrease suicidal thoughts, and decrease negative thoughts such as excessive guilt, helplessness, and hopelessness. Unfortunately, they may decrease a sense of pleasure derived from activities and have been reported to decrease orgasms in women.

In general, medication should be used for at least 4 weeks up to 6 months. Even though these medications have not been approved for use longer than 6 months, many physicians and patients have continued them indefinitely. Depending on the clinical outcome, consideration of discontinuation should be given after 3 to 6 months, depending on the individual. Medication alone is limited if environmental and personal behaviors remain unchanged. Medication should never be used without ongoing counseling and behavioral therapy.

Depression and treatment may be different in the elderly in the treatment of bipolar disorders and seasonal affective disorders (SAD). Elderly patients may respond to stimulants (e.g., dextroamphetamine) or other agents to increase energy levels. Patients with bipolar disorders, especially those with mania, usually require lithium therapy. Finally, for individuals with SAD, bright-light therapy (there are commercial lights available for this intervention), frequent walks during the day, and a well-planned winter vacation may be helpful.

Patients with a history of major depressive episodes lasting longer than 4 to 6 months should be considered for referral to a psychiatrist. Many of these patients require multiple medications, frequent reevaluation of dosage, and intensive psychological counseling. Individuals with prior suicide gestures and attempts are probably outside the usual scope of practice of a gynecologist and would probably best be managed by a psychiatrist. A history of prior psychotic behavior, manic fugue states, and severe eating disorders should in most cases result in immediate referral. If initial attempts with single medications such as tricyclics, heterocyclics, and SSRIs are unsuccessful, the patient will probably require long and close follow-up referral. Finally, if the physician cannot communicate with the patient, or there is a lack of response, timely referral is probably the best solution.

SUMMARY POINTS

◊ Wellness is the concept of preventive care strategies that encompasses exercise, diet, avoidance of tobacco, moderation of alcohol intake, and receiving necessary immunizations.

◊ Cardiovascular disease is primarily caused by the triad of hypertension, hyperlipidemia, and tobacco abuse. Risk assessment of these factors and age is important in planning and implementing therapy.

◊ Diabetes mellitus is responsible for significant morbidity and mortality, primarily cardiovascular. Screening criteria have recently changed. The incidence of type 2 diabetes will probably increase with the increase in obesity in the United States.

◊ Thyroid disease is more common in women than men. Recent studies suggest that periodic screening of women every 5 years after 35 is cost effective.

◊ Upper respiratory syndromes are usually viral in etiology. Overtreatment with antibiotics has been responsible for emerging resistance in the past decade. The etiology of most bacterial infections of the airways is usually limited to the same organisms.

◊ Gastroesophageal reflux is common and may be treated with H$_2$-receptor antagonists. Peptic ulcer disease is thought to be the result of upsetting the balance between host factors. Recent evidence strongly supports the role of *H. pylori* as the etiologic agent. Gallbladder disease is common in women and requires a high degree of suspicion in may cases. Diarrhea is primarily viral in etiology and, unless associated with systemic disease, is usually self-limited. Constipation is best treated early in life with exercise and increased fluid in the diet. Screening maneuvers for colorectal carcinoma remain controversial; however, fecal occult blood testing is inexpensive and should be considered in patients over the age of 50.

◊ Depression is a common condition that is underdiagnosed. Selective serotonin reuptake inhibitors are effective medications that are changing many of the preconceived perceptions of depression and mental illness.

◊ **REFERENCES**

1. Scroggs JA, Griffin LP, Bayerl M, Schulkin J. Obstetrician-gynecologists as primary care physicians: the perspectives of health maintenance organization medical directors and obstetrician-gynecologists. *Obstet Gynecol* 1997; 90:291–295.
2. Manson JE, Rimm EB, Stampfer MJ, et al. Physical activity and incidence of non-insulin-dependent diabetes mellitus in women. *Lancet* 1991;338:774–778.

3. US Department of Health and Human Services. *Physical activity and health: A report of the Surgeon General.* Atlanta, GA: US Department of Health and Human Services, Centers for Disease Control and Prevention, National Center for Chronic Disease Prevention and Health Promotion, 1996:1–260.

4. Kuczmarski RJ, Flegal KM, Campbell SM, Johnson CL. Increasing prevalence of overweight among US adults: The National Health and Nutrition Examination Surveys, 1960–1991. *JAMA* 1994;272:205–211.

5. United States Preventative Services Task Force. *Recommendations for patient education and counseling.* Baltimore: Williams & Wilkins, 1989: lix–lxii.

6. Folsom AR, Luepker RV, Gillum RF, Jacobs DR, Prineas RJ, Taylor HL, Blackburn H. Improvement in hypertension detection and control from 1973–74 to 1980–81; the Minnesota Heart Survey Experience. *JAMA* 1983;250:916–921.

7. Andre J, Monneau JP, Gueguen R, Deschamps JP. Five-year incidence of hypertension and its concomitants in a population of 11355 adults unselected for disease. *Eur Heart J* 1982;3(Suppl C):53–58.

8. McCarron DA, Henry HJ, Morris CD. Human nutrition and blood pressure regulation: an integrated approach. *Hypertension* 1992;4(Suppl III): 2–13.

9. Havlik RJ, Hubert HB, Fabsitz RR, Feinleib M. Weight and hypertension. *Ann Intern Med* 1983;98:855–859.

10. Mancia G, Bertinieri G, Grassi G, Pomidossi G, Parati G, Gregorini L, Zanchetti A. Effects of blood pressure measurement by the doctor on patient's blood pressure and heart rate. *Lancet* 1983;2:695–698.

11. US Preventative Services Task Force. Screening for high blood cholesterol and other lipid disorders. In: *Guide to Clinical Preventive Services, 2nd ed.* Alexandria, VA: International Medical Publishing, 1996: 15–38.

12. Guidelines for using serum cholesterol, high-density lipoprotein cholesterol, and triglyceride levels as screening tests for preventing coronary artery heart disease in adults. *Ann Intern Med* 1996;124:515–518.

13. Katan MB, Beynen AC. Characteristics of human hypo- and hyper-responders to dietary cholesterol. *Am J Epidemiol* 1987;125:387–399.

14. *National Institutes of Health Publication 93-3095. Second report of the expert panel on detection, evaluation, and treatment of high blood cholesterol in adults.* 0-1–0-10.

15. Jones PH. A clinical overview of dyslipidemias: treatment strategies. *Am J Med* 1992;93:187–198.

16. Anonymous. Report of the expert committee on the diagnosis and classification of diabetes mellitus. *Diabetes Care* 1997;20:1183–1197.

17. Wang C, Crapo LM. The epidemiology of thyroid disease and implications for screening. *Endocrinol Metab Clin North Am* 1997;26:189–218.

18. Ezzat S, Sarti DA, Cain DR, Braunstein GD. Thyroid incidentalomas. *Arch Intern Med* 1994;154:1838–1840.

19. United States Preventative Services Task Force. *Screening for thyroid disease.* Baltimore: William & Wilkins, 1991:105–110.

20. Danese MD, Powe NR, Sawin CT, Ladenson PW. Screening for mild thyroid failure at the periodic health examination. *JAMA* 1996;276: 285–292.

21. Surks MI, Chopra IJ, Marisash CN, Nicoloff JT, Solomon DH. American Thyroid Association guidelines for use of laboratory test in thyroid disorders. *JAMA* 1990;263:1529–1532.

22. Helfand M, Crapo LM. Screening for thyroid disease. *Ann Intern Med* 1990;112:840–849.

23. Shimaoka K, Bakri K, Sciascia M, et al. Thyroid screening program: follow-up evaluation. *NY State J Med* 1982;82:1184–1187.

24. Del Mar C. Managing sore throat: a literature review: II. Do antibiotics confer benefit. *Med J Aust* 1992;156:644–649.

25. Bartelds AIM, Bowers P, Bridges-Webb C, Culpepper L, Froom J, Grob P. Acute otitis media in adults: a report from the international primary care network. *J Am Board Fam Pract* 1993;6:333–339.

26. Schwartz LE, Brown RB. Purulent otitis media in adults. *Arch Intern Med* 1992;152:2301–2304.

27. Evans FO, Sydnor JB, Moore WEC, et al. Sinusitis of maxillary antrum. *N Engl J Med* 1975;293:735–739.

28. Druce HM. Emerging techniques in the diagnosis of sinusitis. *Ann Allery* 1991;66:132–136.

29. Dolan RW, Chowdhury K. Diagnosis and treatment of intracranial complications of paranasal sinus infections. *J Oral Maxillofac Surg* 1995;53: 1080–1087.

30. Gwaltney JM Jr. Acute bronchitis. In: Mandell GL, Bennett JE, Dolin R, eds. *Mandell, Douglas and Bennett's principles and practice of infectious diseases, 4th ed.* New York: Churchill Livingstone, 1995:606–608.

31. US Department of Health and Human Services, National Heart, Lung, and Blood Institute. National asthma education program expert panel on the management of asthma. *Guidelines for the diagnosis and management of asthma.* Washington, DC: US Government Printing Office, 1991.

32. Granton JT, Grossman RF. Community-acquired pneumonia in the elderly patient. *Clin Chest Med* 1993;14:537–553.

33. Woodhead MA, Macfarlane JT, McCracken JS, Rose DH, Finch RG. Prospective study of the aetiology and outcome of pneumonia in the community. *Lancet* 1987;1:671–674.

34. Pomilla PV, Brown RB. Outpatient treatment of community-acquired pneumonia in adults. *Arch Intern Med* 1994;154:1793–1802.

35. Caputo GM, Appelbaum PC, Liu HH. Infections due to penicillin resistant pneumococci. *Arch Intern Med* 1993;115:417–421.

36. Soll AH. Pathogenesis of peptic ulcer and implications for therapy. *N Engl J Med* 1990;322:909–916.

37. Peterson WL. Current concepts: *Helicobacter pylori* and peptic ulcer disease. *N Engl J Med* 1991;324:1043–1048.

38. Feldman M, Burton ME. Drug therapy: histamine2-receptor antagonists-standard therapy for acid-peptic disease. *N Engl J Med* 1990;323: 1672–1680,1749–1755.

39. Everson GT, McKInley C, Kern F Jr. Mechanisms of gallstone formation in women. *J Clin Invest* 1991;87:237–246.

40. Southern Surgeons Club. A prospective analysis of 1518 laparoscopic cholecystectomies. *N Engl J Med* 1991;324:1073–1078.

41. Longstreth GF. Irritable bowel syndrome and chronic pelvic pain. *Obstet Gynecol Surv* 1994;49:505–507.

42. Mitchell CM, Drossman DA. The irritable bowel syndrome: understanding and treating a biopsychosocial illness disorder. *Ann Behav Med* 1987;9:13–18.

43. Drossman DA, Thompson WG. The irritable bowel syndrome: review and a graduated multicomponent treatment approach. *Ann Intern Med* 1992;116:1009–1016.

44. Steinberg JB, Tuggle DW, Postier RG. Adenocarcinoma of the colon in adolescents. *Am J Surg* 1988;156:460–462.

45. Hinton JM, Lennard-Jones JE, Young AC. A new method of studying gut transit times using radio-opaque markers. *Gut* 1969;8:42–47.

46. Waillett WC, Stampfer MJ, Colditz GA, Rosner BA, Speizer FE. Relation of meat, fat, and fiber intake to the risk of of colon cancer in a prospective study among women. *N Engl J Med* 1990;323:1664–1672.

47. Toribara NW, Sleisenger MH. Current concepts: screening for colorectal cancer. *N Engl J Med* 1995;332:861–867.

48. Lieberman DA. Colon cancer screening: the dilemma of positive screening tests. *Arch Intern Med* 1990;150:740–744.

49. Notman MT. Depression in women. Psychoanalytical concepts. *Psychiatr Clin North Am* 1989;12:221–230.

50. McGrath E, Ketia GP, Strickland BR, Russo NF. *Women and depression: risk factors and treatment issues.* Washington, DC: American Psychological Association, 1990.

51. ACOG Technical Bulletin #182, July 1993. Depression in women. *Int J Gynaecol Obstet* 1993;43:203–211.

52. American Psychiatric Association. *Diagnostic and statistical manual of mental disorders, 4th ed (DSM-IV).* Washington, DC: American Psychiatric Association, 1994.

53. Rodin G, Voshart K. Depression in the medically ill, an overview. *Am J Psychiatry* 1986;143:696–705.

54. Depression Guideline Panel. *Depression in primary care: detection, diagnosis, and treatment. No. 5. AHCPR publication no. 93-0552.* Bethesda, MD: US Department of Health and Human Services, Public Health Service, Agency for Health Care Policy and Research, 1993.

CHAPTER 32

Office Gynecology and Diagnostic Practice

◇

William R. Keye, Jr.

In this time of increased involvement of patients in their own care, rapidly developing reproductive technologies, and potentially fatal sexually transmitted diseases (STDs), the importance, and complexity, of the gynecologic history and examination are greater than they have ever been. Women who want to be actively involved in decisions regarding their gynecologic care expect physicians to use the history to obtain information concerning not only medical issues but also their hopes, fears, and goals, so that the most appropriate course of medical or surgical therapy can be charted. With the improving success of *in vitro* fertilization and other forms of assisted reproduction, physicians must be prepared to discuss personal, social, ethical, and moral issues, as well as medical issues, during the course of the medical history. For the protection of patients, their future offspring, and their sexual partners, physicians should also be prepared to inquire about sexual practices and partners during the course of the gynecologic history. Finally, the quality of the medical care provided by a physician, as well as the quality of the relationship between physician and patient, may be largely determined by the quality of the gynecologic history.

Effective history taking requires an understanding of what motivates patients to seek medical care. It also requires that physicians understand and possess good communication skills. This chapter begins with a discussion of these psychosocial and communication issues, progresses to a discussion of the details of a gynecologic history and physical examination, and concludes with a description of office diagnostic procedures.

◇ PATIENT HISTORY

General Principles

Because people seek medical care for different reasons, it is important for physicians to understand why patients come to

their office. A failure to do so may lead to patient dissatisfaction. For example, a patient may come to the gynecologist's office with a stated complaint of pelvic pain and an unstated fear that the pain is being caused by a STD. If the physician focuses on evaluating the pain and provides effective analgesia but does not deal with the patient's real concern regarding infertility, the patient may leave the office pain-free but dissatisfied. Physicians should make several attempts during the course of the history and examination to determine why the patient made the appointment and what issues the patient needs to have addressed during the office visit.

In addition to understanding and meeting patients' needs, physicians must be prepared to provide a medical evaluation in a physically and emotionally comfortable setting. It is their responsibility to allay undue apprehension, dispel false impressions, and make the visit as comfortable and informative as possible, so that patients leave the office calm and in an improved frame of mind. This is achieved by an understanding attitude and a matter-of-fact approach.

Physicians can do several things to reduce patients' anxiety:

◇ The history should be obtained in as comfortable and private a setting as possible. Some patients prefer to be clothed and seated at the same level as the physician, especially if they are meeting for the first time. Other patients may choose to change into an examination robe before seeing the physician if the visit is for a follow-up examination. Under most circumstances, patients should be interviewed alone. Exceptions may be made for children, adolescents, and mentally impaired women or at the specific request to have an attendant or a family member present. Even in these situations, it is usually a good idea to give patients the opportunity of speaking privately.

◇ The initial portion of the interview should be designed to put patients at ease. This often can be accomplished by

517

discussing neutral and nonmedical subjects, such as recent recreational activities, employment, and family. The discussion should be viewed not merely as a means of relaxing patients but also as an opportunity for gathering information about their psychological and social background.

◊ Physicians should not make assumptions about patients' background. For example, a clinician usually assumes that all adult female patients are sexually active and heterosexual. Either assumption or both may not be correct. By asking neutral, open-ended questions (e.g., "Are you sexually active?" "Are you having sex with men?"), physicians let patients know that these assumptions have not been made.

◊ An appropriate length of time should be scheduled to allow patients to tell their story without being hurried or interrupted. Interruptions from phone calls or office staff should be avoided, if at all possible, so that patients have the physician's undivided attention.

◊ Patients should be made to feel that they have the respect of the physician. This means that they will have the opportunity of sharing in the decision-making process, will not be forced to endure unwanted pain, will have what they tell the physician held in strict confidence, and are free to ask questions.

In addition to these aspects of the patient–clinician interaction, patient satisfaction is related to the time required to get an appointment, the patient mix in the reception area, the length of waiting time in the reception or examination room, the attitude of the office staff, and the billing procedures.

Effective Communication

In this age of rapidly expanding medical knowledge, the development of simpler, safer, and more effective techniques of diagnosis and treatment, and an emerging emphasis on preventive health care,[15] it is ironic that there is widespread dissatisfaction in physician–patient relationships. There is increasing evidence that a physician's attitude influences not only patient compliance but also the ultimate effect of therapy. These factors suggest that clinicians must understand the techniques of effective communication.

The first step in effective communication is establishing a good relationship with the patient. Research in human relations has demonstrated that a rapport is most readily established if physicians possess and display certain qualities, including empathy, respect, nonpossessive warmth, genuineness, nonjudgmental acceptance, kindness, and interest. These qualities are common to all effective counselors and can be learned by most clinicians.

Merely possessing the qualities described is not enough; physicians must be able to communicate them to patients through both verbal and nonverbal messages. Physicians convey empathy and respect by listening intently and giving undivided attention. They reinforce these qualities by summarizing their understanding of patients' problems in terms patients can understand.

The communication of warmth, kindness, and interest is, for the most part, nonverbal. Examples of nonverbal communication that convey these qualities include the following measures:

◊ Maintaining eye contact,
◊ Having a relaxed, open posture,
◊ Facing the patient,
◊ Leaning toward the patient,
◊ Showing a facial expression consistent with the patient's predominant emotion,
◊ Having a modulated, nonmechanical tone of voice.

However, forced or excessive expressions of warmth during the early stages of the patient–clinician relationship may be counterproductive.

Once a physician has developed the qualities described and has learned to express them, he or she must put them together to become an effective counselor. The steps involved in doing this are as follows:

◊ Listening effectively,
◊ Creating a nonthreatening atmosphere in which the patient feels free to express herself,
◊ Creating a relationship based on mutual trust and caring,
◊ Responding to the patient in verbal and nonverbal ways that convey empathy, respect, and warmth by reflecting accurately and fully the patient's feelings, communicating acceptance of the patient as a person, and showing attentiveness and caring through nonverbal behavior,
◊ Defining and agreeing with the patient about the exact role of the physician in the counseling situation.

◊ TAKING THE HISTORY

When large numbers of patients are involved, as in a clinic setting or in a busy office, certain basic information (e.g., age, ethnic background, marital status, obstetric history, whatever the patient may want to divulge about the problem for which she is there) is often obtained by interview with a trained assistant or by a questionnaire completed by the patient. The questionnaire is not by itself an adequate way to obtain information from patients. By reviewing the information on the questionnaire with patients, physicians can obtain more detailed information and begin to establish rapport. In addition, the manner in which patients answer these questions may alert physicians to areas that should be probed more deeply.

Overview

The history provides information about the total patient and is perhaps the most important part of the gynecologic evaluation. It enables patients to become acquainted with their physicians in a nonthreatening situation. In most cases, it provides the data to establish a tentative diagnosis before the physical examination. In many respects, physicians taking a history are like detectives who keep the various clues that are pertinent and discard those that are deliberately or inadvertently misleading. If the gynecologic history is sufficiently comprehensive, it should in almost all cases permit a physician to narrow the likely possibilities to one or at most two probable diagnoses. The preliminary opinion may not always be correct, but the history-taking session should not end until a tentative diagnosis has been made.

Like a hospital chart, the office chart is a legal, as well as a medical, record. As such, it is subject to subpoena, and whatever is recorded in it may at some future date need to be defended in court. It should not contain extraneous or casually written material, and the notes should be sufficiently complete so that the case can be readily reconstructed.

The gynecologic history should include the following information:

I. Presenting complaint
   A. Primary problem
   B. Duration
   C. Severity
   D. Precipitating factors
   E. Occurrence in relation to other events (e.g., menstrual cycle, coital activity, gastrointestinal activity, voiding, other pertinent functions)
   F. History of similar symptom
   G. Outcome of previous therapies
   H. Impact on the patient's quality of life, self-image, relationship with family, and daily activities
   I. Role of other stresses in the presenting complaint
II. Menstrual history
   A. Age at menarche
   B. Date of onset of last menstrual period
   C. Timing of menstrual periods
   D. Duration and quantity (i.e., number of pads used per day) of flow
   E. Degree of discomfort
   F. Premenstrual symptoms
   G. Contraception (i.e., current and past methods)
III. Obstetric history
   A. Number of pregnancies
   B. Number of living children
   C. Number of abortions, spontaneous or induced
   D. History of previous pregnancies (i.e., duration of pregnancy, antepartum complications, duration of labor, type of delivery, anesthesia used, intrapartum complications, postpartum complications, hospital, physician)
   E. Perinatal status of fetuses (i.e., birthweights, early growth and development of children, including feeding habits, growth, overall well-being, current status)
   F. History of infertility (evaluation, diagnosis, treatment, outcome)
IV. Past medical history
   A. Allergies
   B. Medications currently used
   C. Past and present medical problems
   D. Hospitalization (reason, date, outcome)
   E. Vaccinations (type, date)
V. Surgical history
   A. Operative procedures (i.e., outcome, complications)
VI. Review of systems
   A. Pulmonary
   B. Cardiovascular
   C. Gastrointestinal
   D. Urinary
   E. Vascular
   F. Neurologic
   G. Endocrinologic
   H. Immunologic
VII. Breast symptoms
   A. Masses
   B. Galactorrhea
   C. Pain
   D. Family history
VIII. Social history
   A. Exercise
   B. Dietary habits (including calcium or folate supplementation)
   C. Drug use
   D. Alcohol use
   E. Smoking habits
   F. Marital status
   G. Number of years married
   H. Sexual history (partners, contraception, protection from STDs)
   I. Occupational history (i.e., exposure to environmental toxins, ionizing radiations, infectious agents)
   J. Emotional, physical, or sexual abuse
IX. Family history
   A. Significant medical and surgical disorders in family members

Presenting Complaint

It is often effective to begin the history with an open-ended question concerning the symptoms that patients may have. This gives them the opportunity of describing their symptoms and concerns in their own words. Less information will be obtained if the interviewer asks only focused, closed-ended questions to which patients can only answer yes or no. Some clinicians find it helpful to have an outline of questions about the gynecologic history to obtain all the necessary information.

The following questions are typical of a gynecologic history:

◊ What were the circumstances at the time the problem began (i.e., time, place, activity, cycles)?
◊ What has been the sequence of events? (Having a calendar to refer to is often helpful.)
◊ Have you had this problem before? Can you describe the previous occurrence and what led to its disappearance?

◇ To what extent is the problem interfering with your daily life and the life of your family?

◇ Have you had previous evaluations or treatments? (Records from previous physicians may be helpful.)

◇ Why did you seek evaluation for the problem now?

◇ What questions do you want answered today? What do you expect and want from today's visit?

Menstrual History

The cycle interval is counted from the first day of menstrual flow of one cycle to the first day of menstrual flow of the next cycle. The range of normal is wide, and a recent change in the usual pattern may be a more reliable sign of a problem than the absolute interval. Although 28-day cycles are the median, only a small percentage of women have cycles of that length. The normal range for ovulatory cycles is between 21 and 35 days.

Estimating the amount of menstrual flow by history is difficult. The average blood loss is 30 ml (range, 10 to 80 ml). The need to frequently change saturated tampons or pads (i.e., more often than one per hour for 6 or more hours) and the passage of many or large blood clots are usually signs of excessive blood flow.

Dysmenorrhea is common. It usually begins just before or soon after the onset of bleeding and subsides by day 2 or 3 of flow. The discomfort is characteristically midline and often is associated with backache and, in primary dysmenorrhea, with systemic symptoms such as lightheadedness, diarrhea, nausea, and headache. Mittelschmerz, or midcycle unilateral pelvic pain at the time of ovulation, is usually mild and seldom lasts for more than 1 or 2 days.

It is important to ask whether or not there is bleeding between menstrual periods and whether this occurs after coitus. Intermenstrual bleeding is a characteristic sign of cervical cancer, although it is also present with benign lesions such as cervical polyps and fibroids or infection.

Finally, physicians should inquire about the presence of premenstrual syndrome (PMS).[17] The symptoms experienced by women with PMS may be physical, emotional, and behavioral. The most common of the physical symptoms are fatigue, headache, abdominal bloating, breast tenderness and swelling, acne, joint pain, constipation, and recurring herpetic or yeast infections. Although these physical symptoms are often uncomfortable, most women with moderate to severe PMS complain most about their premenstrual emotional symptoms, especially depression, anxiety, hostility, irritability, rapid mood changes, altered libido, and sensitivity to rejection. Women with PMS may also experience changes in behavior, including physical or verbal abuse of others, suicide attempts, withdrawal, craving for or intolerance of alcohol, craving for sugar or chocolate, and binge eating.

Many women report that long-standing or severe PMS can cause psychological or social problems that may be as disruptive as the premenstrual symptoms themselves. Psychological reactions to PMS include guilt, shame, decreased self-esteem, unassertiveness, decreased self-confidence, a negative body image, and a sense of hopelessness. In addition, many women with long-standing PMS report that their recurrent emotional and behavioral symptoms have eroded their relationships with co-workers, friends, husbands, and children. Finally, PMS has been an unrecognized factor in poor work records or failed educational pursuits for many women.

Sexual History

Although there are many models for sexual histories, most are not appropriate for the non–sex therapist or in the setting of a brief office visit. A model for office practice has been developed and detailed by Munjack and Oziel,[13] who described two types of sexual histories: a screening history and a problem-oriented history. The screening history is brief and suited for inclusion in the comprehensive medical history that typically is part of a patient's first visit to her gynecologist. The problem-oriented history is more detailed and designed to investigate problems identified by the screening history.

The screening history is designed to determine whether or not major sexual difficulties exist that need in-depth evaluation and therapy and whether the problem can be dealt with by the physician or should be referred elsewhere for more intensive evaluation. In an attempt to put patients at ease, physicians can begin the sexual history by prefacing questions with statements such as "Most people experience . . ." or "Because sexual problems can develop as part of other gynecologic problems, . . ." If physicians can convey a willingness to help, patients are more likely to discuss problems. In addition, the screening history should begin with a discussion of topics that are unlikely to provoke anxiety. For example, questions about the occurrence of pain during intercourse are less likely to cause anxiety than questions about orgasmic function or noncoital sexual practices.

With these principles in mind, physicians can begin with a general question, such as "Are you having any sexual problems?". If the response is noncommittal, a more specific question, for example, "Are you satisfied with the frequency of sexual relations?", can be posed. Once a problem is identified, physicians can proceed to the problem-oriented sexual history and ask about the date of onset, severity, previous evaluation and treatment, the results of such treatment, conditions that diminish or exacerbate the problem, the patient's response to the problem, and the effect of the problem on the patient's relationship with her partner. To conclude the screening history, physicians should invite patients to discuss concerns that have not been covered by the screening history. Even if a patient denies having any problems, the screening history is of value because it demonstrates the physician's willingness to discuss sexual problems.

As suggested, the problem-oriented history is designed to differentiate organic from psychogenic sexual problems, determine the complexity of the problem, determine the need for referral of the patient to a more sophisticated sexual counselor, and provide information for the formulation of a treatment program if the physician elects to treat the patient.

The problem-oriented sexual history should include the following topics:

◊ Onset of the sexual problem,
◊ Course of the sexual problem,
◊ Conditions that decrease or increase the severity of the sexual problem,
◊ Previous evaluation of the sexual problem and the results of such evaluation,
◊ Previous treatment of the sexual problem and the results of such treatment,
◊ Severity of the sexual problem,
◊ Patient's reaction to the sexual problem,
◊ Impact of the problem on the patient's sexual relationships,
◊ Patient's sexual attitudes and upbringing,
◊ Patient's sexual practices,
◊ Quality of patient's sexual or marital relationship.

A rational treatment or referral plan can be formulated on the basis of discussion of these and related questions.

In addition to a history of sexual dysfunction, it is important to obtain a history of STDs. Physicians should tactfully question patients about past episodes of STDs, sexual practices, number of sexual partners, sociosexual background of sexual partners, use of barrier forms of contraception, use of intravenous drugs, previous blood transfusions, genital lesions, persistent vaginal discharge, or pelvic pain. The discussion of STDs provides an opportunity to discuss modes of prevention, including the practice of safe sex and the use of barrier methods of contraception when the sexual history of a partner is unknown.

Psychosocial History

Health care providers can play a vital role in identifying women who are victims of psychological, physical, or sexual abuse.[1] Unfortunately, women who are abused are often hesitant to acknowledge it. Questions should include the following:

◊ Are you or have you ever been in a relationship in which you have been physically hurt or threatened by a partner?
◊ Have you ever been forced to have sex against your will?
◊ Has your partner ever destroyed things you care about?
◊ Are you or have you ever been in a relationship in which you were treated badly?

If the answer to any of these questions is yes, the physical examination may detect signs of physical abuse. In addition, many abused women may report chronic pain, sleep or appetite disorders, and frequent vaginal and urinary infections. One may become suspicious of a possibly abusive relationship if the patient's partner is present at every office visit, insists on staying close to the patient, and answers all the questions directed to her.

Once abuse is recognized, physicians must acknowledge the problem and direct the woman to an appropriate commu-

nity resource. They should also inquire about the woman's safety before she leaves the office. Some physicians obtain wallet-sized cards or brochures from local agencies that provide support and protection for battered women, and place them in the rest rooms. This provides an option for those women who would not acknowledge abuse when asked by their health care provider.

Depression is another very common condition that may be detected during an annual gynecologic examination. The potential life-threatening nature of depression and the availability of effective antidepressants with few side effects make it even more important to diagnose depression. To diagnose depression, physicians can ask the following questions:

◊ Have you lost interest in the things you used to enjoy?
◊ Do you feel sad, "blue," or "down in the dumps"?
◊ Do you have feelings of guilt or worthlessness?
◊ Do you have thoughts of death or suicide?
◊ Are you sleeping too much, or do you have difficulty falling asleep or staying asleep?
◊ Do you have a loss of energy and feel tired all the time?

An affirmative answer to one or more of these questions may mean the patient is depressed and a candidate for psychotherapy or drug therapy. More than 50% of depressed individuals will respond to antidepressant therapy.

◊ GYNECOLOGIC EXAMINATION

It is important for physicians to know patients' physical condition. A complete physical examination and appropriate laboratory tests are often performed at the first visit.[15] A complete physical examination may or may not be part of a subsequent office visit. For the woman in good health who has recently consulted a family physician or an internist, a complete physical examination may not be needed.

Patients should be encouraged to give feedback to the physician during the examination, especially when the examination is painful. Forewarning patients that they may experience mild to moderate discomfort may be helpful. During the physical examination, another, female participant, usually a nurse or an aide, must be present. Not only can this woman assist the physician, but she can also lend an element of psychological support to the patient. A dialogue between clinician and patient may continue during the examination, with the physician's asking the patient about her symptoms, the location of any pain, and other pertinent questions.

Evaluation of General Appearance

A general impression should be recorded of patients' nutritional state, distribution and proportion of body fat, texture and condition of skin and hair, presence of facial or excessive body hair, acne, abnormal nevi (greater than 5 mm, asymmetric outline, variable pigmentation, and indistinct borders), and any specific physical features.

Examination of the Head and Neck

The patient's hair is examined for cleanliness, texture, and scalp health. The eye examination may include ophthalmoscopy to detect retinal aberrations. The patient's nose, throat, and teeth can also be checked. Finally, the anterior cervical, posterior cervical, and supraclavicular nodes, as well as the thyroid gland, should be palpated.

Examination of the Cardiopulmonary System

Hypertension is the most common chronic disease in women over 50. Therefore, every woman, especially those over 50, should have a blood pressure examination with her annual gynecologic examination.

Careful cardiac auscultation may also be performed as part of the gynecologic examination because many patients eventually undergo surgery or childbirth. Mitral valve prolapse (MVP), the most common cardiac condition diagnosed by auscultation in asymptomatic women, can be problematic during surgery or pregnancy. A prolapsing mitral valve is more common in young women than in men. In most cases, it is not associated with other cardiac defects and consists of a large valve with redundant leaves. Although most women with MVP are asymptomatic, others may experience anxiety, chest pain, palpitations, bacterial endocarditis, or, rarely, sudden death.

Diagnosis of MVP is made by auscultation of a midsystolic nonejection click and a late systolic murmur. Because alterations in venous return influence the auscultatory findings, they may change in nature from examination to examination and may even disappear, only to reappear at a later examination. The diagnosis of MVP, which can be confirmed by two-dimensional echocardiography, is important because of its association with bacterial endocarditis, von Willebrand disease, autoimmune connective tissue disorders, and hyperthyroidism. Women in whom this diagnosis has been made probably should have antibiotic prophylaxis at the time of delivery or during invasive diagnostic and surgical procedures. In addition, they may require antiarrhythmic or even anticoagulant therapy and should be followed or evaluated for the systemic conditions noted.

Examination of the Breasts

The breast examination begins with a breast-oriented history.[8] Patients are asked whether they have noted any lumps, pain, discharge, or other changes in their breasts. They should also be asked about breast surgery, date and results of their last mammogram, current and past hormone use, and family history of breast cancer. Axillary and supraclavicular nodes are then palpated. The breasts should be examined with patients both sitting or standing and lying supine. In the erect position, the nipples and inframammary folds are evaluated for asymmetry. The examiner looks for elevation of one nipple, flattening of one breast, dimpling of the skin, or asymmetry by having patients raise both arms above the head and lean forward, and then contract the pectoral muscles with hands on hips. Then, with patients in the supine position with one arm above the head, all quadrants of each breast are felt with the flat part of the distal phalanges of the fingers. The subareolar area should also be palpated, as 15% of carcinomas occur under the areola. The axillary and supraclavicular areas should be palpated for enlarged or tender lymph nodes. The nipples and adjacent areolar tissue are then compressed in an effort to express fluid from the nipple. The examination of the breasts should conclude with a description of the examination results and a recommendation for follow-up physical or radiologic examinations.

Examination of the Chest

From the back, a curvature of the vertebral column can be assessed by observation and palpation. The chest can also be percussed and auscultated.

Examination of the Abdomen

Patients should be positioned supine with arms against the body to relax the abdominal musculature. If necessary, to obtain adequate relaxation, the knees can be elevated and flexed. In a methodical and consistent manner, all quadrants of the abdomen should be examined. Relaxation of the abdomen to evaluate a suspected mass can be assisted by having patients breathe deeply and then exhale. After all quadrants have been examined, the inguinal nodes should be palpated. Asking about abdominal scars may provide information that was not elicited during the history.

Bulging of the flanks suggests free abdominal fluid, but thin-walled ovarian cysts and irregularly shaped uterine leiomyomata may give a similar clinical picture. Although large ovarian cysts and leiomyomata most commonly cause protrusion of the anterior abdominal wall, there are many confusing exceptions. Palpation for a fluid wave through the lateral quadrants of the abdomen is also a useful procedure. Percussion for areas of flatness or tympany and for shifting dullness may aid in determining whether the distention is caused by intraperitoneal fluid or by intestinal gas. Auscultation is especially useful in differentiating among a large tumor, a distended bowel, or an advanced pregnancy as the cause of abdominal enlargement.

Examination of the Extremities

Examination of the lower extremities supplies important information regarding the cardiovascular system. Edema and varicosities should be noted. In a patient with congenital absence of the vagina, evidence of muscle atrophy in the extremities should be sought because such patients may have nerve root compression secondary to congenital vertebral anomalies. The peripheral pulses and reflexes may also be evaluated at this time. Examination of the calves and ankles for melanomas or dysplastic nevi is advisable.

Pelvic Examination

The first examination of the female genitourinary system often takes place in the neonatal period. An examination is indicated at any age when abnormal bleeding or pelvic symptoms are present, there are questions about primary or secondary sexual development, or sexual activity is being initiated. For teenagers, the first pelvic examination should probably occur at 18 years of age or at the initiation of sexual activity, whichever comes first. Examinations are usually repeated at yearly intervals, at which time a Papanicolaou test (Pap smear) should be performed in addition to a pelvic examination and a screening for breast cancer and hypertension.

The pelvic examination provides physicians with an opportunity to dispel myths and misunderstandings and to educate with respect to pelvic anatomy, physical development, and sexual function. Patients are often reassured if the physician carries on a running dialogue, describing the findings, asking and answering questions, and demonstrating on occasion the physical findings with the aid of a hand-held mirror. To maximize the educational aspects of an examination, clinicians can (1) describe all procedures in advance, (2) keep eye contact with patients during the examination, whenever possible, and (3) explain all findings clearly.

Patient Preparation

The pelvic examination is performed with patients lying on their back with both knees flexed. The buttocks are positioned at the edge of the examining table, and the feet are supported by stirrups. This position allows the necessary exposure of the pelvic organs. Traditionally, patients have been placed with the head and body in a horizontal position. This position does not allow maintaining eye contact and increases patients' sense of vulnerability. The alternative, assuming the availability of an adjustable examination table, is to elevate the head of the table between 30 and 90 degrees. There are no apparent technical disadvantages to this alternate position, and many patients find it easier to relax, actually making the bimanual part of the examination more accurate. Patients should empty the bladder just before the examination.

Equipment

The minimal equipment needed to perform a pelvic examination includes a good light source, a speculum of the correct size, a nonsterile glove, and a water-soluble lubricant. Additional supplies that should be available in the examination room include a variety of speculum sizes; materials to obtain cytologic samples, including fixative; various culture media; large cotton-tipped swabs; pH indicator paper; and a screening test for fecal occult blood. Specialized examinations require other specific equipment.

External Genitalia Examination

The pelvic examination begins with inspection of the vulva. Physicians should note and record evidence of developmental abnormalities, as well as the general state of cleanliness, discharge, hair growth and distribution, and abnormalities of the skin, including tumors, ulcerations, scratch marks, rashes, and minor lacerations or bruises. Vulvar varicosities or hemorrhoids should also be noted. A careful inspection of the skin folds, vulva, and pubic hair may also reveal occult disease or infection. The vulva should be palpated for subcutaneous lesions.

The labia are then spread, and the condition of the hymen and vulvovaginal skin and the size of the clitoris are noted. The examination should be performed in a systematic manner and include the labia majora, labia minora, vestibule, urethral opening, periurethral glands, Bartholin glands, perineum, anus, and perianal areas. With an index finger in the outer vagina and the thumb on the perineum, the labia and urethra are palpated for masses or tenderness. Patients are asked to contract the muscles of the vaginal opening to assess the tone of the levator muscles and the degree of perineal support, and then to strain to reveal the presence of a urethrocele, cystocele, rectocele, enterocele, or vaginal or cervical prolapse.

Vaginal Examination

The vagina should first be inspected with the aid of a speculum. Specula come in various sizes, and an appropriate size should be selected for the individual patient. The largest size that is comfortable often provides the best visualization.

Painless insertion of the speculum may be aided by several techniques. First, the muscles at the opening of the vagina may be relaxed by gentle downward pressure with one or two fingers. The speculum may be moistened with warm water before insertion, but other types of lubricants should be avoided if cultures or cytologic samples are to be collected. The speculum blades should be inserted obliquely, not vertically, through the introitus, immediately rotated to the horizontal plane, and then slowly opened after the vaginal apex is reached. The vaginal walls and cervix should be inspected for lesions. The vaginal discharge should be assessed for volume, color, consistency, and odor. The endocervical mucus should also be examined. Samples for cervical or vaginal cytology, cultures, and direct microscopic examination of the vaginal or cervical discharge should be obtained as indicated. Before the speculum is removed, the cervix should be evaluated for ectropion, erosion, infection, discharge, laceration, polyps, ulcerations, and tumors. As the speculum is removed, with the patient bearing down, the degree of vaginal wall relaxation and uterine prolapse can be assessed. With the speculum removed and the patient still bearing down, one can observe whether or not the patient exhibits stress incontinence.

Bimanual Examination

The technique for the bimanual examination is shown in Figures 1 through 5. After the speculum has been withdrawn, the physician should gently insert the index and middle fingers along the posterior wall of the vagina. At the same time, the other hand is placed on the patient's abdomen in the midline. The first palpable structure is the cervix. Next is the uterine fundus. The bimanual technique can outline its position, size, shape, consistency, and degree of mobility. Uterine or cervical mobility can be further assessed by placing the fingers on one side of the uterus and moving them to the contralateral side. This can be done on both right and left sides to detect chronic or acute inflammatory changes and fixation. The abdominal hand is then placed on one lower quadrant and slowly worked inferiorly and medially to meet the examining fingers of the vaginal hand. In this way, adnexal structures on that side can be appreciated. The degree of adherence of an adnexal structure to the uterus can often be ascertained. Enlargement, consistency, and position of ovaries and tubes can be noted. The ovary is a sensitive structure, and patients differ in tolerance to palpation. The contralateral side should be similarly examined. Finally, the vaginal walls and adjacent structures (bladder and rectum) are palpated. The glove of the examining hand is then replaced with a clean glove for the rectovaginal or rectal examination.

Rectovaginal Examination

The rectal examination is uncomfortable, but it can be made less so if the physician gently places a finger into the anal opening and waits for the anal sphincter to relax before proceeding. The

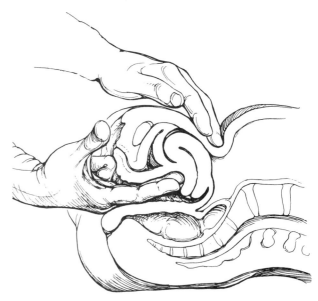

FIG. 2. Bimanual examination, second step. The vaginal fingers are moved into the anterior fornix to permit palpation of the uterine corpus. If the abdominal wall is thin and well relaxed, it is possible to define even minor irregularities in the contour or consistency of the uterus. Third step: With the vaginal fingers still in the anterior fornix and with the aid of the abdominal hand, the uterus is moved gently toward a retroverted position and then from side to side to determine its mobility and the presence or absence of pain on movement of the uterus. (From Duncan AS. In: Bourne A, ed. *British gynaecological practice.* Philadelphia: FA Davis Co, 1955; drawn by G. McHugh; with permission.)

middle finger is inserted into the rectum and the index finger into the vagina. The tone and symmetry of the sphincter are determined. The parametrial tissue is then palpated between the index finger in the vagina and the middle finger in the rectum. Finally, the posterior uterine surface, adnexal areas, uterosacral ligaments, and pouch of Douglas, along with the anorectal area, are palpated. The rectovaginal examination enhances the evaluation of cul-de-sac or ovarian pathology. Particles of hard fecal material may interfere with an accurate examination.

Rectal Examination

Additional information may be gathered from a separate rectal examination. Exerting pressure against the perineum allows introduction of the index finger. Hemorrhoids, polyps, and tumors of the rectum may be felt. The rectal examination can be assisted by placing one hand on the lower abdomen to make it a bimanual procedure. This examination is useful when a vaginal examination is impossible, such as in infants and children.

The rectal wall is palpated throughout its circumference and as far as the finger permits. Almost one-half of all rectosigmoid cancers can be detected by this palpation. The finger can also explore the surface of each pelvic wall, feeling for enlarged nodes or other abnormalities. Any fecal material can be tested for occult blood.[12] Following the rectal examination, the patient is instructed to slide up on the table while the lower

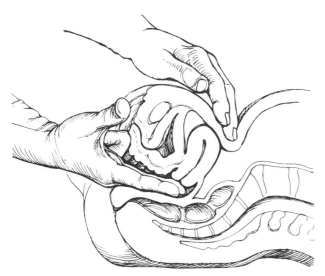

FIG. 1. Bimanual examination, first step. The vaginal fingers feel the consistency and symmetry of the cervix and its axis in relation to the axis of the vagina. They then elevate the uterus toward the abdominal wall, so the total length of the uterus can be determined. (From Duncan AS. In: Bourne A, ed. *British gynaecological practice.* Philadelphia: FA Davis Co, 1955; drawn by G. McHugh; with permission.)

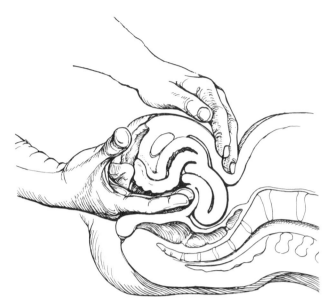

FIG. 3. If the fingertips of the abdominal and vaginal hands come together when carrying out the second step of the bimanual examination, it can be concluded that the uterus is retroverted; the vaginal fingers are then moved to the posterior fornix to outline symmetry, consistency, and mobility of the retroverted corpus. (From Duncan AS. In: Bourne A, ed. *British gynaecological practice*. Philadelphia: FA Davis Co, 1955; drawn by G. McHugh; with permission.)

one-third of the table is replaced. The examiner can answer any questions about the examination and then step out of the room while the patient dresses. Physicians should always wash their hands before examining another patient.

Recording the Findings

The information gained from the pelvic examination can be recorded in the following outline form while the patient dresses:

    I. Perineum
       A. Old lacerations
       B. Lacerations
   II. External genitalia
       A. Stage of development
       B. Color
       C. Evidence of lesions
       D. Bartholin glands
  III. Vestibule
       A. Skene glands
       B. Urethral orifice
       C. Hymenal ring
  IV. Vagina
       A. Presence of leukorrhea
       B. Color
       C. Lesions
       D. Tone
       E. Rugae
   V. Cervix
       A. Shape

       B. Consistency
       C. Mobility
       D. State of parity
       E. Lesions
  VI. Uterus
       A. Position
       B. Mobility
       C. Size
       D. Shape
       E. Consistency
 VII. Adnexa
       A. Position and mobility of ovaries and tubes
       B. Presence of masses or tenderness
VIII. Rectovaginal examination
       A. Degree of confirmation of previous findings
       B. Statement about additional pathology
  IX. Rectal examination
       A. Occult blood

Postexamination Discussion

Back in the consultation room, the findings, diagnoses, and plans for therapy are explained the patient in terms she can understand. It may be helpful to have the patient paraphrase the information to make certain that she understands. This is especially relevant when surgery is contemplated because the nuances of an operation and its results may be unclear to patients. At this time, the use of medications and the duration of their use are explained. The physician should also carefully explain what the patient may expect if any special diagnostic

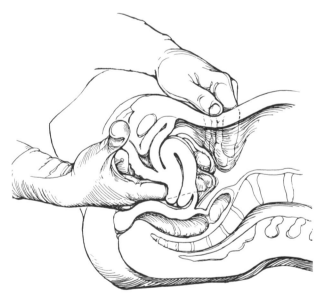

FIG. 4. Bimanual examination, fourth step. To outline the adnexa, the vaginal fingers are moved to the right fornix, and the examiner attempts to bring the abdominal and vaginal fingers together at a point presumed to be superior to the fallopian tube and ovary. (From Duncan AS. In: Bourne A, ed. *British gynaecological practice*. Philadelphia: FA Davis Co, 1955; drawn by G. McHugh; with permission.)

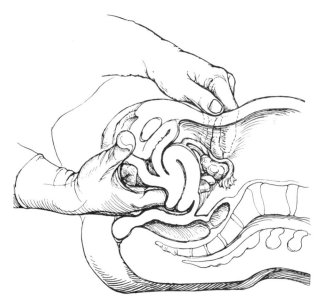

FIG. 5. Bimanual examination, fifth step. When the fingers of the abdominal and vaginal hands are quite close together (it is desirable but not always possible to approximate these fingers), they are then moved gently toward the examiner, so the adnexa slip between the fingers as they can be outlined. (From Duncan AS. In: Bourne A, ed. *British gynaecological practice.* Philadelphia: FA Davis Co, 1955; drawn by G. McHugh; with permission.)

or therapeutic procedures were performed (e.g., heavy leukorrhea after cryosurgery, bleeding after cervical biopsy). In some situations, patients may be instructed to abstain from sexual activity for a specific length of time. The importance of a follow-up examination should be stressed. Prescriptions for medications should be adequately detailed and restrictions on refills explicitly stated.

◊ DIAGNOSTIC PROCEDURES

Pap Smear

The early diagnosis of cervical carcinoma is based on periodic cytologic screening of the cervix. Despite extensive debates regarding the optimum frequency and accuracy of the Pap smear, it has become the standard method of screening for cervical carcinoma.[2] In addition to detecting early cervical cancer, the Pap smear can also assess hormonal status and assist in identifying sexually transmitted pathogens such as herpes simplex, human papillomavirus (HPV), *Chlamydia trachomatis,* and *Trichomonas vaginalis,* as well as benign conditions.[7] The presence of cancer of the cervix may indicate infection with human immunodeficiency virus.[11]

Pap smears should be obtained at periodic intervals in women when they reach the age of 18 or become sexually active, whichever comes first. They should probably be obtained yearly, especially in women who have had coitus with more than one sexual partner, began to have coitus as an adolescent, or have a history of a STD. A Pap smear

should also be performed annually in women who have had a hysterectomy for pelvic cancer or *in situ* disease, although it may not be necessary in women who have had a hysterectomy for benign disease. Recently, some well publicized failures of Pap smears to detect cervical cancer led to an increased interest in technologic enhancements and automated assisted devices to reduce the rate of false-negative smears. However, it is too early in the use of these new devices to know whether or not they will reduce the rate of false-negative Pap smears without increasing the rate of false-positives or raising cost to an unacceptable level. It is important to carefully select the laboratory used for processing, analyzing, and interpreting the smears.

To visualize the cervix, the largest speculum that is comfortable to the patient is used. The speculum is warmed and lubricated with warm water. The cervix is visualized, and a plastic or wooden spatula is used to scrape the squamocolumnar junction and areas on the cervix or vagina that may look suspicious (Fig. 6). In premenopausal women, the squamocolumnar junction is likely to be within the endocervical canal. The spatula is wiped on a clean glass slide, and the slide is sprayed immediately with a fixative (i.e., alcohol and ether) before the cells dry. A second specimen is taken from the endocervix with a cotton-tipped applicator or cytobrush that is placed into the endocervical canal and rotated 360 degrees three to five times. The cytobrush is more effective than a cotton swab in obtaining endocervical cells.[9,18] The cells are then transferred to the slide, and the slide is again sprayed with fixative. The slide, previously labeled to identify its source, is then sent to cytology for evaluation.

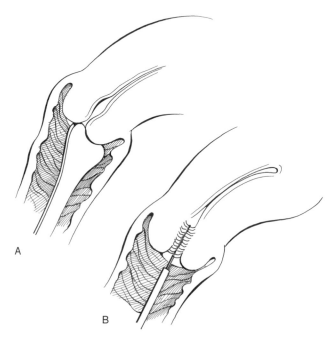

FIG. 6. Pap smear. **A:** Cells obtained from transformation zone using an Ayers spatula. **B:** Cells obtained from the cervix using a cytobrush.

Colposcopy

Colposcopy aids in examining the visible portion of the female reproductive tract (i.e., vulva, vagina, cervix). This technique complements cytologic evaluation and may be able to localize the source of abnormal cells seen on cytology.

Vulvar diseases amenable to colposcopic evaluation include HPV infections, herpes genitalis, and preinvasive cancers. The magnification afforded by the colposcope may aid in the selection of areas for biopsy. The application of 3% acetic acid for 3 to 5 minutes may also help define abnormal areas that typically turn white and display sharp borders (i.e., acetowhite epithelium). The colposcope may also aid in the recognition of clinically inapparent vaginal intraepithelial neoplasia or HPV infection. These lesions are also characterized by acetowhite epithelium.

Colposcopy is most commonly used for evaluating the cervix in patients with an abnormal Pap smear. After it is visualized and excess mucus is gently removed with a dry cotton ball, the cervix is treated with 3% to 5% acetic acid. As noted, flat condylomata or dysplastic areas turn white or develop a vascular pattern with a mosaic appearance or punctuation. The squamocolumnar junction and transformation zone are then thoroughly inspected, and a biopsy of suspicious areas is performed. In addition, nonpregnant patients with an abnormal Pap smear should have an endocervical biopsy. Bleeding occurring as a result of the biopsy can easily be controlled with ferric subsulfate (Monsel solution).

Endometrial Sampling

Advances in devices used for endometrial sampling have simplified the evaluation of abnormal uterine bleeding. Diagnostic dilation and curettage procedures under general or regional anesthesia have been replaced in many situations by outpatient endometrial biopsies, resulting in a savings of money, time, and morbidity. Endometrial sampling is of greatest value in the evaluation of abnormal bleeding when diffuse rather than focal endometrial changes are suspected.

Before obtaining an endometrial sample for biopsy, physicians should have the patient's informed consent. They should then rule out intrauterine pregnancy, cervical or endometrial infection, and cervical stenosis.

The size and position of the uterus are determined by a pelvic examination or by ultrasound, and a speculum is placed into the vagina. If the patient is sensitive to cervical manipulation, a paracervical block can be administered. When endometrial cancer is suspected, an endocervical biopsy sample can be obtained before endometrial sampling. The cervix and upper vagina are then cleansed with an antiseptic such as povidone-iodine.

If the uterus is not anteflexed or retroflexed, a biopsy sample can often be obtained without placing a tenaculum on the cervix. If the degree of flexion is marked, a tenaculum aids in straightening the uterus. It is necessary in some women to anesthetize the anterior cervix with lidocaine 1%

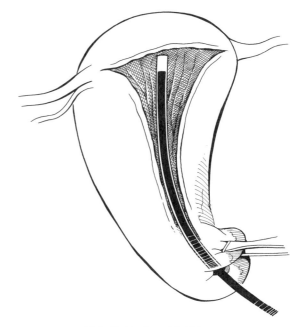

FIG. 7. Endometrial biopsy.

(Xylocaine) to avoid discomfort when the tenaculum is applied to the cervix.

The instrument used to collect the sample is inserted to the top of the fundus, and the length of the uterus noted (Fig. 7). It is not necessary to sound the uterus before obtaining the biopsy sample in most situations. Several samples are then obtained from the endometrial cavity and submitted for histologic evaluation. If cervical stenosis is present, instruments as narrow as 2 to 3 mm in diameter can be used, or the cervical os dilated. There are several instruments available to sample the endometrium. The most commonly used is the Unimar Pipelle Endometrial Suction Curette (Cooper Surgical, Shelton, CT). Others include the Novak Endometrial Suction Biopsy Curette (Miltex Instrument Company, Inc., Lake Success, NY) and Tis–U–Trap Uterine Suction Curette Set (Milex Products, Inc., Chicago IL).

Patients may experience vasovagal syncope during the procedure and cramps or bleeding afterward. Bleeding usually stops within 1 to 2 days after the biopsy.

Vulvar Biopsy

In the past, the toluidine blue test was used to direct vulvar biopsies. The vulva was washed with 1% acetic acid, dried, and then treated with toluidine blue dye. After 2 to 3 minutes, the dye was washed away with 1% acetic acid. Areas of possible vulvar intraepithelial neoplasia retained the dye and thus guided physicians to suspicious areas for biopsy. Because of the high rate of false-positive and false-negative results associated with this method, it has largely been replaced by colposcopy. Colposcopy has been shown to be a sensitive tool for diagnosing vulvar lesions, such as HPV infections.

The only definitive way to exclude invasion is to microscopically examine and perform a biopsy of suspicious areas

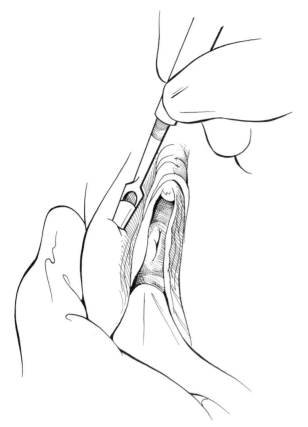

FIG. 8. Vulvar biopsy using Keyes punch.

of the vulva. Vulvar biopsy samples usually are simple to obtain in the office. The area under suspicion is first cleansed with an antiseptic solution and then infiltrated with lidocaine 1% and a 25-gauge needle. Then, a 3- to 6-mm Keyes punch is used to obtain a sample (Fig. 8). Any bleeding that occurs can be controlled with silver nitrate or Monsel solution and gentle pressure. For larger areas, a single interrupted suture achieves hemostasis.

Ovulation Detection and Prediction

The confirmation of ovulation is always an important part of the evaluation of patients with infertility or abnormal uterine bleeding. It is also useful in timing donor and homologous artificial insemination.

Methods used to detect ovulation reflect progesterone secretion by the ovary. Most popular among these is the determination of a biphasic temperature pattern by recording the basal body temperature (BBT). The BBT is the temperature taken immediately on awakening and before activity. Persistent elevation in the BBT of 0.5°F to 1.0°F (0.2°C to 0.4C°) in response to the secretion of progesterone reflects ovulation. However, ovulation has already occurred, and the BBT does not allow prediction of when it will occur. Measures of serum progesterone or the presence of secretory endometrium can also be used to confirm that ovulation has occurred. As with the BBT, these methods provide confirmation of ovulation but

do not make it possible to predict the day of ovulation for the timing of coitus or insemination.

Serial ultrasound studies of follicular growth and disappearance and subsequent formation of a corpus luteum is another method of detecting and timing ovulation. The serial sonographic changes associated with ovulation include a preovulatory follicle of 20 mm or more, a change in the shape of the follicle, thickening of the follicular wall, disappearance of the follicle, and the appearance of fluid in the cul-de-sac. However, these changes can occur without actual ovulation, and ovulation can occur without these characteristic changes. Only direct observation of ovulation at laparoscopy, or pregnancy, provides definite evidence of actual ovulation.

The introduction of home kits for detecting the midcycle surge of luteinizing hormone (LH) in urine has made it possible for patients to predict in advance when ovulation will occur. A peak in urinary LH typically occurs between 8 a.m. and 3 p.m., and ovulation usually occurs 12 to 36 hours later. This makes it possible for infertile couples to time coitus or insemination more accurately than ever before. False-positive results may occur in women with polycystic ovary syndrome and in those taking ovulation-inducing drugs.

Office Hysteroscopy

The development of small hysteroscopes that use carbon dioxide or saline as a distention medium has made it possible to determine in the office setting, often without anesthesia, the cause of abnormal uterine bleeding, the size and shape of the uterine cavity, the presence of urogenital anomalies of the uterus, the location of a misplaced intrauterine device, and the presence of intrauterine adhesions.[14] As a result, dilation and curettage and hysterosalpingography are no longer always the first choice for evaluating abnormal bleeding or intrauterine abnormalities associated with infertility.[3] Office hysteroscopy is of greatest value in evaluating women with abnormal uterine bleeding who have ovulatory menstrual cycles. In such cases, focal rather than diffuse endometrial abnormalities may be present.

The procedure is safe, simple, and quick. It is performed early in the menstrual cycle to avoid an intrauterine pregnancy or a thick endometrium. Patients should give informed consent. The cervix is cleansed with an antiseptic solution, and the hysteroscope is inserted through the cervix (Fig. 9). Insertion of the hysteroscope is facilitated by the performance of a bimanual examination before the hysteroscopy to assess the size, shape, and flexion of the uterus. Flexible diagnostic hysteroscopes typically do not require use of a tenaculum on the anterior cervix. Larger flexible hysteroscopes designed for obtaining biopsies usually require dilation. Injection of a local anesthetic to the anterior cervix and paracervical areas and use of nonsteroidal antiinflammatory drugs reduce the discomfort associated with the procedure for most patients. The endocervical canal, endometrial cavity, and tubal ostia are systematically evaluated, and biopsy samples can be taken of endometrial pathology. Patients should be informed

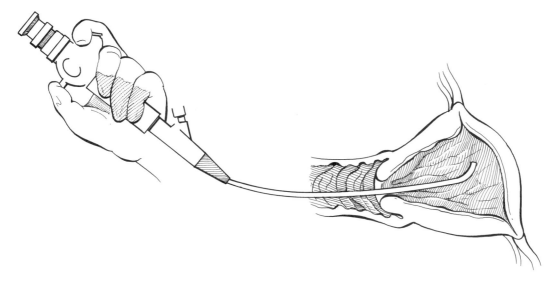

FIG. 9. Office hysteroscopy.

that after the procedure they may experience some uterine cramping or bleeding that should subside within 24 hours.

Transvaginal Ultrasonography

Although there is no substitute for a bimanual pelvic examination, transvaginal ultrasonography may enhance and extend the pelvic examination.[5,6,16] Ultrasound examination cannot replace the physician's physical determination of the mobility and texture of tissues or the presence of tenderness, but it can provide objective confirmation of the size, shape, and location of pelvic organs. The introduction

of lightweight, mobile machines with 5- and 7.5-MHz probes has made office-based ultrasonography a valuable diagnostic technique. Compared with other methods of imaging, ultrasonography is unsurpassed in safety and in providing inexpensive images.

Office-based ultrasonography can be helpful in the following situations:

◊ Evaluating pelvic masses,
◊ Monitoring follicular growth in response to ovulation-inducing drugs,
◊ Diagnosing and sizing uterine leiomyomata,
◊ Differentiating intrauterine from ectopic pregnancies,

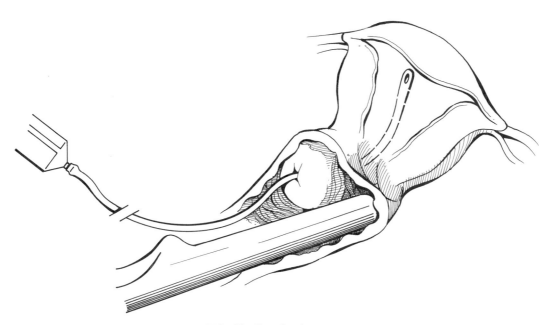

FIG. 10. Sonohysterogram.

◊ Diagnosing pelvic abscesses,
◊ Evaluating the endometrium in women with abnormal uterine bleeding.

A suboptimal examination or confusion resulting from artifacts may have serious consequences, however. The ultrasound image is only as good and useful as the clinical skills used to relate the sonographic findings to the clinical situation under evaluation.

A variation of pelvic ultrasonography is sonohysterography, in which a clear fluid is infused into the uterus while a vaginal ultrasound examination is performed[4,10] (Fig. 10). This technique is a useful adjunct and a less costly alternative to office hysteroscopy in women with abnormal uterine bleeding, Asherman syndrome, and infertility. It can reliably detect irregularities of the endometrium caused by adhesions or polyps but cannot distinguish hyperplasia from neoplasia.

A pelvic examination and baseline vaginal ultrasound examination are performed to evaluate mobility, size, and position of the pelvic organs. A pregnancy test is done if there is any suspicion of pregnancy. The cervix is cleansed with povidone-iodine or another antiseptic solution and a 5.0- to 5.3-French catheter is introduced with a ring forceps into the cervix. H/S Catheter Set for Hysterosalpinography (Ackrad Laboratories, Inc., Cramford, NJ) is commonly used. The speculum is removed, and the ultrasound probe reintroduced into the vagina. Sterile saline is then slowly infused from either a 30- to 60-ml syringe or a bag while the uterus is scanned from cornu to cornu and from the external cervical os to the fundus. Not only can intrauterine lesions be seen, but tubal patency can be ascertained by observing the accumulation of fluid in the cul-de-sac.

SUMMARY POINTS

◊ An effective history and examination require that physicians understand why patients are seeking medical care.
◊ A thorough gynecologic history and examination should include an evaluation of personal health habits and psychosocial issues, including sexuality, abuse, emotional disorders, and drug, alcohol, or tobacco addiction.

◊ A thorough summary of the physician's findings and a discussion of their implications will reduce the patient's anxiety and improve compliance with medial therapies.
◊ Office hysteroscopy and endometrial biopsy are a valuable alternative to dilation and curettage.
◊ Transvaginal ultrasonography may enhance and extend the examination of the pelvis.

◊ REFERENCES

1. American Medical Association. *Diagnostic and treatment guidelines on domestic abuse.* Chicago: American Medical Association, 1995.
2. Austin RM, McLenda WW, eds. College of American Pathologists conference on quality and laboratory issues with the Papanicolaou smear. *Arch Pathol Lab Med* 1997;121:205.
3. Brooks PG, Serden SP. Hysteroscopic findings after unsuccessful dilatation and curettage for abnormal bleeding. *Am J Obstet Gynecol* 1988;158:1354.
4. Chung PH, Parsons AK. A practical guide to using saline infusion sonohysterography. *Contrib Gynecol Obstet* 1997;21
5. Frederick JL, Paulson RJ, Sauer M. Routine use of vaginal ultrasonography in the preoperative evaluation of gynecologic patients. *J Reprod Med* 1991;36:779.
6. Grinfeld L. Ultrasonography in reproductive medicine. *Infertil Reprod Med Clin North Am* 1991;2:643.
7. Heller DS. The Pap smear in identification of inflammatory conditions. *Female Patient* 1997;22:61.
8. Hindle WH. The diagnostic exam. In: Marchant DJ, ed: *Breast disease.* Philadelphia: WB Saunders, 1997:69.
9. Kristensen GB, Holund B, Grinsted P. Efficiency of the cytobrush versus the cotton swab in the collection of endocervical cells. *Acta Cytol* 1989;33:849.
10. Laughead M, Sones LM. Clinical utility of saline solution infusion sonohysterography in a primary care obstetric gynecologic practice. *Am J Obstet Gynecol* 1997;176:1313.
11. Maiman M, Fruchter RG, Clark M, Arrastia CD, Mathews R, Gates EJ. Cervical cancer as an AIDS defining illness. *Obstet Gynecol* 1997;89:76.
12. Mandel JS, Bord JH, Cheirch TR. Reducing mortality from colorectal cancer by screening for fecal occult blood. *N Engl J Med* 1993;328:1365.
13. Munjack DJ, Oziel LI. *Sexual medicine and counseling in office practice: a comprehensive treatment guide.* Boston: Little, Brown and Company, 1980.
14. Nagler F, O'Connor H, Davies A, Badawy A, Mohamed H, Magos A. 2500 outpatient diagnostic hysteroscopies. *Obstet Gynecol* 1996;88:87.
15. Report of the U.S. Preventive Services Task Force. *Guide to clinical preventative services.* Baltimore: Williams & Wilkins, 1996:73.
16. Reuss ML, Kolton S, Tharakan T. Transvaginal ultrasonography in gynecologic office practice: assessment in 663 premenopausal women. *Am J Obstet Gynecol* 1996;175:1189.
17. Rubinow DR. The premenstrual syndrome. *JAMA* 1992;268:1908.
18. Szarewski A, Cuzick J, Nagagam M, Thin RN. A comparison of four cytological sampling techniques in a genitourinary medicine clinic. *Genitourin Med* 1990;66:438.

CHAPTER 33

Ultrasound in Gynecology

◇

Arthur C. Fleischer

There are multiple diagnostic modalities [sonography (US), computed tomography (CT), and magnetic resonance imaging (MRI)] that can be utilized in the evaluation of gynecologic disorders. This chapter emphasizes the use of diagnostic sonography for the initial evaluation of common gynecologic disorders. The roles of magnetic resonance imaging and CT are also included as adjunctive tests in the case of nondiagnostic sonography or as a means to enhance the diagnostic accuracy, particularly in assessing the extent of certain diseases such as endometriosis or neoplasms.

The use of gynecologic sonography has become widespread in both gynecologists' offices and in imaging departments. Its high patient acceptance and relatively low cost make it applicable as an initial means for assessing many gynecologic disorders. Some practitioners have even incorporated transvaginal sonography (TVS) in their routine pelvic assessment, and others use it as a problem solver when a gynecologic disorder is suspected. The TVS is operator dependent, and significant clinical experience with pathoanatomic correlation is required.

In some cases in which pelvic sonography is not diagnostic, however, magnetic resonance imaging (MRI) or computed tomography (CT) can be used to better delineate anatomic abnormalities. These two modalities are available in diagnostic imaging departments and are more costly than TVS. However, their selective use may help improve the diagnostic evaluation, especially in disorders that may have only subtle sonographic findings such as adenomyosis. Both MRI and CT may also be used for staging of certain neoplasms; they are less operator dependent than sonography, and images can be obtained in a variety of scan planes that may not be obtainable with US.

This chapter discusses and illustrates the common uses of these diagnostic modalities in evaluation of a variety of common gynecologic disorders. The subsections are divided according to the most common indications for imaging evaluation of gynecologic disorders. Additional information can be found in several texts that provide more extensive coverage of this topic.[1-4]

◇ SONOGRAPHIC INSTRUMENTATION AND TECHNIQUE

Diagnostic sonography of the pelvic organs can be performed using the transabdominal (TAS) approach in which the uterus and adnexa are imaged through a distended urinary bladder or using transvaginal sonography (TVS), in which the probe is inserted into the vagina for detailed imaging of the uterus and ovaries. The transabdominal approach provides a global depiction of the uterus and adnexa as well as the lower abdomen (Fig. 1). It is best performed as a survey of the pelvic organs, although it is limited by body habitus and overlying bowel or fat. In general, TAS is best utilized for large masses such as fibroid uteri that extend out of the pelvis. The ovaries of some women can be better imaged transabdominally through a fully distended bladder than with a transvaginal probe, in particular those that are anteriorly located. Transvaginal color Doppler sonography affords assessment of flow to and within the uterus and ovaries. It can also be helpful as a means for anatomic distinction between ovarian and uterine masses as well as for the assessment of their vascularity.

Transabdominal sonography affords global depiction of the pelvis and its organs. It should be performed utilizing a distended urinary bladder, which acts to displace bowel superiorly out of the pelvis. However, anatomic detail using transabdominal sonography may be limited by subcutaneous and pelvic fat, which increases artifact and scatters the incident ultrasound beam. Transabdominal sonography is typically performed with a linear or curved linear array transducer operating at 3.5 MHz. The focus should be appropriately set at the level of the uterus and ovaries. Images can be obtained in the sagittal and transverse planes as well as some oblique planes. The real-time capability of TAS is important in assessment of peristaltic bowel and other processes that involve motion such as ureteral jets within the urinary bladder.

The orientation on the screen for TVS is best displayed with the apex of the image at the top of the monitor. However, some prefer the apex image at the bottom. Either way,

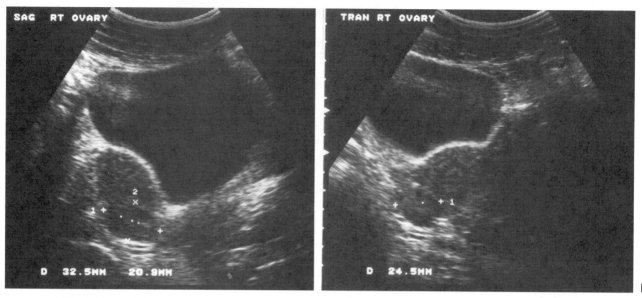

FIG. 1. Transabdominal sonography (TAS). **(A)** Parasagittal image through right adnexal region showing right ovary (between *cursors*) and normal uterus. **(B)** Same as in **A** in the transverse plane showing the transverse dimension of the right ovary (between *cursors*).

the examiner should annotate on the image the orientation of the scan plane and the structures that are being imaged.

The TVS provides more detailed evaluation of the uterus and adnexa than transabdominal sonography. It begins with images of the uterus as the central pelvic landmark in both long and short axis. The operator can then orient the probe into the adnexal regions using the internal iliac vein as a landmark for delineation of the ovarian fossa. There is much variation in the location of the ovaries, particularly in women who have undergone hysterectomy. The probe can be withdrawn into the midvagina and directed anteriorly to provide short-axis views of a uterus that is anteflexed. The retroflexed uterus is easily imaged without major manipulation of the probe because it is in the anatomic plane of the vagina. The operator can use one hand to mildly compress the abdominal wall and evaluate the mobility of these organs. If there are no adhesions, the uterus and ovaries should move smoothly away from each other as the probe is advanced. This has been termed the "sliding organ sign" and, if absent, may suggest the presence of adhesions.[5]

Transvaginal sonography can be performed with a variety of probes including curvilinear, electronic steered, and mechanical sector transducers (Fig. 2). Most transvaginal probes operate at a high frequency, allowing detailed evaluation within the first 10 cm of the field of view. After the probe is wiped with a disinfectant, it should be covered by a condom before insertion. For best patient comfort, the probe should be inserted into the vagina over the operator's fingers, which gently depress the posterior introitus.

The most commonly used TVS probe configurations are those in which transducer elements are rotated (mechanical sector) and those that are made up of multiple send–receive subelements, in which the beam is formed by selective elec-

tronic activation (curvilinear array). The design of the imaging part of the probe, called its "footprint," can also vary according to its size and shape. For most applications, a tightly curved transducer probe that has high line density affords the most detailed image. Transvaginal probes with the smallest footprint and shaft size may be used on postmenopausal women because of the limited distensibility of the vagina.

Hard copy images can be recorded on film, paper, or optical disk. A VCR is needed for videotaping some of the studies involving motion such as sonohysterography. Most scanners are portable. The design of the imaging part of the probe can also vary according to its size and shape. For most applications a tightly curved transducer probe that has high line density affords the most detailed image.

Transvaginal color Doppler sonography (TV-CDS) combines the anatomic information provided by TVS with flow information provided by CDS. This probe and attached equipment are more expensive than the standard transvaginal sonographic scanner. However, TV-CDS can provide additional information that is useful in evaluating some patients with pelvic masses. The TV-CDS involves assessment of flow within the uterus and adnexal structures. The flow to or within a structure can be quantified by analysis of the waveform using either resistive index (RI), which is maximum systolic velocity − minimum systolic velocities, divided by maximum systolic velocity; or the pulsatility index, which is maximum systolic velocity − maximum diastolic velocities, divided by the mean velocity. These parameters are unitless values and angle-independent parameters of relative impedance to forward flow. One must obtain signals between 30° and 60° of the angle of the vessel in order to provide optimal waveforms. Waveforms reflect the change in frequency over time, which is related to velocity. Standard frequency-based color Doppler

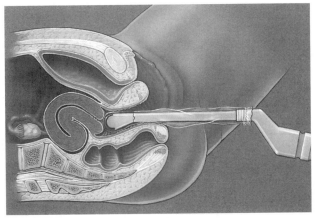

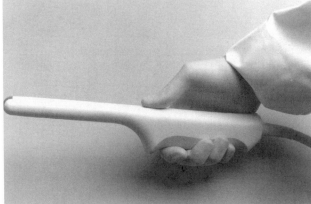

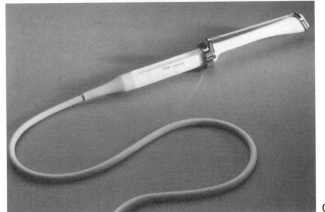

FIG. 2. Transvaginal sonography (TVS). **(A)** Diagram showing transvaginal probe adjacent to cervix in a retroflexed uterus. (Drawing by Paul Gross, MS; This figure is printed in color as Plate 3.) **(B)** Picture of tightly curved curvilinear array transvaginal transducer probe. **(C)** Flat-faced transvaginal probe with needle guide attached to the shaft.

is encoded with red colors indicating flow toward the transducers or blue for away. A new type of processing called amplitude or power Doppler allows determination of overall blood flow. It is more sensitive than frequency based but is degraded by motion.

The technique of TV-CDS is highly operator dependent but can provide important information as to the characterization of blood flow in the uterus and adnexal structures. Depending on the clinical indication, the examination should include evaluation of arterial and venous blood flow to and within the uterus and ovaries. This includes evaluation of the uterine artery and its adnexal branch as well as the main ovarian artery and its branch. Currently there is a range of sensitivity to flow between the scanners from different manufacturers.

◊ ENDOMETRIAL DISEASE

Because of the proximity of the transvaginal probe to the uterus, the endometrium can be accurately depicted in detail in most patients. However, detailed delineation of the endometrium requires the use of proper imaging technique. Because the endometrium is a nongeometric shape, operator error can account for over- or underestimation of its thickness. Thus, it is of the utmost importance to depict the endometrium for measurement purposes in its greatest long-axis plane and maximal thickness in the fundal region, which represents its

bilayer measurement (Fig. 3). The texture of the endometrium (smooth or irregular) should also be determined.

The TVS has an important role in the evaluation of a patient presenting with unexplained uterine bleeding.[6,7] Clinically, it is important to consider the diagnostic possibilities of patients presenting with bleeding in the perimenopausal period as different from those in postmenopausal women. In general, bleeding in premenopausal women is usually associated with anovulation, whereas a variety of pathologies including atrophic endometritis, hyperplasia, and cancer are most common in the postmenopausal woman. In women of childbearing age, the endometrium varies according to the part of the cycle in which they are examined as well as follicular development within the ovary.

In the menstrual phase, the normal endometrium is 3 to 5 mm thick with mildly echogenic texture. As the endometrium develops in the periovulatory period, a multilayered texture can be seen with thicknesses ranging from 5 to 8 mm. The outer echogenic layer represents the basalis, whereas the inner layer is the functionalis. The central echogenic interface is refluxed cervical mucus. In the secretory phase, the endometrium becomes diffusely echogenic and up to 12 to 14 mm in thickness.

In the perimenopausal patient, bleeding is typically associated with anovulatory cycles, endometritis, or uterine fibroids. The effect of fibroids on the endometrium can be assessed by

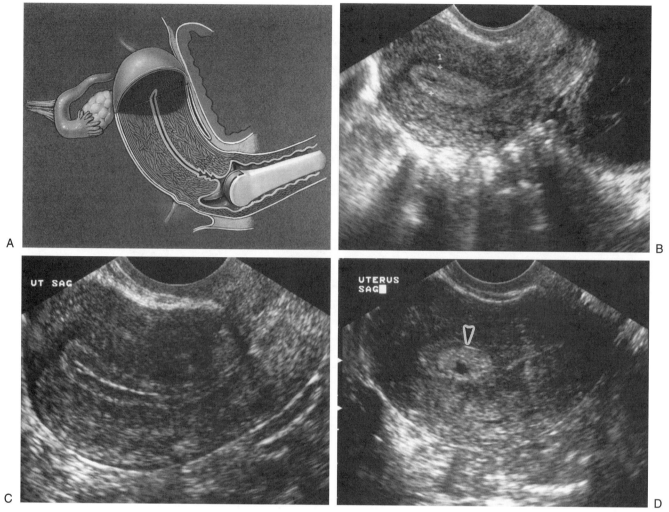

FIG. 3. Endometrial disorders. **(A)** Diagram showing proximity of the endometrium of an anteflexed uterus to the transvaginal probe. The field of view depicting the long axis of the uterus and endometrium is shown. (Drawing by Paul Gross, MS; this figure is printed in color as Plate 4.) **(B)** Transvaginal sonogram showing multilayered endometrium typical of midcycle development. The central echogenic interface represents refluxed mucus, the outer echogenic layer represents basalis, and the inner hypoechoic layer represents functionalis. **(C)** Typical luteal phase endometrium demonstrating increase thickness (between *cursors*) and homogeneous echogenicity. **(D)** Echogenic mass (*arrowhead*) within endometrium containing punctate cystic area representing an endometrial polyp.

their displacement of the endometrium if they are submucosal in location. Endometritis usually produces a thickened endometrium sometimes containing intraluminal fluid. Intraluminal fluid may be seen in postmenopausal women but is usually a benign finding as long as the single-layer thickness of the endometrium is less than 4 mm.

Fibroids disrupt the normal arrangement of the myometrial bundles and are typically hypoechoic or of mixed echogenicity when compared to normal myometrium. Some fibroids contain calcification. The pedicle of a subserosal fibroid can usually be demonstrated during scanning and palpation of the mass relative to the major portion of the uterus. Submucosal fibroids extend into the lumen and typically displace and thin the overlying endometrium. These are best depicted using sonohysterography. Occasionally, fibroids may be present

as solid masses in the adnexal regions, representing either interligamentary or pedunculated varieties.

Transvaginal ultrasound has its greatest role in evaluating peri- or postmenopausal women with unexplained bleeding. In general, endometrial thicknesses less than 5 to 8 mm is normal in nonmedicated postmenopausal women. The actual thickness of the endometrium may be related to body habitus, with larger patients having thicker endometria. The texture of the endometrium is also important to assess because small cystic changes may be found within small polyps or, in patients on tamoxifen, in the subendometrial myometrium layer. In patients with thickened endometrium, TVS can suggest the presence of abnormal histology such as hyperplasia, but it is not histologically specific. Endometrial biopsy or dilation and curettage may be needed for this. The subendometrial area should be assessed in women with endometrial thickening, and if there is irregularity, myometrial invasion might be considered.

Transvaginal ultrasound has a major role in determining which patients should undergo endometrial biopsy. An endometrium less than 5 mm is typical of atrophic endometritis, whereas one greater than 6 mm may represent a variety of abnormal histology.[7] It is emphasized that the endometrium needs to be properly measured because improper scan plane or adjacent fibroids may alter this determination.

The TVS also provides an excellent means of evaluation of patients with unscheduled bleeding who are on hormone replacement. Depending on the regimen used, the endometrial thickness should be less than 8 mm. In some patients who are on combined estrogen/progestin, up to a 3-mm dif-

ference in thickness can be observed depending on when in the "pseudocycle" the patient is imaged.[8] Similarly, patients who take tamoxifen should be serially evaluated by TVS for the presence of endometrial thickening or irregularity because of the increased incidence of hyperplasia and cancer.[9] Some have reported the presence of punctate cystic areas in the inner myometrium of women taking tamoxifen, which may represent reactivated adenomyomas.[10]

Sonohysterography, which involves instillation of saline into the uterine lumen, should be used when there is any suspicion of a polyp or submucosal fibroid on routine TVS (Fig. 4).[11] This technique involves the use of a thin catheter or insemination tube as a means to distend the lumen with saline. Polyps are typically echogenic structures that extend into the

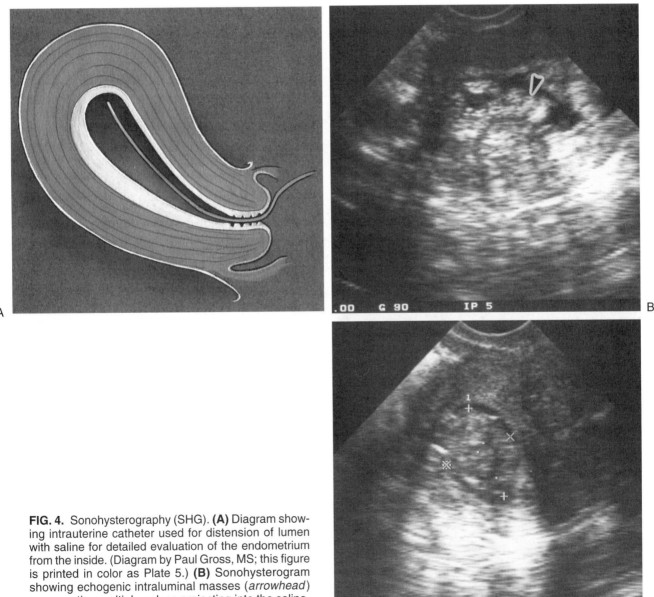

FIG. 4. Sonohysterography (SHG). **(A)** Diagram showing intrauterine catheter used for distension of lumen with saline for detailed evaluation of the endometrium from the inside. (Diagram by Paul Gross, MS; this figure is printed in color as Plate 5.) **(B)** Sonohysterogram showing echogenic intraluminal masses (*arrowhead*) representing multiple polyps projecting into the saline-distended lumen. **(C)** Submucosal fibroid (*cursors*) displacing overlying endometrium.

lumen, whereas submucosal fibroids are usually hypoechoic. The procedure has high patient acceptance and should be performed in the follicular phase of the cycle. In infertility patients, the procedure can detect uterine synechia, which may be associated with infertility. Synechia appear as echogenic thin interfaces that course between the two endometrial layers.

Endometrial cancer may be considered when the endometrium has marked thickening and irregular texture. Most studies report that endometrial cancer is associated with marked thickening over 9 to 10 mm.[6] One may detect the possibility of invasion by evaluation of the hypoechoic interface representing the inner myometrium.[12] Invasive tumors usually distort this layer. In equivocal or difficult cases, contrast-enhanced MRI can be used as a secondary means for further evaluation of myometrial involvement.

◊ PELVIC MASS

Transabdominal and transvaginal sonography provides a means to evaluate the location, internal consistency, and associated disorders in patients with a pelvic mass (Fig. 5). Larger pelvic masses (over 10 cm) may best be delineated using a transabdominal approach. The TVS provides important information about the location of the pelvic mass relative to the ovary and uterus. Color Doppler sonography is a secondary test to assess the vascularity in cases of possible torsion or assessment of the benign or malignant character of a mass.

A general outline of diagnostic considerations according to location and internal consistency is shown in Table 1.

Physiological cysts demonstrate a smooth wall and no internal septations. Their location within the ovary can usually

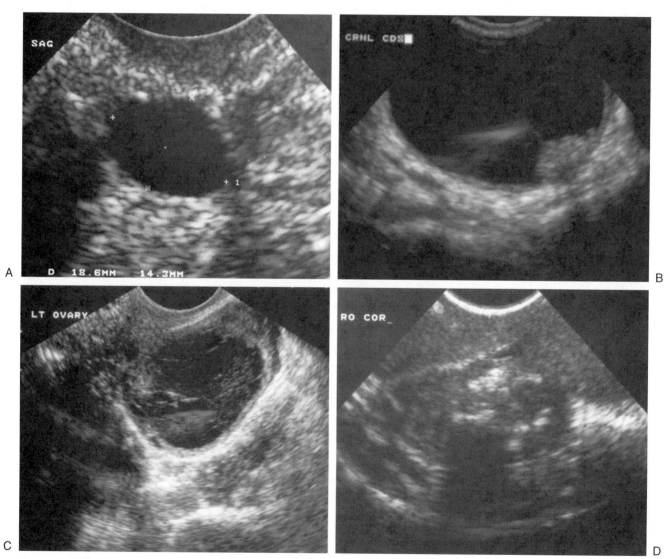

FIG. 5. Pelvic masses. **(A)** Transvaginal sonogram of smooth-walled cyst (between *cursors*) exhibiting the sonographic features of benignity. **(B)** Hemorrhagic corpus luteum with organized hemorrhage containing thin fibrin strands and internal echoes within the mass. **(C)** Papillary excrescence arising from the wall of a mostly cystic ovarian mass. This morphologic feature is highly suggestive of cancer. **(D)** Mass containing several echogenic foci and solid areas indicative of a dermoid cyst.

TABLE 1. *Differential diagnoses of pelvic masses by TAS and TVS*

Location	Internal consistency		
	Cystic	Complex	Solid
Ovarian	Physiological cyst Neoplastic cysts	Dermoid cysts Neoplastic cysts Hermorrhagic cysts Tuboovarian abscess	Metastases Solid ovarian tumors Fibroma
Adnexal Extraovarian	Paraovarian cyst Hydrosalpinx	Endometrioma	Tubal tumor
Uterine Other	Developmental cyst	Degenerated fibroid Arteriovenous malformation Diverticulosis Complicated appendicitis	Pedunculated fibroid Bowel tumor Lymphadenopathy

be documented by TVS. This technique has an important application in postmenopausal asymptomatic women because up to 15% in one series have been shown to have cysts. These cysts may enlarge or regress over a 6-month to 1-year period.[13] Their probability of malignancy can be assessed using laboratory tests such as CA-125.

In the pre- and perimenopausal women, it is important to differentiate cystic masses that may spontaneously regress related to physiological changes from those that continually enlarge. Hemorrhagic corpus luteum cysts typically exhibit thin fibrin strands of echogenic material within a mostly hypoechoic mass contained by a somewhat thick and irregular wall. Low-impedance flow is typical of hemorrhagic corpora lutea. On the other hand, the presence of a papillary excrescence or irregular and thickened internal septations usually is associated with ovarian tumors. The morphologic findings of early ovarian cancers can be subtle, but persistent internal irregularity within a mass in a patient with risk factors suggests the possibility of malignancy.

Although the sonographic morphology of the mass is typically nonspecific, there are a few patterns that demonstrate relatively high specificity. One of these is the "ground glass" appearance of an endometrioma that contains organized clot. The other is the echogenic focus or region seen within typical dermoid cysts. In some dermoid cysts, echoes arising from the hair ball can be shown. With improved resolution, it is not uncommon to see small dermoid cysts that appear as echogenic regions within a normal ovary. If a dermoid cyst is

found in one ovary, it is important to evaluate the contralateral ovary carefully because approximately 15% of patients have bilateral dermoid cysts.

The TV-CDS provides an adjunctive evaluation of patients with pelvic masses to determine potential of malignancy (Table 2). For best results, the TV-CDS findings need to be correlated with morphologic and clinical findings. Although the technique has some limitations, it is helpful in preoperative assessment of patients with pelvic masses. Depending on the patient population in a series, diagnostic accuracies in the 80% to 90% range have been reported.[14,15] Admittedly, there is some overlap of impedance values in some functional ovarian cysts and tumors. Even so, in the proper clinical setting, TV-CDS improves confidence in the differentiation of benign from malignant lesions over that possible with TVS alone.[16]

Malignant lesions tend to have abnormally low-impedance flow, a sign of decreased vascular impedance seen in tumor vessels (Fig. 6). In general, malignancies tend to have low-impedance flow with clusters of vessels in morphologically abnormal areas. The test has better sensitivity in the postmenopausal age group because nonmalignant masses such as those caused by pelvic inflammatory disease or endometriosis, as well as hemorrhagic corpra lutea, may demonstrate low-impedance flow.

When combined with TVS for assessment of morphologic abnormalities, TV-CDS has been shown to have an important role in evaluation of women with risk factors for ovarian cancer. Its incorporation in programs for early detection provides

TABLE 2. *Sonographic features of benign and malignant pelvic masses*

	Benign		Malignant	
	TVS	CDS	TVS	CDS
U.S. morphology	Smooth walled, anechoic		Papillary excrescences, mural nodules, irregular solid areas	
CDS				
Vasculature		Regularly spaced		Irregularly spaced, clustered
Impedance		High		Low
Velocity		Low		High
Size change	Regress or no change		Progress or no change	
Other findings	No ascites; no liver, masses, or lymphadenopathy		Ascites; no liver, masses, or lymphadenopathy	

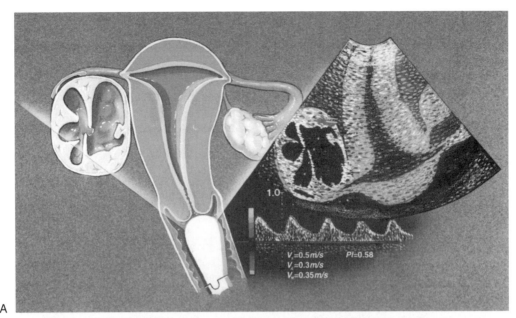

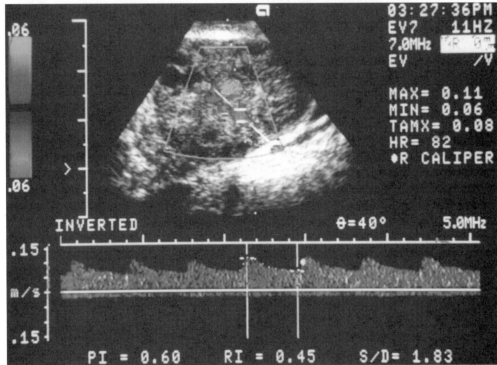

FIG. 6. Transvaginal color Doppler sonography (TV-CDS). **(A)** Diagram showing the components of a transvaginal color Doppler sonogram, which include real-time imaging, display of vessels, with subsequent selection of sample volume for Doppler analysis by evaluation of the Doppler waveform (drawing by Paul Gross, MS). **(B)** Transvaginal color Doppler sonogram showing low-impedance flow (R.I. = 0.45; P.I. = 0.60) within the wall of a corpus luteum. **(C)** Amplitude color Doppler image of hemorrhagic corpus luteum showing no flow within the center of the mass, which contained organized clot. **(D)** Complex mass with low-impedance arterial and increased venous flow within an irregular solid area, highly indicative of ovarian cancer. (These figures are printed in color as Plates 6 through 9.)

a means for detection of tumors in their earliest stages.[14] The major limiting factor in screening for ovarian cancer is its low prevalence. Improved identification of women with risk factors and combining ovarian with endometrial assessment should improve the effectiveness of early detection efforts.

Some studies report the detection of ovarian or endometrial cancer as two per 1000 women screened.[17,18] The data from studies that include large numbers of patients followed over several years will answer questions concerning the efficacy of screening.

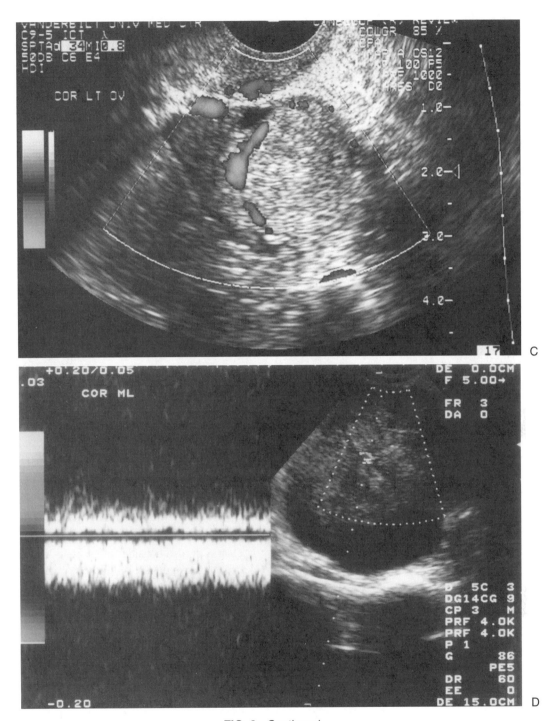

FIG. 6. *Continued.*

◊ PELVIC PAIN

Transvaginal ultrasound has an important role in evaluating patients with pelvic pain (Fig. 7). The TVS can detect ovarian enlargement and the presence of multiple immature follicles in the peripheral part of the ovary typically seen in ovarian torsion. Color Doppler sonography provides added diagnostic assessment to determine the presence of abnormal or normal flow to the ovary. Because venous flow seems to be first affected by torsion, CDS is helpful in determining its presence or absence in an enlarged ovary.[19,20] Absence of venous flow suggests the possibility of torsion in properly performed color Doppler examination. One should be aware that errors in selecting gray scale/color priority settings might erroneously lead one to a diagnosis of torsion. It is therefore important to examine flow in both adnexa to confirm that the absence of flow is a real finding. The CDS findings in ovarian torsion also will depend on the completeness and chronicity of this disorder. Flow within the feeding vessels usually can be detected even though torsion is present. The

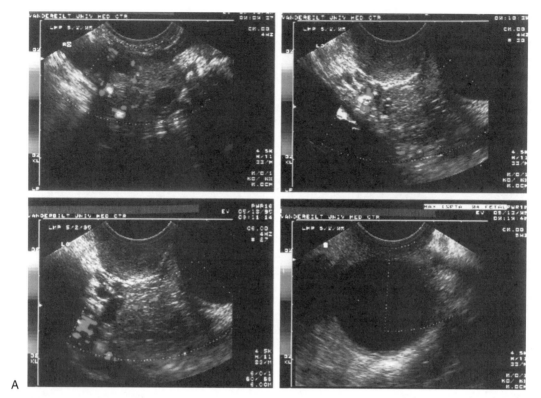

A

FIG. 7. Pelvic pain. **(A)** Composite transvaginal sonogram showing enlarged left ovary (**top right** and **bottom left**) without flow and associated with a paraovarian cyst in left adnexa (**lower right**). The right ovary (**top left**) was normal, showing intraparenchymal flow. The left adnexa was found to be twisted times 3 and was surgically untwisted with good result. (This figure is printed in color as Plate 10.) **(B)** Doppler sonogram of enlarged left ovary containing venous flow. This finding suggests potential viability of this partial ovarian torsion. **(C)** Irregular echogenic area within myometrium suggestive of adenomyosis. **(D)** Sagittal T_2-weighted MR confirming the presence of adenomyosis in the fundal region.

CDS also can be used to confirm the reestablishment of flow after detorsion.

Isolated torsion of the tube is an uncommon disorder. It may be seen in patients who have undergone bilateral tubal ligation. The CDS demonstrates a fusiform structure separate from the ovary that has absent or reversed diastolic flow.

One of the most common causes of pelvic pain is a hemorrhagic cyst. The hemorrhagic component typically demonstrates no flow, whereas the surrounding normal ovary demonstrates arterial and venous flow. Endometriomas may demonstrate various waveforms depending on when the patient is examined. In the menstrual phase, low-impedance flow may be seen as an indication of active hemorrhage within the mass, whereas in other parts of the cycle an endometrioma may demonstrate high-impedance flow because of the presence of organized clot.

Adenomyosis may produce subtle findings on TVS. These include irregular echogenic areas in the subendometrial myometrium. Rarely, actual cystic spaces within the myometrium are seen. The vascularity associated with adenomyosis is diffuse relative to that of a fibroid, which demonstrates peripheral-rim-type flow. Contrast-enhanced MRI can be used to document the presence of adenomyosis.[21]

One must also consider other nongynecologic causes of pain such as appendicitis and renal calculi in evaluating women with this condition. On TVS, appendicitis typically demonstrates a fusiform noncompressible structure in the right lower quadrant that has a thickened (over 6 mm) wall. The best approach for evaluating possible appendicitis is using transabdominal sonography while providing gentle continued pressure on the abdomen. If there is rupture, fluid surrounding the abnormal appendix can be seen. In the acute phases, increased blood flow can be seen around the appendix. The TVS also can localize renal calculi in the distal ureter at the ureteral pelvic junction in some patients.[22] The ureteral jet is seen clearly on CDS, and echogenic structures in the distal ureter can be seen clearly at the base of the bladder.

◊ **INFERTILITY**

Transvaginal ultrasound provides important information in the evaluation of the infertile patient (Fig. 8). This includes serial assessment of follicular maturity as well as evaluation of the thickness and texture of endometrium. The number of follicles and their relative size can be determined, with

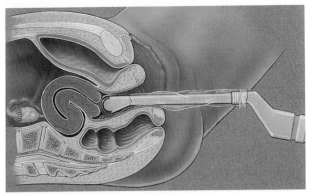

PLATE 3. Transvaginal sonography (TVS). Diagram showing transvaginal probe adjacent to cervix in a retroflexed uterus (drawing by Paul Gross, MS). (This plate is printed in black and white as Figure 33-2A.)

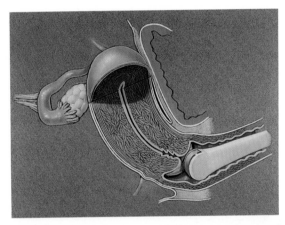

PLATE 4. Endometrial disorders. Diagram showing proximity of the endometrium of an anteflexed uterus to the transvaginal probe. The field of view depicting the long axis of the uterus and endometrium is shown (drawing by Paul Gross, MS). (This plate is printed in black and white as Figure 33-3A.)

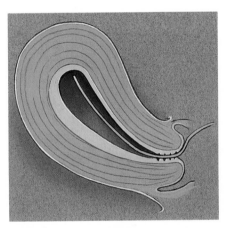

PLATE 5. Sonohysterography (SHG). Diagram showing intrauterine catheter used for distension of lumen with saline for detailed evaluation of the endometrium from the inside (diagram by Paul Gross, MS). (This plate is printed in black and white as Figure 33-4A.)

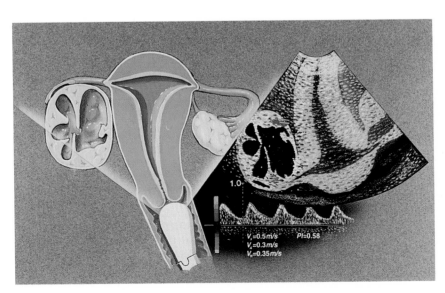

PLATE 6. Transvaginal color Doppler sonography (TV-CDS). Diagram showing the components of a transvaginal color Doppler sonogram, which include real-time imaging, display of vessels, with subsequent selection of sample volume for Doppler analysis by evaluation of the Doppler waveform (drawing by Paul Gross, MS). (This plate is printed in black and white as Figure 33-6A.)

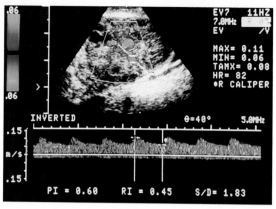

PLATE 7. Transvaginal color Doppler sonography (TV-CDS). Transvaginal color Doppler sonogram showing low-impedance flow (R.I. = 0.45; P.I. = 0.60) within the wall of a corpus luteum. (This plate is printed in black and white as Figure 33-6B.)

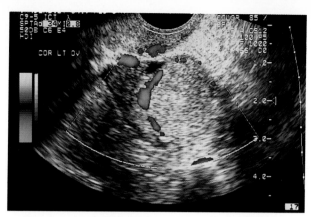

PLATE 8. Transvaginal color Doppler sonography (TV-CDS). Amplitude color Doppler image of hemorrhagic corpus luteum showing no flow within the center of the mass, which contained organized clot. (This plate is printed in black and white as Figure 33-6C.)

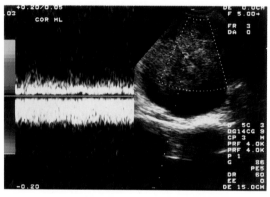

PLATE 9. Transvaginal color Doppler sonography (TV-CDS). Complex mass with low-impedance arterial and increased venous flow within an irregular solid area, highly indicative of ovarian cancer. (This plate is printed in black and white as Figure 33-6D.)

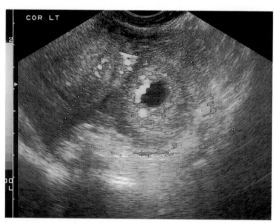

PLATE 11. Ectopic pregnancy. Transvaginal color Doppler sonogram showing vascularity of "tubal ring" of an unruptured ectopic pregnancy. (This plate is printed in black and white as Figure 33-10B.)

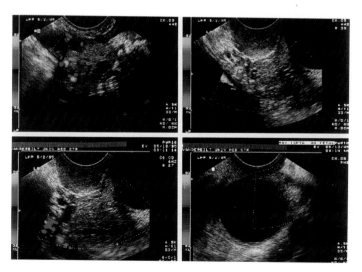

PLATE 10. Pelvic pain. Composite transvaginal sonogram showing enlarged left ovary (top right and bottom left) without flow and associated with a paraovarian cyst in left adnexa (lower right). The right ovary (top left) was normal, showing intraparenchymal flow. The left adnexa was found to be twisted times 3 and was surgically untwisted with good result. (This plate is printed in black and white as Figure 33-7A.)

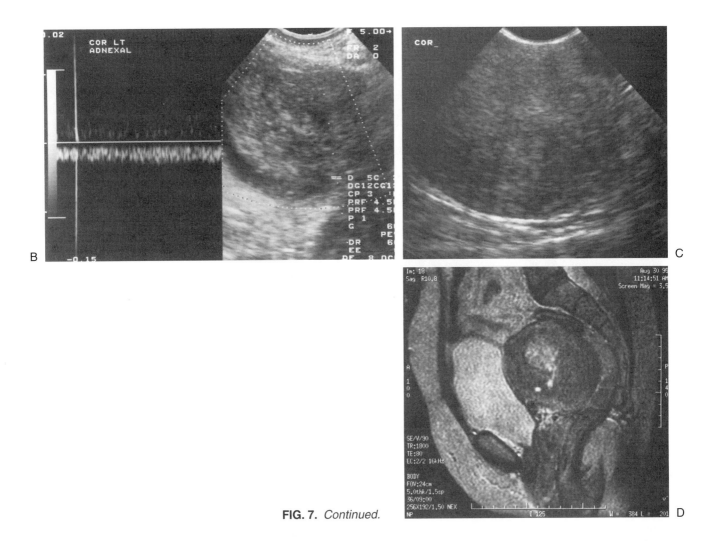

FIG. 7. *Continued.*

FIG. 8. Infertility. **(A)** Mature follicle (between *cursors*) containing a small protrusion from the posterior wall representing the cumulus oophorus. **(B)** Image taken during follicular aspiration showing echogenic needle tip within deflating mature follicle.

mature follicles measuring between 18 and 20 mm and favorable endometrial thicknesses in the periovulatory period between 7 and 11 mm. The multilayered appearance also has been associated with higher rates of implantation.

◊ SONOGRAPHICALLY GUIDED PROCEDURES

The TVS can provide real-time delineation of the location of a needle relative to the area of interest (Fig. 9). For this purpose, a needle guide is attached to the shaft of the probe, which confines the needle course to a prescribed path. This technique can be utilized in follicular aspiration as well as the aspiration of cystic masses. Peritoneal cysts and ovarian remnants as well as tuboovarian abscesses may be drained utilizing this approach. Some have advocated needle aspiration of endometriomas in patients who have had previous surgery.

Transrectal sonography can be used for guided dilation and curettage in patients whose cervix cannot be identified on visual examination. The position of the dilator relative to the external cervical os can be seen. Once the dilator is through the os, transabdominal sonography may be utilized for location within the uterus. Similarly, TAS can be used to identify the location of a uterine tandem used for radiation therapy.

◊ ECTOPIC PREGNANCY

Transvaginal sonography provides an accurate means for detection of ectopic pregnancy (Fig. 10). On TVS, this condition should be suspected in the presence of a rounded structure separate from the ovary in patients in whom an intrauterine pregnancy cannot be detected. The "tubal ring" is an indication of an unruptured ectopic pregnancy when not associated with surrounding fluid. Another finding associated with ectopic pregnancy is echogenic intraperitoneal fluid. One should be able to differentiate a corpus luteum from an ectopic embryo in that the corpus luteum can be traced to be within the outline of the ovary.

Color Doppler sonography may provide an additional means for delineation of ectopic pregnancies.[23] The CDS provides a vascular "road map" separating ovarian from other adnexal structures. The vascularity of ectopic pregnancies varies from hypovascular to hypervascular, and there are no specific waveforms that arise from ectopics. A waveform showing

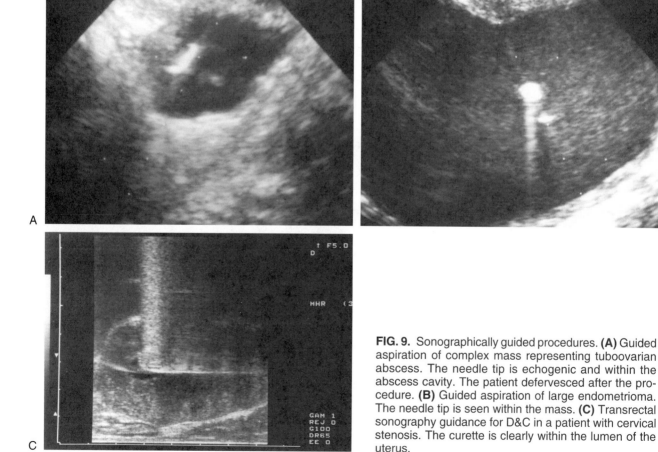

FIG. 9. Sonographically guided procedures. **(A)** Guided aspiration of complex mass representing tuboovarian abscess. The needle tip is echogenic and within the abscess cavity. The patient defervesced after the procedure. **(B)** Guided aspiration of large endometrioma. The needle tip is seen within the mass. **(C)** Transrectal sonography guidance for D&C in a patient with cervical stenosis. The curette is clearly within the lumen of the uterus.

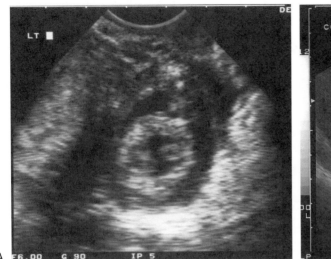
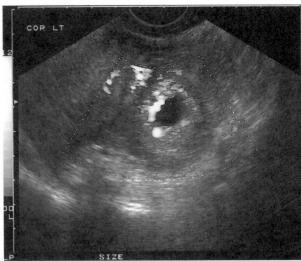

FIG. 10. Ectopic pregnancy. **(A)** Unruptured ectopic pregnancy appearing as a "tubal ring" in left adnexa. **(B)** Transvaginal color Doppler sonogram showing vascularity of "tubal ring" of an unruptured ectopic pregnancy. (This figure is printed in color as Plate 11.)

reversed diastolic flow is seen in ectopics with necrotic trophoblastic tissue.

◊ OTHER IMAGING MODALITIES

Magnetic resonance imaging is an excellent modality for secondary evaluation of a variety of pelvic disorders.[2] These include adenomyosis, endometriosis, and certain pelvic masses such as dermoid cysts. The MRI provides global depiction of pelvic structures in selectable imaging planes, and it can detect lymphadenopathy associated with tumors. Enhanced MRI can also be helpful in assessing the extent of myometrial invasion in patients with endometrial cancer.

Computed tomographic scanning is particularly helpful in the evaluation of the bony pelvis and has improved resolution and reduced scan times by using spiral scanning. Either MRI or CT may be used to delineate intraabdominal abscesses.

The use of sonographic contrast seems promising as a means to evaluate tubal patency with TVS.[24] This is usually performed after sonohysterography, which results in fluid surrounding the ovary. The escape of echogenic contrast out of the frimbriated end of the tube is readily apparent in women with patent tubes.

◊ SUMMARY

This chapter provides an overview of the common applications of pelvic sonography. Pelvic sonography is the initial diagnostic modality of choice in most cases, whereas secondary tests such as color Doppler sonography (CDS), magnetic resonance imaging, and CT scanning provide a means to further enhance diagnostic specificity in difficult or nondiagnostic US studies.

◊ REFERENCES

1. Fleischer A, Javitt M, Jeffery B. *Clinical gynecology.* Philadelphia: Lippincott–Raven, 1997.
2. Hricak H. *MRI of pelvis.* London: Martin Dunitz, 1996.
3. Smelka R, Reinhold C, Ascher S. *MRI of abdomen and pelvis.* New York: Wiley, 1997.
4. Thurman A, Jones M, Cohen D. *Gynecologic obstetric and breast imaging.* Baltimore: Williams & Wilkins, 1997.
5. Timor-Tritsch I. *Transvaginal sonography.* New York: Elsevier, 1988:24.
6. Granberg G, Karlsson B, Wikland M, Grill B. Transvaginal sonography of uterine and endometrial disorders. In: Fleischer A, ed. *Sonography in ob/gyn: principles and practice* Stamford, CT: Appleton & Lange, 1996:851–868.
7. Goldstein SR, Nachtigall M, Snyder JR, et al. Endometrial assessment by vaginal ultrasonography before endometrial sampling in patients with postmenopausal bleeding. *Am J Obstet Gynecol* 1990;163:119.
8. Levine D, Gosink B, Johnson L. Change in endometrial thickness in postmenopausal women undergoing hormone replacement therapy. *Radiology* 1995;197:603.
9. Hann LE, Giess CS, Bach AM, et al. Endometrial thickness in tamoxifen-treated patients: correlation with clinical and pathologic findings. *Am J Roentgenol* 1997;168:657–661.
10. Goldstein SR. Unusual ultrasonographic appearance of the uterus in patients receiving tamoxifen. *Am J Obstet Gynecol* 1994;170:447–451.
11. Parsons A, Lense J. Sonohysterography for endometrial abnormalities: Preliminary results. *J Clin Ultrasound* 1993;21:87.
12. Fleischer A, Dudley B, Entman S, et al. Myometrial invasion: sonographic assessment. *Radiology* 1987;162:307–310.
13. Levine D, Gosink B, Wolf S, Feldesman M, Pretorius D. Simple adnexal cysts: the natural history in postmenopausal women. *Radiology* 1992;184:653–659.
14. Fleischer A, Cullinan J, Peery C, Jones H. Early detection of ovarian carcinoma with transvaginal color Doppler ultrasonography. *Am J Obstet Gynecol* 1996;174:101–106.
15. Kurjak A, Mladen P. New scoring system for prediction of ovarian malignancy based on transvaginal color Doppler sonography. *J Ultrasound Med* 1992;11:631–638.
16. Buy JN, Ghossain MA, Hugol D, et al. Characterization of adnexal masses: combination of color Doppler and conventional sonography compared with spectral Doppler analysis alone and conventional sonography alone. *Am J Roentgenol* 1996;166:385–393.
17. Kurjak A, Shalan H, Kupesic S, et al. An attempt to screen asymptomatic women for ovarian and endometrial cancer with transvaginal color and pulsed Doppler sonography. *J Ultrasound Med* 1994;13:295–301.

18. Schulman H, Conway C, Zalud I, Farmakides G, Haley J, Cassata M. Prevalence in a volunteer population of pelvic cancer detected with transvaginal ultrasound and color flow Doppler. *Ultrasound Obstet Gynecol* 1994;4:414–420.

19. Fleischer A, Kepple D. *Transvaginal sonography: A text atlas, 2nd ed.* Philadelphia: Lippincott–Raven, 1995.

20. Fleischer A, Stein S, Cullinan J, Warner M. Color Doppler sonography of adnexal torsion. *J Ultrasound Med* 1995;14:523–528.

21. Rheinhold C, McCarthy S, et al. Diffuse adenomyosis: comparison of endovaginal US and MR imaging with histopathologic correlation. *Radiology* 1996;199:151–158.

22. Laing F, Benson C, DiSalvo D. Distal ureteral calculus detection with vaginal US. *Radiology* 1994;192:545.

23. Emerson DS, Cartier MS, Altieri LA, et al. Diagnostic efficacy of endovaginal, color Doppler flow imaging in an ectopic pregnancy screening program. *Radiology* 1992;183:413–420.

24. Fleischer AC, Vasquez JM, Cullinan JA, Eisenberg E. Sonohysterography combined with sonosalpingography: correlation with endoscopic findings in infertility patients. *J Ultrasound Med* 1997;16: 381–384.

25. Wolf SI, Gosink BB, Feldesman MR, et al. Prevalence of simple adnexal cysts in postmenopausal women. *Radiology* 1991;180:65–71.

CHAPTER 34

Pediatric and Adolescent Gynecology

◊

Paula J. Adams Hillard

Pediatric and adolescent gynecology are frequently viewed as a single focused aspect of gynecology. In fact, these two areas are reasonably distinct, with the logical dividing date of menarche. Premenarchal girls differ from menarchal adolescents in anatomy, etiologies of similar symptoms, and the spectrum of likely and common syndromes. In addition, they require a different approach to patient management in both the office and the operating room. However, one common feature that is frequently neglected by the adult gynecologist is the need to involve a parent, parents, or other adult caretakers in the care. In this chapter, the two foci of pediatric and adolescent gynecology are addressed separately, although where relevant, the differences between premenarchal (or sometimes prepubertal) girls and adolescents, as well as the differences between these young women and older women, are addressed and highlighted.

◊ PEDIATRIC GYNECOLOGY

Infancy

The obstetrician/gynecologist in training should be encouraged to observe the normal genitalia of the female infants that he/she delivers. Under the influence of maternal estrogens, the labia are generous in size, and the hymen is prominent and fimbriated or redundant in appearance. The female infant will often experience an estrogen-withdrawal bleeding episode within several days after birth. Mothers should be informed of this normal phenomenon in an effort to preclude maternal anxiety and even unnecessary visits to the pediatric emergency department. In a series of pediatric patients seen in the emergency department of our Children's Hospital for vaginal bleeding, the vast majority of those under the age of 2 were seen for this indication. These ED visits are completely avoidable through parental education.

Observation of the female infants' genitalia at birth allows the detection of various developmental and congenital abnormalities, some of which may be life-threatening. Chromo-

somal abnormalities, enzyme deficiencies (including 17- or 21-hydroxylase deficiency as causes of congenital adrenal hyperplasia), and prenatal masculinization of a female fetus resulting from maternal androgen-secreting ovarian tumors or, rarely, drug exposures can all result in genital abnormalities. The etiology of these problems, as well as intersex disorders that may be discovered in an older child, can be complex. This situation of ambiguous genitalia represents a social and potential medical emergency that is best handled by a team of specialists, which may include urologists, neonatologists, endocrinologists, and pediatric gynecologists. The parents should be informed that the baby's genitals are not fully developed and, therefore, a simple examination of the external genitalia cannot determine the actual sex. The parents should be told that data would be collected but that it may take several days to determine the baby's intended sex.

One additional benefit of an observation of female infants' genitalia at the time of birth is the early diagnosis of genital anomalies such as an imperforate hymen (which can be seen with a resultant mucocele, a collection of vaginal mucus behind the thin hymenal membrane), vaginal agenesis, vaginal septum, or hymenal anomalies such as bands. Hymenal abnormalities occur in <1% of newborn females. Normal hymenal variations include hymenal bumps, ridges, or bands; imperforate or cribriform configurations are rare. If there is any doubt about hymenal patency, a rectal thermometer may be used to gently test it. Obstructive lesions including imperforate hymen, vaginal agenesis, or vaginal septa may result in hematometra or hematocolpos with resultant pain or even, rarely, urinary tract obstruction after menarche. These problems can be avoided with surgical correction, most appropriately timed after the onset of puberty and estrogenic stimulation of the genital tract but before the development of symptoms of obstruction, which may also result in endometriosis. Care must also be taken to delineate the exact anatomic nature of the obstruction; opening a thin imperforate hymen is a relatively easy surgical procedure, whereas the correction of other types of obstructive lesions such as vaginal septa requires careful planning. Magnetic resonance imaging performed in pubertal individuals is currently felt to provide the most information about the precise anatomy of these obstructive lesions.

Labial agglutination may occur during the first few years of life as a result of chronic vulvar irritation. The treatment consists of a short course of externally applied estrogen cream for several weeks. The area of agglutination will become thin and may spontaneously separate or can easily be separated in the office with the use of topical lidocaine jelly or EMLA cream. Attention must be given to the prevention of subsequent adhesions, as they clearly have a risk of recurring. One option is to recommend the use of a topical emollient, such as vitamin A and D ointment, to prevent the labia from adhering to one another. This topical treatment should be continued until there are signs of endogenous estrogen production (breast budding). With pubertal development and estrogen stimulation, the risk of recurrence becomes vanishingly small.

Vulvar Anatomy and Bacteriology

In the prepubertal child, the labia minora are thin, and the vaginal orifice is in close proximity to the anus (Figs. 1 and 2). The unestrogenized vulva and vestibule normally appear mildly erythematous and may appear to be infected; in addition, they are quite sensitive to chemical irritants. Smegma around and beneath the prepuce resembles patches of candidal vulvitis to the inexperienced examiner. The normal vaginal bacterial ecology has not been well defined, although the normal flora do differ from the flora found in the well-estrogenized vaginas of postmenarchal women. Several studies attempting to define the normal flora do not separately characterize the subjects by

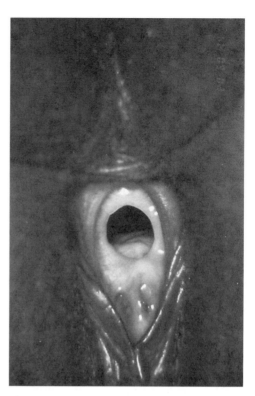

FIG. 2. Colposcopic photograph (10×) of a 7-year-old girl shows an annular hymen, with tissues present all the way around the vaginal opening. (From Pokorny SF. *Pediatric and adolescent gynecology*. New York: Chapman and Hall, 1996.)

estrogen status. Anaerobes predominate among the vaginal microflora of prepubertal girl.[13] Once a child is out of diapers, candidal infections are uncommon.

Vulvovaginitis is the most common cause of vulvar symptoms in the prepubertal age group. The physical proximity of the vagina and vulva to the anus can result in overgrowth of enteric bacteria that can cause a primary vulvitis and a secondary vaginitis. Vaginal foreign bodies are another source of bacterial overgrowth and often produce a blood-tinged or bloody purulent discharge. The most common foreign body in young children is a small piece or pieces of toilet paper, although a curious child can place any number of different small objects within the vagina.[19]

It is often difficult for a young child to describe vulvar sensations. Parents may note that the child cries during urination, scratches herself, or touches herself frequently. Often, the child's pediatrician will have evaluated the child for UTI and pinworms. Vulvovaginal complaints of any sort in a young child should prompt the consideration of possible sexual abuse. Sensitive but direct questioning of the parent or caretaker and the child herself should be a part of any evaluation. The parent should be asked about any significant changes in behavior (such as the recent onset of nightmares) that may accompany sexual abuse. Questioning the child who is verbal can be a useful "teachable moment" in which the physician explains the concept of the genital area as a "private zone," and the idea that touching in this area should be reported to a

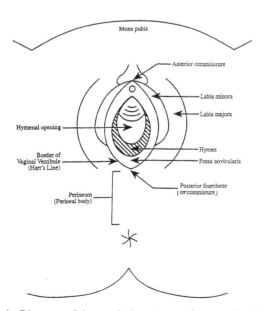

FIG. 1. Diagram of the genital anatomy of a prepubertal girl. This drawing shows a crescentic hymen. (From Pokorny SF. *Pediatric and adolescent gynecology*. New York: Chapman and Hall, 1996.)

parent. If the history is suspect, the injuries or physical findings are inconsistent with the history, or the child notes that an adult touched or hurt her, a report must be made to the appropriate social services agency.

Chronic skin conditions such as lichen sclerosus, seborrheic dermatitis, and atopic dermatitis may occur in young children. Lichen sclerosus has a characteristic whitish cigarette paper type of appearance with a keyhole distribution around the vulva and anus. Topical low- or medium-potency corticosteroids such as hydrocortisone or betamethasone can be effective in relieving symptoms. When this condition begins in childhood, it may regress with puberty, although this is not invariable.

Examination of the Prepubertal Child

The genital examination of the prepubertal child should be approached quite differently from the gynecologic examination of an adolescent or adult.[18] Frequently it is helpful to examine a toddler on her mother's lap while the mother elevates and or abducts the child's hips. An older child can sit straddling her mother's lap while mother, fully clothed, places her legs in the stirrups. The frog-leg or knee-chest positions can also be helpful. Care should be taken to inform the child of the necessary steps of the exam. Visualization of the vaginal vestibule is aided by lateral traction on the labia and buttocks. Conversing with the child will allow her to relax, and the hymen can be visualized. Initial reports attempting to correlate the normal hymenal diameter with chronological age and suggesting a diameter beyond which sexual abuse was likely were found to be inaccurate, as the visualized diameter depends on the child's cooperation and relaxation. A Valsalva maneuver can be helpful in the exam; the child can be asked to pretend she is blowing up a balloon or blowing out her birthday candles. This will often allow visualization of the distal 1 to 2 cm of the vagina. An otoscope can also be used to visualize the vagina in a cooperative child. A vaginal speculum is neither appropriate nor indicated in the examination of the prepubertal child in the office.

Vulvovaginitis: Diagnosis and Treatment

The first step in treatment of prepubertal vulvovaginitis involves attention to vulvar hygiene and toileting, including the avoidance of vulvar irritants such as topical medications, shampoo, and deodorant soap. Vaginal cultures, including cultures for gonorrhea and *Chlamydia,* are indicated when vaginal discharge persists after attention to hygiene. Pokorny has described an atraumatic method for obtaining cultures, consisting of a catheter within a catheter, through which nonbacteriostatic saline can be injected, aspirated, and sent for culture.[21] This method of taking cultures is generally better tolerated than using a cotton- or dacron-tipped swab. This same technique can be used to irrigate the vagina to remove small pieces of toilet paper. Pediatric vaginitis is usually caused by multiple organisms that are present in the perineum

and vulva, although a single organism such as *Streptococcus* or *Shigella* may be causative. Culture reports may indicate "normal vaginal flora" in the majority of cases, although, as has been indicated, it is not entirely well established what constitutes normal flora in this age group. Overgrowth of a single organism is more likely to be found when the symptoms have a fairly abrupt onset or are associated with an upper respiratory infection.

A short course of broad-spectrum antibiotics can eliminate the overgrowth of enteric bacteria, and topical estrogen cream increases the cornification of the vaginal epithelium, making it more resistant to infection. Ongoing attention to hygiene is necessary, as recurrent infections are common. Recurrences can be minimized by the weekly use of an antibacterial soap (PhisoHex) in the bath water. Antifungal therapies are frequently prescribed by pediatricians or physicians unfamiliar with the common causes of pediatric vulvovaginitis and are generally ineffective.

Vaginal Bleeding

Vaginal bleeding in a prepubertal child warrants a careful investigation. A common cause is a vulvar irritation as a result of vulvovaginitis or lichen sclerosus, although other causes should be considered if an obvious vulvar lesion is not present. A vaginal foreign body should be considered, as should rare causes of bleeding such as a vaginal tumor. The vagina should be visualized, and if this cannot be done in the office, an examination under anesthesia is indicated. The possibility of sexual abuse must also be assessed. Onset of bleeding without other signs of pubertal development is abnormal and must be investigated. Precocious puberty should be considered, and the exam should include looking for signs of estrogen stimulation (breast budding) and adrenarche. Data from a large study involving pediatric office practices indicate that African-American girls have an earlier onset of pubertal development than do Caucasians.[14] Precocious puberty has traditionally been defined as pubertal development occurring before age 8. Data from pediatric office practices reveal that 27% of African-American girls and 7% of white girls had signs of breast budding or pubic hair development at age 7. Thus, the definition for precocious puberty should be reassessed in light of these data. Serious causes of precocious puberty, including hormonally active ovarian tumors or CNS lesions, should be actively investigated.

Acute trauma and bleeding may result from a straddle injury or from sexual assault. Unintended trauma most commonly results in injury to the anterior vulva or laterally to the labia.[4] Straddle injuries may result in the formation of a large vulvar hematoma, which may require evaluation. Penetrating injuries with transection of the hymen are most commonly the result of sexual assault.[20] Any bleeding vulvar laceration requires a careful examination to assure that there are no vaginal lacerations and to completely repair the injury. This may require an examination under anesthesia or the use of conscious sedation in the Emergency Department.

◊ ADOLESCENT GYNECOLOGY

Normal and Abnormal Puberty

The average age of menarche in the United States is 12.8 years (Fig. 3). Menstrual cycles in the first two gynecologic years are frequently anovulatory, although the cycle length is typically regular within a range of about 22 to 45 days. Mean duration of bleeding is less than 7 days.[28] Patient estimate of quantity of menstrual flow is typically unreliable, and adolescents may have less basis for comparison than older women. Measurement of hemoglobin/hematocrit provides objective evidence of heavy bleeding.

First Gynecologic Visit

The American College of Obstetricians and Gynecologists Guidelines for Women's Healthcare indicates that the adolescent's first visit to an obstetrician/gynecologist should take place sometime between the ages of 13 and 15. This is in recognition of the role that obstetrician/gynecologists can potentially play in providing preventive guidance, screening, and preventive services to adolescents. Obstetrician/gynecologists are uniquely suited to provide these services in that the consequences of adolescent risk-taking behaviors include unintended pregnancies, STDs, ectopic pregnancies, PID, and infertility—all conditions with which the gynecologist is familiar. This initial visit is an ideal opportunity to discuss normal adolescent development and concerns related to adolescents with the adolescent's parents and the adolescent herself. At this visit, issues of confidentiality should be discussed with the adolescent and her parents. Numerous studies have concluded that without assurances of confidentiality, many teens will not divulge their health concerns, particularly those that relate to sex, substance use, and other risk-taking behaviors.[7,12] The initial visit does not necessarily need to include a pelvic examination. The ACOG Guidelines state that the provision of additional services beyond guidance and screening should be based on information obtained at this visit. If the adolescent has had intercourse, a pelvic exam, Pap test, and screening for STDs are appropriate. In at least two surveys, adolescents have indicated their desire to discuss health issues such as STDs, contraception, and sexual abuse.[27] These surveys have also indicated that these issues were infrequently addressed by clinicians.

The first pelvic examination requires careful attention to education and gentle technique. It is more important that this exam be atraumatic than that it confirm uterine or ovarian dimensions. The exam should be tailored to the needed information. If an adolescent has not been sexually active but is experiencing severe dysmenorrhea, the bimanual and rectovaginal components of the exam are more important than a speculum examination of the cervix. If a speculum exam is deemed appropriate and necessary, as with an adolescent who has had intercourse and thus requires a Pap smear and cervical cultures, an appropriately sized speculum is indicated. The Huffman or "virginal" speculum is quite narrow and can be used with a narrow or rigid hymen. However, visualization of the cervix with the Huffman speculum often requires manipulation that may be more uncomfortable than that required with the more frequently used Pederson speculum. The Pederson speculum should be the most frequently used speculum for adolescents and can be used comfortably for almost all teens. The Graves speculum, which is commonly used for adults, may be necessary for some obese or parous adolescents or when cervical procedures (colposcopy and biopsy) are indicated. Adolescents should be informed about the need for an examination; the amount of information that is provided before the exam should be tailored to the adolescent's wishes. Some adolescents want to know only the basics of the exam, but others want a step-by-step explanation. The adolescent should be offered the opportunity to have a parent or friend accompany her during the exam. The exam itself should be performed slowly and gently with forewarning of each successive step of the exam. Pap smears are indicated for adolescents who have been sexually active, and routine screening for STDs is also recommended by the CDC.

The Guidelines for Adolescent Preventives Services (GAPS) recommendations are a set of recommendations arrived at by a panel of experts from a number of different disciplines.[3] They are based on the rationale that (1) the primary health threats to adolescents are behavioral rather than biomedical, (2) an increasing number of adolescents are involved in behaviors with the potential for serious consequences, and (3) adolescents are engaging in these behaviors at earlier ages.[11] The comorbidities that adolescents experience are related to the risk-taking behaviors of unsafe sexual practices, substance use/abuse, and violence. The GAPS report concludes that many adolescents are engaged in multiple

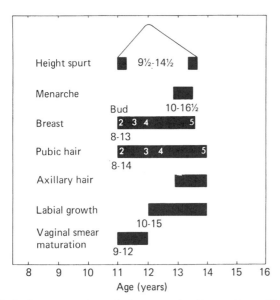

FIG. 3. Sequence of events that occur in girls at puberty. Numbers under each event represent the normal range of ages within which the event may occur. (From Tanner JM. *Growth at adolescence, 2nd ed.* Oxford: Blackwell Scientific, 1962.)

health risks simultaneously, and most adolescents engage in some type of behavior that is a threat to their health and well-being. The ACOG guidelines were developed in an effort to screen for and detect the risk-taking behaviors that result in significant morbidities for adolescents and to provide early or preventive interventions and services.

Abnormal Bleeding

Acute adolescent menorrhagia is most frequently associated with anovulation in the absence of specific anatomic abnormalities or underlying disease. Although the most frequent cause of bleeding is functional abnormalities of ovulation and hormonal feedback, other causes such as coagulopathy or underlying hepatic or renal disease occur in up to 20% of patients.[8] Pregnancy-related bleeding (ectopic pregnancy or spontaneous abortion) must be ruled out through both history (a confidential sexual history obtained privately) and with a sensitive pregnancy test. The potential medical consequences of missing a pregnancy-related complication dictate that a pregnancy test be performed in *all* cases of abnormal bleeding. A pelvic examination is almost always indicated but is essential if bleeding is accompanied by significant pelvic pain, the adolescent has a history of sexual activity (either voluntary or involuntary), or the pregnancy test is positive. If the young adolescent has not previously had a pelvic examination, attention must be paid to doing the exam in a gentle and atraumatic manner. The emergency department is not an optimal setting for the first exam, as appropriately sized specula are frequently not available; in addition, the adolescent and her parents are almost invariably extremely anxious because of the presence of heavy bleeding. A pelvic ultrasound can sometimes provide as much or more information than a difficult exam in a very anxious young teen.

An individual with menorrhagia and signs of hirsutism should be evaluated with hormonal testing for disorders of androgen excess, and appropriate hormonal therapy prescribed. For individuals without ovarian or adrenal androgen-producing tumors, oral contraceptives will provide menstrual management and decrease acne and hirsutism.[16]

Acute adolescent menorrhagia should be managed similarly to acute menorrhagia occurring in older women, with hormonal therapy. High-dose combination oral contraceptives should be given in a tapering fashion if the patient is hemodynamically stable and does not require fluid resuscitation or transfusion. Parenteral estrogens can be given acutely if hospitalization is required or there is concern about the possible need for a D&C to stop acute hemorrhage. Oral progestins are then added to the regimen, or a combination oral contraceptive pill is prescribed. Oral contraceptives (OCs) should be continued for a minimum of 3 months and may be continued on an ongoing basis if the adolescent chooses to do so. Alternatively, after several months of therapy with OCs, the pills can be discontinued; when this option is chosen, the physician should give careful guidelines to the teenager and her mother about the subsequent occurrence of frequent menses (occur-

ring more frequently than every 21 days), prolonged cycles (menses occurring less frequently than every 42 to 45 days), or bleeding lasting longer than 7 days. The use of oral contraceptives as medical therapy must be explained carefully to the parents, who frequently have concerns about the potential risks of "hormones" or who may fear that the use of OCs as medical therapy will provide an excuse for the initiation of sexual activity. In addition, mothers of teenagers may be familiar with higher-dose OCs, which were used during their own youth, and thus need reassurance about the fact that the ongoing use of OCs will include a low-dose pill.

Amenorrhea

Primary amenorrhea is defined as the absence of menses by age 16. In practice, the young woman who shows no signs of breast development by age 12 should be evaluated for pubertal abnormalities. In one large series from a tertiary referral center, ovarian failure was the most common cause of delayed sexual development. Congenital absence of the uterus and vagina and physiological delay of puberty were also frequently diagnosed etiologies. Other etiologies were diverse and numerically less frequent. Only 14% of all patients presenting with abnormalities of pubertal development had subsequent normal reproductive potential. All of these patients were in the physiological delay category.[23] Thus, the authors concluded that pubertal aberrancy should not be considered a benign entity because it is associated with morbidity, mortality, and significant compromise of reproductive potential.

Pregnancy must always be considered as an etiology of amenorrhea, whether it is secondary or primary amenorrhea. The adolescent should be questioned privately and without her parents about a history of sexual intercourse, whether voluntary or involuntary. Just as with excessive bleeding, the consequences of missing the diagnosis of pregnancy are medically serious, and a pregnancy test should always be performed to confirm the history. In one study in which pregnancies were diagnosed in a pediatric emergency department, 10% had denied sexual activity. The clinician's clinical skills will be tested in the situation of an unexpected diagnosis of pregnancy. The adolescent should be strongly encouraged to tell her parent(s) or a responsible adult. Counseling about pregnancy options should take place. The clinician must be aware of any state laws that mandate parental notification or consent when an adolescent chooses abortion.

Anatomic abnormalities ranging from Mayer-Rokitansky-Kustner-Hauser syndrome (Müllerian agenesis) to obstructing or partially obstructing vaginal septa to imperforate hymen are associated with primary amenorrhea and thus are most frequently diagnosed during adolescence.[15] Treatment options include both surgical and nonsurgical management but should also include attention to the psychological ramifications of this diagnosis.

Exercise-induced amenorrhea is associated with hypoestrogenemia and can contribute to osteopenia and risk of fracture. Modification of exercise levels, intervals of less vigorous training, or injuries precluding exercise may result in return of menses. Attention to the risk of osteopenia is imperative during adolescence, when bone accretion is normally occurring. Estrogen replacement or oral contraceptives may result in a normalization of bone metabolism.[9]

Eating disorders are frequently associated with menstrual dysfunction. The psychiatric definition of anorexia nervosa includes amenorrhea as one criterion. Amenorrhea may even precede severe weight loss. Anorexia nervosa should be managed by a clinician familiar with the medical effects of the disorder, and counseling is always indicated. When the adolescent is in counseling, attention can be placed on the amenorrhea, and appropriate hormonal therapy provided. There is some evidence that the bone loss associated with anorexia nervosa may not be rapidly or completely reversible with the use of estrogen supplementation. In one study, approximately 50% of women with bulimia had menstrual abnormalities. Thus, eating disorders should be considered as a possible cause when adolescents present with menstrual irregularities.

Dysmenorrhea

Primary dysmenorrhea, beginning with the onset of ovulatory menstrual cycles, is common, occurring in up to 90% of adolescents.[6] The use of nonsteroidal antiinflammatory drugs (NSAIDs) is usually helpful in relieving the prostaglandin-mediated symptoms, and many adolescents with dysmenorrhea have tried over-the-counter medications, although not always in appropriately therapeutic doses. Adolescents may be unaware that these drugs are more effective in relieving dysmenorrhea than other over-the-counter analgesics. Adolescents with severe dysmenorrhea and associated menstrual molimina that affect the performance of adolescent activities (particularly school attendance but also athletic endeavors) can benefit from the medical use of oral contraceptives. Parents may need to be informed of the potential noncontraceptive benefits of these medications, the rare risk of serious complications, the lack of association with long-term adverse medical events, and the fact that OC use does not accelerate the initiation of sexual activity in this age group.

Adolescents who have persistent dysmenorrhea in spite of the use of NSAIDS and oral contraceptives should be evaluated for other causes of pelvic pain, such as irritable bowel syndrome, but also including endometriosis. At one time, it was felt that endometriosis did not occur in adolescents. However, when complaints of severe dysmenorrhea are carefully investigated with appropriate laparoscopy, endometriosis can be found in a significant percentage of teens. The percentage of adolescents with chronic pain who have endometriosis is not well established. Various series of adolescents undergoing laparoscopy for chronic pain (generally defined as pain unresponsive to oral contraceptives and NSAIDs) reveal that up to 75% of teens with this complaint have endometriosis.[22] However, the percentage of teens with endometriosis found at laparoscopy depends on the indications for the surgical procedure and the criteria for diagnosis. Tra-

ditionally, visual confirmation was deemed sufficient; however, when strict criteria are used for diagnosis, endometriosis is not always confirmed. Endometriosis in adolescents is most frequently minimal or mild and may be atypical, with clear, white, or red lesions rather than the typical "powder-burn" lesion seen most frequently in older women.[10] It has been suggested that there is an age-related change in the appearance and color of endometriotic lesions. There is good evidence supporting the familial occurrence of endometriosis; the evidence is most consistent with a polygenic/multifactorial etiology. An asymptomatic individual with a first-degree relative who has endometriosis has a 7% risk of developing the disease.[25]

Pelvic Masses

Pelvic masses in adolescents may be detected as a result of symptoms (pain, pressure, urinary symptoms) or signs (the presence of a pelvic or abdominal mass). Pelvic masses in adolescents are most likely to be ovarian rather than uterine, although pregnancy should always be considered a possibility and ruled out with a sensitive pregnancy test.

Fewer than 5% of ovarian malignancies occur in children and adolescents. Ovarian tumors account for only 1% of all tumors in these age groups. Germ cell tumors make up half to two-thirds of ovarian neoplasms in individuals younger than 20. A review of studies conducted from 1940 until 1975 concluded that 35% of the neoplasms occurring during childhood and adolescence were malignant.[5] In girls younger than 9 years of age, approximately 80% of the ovarian neoplasms were found to be malignant. Germ cell tumors make up approximately 60% of ovarian neoplasms, compared with only 20% in adults. The mature cystic teratoma is the most frequent neoplastic tumor of children and adolescents, accounting for more than one-half of ovarian neoplasms in women younger than 20.[5] Because neoplastic tumors are rare, these studies come from tertiary care centers and may not be representative of the distribution of masses found in the community. Some reports include only neoplastic masses, whereas others include nonneoplastic masses. One community survey of ovarian masses revealed that the frequency of malignancy was much lower; only 10% of masses were neoplastic, and only 6% of all masses were malignant. Another series reported that nonneoplastic masses in individuals younger than 20 constituted two-thirds of the total; even in girls younger than 10, 60% of the masses were nonneoplastic, and two-thirds of the neoplastic masses were benign. Functional follicular cysts can occur in all ages and have been reported in female fetuses, newborns, and prepubertal children. Unilocular cysts will resolve spontaneously, and surgical therapy should be reserved for symptomatic masses, suspected torsion, or masses that include a solid or multiloculated appearance on ultrasound. Attention to the long-term effects of ovarian function and future fertility dictate a conservative approach to ovarian masses in young girls; preservation of ovarian tissues with oophorocystectomy is a priority for benign tumors. Functional cysts in prepubertal girls may be associated with sexual precocity.

Unintended Pregnancy

The latest data from the National Survey of Family Growth, 1995, indicate that more than 50% of adolescents have had intercourse.[2] Although most of the youngest teens have *not* had intercourse, the percentage of young teens who have had intercourse has been increasing. Some of the adolescents report the experience of involuntary intercourse; the younger the age at initiation of intercourse, the more likely the experience was involuntary. Seventy-four percent of those who reported first intercourse at age 13 or younger reported that they had experienced involuntary intercourse.[26] At least 75% of adolescent pregnancies are unintended. Most (approximately 80%) adolescents use a method of contraception but do not always use the method consistently, correctly, and continuously.

Developmental factors contribute to adolescents' risk for unintended pregnancy. During early and midadolescence, concrete thinking is developmentally normal, and the "personal fable" and magical thinking mitigate against the reality that pregnancy could happen to the individual. Middle adolescents enjoy showing off their new "adult" bodies, frequently seek peer group approval, and feel invulnerable. However, they also have increased mobility and independence coupled with less adult presence and protection. These factors frequently lead to risk-taking behaviors and experimentation with driving, substance use, and sexual activity. These teens may be unable to anticipate or prevent the consequences of these activities because of inexperience in abstract thinking. While they are developing the ability to perceive causal relationships and future consequences, this ability is variably applied, particularly in stressful situations such as an intimate or sexual relationship. There may be discordance among an individual adolescent's physical, social, sexual, and cognitive development. Thus, adolescents may not be developmentally equipped to use contraceptives effectively. Therefore, postponing sexual intercourse is the preferred form of sexual behavior for many or most adolescents until they are developmentally capable of responsible sexual behavior.

About one-third of adolescents waited a year after initiating intercourse before seeking medical contraceptive services, and another third had not sought medical care.[26] An increasing percentage of adolescents are using contraception at first intercourse. In 1982, 52% used no method of contraception at the time of first intercourse; in 1988, 35% reported using no method; and in 1995, 23% did not use any method of contraception.[2] Oral contraceptives are the most popular method of contraception among adolescents, and condoms are the next most popular method.[2]

Adolescents generally have higher failure rates of various methods of contraception during typical use, primarily because of problems of compliance—defined for contraception as the use of a method in both a consistent and ongoing manner. Failure rates among adolescents using oral contraceptive pills can be as high as 15% to 18%; as many as 50% or more adolescents have discontinued the method by the end of 1 year. Missed pills are frequently a problem for women of all ages

but are particularly frequent among the youngest adolescents. In one study, only one-quarter of adolescents 14 or younger took their oral contraceptive pill every day.[17] For many adolescents, the longer-term methods of contraception—depot medroxyprogesterone acetate or the implantable subdermal levonorgestrol rods—may be more appropriate methods, given the problems of compliance.

Sexually Transmitted Diseases

Biological factors that impact an adolescent's risk of STD acquisition or complications include the active cervical metaplasia and ectopy, which may increase the risk of *Chlamydia* or HPV acquisition.

Aspects of adolescent development also affect the risks for STDs. The feeling of invulnerability may result in decreased use of condoms or denial of symptoms. In addition, the clinical presentation of STDs may be affected by both an excessive attention to hygiene (e.g., douching) and excessive neglect of perineal hygiene. When infection is suspected, the adolescent typically reacts with embarrassment and fear, which result in delays in seeking treatment. Once an STD is diagnosed, adolescents may fail to complete therapy, especially if symptoms decrease; they also frequently fail to keep follow-up appointments and have difficulty informing or may fail to inform their partners of the STD acquisition.

Behavioral factors placing adolescents at increased risk include the fact that they may be more likely to have multiple sexual partners rather than single, long-term relationships; adolescents may have either concurrent partners or engage in serial monogamy with sequential partners. They may be more likely to engage in unprotected intercourse and may select partners at higher risk for STDs.

Adolescents have the highest rates of gonorrhea and HPV of any age group.[1] Routine screening for *Chlamydia* is recommended by the CDC for all sexually active adolescents, regardless of other risk factors. *Chlamydia* screening has been shown in a randomized clinical trial to be associated with a lower risk of PID among those screened when compared to those individuals who received the usual standard of care.[24] When one controls for rates of sexual activity (approximately 50% for adolescents 15 to 19), adolescents have the highest rates of PID.

Clinicians should be aware that in the United States, all adolescents could legally consent to the diagnosis and treatment of STDs and have the right to these services without parental consent or knowledge. Barriers to STD prevention in adolescents and young adults include financial constraints, lack of transportation, discomfort with facilities and services designed for adults, and concerns about confidentiality.

Hepatitis B is the only completely preventable STD. The ACIP now recommends the hepatitis B vaccination series at age 11 to 12. However, a cohort of adolescents currently exists who did not receive the vaccine at this age. The American Academy of Pediatrics and the American College of Obstetricians and Gynecologists both recommend that all adolescents receive the vaccine as a "catch-up."

The treatment of STDs among adolescents is identical to treatment in adults. The differences in STD presentation in adolescents relate to the developmental and risk-profile differences noted above, which place adolescents at increased risk. In addition, problems of compliance with medication are frequent; single-dose therapies may thus be more appropriate for teens with uncomplicated gonorrhea or *Chlamydia* crevices.

SUMMARY POINTS

◊ This chapter has outlined and summarized the basic aspects of pediatric and adolescent gynecology, highlighting the differences from the manner in which conditions are evaluated and managed in adults. Psychosocial and behavior factors greatly influence the health of adolescents. Preventive guidance and screening may be able to prevent or minimize the health morbidities.

◊ The gynecologic care of children and adolescents requires attention to a set of pathologic entities and treatments as well as psychosocial issues that are different from those that apply to the care of adults.

◊ A mixed bacterial vaginitis is the most common cause of vulvovaginal symptoms in prepubertal children; sexual abuse must always be considered as a possible etiology.

◊ Labial agglutination can be managed with topical estrogen cream; prevention of recurrence with a topical emollient is important.

◊ Most health threats in adolescents are related to risk-taking behaviors such as premature sexual intercourse, alcohol, and other substance abuse.

◊ Contraceptive compliance is difficult for adolescents and is the major factor that leads to higher failure rates during typical use for this age group than for older individuals.

◊ Adolescents with dysmenorrhea unresponsive to nonsteroidal antiinflammatory drugs and oral contraceptives may have pelvic endometriosis.

◊ REFERENCES

1. 1998 guidelines for treatment of sexually transmitted diseases. *MMWR* 1998;47:118.
2. Abma J, Chandra A, Mosher W, Peterson L, Piccinino L. Fertility, family planning, and women's health: New data from the 1995 National Survey of Family Growth. National Center for Health Statistics. *Vital Health Stat* 1997;23:1–125.
3. American Medical Association. *Guidelines for adolescent preventive services (GAPS)*. Chicago: American Medical Association, 1992.
4. Bond GR, Dowd MD, Landsman I, Rimsza M. Unintentional perineal injury in prepubescent girls: a multicenter, prospective report of 56 girls. *Pediatrics* 1995;95:628–631.
5. Breen JL, Maxson WS. Ovarian tumors in children and adolescents. *Clin Obstet Gynecol* 1977;20:623.
6. Campbell MA, McGrath PJ. Use of medication by adolescents for the management of menstrual discomfort. *Arch Pediatr Adolesc Med* 1997; 151(9):905–913.
7. Cheng TL, Savageau JA, Sattler AL, DeWitt TG. Confidentiality in health care: A survey of knowledge, perceptions, and attitudes among high school students. *JAMA* 1993;269:1404–1407.
8. Claessens E, Cowell CA. Acute adolescent menorrhagia. *Am J Obstet Gynecol* 981;139:277.
9. Cumming DC. Exercise-associated amenorrhea, low bone density, and estrogen replacement therapy. *Arch Intern Med* 1996;156:2193–2195.
10. Davis GD, Thillet E, Lindemann J. Clinical characteristics of adolescent endometriosis. *J Adolesc Health* 1993;14(5):362–388.
11. Elster AB, Kuznets NJ. *AMA guidelines for adolescent preventive services (GAPS): Recommendations and rationale*. Baltimore: Williams & Wilkins, 1994:1–191.
12. Ford CA, Millstein SG, Halpern-Felsher B, Irwin CE. Influence of physician confidentiality assurances on adolescents' willingness to disclose information and seek future health care: A randomized controlled trial. *JAMA* 1997;278:1029–1034.
13. Hammerschlag MR, Alpert S, Onderdonk AB, et al. Anaerobic microflora of the vagina in children. *Am J Obstet Gynecol* 1978;131:853–856.
14. Herman-Giddens ME, Slore EJ, Wasserman RC, et al. Secondary sexual characteristics and menses in young girls seen in office practice: A study from the pediatric research in office settings network. *Pediatrics* 1997;99:505–512.
15. Lindenman E, Shepard MK, Pescovitz RH. Mullerian agenesis: An update. *Obstet Gynecol* 1997;90:307–312.
16. Lucky AW. Hormonal correlates of acne and hirsutism. *Am J Med* 1995; 98:89S–94S.
17. Oakley D, Sereika O, Bogue E-L. Quality of condom use of reported by female clients of a family planning clinic. *Am J Public Health* 1995;85 :1526–1530.
18. Pokorny SF. The genital examination of the infant through adolescence. *Curr Opin Obstet Gynecol* 1993;5:753–757.
19. Pokorny SF. Long-term intravaginal presence of foreign bodies in children. A preliminary study. *J Reprod Med* 1994;39:931–935.
20. Pokorny SF, Pokorny WJ, Kramer W. Acute genital injury in the prepubertal girl. *Am J Obstet Gynecol* 1992;166:1461–1466.
21. Pokorny SF, Stormer J. Atraumatic removal of secretions from the prepubertal vagina. *Am J Obstet Gynecol* 1987;156:581–582.
22. Reese KA, Reddy S, Rock JA. Endometriosis in an adolescent population: the Emory experience. *J Pediatr Adolesc Gynecol* 1996;9(3): 125–128.
23. Reindollar RH, Byrd JR, McDonough PG. Delayed sexual development: a study of 252 patients. *Am J Obstet Gynecol* 1981;140:371–380.
24. Scholes D, Stergachis A, Heidrich FE, Andrilla H, Holmes KK, Stamm WE. Prevention of pelvic inflammatory disease by screening for cervical chlamydial infection. *N Engl J Med* 1996;334:1362–1366.
25. Simpson JL, Elias S, Malinak LR, Buttram VCJ. Heritable aspects of endometriosis. I. Genetic studies. *Am J Obstet Gynecol* 1980;137(3): 327–311.
26. The Alan Guttmacher Institute. *Sex and America's teenagers*. New York: The Alan Guttmacher Institute, 1994:1–88.
27. The Commonwealth Fund Commission on Women's Health. *The Commonwealth Fund survey of the health of adolescent girls*. New York: The Commonwealth Fund, 1997.
28. Treloar AE, Boynton RE, Behn BG, Brown BW. Variation of the human menstrual cycle through reproductive life. *Int J Fertil* 1967;12:77–126.

CHAPTER 35

Contraception and Sterilization

◇

Ronald A. Chez
Irvin Strathman

The ability of a sexually active woman to control her fertility is an essential aspect of her overall well-being. To prevent pregnancy, couples can use a temporary modality, contraception, or a permanent one, sterilization. If an undesired pregnancy occurs and the fetus has not reach a stage of viability, pregnancy termination or induced abortion may be an option.

◇ CONTRACEPTIVE USE IN THE UNITED STATES

In 1995, sterilization was the dominant method used for contraception by couples. Eleven percent of men and 28% of women were sterilized. The latter number approached 50% in women 40 to 44 years of age. Birth control pills were used by 27% of women of reproductive age, hormone injections by 3%, and hormone implants and intrauterine devices (IUDs) each by 1%. Twenty percent of couples used male condoms.

The 1995 data also indicate that one-third of sexually active women did not use contraception and that one-fourth of women did not use some form of birth control at the time of their first intercourse. Further, it is estimated that one-half of women who do use some form of contraception do so either inconsistently or incorrectly. As a result, more than one-half of the estimated 6 million conceptions in the United States each year are unintended. In women 40 years of age and older, the number is more than 75%; it exceeds 90% in women less than 20 years of age. Unintended pregnancy in teenagers has the characteristics of a public health epidemic.

◇ CONTRACEPTIVE EFFECTIVENESS

Contraceptive efficacy is calculated as the number of pregnancies that occur during a specific time interval of contraceptive use. There are several ways to determine contraceptive efficacy in clinical studies. The Pearl index defines contraceptive failure as the number of pregnancies per 100 woman-years of exposure. The denominator contains each subject's total months or total cycles of exposure during the time she is the study. When the quotient is in months, it is multiplied by 1200; when it is in cycles, 1300 is used.

The life table analysis method calculates a separate failure rate for each month of use. A cumulative failure rate is derived by combining the rates from each month over the time of the study. Methodologic flaws frequently impede comparison of the data from one study to another. These problems include lack of random assignments, demographic characteristics of the subjects, sexual habits of the subjects, consistency and correctness of method use, how and when in gestation pregnancy is detected, and the duration of the study, including follow-up and drop-out rates of the study group.

Nevertheless, it is possible to provide patients reliable information about effectiveness suitable for family planning purposes. Table 1 lists the percentages of women who experienced an unintended pregnancy in the first year of use according to the method used. The term *method effectiveness* refers to conception occurring with the correct use of the contraceptive modality; it is defined as a method failure. The term *use effectiveness* refers to conception occurring with both correct and incorrect use of the contraceptive method. It can also include failure secondary to inadequate or absent provision of services.[18]

The difference between use effectiveness and method effectiveness is small with family planning modalities not related to coitus (i.e., birth control pills, contraceptive implants, hormone injections, IUDs). Contraceptive methods that are coitally related and require consistent and proper use (i.e., diaphragm, condom, foam, rhythm, withdrawal) are less effective in actual use.

Additional factors influence contraceptive effectiveness. Contraceptive failure rates are lower when users wish to prevent pregnancy rather than extend the interval between

TABLE 1. *Estimated percentage of women who experience an unintended pregnancy in first year of contraceptive use*

Method	Effectiveness	
	Method	Use
No method (chance)	85.0	85.0
Periodic abstinence		20.0
Calendar method	9.0	—
Postovulation	3.0	—
Symptothermal	2.0	—
Ovulation detection	1.0	—
Withdrawal	4.0	19.0
Condom, male	3.0	12.0
Condom, female	5.0	21.0
Diaphragm	6.0	18.0
Cervical cap, nulliparous women	9.0	18.0
Cervical cap, parous	26.0	36.0
Spermicides	6.0	21.0
Intrauterine device, copper	0.6	0.8
Intrauterine device, progesterone	1.5	2.0
Oral contraceptives, combination	0.1	—
Oral contraceptives, progestin alone	0.5	—
Levonorgestrel implants (Norplant)(six rods)	0.1	0.1
Depot medroxprogestrone acetate (Depo-Provera)	0.3	0.3
Tubal sterilization	0.4	0.4
Vasectomy	0.1	0.2

(Adapted from Hatcher RA, Trussell J, Stewart F, et al., eds., *Contraceptive technology*, 16th ed. New York: Irvington Publishers, 1994:113.)

wanted births; this is particularly true of coitus-related methods. In addition, contraceptive failure rates are lowest in women older than 30 years who have achieved higher socioeconomic status and educational level and are using the contraceptive modality to prevent pregnancy. Finally, the availability of emergency contraception and access to safe abortion services in the event of contraceptive failure also affects patients' motivation to use contraception in an effective manner.

◊ CHOOSING A METHOD

On average, a woman's potential years of fertility extend from 2 years after her menarche to within several years of her menopause. Women who are sexually active experience a series of stages that include menarche, age of first intercourse, age of marriage and first birth, age when the desired family size is achieved, and the age of sterility or menopause. During each of these, a woman's interests, needs, and reproductive goals can change. Therefore, the appropriate method of contraception can also change.

Many factors influence a woman's final decision as to which method she chooses. These include her attitude about delaying rather than preventing pregnancy, the need for prompt reversibility of the method, whether the method should be independent of coitus, and the appropriateness of the method relative to her religious and cultural beliefs. Other factors are the stability of the sexual relationship, the number of sexual partners, her partner's attitude toward contraception, the frequency of coitus, and the ability to predict and prepare for coitus.[9] Institutional or societal barriers also affect decision making. They include the availability of and initial access to contraceptive methods, cost of the methods initially and continually, medical requirements for follow-up and monitoring, and the attitude and behaviors of the providers.

Thus, dialogue and counseling are integral to the family planning process. A focused history that incorporates questions relative to the patient's needs and goals identifies information pertinent to the preceding paragraphs. The interpersonal skills of the provider are essential to the success of this process. These skills include the ability to actively listen, effectively question, and respond to questions asked and competence in reflecting the patient's feelings through summarizing and paraphrasing and giving clear information. The goal is to facilitate the patient's choosing and receiving the method best suited to her current childbearing needs.[13]

◊ PERIODIC ABSTINENCE

Abstinence from intercourse during the days of the menstrual cycle when an ovum can be fertilized is a nonpharmacologic, nonmechanistic means to regulate fertility. This interval of abstinence can be determined by the calendar rhythm method, basal body temperature method, cervical mucus method, or symptothermal method.

Calendar Rhythm Method

The rationale for the calendar rhythm method is based on three assumptions: (1) A human ovum is capable of being fertilized for only about 24 hours after ovulation; (2) spermatozoa can retain their fertilizing ability for only 48 hours after coitus; and (3) ovulation usually occurs 12 to 16 days before the onset of the subsequent menses. In this method, the period of abstinence is determined by calculating the woman's previous cycle lengths. Her fertile period is calculated by subtracting 18 days from the length of her shortest cycle and 11 days from the length of her longest cycle. The couple abstains from coitus during this calculated fertile period. For most women with regular menstrual cycles, abstinence is required for nearly one-half of the days of the menstrual cycle. Women with irregular menstrual cycles cannot use the method. This method is no longer recommended because the use–pregnancy rates are high, as most couples do not wish to abstain for the relatively long interval required.

The term *natural family planning* has replaced "rhythm" to describe newer techniques whereby women rely on physiologic changes in the menstrual cycle to determine their fertile period. These methods require training of the couple. They are most effective when the couple is highly motivated, share the responsibility, openly communicate, and do not risk breaking the rules.

Basal Body Temperature Method

The temperature method requires that a woman's basal body temperature be recorded each day. A rise of 0.5°C above the mean temperature of the preovulatory phase for 3 days is indicative of postovulatory progesterone production by the corpus luteum. A couple is required to abstain from intercourse from the onset of menses until the third consecutive day of elevated basal temperature. Because abstinence is required for the entire preovulatory phase of the menstrual cycle and for the entire cycle if ovulation does not occur, the temperature method alone is not commonly used.

Cervical Mucus Method

The cervical mucus method is based on recognition of the changes in the quality and quantity of cervical mucus that appears at the vaginal introitus throughout the menstrual cycle in response to changes in circulating estrogen and progesterone. With this method, abstinence is required during menses, then every other day until the first day that cervical mucus is observed. Abstinence is then required every day thereafter until 3 days after the last day of wet, slippery mucus (i.e., peak mucus day) or in the presence of vaginal bleeding.

Symptothermal Method

The symptothermal method combines multiple indices to determine the fertile period. Abstinence starts when the first day of the fertile period is identified by the calendar or cervical mucus method and continues until the basal temperature or cervical mucus method identifies the last fertile day. The symptothermal method is more difficult to learn, but it is more effective, and the 1-year continuation rates are higher than in those methods that rely on a single index.

One deterrent to the use of natural family planning is the need to abstain from sexual intercourse for many days each menstrual cycle. To reduce the number of days of abstinence, simple, self-administered enzyme immunoassays for urinary estrogen and pregnanediol glucuronide that can be performed at home have been developed. These tests should more accurately define the limits of the fertile period.[14]

◊ MECHANICAL BARRIER METHODS

Mechanical barrier methods of family planning—the male condom, the female condom, and the diaphragm—can be highly effective methods of contraception. In addition to contraception, condoms made of latex or polyurethane have the advantage of reducing the rate of transmission of sexually transmitted diseases (STDs) including gonorrhea, chlamydiosis, trichomoniasis, and bacterial vaginosis. Condoms also prevent the transmission of herpesviruses and the human immunodeficiency virus (HIV). Users of condoms and diaphragms have less cervical neoplasia. This may be secondary to decreased transmission of human papillomavirus (HPV), some strains of which have been associated with cervical neoplasia.[5]

Male Condom

The condom should cover the entire length of the erect penis and be applied before any vaginal insertion. If it is not manufactured with a nipple reservoir on its end, a space should be left for the ejaculate. Adequate water-based lubrication will help prevent tearing and will not increase slippage. Oil-based lubricants should not be used because they cause latex to deteriorate. On withdrawal from the vagina, the condom should be held against the base of the penis to minimize spillage of semen.

Diaphragm

The diaphragm is a shallow latex cup with a spring mechanism in its rim to hold it in place in the vagina. Diaphragms are manufactured in various diameters. The properly fitted diaphragm lies just posteriorly to the symphysis pubis and deeply into the posterior vaginal fornix, so that the cervix is completely covered by and preferably behind the center of the membrane. The largest diaphragm that fills this space comfortably should be selected. If the diaphragm is too small, there is an increased possibility of its being dislodged during coitus. A diaphragm that is too large may produce vaginal ulceration and discomfort from rim pressure. The correct diaphragm size is determined by vaginal examination and measurement of the diagonal length of the vaginal canal. After a proper size is determined, the woman practices removing and reinserting the diaphragm in the office to assess that she can place the diaphragm properly.

The diaphragm can be inserted up to 4 hours prior to intercourse and should be left in place for a minimum of 8 hours after the last ejaculation. It is used with contraceptive cream or jelly that lines the rim and is placed inside the cup at insertion. Effectiveness of the diaphragm method is directly related to the age of the user, experience with its use, continuity of use, and whether or a spermicide was used concomitantly.[4]

Female Condom

The female condom is a lubricated, 17-cm-long, polyurethane sheath attached to two flexible rings. One ring is attached to the open end of the sheath that covers the labia and perineum; the other ring is at the sealed end of the sheath inside the vagina. This method can be as effective as male condoms. Compared with male condoms, it has advantages including insertion in advance of sexual foreplay and coitus, the woman's control of the method, and less disruption of sexual activity during the man's detumescence phase.[13,23]

◊ CERVICAL CAP

The cervical cap is a cup-shaped device made of latex that fits over the base of the cervix. The cap can be inserted up to 8 hours before coitus and may be left in place for up to 48 hours. As with the diaphragm, contraceptive effectiveness is increased if the cup is partially filled with spermicide. The cervical cap is manufactured in four sizes. A proper fit usually requires a relatively normal cervical length and shape. Use of this cap requires more training for both the provider and the user than does use of the diaphragm.[19]

◊ SPERMICIDES

Vaginal foams, creams, suppositories, jellies, and films all have to be inserted in the vagina just before each coital act. Their mechanism of action is via a spermicidal agent, usually the surface-active agent nonoxynol-9. Nonoxynol-9 is also a microbicide. Its use reduces the risk of becoming infected with STDs of both bacterial and viral origin. However, clinical data on its effect on human transmission of HIV are inconsistent and require further study. Users of spermicidal jelly or foam with or without a barrier method have more urinary tract infections than nonusers, apparently secondary to excessive *Escherichia coli* vaginal colonization. A current challenge is to find products that have spermicidal and microbicidal, including antiviral, properties without affecting the normal vaginal flora.

The periconceptional use of spermicides is not associated with adverse pregnancy outcomes. Specifically, there is no increased risk of congenital malformation in neonates or karyotype abnormalities in spontaneous abortuses of women who conceived while using vaginal spermicides.

◊ ORAL CONTRACEPTION

More than 30 combination oral contraceptive (OC) formulations and two progestin-only formulations are currently available for use in the United States. These combination OCs contain one of two synthetic estrogens, ethinyl estradiol or mestranol (Fig. 1), and one of seven progestins: norethindrone, norethindrone acetate, ethynodiol diacetate, norethynodrel, and norgestrel or its active isomer levonorgestrel, desogestrel or norgestimate (Fig. 2). These progestins are all 19-nortestosterone derivatives.

Combination OCs are ingested daily for 21 consecutive days followed by a 7-day steroid-free period to allow with-

drawal bleeding to occur. The pills initially marketed were monophasic in design; that is, the same dose of the two steroids was taken daily. In the 1980s, combination OCs that contained two or three different amounts of the same estrogen and progestin during the 21-day medication period were marketed. These formulations have been described as biphasic or triphasic and are generally known as multiphasic. In concept, the phasic formulations provide reduced total dose of steroid, while maintaining efficacy and cycle control. The progestin-only formulations consist of progestin without estrogen. The tablets that contain only progestin are ingested daily without a steroid-free interval.

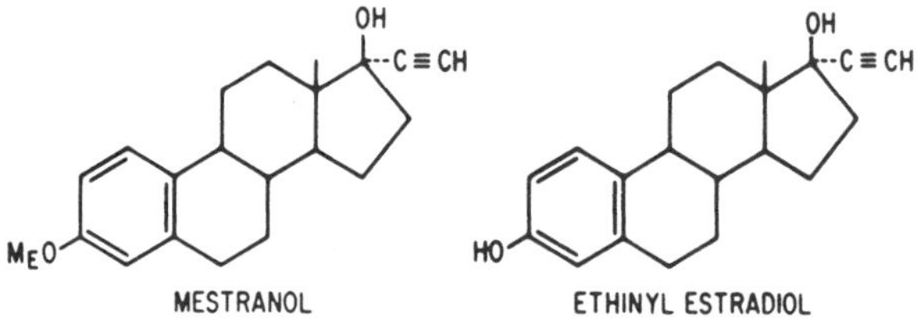

OCs have been marketed in the United States since 1962. Initially, they contained amounts of progestin 10 times higher and amounts of estrogen three to six times higher than current pills. In the United States, most OCs contain estrogen in doses of 20 to 35 μg and relatively equipotent doses of the various progestins. This reduction in dosage has made OCs safer in terms of adverse side effects, while still retaining contraceptive efficacy. OC formulations containing 30 to 35 μg of ethinyl estradiol per tablet account for more than 95% of prescriptions in the United States. Formulations with more than 50 μg of estrogen are no longer marketed in the United States.

The high effectiveness of combination OCs results from their multiple effects on the reproductive system. The midcycle surge of gonadotropins is consistently inhibited, thus blocking ovulation. This exogenous hormonal administration renders cervical mucus thick, viscid, and scanty in amount, retarding sperm penetration. Uterine and tubal motility is altered, which affects the transport of both ova and sperm. Production of glycogen by the endometrial glands is diminished, impairing the survival of the blastocyst in the uterine cavity. Ingestion of OCs does not produce a hypoestrogenic state. Levels of circulating endogenous estrogens during an OC cycle are similar to levels during the early follicular phase of the normal menstrual cycle.

Progestin-only preparations do not consistently inhibit ovulation; therefore, they are less effective than combination OCs. Ingestion of the progestin-only preparations at the same time each day helps sustain blood steroid levels at the daily nadir so that they do not fall below the contraceptive-effective level.

OCs produce metabolic alterations in addition to those involving the reproductive axis. Some metabolic changes are dose-related to the estrogen component of the birth control pill, and others are related to the progestin component (Table 2). With currently available low-dose OCs, measured changes in the classical laboratory are small, usually within the normal range, and estrogen and progestin effects tend to offset each other. With the exception of patients who have risk factors for thromboembolic disease or have hypertension, these metabolic changes have no clinical relevance.

Related to the synthetic estrogen is an increase in hepatic proteins, including clotting factors (i.e., fibrinogen, factor VII, factor X) and angiotensinogen. Clinically, the former changes may contribute to the risk of thromboembolic disease, and the increase in angiotensinogen may contribute to

FIG. 1. Formulas of the two estrogens used in combination oral contraceptives.

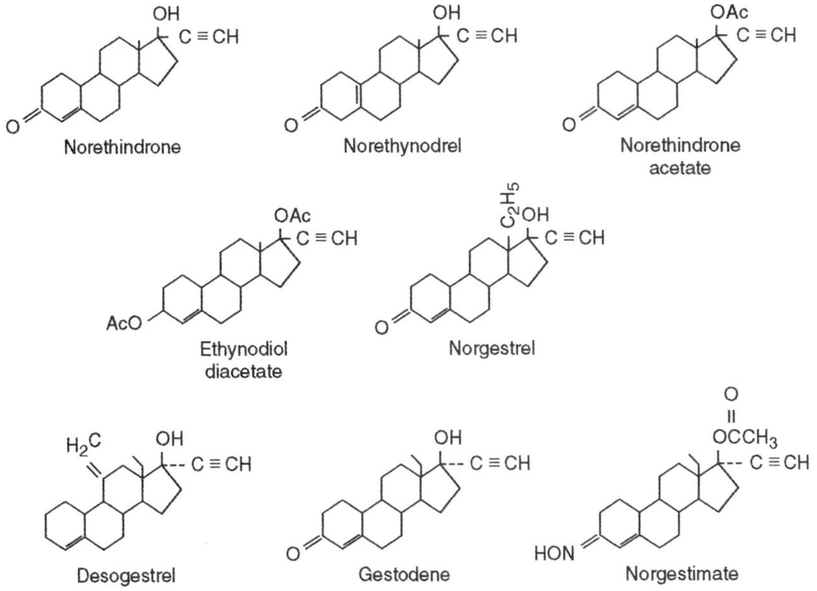

FIG. 2. Formulas of eight progestins used in combination oral contraceptives.

hypertension. Only a small percentage of women taking OCs develop high blood pressure. The elevated blood pressure that occurs in some women during their use of OCs is a reversible phenomenon that disappears when the birth control pills are discontinued.

Related to the progestin are an increase in circulating levels of glucose and insulin and a relative peripheral insulin insensitivity. The alterations in glucose metabolism are dose-related. The current progestin dosing either produces no change or slightly improves carbohydrate metabolism.

Lipid metabolism can be altered by both estrogens and progestins. Estrogens produce beneficial changes in the lipid profile, increasing the antiatherogenic fraction (i.e., high-density-lipoprotein cholesterol [HDL-C]) and decreasing the atherogenic fraction (i.e., low-density-lipoprotein cholesterol [LDL-C]). Progestins have the potential to produce changes in lipid metabolism that are opposite to those resulting from estrogen. Under their influence, HDL-C decreases and LDL-C increases. Thus, the effect of a specific OC formulation on lipids is the result of the dose and potency of both the estrogen and the progestin components. The changes in circulating blood lipid levels that occur with low-dose OCs appear to be of laboratory interest only. Almost all changes remain within the range of normal. Further, no clinical association has been found between changes in these levels and adverse effects in users.

Some women have minor adverse effects associated with OC use. These symptoms are not a threat to overall health and usually resolve with continued use or change to a different formulation. Symptoms produced by the estrogen component are nausea, breast tenderness, fluid retention, and depression. Estrogens affect tryptophan metabolism, decreasing serotonin levels. This change can be associated with depression in some women and somnolence and mood changes in others. Symptoms produced by the progestin component include weight gain, acne, amenorrhea, and nervousness. The progestins are anabolic in nature and can increase

body weight. Estrogens decrease sebum production, and progestins increase sebum production. Progestins decrease the synthesis of estrogen receptors by endometrial cells. The suppression of endometrial growth in some women will result in failure to have withdrawal bleeding. Although amenorrhea during OC use is not of medical significance, it removes the monthly signal of bleeding that reassures a woman that she is not pregnant.

Breakthrough bleeding and chloasma are adverse effects attributed to both components of combination OC pills. Breakthrough bleeding results from too little estrogen or too much progestin, or both. Amenorrhea and breakthrough bleeding can be alleviated by an increase in the amount of estrogen in the formulation or by a more estrogenic formulation. Chloasma, pigmentation of the malar eminences of the face, is accentuated by sunlight and usually takes a long time to disappear after OC use is discontinued.

Earlier studies reported an increased incidence of cholelithiasis associated with OCs. However, recent findings in studies with lower-dose pills indicate a minimal risk of gallbladder disease.

For over 20 years, public media misinformation, adverse publicity, and excessive focus on infrequent adverse side effects have alarmed women using or considering using the pill. Current surveys show that women continue to be anxious about the risks of OC use and stroke, heart attack, and cancer.

Cardiovascular Disease

Clinical safety markedly exceeds risk with current low-dose OCs. Concerns about cardiovascular risk are not relevant except in women older than 35 years who are smokers; they should discontinue their use. Further, the use of OCs by healthy, nonsmoking women 40 years of age and older may have benefits that outweigh the possible health risks associated with both pregnancy and alternative methods of re-

TABLE 2. *Metabolic effects of contraceptive steroids*

Affected structure	Chemical effects	Clinical effects
Estrogen—ethinyl estradiol		
Proteins		
Albumin	↓	None
Amino acids	↓	None
Globulins	↑	
Angiotensinogen		↑ Blood pressure
Clotting factors, I, VII, X		Hypercoagulation
Carrier proteins (CBG, TGB, transferrin, ceruloplasmin)		None
Carbohydrates		
Plasma insulin	None	None
Glucose tolerance	None	None
Lipids		
Cholesterol	None	None
Triglycerides	↑	None
HDL-cholesterol	↑	Antiatherogenic
LDL-cholesterol	↓	Antiatherogenic
Electrolytes		
Sodium excretion	↑	Fluid retention
Tryptophan Metabolism	↓	Depression
		Mood changes
		Sleep disturbances
Vitamins		
B complex	↓	None
Ascorbic acid	↓	None
Vitamin A	↑	None
Skin		
Sebum production	↓	Less acne
Pigmentation	↑	Chloasma
Target Tissues		
Breasts	↑	Breast tenderness
Endometrial receptors	↑	Hyperplasia
Gestagens—19-nortestosterone derivatives		
Proteins	None	None
Carbohydrates		
Plasma insulin	↑	None
Glucose tolerance	↓	None
Lipids		
Cholesterol	↓	None
Triglycerides	↓	None
HDL-cholesterol	↓	Atherogenic
LDL-cholesterol	↑	Atherogenic
Nitrogen Retention	↑	↑ Body weight
Skin		
Sebum production	↑	↑ Acne
Androgens	↑	Nervousness
Target Tissue		
Endometrial receptors	↓	↓ Endometrial cancer

↓, decreased; ↑, increased; CBG, corticosteroid-binding globulin; HDL, high-density lipoprotein; LDL, low-density lipoprotein; TBG, thyroxine-binding globulin.

versible contraception. Many clinicians continue oral contraception in these women until the menopause is reached.

Myocardial Infarction

The data in the initial studies that reported an increased risk of acute myocardial infarction (MI) in current OC users compared to controls were obtained from women receiving much larger amounts of synthetic steroids than those prescribed today. In those studies, variables were identified that were associated with a significantly higher risk of MI when the pill was used. These variables included being older than 35 years of age, smoking, hypertension, diabetes mellitus, and hyperlipidemia.[24] The more of these risk factors that were present, the greater was the risk for MI. The overwhelming majority of women of reproductive age do not have any of these factors. In addition, more recent studies using low-dose OCs did not find an increased risk of serious cardiovascular disease in healthy, nonsmoking women who elected to use the pill until they reached the menopause. Separately, all epidemiologic studies have concluded there is no increased risk of MI in former pill users and that the incidence of the problem is not correlated with the duration of use of the method. Thus, any increased risk of arterial vascular disease is caused by a thrombotic process and not atherogenesis.

Stroke

As is MI, stroke is relatively rare in young women, and thus epidemiologicdies require large numbers of subjects. Data from both case–control and cohort studies identified a temporal relationship between the original higher-dose OCs and ischemic stroke and a less certain association with hemorrhagic stroke. Normotensive, nonsmoking women younger than 35 years who use the current low-estrogen combination pills and past users of the pill do not have an increased risk of hemorrhagic or ischemic stroke.[25]

Venous Thromboembolism

The occurrence of venous thromboembolism is rare in young women and may be estrogen dose–related in pill users. The recent introduction of the new progestins norgestimate, desogestrel, and gestodene has refocused concerns about this relationship.[22] Current estimates are that progestin combinations with gestodene and desogestrel are associated with 20 to 30 incidents of nonfatal venous thrombosis per 100,000 users, compared to 10 to 15 per 100,000 users of other progestin combinations and 4 cases per 100,000 reproductive-age women who are nonusers and not pregnant. Pregnant women have an incidence of nonfatal thrombosis of 60 per 100,000. Of note, increasing body mass index is a risk factor.

There has been considerable controversy as to the validity of these estimates. In addition to questions of biologic plausibility, generic questions of prescription bias, diagnosis and referral bias and the confounding of other factors such as smoking have been raised. Moreover, the thrombogenic potential of these compounds may relate to inherited activated protein C resistance. If initial observations are confirmed, screening for activated protein C resistance may prove useful in avoiding thromboembolism in OC users.

Neoplasia

American women using OCs for 8 years have a slight increase in cervical, liver, and breast cancer. They also have a significant reduction in endometrial and ovarian cancer. The estimated number of additional or fewer cases per 100,000 users ranges from 197 to 41 in each instance.[20]

Breast Cancer

There have been at least 54 epidemiologic studies of breast cancer and OC use.[6] Confounding variables in these studies included the natural history of breast cancer with a rapid increase in incidence between ages 35 and 50 years, a positive family history, the relationship of breast cancer to gravidity and parity, and the age of last pill use. Duration of use appears to have a minimal influence. Current OC users have an increased relative risk of 1.24, compared to controls. This risk declines to 1.0 after 10 years of nonuse. There is a slightly higher relative risk of 1.59 in women who started using the pill before age 20 years, but this difference in risk disappears after 5 years on nonuse. Age of stopping the pill is also a factor related to cumulative incidence. Women who stop the pill at age 25 years experience an excess of breast cancer of 1 per 10,000 users at age 35 years, but the incidence is the same as that of women in the general population at age 45 years. Women who stop at age 40 years have an estimated excess incidence of 1 in 526 at age 50 years and 1 in 714 at age 60 years.

Female Genital Cancer

It is uncertain whether OCs increase the risk of cervical neoplasia, act as a cocarcinogen for its development, or have no effect on its incidence. Any association of an increased risk of cervical dysplasia and cervical cancer in OC acceptors may be modulated by confounding factors, including age of first coitus, number of sexual partners, greater exposure to HPV, more frequent cytologic screening among birth control pill users, and protection by barrier or spermicide use in the control group. Some case–control studies that have corrected for these confounding factors have concluded that women who have used OCs longer than 5 years still have an increased risk of developing cervical cancer, compared with controls, and others studies have not so concluded. As do all sexually active women, OC users require at least annual screening of cervical cytology.

Almost all the studies examining endometrial cancer in OC users have concluded that the use of the exogenous steroids offers protection against this form of cancer. Women who use OCs for at least 1 year experience a 50% reduction in their risk for endometrial cancer that persists for at least a decade after use ceases. This protection is greater for nulliparous than parous women.

The risk of ovarian cancer, specifically epithelial ovarian cancer, is also reduced by OC use. The relative risk of an OC user's developing ovarian cancer is 0.6, with the magnitude of protection directly related to the duration of use. As little as 6 months of pill use provides the user with protection from ovarian cancer that persists for at least a decade after OC use is discontinued. This reduction in the risk of ovarian cancer

occurs only in pill users of low parity (i.e., four or fewer), who are at the greatest risk of developing this type of cancer.

Other Neoplasms

Development of a benign hepatocellular adenoma is a rare occurrence, with an annual incidence of 1 in 30,000 to 250,000 users. The incidence is increased in women who have used the pill longer than 5 years. If use of the pill is stopped, the adenoma spontaneously regresses and disappears. The incidence of pituitary adenomas is not increased in OC users.

Some epidemiologic studies have shown an increased risk of malignant melanoma in birth control pill users, others have demonstrated no effect, and still other studies have reported a decreased risk. The results may be influenced by the confounding factor of sunlight exposure.

Contraindications to Oral Contraceptive Use

The risks associated with OC use far outweigh the contraceptive and noncontraceptive benefits of using the pill for some women. Women with high-risk factors for either venous or arterial vascular disease should not use OCs. These high-risk factors include the following:

◊ History of deep vein thrombosis, pulmonary embolism, or congestive heart failure,
◊ Cerebrovascular or coronary artery disease,
◊ Untreated hypertension,
◊ Diabetes with vascular complications,
◊ Age greater than 35 years and cigarette smoking.

Other absolute contraindications to birth control pill use include estrogen-dependent neoplasia, breast cancer, undiagnosed abnormal genital bleeding, pituitary prolactinoma, known or suspected pregnancy, active liver disease, intestinal malabsorption syndrome, and current use of rifampin (because of its effect on liver metabolism of sex steroids). The contraindications to OC use do *not* include a history of pregnancy-induced hypertension, the presence of superficial varicose veins, a history of liver disease with normal hepatic function tests, sickle cell trait or disease, or asymptomatic mitral valve prolapse. The relative contraindications to OC use include migraine headaches, oligomenorrhea, and depression, since these conditions can be exacerbated in some patients.

Noncontraceptive Benefits of Oral Contraceptive Use

Many patients and physicians are unaware of the considerable noncontraceptive health benefits associated with OC use. The benefits resulting from the consistent inhibition of ovulation include lowered incidences of functional ovarian cysts, ovarian cancer, dysmenorrhea, and premenstrual syndrome. The benefits resulting from inhibition of estrogen receptor synthesis in target cells by synthetic progestins in pills are reduced incidences of endometrial cancer, benign breast disease, and menstrual blood loss. A reduction in menstrual blood flow results in less iron deficiency anemia. An additional benefit of OC use is a lower incidence of clinical acute salpingitis caused by gonorrhea or a chlamydial infection (even though the incidence of chlamydial cervicitis is increased), as well as fewer cases of rheumatoid arthritis, ectopic pregnancy, and osteoporosis.

Pregnancy after Discontinuation of Oral Contraceptives

About 20% of women who discontinue OCs to conceive have up to a 6-month delay in return of fertility, compared with women who stop nonhormonal methods. There is no difference in the rate of fertility after 1 year; nor are there differences in the rates of spontaneous abortion, chromosomal abnormalities in the abortuses, and birth defects from those in women in the general population.

If OCs are inadvertently ingested early in pregnancy, there is no significantly increased risk of congenital malformations among the offspring of these pregnancies. Because estrogen inhibits the action of prolactin in breast tissue receptors, the postpartum use of combination OCs decreases the amount but not the quality of milk produced by women who breast-feed their babies. Progestin-only formulations do not decrease the amount of breast milk, and their use should be considered for mothers who are breast-feeding and want to use an OC.

◊ LEVONORGESTREL IMPLANTS

Levonorgestrel implants (Norplant System) were approved by the U.S. Food and Drug Administration (FDA) for contraceptive use in the United States in 1990. The system consists of six silicone rubber rods, each measuring 34 mm long and 2.4 mm in diameter and containing 36 mg of levonorgestrel. The rods are inserted subcutaneously, usually in the woman's upper inner arm, where they are visible under the skin and can be readily palpated. Release of the progestin by diffusion provides effective contraception for 5 years. The mechanism of action is a combination of suppression of the luteinizing hormone surge with suppression of ovulation, development of viscous and scant cervical mucus (preventing sperm migration through the canal), and interference with endometrial growth and development. The contraceptive efficacy of the method is equivalent to that of surgical sterilization.

The advantages of this method are the longevity of its high effectiveness, nonrelation of its use to coitus, absence of exogenous estrogen, no adverse effects on breast milk production (favoring its use in postpartum lactating women), prompt return to the previous state of fertility on removal, and lack of apparent impact on lipid, carbohydrate, or protein metabolism. The major disadvantage is the presence of irregular menstrual and intermenstrual vaginal bleeding in more than two-thirds of women in the first several years of use; this

tends to revert to regular cycling.[1] Other reported adverse effects may include weight gain, headaches, and acne. The initial expense of the method is high, but no further expense for the method is incurred for 5 years. Importantly, both insertion and removal of the rods require minor surgery with a sterile field and local anesthesia. Training is required for both procedures, and the associated complication rates and the length of time to perform the procedure are a function of the clinician's experience. Systems using only one or two slightly longer rods are in clinical trials.

◊ DEPOT MEDROXYPROGESTERONE ACETATE

Depot medroxyprogesterone acetate (DMPA; Depo-Provera) is a C21-17 acetoxyprogestogen that is injected as microcrystals in an aqueous suspension. It was approved as a contraceptive in the United States in 1992. Its mechanism of action includes inhibition of ovulation by suppression of gonadotropin-releasing factors from the hypothalamus, production of an atrophic endometrium, and decreased sperm penetration of the cervical mucus. A single intramuscular injection of 150 mg of DMPA provides at least 13 weeks of contraceptive efficacy equivalent to that of the combination of OC and surgical sterilization. Therefore, the dosing schedule is at 3-month intervals.

No clinically relevant changes in carbohydrate, lipid, and protein metabolism are found in users. The existing evidence does not suggest a teratogenic risk if pregnancy occurs. Nor is there an overall increased risk of breast, cervical, ovarian, or liver cancer; there is a decreased risk of endometrial cancer in DMPA users.

The negative effects of this method are menstrual cycle dysfunction and weight gain. Unpredictable episodes of vaginal spotting and bleeding are found in almost all women. Amenorrhea occurs in more than 50% of patients by the end of 1 year. Return to fertility is initially delayed after discontinuation of use because of the long duration of action of the depot suspension. Long-term fertility is not different from that of nonusers. Users experience an average 5-lb (2.27-kg) weight gain in the first year of use. This gain continues in lesser increments each subsequent year.[16]

Candidates for this method include women who desire long-interval birth spacing who cannot use estrogen-containing preparations for medical reasons or related adverse effects, postpartum lactating women (because there is no effect on milk quantity or quality), and women for whom compliance with a method associated with coitus or requiring daily attention is difficult or not feasible.

◊ INTRAUTERINE DEVICES

Although the IUD is a highly effective method of contraception, it is used by fewer than 2% of American women of reproductive age. The reasons for the low rate of utilization include physician fear of medicolegal liability, lack of physician and public understanding of the method's benefits, overstatement of its risks, and lack of physician insertion skills.

Four types of IUDs have been approved by the FDA for use in the United States. Two of these were withdrawn from the market by the manufacturers when the cost of defending the device against litigation was deemed too expensive. The litigation was stimulated by a series of septic abortion–related deaths in women using Dalkon Shield IUDs in the mid-1970s. Other devices did not show evidence this association but were tarnished by the attendant publicity.

The two IUDs now available in the United States are shown in Figure 3. One releases progesterone (65 μg per day) from a reservoir on its stem. There is sufficient steroid to last for 400 days; therefore, this IUD must be replaced each year. This device is associated with less blood loss than the copper-releasing IUD, but also a higher incidence of ectopic pregnancy if conception occurs. The other IUD is the copper T 380A, introduced to the United States in 1988. This device has 308 mg of copper covering parts of its stem and arms, resulting in a total surface exposure of 380 mm². Contraceptive effectiveness continues for 10 years, after which it must be replaced. The net cumulative pregnancy rate of the copper T380A IUD after 10 years of use is only 2.6%. Additional benefits of this method are that it is not associated with systemic side effects, it does not interrupt coitus, it does not interfere with lactation, there is a prompt return to fertility upon its removal, a clinician is required to remove it, and no further contraceptive efforts are required of the couple.

Controversy exists as to whether an IUD acts as an abortifacient. Most data indicate that copper IUDs prevent fertilization by altering or inhibiting sperm migration and ovum transport. Cytolysis of both sperm in the uterus and unfertilized ova in the fallopian tube is found.[21]

The disadvantages of this method include the risk of perforation at the time of IUD insertion and increased vaginal bleeding and pain at menses. IUD insertions are usually performed to coincide with menses to reduce the likelihood of pregnancy. However, the IUD may be safely inserted on any day of the menstrual cycle or 4 to 8 weeks after delivery without increasing the incidence of adverse effects. The rate of uterine fundal perforation at insertion approximates 1 in 1500 insertions. It usually results from failure to accurately determine the position of the uterus by palpation before passage of a sound through the cervical canal to the top of the fundus. IUDs that are properly inserted entirely within the endometrial cavity do not migrate through the myometrium into the peritoneal cavity.

Nearly 50% of copper IUD removals are for excess bleeding or pain at menses. After insertion of a copper-bearing IUD, the average mean menstrual blood loss increases to 50 to 60 ml. In women using the progesterone-releasing IUD, the mean blood loss per menstrual cycle decreases to 25 ml. Some patients have dysmenorrhea that does not respond to antiinflammatory analgesics.

Controversy has also surrounded the question of whether IUD use increases the risk for acute salpingitis. Studies that reported an increase were flawed by the inaccuracy of the diagnosis of salpingitis, when based only on physical examination, a preponderance of Dalkon Shield IUDs in some studies, and a control group of women who used methods of contraception that protect against salpingitis (i.e., barrier methods and OCs). The data from a World Health Organization–sponsored, retrospective, 23-country study are depicted in Figure 4. The risk of acute pelvic inflammatory disease (PID) was highest during the 20 days after insertion, with an incidence of about 1 per 1000 woman-years. This rate subsequently fell and did not increase for up to 8 years of use.[8] The type of IUD did not influence the results. Since the bacteria delivered to the endometrial cavity during the IUD insertion procedure explain the initial increased risk of salpingitis in IUD users, these data emphasize the importance of meticulous aseptic technique at the time of insertion and use of the IUD for its maximum life span before it is replaced and a new insertion performed.

The major risk for subsequent PID in an IUD user is exposure to STDs. Thus, the copper IUD is an appropriate

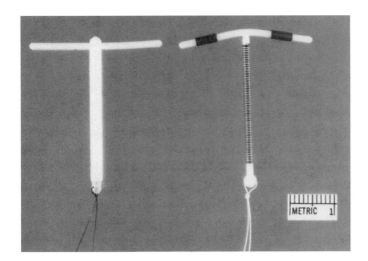

FIG. 3. Intrauterine devices (IUDs) manufactured and approved for use in the United States include the copper T380A **(right)** and the progesterone-releasing IUD **(left)**.

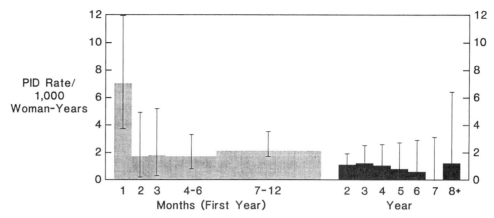

FIG. 4. Incidence of pelvic inflammatory disease (PID) by duration of intrauterine device use. The 95% confidence intervals are shown. (Adapted from ref. 8.)

method of contraception for parous women in a stable monogamous sexual relationship who have completed their families and do not desire sterilization or have contraindications to OC use.

If pregnancy occurs and the string of the *in utero* IUD is visible, it should be removed to reduce the otherwise two- to fourfold increased incidence of spontaneous abortion and premature labor and delivery. A patient with a copper or progesterone-releasing IUD *in utero* that has a monofilament appendage does not have an increased risk of septic abortion. If the appendage is not visible and it cannot be retrieved without disrupting the pregnancy, it should be removed at the time of delivery. The presence of the IUD or copper does not increase the risk of congenital anomalies in the fetus.

Although IUD use does not increase the risk of ectopic pregnancy, it does offer greater protection against an intrauterine pregnancy than against an extrauterine pregnancy. As a result, the ratio of extrauterine to intrauterine pregnancy is greater when conception occurs in an IUD user than when it occurs in a woman who is not an IUD user.[15]

In some countries, a levonorgestrel-releasing IUD is available. It provides highly effective contraception for at least 5 years. Noncontraceptive benefits include a marked reduction in the incidence of ectopic pregnancy, a reduction in dysmenorrhea, a relatively low incidence of PID, and decreased menstrual blood flow. Approximately one-third of users become amenorrheic after 1 year.

◊ STERILIZATION

For most patients, sterilization for contraceptive purposes is a voluntary, elective procedure. Sterilization should be considered as a method of family planning only for those who desire a permanent method. Although both male and female sterilization procedures sometimes can be surgically reversed, the surgery is technically more difficult than the original sterilization procedure, and there are considerable costs that usually are not reimbursed by third-party payers. Success rates for reversal vary according to the method of steriliza-

tion, the age of the patient, and portion of the tube involved. They tend to be better for tubal reanastomosis than for reanastomosis of the vas deferens.

Counseling is mandatory prior to sterilization and must include a description of the procedure and explanation of the risks of surgery and anesthesia, as well as explanation of the benefits. Patients also should be reminded that sterilization does not provide protection against STDs. Discussion of the possibility of regretting sterilization is appropriate. Requests for reversal of the procedure more often are made by younger women, those with lower parity, after a divorce with remarriage, and after the loss of one or more children.[12]

Vasectomy

Vasectomy is performed by incision or puncture of the scrotal sac, identification and transection of the vas deferens, occlusion of both severed ends by suture ligature or fulguration, replacement of the divided vas deferens in the scrotal sac, and closure. This procedure is usually performed under local anesthesia in an outpatient facility. Hematoma formation and sperm granulomas are potential complications associated with vasectomy. The occurrence of spontaneous reanastomosis is rare and inversely related to the time interval after vasectomy. Vasectomy does not increase the risk of prostate or testicular cancer, nor are there associated adverse effects on health, including cardiovascular disease.

After the sterilization procedure, some sperm still remain in the ejaculatory ducts. The man is not considered sterile until he has produced two sperm-free ejaculates 1 month apart as documented by semen analysis. This usually requires 15 to 20 ejaculations. Neither the volume nor the appearance of the ejaculate changes after vasectomy.

Female Sterilization

Approximately 1 million American women a year are sterilized by either procedures on the fallopian tubes or hysterectomy. Female sterilization is an intraperitoneal procedure that is usually performed under general or regional anesthesia. Therefore, more risks are involved with female sterilization than with vasectomy.[10] The timing of and route and method used for female sterilization vary. It can be performed in the first hours or days of the postpartum period through a small transverse infraumbilical incision without extending the length of hospitalization. Interval tubal sterilization procedures are performed at a time other than the puerperium. Access to the tubes is obtained by laparoscopy, laparotomy, or colpotomy. The methods of fallopian tube sterilization include mechanical occlusion with clips, bands, or Silastic rings, segmental destruction with bipolar or unipolar electrocoagulation, and suture ligation with partial salpingectomy. The Pomeroy technique is illustrated in Figure 5.[3]

The failure rate of female sterilization has been examined by the United States Collaborative Review of Sterilization.[17] Rates vary according to the procedure performed. The highest 10-year cumulative probability of pregnancy per 1000 tubal ligations was 36.5; this occurred with the spring clip method. Rates with other methods, in decreasing order, were bipolar coagulation (25), interval partial salpingectomy (20), and silicone rubber band (18). The lowest rate of 7.5 per 1000 procedures was with unipolar coagulation and with postpartum partial salpingectomy. The success of reversal procedures directly relates to the failure rates of each method.[17]

Importantly, the failure rate does not vary from year to year and is cumulative over the 10 years. It is also greater in women who were ages 18 to 27 years at the time of the sterilization. One-third of pregnancies in sterilized women are ectopic. There are no data to support a cause-and-effect relationship between tubal sterilization and changes in libido, ability to enjoy sex, adverse effect on lactation, or change in menstrual cycle patterns.

◊ EMERGENCY CONTRACEPTION

Emergency contraception is therapy offered to women who experience an act of unprotected sexual intercourse. It is synonymous with the terms "morning after pill" and "postcoital contraception." The methods that have been used for this purpose include combination OCs, conjugated and synthetic estrogens, progestin-only pills, danazol (Danocrine), insertion of a copper IUD, and antiprogestin medication. At present, combination OCs and insertion of a copper IUD are the two most effective and most readily available methods in the United States.[2]

Combination Oral Contraceptive Pill Method

In his original studies, Yuzpe used two OC pills that together provided 0.1 mg of ethinyl estradiol and 1.0 mg of DL-norgestrel. Two doses were taken 12 hours apart, with the first dose ingested within 72 hours of coitus. The equivalent steroids in this combination now can be obtained through a number of lower-dose OCs, all of which contain ethinyl estradiol and levonorgestrel, the active form of DL-norgestrel. Although this use of these medications has not been approved for marketing, emergency contraception has been affirmed and encouraged as an unlabeled indication by the Commissioner of the FDA.

Reproductive-age women who present within 72 hours of unprotected sexual intercourse, independent of the time of menstrual cycle, are candidates for this method. Other than pregnancy, the absolute and relative contraindications to the prescription of a combination OC for contraception do not apply for emergency contraception. There have been no reports of major cardiovascular, neurologic, or increased adverse side effects with the prescribed regimen.

The emergency contraceptive method described results in a 75% reduction in the number of pregnancies from what would be expected relative to the time of exposure and the calculated day of ovulation. There is no apparent difference in efficacy relative to when in the 72 hours the first dose is ingested. There appears to be a reduced efficacy after 72 hours, but there are limited data from which to draw conclusions.

Approximately 50% of patients will experience nausea after the first or second dose. The intensity of the nausea can be reduced by using antiemetic prophylaxis approximately 1 hour before the dose. About 20% of patients will vomit. There are no data to support repeating the dose if vomiting occurs. In addition, some patients will experience breast tenderness, headache, and dizziness.

Almost all patients have their next menstrual cycle within 21 days of dosing. If not, follow-up care to assess for pregnancy is indicated. There are insufficient data to indicate a teratologic effect with the combination OC pill method of

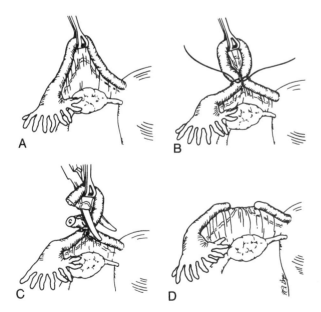

FIG. 5 A–D. Modified Pomeroy technique of female sterilization. (From Sciarra JJ. Surgical procedures for tubal sterilization. In: Sciarra JJ, Zatuchni GI, Daly MJ, eds. *Gynecology and Obstetrics*, vol. 6. Philadelphia: JB Lippincott, 1990:3; with permission.)

emergency contraception. However, the fact that women who are unknowingly pregnant and continue to take OCs on a daily basis do not have an increased incidence of congenital anomalies may be pertinent.

The mechanisms of the combination OC pill method of emergency contraception are not clearly established. It is known that it can inhibit or delay ovulation. There are conflicting reports on whether the endometrium is made unsuitable for implantation.

Patients who receive a combination OC pill for emergency contraception should also be assessed for the need to provide counseling for both a method of continuing contraception and for safe sex.

Packaging of the appropriate number of combination OC pills for the specific purpose of emergency contraception is available in other countries and may soon be available in the United States. A progestin-only pill containing 0.75 mg of levonorgestrel is also available in other countries. Two doses are taken 12 hours apart with the first dose ingested within 48 hours of intercourse. Less nausea and vomiting are associated with this method without a decrease in efficacy.

Copper Intrauterine Device Method

A copper IUD inserted within 5 days after sexual intercourse can also be used as an emergency contraceptive. Its efficacy is almost 100% and has the advantage that the patient continues with a reliable method of reversible contraception.

◊ PREGNANCY TERMINATION

The termination of a pregnancy can be accomplished by either surgical or medical means. In the first trimester, the surgical approach entails dilation of the cervical canal and suction or sharp curettage of the decidua and products of conception. In the second trimester, dilation of the cervix with hydrophilic dilators, such as laminaria tents inserted for several hours prior to instrumentation of the uterine cavity, will decrease trauma and injury to the cervix.

The immediate complications of surgical evacuation of the uterus at any gestational age include hemorrhage, infection, retained products of conception, cervical laceration, perforation of the uterus with bowel injury, and risks associated with anesthesia. All of these are increased as the length of gestation increases. Sharp curettage performed for pregnancy termination is the most common antecedent history for the development of intrauterine synechiae and its associated menstrual dysfunction and infertility.

Medical methods for induced abortion up to 63 days' gestation include oral mifepristone (RU 486) or intramuscular methotrexate followed by placement of intravaginal misoprostol (Cytotec). Mifepristone is a 19-norsteroid with a high affinity for progesterone receptors. It is a progesterone antagonist without agonist properties or estrogenic activity. Misoprostol is a prostaglandin. The effectiveness rate of these two methods is 95%.[7,11]

SUMMARY POINTS

◊ Each family planning decision, whether it involves contraception, sterilization, or pregnancy termination, must be individualized to the patient's and couple's needs and circumstances.

◊ All methods of family planning involve risks and benefits, advantages and disadvantages. Some adverse effects are relatively frequent and not serious, whereas others are rare but quite serious.

◊ Each method is associated with absolute or relative contraindications to its use. For most patients, the risk of contraception is less than the risk of pregnancy, but to some extent each family planning decision is a compromise.

◊ Several family planning methods have both contraceptive and noncontraceptive health benefits.

◊ Only after the benefits and risks of each modality are compared with the other available methods and with the risks of selecting no method, including resultant unwanted pregnancy, can a family planning decision be formulated.

◊ REFERENCES

1. Alvarez-Sanchez F, Brache V, Thevenin F, Cochon L, Faundes A. Hormonal treatment for bleeding irregularities in Norplant implant users. *Am J Obstet Gynecol* 1996;174:919–922.
2. American College of Obstetricians and Gynecologists (ACOG). *Emergency oral contraception. ACOG practice patterns no. 3.* Washington, DC: ACOG, 1996.
3. American College of Obstetricians and Gynecologists (ACOG). *Sterilization. Technical bulletin no. 222.* Washington, DC: ACOG, 1996.
4. Bounds W, Guillebaud J, Dominik R, Dalberth BT. The diaphragm with and without spermicide: a randomized, comparative efficacy trial. *J Reprod Med* 1995;40:764–774.
5. Cates W Jr. Barrier methods. *Network* 1996;16:4–27.
6. Collaborative Group on Hormonal Factors in Breast Cancer. Breast cancer and hormonal contraceptives: collaborative reanalysis of individual data on 53,297 women with breast cancer and 100,239 women without breast cancer from 54 epidemiological studies. *Lancet* 1996;347: 1713–1727.
7. El-Refaey H, Rajaasekar D, Abdalla M, Calder L, Templeton A. Induction of abortion with mifepristone (RU 486) and oral or vaginal misoprostol. *N Engl J Med* 1995;332:983–987.
8. Farley TMM, Rosenberg MJ, Rowe PJ, et al. Intrauterine devices and pelvic inflammatory disease: an international perspective. *Lancet* 1992; 339:785–789.
9. Forrest JD. Timing of reproductive life stages. *Obstet Gynecol* 1993; 82:105–111.
10. Gentile GP, Kaufman SC, Helbig DW. Is there any evidence for posttubal sterilization syndrome? *Fertil Steril* 1998;69:179–186.
11. Hausknecht RU. Methotrexate and misoprostol to terminate early pregnancy. *N Engl J Med* 1995;333:537–540.
12. I-Cheng C, Jones DB. Incidence, risk factors, and prevention of poststerilization regret in women: an updated international review from an epidemiological perspective. *Obstet Gynecol Surv* 1994;49:722–732.
13. IMAP Statement on Contraceptive Counselling. *IPPF Med Bull* 1994;28:1–2.

14. IMAP Statement on Periodic Abstinence for Family Planning. *IPPF Med Bull* 1996;30:1–2.
15. Mol BWJ, Ankum WM, Bossuyt PMM, Van der Veen F. Contraception and the risk of ectopic pregnancy: a meta-analysis. *Contraception* 1995;52:337–341.
16. Nelson AL. Counseling issues and management of side effects for women using depot medroxyprogesterone acetate contraception. *J Reprod Med* 1996;41:391–400.
17. Peterson HB, Xia Z, Hughes JM, Wilcom LS, Tylor LR, Trussell J. The risk of pregnancy after tubal sterilization: findings from the U.S. Collaborative Review of Sterilization. *Am J Obstet Gynecol* 1996;174:1161–1170.
18. Potter LS. How effective are contraceptives? The determination and measurement of pregnancy rates. *Obstet Gynecol* 1996;88:13S–23S.
19. Richwald GA, Greenland S, Gerber MM, Potik R, Kersey L, Comas MA. Effectiveness of the cavity-rim cervical cap: results of a large clinical study. *Obstet Gynecol* 1989;74:143–148.
20. Schlesselman JJ. Net effect of oral contraceptive use on the risk of cancer in women in the United States. *Obstet Gynecol* 1995;85:793–801.
21. Spinnato JA II. Mechanism of action of intrauterine contraceptive devices and its relation to informed consent. *Am J Obstet Gynecol* 1997;176:503–506.
22. Spitzer WO, Lewis MA, Heinemann LAJ, Thorogood M, MacRae KD. Third-generation oral contraceptives and risk of venous thromboembolic disorders: an international case-control study. *BMJ* 1996;312:83–90.
23. Trussell J, Sturgen K, Strickler J, Dominik R. Comparative contraceptive efficacy of the female condom and other barrier methods. *Fam Plann Perspect* 1994;26:66–72.
24. World Health Organization Collaborative Study of Cardiovascular Disease and Steroid Hormone Contraception. Acute myocardial infarction and combined oral contraceptives: results of an international multicentre case-control study. *Lancet* 1997;349:1202–1209.
25. World Health Organization Collaborative Study of Cardiovascular Disease and Steroid Hormone Contraception. Acute myocardial infarction and combined oral contraceptives: ischaemic stroke and combined oral contraceptives: results of an international, multicentre, case-control study. *Lancet* 1997;348:498–510.

CHAPTER 36

Induced Abortion

———— ◇ ————

Suzanne R. Trupin

Approximately 1.4 million abortions are performed annually in the United States. Worldwide 20 to 30 million legal abortions are preformed annually, with another 10 to 20 million reportedly being done illegally. Regardless of contraceptive availability, about half the 6 million pregnancies occurring each year are reportedly unplanned. Of these pregnancies, approximately half are terminated by induced abortion. This rate has remained fairly constant since 1980. The typical patient seeking an abortion has been young, white, unmarried, and poor (Table 1 and Figs. 1 to 3).

◇ LEGALIZATION OF ABORTION

Since the landmark 1973 Supreme Court decision legalizing abortion, hundreds of laws, federal and state, have been proposed or passed, making this the most actively litigated and highly publicized area in the field of medicine. Many of these laws are enjoined by court order and thus not enforceable. They span a variety of controversial rulings: provisions to establish viability before termination, parental or spousal notification, mandatory waiting periods, mandatory counseling wording, denial of public funding, denial of public funds for counseling ("gag orders"), and provisions against specific abortion techniques. Laws in some states criminalize these procedures; performing a specific abortion would constitute a felony offense by the provider. Thirty states have forced parental consent or notification. Nine state courts block these laws. Thirty-four states ban abortion coverage for low-income women, and 12 states have blocked these laws.

Before *Roe v Wade*

Before the 19th century, most states had no specific abortion laws. The provisions of British common law took precedence, and women had the right to terminate a pregnancy prior to viability. Beginning with a Connecticut statute followed by a 1829 New York law, the next 20 years saw the enactment of a series of laws restricting abortion, punishing providers, and in some cases punishing the woman herself. The first federal law on the subject was the notorious Comstock Law of 1873 that permitted a special agent of the postal service to open mail dealing with abortion or contraception in order to suppress the circulation of "obscene" materials. From 1900 until the 1960s, abortions were prohibited by law. However, the Kinsey report noted that 9 of 10 premarital pregnancies were electively aborted. Public and physician opinion began to be shaped by the alarming reports of increased numbers of unsafe illegal abortions. In 1965, there were 265 deaths due to illegal abortions. Twenty percent of all pregnancy-related complications in New York and California were due to abortions (Grimes and Cates, 1979). A series of Supreme Court decisions granted increased rights to women and assured their right to autonomy in this process. No decision was more important than *Griswold v Connecticut*, which in 1965 constitutionally established a woman's right to privacy.

Roe v Wade

In response to overwhelming political support for abortion, *Roe v Wade* was the culmination of the work of a wide consortium of individuals and groups who collectively crafted a strategy to repeal the abortion laws. In 1969, abortion rights supporters held a conference to formalize their goals and formed the National Association for the Repeal of Abortion Laws (NARAL). The movement lawyers were committed to universal access to rights at a time when states were gradually liberalizing pertinent laws. Lawyers Linda Coffee and Sarah Weddington met the Texas waitress, Norma McCorvey, who wished to have an abortion but was prohibited by law. She would become plaintiff "Jane Roe." Although the ruling came too late for McCorvey's abortion, her case was successfully argued before the Supreme Court in a decision that instantly granted the right of a woman to seek an abortion.

In 1973, in an opinion written by the Nixon Supreme Court appointee Harry Blackmum, the court ruled that a woman had

TABLE 1. *Legal abortions, abortion ratios, and abortion rates in selected years from 1972 to 1995 and characteristics of women who obtained legal induced abortions in those years*

Characteristics	1972	1980	1990	1995
Reported legal abortions	586,760	1,297,606	1,429,577	1,210,883
Abortion ratio	180	359	345	311
Abortion rate	13	25	24	20
		Percentage distribution		
Residence				
In-state	56.2	92.6	91.8	91.7
Out-of-state	43.8	7.4	8.2	8.3
Age group				
<20	32.6	29.2	22.4	20.1
20–24	32.5	35.5	33.2	32.5
>24	34.9	35.3	44.4	47.4
Race				
White	77.0	69.9	64.8	59.5
Black	23.0	30.1	31.8	35.0
Other			3.4	5.5
Ethnicity				
Hispanic	—	—	9.8	15.4
Non-Hispanic	—	—	90.2	84.6
Type of procedure				
Curettage	88.6	95.5	98.8	98.9
Suction	65.2	89.8	96.0	96.6
Sharp	23.4	5.7	2.8	2.3
Instillation	10.4	3.1	0.8	0.5
Other	1.0	1.4	0.4	0.6
Weeks gestation				
<9	34.0	51.7	51.6	54.0
9–10	30.7	38.4	25.3	23.1
11–12	17.5	12.2	11.7	10.9
13–15	8.4	5.1	6.4	6.3
16–20	8.2	3.9	4.0	4.3
>20	1.2	0.9	1.0	1.4

(From Henshaw and Kost, 1996, with permission.)

a right to induced abortion during the first two trimesters of pregnancy. He cited the safety of the procedures and the fundamental right of women to be free from the states' legislating concerning their medical decisions in the first trimester of pregnancy. Blackmum, writing for the majority, sidestepped the question of viability, specifically stating that scholars in many respected disciplines could not resolve this issue. Therefore, he felt that the court need not resolve this either. Since this ruling, the states have regained much control, and serious restrictions have been placed on abortion services. The Hyde amendment in 1976 prohibited use of federal funds for abortions, except in the case of maternal life endangerment. Since then, it is estimated that up to one-third of public funding recipients are unable to obtain an abortion due to lack of funds.

Viability Determinations

Loosely defined, the term *viability* is the fetus' ability to survive extrauterine life with or without life support. A number of landmark Supreme Court decisions dealt with this question. In *Webster v Reproductive Health Services* (1989), the court upheld the state of Missouri's requirement for preabortion viability testing after 20 weeks' gestation. However, no reliable or medically acceptable tests exist for this prior to 28 weeks. The preamble to this law states that life begins at conception and the unborn are entitled to the same constitutional rights as all others. By 1992, in a ruling controversial because of its inclusion of mandatory waiting periods, elaborate consent processes, and record-keeping regulations, *Planned Parenthood v Casey* tried to account for the variability of viability by putting in language recognizing that some fetuses never attain viability (e.g. anencephalics). In

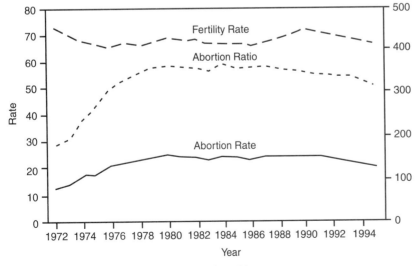

FIG. 1. Fertility rate and abortion ratio and rate, by year—United States, 1972–1995. (From Koonin LM, MacKay AP, Berg CJ, Atrash HK, Smith JC. Pregnancy-related mortality surveillance—United States, 1987–1990. *MMWR CDC Surveillance Summaries* 1997;46 (No. SS-4), 10.)

* Number of live births per 1000 women aged 15–44 years.
† Number of legal induced abortions per 1000 live births.
§ Number of legal induced abortions per 1000 women aged 15–44 years.

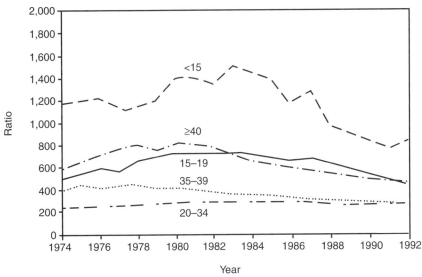

FIG. 2. Abortions ratios, by age group, of women who obtained a legal abortion—United States, 1974–1992. (Koonin LM, Smith JC, Ramick M, Green CA. Abortion surveillance—United States, 1992. *MMWR CDC Surveillance Summaries* 1996;45 (No. SS-3), 1–36.)

* Number of abortions per 1,000 live births.
† In years

Colautti v Franklin, the court overturned a Pennsylvania law requiring physicians to follow specific directives in certain medical circumstances and recognized physician judgment as sacrosanct and important.

Parental Consent

Parental consent is not required in the case of carrying a pregnancy to term, seeking contraception, or being treated for a variety of conditions, including sexually transmitted diseases. In two decisions handed down in 1991, *Hodgson*

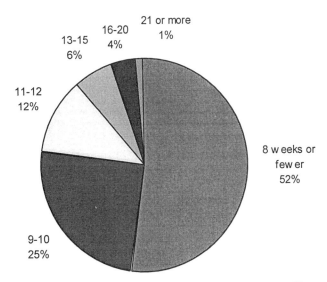

FIG. 3. Abortions performed per week of gestation. (Data from: Henshaw SK, Kost K. Abortion patients in 1994–1995: characteristics and contraceptive use. *Fam Plann Perspect* 1996;28:104–107, 158; and Facts in Brief-Induced Abortion. Alan Guttmacher Institute, 120 Wall Street, New York, NY 10005, http://www.agi-usa.org. January, 1997.)

v Minnesota and *Ohio v Akron Center for Reproductive Health,* the Supreme Court held that it is legal to have parental notification laws for abortions. These provisions often include waiting periods and fairly limited provisions for judicial bypass. Sociologic research shows that most minors do involve their parents in their decision to abort. However, these laws have fostered a new ominous trend: minors obtaining abortions significantly later in their pregnancies and often traveling very far to states with no such law (Joyce et al., 1997).

Intact Dilation and Extraction

The recently crafted political term "partial-birth abortion" loosely means "partially vaginally delivering a living fetus before killing the fetus and completing the delivery" (Planned Parenthood Fact Sheet, 1997). This delineation is so overly broad that both legal and expert gynecologic testimony claim this definition encompasses virtually all methods of second trimester abortion including dilation and extraction and inductions. In 19 states, laws have banned these procedures; in only eight states are they enforced. In his first administration, President Clinton vetoed two bills banning such abortions.

Providers

Providers of elective induced abortions are generally obstetricians and gynecologists. However, many studies have illustrated the safety of allowing a variety of practitioners of various disciplines, both physician and nursing, to perform these procedures. Various factors over the years have influenced the number of providers. Abortion is the only common surgical procedure that is elective in obstetric and gynecologic residencies. Thus, few board-certified gynecologists are actually qualified to perform the procedure. Increasing violence against providers and clinics has further decreased providers' willingness to provide abortion services (Grimes, 1991). There has been a "graying" of providers who continue to be committed to performing abortions. Most represent an older population of clinicians who became committed to access to safe, legal abortions after caring for young women who suffered or died from complications of an illegal abortion. The lack of abortion providers is underscored by the fact that 80% of counties in the United States have no abortion services.

◊ ABORTION COUNSELING

Some patients find the decision to have an abortion an easy one; for others it takes time. Preoperative counseling for abortions should include a discussion of all options regarding the pregnancy. It is important to remind patients that their current ethical framework may not always be consistent with future views. Discussion should focus on the decision-making process and patients' support system. Of utmost importance is to ensure that patients are not being coerced in their decision. Counseling sessions should provide medical information, review the pertinent medical history, and discuss previous procedures. Patients should be informed of the risks of the procedure, and full disclosure of information includes discussing the risks of continuing the pregnancy. If a patient withdraws consent to proceed during the abortion process, verbal or written consent must be reestablished before the abortion can proceed. Preoperative counseling should also explore the subjects of future contraception and protection against sexually transmitted diseases.

◊ ETHICAL ISSUES IN INDUCED ABORTION

The public debate on abortion has gained progressive furor with the rapid advances in scientific technology and the public activism of individuals and groups who use civil disobedience and violence directed at providers to achieve their stated goals of eliminating access to legal abortion. Bioethicists suggest that sonography and the high-resolution images it provides, together with advances in neonatal technology that have improved fetal survival early in gestation, have contributed to the perception that the fetus is an individual entitled to legal protection. The dearth of adoptive children and progressive increase in infertility are cited by others as motivating factors for activists' stance against abortion. Scientific advances in areas of fetal tissue use, assisted reproductive technologies, and selective reduction procedures have illustrated the discord existing between the legal, ethical/moral, and religious platforms concerning abortion. Although data are scant, some couples use abortion for sex selection. Scholars have had difficulty in constructing a framework that allows acceptable application of these technologies yet excludes the so-called "purely elective" or "contraceptive" use of abortion to which many object (Fig. 4).

◊ INDICATIONS FOR ABORTION

Medical Indications

Medical indications for abortion have narrowed with advances in perinatal care. Most perinatologists and abortion counselors prefer to put the risks in statistical perspective, if data are available, and leave the final decision to the patient, as opposed to the concept of recommending abortion. In-

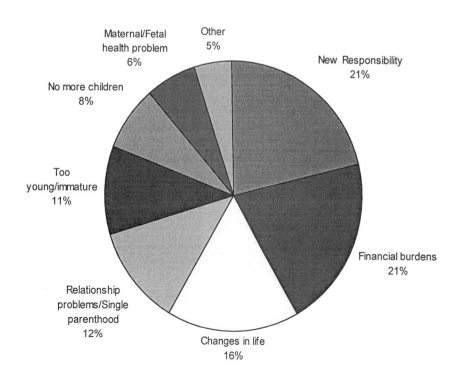

FIG. 4. Most important concerns driving the decision to abort. (From Torres and Forrest, 1988, with permission.)

duced abortion is generally safer than proceeding to term. In the 1980s, it was estimated that maternal mortality was reduced sevenfold by a first-trimester abortion, and recent data indicate that it may be even safer; consequently, any discussion of risk must always be put in perspective (Table 2). Maternal conditions that may be considered under medical indications include renal failure, diabetic retinopathy, sickle cell disease, cardiac disease, neoplasia, autoimmune disease, and psychiatric disease. Cardiac conditions that may result in maternal mortality include severe mitral stenosis, coarctation of the aorta with vascular involvement, uncorrected tetralogy of Fallot, aortic stenosis, previous myocardial infarction, myocardial infarction during pregnancy, artificial heart valves, and Marfan syndrome with aortic involvement. A cardiac condition with potentially greater mortality is Eisenmenger syndrome with pulmonary hypertension. Other medical indications include intrauterine infections and preterm premature rupture of membranes. No woman who understands her risks should categorically be told to abort her pregnancy. Nondirective counseling in this area is essential (Berg and Smith, 1997).

Fetal Indications

Prenatal diagnosis has progressed, but most conditions diagnosed have no real means of treatment other than abortion. Fetal indications for induced abortion include those anatomic conditions incompatible with life (e.g., anencephaly) and major congenital abnormalities (e.g., hypoplastic left heart) (Table 3). When the condition is diagnosed in time to have an abortion, 50% to 80% of patients selected abortion, although even severe cardiac conditions can theoretically be treated by cardiac transplantation. Few providers nationally will provide abortion in the third trimester up to approximately 32 to 34 weeks. There is a vigorous debate about what constitutes the current the standard of care and whether or not appropriate counseling for these conditions should include offering referral to these facilities.

◊ SURGICAL ABORTION

Preoperative preparation for most women after the targeted history and consent process can be fairly simple. The pregnancy is assessed to see whether or not it falls within the gestational age limits of the facility; evaluation also includes ad-

TABLE 2. *Case-fatality rates for induced abortion and pregnancy*

Vacuum curettage[a] ≤ 12 weeks	0.05
Dilation and evacuation 13–15 weeks[a]	2.00
Dilation and evacuation 16–20 weeks[a]	6.5
Dilation and evacuation > 21 weeks[a]	11.9
Overall maternal mortality[b]	10–20

[a]Deaths per 100,000 induced abortions.
[b]Maternal deaths per 100,000 live births range accounting for reporting variances.

TABLE 3. *Anomalous fetuses*

Nonviable[a]	Viable
Hypoplastic left heart	Down syndrome
Trisomy 13	Spina bifida
Trisomy 18	Hydrocephalus/Dandy-Walker syndrome
Renal agenesis	Diaphragmatic hernia
Thanatophoric dysplasia	Achondroplasia
Alobar holoprosencephaly	Most cardiac anomalies
Hydranencephaly	Cleft/lip palpate
	Hydronephrosis
	Clubfoot or other limb deformity
	Cystic hygroma
	Esophageal atresia/fistula
	Duodenal atresia
	Omphalocele

This list is not exhaustive
[a]A nonviable fetus is one in which death is already a certain or near-certain outcome, or in which there is a certain or near-certain absence of cognitive developmental capacity.
(Data from Chervenak et al., 1995; and Crane et al., 1994.)

equate cervical visualization, uterine palpation, testing for infection, and assessment of suitability of local or general anesthesia. Laboratory analysis should include assessment of the hemoglobin or hematocrit and establishment of a patient's Rh factor status. Some practitioners test for *Chlamydia trachomatis* and *Neisseria gonorrhoeae*, but costs are generally prohibitive for the additional tests for syphilis, human immunodeficiency virus disease, and/or hepatitis, although this is clearly a population at risk. Pap smear screens are recommended per usual protocols but are not necessary for the abortion.

Ultrasound establishes the correctness of the dates of the pregnancy, as well as confirming fetal number, placental localization, and the presence of uterine anomalies and fibroids; it also screens for nonpalpable ovarian masses. Extensive fetal anatomic surveys are usually limited to patients considering pregnancy continuation. Sonography can be utilized to guide the performance of the procedure (Fig. 5) and to confirm that the tissue evacuation is complete.

Anesthesia for first-trimester and early-second-trimester procedures is typically local infiltration paracervically with lidocaine 1% (Xylocaine) or chloroprocaine (Nesacaine). Preoperative preparation may include acetaminophen or a nonsteroidal antiinflammatory drug (NSAID). Conscious sedation can be given with midazolam (Versed), 2.5- to 5.0-ml doses, which is easily reversed by flumazenil (Romazicon); rapid-acting narcotics are also occasionally used.

Cervical Dilation

Forceful cervical dilation can cause cervical lacerations, damage, or permanent incompetence, all of which are extremely rare with modern technology. Early-first-trimester procedures often require no dilatation for the multiparous patient and little dilatation with primigravidas. For procedures performed at less

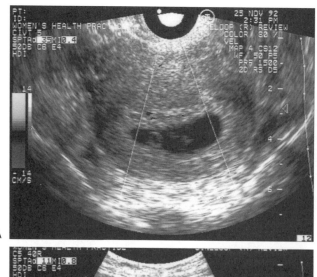

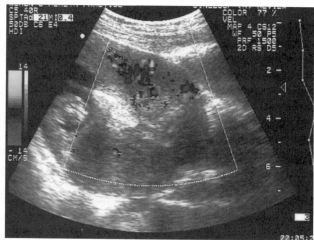

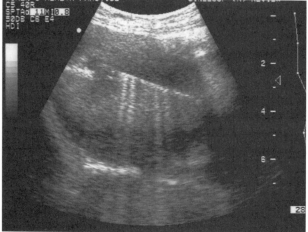

FIG. 5. A: Sonographic guidance of termination. **B:** Sonographic appearance of a suction cannula. **C:** Sonographic visualization.

than 9 to 12 weeks since the last menstrual period (LMP), dilation is accomplished with progressive use of cervical dilators: Pratt-type or plastic Denniston dilators used serially to enlarge the cervical canal. Beyond this time of gestation, medical and/or mechanical aids for dilation are very helpful. Most commonly employed is the seaweed *Laminaria japonica* (in singles or multiples), which expands over 3 to 24 hours to enhance dilation (Fig. 6). Successive applications of increasing numbers of laminaria can be effective and used for longer than 24 hours. Once the dilators are inserted, patients should understand that the abortion process needs to be completed (Munsick, 1996). Failure to dilate the cervix is rare, but if the os is so stenotic that it cannot admit even a no. 3 dilator, preoperative use of misoprostol (Cytotec), 400 to 800 µg intravaginally, can be helpful, as is waiting until the pregnancy progresses.

First-Trimester Abortion

Early abortions are almost exclusively performed by suction curettage. The earliest surgical abortions are performed at 3 to 5 weeks after LMP. In some institutions, early abortion is performed before sonographic visualization of the gestational sac, but most early abortions are performed after the intrauterine nature of the pregnancy is confirmed. Prior to visual-

ization of the sac on vaginal sonography, human chorionic gonadotropin (hCG) titers greater than 1500 IU/ml suggest ectopic gestation. Grasping the anterior lip with a single-tooth tenaculum stabilizes the cervix, and local anesthetic is infiltrated submucosally in the paracervical region. The cervix is dilated commensurately with the length of gestation and the need of cannula aperture. For a 7- to 9-week post-

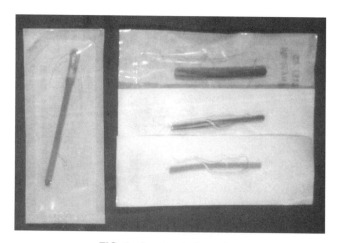

FIG. 6. *Laminaria japonica.*

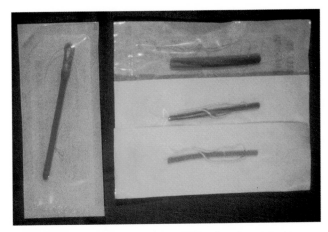

PLATE 12. *Laminaria japonica*. (This plate is printed in black and white as Figure 36-6.)

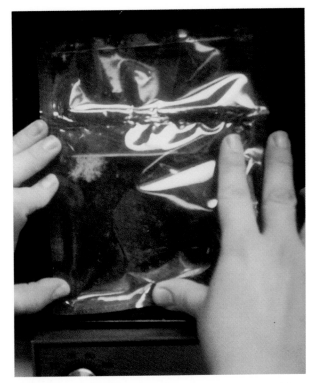

PLATE 13. Visualization of villi. (This plate is printed in black and white as Figure 36-7.)

LMP gestation, cannulas of 5 to 9 mm in width are utilized; they can be soft, flexible cannulas or rigid, either straight or bent. Use of uterine sounds should be avoided, as they increase the incidence of uterine perforation, and depth can be assessed by other means. The actual evacuation is accomplished by suction generated by a self-locking syringe or a machine aspirator at pressures of 60 to 70 mm Hg. Completeness of the procedure is established by the appearance of bubbles in the suction cannula and the characteristic uterine sound of the catheter against a denuded uterine wall. Washing the villi and observing them through backlighting can enhance tissue visualization (Fig. 7). Visual confirmation of tissue must be done before the patient leaves the facility. Histologic evaluation of the products of conception can identify the rare molar gestation. In cases of known fetal anomalies, this is even more important. Blood loss is extremely low, varying from 15 to 50 ml in most cases.

Second-Trimester Abortion

Dilation and evacuation (D&E) is the most common and safest method of second-trimester abortion (Hern et al, 1993). The procedure requires additional dilation of the cervix (up to 2 to 3 cm), and some of the evacuation needs to occur with the use of forceps. The forceps are most safely manipulated in the lower portion of the uterus. Occasional use of uterotonic agents enhances the ability to reach the products of conception. Blood loss with these procedures is typically in the 100- to 300-ml range. Vasopressin, 4 U, at the time of paracervical block significantly reduces bleeding (Schulz et al, 1985).

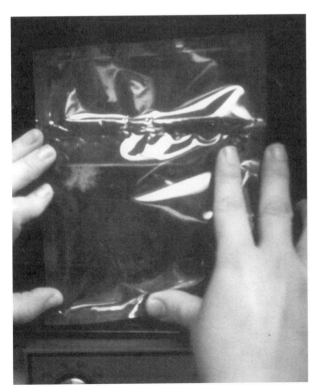

FIG. 7. Visualization of villi.

Saline- and Prostaglandin-induced Abortions

After 16 weeks' gestation, abortions can be performed with intrauterine abortifacient injection. Several solutions have been used, including hypertonic glucose, saline, urea, or uterotonics such as prostaglandins or oxytocin. The uterus is relatively resistant to oxytocin induction at this point. Recent articles suggest that oxytocin may be as effective as prostaglandins; however, higher doses of oxytocin are typically required (Owen et al., 1992). The widely used prostaglandins (PG) are PGE_2 (dinoprostone) suppositories (20 mg) or 15-methyl-$PGF_{2\alpha}$ (carboprost (250 µg) and tromethamine) (83 µg) for intramuscular injection. While saline and urea are hypertonic, the instillation procedure kills the fetus; isolated reports of fetal survival in cases of prostaglandin induction exist. Induction techniques may offer some advantages for the postmortem evaluation of fetal anatomic abnormalities, but approximately 97% of anomalies are able to be evaluated after D&E (Klaff, 1995). Preoperative karyotyping may assure an accurate chromosomal evaluation.

Postoperative Care

Antibiotic prophylaxis against infection reduces the incidence of postoperative cervicitis, salpingitis, and endometritis, since cultures are not typically available preoperatively (Sawaya et al., 1996). Doxycycline and erythromycin are excellent for their broad spectrum of coverage; if the patient is allergic to these, metronidazole or ampicillin in a short course of 3 to 7 days can be considered as alternatives, depending on the patient's access to follow-up. Postoperative pain is typically mild and responds to acetaminophen. An alternative regimen includes the use of of an NSAID, which has the unwanted side effect of masking a postoperative fever. Rh_0(D) immune globulin should be administered to the Rh-negative patient on the day of the procedure. An intrauterine device can be inserted on the day of the procedure, although the expulsion rate is slightly higher than if it is inserted after complete uterine involution. Medroxyprogesterone acetate (Depo-Provera) injections or levonorgestrel implants (Norplant System) can be initiated on the day of the procedure.

Postoperative appointments 1 to 3 weeks later can ensure timely involution, confirm the induced abortion has been completed, evaluate for complications, reassess psychological status, and continue contraceptive and gynecologic care (Fig. 8). However, compliance with follow-up visits is low.

◊ MEDICAL ABORTION

Medical abortions can benefit abortion patients by reducing the risk of cervical laceration and uterine perforation; they also allow women to undergo an abortion without an invasive surgical procedure. This is a significant benefit in areas of the country with no abortion providers. Ancient civil and naturalist practitioners over many centuries have administered herbal abortifacients. They are, however, ineffective and dangerous, and at least one woman has died from

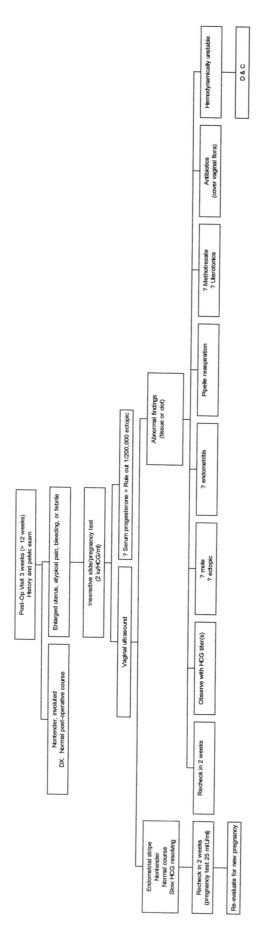

FIG. 8. Postoperative management flowsheet.

pennyroyal administration. Women of childbearing age should be specially cautioned about these compounds. By the 1970s, prostaglandins were used and efficacy was excellent, but there were side effects of vomiting and diarrhea. Prostaglandin analogs were developed, many of which had fairly high rates of success, but side effects still remained severe, and some patients still had to undergo surgical abortion to complete the process or stop bleeding.

Mifepristone (RU 486)

In 1988, the French released the progesterone antagonist RU 486, later named mifepristone, for use as an abortifacient. Originally, it was used by itself and later in combination with a prostaglandin analog. Mifepristone has a potent receptor affinity for the progesterone receptor, making it an effective antiprogesterone. The dosage of prostaglandin required is so low that side effects are minimized. Many analogs have been successfully tried, but only misoprostol is approved by the Food and Drug Administration (FDA) in the United States, although not for this indication. The fundamental principle is that progesterone support in early pregnancy is essential, and blocking this support causes expulsion of the conceptus. Abortions using mifepristone are available in France, China, Sweden, and the United Kingdom, and there have been several clinical trials in the United States (Grimes, 1997).

Regimens vary widely. In women up to 49 days' gestation, mifepristone, 200 to 600 mg in a single dose, is administered, followed 36 to 60 hours later by either gemeprost (not available in the United States), 1 mg vaginally, or sulprostone (also not available in the United States), 250 µg intramuscularly. Within a few hours after the prostaglandin is administered, over 50% of patients have aborted, and within 24 hours afterward, over 85% have aborted, although bleeding may persist for up to 60 days. Continuing pregnancy rates are low, and fewer than 1% of patients require curettage due to hemorrhage. Subsequently, regimens have been studied in which mifepristone is followed with misoprostol, which has been administered both orally and vaginally in doses of 200 to 800 µg.

Methotrexate

Methotrexate is an antimetabolite that blocks dihydrofolate reductase, an enzyme essential for the production of the DNA nucleotide thymidine. As rapidly dividing cells are most affected, methotrexate has been used clinically for the treatment of molar gestation, ectopic pregnancy, and early medical abortion. Although methotrexate is not FDA-approved for this indication, medical protocols for abortion have been extensively studied. Toxicity is dose-dependent. At the low doses used in regimens for ectopic pregnancy, methotrexate's side effects are primarily gastrointestinal, with nausea, vomiting, and diarrhea, although there have been isolated reports of marrow suppression

(leukopenia) and alopecia. At high doses, it can cause renal toxicity or gastrointestinal-lining damage. Methotrexate in the 50- to 150-mg range should not produce ovarian toxicity and has no long-term toxicity with regard to reproductive function. The protocols are more complex than those for surgical abortions, requiring more evaluation and more provider visits; failure rates are also higher (Fig. 9).

After a complete blood cell count and blood and liver chemistry profiles in patients at less than 63 days' gestation, methotrexate, 50 mg/m$_2$, is administered intramuscularly. Then, 1 to 7 days later, misoprostol, 800 mg, is inserted vaginally. Sonography is performed after the heavier bleeding expected in 1 to 2 days. Unsuccessful abortion completion at this point may be treated with another application of vaginal misoprostol. Some patients take as many as 4 weeks to complete the abortion, and 4% to 6% of women will require surgical abortion. Success rates are 90% to 93%, with complication rates similar to those with mifepristone. Medical abortion is a slow and relatively ineffective procedure, compared to surgical abortion, and should be reserved for a select population. Access to a provider who can perform a surgical abortion is essential for the safety of this procedure.

◊ COMPLICATIONS OF ABORTION

Abortion procedures are extremely safe in the United States, with serious complications developing in only 1 in 100 patients and death occurring in 1 in 100,000. The safest abortions are those performed at 7 to 10 weeks post-LMP. Death rates for D&E have been reported at approximately 7 per 100,000 (Lawson et al., 1994). Concomitant sterilization, preexisting medical conditions, and general anesthesia increase complications. The Centers for Disease Control and Prevention defines major complications of abortion as hemorrhage requiring transfusion, infection with 2 or more days of fever with a peak of at least 104°F (40°C), hospitalization of 11 days or more, or major unintended surgery. Other immediate complications include acute cervical laceration, failure to dilate the cervix, failure to obtain tissue, postoperative pain, acute uterine hematometria, and, rarely, pulmonary embolism (Tables 4 and 5). Immediate complications can include symptomatic breast engorgement, moderate to severe pain, and allergic reactions to medications. More delayed complications include retained products of conception, infections, and continuing pregnancy. Longer-term complications might include weakening of the cervix, intrauterine adhesions, or Rh sensitization. Rates of all complications are extremely low.

Uterine Hemorrhage

Rates of uterine hemorrhage (more than 500 ml blood loss) are low, less than 5% of cases, and the need for transfusion is exceedingly rare. Uterine atony can be decreased by complete evacuation of the uterus, use of vasopressin injection in the paracervical block (4 U or 0.2 ml), or use of postoper-

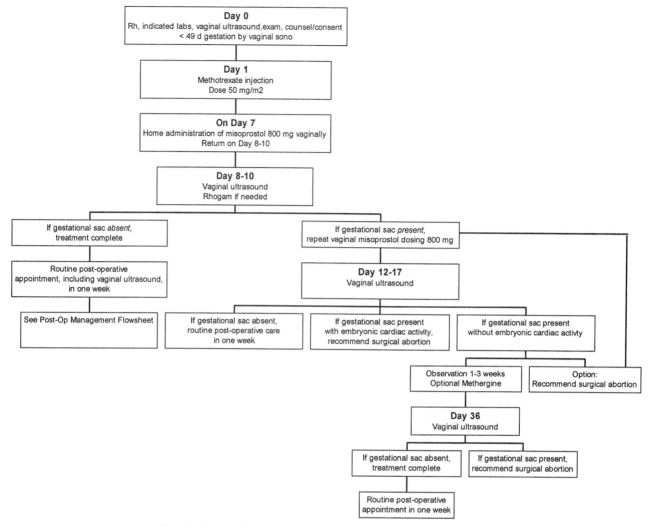

FIG. 9. Nonsurgical (methotrexate/misoprotol) abortion flowsheet.

ative oral or intramuscular methylergonovine maleate (0.2 mg) (Woodward, 1983). Failure to respond can be treated with carboprost tromethamine, and continued atony can be treated with intrauterine Foley balloon distention to tamponade the uterine cavity.

Uterine Perforation

Uterine perforation occurs in approximately 1 in 250 terminations (Kaali et al., 1989) and is usually recognized by an experienced provider at the time of the procedure. In first-trimester fundal perforations, observation is all that is required. If the nature and extent of the perforation are unknown or if suction was applied during the perforation, evaluation by laparoscopy is necessary. In early-first-trimester abortions, the procedure may be safely completed in experienced hands with sonographic guidance of the catheters. A perforation during D&E is a more serious complication, and the amount of bleeding may necessitate a laparotomy. Darney et al. (1990) established that 14 of 15 perforations during D&E were associated with major organ

injury. Organs damaged include the uterus, bowel, and bladder. Surgical interventions, when necessary, should not be delayed.

Endometrial Adhesions

Asherman syndrome should be suspected in a patient with no menses for several cycles following abortion. This is a rare complication and may be avoided through the prevention of endometritis and the avoidance of postevacuation sharp curettage.

Retained Tissue

Evaluation of the products of conception at the time of abortion can significantly reduce the number of cases of retained tissue. There have been case reports of very delayed retention of incompletely removed tissue, but consideration of a new pregnancy must be given in these cases. Persistence of a positive pregnancy test can signal retained products of conception, but careful postoperative evaluation by those expe-

TABLE 4. *Complications of abortion and complication rates*

Complication[a]	Percentage[b]
Immediate	
Failure to dilate cervix	0.1
Perforation	0.09–0.5
Acute hematometria	0.1–1.0
Anesthetic reaction, mild/severe	0.2
Breast engorgement	0.05
Hemorrhage (>500 ml)	0.05–4.9
Pain (moderate-severe)	0.5–5.0
Allergic reaction to medications	0.0–0.05
Transfusion	0.06
Delayed	
Retained products of conception	0.5–1.0
Endometritis/salpingitis	1.0–5.0
Infection	0.5–1.0
Transient fever	2.0
Persistent positive HCG (>3 weeks)	0.5–5.0
Continuing pregnancy	0.05
Post-abortion molar gestation	0.01–0.05
Longterm	
Cervical injury	0.1–1.6
Ashermanns, complete/partial	0.1–2.3
Infertility	1.0–2.0
Chronic pelvic inflammatory disease	1.0–2.0
Psychologic sequelae	0.5–1.0

[a]Rates of serious complications <1/100.
[b]Estimates based on cumulative data in medical literature.

rienced with the normal involution process typically reveals that this is a self-limited process. Normal resolution of the pregnancy test depends on the length of the pregnancy at the time of abortion and the sensitivity of the hCG tests used. Sonography can be helpful, but many pregnancies have some intrauterine fluid accumulation that appears within a few hours of abortion and does not dissolve for several days in a first-trimester pregnancy (Haddad et al., 1992). Retained products of conception may be most effectively handled by endometrial aspiration (3- to 5-mm suction pipettes), which is also useful for treatment of hematometria and can be diagnostic for retained tissue. Alternatives that may be useful in selected cases are observation, uterotonics, or repeat suction curettage. In some cases, the retained tissue can cause uterine hemorrhage and increase the incidence of postabortal infection.

TABLE 5. *Abortion-related deaths: United States 1987–1990*

Complication	Percentage	Number
Hemorrhage	18.5	10
Embolism	11.1	6
Pregnancy-induced hypertension	1.2	1
Infection	49.4	25
Anesthesia	8.6	4
Other/unknown	11.1	6

(From *MMWR* 1997; 46(SS-4).)

Infectious Complications

Endometritis can occur with or without retained products of conception. Clinical signs are abdominal pain, increased cramping, fever, and increased bleeding. Endometritis is difficult to diagnose but can be presumed when tenderness, especially associated with febrile morbidity (fever greater than 100.4°F [38°C]) or an elevated white blood cell count, is present. It is expected to occur in about 0.5% of suction curettage procedures, 1.5% of D&E procedures, and 5% of uterine instillations, in spite of prophylactic antibiotics. The organisms most likely responsible for endometritis are vaginal flora. A broad-spectrum oral antibiotic is usually sufficient therapy; repeat curettage may be indicated.

Psychological Consequences of Abortion

Improvement in emotional health postabortion is the most consistent statistically documented response. Symptoms of depression are likely to be a continuation of prior feelings. Patients are more likely to be depressed before rather than after an abortion, and while approximately one-third of women report postabortion feelings of guilt, these feelings are typically mild (Adler et al., 1990). In abortion denied, the children are rarely put up for adoption.

◊ CONCLUSION

An estimated 1.2 to 1.6 million abortions have occurred in the United States in each of the past 10 years. The complications are very few, and the death rates in the United States remain less than 1 per 100,000. It is important for health care providers to understand the process of induced abortion and to recognize the potential risks, benefits, and complications of this procedure. Extensive research indicates that induced abortions continue to be a procedure requested by women regardless of religious conviction or historical time frame. It is an obligation of the medical profession to keep it safe.

◊ RECOMMENDED READINGS

Legalization
Abortion surveillance: preliminary analysis—United States, 1995. *MMWR Morb Mortal Wkly Rep* 1997;46:1133–1137.
Council on Scientific Affairs, American Medical Association. Induced termination of pregnancy before and after Roe v Wade: trends in the mortality and morbidity of women. *JAMA* 1992;268:3231–3239.
Ellerton C. Mandatory parental involvement in minors' abortion: effects of the laws in Minnesota, Missouri, and Indiana. *Am J Public Health* 1997; 87:1367–1374.
Facts in Brief-Induced Abortion. Alan Guttmacher Institute, 120 Wall Street, New York, NY 10005, http://www.agi-usa.org. January 1997.
Gorney C. *Articles of faith: a frontline of the abortion wars.* New York: Simon & Schuster, 1998.
Grimes DA, Cates W Jr. Complications from legally-induced abortion: a review. *Obstet Gynecol Surv* 1979;34:177–191.
Grimes DA, Forrest JD, Kirkman AL, Radford B. An epidemic of antiabortion violence in the United States. *Am J Obstet Gynecol* 1991;165: 1263–1268.
Henshaw SK, Kost K. Abortion patients in 1994–95: characteristics and contraceptive use. *Fam Plann Perspect* 1996;28:104–107,158.

Henshaw SK, Van Vort J. Abortion services in the United States, 1991 and 1992. *Fam Plann Perspect* 1994;26:100–106,112.

Joyce T, Henshaw SK, Skatrud JD. The impact of Mississippi's mandatory delay law on abortions and births. *JAMA* 1997;278:653–658.

Joffe C. *Doctors of conscience: the struggle to provide abortion before and after Roe v Wade.* Boston:Beacon Press, 1996.

Koonin LM, MacKay AP, Berg CJ, Atrash HK, Smith JC. Pregnancy-related mortality surveillance—United States, 1987–1990. *MMWR CDC Surveillance Summaries* 1997;46 (No. SS-4), 17–36.

Koonin LM, Smith JC, Ramick M, Green CA. Abortion surveillance—United States, 1992. *MMWR CDC Surveillance Summaries* 1996;45(No. SS-3), 1–36.

McFarlane DR. U.S. abortion policy since Roe v Wade. *Am J Gynecol Health* 1993;7(4):98–106.

Meier KJ, McFarlane DR. State family planning and abortion expenditures: their effect on public health. *Am J Public Health* 1994;84: 1468–1472.

MMWR 1997;46(S8-4):23.

Omenn GS, Fielding JE, Lave LB. Annual review of public health abortion: a legal and public health perspective. *Annu Rev Public Health* 1991; 12:361–382.

Perry AM. Should legislatures practice medicine?. *N Engl J Med* 1997;337: 1240 (letter); discussion 1241.

Reagan L. *When abortion was a crime.* Berkeley, CA: University of California Press, 1998.

Risen J, Thomas J. *Wrath of angels: the American abortion war.* New York: Basic Books, 1998.

Rosenfield A. Women's reproductive health. *Am J Obstet Gynecol* 1993; 169:128–133.

Solinger R. *Abortion wars: a half century of struggle, 1950–2000.* Berkeley, CA: University of California Press, 1998.

Counseling

Baker A. *Abortion and options counseling: a comprehensive reference.* Granite City, IL: The Hope Clinic of Granite City, 1995.

Chervenak FA, McCullough LB, Campbell S. Is third trimester abortion justified? *Br J Obstet Gynaecol* 1995;102:434–435.

Crane JP, Lefevre ML, Winborn RC, et al. A randomized trial of prenatal ultrasonography screening: impact on detection, management, and outcome of anomalous fetuses. *Am J Obstet Gynecol* 1994;171: 392–399.

Ross S. Abortion must not be advocated as preventive solution to unwanted pregnancy. *BMJ* 1997;314:1623–1624 (letter).

Torres A, Forrest JD. Why do women have abortions? *Fam Plann Perspect* 1988;20:169–176.

Indications

Berg TG, Smith CV. Pregnancy contraindications: which are absolute? *OBG Management* 1997:50–59.

Surgical Abortion

Baxi L. Midtrimester elective abortion. *Am J Obstet Gynecol* 1997;176: 952–953 (letter; comment on *Am J Obstet Gynecol* 1996;175: 889–892).

Berkowitz RL, Stone JL, Eddleman KA. One hundred consecutive cases of selective termination of an abnormal fetus in a multifetal gestation. *Obstet Gynecol* 1997;90:606–610.

Edwards J, Carson SA. New technologies permit safe abortion at less than six weeks gestation and provide timely direction of ectopic gestation. *Am J Obstet Gynecol* 1997;176:1101–1106.

Evans MI, Hume RF Jr, Polak S, et al. The geriatric gravida: multifetal pregnancy reduction, donor eggs, and aggressive infertility treatments. *Am J Obstet Gynecol* 1997;177:875–878.

Hakim-Elahi E, Tovell HM, Burnhill MS. Complications of first trimester abortion: a report of 170,000 cases. *Obstet Gynecol* 1990;76:129.

Hern WM, Zen C, Ferguson KA, Hart V, Haseman MV. Outpatient abortion for fetal anomaly and fetal death from 15–34 weeks' gestation: techniques and clinical management. *Obstet Gynecol* 1993;81:301–306.

Howie FL, Henshaw RC, Naji SA, Russell IT, Templeton AA. Medical abortion or vacuum aspiration? Two-year follow up of patient preference trial. *Br J Obstet Gynaecol* 1997;104:829–833.

Klatt GC. The pathologic examination of fetal specimens from dilatation and evacuation procedures. *Am J Clin Pathol* 1995;103:415–418.

Kyle PM, Sepulveda W, Blunt S, Davigo G, Cox PM, Fisk RS. High failure rate of postmortem karyotyping after termination for fetal abnormality. *Obstet Gynecol* 1996;88:859–862.

Munsick RA, Fineberg NS. Cervical dilation from multiple laminaria tents used for abortion. *Obstet Gynecol* 1996;87:726–729.

Owen J, Hauth JC, Winkler CL, Gray SE. Midtrimester pregnancy termination: a randomized trial of prostaglandin E_2 versus concentrated oxytocin. *Am J Obstet Gynecol* 1992;167:1112–1116.

Paintin D. Abortion after 24 weeks. *Br J Obstet Gynaecol* 1997;104:398–400 (comment on *Br J Obstet Gynaecol* 1997;104:478–487).

Prasad CJ, Ireland KM. The effectiveness of cytologic evaluation of products of conception. *Arch Pathol Lab Med* 1992;116:1159–1162.

Savage W. Do fetuses feel pain? Surgical terminations of pregnancy take place under general anesthesia. *BMJ* 1997;314:1201 (letter).

Sawaya GF, Grady D, Kerlikowske K, Grimes DA. Antibiotics at the time of induced abortions: the case for universal prophylaxis based on a meta-analysis. *Obstet Gynecol* 1996;87:884–890.

Shulz KF, Grimes DA, Christensen DD. Vasopressin reduces blood loss from second-trimester dilatation and evacuation abortion. *Lancet* 1985; 2:353–356.

Medical Abortion

Creinin MD, Edwards J. Early abortion: surgical and medical options, current problems in obstetrics. *Gynecol Fertil* 1997;20:1–32.

Creinin MD, Vittinghoff E, Schaff E, Klaisle C, Darney PD, Dean C. Medical abortion with oral methotrexate and vaginal misoprostol. *Obstet Gynecol* 1997;90:611–616.

Grimes DA. Medical abortion in early pregnancy: a review of the evidence. *Obstet Gynecol* 1997;89:790–796.

Ho PC, Ngai SW, Liu KL, Wong GC, Lee SW. Vaginal misoprostol compared with oral misoprostol in termination of second-trimester pregnancy. *Obstet Gynecol* 1997;90:735–738.

Novoa JC, Novoa JC Jr. New technologies? *Am J Obstet Gynecol* 1997;177: 1270 (letter).

Complications

Adler NE, David HP, Masor BN, et al. Psychological responses after abortion. *Science* 1990;248:41–44.

Brind J, Chinchilli VM. Induced abortion and the risk of breast cancer. *N Engl J Med* 1997;336:1834 (letter; comment on *N Engl J Med* 1997; 336:81–85); discussion 1835.

Brodie HK, Banner L. Normatology: a review and commentary with reference to abortion and physician-assisted suicide. *Am J Psychiatry* 1997; 154(6; suppl):13–19 (review article).

Dagg PK. The psychological sequelae of therapeutic abortion—denied and completed. *Am J Psychiatry* 1991;148:578–585.

Darney PD, Atkinson E, Hirobayashi K. Uterine perforation during second trimester abortion by cervical dilation and instrumental extraction: a review of 15 cases. *Obstet Gynecol* 1990;75:441–444.

Ferris LE, McMain-Klein M, Colodny N, Fellows GF, Lamount J. Factors associated with immediate abortion complications. *CMAJ* 1996; 154: 1677–1685.

Grimes DA, Cates W Jr. Complications from legally induced abortion: a review. *Obstet Gynecol Surv* 1979;34:177–191.

Haddad S, Ruach M, Ohel G. Sonographic demonstration of endometrial fluid collection following termination of pregnancy. *Obstet Gynecol* 1992;79:703–704.

Henriques CU, Wilken-Jensen C, Throrense P, Moller BR. A randomized controlled trial of prophylaxis of post-abortal infection: ceftriaxone verses placebo. *Br J Obstet Gynaecol* 1994;201:610–614.

Iles S, Gath D. Psychiatric outcome of termination of pregnancy for fetal abnormality. *Psychol Med* 1993;23:407–413.

Kaali SG, Szigetvari IA, Bartfai GS. The frequency and management of uterine perforations during first trimester abortions. *Am J Obstet Gynecol* 1989;161:406–408.

Koonin LM, MacKay AP, Berg CJ, Atrash HK, Smith JC. Pregnancy-related mortality surveillance—United States, 1987–1990. *MMWR CDC Surveillance Summaries,* 1997;46 (No. SS-4), 10.

Lawson HW, Frye A, Atrash HK, et al. Abortion mortality, United States 1972–1987. *Am J Obstet Gynecol* 1994;171:1365–1372.

Mitchison S. Suicides after pregnancy: study did not show association between induced abortion and suicide. *BMJ* 1997;314:902 (letter; comment on *BMJ* 1996;313:1431–1434); discussion 902–903.

Senghas RE, Dolan MF. Induced abortion and the risk of breast cancer. *N Engl J Med* 1997;336:1834 (letter); discussion 1835.

Stotland NL. The myth of the abortion trauma syndrome. *JAMA* 1992;268: 2078–2079.

Woodward G. Intraoperative blood loss in midtrimester dilatation and extraction. *Obstet Gynecol* 1983;62:69–72.

CHAPTER 37

Pelvic Infections and Sexually Transmitted Diseases

◇

David A. Eschenbach

The female reproductive tract is susceptible to a large number of infectious agents, and pelvic infections are common. Many pelvic infections are sexually transmitted (Table 1). This chapter provides data on usual presentations and updated treatment of pelvic infections.

The impact of pelvic infections on the physical condition of women ranges from minor annoyance to serious illness and, in some instances, even death. The cost of treating pelvic infections is enormous if direct medical costs and indirect costs, including time lost from work, are calculated. Using pelvic inflammatory disease (PID) as an example, it has been estimated that by the year 2000, one of every four women who reached reproductive age in the 1970s will have had an episode of PID. Of women with PID, 25% will have been hospitalized, 25% will have had major surgery, and 20% will have tubal sterility.

Normally sterile upper genital tract sites (endometrium, fallopian tubes, ovaries) are subject to ascending infection from lower genital tract microorganisms. Some agents preferentially infect certain sites and give rise to characteristic symptoms; other agents cause few symptoms until major pathologic changes occur or until congenital neonatal infection or male-partner infection ensues. Clinicians should have special knowledge of the infections caused by *Neisseria gonorrhoeae, Chlamydia trachomatis,* group B streptococci, *Treponema pallidum,* anaerobic bacteria, bacteria associated with bacterial vaginosis, and *Mycobacterium tuberculosis*; these infection either are common or potentially produce severe sequelae. It is now appreciated that most viral infections of the genital tract are asymptomatic. Several viruses can produce severe disease in both adults and neonates, including herpes virus, cytomegalovirus, hepatitis B virus, human papillomavirus, and human immunodeficiency virus (HIV).

◇ VULVA

Herpes

Type-specific serologic assays indicate that one-third of women 20 to 45 years of age have been exposed to herpes simplex virus type 2 (HSV-2). Between 60% and 85% of women with HSV-2 antibodies have never had a recognized genital infection. Despite the frequency of asymptomatic infection, HSV infection is a common cause of vulvar ulcers. Other causes of genital ulcers include syphilis and chancroid. Ulcers from HSV usually occur 3 to 7 days after exposure. Symptomatic primary (first) genital infections typically consist of multiple vesicles that rapidly produce ulcerations of the vulva, which can be exceedingly painful. The cervix and vagina may also be involved, producing a gray necrotic cervix and profuse leukorrhea. External dysuria is common, and bilateral inguinal lymphadenopathy is usual. Vulvar lesions may last for 3 or more weeks before healing is complete. Constitutional symptoms of fever, malaise, headache (i.e., aseptic meningitis), and urinary retention (i.e., myelitis) may persist for a week.

After primary infection, latent HSV usually localizes in the sacral ganglion and perhaps the dermis. Periodic asymptomatic shedding occurs, particularly in the first 6 months after primary infection. The virus can be isolated on 1% of the days when there are no symptoms or physical evidence of infection. Most patients develop a secondary (i.e., recurrent) infection from latent virus weeks to months after the primary infection. Secondary lesions are usually less painful and more localized and last for a shorter time (3 to 7 days) than the lesions of primary infection. Systemic manifestations are unusual with secondary infection.

Between 75% and 85% of genital infections are caused by HSV-2, with the remainder caused by HSV-1, the primary cause of oral herpes. The two types of herpes infections are

579

TABLE 1. *Sexually transmitted infections*

Organisms	Diseases
Bacteria	
Neisseria gonorrhoeae	Gonorrhea
Chlamydia trachomatis	Chlamydiosis
Treponema pallidum	Syphilis
Haemophilus ducreyi	Chancroid
Calymmatobacterium granulomatis	Granuloma inguinale
Gardnerella vaginalis, anaerobes	Vaginitis
Group B β-hemolytic streptococcus	Group B streptococcal infection
Mycoplasmas	
Mycoplasma hominis	Mycoplasmosis
Ureaplasma urealyticum	Mycoplasmosis
Viruses	
Herpesvirus hominis (herpes simplex virus)	Genital herpes
Cytomegalovirus (CMV)	CMV infection
Hepatitis B virus	Hepatitis B
Human papillomavirus	Condyloma acuminatum
Molluscum contagiosum virus	Molluscum contagiosum
Human immunodeficiency virus	Acquired immunodeficiency syndrome
Protozoa	
Trichomonas vaginalis	Vaginitis
Entamoeba histolytica	Proctitis
Fungi	
Candida albicans	Vaginitis
Parasites	
Sarcoptes scabiei	Scabies
Phthirus pubis	Pediculosis pubis

clinically indistinguishable. Vesicles and ulcers contain many highly infectious virus particles, and viral shedding occurs until the lesions disappear. Therefore, direct contact with either genital or oral HSV lesions leads to a high rate of infection. Transmission usually occurs from contact with ulcerative lesions. Transmission is greatest during a primary infection, intermediate during a secondary infection, and probably least with asymptomatic shedding.

The diagnosis of herpes can be made clinically if typical, painful, multiple vulvar ulcers are present. However, many HSV lesions are atypical. Laboratory confirmation of atypical lesions and lesions that appear during pregnancy is best attained by virus isolation, which can usually be achieved within 48 hours or by polymerase chain reaction (PCR) identification. Other direct HSV identification methods, including Papanicolaou smear, fluorescein tagging, and immunoperoxidase staining, are only 50% sensitive in identifying HSV. Accordingly, a negative direct Pap smear does not exclude HSV infection. Complement fixing and neutralizing antibodies appear within 1 week of the onset of infection; failure of an experienced laboratory to identify antibodies within 3 weeks is evidence against HSV infection. High antibody levels do not protect against recurrent HSV infection, although anti-

body passively transferred to the fetus appears to offer considerable protection against neonatal infection.

The rising incidence of herpes infection and the potentially serious fetal infection caused by HSV make this an important infection in pregnancy. New guidelines for herpes are discussed in Chapter 25.

Women with cervical cancer have a higher prevalence of antibody and usually a higher antibody titer than controls without cancer. However, HSV does not appear to cause cervical cancer.

Oral acyclovir (Zovirax), 400 mg three times daily for 5 days, or valacyclovir (Valtrex), 500 mg twice daily for 5 days, shortens the ulcerative phase. Topical acyclovir therapy is considerably less effective than oral therapy. Acyclovir does not eradicate HSV or prevent recurrence. Patients with six or more yearly recurrences may benefit from oral acyclovir, 200 mg two to five times daily, or valacyclovir, 500 mg daily for up to 12 months. The expense of this drug limits its routine use. Local therapy of genital herpes is limited to pain relief. Most local treatment modalities either do not penetrate into virus-containing cells or are administered after epithelial damage has occurred. Corticosteroids and antibacterial and antifungal ointments are without benefit, and because they prevent drying, they tend to delay healing. Wet-to-dry therapy is often helpful (i.e., 10-minute sitz bath three or four times daily followed by drying with a lightbulb or hair dryer).

Human Papillomavirus

Human papillomavirus (HPV) is a DNA virus that is distinct from the papovaviruses that cause the common wart. HPV thrives in the moist genital area and usually is sexually transmitted. HPV infection is common and typically subclinical. HPV DNA was found in the genitalia in 30% to 45% of women with PCR DNA amplification. The vulva was positive for HPV DNA in more than 40%, and the cervix in over 30%. Only 1% of the women had visible warts, and only 9% had a history of genital warts. The average incubation period for visible warts is 3 months. Genital warts most commonly occur on the labia and posterior fourchette (Fig. 1). They originally appear as individual lesions, although, if neglected, large confluent growths can attain up to several centimeters in diameter. Vaginal and cervical warts are even more common than labial warts, although most of these are flat lesions visible only by colposcopy. Over 70 HPV types have been identified. Visible genital warts are usually caused by HPV types 6 and 11; 3% of college women had these types. The flat-wart variant is caused by HPV types 16, 18, 31, 33, and 35 (found in 22% of college women tested) and is visible only by colposcopy. A biopsy needs to be done of flat or atypical-appearing cervical warts to exclude cervical neoplasia; treatment should be delayed until the nature of the lesion is determined. HPV types 16, 18, 31, 39, 45, 51, and 52 are associated with high-grade cervical dysplasia and cervical cancer where the HPV DNA is integrated into the cancer cell. Women with flat warts should have frequent Pap smears.

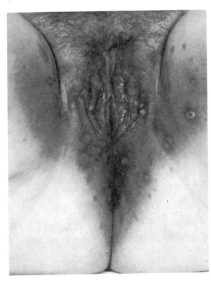

FIG. 1. Condylomata acuminata of the vulva.

Vulvar warts must be differentiated from the less verrucous, flatter growths of syphilitic condyloma latum (Fig. 2) and carcinoma *in situ* of the vulva; darkfield examination or punch biopsies may be required to differentiate these lesions. Small to medium-sized verrucous lesions can usually be treated with cryotherapy, podophyllin in tincture of benzoin, podofilox (Condylox), or trichloroacetic acid. Small amounts of podophyllin (0.25 ml) should be used to avoid severe burns. Podophyllin is contraindicated during pregnancy, as

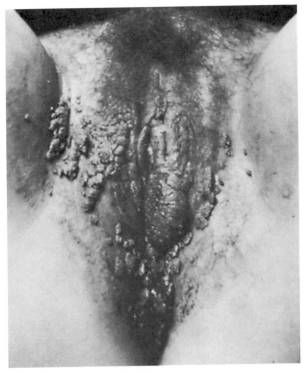

FIG. 2. Condylomata lata of the vulva and perineum. (From Curtis AH, Huffman JW. *A textbook of gynecology,* 6th ed. Philadelphia: WB Saunders, 1950; with permission.)

large amounts have produced coma in adults and fetal death in pregnancy. A biopsy should be done on atypical lesions before therapy is initiated because podophyllin causes bizarre histologic changes that persist for months. Cryotherapy, trichloroacetic acid, or laser ablation can be used on vaginal warts during pregnancy. Recurrence rates of 50% probably relate to the failure of these methods to kill the virus in adjacent untreated areas. 5-Fluorouracil can be used intravaginally, but caution is needed because severe burns have occurred, which limit its routine use. Large warts may not respond to surgical or laser removal alone but also may require regional interferon therapy.

Vestibulitis

Patients with vestibulitis characteristically have pain with vaginal penetration (i.e., intercourse or tampon insertion) and, in extreme cases, have difficulty sitting or wearing tight clothing. This condition is frequently treated as vaginitis because acidic vaginal discharge increases local irritation. Patients typically have an erythematous area, most commonly at the 4-o'clock and 7-o'clock positions just outside the hymenal ring. There is no clear evidence that HPV or bacteria cause the inflammation, but 20% of patients note symptoms after a severe episode of candidiasis. Treatment is often not effective, but regimens include topical corticosteroids (i.e., without an alcohol base), local corticosteroid injection, oral tricyclic antidepressants, and, in severe cases, skinning vulvectomy.

Furunculosis

Hair follicles or areas of hidradenitis in the vulva may become infected by staphylococci or other bacteria, giving rise to pustules. This condition must be distinguished from herpetic and syphilitic lesions. The diagnosis can be made by culture or by the finding of gram-positive cocci in Gram stains of pus. If only a few small lesions are present, treatment with hot, wet compresses or hexachlorophene scrubbing can be used. If a larger area is involved, administration of antistaphylococcal antibiotics is required until infection subsides, which may take weeks. Daily low-dose suppressive antibiotic therapy (e.g., erythromycin, 250 mg) may be used to prevent frequent recurrences.

Bartholinitis

Two stages of Bartholin gland infection occur. The first is an acute infection of the duct and gland, usually caused by either *N. gonorrhoeae* or *C. trachomatis*. If infection causes obstruction of the ducts, an abscess stage can result. Anaerobic bacteria can be isolated from most abscesses. Rarely, synergistic vulvar gangrene has resulted from bartholinitis.

Cultures and a Gram stain of material expressed from the duct may identify gonococci. Cervical gonococcal and chlamydial cultures should be obtained, and if the patient has gonorrhea, treatment for it should be administered, followed by tetracycline, as discussed later in this chapter. Patients with an abscess usually require abscess marsupialization or incision with placement of a catheter in the abscess cavity for 3 to 6 weeks to establish a new duct. Simple incision and drainage should be avoided, since it leads to inadequate drainage and recurrent abscess or cyst. Recurrent infection from vaginal flora and mucus cyst formation are common sequelae of bartholinitis.

Chancroid

The soft chancre of chancroid is a painful ulcer with a ragged, undermined edge and a raised border. In contrast, the syphilitic chancre is painless and indurated. "Kissing ulcers" on opposing surfaces of the vulva occur. Tender, unilateral adenopathy is common, and node suppuration occurs in about 50% of patients with lymphadenopathy. The incubation period of this sexually transmitted disease (STD) is 2 to 5 days. The infection is caused by *Haemophilus ducreyi,* a gram-negative bacterium that forms a school-of-fish pattern when seen in the Gram-stain preparation. The organism is fastidious, and it is best identified by culture of material from aspi-

rated lymph nodes or from the chancre onto specific selective media. The differential diagnosis includes syphilis, genital herpes, and lymphogranuloma venereum.

Preferred treatment is azithromycin (Zithromax), 1 g orally, or ceftriaxone sodium (Rocephin), 250 mg intramuscularly, in single doses, or erythromycin, 500 mg four times daily for 7 days. Amoxicillin/clavulanate potassium (Augmentin) and ciprofloxacin (Cipro) are alternative regimens.

Granuloma Inguinale

Granuloma inguinale is rare in temperate climates and is usually considered an STD, although gastrointestinal transmission can occur. The initial papular lesion typically ulcerates and develops into a soft, red, painless granuloma that may be covered by a thin, gray membrane. The granuloma may spread over the course of many months to involve the anus and rectum (Fig. 3). Lymph nodes are moderately enlarged and painless, but they do not suppurate. The infection can become chronic, and long-standing disease may cause genital

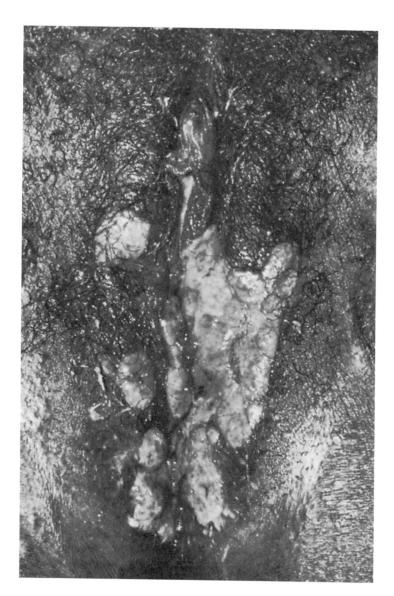

FIG. 3. Vulval granuloma inguinale of relatively recent origin. Some lesions are separate, others confluent. The margin of lesion is raised and scrolled; the base is granular and covered imperfectly by thin, gray slough. (From Demis DJ, Crounse RG, Dobson RL, McGuire J, eds. *Clinical dermatology,* vol 3. Hagerstown, MD: Harper & Row, 1972; with permission.)

scarring and depigmentation, as well as lymphatic fibrosis with consequent genital edema. Cancer has been reported in granulomatous areas, but this is unusual.

Infection is caused by a gram-negative bacillus, *Calymmatobacterium granulomatis,* that is difficult to culture because it is an intracellular parasite. The identification is usually made from scraped material or a biopsy specimen obtained from the periphery of the lesion. Bipolar-staining bacteria are best identified within mononuclear cells (i.e., Donovan bodies) by Wright or Giemsa staining.

Therapy of choice is a 3-week course of tetracycline. Trimethoprim/sulfamethoxazole, erythromycin, and the quinolones are alternatives.

Lymphogranuloma Venereum

The incubation period for lymphogranuloma venereum (LGV) is 2 to 5 days. Thereafter, a transient, primary, painless genital or anorectal ulcer develops. Multiple, large, confluent inguinal nodes develop 2 to 3 weeks later and eventually suppurate. Acute infection may cause generalized systemic symptoms. If untreated, the infection enters a tertiary phase that can lead to extensive lymphatic obstruction. This development, together with continued infection, causes fistulas and ulceration of the anal, urethral, or genital area. Women with LGV are particularly susceptible to rectal stricture. Edema and elephantiasis of the external genitalia and lower extremities are other serious sequelae.

The infection is caused by the sexually transmitted organism *C. trachomatis,* an intracellular bacterium. Usually, only L_{1-3} *Chlamydia* immunotypes, which produce accelerated *in vitro* tissue destruction, typically cause LGV. The diagnosis can be made by culturing chlamydiae from genital lesions or lymph nodes. The most specific and sensitive serologic test is the microimmunofluorescent antibody test, in which the specific L immunotypes are identified. The results of complement fixation (CF) tests are positive in 95% of patients with LGV, but the CF test lacks specificity; test results are often falsely positive in patients who do not have LGV but have previously been exposed to other chlamydial infections.

LGV responds to 3-week regimens of doxycycline, erythromycin, or sulfisoxazole (Gantrisin). Large lymph nodes should be aspirated to avoid chronic drainage. Surgical excision of scarred areas may be necessary.

◊ ACUTE URETHRAL SYNDROME

Acute cystitis is present in approximately 50% of women with symptoms of dysuria and urinary frequency. In the past, cystitis had been defined by pyuria and midstream urine cultures that contain more than 10^5 organisms per milliliter of coliform or staphylococcal organisms. The cause of symptoms in the remaining women was unknown. It is now apparent that about one-half of the remaining symptomatic women also have cystitis; these patients have less than 10^5 coliforms or *Staphylococcus saprophyticus* organisms per milliliter isolated from urine obtained by suprapubic

aspiration or urethral catheterization. Virtually all of these women have pyuria, defined as eight or more leukocytes per high-power field of urine. Pyuria occurs among another 25% of women with recent onset of internal dysuria and urinary frequency. Pyuria occurring with negative urine cultures is termed *acute urethral syndrome*, and these patients usually have *C. trachomatis*. The remaining 25% of patients with these symptoms have no pyuria, bacteriuria, or chlamydial infection. Some women with external dysuria (i.e., labial pain with urination) have candidal or herpetic vulvitis. Although many women with recently acquired gonorrhea develop transient dysuria, *N. gonorrhoeae* is only occasionally isolated from women with dysuria.

Treatment of acute urethritis consists of therapy for the infectious agent, whether it is coliform or *S. saprophyticus* cystitis, or *C. trachomatis* urethritis.

◊ VAGINITIS

Vaginitis is the most common reason for a gynecologic visit. Symptoms of vaginitis include increased vaginal discharge, vulvar irritation and pruritus, external dysuria, and a foul discharge odor. Women with infectious vaginitis have either abnormal organisms (i.e., trichomonads) or a quantitative increase in normal flora (i.e., *Candida, Gardnerella vaginalis,* anaerobes). At least four types of infectious vaginitis are found: candidal, trichomonal, bacterial vaginosis, and, in children, gonococcal. Every effort should be made to establish the diagnosis of one of these specific infections and to avoid the diagnosis of a nonspecific vaginitis. The establishment of a specific diagnosis is mandatory because the selection of effective therapy depends on a correct diagnosis. Treatment of nonspecific vaginitis inevitably fails.

Other conditions that may cause excessive vaginal discharge include cervicitis, normal cervical mucus from cervical ectopy, vaginal foreign bodies (most commonly, retained tampons), and allergic reactions to douching or vaginal contraceptive agents. Atrophic vaginitis among postmenopausal women may produce burning and dyspareunia, but an infectious cause has not been established.

A small amount of vaginal discharge may be normal, particularly at the midcycle, when large amounts of cervical mucus production may produce a clear vaginal discharge. A normal vaginal discharge should not have a foul odor or produce irritation or pruritus.

Examination

The external genitalia may be normal or edematous, erythematous, excoriated, or fissured. Local vulvar disease, especially vestibulitis, must be excluded from a secondary effect of vaginitis.

On speculum examination, the vaginal mucosa may be erythematous. Discharge characteristics that are important to observe are viscosity, floccular appearance, color, and odor. Vaginal pH status should always be determined. A potassium hydroxide (KOH) odor test and a microscopic examination consisting of a normal saline and 10% KOH wet mount should be done. A drop of each solution is mixed with discharge. Before placing a cover glass over the two separate drops, the KOH portion is tested for the presence of a fishy amine odor. Microscopic examination of the KOH portion is made for hyphae under the 100× objective, and examination of the saline portion is made for trichomonads and clue cells under the 400× objective. Multiple causes of vaginitis are frequent.

Vaginal cultures are not particularly helpful except when used selectively to identify *Candida*. Microscopy is specific, but only 80% sensitive in identifying various types of vaginitis. When infectious vaginitis is suspected in patients in whom a specific diagnosis cannot be established, a repeat examination should be performed 2 weeks later.

Candidiasis

The most prominent symptom of candidiasis is vulvar and vaginal pruritus. External irritation and dysuria are common. Increased vaginal discharge is infrequent. Vulvar signs of edema, geographic erythema, and fissures may be present. Classically, the vaginal walls are red and contain adherent, dry, white, curdy plaques. However, most women with candidiasis, have little discharge and no erythema.

Candida albicans causes about 90% of vaginal yeast infections. Noncandidal species can also cause infection. These saprophytic fungi are isolated from the vagina in 15% to 25% of asymptomatic women. Although the mere presence of vaginal candidae does not always identify an infection, large numbers of organisms lead to symptomatic vaginitis. However, severe inflammation will develop in some women with only a few organisms. Candidiasis occurs because of changes in host resistance or local bacterial flora that allow the organisms to proliferate. The most widely accepted risk factors for candidiasis include pregnancy, diabetes, and use of immunosuppressive drugs and broad-spectrum antibiotics. Frequent vaginal intercourse and vaginal douching have recently been associated with candidiasis. Because cellular, not humoral, immunity is required to resist candidal infections, pregnant women and patients receiving immunosuppressive drugs that decrease cellular immunity are predisposed to candidiasis. Candidal overgrowth is also favored by high urine glucose levels that can occur in diabetes or pregnancy or during candy binges. Broad-spectrum antibiotics cause suppression of the normal vaginal and gastrointestinal bacterial flora, allowing fungal overgrowth. The role of oral contraceptives in candidal infection remains controversial. Oral contraceptives cause both carbohydrate alterations and an increased prevalence of candidae in the vagina, but the incidence of symptomatic candidal infection among oral contraceptive users is usually no higher than that among nonusers. A small subset of users may develop recurring infections, but it usually is not necessary to discontinue oral contraceptive use.

Candidiasis is best diagnosed by KOH wet-mount examination. Vaginal plaques, vaginal discharge, or vulvar scrapings from the edge of the erythematous border is mixed with 10% KOH (Fig. 4). The mycelial form is usually found only during an infection; mycelia can be identified by KOH wet

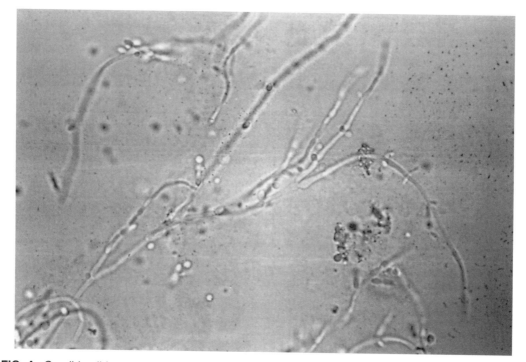

FIG. 4. *Candida albicans* growing as hyphae and pseudohyphae within infected tissue (×320). (From Monif GRG. *Infectious diseases in obstetrics and gynecology.* Hagerstown, MD: Harper & Row, 1974; with permission.)

mount in 80% of cases. The pH of vaginal discharge is normal (i.e., 4.7 or less). Fungi can readily be recovered on various media. Because they are part of the normal vaginal flora, culture positivity does not necessarily indicate infection. However, a culture for *Candida* only should be done on KOH wet mount–negative patients with symptoms or signs of candidiasis. Up to 50% of women with candidiasis have a negative wet mount, but a positive *Candida* culture.

Local vaginal therapy is used because most antifungal preparations are not absorbed from the intestinal tract. Various intravaginal azole agents used for 3 to 5 days are effective, including miconazole, clotrimazole, butoconazole (Femstat), tioconazole (Vagistat-1), and terconazole (Terazol). These agents should be administered to women with primary and infrequent candidal vaginitis. Azole drugs are not absorbed to any degree from the vagina, and the same local regimens can be used safely in pregnancy. The vaginal insertion of boric acid powder in capsules is also effective. A one-time dose of fluconazole (Diflucan), 150 mg orally, or itraconazole (Sporanox), 400 mg initially then 200 mg for 2 days, is also effective for those with mild symptoms, but patients with severe symptoms need repeated doses in 4 days. Prolonged 2-week intravaginal therapy may also be necessary for severe symptoms. Oral nystatin administration to decrease gastrointestinal colonization does not markedly improve therapeutic cure rates or diminish recurrence rates. About 15% of male sexual contacts of women with candidiasis have symptomatic balanitis; symptomatic males should be identified and treated to prevent recurrent female infection.

The number of non-*albicans* candidal infections is increasing. These infections respond poorly to azole therapy, including fluconazole. Boric acid or nystatin therapy works best. Even gentian violet 1% aqueous solution has a limited place in such patients.

Patient with frequently recurrent candidiasis represent the most difficult problem in treatment. Extended 2- to 3-week vaginal therapy, male therapy, and reduction of sugar intake are usually ineffective. A glucose tolerance test and HIV testing should be performed in recurrent or resistant cases to exclude unrecognized diabetes and HIV infection. In addition, some women with candidiasis have other concurrent vaginal infections; a repeat physical and wet-mount examination may clarify the problem.

Patients with frequently recurring candidiasis (four or more times a year) should receive suppressive anticandidal therapy. First, standard anticandidal therapy is undertaken for 2 weeks, followed by suppressive therapy with an intravaginal azole or boric acid, twice weekly or daily for 5 days once a month, or oral fluconazole, 150 mg weekly. Suppressive treatment should continue for at least 1 year; recurrent candidiasis is usually reduced to no or one infection yearly.

Trichomoniasis

Characteristic symptoms of trichomoniasis include a profuse, yellow, malodorous, often uncomfortable vaginal discharge

and vulvar irritation. *Trichomonas vaginalis* is a common sexually transmitted organism, present in 3% to 15% of asymptomatic women and in up to 20% of women who attend clinics for STDs. The organism is most likely identified among symptomatic women with recently acquired the infection. However, about 50% of women with trichomoniasis are asymptomatic. Most male contacts of women with trichomoniasis asymptomatically carry the organism in the urethra and prostate.

A classic profuse, frothy, yellow vaginal discharge is present in only about one-third of women. The vulva may be edematous and inflamed by the discharge. Sometimes, subepithelial redness of the cervix (i.e., strawberry cervix) is seen with the naked eye; smaller red areas are more commonly identified colposcopically. The discharge in women with symptomatic trichomoniasis often has a pH greater than 4.7 and forms an amine odor with 10% KOH. Motile trichomonads are demonstrated in the saline wet-mount smear (Fig. 5). Trichomonads are larger than white blood cells (WBCs) and are identified by their jerky motility. The wet mount usually also contains many polymorphonuclear leukocytes. Although the wet mount can identify trichomonads with 80% sensitivity among symptomatic women, overall less than 50% of women with trichomoniasis by culture have the organisms identified by wet mount. Trichomonads can be identified in a Pap smear by their characteristic flagellate appearance.

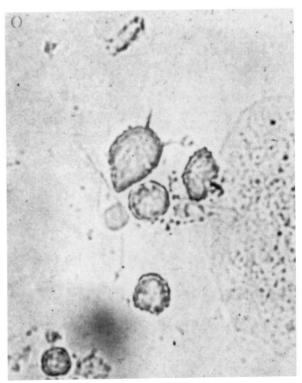

FIG. 5. Characteristic configuration of a trichomonad seen in wet smear at high-power magnification. (From Monif GRG. *Infectious diseases in obstetrics and gynecology.* Hagerstown, MD: Harper & Row, 1974; with permission.)

T. vaginalis is an anaerobic protozoan. A culture of this organism is easy to perform but not readily available, and culture should be limited to cases in which the diagnosis is suspected but cannot be confirmed by wet mount. Screening cultures in asymptomatic women are not recommended, except for certain high-risk populations. Women with trichomoniasis should also be cultured for *N. gonorrhoeae* because up to one-half of women with gonorrhea have also had trichomoniasis. Trichomoniasis frequently causes symptoms that lead patients with gonorrhea to present for care.

T. vaginalis resides not only in the vagina but also in the urethra, bladder, and Skene glands, so therapy needs to be systemic, rather than local. Metronidazole is effective in treating trichomoniasis; the preferred regimen is 2 g in one dose because of complete patient compliance and high effectiveness. Extended 7-day metronidazole therapy, 500 mg twice daily, does not increase the 95% cure rate of a single dose. Simultaneous treatment of the male sexual partner is recommended. Recurrent trichomoniasis is usually attributable to either a lack of compliance or reexposure to an untreated sexual partner. Increasing *in vitro* and *in vivo* resistance of the trichomonad to metronidazole has been reported, and metronidazole, 3-g daily split orally and intravaginally for 7 days, is occasionally necessary for a cure.

Metronidazole therapy is controversial because of its tumor-causing potential in humans. In animals, large doses (equivalent to 350 to 1000 human doses) cause tumors. The drug also causes the mutation of salmonellae associated with carcinogenic potential. No increased tumor rates were found in small series of women evaluated for up to 10 years after metronidazole therapy for trichomoniasis. These data are only slightly reassuring that the drug does not cause cancer, because longer, larger studies are needed to exclude this possibility. Metronidazole should be avoided in pregnancy, particularly during the first 20 weeks. However, other drugs that may be used during pregnancy lack efficacy, including iodine preparations, which are also absorbed in high enough levels to suppress the fetal thyroid. An association between *T. vaginalis* and prematurity needs further study. For nonpregnant women, the short-term use of a drug with at most a minimal carcinogenic potential seems justified, especially since this is the only agent that eradicates *T. vaginalis*. Persistent discharge after adequate treatment for trichomoniasis should lead to repeat cultures for both candidiasis and gonorrhea.

Bacterial Vaginosis

The term *bacterial vaginosis* describes the vaginal condition resulting from overgrowth of both anaerobic bacteria and *G. vaginalis*. Both anaerobes and *G. vaginalis* are normal inhabitants of the vagina, but overgrowth of the normal *Lactobacillus*-dominant flora by these bacteria results in a thin, homogeneous, fishy-smelling, gray vaginal discharge that adheres to the vaginal walls and often is present at the introitus. In contrast to the findings in most other kinds of vaginitis, the vaginal epithelium appears normal, and WBCs are usually not present. The fishy amine odor produced by anaerobes is accentuated when 10% KOH is added to the discharge.

The diagnosis of bacterial vaginosis is based on the presence of three of the following four characteristics of the discharge: pH greater than 4.7, a homogeneous thin appearance, a fishy amine odor with the addition of 10% KOH, and clue cells. Clue cells are vaginal epithelial cells to which organisms are attached. The cell border of these cells is so obscured by adherent bacteria that it cannot be identified. In bacterial vaginosis, 2% to 50% of the epithelial cells are clue cells. Polymorphonuclear leukocytes and lactobacilli are notably absent. Gram stains can also be used for diagnosis based on a reduction in *Lactobacillus* morphotypes and an increase in small gram-negative rods and gram-positive cocci. Cultures are not helpful because anaerobes and *G. vaginalis* can be recovered from normal women. In fact, up to 40% of asymptomatic normal women without vaginitis carry *G. vaginalis*. The distinguishing feature of bacterial vaginosis is the 10- to 1000-fold increased concentration of anaerobic bacteria and *G. vaginalis*.

Factors leading to the overgrowth of anaerobes and *G. vaginalis* have not been identified. Sexual transmission of the infection has long been considered a risk factor, but this has not been proven. *G. vaginalis* can usually be recovered from the urethra of the male sexual contact, but treatment of sexual contacts does not prevent recurrence.

Treatment is not advocated for most asymptomatic women with bacterial vaginosis because it can spontaneously disappear. However, the 10- to 1000-fold increase in the concentration of potentially virulent bacteria in the vagina appears to cause upper genital tract infection after surgery. An increased relative risk (RR) of postoperative infection has been reported in patients with bacterial vaginosis following cesarean section (RR = 6), hysterectomy (RR = 3 to 4), and induced-abortion PID (RR = 3). Bacterial vaginitis has also been assoiated with spontaneous PID and postpartum endometritis after vaginal delivery. Treatment of bacterial vaginosis is particularly beneficial for those undergoing elective surgery. Bacterial vaginosis in pregnancy has also been related to premature delivery (RR = 2 to 4), amniotic fluid infection (RR = 2 to 3), and chorioamnionitis (RR = 2 to 3); treatment of women with prior preterm delivery has reduced the incidence of preterm delivery.

Metronidazole, 500 mg twice daily for 7 days, and clindamycin, 300 mg twice daily for 7 days, are the most effective oral regimens for bacterial vaginosis. Topical metronidazole 0.75% gel and clindamycin 2% cream are as effective as oral therapy. Oral ampicillin, 500 mg every 6 hours for 7 days, cures 60% of cases. Metronidazole and clindamycin are particularly effective against the anaerobes. Fluoroquinolones, tetracycline, sulfonamides, and erythromycin are ineffective. Treatment of the male sexual contact with metronidazole can be advocated only when bacterial vaginosis recurs, but effectiveness is unproven.

Toxic Shock Syndrome

Toxic shock syndrome is an acute illness caused by toxin-producing *Staphylococcus aureus*. About 6% of women carry *S. aureus* in the vagina, but only 2% of women have the type of organism capable of producing the toxic shock toxin. The syndrome is highly associated with menstruation and probably with tampon use, but it has also occurred from *S. aureus* infection of the breast and endometrium after delivery and from abdominal surgical wounds. Characteristic features include a high fever (greater than 102°F [38.9°C]), a diffuse rash, hypotension, skin desquamation (usually 1 to 2 weeks later), and a wide variety of systemic effects, including gastrointestinal (vomiting, diarrhea), muscular (myalgia), mucous membrane (hyperemia), renal (elevated blood urea nitrogen or creatinine level), hepatic (enzyme abnormalities), hematologic (thrombocytopenia), and neurologic (disorientation, coma). Vaginal or specific-site cultures recover *S. aureus*. Blood, throat, and cerebrospinal fluid cultures, together with serologic tests for Rocky Mountain spotted fever, leptospirosis, and measles, are usually indicated to exclude diseases with similar clinical presentations.

A vaginal tampon, if present, should be removed. Patients should be hospitalized and, when indicated, given large fluid volumes for blood pressure maintenance. β-Lactamase-resistant antibiotics are recommended, and if other causes of bacterial sepsis, such as meningococcemia, cannot be excluded, additional antibiotics are necessary. Other life-supporting measures, such as intubation, vasopressor administration, and dialysis, are often necessary. The case-fatality ratio has been reduced from 15% to 3% with supportive therapy. Antibiotics are not of proven benefit in the acute stage, but they do reduce recurrence rates from 30% to 5%.

Although the effectiveness is uncertain, it is prudent for all women to avoid the prolonged and overnight use of tampons or intravaginal contraceptive devices. It is recommended that postpartum women not use tampons for 6 to 8 weeks after delivery. Women who have had toxic shock syndrome should be warned of recurrent episodes and advised against resuming tampon use.

◊ SYPHILIS

Physicians must constantly be aware of possible syphilitic infection, particularly in populations with high rates of HIV infection. Most women with syphilis are asymptomatic and have only serologic evidence of infection. *T. pallidum* organisms rapidly enter lymphatics after exposure, but a primary chancre lesion usually takes about 3 weeks to develop. The classic chancre ulcer is painless and firm with sharply defined, raised edges; however, most syphilitic ulcers are atypical. Any suspicious genital ulcer should be studied by darkfield examination. Serous material expressed from the ulcer base is mixed with saline solution, and because *T. pallidum* is an anaerobe, this mixture must be immediately placed under a cover-slip with the edges occluded by petroleum jelly. Identification of typical spirochetes by darkfield microscopy establishes the diagnosis of primary syphilis. Serologic tests are usually nonreactive when the chancre first appears but become reactive 1 to 4 weeks later.

Secondary syphilis appears 6 or more weeks later and is characterized by a symmetric, macular, papular, or papulosquamous rash and generalized, nontender lymphadenopathy. Condylomata lata (see Fig. 2) are highly infectious, hypertrophied, wart-like lesions of secondary syphilis that usually occur in moist areas, such as the vulva or perineum; they must be distinguished from other vulvar lesions. Superficial, painless mucosal erosions of the mouth or vagina, called mucous patches, develop in one-third of patients. Systemic symptoms of fever, weight loss, and malaise may occur. Serologic tests are positive in the secondary stage.

Untreated patients then enter a latent phase of syphilis during which clinical and physical manifestations are absent. Diagnosis in this phase is established by serologic tests. Intermittent spirochetal bloodstream invasion may occur early (the first 4 years) in the latent phase. In pregnancy, the risk of congenital fetal infection in the primary and secondary phases of syphilis is 80% to 95%; the risk during the early latent phase is 70%. During the late latent phase, immunity develops, which reduces blood invasion, and the risk of congenital syphilis decreases to 10%. Congenital syphilis is again increasing to 1 in 10,000 liveborn infants. Fetal or perinatal death occurs in 40% of those with congenital syphilis. About one-third of adult patients with untreated late syphilis manifest central nervous system or cardiovascular symptoms of tertiary syphilis.

Darkfield examination of ulcer material from possible syphilitic ulcers should be done on 3 consecutive days. VDRL or rapid plasma reagin (RPR) and fluorescent treponemal antibody (FTA) serology should be performed for a patient with a suspicious lesion. If the serologic results are nonreactive and spirochetes cannot be demonstrated by darkfield examination, serologic tests should be repeated in 1 month.

VDRL and RPR tests detect a nontreponemal, nonspecific reagin antibody. The tests can be titrated, and the titer either falls or disappears after therapy for early or secondary syphilis. Thus, the VDRL test can be used to judge the activity of either a first episode or reacquired infection in a patient with documented syphilis. Treated patients with latent syphilis may retain high, stable VDRL titers. Acute bacterial or viral infections can give rise to acute false-positive serologic reactions that last for up to 6 months. Several conditions, such as aging, addiction to drugs, autoimmune disease, and pregnancy, may give rise to chronic, nonspecific, false-positive VDRL reactions. False-positive VDRL titers usually are 1:8 or less. In contrast, the FTA test involves a specific anti-treponemal antibody, and false-positive FTA reactions are rare. Patients with a positive VDRL reaction must have a confirmatory FTA test to exclude a false-positive VDRL reaction. Patients with a false-positive VDRL reaction will have a negative FTA reaction. In patients with syphilis, the FTA test remains positive indefinitely, and because the test is not titrated, repeat FTA testing should not be done in a known positive patient.

The treatment schedules for syphilis currently recommended by the U.S. Public Health Service's Centers for Disease Control and Prevention (CDC) are as follows:

◊ *Early syphilis:* Early syphilis is defined as primary, secondary, or latent syphilis of less than 1 year's duration. The drug of choice is penicillin G benzathine, 2.4 million U total intramuscularly, because it provides effective treatment in a single dose. Alternative choices for penicillin-allergic patients include 2-week regimens of doxycycline, 100 mg twice daily, or tetracycline, 500 mg four times daily. Ceftriaxone, 250 mg daily intramuscularly for 10 days, may be used if close follow-up can be ensured.

◊ *Syphilis of longer than 1 year's duration:* Penicillin G benzathine, 2.4 million U intramuscularly each week for 3 successive weeks (7.2 million U total), is the drug of choice in this situation. Alternative choices for the penicillin-allergic include doxycycline and tetracycline for 4 weeks. Intravenous aqueous penicillin G or penicillin G procaine is recommended for neurosyphilis. Erythromycin is not recommended for neurosyphilis. Tetracycline must not be used in pregnancy. Spinal tap to exclude asymptomatic neurosyphilis is recommended for those with neurologic or ophthalmologic signs, other evidence of active disease (aortitis, gummas), HIV infection, treatment failure, and infection for more than 1 year with a titer of 1:32 or greater. Neurosyphilis and syphilis in HIV-positive patients should be treated by infectious disease specialists.

◊ *Syphilis in pregnancy:* Treatment using penicillin is the same as for the corresponding stage of syphilis among nonpregnant women. For penicillin-allergic pregnant patients, tetracycline is not used because of toxicity, and erythromycin is not used because of high failure rates to cure the fetus. Penicillin is so superior to other antibiotics for treating syphilis in pregnancy that penicillin-allergic pregnant patients should be desensitized. The Jarisch-Herxheimer reaction commonly occurs, and pregnant women should be hospitalized in anticipation of this possibility. The reaction is ascribed to the sudden massive destruction of spirochetes by antibiotics; it is marked by fever, myalgia, tachycardia, and occasionally hypotension. The reaction usually begins within 24 hours and subsides spontaneously in the next 24 hours. All patients need to be followed with quantitative serologic tests to monitor treatment results, and HIV testing should be offered to all patients with syphilis. All sexual partners need to be contacted and tested for syphilis.

◊ CERVICITIS

Acute cervicitis is defined as the presence of yellow cervical mucopus or an increased number of WBCs in cervical mucus. Symptoms are usually limited to a purulent vaginal discharge.

Physical findings include mucopus in the endocervical canal or bleeding after swabbing of the cervix. Organisms that infect the cervical columnar epithelium, *C. trachomatis* or *N. gonorrhoeae*, can be isolated separately or in combination from about one-half of women with purulent cervicitis. Unknown organisms cause the other cases. The diagnosis can also be established by the finding of more than 10 WBCs per 1000× microscopic field.

Infectious ulcers of the cervix caused by herpesvirus, syphilis, and chancroid must be distinguished from erosion and the other conditions described in Chapter 48. Depending on the nature of the lesion, Gram stain, Pap smear, culture, darkfield examination, colposcopy, and in some cases biopsy may be required.

If *N. gonorrhoeae* is found by Gram stain or culture, treatment should be the same as for gonococcal infections, including treatment for coexisting *C. trachomatis*. If *N. gonorrhoeae* is not found, doxycycline, tetracycline, or azithromycin regimens used for *C. trachomatis* are recommended. Ampicillin can also be used for patients without *C. trachomatis*.

◊ ENDOMETRITIS

Lymphocytes and neutrophils normally appear in the endometrium in the second half of the menstrual cycle; their presence does not necessarily constitute endometritis. However, plasma cells are not normally in the endometrium, as they represent an immune response, usually to a bacterial antigen.

Endometritis produces nonspecific symptoms, and it should not be diagnosed unless plasma cells or a specific causative infection is found. Endometritis may occur in the following situations:

◊ Puerperal endometritis (see Chapter 26),
◊ Chlamydial or gonococcal endometritis, often occurring among patients with salpingitis,
◊ Endometritis after instrumentation or surgery,
◊ Tuberculous endometritis,
◊ Purulent endometritis, occurring in pyometra caused by a cervical stricture or after radium insertion,
◊ Endometritis occurring characteristically in the presence of an intrauterine device (IUD).

The chronic endometritis associated with the use of IUDs is well documented; it results from organisms attached to the IUD surface rather than from the foreign body *per se.* Transfundal endometrial cultures of hysterectomy specimens from women who had used tailed IUDs for more than a few weeks uniformly recovered bacteria, while cultures from women who had used no IUD were sterile. Bacteria that can be recovered are usually of low pathogenicity, but more virulent intrauterine bacteria occasionally cause malodorous discharge and salpingitis. In addition, an anaerobe, *Actinomyces israelii,* has been found in Pap smears from about 5% of women using IUDs, but not in non–IUD users. This organism appears to colonize the IUD, and when it is found on a Pap smear, asymptomatic patients should be warned of abnormal discharge or abdominal pain, representing infection. If symptomatic infection occurs, the IUD should be removed, and patients treated with ampicillin for 2 to 4 weeks. Asymptomatic patients should not have the IUD removed because of *A. israelii*.

Chronic plasma cell endometritis in nonpregnant non–IUD users is often related to endometrial infection with *C. trachomatis* and to a lesser extent *N. gonorrhoeae*. Plasma cell endometritis occurs in about 50% of women with acute cervicitis and over 80% of women with acute salpingitis. Symptoms are abnormal uterine bleeding and mild uterine tenderness. Untreated endometritis can progress to clinically evident salpingitis.

◊ GONORRHEA

Gonorrhea is caused by the gram-negative diplococcus *N. gonorrhoeae*. These organisms attach only to columnar or transitional cells by pili and are rapidly brought intracellularly by pinocytosis. They attract leukocytes, giving rise to the commonly associated purulent discharge. Gonorrhea is usually sexually transmitted, although organisms can be acquired by neonates in their passage through an infected cervix, causing gonorrheal ophthalmia.

Course of the Disease

N. gonorrhoeae in the lower genital tract infects the urethra, Bartholin glands, and endocervix. The anus and rectum can also be infected either from cervical infection or during anal coitus. Urinary frequency, dysuria, and a purulent vaginal discharge are the first symptoms to appear 2 to 5 days after exposure. Many women do not seek medical attention if these symptoms are mild. The discharge occasionally is locally irritating and causes vulvar edema and soreness. Pharyngitis may result from gonorrheal pharyngeal infection. In 2% of infected women, disseminated gonococcal infection occurs, causing fever, septicemia, dermatitis, arthritis, endocarditis, or meningitis, in various combinations. Untreated gonorrhea is associated with premature delivery and premature rupture of membranes.

In 10% to 17% of women with untreated gonorrhea, the organisms ascend to produce upper genital tract infection or acute PID (Fig. 6). Acute PID is the most common serious sequela of gonorrhea. The mechanical and antibacterial properties of cervical mucus probably provide a barrier against upward extension, but during menstruation the mucus barrier is lost, and gonococci can disseminate in menstrual blood medium to the uterus and fallopian tubes. A transient endometritis occurs as the organisms pass through the uterine cavity and reach the fallopian tubes, where they produce an acute and usually bilateral inflammatory reaction of tubal mucosa. The tubes characteristically become swollen and reddened as the muscularis and serosa become inflamed. If exudate drips from the fimbriated ends of the tubes, a pelvic peritonitis is produced that ultimately can cause peritoneal adhesions. The swollen and congested fimbriae may adhere to one another and produce tubal occlusion.

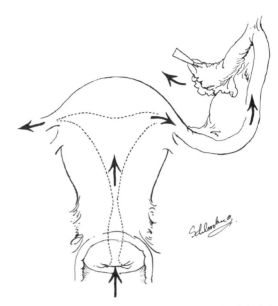

FIG. 6. Mode of transmission of gonococcal pelvic infection. Portal of entry is external genitalia. Organism enters cervix, following mucous membrane, passes up through uterine cavity, and attacks fallopian tube. Pelvic peritonitis results from escape of pus from tubal fimbria. (From Wharton LR. *Gynecology and female urology*. Philadelphia: WB Saunders, 1943; with permission.)

The process can take any of the following courses. With prompt, appropriate antibacterial therapy, the infection may subside with little permanent damage to the reproductive tract. The fimbriae may occlude, producing permanent tubal infertility. The swollen and congested fimbriae may adhere to one another or to the ovary, trapping the exudate in the tube and giving rise to pyosalpinx or, if the ovary becomes infected, a tuboovarian abscess. The mucosal folds may adhere to one another, forming gland-like spaces that are filled at first with exudate and later, as the process becomes chronic, with watery secretion in follicular salpingitis (Fig. 7). If the infection subsides after agglutination of the fimbriae and closure of the distal tube, watery secretion accumulates and distends the tube, forming a hydrosalpinx (Fig. 8).

Symptoms and Signs

At least 50% of women with *N. gonorrhoeae* infection have no symptoms. The most common symptoms, when they occur, are dysuria, urinary frequency, and a purulent vaginal discharge. Except for the discharge, which can be milked from the urethra or is present in the vagina or cervix, there are few signs of acute gonococcal infection in women. Bilateral, mild to severe lower abdominal pain may occur with acute salpingitis. Pelvic peritonitis can cause pain on movement of the cervix. Direct and rebound tenderness, muscle guarding that prevents abdominal palpation in the lower quadrants, and tender adnexa are present to various degrees on bimanual examination. However, a sizable proportion of women with salpingitis experience either mild or no symptoms. In subacute salpingitis, infection continues with signs and symptoms

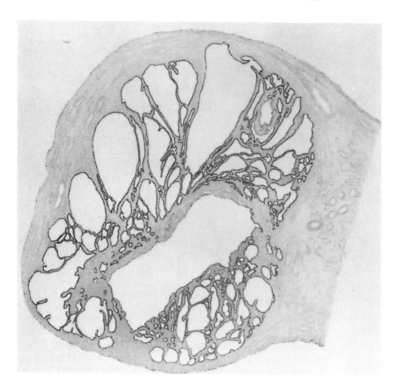

FIG. 7. Follicular salpingitis, an end stage of gonorrheal salpingitis. Mucosal folds are adherent, giving rise to innumerable round or irregular cyst-like cavities lined by cuboidal epithelium. (From Kelly HA. *Operative gynecology,* vol 2. New York: Appleton, 1898: plate XI; drawing by Max Brodel, with permission.)

that are even less overt than those of the acute stage. In the end stage of salpingitis, the uterus and the adnexa are usually fixed by pelvic peritoneal adhesions. The adnexa are often either adherent to the posterior aspect of the uterus or prolapsed in the cul-de-sac, which may pull the uterus into a retroverted position. Notable features are dyspareunia, sterility, and chronic, aching pelvic pain that increases before menstruation.

Diagnosis

The diagnosis of gonorrhea depends on a culture of *N. gonorrhoeae.* Identification of *N. gonorrhoeae* by DNA tests is available but expensive. The finding of intracellular gram-

negative diplococci in the Gram stain of exudate from the cervix or urethra points to gonorrheal infection. Gram stains for gonorrhea are insensitive. Gonococcal cultures should be performed on women with positive Gram stains, symptoms or signs suggestive of gonorrhea (e.g., cervicitis, undiagnosed vaginitis, dysuria), other STDs, bartholinitis or skenitis, acute lower abdominal pain suggestive of acute salpingitis, or suspected disseminated gonococcal infection, as well as on women who have had contact with men with gonorrhea.

The sites to be cultured are in order of importance: cervix, anal canal, pharynx, and urethra. Vaginal discharge should be wiped away from the cervix before mucus is obtained for cul-

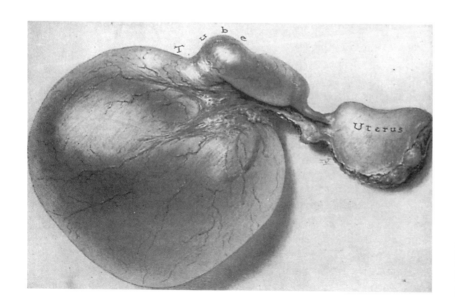

FIG. 8. Hydrosalpinx. (From Curtis AH, Huffman JW. *A textbook of gynecology,* 6th ed. Philadelphia: WB Saunders, 1950; with permission.)

ture or Gram stain. Genital samples must be cultured on Thayer-Martin or similar media containing antimicrobial agents that inhibit growth of the normal bacterial and fungal flora. Because 40% to 50% of women with *N. gonorrhoeae* also have *C. trachomatis,* patients with gonorrhea should also receive a test for chlamydial infection.

Because gonorrhea is an STD, it usually is present in the male partner. That more than 40% of the male contacts of women with gonorrhea are asymptomatic carriers who would otherwise not seek treatment underscores the importance of identifying and treating male sexual contacts.

Drug Therapy of Uncomplicated Lower Genital Tract Gonorrhea

The CDC-recommended treatment schedules for gonorrhea reflect increased resistance to penicillin and tetracycline, frequent coexistence of chlamydial infection with gonorrhea, potentially serious complications, and frequently no testing for *C. trachomatis.* Penicillin is no longer recommended to treat gonorrhea. β-Lactamase production by extrachromosomal plasmids that destroys β-lactam antibiotic activity has been present in an increasing number of gonococcal strains. Smaller numbers of strains with chromosomal resistance and with plasmid-mediated tetracycline resistance are also present.

The recommended regimens are shown in Table 2. A loading dose of ceftriaxone or cefixime (Suprax) is used to inhibit *N. gonorrhoeae.* Penicillin-allergic patients should receive spectinomycin (Trobicin) After the loading dose, a follow-up regimen is used to inhibit *C. trachomatis.* Tetracyclines should not be given to pregnant women. Special antibiotic regimens are recommended for patients with complicated gonococcal infections. These regimens are published in the widely circulated CDC reports.

The first-choice regimens are so effective that test-of-cure cultures are not recommended. A rescreening culture in 1 to 2 months is recommended instead. Patients treated with alternative regimens should have a test-of-cure culture in 4 to 7 days after therapy.

Patients with gonorrhea should have serologic tests for syphilis. Those with incubating syphilis (i.e., seronegative, without clinical signs of syphilis) are likely to be cured by all the regimens mentioned, except for spectinomycin and the fluoroquinolones. Patients treated with these regimens need a follow-up serologic test for syphilis.

◊ CHLAMYDIAL INFECTION

C. trachomatis is a sexually transmitted bacterium that is often associated with gonorrhea. These organisms infect the same tissues and produce the same symptoms and diseases as gonorrhea. Chlamydial infection causes urethritis, bartholinitis, cervicitis, endometritis, salpingitis, Fitz-Hugh–Curtis syndrome (i.e., perihepatitis), and LGV. It is also associated with premature delivery. Neonates born of mothers with chlamy-

TABLE 2. *Treatment regimens for gonorrhea and chlamydiosis*

Gonorrhea
Recommended loading dose regimen (choice of one plus treatment for chlamydiosis)
 Ceftriaxone (Rocephin), 125 mg IM
 Cefixime (Suprax), 400 mg PO
 Ciprofloxacin (Cipro), 500 mg PO
 Ofloxacin (Floxin), 400 mg PO
Alternative regimen (choice of one)
 Spectinomycin (Trobicin), 2 g IM
 Ceftizoxime (Cefizox), 500 mg IM; cefotaxime (Claforan), 500 mg IM; cefotetan (Cefotan), 1 g IM; or cefoxitin (Mefoxin), 1 g IM
 Cefuroxime axetil (Ceftin), 1 g PO; or cefpodoxime proxetil (Vantin) 200 mg PO
 Ciprofloxacin, 500 mg PO; or Enoxacin (Penetrex), 400 mg PO; lomefloxacin (Maxaquin), 400 mg PO; or norfloxacin (Noroxin), 800 mg PO; all in a single dose

Chlamydiosis
Follow-up regimen to treat Chlamydiosis (choice of one)
 Azithromycin (Zithromax), 1 g PO, in a single dose
 Doxycycline, 100 mg PO, b.i.d. for 7 d
Alternative regimen (choice of one)
 Ofloxacin, 300 mg PO, b.i.d. for 7 d
 Erythromycin (see "Penicillin-allergic or pregnant patients" below)
 Sulfisoxazole 500 mg orally 4 times daily for 10 days (inferior to other regimens)

Penicillin-allergic or pregnant patients (choice of one)
Preferred regimen
 Azithromycin, or
 Erythromycin base, 250 mg PO, q.i.d. for 14 d; or azithromycin
 Erythromycin ethylsuccinate, 800 mg PO, q.i.d. for 7 d or 400 mg q.i.d. for 14 d
Alternative regimen
 Amoxicillin, 500 PO t.i.d. for 10 d

dial cervical infection have up to a 40% risk of chlamydial conjunctivitis and a 20% risk of chlamydial pneumonia. As with gonococcal infection, male sexual contacts have both symptomatic and asymptomatic urethritis.

C. trachomatis is an obligate intracellular bacterium. After attachment to columnar or transitional epithelial cells, these organisms are engulfed by pinocytosis and remain within a phagosome membrane that protects them from host defense mechanisms. They replicate until they replace most of the cell and, ultimately, cause the cell to rupture. Infective particles are released into the extracellular space, and the process is repeated. Replication time is a relatively slow 24 to 48 hours, explaining the characteristically long latent period between the time of exposure and the onset of symptoms, which ranges from weeks to months.

Chlamydial infections are assuming increasing importance. In most Western societies, *C. trachomatis* is three to five times more common than *N. gonorrhoeae,* because it is not routinely sought in asymptomatic patients. Chlamydial infection is most often asymptomatic and hence frequently not identified until overt infection occurs. Infection is particularly common among teenagers. *C. trachomatis* has been particularly associated with serious sequelae, including tubal infertility and ectopic pregnancy. It appears capable of producing permanent tissue damage more readily than *N. gonorrhoeae*. Permanent tissue damage appears largely related to the immune response to infection. Reinfection, chronic infection, and infection in the presence of antibody to chlamydial heat shock protein is particularly associated with tissue damage.

Chlamydial infection should be suspected with acute urethritis, mucopurulent cervicitis, and salpingitis. The rate of chlamydial salpingitis approximates that of gonorrhea. Chlamydial infections can be diagnosed by culture, by a direct monoclonal antibody slide test, or by an enzyme-linked immunosorbent assay. Each older diagnostic method has advantages and disadvantages. However, new DNA methods utilizing ligase chain reaction or PCR offer both sensitivity and specificity not achieved with older tests. Samples should be taken from the cervix and perhaps from the urethra. Urine appears the preferable site for DNA tests. Diagnosis by serology and Pap smear is not reliable.

Azithromycin and doxycycline are the most effective drugs to treat chlamydial infection (see Table 2). Ofloxacin (Floxin), erythromycin, and sulfisoxazole (the least effective) are alternatives. Azithromycin is preferred, but amoxicillin may be used in pregnancy. Cephalosporins and aminoglycosides are not effective for chlamydial infection.

◇ GENITAL MYCOPLASMAS

Genital mycoplasmas have often been thought of as organisms in search of a disease because they are ubiquitous and not highly virulent. *Mycoplasma hominis* is recovered from the vagina in 15% to 70% of women, and *Ureaplasma urealyticum* is recovered from 40% to 95% of women. The importance of a third isolate, *Mycoplasma genitalium*, is unknown. These organisms are phylogenetically positioned between bacteria and viruses.

The most convincing role for mycoplasma in human female infections is as a pathogen in postpartum fever. Mycoplasmas have been recovered from the blood of 10% to 15% of women with postpartum fever, and antibodies to *M. hominis* have been demonstrated in 50% of such women. Their role in salpingitis is less clear. Mycoplasmas can be recovered from the tubes of 5% to 15% of women with salpingitis. In primate model studies, *M. hominis* produces an adnexitis but not salpingitis.

Maternal *U. urealyticum* had been associated with low birthweight, but this association appears to result from concomitant risk factors, not *U. urealyticum* itself. Treatment of *U. urealyticum* does not reduce preterm births. These organisms have been associated with chorioamnionic infection and may cause cerebrospinal fluid and lung infection in premature neonates. Recovery of *U. urealyticum* from fetal tissue of midtrimester spontaneous abortuses also suggests a relationship with abortion. The role of *U. urealyticum* in fertility

is not settled. In some studies, mycoplasmas were more frequently isolated from infertile than fertile women, and antibiotic treatment was associated with higher pregnancy rates. However, these observations have not been confirmed in most reports.

Both mycoplasmas are sensitive to tetracyclines. Erythromycin inhibits *U. urealyticum in vitro* but not *M. hominis*. However, neither antibiotic very effectively eradicates mycoplasmas from the vagina.

◇ ANAEROBIC BACTERIA

Anaerobic bacteria are highly associated with pelvic infections. Application of modern anaerobic culture techniques accounts for most of the increased recognition of these infections. Multiple anaerobic species, usually together with one or more aerobic bacteria, typically combine to form a polymicrobial infection. Intraabdominal abscess and postoperative, postpartum, and bacterial vaginosis infections are the most important examples of anaerobic infection.

Anaerobic bacteria are part of the normal vaginal flora. Although many mechanisms by which anaerobic bacteria become pathogenic are unknown, two mechanisms known to cause anaerobic infection include (1) reduction of the redox potential that occurs with tissue trauma from surgery and (2) antibiotic selection that preferentially inhibits aerobic bacteria. Clinicians can virtually assume the presence of anaerobes when infection is associated with a foul-smelling odor and abscess formation; only anaerobes produce odorous metabolic products. Anaerobes are virtually always isolated from an abscess if modern anaerobic techniques are used before antibiotic therapy. Anaerobic infections can also produce gas and cause thromboembolism.

The anaerobic bacteria most commonly found in genital infections include anaerobic gram-positive cocci (*Porphoromonas* and *Peptostreptococcus* species), gram-negative rods (*Prevotella* [*P. melaninogenicus*, *P. bivius*], *Bacteroides* [*B. fragilis*], and *Fusobacterium* species), and gram-positive rods (*Clostridium* species).

Cultures should be obtained before antimicrobial therapy is begun. Because anaerobes are part of the normal flora, deep tissue cultures are required that are not contaminated by surface bacteria. Forty-eight or more hours are required for anaerobe recovery, so antibiotic selection is usually based on clinical signs. Anaerobic infection should be particularly suspected with abscess formation, a foul odor, gas formation, tissue necrosis, sterile cultures from obviously infected sites, and thromboembolism. Antibiotic sensitivity testing is only a rough guide to antibiotic susceptibility, but *in vitro* and *in vivo* experience has shown that clindamycin, metronidazole, imipenem/cilastatin sodium (Primaxin), second- and third-generation cephalosporins (cefoxitin sodium [Mefoxin], cefotaxime sodium [Claforan]), and extended-spectrum penicillins (ticarcillin disodium/clavulanate potassium [Timentin], amoxicillin/clavulanate potassium) are effective in treating anaerobic infections.

◊ SALPINGITIS

Acute primary salpingitis results when pathogenic bacteria in the cervix invade the fallopian tubes. *N. gonorrhoeae, C. trachomatis,* normal flora aerobic and anaerobic bacteria, and perhaps genital mycoplasmas cause the majority of tubal infections. Virtually all primary salpingitis occurs among sexually active, menstruating, nonpregnant women. Gonococcal and chlamydial infections account for 50% to 60% of cases. Tuberculous, parasitic, or fungal salpingitis is rare in industrialized countries. Salpingitis usually occurs without instrumentation or trauma to the genital tract; however, approximately 15% of cases occur after instrumentation (e.g., IUD insertion, dilation and curettage, abortion, hysterosalpingography). Perisalpingitis secondary to acute appendicitis or other intraabdominal bacterial infection accounts for less than 1% of cases.

Acute salpingitis is a common event. Annually, it develops in up to 1% of women between 15 and 39 years of age. Young, sexually active women between 15 and 24 years of age have the highest rate of infection. This rate of infection has tremendous national consequences. At least $1 billion is required to treat the 800,000 women in whom acute salpingitis is diagnosed in the United States annually, and $40 billion is spent to diagnose and treat tubal infertility.

Epidemiology

Most women are infected with sexually transmitted organisms. The rate of salpingitis is increased in women with multiple sexual partners. The high rate of salpingitis in younger women is due to their increased rates of gonorrhea and chlamydial infection. Routine screening for *C. trachomatis* and *N. gonorrhoeae* has reduced salpingitis in Europe and the United States. Sexually active women at increased risk for STDs, especially women younger than 25 years and with multiple sexual partners, should be annually screened for chlamydial infection and gonorrhea. Such screening will prevent salpingitis and subsequent tubal infertility and ectopic pregnancy more effectively than any other measure. Previous salpingitis also predisposes women to subsequent salpingitis, probably because mucosa damaged from prior infection is more susceptible to infection than normal tissue. Patients with previous uncomplicated gonorrhea have a high rate of subsequent salpingitis, in part because of increased rates of subsequent gonorrheal infection. Prior chlamydial infection predisposes patients to salpingitis if a subsequent chlamydial infection occurs. Repeated chlamydial infections produce a hyperimmune response that increases the chance and severity of tissue damage.

The presence of an IUD is an independent risk factor for salpingitis. IUD users have a two- to fourfold increased rate of both salpingitis and tubal infertility, compared to non–IUD users. The highest rate of salpingitis in IUD users occurs within a few weeks of insertion as a result of the introduction of cervical bacteria into the endometrial cavity along with the IUD. Most infections in IUD users, however, occur long after insertion, probably because bacteria wick along the IUD tail from the vagina to the uterus and adhere to the IUD surface. IUDs also appear to enhance anaerobic bacterial growth, and their use is associated with actinomyces and bacterial vaginosis infection. Because IUD use is also associated with tubal infertility, an IUD should not be inserted in women who desire future pregnancy. In contrast, barrier or oral contraceptive methods appear to protect against salpingitis. The protective effect of oral contraceptives on salpingitis appears to exist only for patients with chlamydial infection, possibly due to a down-regulation of the hyperimmune response and thus inflammation caused by the organisms.

The role of male contacts with untreated gonococcal or chlamydial urethritis is often ignored by gynecologists. Only 25% of male contacts of women with gonococcal salpingitis have been treated by the time the female partner develops symptomatic salpingitis. Over 50% of the male contacts with gonococcal urethritis are asymptomatic, and *N. gonorrhoeae* is isolated from 40% of these asymptomatic males. Men with nongonococcal urethritis represent reservoirs of chlamydial salpingitis. To reduce the rate of new and recurrent salpingitis, all male contacts of women with any type of salpingitis should be examined and cultured. If infectious organisms are found, males should be appropriately treated. It is also particularly important to culture and treat male contacts of asymptomatic women with gonorrhea or chlamydial infection.

Bacteriology

Neisseria gonorrhoeae

In most studies in the United States, *N. gonorrhoeae* is recovered from 40% to 50% of women with acute salpingitis. However, gonococcal prevalence varies greatly: *N. gonorrhoeae* is isolated from less than 20% of salpingitis cases in Sweden and from 80% of cases in certain urban populations in the United States. In women with both cervical gonorrhea and salpingitis, *N. gonorrhoeae* is the most frequent intraabdominal isolate, but the sole isolate in only 30% of these cases. The remainder have either no organisms or other organisms isolated alone or together with *N. gonorrhoeae* in the abdomen. Chlamydial infection frequently coexists with gonorrhea; in some studies, more than 50% of women with gonorrhea also had *C. trachomatis* in the cervix. Positive tubal gonococcal cultures are usually obtained during the early stages of infection. During the later stages of infection, the organisms are either present only within epithelial cells or inhibited by leukocytes, two factors that make their isolation more difficult.

Chlamydia trachomatis

C. trachomatis is as important as the gonococcus in causing acute salpingitis. Recent reports indicate that 30% to 60% of women with salpingitis have *C. trachomatis,* and in most of these women the organisms can be isolated from the fallopian tube. Application of new DNA tests for *C. trachomatis* may identify even more infections. Chlamydial salpingitis has been underdiagnosed because many patients with mild symptoms are not identified and not included in studies of salpingitis. Recently, it became evident that women with mild symptoms and signs can have not only salpingitis but also severe tubal damage. Chlamydial salpingitis often produces mild symptoms and signs but may produce more severe tubal damage, compared to gonococcal salpingitis.

Nonsexually Transmitted Aerobic and Anaerobic Bacteria

Nonsexually transmitted aerobic and anaerobic bacteria are normally present in cervical and vaginal flora and particularly include organisms associated with bacterial vaginosis. These organisms can be a direct cause of salpingitis, but they may also cause secondary infection in combination with *N. gonorrhoeae* and *C. trachomatis,* IUD use, or instrumentation. Polymicrobial infection with these agents is common in salpingitis. In such cases, many different gram-positive and gram-negative aerobic and anaerobic organisms are isolated, particularly *Porphoromonas, Prevotella,* and *Bacteroides* species, including *B. fragilis.* Anaerobic organisms are especially common in serious infections, and they are virtually always found in abscesses.

Mycoplasmas

Genital mycoplasmas have been recovered from the tubes or cul-de-sac in 2% to 20% of patients with salpingitis. In addition, more than 20% of patients with salpingitis have changes of mycoplasmal antibody titer suggestive of invasive infection. These organisms lack the virulence of *N. gonorrhoeae* and *C. trachomatis,* and they appear to cause an adnexitis rather than salpingitis.

Pathogenesis

Salpingitis occurs when vaginal and cervical bacteria ascend into the endometrium and fallopian tubes. The ascent of bacteria can probably occur during menses, as evidenced by pain that occurs within 7 days of the onset of menses in one-half to two-thirds of patients with gonococcal salpingitis. This finding suggests that gonococci are disseminated from the cervix at menstruation. Virulent gonococci proliferate at menstruation, and less virulent gonococci are present at other times of the cycle. Other risk factors for salpingitis exist. Virulent bacteria in the cervix are more likely to cause salpingitis than nonvirulent bacteria. *C. trachomatis* and *N. gonorrhoeae* are two virulent organisms capable of causing salpingitis, but virulence is occasionally evidenced by bacteria in the normal flora as well.

Specific bactericidal antibodies to *N. gonorrhoeae* appear to reduce salpingitis. Clinically recognized salpingitis develops in only 10% to 17% of women with cervical gonorrhea, and most of these women probably develop tubal infection

during the first one or two menstrual periods after gonococcal acquisition, before specific bactericidal antibodies have developed.

C. trachomatis may not depend on menses for ascent into the upper genital tract. Endometritis caused by *C. trachomatis* appears to be a common chronic intermediate infection that exists through several menstrual cycles. Tubal damage from chlamydial infection often occurs from the immune response to infection. As mentioned, repetitive chlamydial infections elicit a hyperimmune response that accelerates tissue damage. The presence of chlamydial heat shock protein may contribute to an acceleration of tissue damage.

The usual route of infection with either organism is the contiguous spread from the cervix to the endometrial cavity and fallopian tubes. Lymphatic or hematogenous dissemination of organisms from the uterus to the adnexa is uncommon in nonpregnant women. When the bacteria reach the uterus, they invade the fallopian tubes by contiguous spread along the mucosa (see Fig. 1), although it is possible for organisms may be transported to the fallopian tubes by cilia or even carried by their attachment to spermatozoa or to other organisms.

Fitz-Hugh–Curtis Syndrome

Perihepatitis consisting of liver capsule inflammation without damage of the liver parenchyma has been referred to as Fitz-Hugh–Curtis syndrome (Fig. 9). Swelling of the liver capsule produces pain with inspiration, usually in the right upper quadrant. A purulent or fibrinous exudate appears on the capsular surface, but violin-string adhesions between the liver capsule and the anterior abdominal wall is a late manifestation of capsular inflammation.

Perihepatitis was formerly believed to be caused solely by *N. gonorrhoeae,* but *C. trachomatis* also causes this syn-

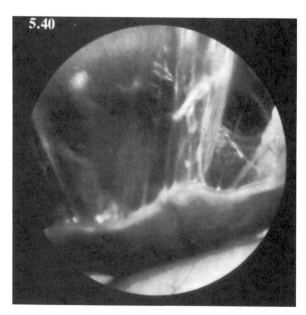

FIG. 9. Liver adhesions in Fitz-Hugh–Curtis syndrome.

drome. Chlamydial heat shock protein is associated with perihepatitis, indicating that the syndrome is another manifestation of a hyperimmune response to chlamydiae. Some organisms travel transperitoneally from the fallopian tubes to reach the liver surface, but organisms may also reach the liver by lymphatic and hematogenous routes. The syndrome occurs virtually exclusively in women, although two men with this syndrome have been reported. Salpingitis is invariably the source, but the syndrome has also followed appendicitis and other causes of peritonitis.

The Fitz-Hugh–Curtis syndrome is frequently misinterpreted as cholecystitis, viral pneumonia, or pyelonephritis. Liver enzyme levels may be mildly elevated. The syndrome causes symptoms in 5% to 10% of women with salpingitis, but another 5% of women have asymptomatic perihepatitis. This later group may have the violin-string adhesions recognized as an incidental finding at a subsequent surgery. Many women with Fitz-Hugh–Curtis syndrome note the onset of lower abdominal pain before or with the upper abdominal pain, but some have such severe upper abdominal pain that they fail to complain of lower abdominal pain. Given the frequency of salpingitis and the infrequency of acute cholecystitis in women 15 to 30 years of age, Fitz-Hugh–Curtis syndrome is a more likely cause of upper quadrant pain than cholecystitis and should be suspected in any woman with pleuritic upper quadrant pain and physical signs of salpingitis. Laparoscopy is useful to diagnose unclear cases.

Diagnosis

The largest unsolved problem with salpingitis is the lack of sensitive and specific diagnostic criteria. For more than one-half of women, salpingitis does not cause sufficiently typical symptoms to be diagnosed. Patients with mild abdominal pain and other mild manifestations are often not identified. About two-thirds of women with salpingitis severe enough to cause infertility from tubal obstruction have never had a recognized episode of salpingitis (Table 3). An emphasis must be placed on increasing the sensitivity for the diagnosis. The

TABLE 4. *Laparoscopic observations in patients with a clinical diagnosis of pelvic inflammatory disease*

Diagnosis	Jacobson and Westrøm	Chaparro et al.	Sweet et al.	Total (%)
Salpingitis	532	103	25	661 (62)
Normal findings	184	51	0	235 (22)
Ovarian cysts	12	39	0	51 (5)
Ectopic pregnancy	11	27	1	39 (4)
Appendicitis	24	2	1	27 (3)
Endometriosis	16	0	0	16 (1)
Other	35	1	1	37 (3)
Total	814	223	28	1066 (100)

(From Eschenbach DA. *Obstet Gynecol* 1980;55:142S; with permission.)

problem is that the spectrum of clinical severity among patients with salpingitis is very broad. Although severe manifestations are usually recognized as salpingitis, they occur in only 30% of patients. Insistence on rigid criteria, such as fever, severe tenderness, leukocytosis, and an elevated erythrocyte sedimentation rate (ESR), leads to a failure of diagnosis in nonovert cases.

On the other hand, a clinical diagnosis of salpingitis that relies on the history, physical examination, and nonspecific laboratory tests also has a large false-positive error rate. Several studies have demonstrated that a clinical diagnosis of salpingitis can be confirmed by laparoscopy in only 60% of patients (Table 4); about 20% of patients had no disease observed, and another 15% had other pelvic conditions, most commonly ovarian cyst, ectopic pregnancy, appendicitis, or endometriosis.

History

The important points in the history of patients with presumed PID are listed in Table 5. Most of these findings, however, do not distinguish women with salpingitis from those with other

TABLE 3. *Proportions of patients with tubal occlusion from salpingitis who have no history of salpingitis*

Study	Infertile patients with tubal occlusion	No history of salpingitis (%)
Punnonen et al. (1979)	23	9 (37)
Moore et al. (1982)	33	15 (45)
Jones et al. (1982)	77	62 (81)
Kane et al. (1984)	70	42 (60)
Conway et al. (1984)	48	36 (75)
Brunham et al. (1985)	18	11 (61)
Total	269	175 (65)

(From Wølner-Hanssen P, Kiviat NB, Holmes KK. Atypical pelvic inflammatory disease: subacute, chronic or subclinical upper genital tract infection in women. In: Holmes KK, Mårdh P-A, Sperling PF, et al., eds. Sexually transmitted diseases. New York: McGraw-Hill, 1990.)

TABLE 5. *Clinical findings in 176 women with suspected acute pelvic inflammatory disease (PID)*

Finding	When PID present (%) (n=134)	When PID not present (%) (n=142)
Mean duration of symptoms (days)	11	24
Abnormal vaginal bleeding	16	26
Nausea/vomiting	28	31
Mean temperature on admission	37.6°C	37.3°C
Abdominal rebound/guarding	61	52
Cervical motion tenderness	80	69
Adnexal tenderness	90	79
Adnexal mass, fullness	19	12

(From Morcos et al., 1993, with permission.)

causes of pelvic pain. Lower abdominal pain is the most consistent symptom in women with overt salpingitis, although it may be mild or even absent. Acute pain is present for less than 15 days in 85% of patients who present with PID. Most women with gonococcal salpingitis usually have acute onset of pain during menses; in chlamydial salpingitis, the onset of pain is often insidious and not associated with menses. The abdominal pain is usually continuous and most severe in both lower quadrants. It is increased by movement, the Valsalva maneuver, and intercourse. Abnormal vaginal bleeding occurs in 15% to 35% of women with salpingitis. Symptoms of appendicitis and ectopic pregnancy overlap with those of PID. The risk of STD can be helpful in forming a tentative opinion: An increased risk of PID would be expected for women with multiple sexual partners, other STDs, symptomatic male partners, and prior gonorrhea or PID.

Physical Examination

Most patients with salpingitis have lower abdominal, cervical, and bilateral adnexal tenderness. Cervical motion tenderness is a sensitive indicator of salpingitis. None of these findings is specific; patients with other disease or with no apparent disease may have similar physical findings. Other associated findings lack the sensitivity to be useful. For example, although a temperature of 100.4°F (38°C) or higher is present more often in patients with than in those without salpingitis, only 45% of patients with laparoscopically confirmed salpingitis have a temperature greater than 100.4°F. Other clinical findings in patients with a final diagnosis of PID are shown in Table 5.

Laboratory Tests

Such nonspecific tests as the peripheral WBC count and the ESR can be helpful only if the results are abnormal, but they are often normal. Of patients with laparoscopically confirmed salpingitis, 50% have a normal WBC count and 25% have a normal ESR. C-reactive protein levels may be more useful.

Laboratory signs such as yellow cervical mucopus and a cervical Gram stain with an increase of polymorphonuclear leukocytes to more than 30 per high-powered field appear to offer a more specific indication of salpingitis in patients with pelvic tenderness. It is mandatory to obtain a culture for gonorrhea and a test for chlamydial infection. Cervical culture for other organisms is not recommended.

Endometrial Biopsy

Endometrial biopsies are easy to obtain. Histologic evidence of endometritis is based on finding plasma cells and polymorphonuclear leukocytes migrating through the epithelium. Histologic endometritis has a 90% sensitivity and specificity for diagnosing salpingitis, compared to laparoscopy.

Ultrasound and Computed Tomography

Abnormal vaginal ultrasound findings have correlated with a diagnosis of salpingitis made by laparoscopy, but these findings remain too insensitive with mild tubal abnormalities and too nonspecific for a certain diagnosis. Ultrasound is useful for distinguishing an abscess from an inflammatory mass within the adnexa, defining a mass in obese or excessively tender patients, and following the size of a mass with treatment. Computed tomography has successfully been used for the same purposes; it may be especially helpful if ultrasound is difficult to perform, as in peritonitis or a recent abdominal incision.

Laparoscopy

Laparoscopy provides the most accurate way to diagnose salpingitis. It should be used when the diagnosis is unclear, particularly in patients with severe peritonitis, to exclude a ruptured abscess and appendicitis. It is estimated that for every 100 times a clinical diagnosis of PID is made without visual confirmation, three patients with appendicitis are treated for PID, resulting in a critical delay in the correct diagnosis. Pain and tenderness resulting from acute PID should abate 3 or 4 days after antibiotics are started. Patients without a reduction of tenderness on antibiotic therapy and those with mild clinical findings also benefit from laparoscopy. About 20 of 100 women with a clinical diagnosis of PID have no abnormality at laparoscopy. In all cases in which laparoscopy is performed, regardless of the findings, culture samples should be taken from the fimbriated ends of the tubes. A small number of patients may have endosalpingitis and normal-appearing tubes.

Open laparoscopy is used to identify and percutaneously drain pelvic abscesses. The abscess is visualized, and a 14-French catheter is placed into the abscess, which is drained of pus and carefully rinsed with sterile bacteriostatic water. A closed drainage system is then connected to the catheter for 1 to 3 days until drainage ceases. About 90% of abscesses can successfully be treated by percutaneous drainage.

Examination of the Male Partner

Examination of the male sexual partner can help establish the diagnosis of PID. At least 80% of male contacts of women with PID will not have been treated by the time PID occurs in the female partner. If there is no urethral discharge, a Gram stain and urethral material for *N. gonorrhoeae* and *C. trachomatis* identification should be obtained.

Treatment

Adequate treatment of salpingitis includes an assessment of severity, antibiotic therapy, additional general health measures, close patient follow-up, and treatment of the male sexual partner. Most patients, except for those with the mildest manifestations, should be hospitalized. Specific indications for hospitalization include severe manifestations of salpingitis (i.e., severe peritonitis, severe nausea, or fever higher than 100.4°F [38°C]), a suspected abscess, outpatient antibiotic failure, and an uncertain diagnosis with severe symptoms.

Patients should be examined within 2 to 3 days and again at 7 and 21 days after treatment to verify a satisfactory response. If an IUD is in place, it should be removed 24 to 48 hours after therapy is started. Ideally, the antibiotic should be selected according to the organism isolated, but in salpingitis empiric therapy is used. The treatment regimens recommended by the CDC were designed to treat gonococcal and chlamydial salpingitis and anaerobic salpingitis. Inpatient regimens include at least 4 days of intravenous doxycycline and either cefoxitin or cefotetan disodium (Cefotan), or intravenous clindamycin and gentamicin, followed by oral clindamycin or doxycycline for a total of 14 days. The clindamycin regimen is also effective for patients with chlamydial infection. Outpatient regimens include a loading dose of an antibiotic recommended for gonorrhea and doxycycline, 100 mg twice daily for 14 days. A second outpatient regimen includes 14 days of ofloxacin, 400 mg twice daily, plus clindamycin, 450 mg four times daily, or metronidazole, 500 mg twice daily. It is also possible to use other antibiotic regimens with similar antimicrobial activity. Gonococcal salpingitis responds more rapidly to antibiotics than nongonococcal salpingitis. The recommended agents must be used in full doses because partially treated, subacute salpingitis may follow the use of lower doses.

Hospitalized patients with peritonitis but no adnexal abscess usually respond rapidly to the regimens. In the presence of an adnexal abscess, even if systemic manifestations are mild, antibiotics should be selected that inhibit B. fragilis because of its frequency in pelvic abscesses. Clindamycin, metronidazole, cefoxitin, or imipenem/cilastatin should be used to treat a known or suspected pelvic abscess.

Abdominal surgery is indicated for a ruptured abscess. Colpotomy drainage is usually preferable for an unruptured midline abscess present in the cul-de-sac. If laparotomy is performed for a presumptive diagnosis of appendicitis but instead acute salpingitis is found, the procedure should be limited to taking a tubal culture and closure of the abdomen. If laparotomy is required for such problems as an unresolved abscess or adnexal mass, surgery should be limited to the most conservative procedures that will be effective. Unilateral abscesses respond to unilateral salpingo-oophorectomy if appropriate antibiotic regimens are used; routine hysterectomy and bilateral salpingo-oophorectomy are seldom needed to treat acute salpingitis in young women. As mentioned, even percutaneous drainage of abscesses is usually successful.

When chronic pain occurs, surgery should be deferred as long as possible to allow maximum healing. Analgesics and oral contraceptives to prevent ovulation may suffice until the swelling and fixation are reduced. Surgery may be indicated for persistent pain that does not respond to conservative measures, for recurrent attacks of pelvic pain, or for a pelvic mass that does not resolve. Laparoscopy with lysis of adhesions usually suffices, but adnexectomy or, rarely, even hysterectomy is required. Surgery is also necessary for infertile patients.

◊ OOPHORITIS

Most cases of oophoritis are secondary to salpingitis. The ovary becomes infected by purulent material escaping from the fallopian tube. If the tubal fimbriae are adherent to the ovary, the tube and ovary together may form a large retort-shaped tuboovarian abscess. Antibacterial therapy, as previously outlined, is immediately indicated, and surgery is mandatory if the mass is considered to be leaking or ruptured or if it fails to resolve. Ovarian abscess after gynecologic surgery is particularly resistant to antimicrobial treatment.

Oophoritis may occur without accompanying salpingitis in infections such as mumps and septicemia. Oophoritis of this type usually results in lower abdominal pain that lasts for only a few days during the course of an acute infectious illness. The ovarian infection usually subsides without incident, although abscesses may occur. If bimanual examination is not satisfactory, ultrasound scans may be used to detect abscesses.

◊ GENITAL TUBERCULOSIS

Female genital tuberculosis remains relatively uncommon in the United States. Fewer than 1% of salpingitis cases can be attributed to M. tuberculosis. Pulmonary tuberculosis remains a problem in many impoverished areas, and its rate is rising because of an increasing number of female patients with HIV infection. Although the spread of tuberculosis from the primary pulmonary infection to the pelvis usually occurs early during tubercular infection, early detection of genital infection is seldom feasible. Genital tuberculosis develops in about 10% of patients with pulmonary tuberculosis.

Pathogenesis

Virtually all genital infections are secondary to a pulmonary infection, which usually spreads by the bloodstream from the lungs to the fallopian tubes within 1 year of the primary pulmonary infection (Figs. 10 and 11). Direct extension then occurs from the tube in several directions: to the pelvic peritoneum and ovary, to the endometrium, and to the cervix. Less commonly, lymphatic extension to the genitalia can occur from abdominal sources or by direct extension from the intestinal tract. Genital tuberculosis is seldom caused by an ascending infection from a sexual partner with tuberculous epididymitis.

The initial tubal lesion may remain localized for a considerable time (in some cases years), or it may extend to the interior tubal mucosa. Endosalpingitis results either in an exudative phase, in which ulcer formation at the site of caseous degeneration produces a typical moth-eaten pattern hysterosalpingography, or in an adhesive phase, in which large tubercles are present within the tubes. Dense perisal-

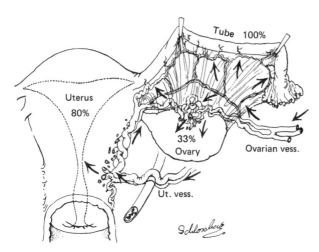

FIG. 10. Mode of transmission of tuberculous pelvic infection. Tubercle bacillus invades pelvic organs by way of bloodstream from distant focus in the lung or other organ. (From Wharton LR. *Gynecology and female urology.* Philadelphia: WB Saunders, 1943; with permission.)

pingeal adhesions are characteristic. In contrast to bacterial salpingitis, tubal occlusion, particularly fimbrial closure, does not occur early in tuberculous disease, and the tubes may remain patent despite relatively marked destruction of the tubal wall.

Tubal infection is present in virtually all women with genital tuberculosis. Endometrial infection is present in 50% to 80% of cases. Because of menstrual sloughing, infected endometrium is shed monthly; after menstruation, the endometrium is again infected from tubal seeding. Myometrial infection can occur but only in the most advanced cases. Cervical infection occurs in only 10% to 25% of patients, resulting in either a papillomatous lesion or an ulcerative lesion that can grossly resemble cervical carcinoma.

Clinical Forms

Latent Genital Tuberculosis

In the latent form, genital tuberculosis appears to be partially or completely arrested after an initial tubal infection, and patients have few or no pelvic complaints. Pelvic physical findings are normal. The diagnosis is usually made in the course of an investigation of infertility (i.e., endometrial biopsy or dilation and curettage) or by chance at laparotomy. In these cases, a precarious balance exists between the disease and the host defense mechanisms. Active but latent infections have been documented 30 years after an initial infection.

Tuberculous Salpingitis

Tuberculous salpingitis is a more advanced infection that may develop immediately after the primary hematogenous tubal spread, or it may follow a prolonged latent phase. The tubes are grossly enlarged by the inflammatory reaction. Al-

though the symptoms and findings can be identical to those of acute bacterial salpingitis, the clinical manifestations are usually more indolent and prolonged. Additionally, tuberculous salpingitis does not respond to the antibiotic therapy used for other forms of salpingitis. Despite these differences, tuberculosis is often discovered only by histologic examination of an excised tube.

Tuberculous Peritonitis

In tuberculous peritonitis, widespread infection of all peritoneal surfaces produces ascites, adhesions, and innumerable small nodules (i.e., tubercles) throughout the abdomen. The serosal surfaces of the pelvic organs are typically involved, and the tubes are often patent. This form results from hematogenous or lymphatic spread.

Diagnosis

A history of pulmonary tuberculosis is often elicited from patients with genital tuberculosis, but simultaneous active pulmonary infection is uncommon. A normal chest film does not exclude genital tuberculosis because pulmonary lesions are found in only 30% to 50% of cases. The most common complaints are sterility and pelvic pain. Deteriorating health and menstrual abnormalities may also occur. Menorrhagia may be associated with the abdominal pain, but amenorrhea or oligomenorrhea may also occur in patients with tuberculous peritonitis. Most women with genital tuberculosis are in their 20s and 30s, but because of the frequent tendency for long latency periods, the disease may become active even after

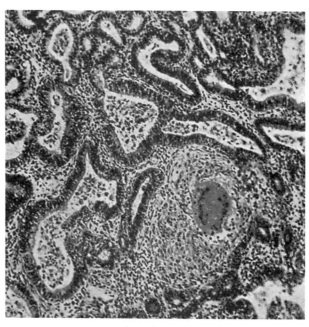

FIG. 11. Tuberculosis of fallopian tube (×105). (From Curtis AH, Huffman JW. *A textbook of gynecology,* 6th ed. Philadelphia: WB Saunders, 1950; with permission.)

menopause. The clinical picture of tubal tuberculosis may be similar to that of acute bacterial salpingitis. In some cases, the clinical picture may be unusual, and when one is confronted with a pelvic problem that does not conform to expected rules, the first consideration should be ectopic pregnancy and the second should be pelvic tuberculosis. Pelvic tuberculosis should be strongly considered if salpingitis occurs in a woman who is considered to be virginal.

A first-strength purified protein derivative tuberculin skin test is important because a negative result virtually rules out the possibility of tuberculosis. Diagnosis can best be established by an endometrial biopsy, which should be performed in the week preceding menstruation, when the endometrium is thickest and is most likely to contain tubercles. A portion of the specimen should be cultured, and the remainder submitted for histologic examination. Repeated cultures of the menstrual flow can also be used. If cultures of either biopsy specimens or menstrual blood are negative, a curettage may be productive. Antimicrobial susceptibility testing should be performed to predict drug resistance.

Endometrial biopsy, curettage, and culture of menstrual flow or endometrial tissue can provide an exact diagnosis of genital tuberculosis if the results are positive; if the results are negative, the presence of the disease cannot be excluded. If these measures fail to verify a diagnosis in a patient whose history and pelvic findings suggest genital tuberculosis, diagnostic laparotomy is justified. Diagnostic laparoscopy may be performed if there is minimal likelihood of tuberculous peritonitis, but caution must be used because of the possibility of perforating a loop of adherent bowel. Hysterosalpingography may reveal a characteristic tubal pattern, but it may also cause severe exacerbation of disease and should not be used if there is a possibility of this disease.

The incidental discovery of reproductive tract tuberculosis may be the first indication that the patient has tuberculosis. In such patients, an effort must be made to determine whether or not other sites (e.g., lungs, urinary tract, bone, and gastrointestinal tract) may also be infected.

Treatment

Three drug therapies are isoniazid, 300 mg daily, rifampin, 600 mg daily, and pyrazinamide, 1500 mg daily, for 18 to 24 months. In areas of high resistance, streptomycin or ethambutol (Myambutol) is added as a fourth drug. Patients without adnexal masses should have an endometrial biopsy for culture and microscopic examination 6 and 12 months after the start of therapy. Persistent organisms need to be susceptibility-tested to identify drug-resistant strains. Laparotomy is performed if adnexal masses persist for 4 months; rifampin or streptomycin should be given preoperatively. Bilateral salpingectomy and removal of other tuberculous foci may be performed in young women with minimal disease, but bilateral salpingo-oophorectomy and total hysterectomy are indicated in those who have advanced disease or are of advanced age. Pregnancy after tubal tuberculosis is rare, even

in women with minimal disease. If the tubes are damaged by genital tuberculosis, efforts to improve fertility by tubal operations are usually futile.

SUMMARY POINTS

◊ STDs are common, particularly in young sexually active poor women with multiple sexual partners. However, most STDs occur among the larger population of women not in groups at high risk for STDs.

◊ STDs are often asymptomatic for both women and their sexual partners.

◊ Most of the classic symptoms associated with various STDs are common in women without infection and, conversely, not present in many women with STDs.

◊ Many of the signs present in women with STDs are common and present in women with no identifiable infection. Specific laboratory tests are usually required to confirm infection.

◊ Treatment of STDs best utilizes a combination of antimicrobial therapy directed at the patient and her partner, education about reducing exposure, and, when appropriate, careful follow-up examination and testing.

◊ RECOMMENDED READING

Bauer HM, Ting Y, Greer CE, et al. Genital human papillomavirus infection in female university students as determined by a PCR-based method. *JAMA* 1991;265:472.

Boardman LA, Peipert JF, Brody JM, et al. Endovaginal sonography for the diagnosis of upper genital tract infection. *Obstet Gynecol* 1997;90:54.

Eschenbach DA, Wolner-Hanssen P, Hawes SE, et al. Acute pelvic inflammatory disease: associations of clinical and laboratory findings with laparoscopic findings. *Obstet Gynecol* 1997;89:184.

Hillier SL, Krohn MA, Rabe LK, et al. The normal flora, H$_2$O$_2$-producing lactobacilli and bacterial vaginosis in pregnant women. *Clin Infect Dis* 1993;16(suppl 4):S273.

Kimani J, McClean IW, Biyayo JJ, et al. Risk factors for *Chlamydia trachomatis* pelvic inflammatory disease among sex workers in Nairobi, Kenya. *J Infect Dis* 1996;173:1437.

Koutsky LA, Galloway DA, Holmes KK. Epidemiology of genital human papillomavirus infection. *Epidemiol Rev* 1988;10:122.

Korn AP, Landers DV, Green JR. Pelvic inflammatory disease in human immunodeficiency-virus infected women. *Obstet Gynecol* 1993;82:765.

Kulhanjian JA, Soroush V, Au DS, et al. Identification of women at unsuspected risk of primary infection with herpes simplex virus type 2 during pregnancy. *N Engl J Med* 1992;326:916.

Larsson P-G, Platz-Christensen J-J, Thejls H, et al. Incidence of pelvic inflammatory disease after first-trimester legal abortion in women with bacterial vaginosis after treatment with metronidazole: a double-blind, randomized study. *Am J Obstet Gynecol* 1992;166:100.

Martin DH, Mroczkowski TF, Dalu ZA, et al. A controlled trial of a single dose of azithromycin for the treatment of chlamydial urethritis and cervicitis. *N Engl J Med* 1992;327:921.

Morcos R, Frost N, Hnat M, et al. Laparoscopic versus clinical diagnosis of acute pelvic inflammatory disease. *J Reprod Med* 1993;38:53.

Njirjesy P, Seeney SM, Terry Grody MH, et al. Chronic fungal vaginitis: the value of cultures. *Am J Obstet Gynecol* 1995;173:820.

Plummer FD, D'Costa LJ, Nsanze H, et al. Epidemiology of chancroid and *Haemophilus ducreyi* in Nairobi, Kenya. *Lancet* 1983;2:1293.

Quinn TC, Gaydos C, Shepherd M, et al. Epidemiologic and microbiologic correlates of *Chlamydia trachomatis* infection in sexual partnerships. *JAMA* 1996;276:1737.

Schacter J, Moncada J, Whidden R, et al. Noninvasive test for diagnosis of *Chlamydia trachomatis* infection: application of ligase chain reaction to first-catch urine specimens of women. *J Infect Dis* 1995;172:1411.

Schaefer G. Female genital tuberculosis. *Clin Obstet Gynecol* 1976;19:223.

Scholes D, Stergachis A, Hendrick P, et al. Prevention of pelvic inflammatory disease by screening for cervical chlamydial infection. *N Engl J Med* 1996;334:1399.

Shands KN, Schmid GP, Blum DBB, et al. Toxic shock syndrome in menstruating women: association with tampon use and *Staphylococcus aureus* and clinical features in 52 cases. *N Engl J Med* 1980;303:1436.

Sobel JD. Recurrent vulvovaginal candidiasis: a prospective study of the efficacy of maintenance ketoconazole therapy. *N Engl J Med* 1986;315:145.

Soper DE, Bump RC, Hurt WG. Bacterial vaginosis and *Trichomonas vaginalis* are risk factors for cuff cellulitis after abdominal hysterectomy. *Am J Obstet Gynecol* 1991;163:1016.

Taylor-Robinson D. Infections due to species of *Mycoplasma* and *Ureaplasma:* an update. *Clin Infect Dis* 1996;23:671.

Public Health Service, Centers for Disease Control. 1993 Sexually transmitted disease treatment guidelines. *MMWR* 1993;42:1.

Walker CK, Kohn JG, Washington AE, et al. Pelvic inflammatory disease: metaanalysis of antimicrobial regimen efficacy. *J Infect Dis* 1993;168:969.

Watts DH, Krohn M, Hillier SL, et al. Bacterial vaginosis as a risk factor for postcesarean endometritis. *Obstet Gynecol* 1990;75:52.

Westrøm L, Joesoef R, Reynolds G, et al. Pelvic inflammatory disease and infertility: a cohort study of 1844 women with laparoscopically verified disease and 657 control women with normal laparoscopic findings. *Sex Transm Dis* 1992;19:158.

CHAPTER 38

Menstruation and Disorders of
Menstrual Function

◇

Charles B. Hammond
Daniel H. Riddick

Menstrual dysfunction is a symptom of an underlying abnormality of the reproductive system. The abnormality may be developmental, endocrinologic, or the result of an acquired anatomic lesion. It may also be caused by ovarian failure, normally timed (menopause) or premature. An appreciation of the pathophysiological conditions underlying abnormalities of menstruation as well as a rational approach to evaluation and therapy require a complete understanding of the normal anatomy, embryology, and endocrinology of the reproductive system. This chapter deals with normal menstruation and the abnormalities of menstrual function that are frequently encountered in gynecologic practice.

◇ NORMAL MENSTRUATION

For successful reproduction, the human endometrium must receive and respond to appropriate hormonal signals that prepare it for embryo implantation. When conception does not occur, these messages initiate mechanisms that lead to orderly shedding and controlled regeneration of this tissue. An understanding of the hormonal and endometrial events resulting in normal menstruation is necessary to diagnose and treat the menstrual abnormalities so frequently encountered by the gynecologist. This section details the unique biochemical, vascular, and hemostatic mechanisms that are initiated in the endometrium.

The follicular phase of the menstrual cycle is a period of rapid endometrial growth induced by increasing ovarian estradiol production. At the time of menstruation, most of the functional layer of the endometrium sloughs and is replaced by a fibrinous eschar punctured by remnants of endometrial glands and the recently occluded spiral arterioles.[1] Regrowth of the endometrial glands and stroma begins in the region of the glandular stumps and quickly radiates outward. The fi-

brinolytic activity of the endometrium, maximal at this stage of the cycle, aids in the dissolution of the fibrin clot and in the orderly proliferation of stromal and epithelial cells. The process of sloughing of the endometrium, clearing of the fibrinous mesh, and the total reepithelialization of the desquamated region is completed within 4 to 6 days of the initiation of menstruation.[2]

The endometrium continues to increase in thickness throughout the follicular phase with the superficial, or functional, layer being the primary site of mitotic activity. Endometrial depth is maximal in the late follicular phase, with further increase in thickness inhibited by postovulatory progesterone production by the corpus luteum. Although the histologic appearance of the endometrium continues to change during the luteal phase, the mitotic activity in the functional layer is markedly curtailed.[3] After proliferation of the stroma and glandular epithelium has halted, angiogenesis in the functional layer of the endometrium continues under the influence of progesterone. By the end of the luteal phase, a well-differentiated microvasculature has developed within the functional layer, consisting of spiral arterioles, capillaries, and venules.[4] The completion of a superficial vasculature in the endometrium is a prerequisite to successful embryonic implantation and development. Disruption of the endometrial microvasculature during menstruation requires that specific hemostatic mechanisms be initiated to limit menstrual blood loss.

There is no doubt that menstruation is initiated by the precipitous fall in progesterone that occurs. The precise biochemical and cellular events leading to the orderly shedding of the endometrium remain to be described. Much of what is known concerning the initiation of menstruation comes from the classic experiments of Markee.[5] Using the rhesus monkey as a model, Markee implanted endometrium in the anterior chamber of the eye. This allowed for direct observation of the endometrium in various endocrinologic states. The endometrium was noted to alternately blanch and blush, implying that the vasculature constricts and dilates rhythmically. With the abrupt withdrawal of progesterone, the endometrium decreased in thickness, and a prolonged episode of vasoconstriction was observed. These events were followed by vasodilation and hemorrhage into the surrounding tissue. From these observations, Markee concluded that a vasoconstrictor substance was released into the endometrium in response to progesterone withdrawal, which initiated menses.

The vasoactive substance described by Markee has not been identified conclusively. The discovery of prostaglandins in endometrium and the subsequent description of the vascular effects of these compounds led to the conclusion that prostaglandins of the F and E series are important in endometrial physiology.[6] Specifically, prostaglandin $F_{2\alpha}$ has been shown to be a potent vasoconstrictor, whereas prostaglandin E_2 is a vasodilator. It has been implied that there are increased levels in menstrual blood in women with menorrhagia and dysmenorrhea. Further support of the role of prostaglandins in regulating menses is provided by the observation that the potent inhibitor of prostaglandin synthesis and action, mefenamic acid, decreases menstrual blood loss in women with essential menorrhagia.[7] Despite these lines of evidence, the specific physiological roles of prostaglandins and other agents in normal and pathologic endometrial function remain to be elucidated.

The development of a microvascular system in the functional layer of the endometrium has obvious reproductive significance. Of equal importance is the role that this vascular system plays in the initiation of menstruation and the specific mechanisms that are involved in obtaining hemostasis. The vascular and hemostatic events preceding and during menses have been studied by Bartelmez and, subsequently, by Christiaens and associates using uteri extirpated at the time of menstruation.[8,9] Histologic observations reveal shrinkage of the functional layer of the endometrium and breaks in the walls of the spiral arterioles, first appearing in the immediate premenstrual phase. This is followed by extravasation of blood into the functional layer, a process that may lead directly to tissue desquamation. The shedding of the functional layer of the endometrium results in disruption of vascular integrity and bleeding into the uterine cavity.

The establishment of hemostasis in menstrual endometrium is achieved through several mechanisms. During the first 24 hours, hemostatic plugs consisting of degranulated platelets are noted to be partially or completely occluding the spiral arterioles. The plugs differ from those that develop elsewhere in the body because they are relatively devoid of fibrin and may not be totally occlusive. The right fibrinolytic environment in the endometrium may account for these unique findings. The formation of platelet aggregates is clearly important because women with disorders of platelet function (e.g., von Willebrand disease) frequently suffer from menorrhagia. Observations from hysterectomy specimens obtained after

TABLE 1. *Definition of abnormal uterine bleeding*

Oligomenorrhea: bleeding at intervals of greater than 40 days that usually is irregular
Polymenorrhea: bleeding at intervals of less than 22 days that may be regular or irregular
Menorrhagia: bleeding that is excessive in both amount and duration at regular intervals
Metrorrhagia: bleeding of usually normal amount but at irregular intervals
Menometrorrhagia: bleeding that is excessive in amount, is prolonged in duration, and may occur at regular or irregular intervals
Hypomenorrhea: regular uterine bleeding in decreased amount
Intermenstrual bleeding: bleeding that occurs between what is otherwise regular menstrual bleeding

the first 24 hours of menstruation reveal the completion of endometrial desquamation and a decrease in the presence of hemostatic plugs. It is assumed that hemostasis is maintained during this time by progressive vasoconstriction in the vasculature of the basal layer. Prompt regeneration of the functional layer with the reestablishment of vascular integrity completes the process.[3,4]

Normal menstruation is a complex process involving physiological events both understood and yet to be defined. The generation of a functional endometrium capable of either sustaining an embryo or shedding in an orderly manner requires precise endocrinologic signals coupled with appropriate endometrial responses. Even subtle derangement of these physiological events may lead to abnormalities of menstruation that require medical evaluation and treatment. Large epidemiologic studies have found that the mean duration of menses is 5.2 days with blood loss ranging from 35 to 43 ml per cycle.[10] Although the precise definition of excessive menstrual blood loss is more than 80 ml per cycle, a menstrual pattern that disrupts a person's normal routine deserves investigation. A list of the abnormalities of menstruation and their definitions appears in Table 1. The remainder of this chapter addresses the appropriate evaluation and treatment of these and other conditions associated with menstrual function.

◊ AMENORRHEA

Amenorrhea, or the absence of menstruation, is a symptom, not a disease, and is a common reason for medical consultation. Primary amenorrhea is defined as the failure of menarche to occur before 16 years of age. The cessation of menses for at least 12 months in a postmenarchal woman is classified as secondary amenorrhea. In general, the distinction between primary and secondary amenorrhea is of little importance because there is considerable overlap in the etiology of these conditions. The specific cause of amenorrhea can be efficiently determined by first completing a thorough history and physical examination, followed by selected laboratory and radiologic tests. Pregnancy must always be considered a possibility in women with secondary amenorrhea, and urine or serum

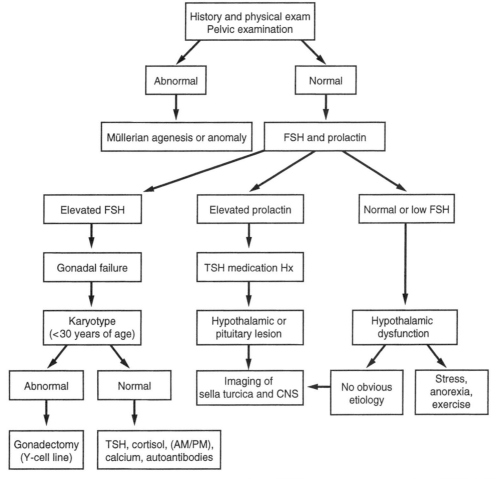

FIG. 1. Algorithm for the evaluation of amenorrhea. CNS, central nervous system; FSH, follicle-stimulating hormone; TSH, thyroid-stimulating hormone.

testing for human chorionic gonadotropin (hCG) should be performed early in the evaluation. Rarely, either provocative pituitary testing or a progestin challenge may be required to arrive at a diagnosis. It is useful to categorize the cause of amenorrhea into four subgroups: hypothalamic dysfunction, pituitary dysfunction, ovarian failure, and anatomic abnormalities of the reproductive tract. In all four diagnostic groups, secondary sexual characteristics may or may not be present. An algorithm for the evaluation of amenorrhea is shown in Fig. 1.

◊ HYPOTHALAMIC DYSFUNCTION

Hypothalamic causes of amenorrhea may be structural or functional. The latter are diagnoses of exclusion.[11] If an organic cause cannot be identified by full testing, including radiologic imaging, chemical dysfunction is blamed. In general, such patients with either type have lower levels of FSH and LH, but this may not be obvious on basal testing. Patterns of gonadotropin secretion may be altered by hypothalamic GnRH secretion pattern changes. Several groups of disorders are discussed in the sections that follow.

Hypothalamic Disorders

Several congenital syndromes associated with abnormal hypothalamic–gonadal function have been described. These conditions present with primary amenorrhea and an absence of secondary sexual characteristics. The most common of these rare disorders results from a failure in the development of the central structures of the hypothalamus. First described in boys, Kallmann syndrome has subsequently been identified in girls. The arcuate nucleus and olfactory bulbs are affected, leading to deficient gonadotropin-releasing hormone (GnRH) secretion in association with anosmia. In the absence of normal, pulsatile GnRH secretion, the pituitary gland fails to secrete sufficient gonadotropin to stimulate ovarian function. The administration of pulsatile GnRH results in normal gonadal function, confirming that the site of the abnormality is in the arcuate nucleus or its connections within the hypothalamus.[12] In theory, the lack of secondary sexual characteristics and eunuchoid growth associated with this disorder can be treated with pulsatile GnRH; this is impractical, however. The condition is best treated with estrogen therapy followed by cyclic estrogen and progestin once adequate breast development is achieved. When pregnancy is desired, ovulation induction can be accomplished either with GnRH administration or with the use of human menopausal gonadotropins.

Two additional syndromes of hypothalamic dysfunction resulting in incomplete pubertal development and the associated primary amenorrhea are the Prader-Willi and the Laurence-Moon-Biedl syndromes. Both of these rare conditions should be suspected from historical information and physical findings. Hypothalamic dysfunction in the Prader-Willi syndrome is associated with massive obesity, carbohydrate intolerance, hypotonia, and mental retardation. The associated abnormalities with the Laurence-Moon-Biedl syndrome are polydactyly, obesity, mental retardation, and retinitis pigmentosa. An autosomal recessive inheritance is associated with the latter syndrome.

Various systemic stresses may be associated with abnormal hypothalamic function, reduced gonadal function, and amenorrhea. These include significant weight loss, excessive exercise, and severe emotional distress. When these conditions occur before menarche, pubertal delay and primary amenorrhea result. In postmenarchal women, secondary amenorrhea may be the only presenting complaint. A complete history and physical examination should suggest the appropriate diagnosis. Treatment is directed toward altering the patient's behavior; when it is successful, spontaneous resumption of gonadal function usually occurs. Weight loss associated with the eating disorders anorexia nervosa and bulimia may be life-threatening and extremely difficult to treat. Not infrequently, women suffering from these disorders require psychiatric care. When amenorrhea is associated with athletic training, it may be impractical to cease exercising to allow for normalization of hypothalamic function. Because it has been documented that these women are at risk of stress fractures secondary to loss of bone mass, hormone replacement therapy with cyclic estrogen and progestin or oral contraceptives is warranted.[13]

Destructive processes or neoplastic lesions that involve the hypothalamus can present as either primary or secondary amenorrhea. Magnetic resonance imaging (MRI) of the head should be obtained in women with amenorrhea associated with neurologic findings or complaints. In addition, a hypothalamic lesion should be suspected when serum gonadotropin concentrations are low and a complete history and physical examination fail to reveal an obvious cause. Various CNS tumors can present in this manner, including hamartomas, craniopharyngiomas, and gliomas. These lesions may also be associated with an increased serum prolactin level because destruction of the hypothalamic–pituitary portal circulation may release the pituitary lactotroph from hypothalamic suppression. Infiltrative or infective disorders such as sarcoidosis and encephalitis may also be associated with hypothalamic failure.

◊ PITUITARY DYSFUNCTION

Amenorrhea may result from either a destructive process or a tumor creating pituitary dysfunction or from pituitary tumors that secrete an excess of a particular trophic hormone. In this clinical setting, serum gonadotropin concentrations are low, whereas levels of other hormones produced in the pituitary gland vary, depending on the specific pathologic condition. As an initial screening test, a determination of serum prolactin should be obtained because the level of this hormone is elevated in most women with amenorrhea based on abnormal pituitary function. A careful history and physical examination may uncover other signs or symptoms of pituitary disease that require the measurement of thyroid-stimulating hormone (TSH), growth hormone (GH), or adrenocorticotropic hormone (ACTH) in serum for confirmation. Radiologic imaging of the pituitary gland may be necessary to arrive at the correct diagnosis and determine appropriate therapy.

Pituitary Disorders

Amenorrhea secondary to abnormal pituitary function frequently is associated with elevated serum concentrations of prolactin (i.e., hyperprolactinemia). A common source of high prolactin levels is a benign pituitary adenoma composed of autonomously functioning lactotrophic cells. These tumors may present with galactorrhea and amenorrhea, although larger lesions may also produce headaches and visual disturbances. Other patients may have only amenorrhea without breast secretion. Amenorrhea and hyperprolactinemia resulting from a pituitary tumor is called the Forbes-Albright syndrome. If a prolactin-producing adenoma should arise before menarche, an arrest or delay of pubertal development and primary amenorrhea will be the presenting symptoms. Galactorrhea occurs only if breast development has been completed before the onset of the hyperprolactinemia. In most cases of hyperprolactinemia, secondary amenorrhea with normal pubertal development is found on clinical evaluation.

Various conditions other than pituitary adenoma may present with hyperprolactinemia. Most psychotomimetic and other drugs can induce a mild elevation in serum prolactin levels, resulting in amenorrhea. In this clinical setting, further evaluation can be obviated if the neurologic examination is normal and the serum concentration of prolactin is less than 100 ng/ml. Prompt resumption of menstruation occurs in these women with discontinuation of the drug. If the causative medication is necessary, hormone replacement with cyclic estrogen and progestin is warranted. Hypothyroidism may also be associated with hyperprolactinemia and should be ruled out by obtaining a TSH level. Physical stress, exercise, and recent food intake may temporarily elevate prolactin levels. To assure an accurate diagnosis, prolactin concentrations should be measured in a fasting state in the morning. Borderline levels must be corroborated by repeating the evaluation.

Once pharmacologic and physiological causes of hyperprolactinemia have been ruled out, the evaluation must determine the presence or absence of a pituitary tumor. Radiologic investigation is used to locate the lesion and document whether a microadenoma (i.e., diameter < 10 mm) or macroadenoma (i.e., diameter > 10 mm) is the source of the elevated prolactin level. The cone-down view of the sella turcica is an x-ray study that has the advantage of being readily available and inexpensive. These advantages are offset by the relative insensitivity of this technique because only tumors greater than 10 mm are detected consistently. In addition, anatomic variation in the sella may be confused with the erosion caused by tumor growth. Despite these limitations, the cone-down view of the sella is useful when clinical management will be altered only by the presence of a large tumor.

In most settings in which a pituitary tumor is suspected, radiologic imaging should be obtained with either a computed tomography (CT) or MRI study. These procedures are more expensive than simple radiography but are capable of detecting small lesions. An additional benefit is the ability of CT and MRI to evaluate the patient for suprasellar extension of the tumor. Because modern management of pituitary adenomas depends on the size and precise location of the tumor, initial evaluation of hyperprolactinemia and amenorrhea should include either a CT scan with injection of intravenous contrast material or an MRI.

Hyperprolactinemia may be associated with amenorrhea in the absence of a pituitary tumor. In this setting, treatment may include cyclic estrogen and progesterone therapy, low-dose oral contraceptive pills, or the administration of the dopamine agonists bromocriptine or cabergoline. The choice of therapy depends on the patient's goals, with medication being the only alternative for women who desire the resumption of ovulatory cycles so that conception is possible. Estrogen replacement or resumption of ovulatory cycles is necessary because these patients are at risk for the sequelae of hypoestrogenism.

Women with a microadenoma and no neurologic symptoms may also be offered either hormone replacement or dopamine agonist therapy. The latter treatment is required if conception is desired, although some of these patients will ovulate in response to gonadotropin therapy. When a patient presents with macroadenoma with or without suprasellar extension, aggressive treatment with a dopamine agonist is required. The majority of such lesions regress promptly with resolution of symptoms. As a general rule, all women with hyperprolactinemia, regardless of the mode of therapy, should be followed with serum prolactin determinations. In addition, CT scans should be obtained at intervals until the stability of a given tumor can be assured. These measures are necessary because the biological behavior of prolactin-producing adenomas is variable and must be determined for each individual tumor. Surgical approaches (including transsphenoidal approaches) and radiation therapy, commonly used in the past, should be reserved for selected cases of large or unresponsive tumors. Despite adequate therapy, there may be recurrence or persistence of the tumor or resultant panhypopituitarism.

Amenorrhea secondary to abnormal pituitary gland function can also occur with low prolactin levels. Pituitary failure after a severe postpartum hemorrhage with necrosis of the gland is referred to as Sheehan's syndrome. Hypopituitarism may also occur after head trauma or destructive neoplastic processes. Symptoms of slowly progressive lethargy and cachexia usually are present. Suspicion of this life-threatening condition should lead to provocative testing of the pituitary gland. Treatment requires replacement of the adrenal and thyroid hormones found to be deficient. Rarely, amenorrhea may be caused by pituitary adenomas that produce either ACTH or GH. Diagnosis usually is made obvious by the patient's presenting symptoms, which are consistent with Cushing syndrome.

◊ OVARIAN FAILURE

In the course of evaluating amenorrhea, elevated levels of serum gonadotropins may be detected. When the serum FSH concentration is greater than 40 mIU/ml on two occasions, the diagnosis of gonadal failure is confirmed. The rise in FSH is secondary to the loss of inhibition of gonadotropin secretion resulting from low sex steroid synthesis and a lack of inhibin production by the granulosa cells. Hypergonadotropic hypogonadism is a heterogeneous disorder presenting with primary amenorrhea in about 15% of cases and secondary amenorrhea in the remaining 85%. In women with primary amenorrhea and elevated gonadotropin levels, the condition is associated with incomplete pubertal development and should be considered irreversible. This contrasts with cases that present with secondary amenorrhea, in which some ovarian function may be preserved. Rebar and Connolly, in a review of 115 cases of hypergonadotropic hypogonadism, noted that 48% of women with secondary amenorrhea responded to a progestin challenge with withdrawal bleeding. Further, 23 of 97 patients exhibited evidence of ovulation sporadically, and 8% conceived after the diagnosis of gonadal failure was made. These observations have resulted in the reevaluation of the previous dogma that this condition is always permanent.[14]

Hypergonadotropic amenorrhea must be evaluated completely because associated conditions warrant specific therapy. In women who present before 30 years of age, a karyotype should be obtained. Various sex chromosomal abnormalities may lead to premature gonadal failure, with those involving a Y chromosome-bearing cell line requiring gonadectomy. Immunologic or endocrine dysfunction may also occur in these patients. Thyroid and adrenal disease are the most common; therefore, evaluation should include TSH, T_4, antithyroglobulin, antimicrosomal antibodies, and morning cortisol determinations. In addition, serum calcium and phosphorus concentrations may be drawn to exclude the rare case of abnormal parathyroid function. The detection of associated endocrinopathies requires close follow-up and specific hormone replacement therapy. Many women with premature gonadal failure exhibit signs of osteoporosis, and bone density may be determined. The initial evaluation should include an antinuclear antibody test because hypergonadotropic amenorrhea and connective tissue diseases can occur concomitantly. Ovarian biopsy is no longer considered appropriate as a routine in this evaluation.

Specific Etiologies

Cytogenetic abnormalities that involve the sex chromosomes may result in hypergonadotropic amenorrhea. Termed gonadal dysgenesis, this condition is the result of accelerated loss of ovarian follicles occurring during embryogenesis or in the first few years of life. In the absence of follicles, the ovaries are composed only of stromal tissue and appear as fibrous bands referred to as streak gonads. The most common form of gonadal dysgenesis, Turner syndrome, is caused by monosomy X. In addition to streak gonads, short stature, webbed neck, coarctation of the aorta, high arched palate, shield-shaped chest, widely spaced nipples, increased carrying angle of the upper extremities (i.e., cubitus valve), shortened fourth metacarpal bones of the hand, low hairline on the neck, and various renal abnormalities are all associated with this condition. Patients with an XO karyotype uniformly present with primary amenorrhea and an absence of secondary sex characteristics. Amenorrhea associated with the mosaic form of Turner syndrome may occur after pubertal development and menarche are complete. An excess of X chromosomes (e.g., 47,XXX) or deletions of only one portion of one X chromosome are also found in women with premature gonadal failure. A specific form of gonadal dysgenesis occurs in phenotypically normal women with 46,XY karyotype and is referred to as Swyer syndrome. As previously mentioned, the presence of a Y chromosome requires that gonadectomy be performed to avoid the potential development of a gonadoblastoma.

Chemotherapy, particularly with alkylating agents, and pelvic irradiation therapy can result in temporary or permanent premature ovarian failure. In general, the older the woman is at the time of therapy, the more likely that the hypergonadotropic amenorrhea will be permanent. Young cancer patients receiving radiation treatment may possibly avoid permanent gonadal failure through appropriate shielding or surgical transposition of the ovaries out of the radiation field. No effective measures exist that can prevent ovarian failure in association with some types of chemotherapy, although oocyte harvest and cryopreservation is a theoretical mechanism to allow future fertility.

Hypergonadotropic amenorrhea may also be associated with several rare disorders. Defects in the 17α-hydroxylase enzyme and the enzymatic deficiency leading to galactosemia present with primary amenorrhea. In addition, viral illness that affects the ovaries may result in premature gonadal failure. Congenital thymic aplasia and other uncommon autoimmune disorders may be associated with hypergonadotropic amenorrhea as well. Finally, this condition can be idiopathic, with the complete evaluation of a patient with amenorrhea and elevated gonadotropin levels yielding no definable cause.[15] A useful classification system of hypergonadotropic amenorrhea is listed in Table 2.

Treatment of patients with amenorrhea associated with elevated gonadotropin levels involves estrogen replacement and therapy directed toward concurrent disorders. When secondary sex characteristics are absent, conjugated estrogens

TABLE 2. *Classification of hypergonadotropic amenorrhea[a]*

I. Cytogenetic alterations
  A. Reduced germ cell number
  B. Accelerated atresia (?)
  C. Structural alterations or absence of an X chromosome
  D. Trisomy X with or without mosaicism
  E. In association with myotonia dystrophica
II. Enzymatic defects
  A. 17α-Hydroxylase deficiency
  B. Galactosemia
III. Physical insults
  A. Chemotherapeutic (especially alkylating) agents
  B. Ionizing radiation
  C. Viral infection
  D. Cigarette smoking
  E. Surgical extirpation
IV. Immune disturbances
  A. In association with other autoimmune disorders
  B. Isolated
  C. Congenital thymic aplasia
V. Defective gonadotropin secretion or action (?)
  A. Secretion of biologically inactive gonadotropin
  B. α- or β-subunit defects
  C. Gonadotropin receptor or postreceptor defects
VI. Idiopathic

[a]From ref. 15, with permission.

are administered in increasing doses until 2.5 to 3.75 mg is taken daily. This regimen is continued until breast development has progressed or menstrual spotting begins. At this point, the estrogen dose is reduced to 1.25 mg daily with 10 days per month of concurrent administration of 10 mg of medroxyprogesterone acetate. Women who present with secondary hypergonadotropic amenorrhea may be treated with usual estrogen–progestin replacement regimens.

◊ **ANATOMIC ABNORMALITIES**

In women with normal development of secondary sexual characteristics and primary amenorrhea, the pelvic examination becomes the most important element of the evaluation. If a normal vagina, cervix, and uterus are present, then hypothalamic, pituitary, and ovarian causes of the amenorrhea must be explored. When the pelvic examination is abnormal, incomplete Müllerian development is the most likely cause. To determine the appropriate therapy, a careful study of the reproductive tract is necessary to define abnormalities. This may require the use of pelvic ultrasound, CT scan, or MRI. In rare instances, examination under anesthesia or laparoscopy is necessary to understand a particular patient's anatomy. The surgical approach needed and the potential for success are determined by the specific Müllerian anomaly present.

Women with a normal uterus, endometrium capable of responding to estrogen, and obstruction of the outflow tract present with cyclic pain and primary amenorrhea. This constellation of findings most commonly is associated with an imperforate hymen. Examination reveals a bulging hymen just inside the introitus, and ultrasound demonstrates an obvious hematocolpos. Surgical therapy is directed toward making a cruciate incision in the hymen, eliminating the obstruction. This procedure is uniformly successful.

Incomplete canalization of the vagina results in a transverse vaginal septum and outflow tract obstruction. Again, the treatment is to establish a path for egress of menstrual flow by excising the septum. This usually is more difficult than treating an imperforate hymen because a transverse vaginal septum is a much thicker band of tissue. Success is assured, however, through a careful surgical approach by an experienced surgeon. A split-thickness skin graft may be required if a large segment of the vaginal mucosa is denuded.

Atresia of the cervix is a rare abnormality that presents in a similar manner. There is no successful surgical approach to correct this lesion, and abdominal hysterectomy is recommended to alleviate the cyclic pain. With all Müllerian anomalies that create an outflow tract obstruction, endometriosis frequently is found if laparoscopy is performed. Therefore, laparoscopy should be considered if symptoms of pelvic pain are noted in these patients.

A markedly foreshortened vagina ending blindly may be noted in association with primary amenorrhea and a lack of cyclic pain. Further investigation documents the absence of Müllerian structures, termed Müllerian agenesis. This clinical entity is also referred to as the Mayer-Rokitansky-Kuster-Hauser syndrome and is frequently associated with renal and skeletal anomalies. Reproduction is not possible, and corrective efforts should be directed toward creating a functional vagina. This can be successfully accomplished using progressive vaginal dilation or by a surgical approach creating a neovagina with a skin graft. Another cause of this type of pelvic abnormality (absence of vagina, cervix, and uterus) is the androgen insensitivity syndrome. In this problem, androgen receptors are ineffective, and the patient has intraabdominal testes, yet good breast development. Scanty hair is often noted. This diagnosis is usually made by karyotype. Management is by gonadal extirpation and neovaginal creation as above.

Asherman's syndrome is an unusual cause of secondary amenorrhea that results from obliteration of the endometrial cavity by scar tissue. In the clinical setting of secondary amenorrhea with normal ovarian function and a failure to have withdrawal bleeding after a progestin challenge, hysterosalpingography (HSG) confirms the diagnosis. Asherman's syndrome results from an injury to the endometrium when inflammation or infection is present and estrogen levels are low. This usually occurs when a dilation and curettage (D&C) is performed for postpartum hemorrhage. Hysteroscopy with lysis of the adhesions can often restore normal menstruation and reproductive potential.[16]

◊ ABNORMAL UTERINE BLEEDING

Abnormal uterine bleeding frequently prompts women to seek medical attention. Excessive menstrual blood loss is the single most common indication for hysterectomy and ac-

counts for significant lost productivity by the female population. Various strict criteria have been applied to the diagnosis of abnormal uterine bleeding. In practice, a significant change in menstrual pattern or amount of bleeding that necessitates an alteration in lifestyle should be investigated. A complete history and physical examination combined with appropriately selected laboratory tests and imaging procedures almost always yields an accurate and specific diagnosis. With this information, most cases of abnormal uterine bleeding can be treated either medically or by minimally invasive surgical techniques, avoiding hysterectomy. As with amenorrhea, the evaluation should begin by excluding pregnancy as a cause of unusual menstrual bleeding before initiating other testing. An algorithm for the evaluation of abnormal uterine bleeding is shown in Fig. 2.

Evaluation

After the possibility of a pregnancy has been eliminated, a complete history and careful pelvic examination must be performed early in the diagnostic evaluation of abnormal uterine bleeding. When uterine or adnexal pathology is suspected, confirmation and further definition should be obtained through the use of pelvic ultrasonography. The finding of uterine leiomyomata in association with disorders of menstruation is exceedingly common. Because the therapeutic options depend on the number, size, and locations of the fibroid tumors, evaluation should be directed toward collecting this information (see Treatment). Transvaginal or pelvic ultrasonography or hysterography may be useful in this regard,[17] but the more expensive imaging techniques, CT scan and MRI, are seldom necessary.

During the course of evaluating abnormal uterine bleeding, adnexal pathology may be encountered. The sonographic characteristics of the mass are useful in determining the appropriate diagnostic testing and therapy. A small unilocular cyst may be followed expectantly because the majority resolve spontaneously. A multiloculated cyst or mass with solid components should be investigated further. A serum CA-125 concentration may provide useful information, but prompt surgical exploration and a histologic diagnosis are required. If cancer is suspected, preoperative evaluation of the gastrointestinal tract, kidneys, and liver can efficiently be completed using CT scanning or MRI.

When the pelvic examination does not clarify the diagnosis, increasing use of pelvic (uterine) ultrasound has been useful. Transvaignal ultrasound or sonohysterography may reveal endometrial polyps or lesions, or even simple measurement of an excessively thick endometrial stripe may suggest a cause. In such patients, office hysteroscopy or D&C may be appropriate.[17] A determination should be made as to whether or not abnormal uterine bleeding is associated with ovulatory cycles. A history of menstrual bleeding occurring at regular intervals preceded by moliminal symptoms such as breast tenderness, bloating, and pelvic tenderness is highly predictive of normal ovulatory function. Conversely, irregu-

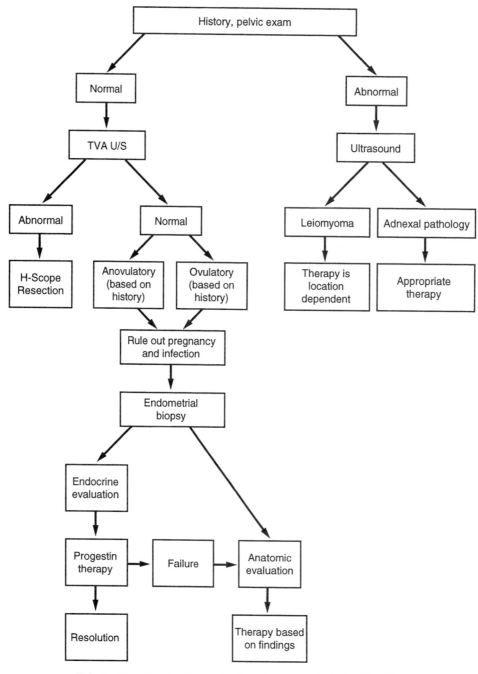

FIG. 2. Algorithm for the evaluation of abnormal uterine bleeding.

lar bleeding in the absence of prodromal symptoms usually is the result of endocrine dysfunction leading to anovulation. If the distinction between ovulatory and anovulatory bleeding is not apparent from historical information, then objective data must be obtained. The basal body temperature graph, determination of serum progesterone concentration, and endometrial biopsy may all be used to determine if ovulation has occurred. Ovulation is suggested if the temperature curve is biphasic and is better documented when the serum progesterone level is greater than 2 ng/ml or when secretory transformation of the endometrium is noted on biopsy.

Anovulatory uterine bleeding is a symptom of an endocrine disturbance. The appropriate evaluation in this clinical setting must determine the source of the underlying endocrinopathy. Tests of thyroid, hypothalamic, pituitary, and adrenal function are warranted. In general, an abnormality that can cause amenorrhea may, in a less severe form, result in anovulation and abnormal uterine bleeding. Therefore, the evaluation should include determination of serum concentrations of TSH, FSH, LH, prolactin, and dehydroepiandrosterone. When anovulatory bleeding is associated with signs of androgen excess, as noted on physical examination, serum testosterone and 17-hydroxyprogesterone levels must also be obtained. In the hirsute patient, elevation of serum 17-hydroxyprogesterone concentration indicative of adult-onset 21-hydroxylase deficiency may be evident only if provocative adrenal testing with ACTH is performed.

In most cases, anovulatory uterine bleeding is associated with chronic oligoanovulation or polycystic ovary syndrome. This latter condition is associated with tonic estrogen production in the absence of ovulation and progesterone secretion. The endometrium is chronically stimulated, inducing proliferation without secretory transformation and orderly shedding. Chaotic, dysfunctional uterine bleeding, which at times may be heavy, ultimately results. An endometrial evaluation must be performed in these women to determine the presence or absence of hyperplastic or neoplastic disorders of the endometrium.

The histologic classification of endometrial hyperplasia is important to predict the potential for malignant transformation and to determine the most appropriate therapy. Simple hyperplasia is defined as increased crowding of the endometrial glands. The glands may exhibit irregular outlines and be dilated, but cytologic atypia is absent. In cases of complex (proliferative) hyperplasia, the glands display irregular outlines, are tortuous, and appear crowded back to back without intervening stroma. Cytologic atypia can occur with either simple or complex hyperplasia and is characterized by an atypical nuclear appearance and a loss of cellular polarity within the epithelium of the glands. Progression to frank endometrial carcinoma is often seen in patients with atypical hyperplasia.[18,19]

Abnormal uterine bleeding that occurs during the extremes of a woman's reproductive life typically is the result of anovulation. In the adolescent, prolonged episodes of uterine bleeding may occur during the transition to regular, ovulatory menstrual cycles. The possibility of pregnancy should be eliminated and the potential for pelvic infection ascertained. In the absence of either of these conditions, therapy can be based on the assumption that the bleeding is secondary to anovulation without subjecting these young women to endometrial biopsy or further diagnostic testing. During the perimenopause, disturbing abnormal uterine bleeding frequently results from waning ovarian function. Before the initiation of therapy, a careful pelvic examination and endometrial biopsy must be performed because anatomic and endometrial abnormalities are relatively common in this age group.

Women with abnormal uterine bleeding may have historical or objective findings that are consistent with an unusual bleeding pattern superimposed on normal, ovulatory ovarian function. In this clinical setting, the possibility of a pregnancy must be excluded by obtaining a serum level of hCG. When abnormal uterine bleeding is associated with pregnancy, a thorough evaluation should proceed promptly to determine the potential for an ectopic gestation. The appropriate diagnostic studies and therapy of pregnancy complications are detailed elsewhere in this text.

In the absence of pregnancy, ovulatory abnormal uterine bleeding can be associated with endometritis. The diagnosis

may be obvious based on uterine tenderness and a history consistent with sexually transmitted disease. Confirmatory cervical cultures for *Neisseria gonorrheae* and *Chlamydia trachomatis* should be obtained before antibiotic treatment is initiated. The lack of these findings on physical examination does not eliminate endometritis as a potential cause of uterine bleeding. An endometrial biopsy is the most specific and sensitive test for determining the presence of this disorder. The diagnosis of endometritis is confirmed by the presence of plasma cells within the endometrial glands and stroma.[20] Thus, an endometrial biopsy is an important component of the evaluation of abnormal uterine bleeding in ovulatory women even when other findings are not indicative of pelvic infection.

Anatomic abnormalities of the myometrium, endometrium, or endocervix are common causes of uterine bleeding in ovulatory women. The emphasis of the evaluation should shift toward detecting these lesions when the possibilities of pregnancy and endometritis have been eliminated. As noted previously, findings on pelvic examination consistent with leiomyomata can be clarified further with the use of pelvic ultrasound. However, because submucous leiomyoma and polyps of the endometrium and endocervix may escape detection by even the most skilled and experienced examiner, further evaluation designed to detect subtle anatomic lesions should be completed even if the pelvic examination is normal.

Formerly, the D&C was the procedure of choice to evaluate abnormal uterine bleeding. This intervention provides ample tissue for the histologic diagnosis of endometrial abnormalities. Blind exploration of the uterine cavity, however, has an unacceptably high false-negative rate, failing to detect small but clinically significant lesions. Information concerning the uterine cavity can be obtained with imaging techniques or by direct visualization using the hysteroscope. The combination of an office endometrial biopsy and an appropriate method to determine the anatomic integrity of the myometrium and endometrium should replace the blind D&C in the evaluation of uterine bleeding.

The hysteroscope is a valuable aid in the accurate diagnosis of anatomic lesions that affect the endometrial cavity. Several excellent studies have addressed the relative effectiveness of the blind D&C and hysteroscopy for the diagnosis of abnormal uterine bleeding. Three studies in particular are worthy of mention. In 1981, Valle published his experience with 553 women who had hysteroscopy for uterine bleeding. In almost one-half of the cases, 259, an anatomic lesion was noted at hysteroscopy. These lesions included submucous fibroids and endometrial polyps, only 15% of which were identified by prior, blind curettage.[21] Gimpelson and Rappold also noted a failure of the blind D&C to detect intrauterine anatomic lesions that were easily identified with hysteroscopy. Of the 10% of women in their series with polyps or fibroids, only one was diagnosed on D&C.[22] Finally, Brooks and Serden performed hysteroscopy on 29 women who had had a blind D&C within the preceding year, all with persistent bleeding. Twenty-four of the women had anatomic abnormalities detected by direct visualization, but only three had had a similar diagnosis made by curettage.[23] These studies, in addition to other data in the literature, lead to the conclusion that hysteroscopy provides increased diagnostic yield when compared with blind D&C in the evaluation of abnormal uterine bleeding. The increased yield is most evident in the detection of anatomic abnormalities.

Diagnostic hysteroscopy can be accomplished in the office or operating room. Hysterosalpingoscopy is another sensitive technique to detect abnormalities of the uterine cavity. The ability of this technique to detect subtle lesions is enhanced when a film is obtained early in the process of filling the cavity with contrast material. The difficulty with using HSG in the evaluation of abnormal uterine bleeding is that the technique lacks specificity. The rate of false-positive results may be as high as 30%. In the clinical setting of ovulatory abnormal uterine bleeding, the HSG is a reasonable screening examination. The absence of intracavitary lesions is reassuring, and abnormal studies can be followed by hysteroscopy to confirm the findings and initiate treatment.

Transvaginal ultrasonography (TVS) with and without fluid injection into the uterus (sonohysterography) is another technique that is useful in the evaluation of abnormal uterine bleeding. When the pelvic examination is consistent with uterine leiomyomata, the number and location of the tumors can be determined with TVS. This procedure has been compared with hysteroscopy for accuracy in the identification of submucous myomas, the type of fibroids most often associated with uterine bleeding. In a series of 71 women with symptomatic uterine myomas, TVS had a sensitivity of 100% and a specificity of 94%. The predictive value of an abnormal ultrasound scan was 81%, and that of a normal TVS was 100%.[24] Questions concerning the lower size limit of lesions that can be detected with this technique and the predictive value of positive and negative results in larger populations remain to be answered. The TVS is clearly a useful adjuvant in the anatomic evaluation of patients with abnormal uterine bleeding.

A thorough evaluation, including an endometrial biopsy, anatomic studies, and a history and physical examination, may be completed without identifying a specific cause of abnormal uterine bleeding. In these cases, a coagulation disorder should be ruled out by obtaining a prothrombin time, bleeding time, partial thromboplastin time, and platelet count. When these tests prove to be normal, the symptoms of uterine bleeding may be secondary to adenomyosis, a diagnosis made by exclusion or at the time of hysterectomy. It is possible that the entire evaluation will fail to identify the source of abnormal bleeding. In these instances, it is assumed that the abnormality exists within the many biochemical events occurring in the endometrium that lead to controlled, self-limited menstrual bleeding. Further understanding of these abnormal events is not available.

Treatment

The successful treatment of abnormal uterine bleeding depends on making an accurate diagnosis. In the case of bleeding associated with anovulation, a careful search may identify an underlying endocrinopathy. Treatment directed toward eliminating the primary disorder usually results in the resumption of regular menses. When chronic oligoovulation is present, therapy must be preceded by an endometrial biopsy. In the absence of hyperplasia or neoplasia, cyclic oral contraceptives or progestins administered in a dose of 10 mg of medroxyprogesterone acetate 10 days out of a month are uniformly successful. If medroxyprogesterone is not well tolerated, 2.5 to 5.0 mg of norethindrone 10 days of the month may be used instead. When abnormal uterine bleeding persists despite cyclic progestin treatment, a search for an anatomic cause must be initiated.

The endometrial biopsy may reveal simple or complex hyperplasia with or without atypia. In these cases without atypia, progesterone withdrawal after 10 days of treatment should be followed by 10 to 20 mg of medroxyprogesterone daily for 2 to 3 months. Repeat endometrial biopsy off of therapy usually confirms the disappearance of the histologic abnormality. Cyclic treatment with medroxyprogesterone can then be initiated as outlined. Most authors recommend hysterectomy when the endometrial histology reveals cytologic atypia because these lesions are likely to progress to adenocarcinoma. When adenocarcinoma of the endometrium is identified, complete staging followed by total abdominal hysterectomy with bilateral salpingo-oophorectomy are warranted.

Anovulatory bleeding occurring at the extremes of reproductive age requires specific treatment. The adolescent usually presents after many days of menstrual bleeding that has failed to cease spontaneously. In this instance, the uterine bleeding arises from a denuded, rather than a hypertrophied and disordered, endometrium. Proliferation of the remaining endometrium with estrogen, not stabilization with progestin, is required. In severe cases, conjugated estrogen can be administered in a dose of 12.5 mg intravenously and repeated in 12 hours. This treatment usually results in the prompt cessation of bleeding. Combination oral contraceptives can then be begun to control subsequent menstruation. In cases in which the bleeding is less severe, oral ethinyl estradiol (20 to 40 µg) can be substituted for the intravenous doses.[25] During the perimenopausal years, abnormal uterine bleeding may occur in association with a moderate elevation in FSH levels. Endometrial and anatomic abnormalities must be eliminated as potential causes. When these pathologic entities are not present, bleeding can be controlled by initiating routine, cyclic estrogen and progestin replacement therapy. If no contraindications exist, low-dose oral contraceptives may be substituted.

The hysteroscope has proved to be particularly useful for the management of abnormal uterine bleeding. Although originally described as a diagnostic tool, the hysteroscope is now recognized as a valuable therapeutic instrument. This transition occurred after technical improvements in fiber optics and the discovery of techniques using distending media, which consistently provided the surgeon the visibility required to perform intrauterine procedures. The use of surgical adjuvants in operative hysteroscopy (e.g., Nd:YAG laser, resectoscope) has further broadened the applications of this instrument to gynecologic disease. Techniques for the removal of endometrial polyps and pedunculated intrauterine myomas under direct visualization are well established.[26] When these small lesions are present, excision uniformly results in correction of the abnormal uterine bleeding.

As noted previously, the complete evaluation of abnormal uterine bleeding may fail to identify a specific source. Chronic menometrorrhagia of unknown cause is a frequent indication for hysterectomy. An alternative approach in this clinical setting is to destroy the endometrium hysteroscopically. This procedure is referred to as an endometrial ablation. Candidates for an endometrial ablation include women with significant uterine bleeding who have completed childbearing and in whom all nonsurgical therapy has failed. Hyperplasia and neoplasia must be excluded by endometrial sampling before the procedure. In addition, the potential presence of anatomic lesions should be eliminated by preoperative evaluation.

In 1981, Goldrath and colleagues published their initial experience with hysteroscopic treatment of chronic menometrorrhagia, using the Nd:YAG laser.[27] Prior attempts at endometrial destruction in these patients with chemicals or cryocautery had met with only limited success. The 3- to 5-mm depth of coagulation achieved with the Nd:YAG laser is ideal because the basalis layer of the endometrium must be destroyed to assure a continued beneficial effect. Further, the thickness of the normal myometrium ensures a significant margin of safety, protecting intraabdominal structures from inadvertent injury. The endometrial ablation procedure is ideal for women with complicating medical conditions such as chronic renal failure, heart disease, and abnormalities of coagulation, in whom a laparotomy carries a significant risk. Subsequent reports have confirmed the effectiveness of this procedure.[28]

The resectoscope, identical to the instrument used by urologists, can also be used to treat uterine bleeding. When equipped with a cautery electrode or roller ball, the resectoscope can be used to perform the endometrial ablation procedure. Although no study has directly compared the two energy sources, most authorities consider the cautery and the Nd:YAG laser equivalent for this purpose. Although the roller ball has been widely touted as being much faster, a competent hysteroscopist can complete the procedure with equal speed using either energy source. Only the nonelectrolyte solutions glycine and sorbitol can be used as distention media with the resectoscope.[29]

After the initial evaluation is completed, and before ablation is done, the patient is placed on danocrine (800 mg/day) or GnRH agonist for 4 to 6 weeks preoperatively to ensure atrophy of the endometrium. Either general or regional anesthesia can be used. The patient is placed in the dorsal lithotomy position and prepared in the usual manner. The draping must include a fluid collection device attached to the buttock. A tenaculum is placed on the anterior lip of the cervix, which is then dilated to easily accommodate the operating hysteroscope. Uterine distention can be accomplished with the continuous infusion of normal saline solution, lactated Ringer solution, glycine, or dextran 70 (Hyskon). We use either lactated Ringer solution or glycine to avoid the bubbles that are created when the laser or electrosurgical energy is used with the more viscous dextran 70.

The hysteroscope is cleared of air and inserted with the distention media flowing. The procedure can be completed either under direct vision or with the surgeon working from the image on the video monitor. In both cases, care must be taken to avoid eye injury with the use of a protective lens on the hysteroscope and proper safety glasses if the Nd:YAG laser is used. The entire endometrial surface must be treated to ensure an adequate outcome. Care must be taken to avoid treatment of the endocervical canal because this can result in injury to the descending branch of the uterine artery and postoperative hemorrhage. When this procedure is performed by an experienced gynecologic endoscopist, the operating time should be between 30 and 45 minutes.

The volume of distending medium infused and recovered during the procedure must be closely monitored. The difference in the two measurements is the volume of fluid that has been absorbed by the patient. If the fluid deficit reaches 2000 ml, the procedure should be terminated because fluid overload with pulmonary edema is a potential complication of this procedure. About 50% of the patients treated with an endometrial ablation will have amenorrhea, 40% will have hypomenorrhea, and 10% will continue to have menorrhagia. In those patients in whom the endometrial ablation fails, a repeat procedure frequently is successful.

Abnormal bleeding associated with uterine leiomyomata may be treated by a variety of methods. Selection of the therapeutic approach depends on the location of the myoma and the patient's desire for childbearing potential. When fertility is not an issue and the tumors are multiple and intramural, the most appropriate treatment is hysterectomy. Laparotomy with myomectomy can successfully treat menorrhagia associated with intramural and subserosal fibroids in more than 90% of cases if retention of reproductive potential should be desired.

Submucous leiomyomata can be treated using the resectoscope in most cases. The technique, first described by Neuwirth, involves using a cutting loop in place of the coagulation electrode described previously.[30] The loop is extended over the lesion and, with the current activated, drawn back toward the surgeon. Sequential resection of the intracavitary lesion results. It is critically important that the energy not be activated while the electrode is moving away from the operator because this may lead to perforation and damage to intraabdominal organs. This minimally invasive technique can be performed as an outpatient procedure and is successful in over 90% of women.[31] The resolution of menorrhagia achieved with either endometrial ablation or resection of a submucous myoma has been shown to be permanent in most cases (Table 3).[32] In women with abnormal uterine bleeding secondary to fibroid tumors, preoperative treatment with a GnRH agonist results in cessation of blood loss, allowing for correction of anemia when present.[33]

TABLE 3. *Long-term effectiveness of hysteroscopic treatment of menorrhagia*[a]

Procedure	Number of patients	Follow-up	Recurrent symptoms (%)	Repeat surgery (%)	Hysterectomy (%)
Ablation	62	8 yr	22.5	8.1	4.8
Resection	94	9 yr	24.5	15.9	8.5

[a]Data from ref. 32.

◊ PREMENSTRUAL SYNDROME

Most women with ovulatory ovarian function experience molimenal symptoms during the luteal phase of the menstrual cycle. In about 10% of women, premenstrual symptoms are severe enough that medical attention is sought.[34] Although no specific definition of premenstrual syndrome (PMS) is universally accepted, most experienced clinicians require three findings to make the diagnosis. First, a symptom complex consistent with PMS must be present. Second, symptoms must occur exclusively during the luteal phase of ovulatory menstrual cycles. Finally, the symptoms must be severe enough that the person's life is disrupted.[35] As with other disorders associated with menstruation, a complete evaluation leading to a specific diagnosis of PMS enhances the possibility that therapy will be successful.

The symptoms associated with PMS are diverse, with each patient describing a unique set of complaints. Alterations in mood, social behavior, and cognitive function are common. Somatic complaints usually are part of the symptom complex (Table 4). Most women seeking treatment describe multiple symptoms, all occurring during the characteristic time in the cycle. Psychological disorders, including depression and anxiety, frequently are confused with PMS and must be ruled out before initiating therapy. These patients fail to display the cyclicity of symptomatology present with true PMS. The diagnosis can be made with the greatest accuracy by having the patient keep a menstrual calendar, carefully recording daily symptoms. A review of 2 months of symptom charts usually is sufficient.

The precise cause of PMS is unknown, but studies have begun to expand our understanding of this complex disorder. Early theories that the pathophysiology of PMS is related to a simple deficiency of progesterone have been abandoned. In an investigation of 18 women studied over two cycles with daily

hormone determinations, the most severe symptoms were noted at times when the serum estradiol and progesterone concentrations were at their peak.[36] Clearly, factors other than absolute amounts of ovarian steroids are important in producing symptoms. Alternative hypotheses include derangements in the relative amounts of estrogen and progesterone produced, changes in production of other ovarian hormones, and altered CNS effects of ovarian steroids in affected women.

A growing body of evidence indicates that the neuroendocrine mechanisms are important in the pathophysiology of PMS. Serotonin is a neurotransmitter present in the CNS that has been shown to be important in the genesis of mood. Peripheral markers of serotonin production are altered in women with affective disorders, implying decreased synthesis within the CNS. Similar changes in serotonin synthesis have been noted during the luteal phase in women suffering from PMS.[37] The connection between this neurotransmitter and PMS is further strengthened by the observation that medications that act by increasing release or decreasing reuptake of serotonin are effective in alleviating symptoms.[37,38] γ-Aminobutyric acid (GABA) has a general suppressive effect on brain function. The activation of the GABA-A receptor results in a decrease in anxiety levels and is known to be the mechanism of action of benzodiazepines. Metabolites of progesterone also interact with the GABA-A receptor and may provide a mechanism through which altered ovarian function might influence mood. Medications that act as GABA agonists have been shown to be effective in treating the anxiety associated with PMS.[39]

Successful treatment of PMS depends on careful diagnosis and charting of each person's symptoms. Simple interventions, such as exercise, alteration of diet, avoidance of salt, alcohol, and caffeine, may result in dramatic improvement and should be given an adequate trial. Changes in lifestyle that reduce stress may also provide relief. In women in whom symptoms of anxiety predominate, a trial of the anxiolytic agents buspirone or alprazolam administered during the luteal phase can be initiated. When depression is a major symptom, continuous therapy with clomipramine, nortriptyline, or fluoxetine has been shown to be more effective than placebo in blinded studies.[40] These centrally active agents should only be used by practitioners familiar with their use.

The mainstay of treatment for PMS involves the use of agents that suppress ovarian function. Oral contraceptive pills may provide a simple and inexpensive solution in many instances. Alternatives include the use of high doses of progestins or the administration of GnRH agonists. Medroxyprogesterone acetate in doses of 30 mg daily suppresses

TABLE 4. *Symptoms of premenstrual syndrome*

Psychological	**Somatic**
Irritability	Mastalgia
Emotional lability	Bloating
Anxiety	Headache
Depression	Fatigue
Hostility	Insomnia
Cognitive	**Social behavior**
Inability to concentrate	Craving carbohydrates
Confusion	Withdrawal
	Arguing

ovulation and affords relief of symptoms to some women. The frequency of abnormal uterine bleeding and progestin-related adverse effects associated with this treatment limit its usefulness. The GnRH agonist leuprolide acetate consistently provides relief from the symptoms of PMS. However, the profound hypoestrogenism, with the potential for osteoporosis and increased risk of cardiovascular disease, induced by this drug makes it less appealing. In an effort to counteract these drawbacks, Mortola and associates have pioneered the combined use of GnRH agonist suppression with estrogen and progesterone replacement therapy with excellent results,[40] although this therapy is very expensive and probably not useful for very long-term use.

◊ DYSMENORRHEA

Dysmenorrhea, or painful menstruation, may present as an isolated disorder or in association with other conditions. The primary focus usually occurs in nulliparous young women with a normal pelvic examination. In this setting, the cause of the dysmenorrhea is increased prostaglandin $F_{2\alpha}$ production by the endometrium, leading to myometrial contractions. When a careful history confirms the classic presentation and chronic nature of the symptoms, further evaluation, other than a pelvic examination, is not necessary. Treatment may be initiated with nonsteroidal antiinflammatory agents, which block prostaglandin synthesis through inhibition of the enzyme cyclooxygenase and are often effective. Therapy is most successful when begun before the onset of menstruation and continued until the patient's symptoms have abated. Endometrial prostaglandin synthesis is also inhibited by progesterone. Therefore, treatment with oral contraceptive pills is also effective with the additional benefit of lessening and regulating the flow. In the case of an abnormal pelvic examination, treatment would be withheld until further evaluation has been completed.

When the therapeutic measures outlined fail, or if dysmenorrhea should develop in a woman with a history of asymptomatic menses, further evaluation of the dysmenorrhea is warranted. In this clinical setting, the dysmenorrhea may be a symptom of pelvic endometriosis. When conservative measures fail to effect relief, laparoscopy should be performed to confirm the diagnosis and initiate treatment. Symptomatic endometriosis can occur in any woman between menarche and menopause. Laparoscopy should not be withheld because of the clinician's perception that the patient is too young or too old to suffer from this condition.

Dysmenorrhea may occur in women with increasing menometrorrhagia. A careful evaluation should be initiated to detect lesions within the uterine cavity that may be precipitating both symptoms. In this regard, hysteroscopy, HSG, and TVS are useful. Careful inspection of the cervix may reveal cervical stenosis or an endocervical polyp as the cause of dysmenorrhea. Stenosis may not be suspected if the history includes prior treatment for cervical dysplasia. Treatment of dysmenorrhea in association with these conditions is surgical, directed toward removing the anatomic lesion or attempting to correct a stenotic endocervical canal. In women with dysmenorrhea that is refractory to all conservative measures, hysterectomy may be warranted if fertility is not an issue. If childbearing potential is desired, a presacral neurectomy may be necessary in women with severe symptoms.

SUMMARY POINTS

◊ The mean duration of normal menses is 5.2 days with blood loss ranging from 35 to 43 ml per cycle. Uterine bleeding is considered abnormal if it occurs more often than every 21 days, lasts longer than 8 days, or if it is intermenstrual.

◊ The four major groupings of causes of amenorrhea are hypothalamic, pituitary, ovarian, and anatomic abnormalities.

◊ Abnormal uterine bleeding may be evaluated easily in the office by endometrial biopsy, transvaginal ultrasound (with and without fluid instillation), and hysteroscopy.

◊ Hysteroscopic myomectomy or polypectomy and endometrial ablation offer options to hysterectomy for some patients with abnormal uterine bleeding.

◊ REFERENCES

1. Ludwig H, Spornitz UM. Microarchitecture of the human endometrium by scanning electron microscopy: menstrual desquamation and remodeling. In: Bulletti C. Gurpide E, eds. *The primate endometrium.* New York: New York Academy of Sciences, 1991:28.
2. Nogales-Ortiz F, Puerta J Nogales FF Jr. The normal menstrual cycle. Chronology and mechanism of endometrial desquamation. *Obstet Gynecol* 1978;259–251.
3. Padykula HA. Regeneration in the primate uterus: the role of stem cells. In: Bulletti C, Gurpide E, eds. *The primate endometrium.* New York: New York Academy of Sciences, 1991:47.
4. Kaiserman-Abramof IR, Padykula HA. Angiogenesis in the postovulatory primate endometrium: the coiled arteriolar system. *Anat Rec* 1989; 224:479.
5. Markee JE. Menstruation in intraocular endometrial transplants in the rhesus monkey. *Contrib Embryol Carnegie Inst* 1940;28:219.
6. Bonney RC, Higham JM, Watson H, et al. Phospholipase activity in the endometrium of women with normal menstrual blood loss and women with proven ovulatory menorrhagia. *Br J Obstet Gynaecol* 1991; 98:363.
7. Guillebaud J, Anderson ABM, Turnbull AC. Reduction by megefamic acid of increased menstrual blood loss associated with intrauterine contraception. *Br J Obstet Gynaecol* 1978;85:53.
8. Bartelmez GW. The phases of the menstrual cycle and their interpretation in terms of the pregnancy cycle. *Am J Obstet Gynecol* 1957;74:931.
9. Christiaens GCML, Sixma JJ, Haspels AA. Morphology of haemostasis in menstrual endometrium. *Br J Obstet Gynaecol* 1980;87:425.
10. Rybo G. Menstrual blood loss in relation to parity and menstrual pattern. *Acta Obstet Gynecol Scand* 1966;45:25.
11. Laughlin GA, Dominguez CE, Yen SSC. Nutritional and endocrine-metabolic aberrations in women with functional hypothalamic amenorrhea. *J Clin Endocrinol Metab* 1998;83:25–32.
12. Schwanzel-Fukada M, Pfaff DW. Origin of luteinizing hormone releasing hormone neurons. *Nature* 1989;45:25.

13. Myburg KH, Hutchins J, Fataar AB, et al. Low bone density is an etiologic factor for stress fractures in athletes. *Ann Intern Med* 1990; 113:754.

14. Rebar RW, Connolly HV. Clinical features of young women with hypergonadotropic amenorrhea. *Fertil Steril* 1990;53:804.

15. Rebar RW, Cedars MI. Hypergonadotropic forms of amenorrhea in young women. *Endocrinol Metab Clin North Am* 1992;21(1):173.

16. Hurts BS. Laparoscopic myomectomy. In: Azziz R, Murphy AA, eds. *Practical manual of operative laparoscopy and hysteroscopy.* New York: Springer-Verlag, 1997.

17. Al-Azzawi F. Hysteroscopy or ultrasound? *Curr Opin Obstet Gynecol* 1996;8:246–256.

18. Kurman RJ, Kaminski PF, Norris HJ. The behavior of endometrial hyperplasia: A long-term study of untreated hyperplasia in 170 patients. *Cancer* 1985;56:403.

19. Evans-Metcalf ER, Brooks SE, Reale FR, Baker SP. Profile of women 45 years of age and younger with endometrial cancer. *Obstet Gynecol* 1998;91:349–354.

20. Paavonen J, Kiviat N, Brunham RC. Prevalence and manifestations of endometritis among women with cervicitis. *Am J Obstet Gynecol* 1985; 152:280.

21. Valle RF. Hysteroscopic evaluation of patients with abnormal uterine bleeding. *Surg Gynecol Obstet* 1981;153:521.

22. Gimpelson RJ, Rappold HO. A comparative study between panoramic hysteroscopy with directed biopsies and dilatation and curettage. *Am J Obstet Gynecol* 1988;158:489.

23. Brooks PG, Serden SP. Hysteroscopic findings after unsuccessful dilatation and curettage for abnormal uterine bleeding. *Am J Obstet Gynecol* 1988;158:1354.

24. Fedele L, Bianchi S, Dorta M, et al. Transvaginal ultrasonography versus hysteroscopy in the diagnosis of uterine submucous myomas. *Obstet Gynecol* 1991;77:745.

25. Claessens EA, Cowell CA. Acute adolescent menorrhagia. *Am J Obstet Gynecol* 1981;139:277.

26. Hallez J-P. Myomectomy by endo-uterine resection. *Curr Opin Obstet Gynecol* 1996;8:250–260.

27. Goldrath MH, Fuller TA, Segal S. Laser vaporization of the endometrium for the treatment of menorrhagia. *Am J Obstet Gynecol* 1981;140:14.

28. O'Conner H, Broadbent JAM, Magos AL, McPherson K. The Medical Research Council randomized trial of endometrial resection versus hysterectomy in the management of menorrhagia. *Lancet* 1997;349: 897–901.

29. Vancaillie TC. Electrocoagulation of the endometrium with the ball-end resectoscpe. *Obstet Gynecol* 1989;70:668.

30. Neuwirth RS. Hysteroscopic management of symptomatic uterine fibroids. *Obstet Gynecol* 1983;62:509.

31. Loffer FD. Removal of large symptomatic intrauterine growths by the hysteroscopic resectoscope. *Obstet Gynecol* 1990;76:836.

32. Derman SG, Rehnstrom J. Neuwirth RS. The long-term effectiveness of hysteroscopic treatment of menorrhagia and leiomyomas. *Obstet Gynecol* 1991;77:591.

33. Friedman AJ, Barbieri RL, Benacerraf BR, Sciff I. Treatment of leiomyomata with intranasal or subcutaneous leuprolide, a gonadotropin-releasing hormone agonist. *Fertil Steril* 1987;48:560.

34. Andersch B, Wendstam C, Hahn L, Ohman R. Premenstrual complaints. I. Prevalence of premenstrual symptoms in a Swedish urban population. *J Psychosom Obstet Gynecol* 1986;5:39.

35. Johnson SR. Clinicians approach to the diagnosis and management of premenstrual syndrome. *Clin Obstet Gynecol* 1992;35:637.

36. Hammarback S, Damber J-E, Backstrom T. Relationship between symptom severity and hormone changes in women with premenstrual syndrome. *J Clin Endocrinol Metab* 1989;68:125.

37. Rapkin AJ. The role of serotonin in premenstrual syndrome. *Clin Obstet Gynecol* 1992;35:629.

38. Backstrom T. Neuroendocrinology of premenstrual syndrome. *Clin Obstet Gynecol* 1992;35:612.

39. Rausch JL, Weston S, Plouffe L. Role of psychotropic medication in the treatment of affective symptoms in premenstrual syndrome. *Clin Obstet Gynecol* 1992;35:667.

40. Mortola JF, Girton L. Fischer U. Successful treatment of severe premenstrual syndrome by combined use of gonadotropin-releasing hormone agonist and estrogen/progestin. *J Clin Endocrinol Metab* 1991;71:252A.

CHAPTER 39

Androgen Excess

◇

Charles B. Hammond
Marc A. Bernhisel

Androgen excess is a pathologic state in women manifested primarily by masculine somatic changes. Hirsutism, the most common finding associated with androgen excess, is defined as excessive hair growth, characteristically of dark color and coarse texture, that occurs in the androgen-dependent areas of the skin.[43] Hirsutism is frequently accompanied by the development of acne vulgaris, a consequence of androgen stimulation to the pilosebaceous unit. The parameters of excess hair growth are often viewed against a culturally or ethnically determined norm.[40] True androgen excess commonly results in ovulatory dysfunction, menstrual abnormalities, and infertility.

Virilization, the most severe form of androgen excess, is characterized by the regression of female characteristics and the acquisition of male characteristics. Signs and symptoms of virilism include severe hirsutism, male-pattern hairline regression, acne, increased muscle mass, clitoromegaly, and deepening of the voice. Virilism is always associated with a pathologic state of severe androgen excess and often associated with neoplasia.

This chapter reviews the synthesis and metabolism of the androgen steroids, their roles in normal and abnormal physiology, and the clinical diagnosis and treatment of patients with androgen excess states.

◇ ANDROGENS

Androgens are a unique group of steroid structures that normally function to stimulate primary and secondary male sexual characteristics, as well as some female secondary sexual characteristics. *In utero,* androgens are an integral factor in the development of the male reproductive tract. This development begins as early as 6 weeks' gestation and occurs in response to androgen secretion by the testes. The wolffian (i.e., mesonephric) duct, stimulated by androgens, develops into the epididymis, vas deferens, and seminal vesicles. Continued androgen elaboration from the fetal testicular Leydig cells results in the differentiation of the bipotential genital tubercle and urogenital sinus into the penis, scrotum, and penile urethra.

Androgens function in both sexes at puberty to initiate pubarche and adrenarche. In males, increased secretion of testosterone and dihydrotestosterone complete the maturation of the male reproductive tract both morphologically and physiologically. These, together with adrenal androgens, stimulate pubertal hair growth in males. In females, adrenal androgens are primarily produced in the zona reticularis as a byproduct during the enzymatic change of cholesterol to cortisol. The androgens produced stimulate pubertal hair growth in the mons pubis and axilla. Androgens derived from the stroma and theca within the ovary serve as obligate precursors in the synthesis of estrogens, which are produced in the follicle-stimulating hormone (FSH)-mediated process of aromatization.

◇ STEROIDOGENESIS

Steroidogenesis occurs in specialized tissues, largely in response to specific regulatory hormones. For example, adrenocorticotropic hormone (ACTH), the regulatory hormone of adrenal cortisol production, has a high binding affinity to an adrenal plasma membrane receptor and reacts there with adenyl cyclase to activate cyclic adenosine monophosphate formation. This ultimately results in the production of free cholesterol. In the adrenal gland, a specific membrane receptor binds the cholesterol–lipoprotein complex (low-density lipoprotein [LDL]) and converts it into free cholesterol or its esterified storage form. Cholesterol, a 27-carbon (C-27) sterol, is the basic structural molecule of all steroid classes (i.e., glucocorticoids, mineralocorticoids, sex steroids). Cholesterol is converted into steroids in both the adrenal and the ovary in an enzyme-dependent, hormone-regulated manner. These enzymatic modifications of cholesterol occur in the cytosol, mitochondria, and microsomes of the specialized tissue cells. The first and rate-limiting step in cholesterol metabolism is the conversion to the C-21 pregnenolone by a process of serial hydroxylations, resulting ultimately in side-chain cleavage. Pregnenolone is metabolized by one of two alternative pathways—pathway Δ^5 and pathway Δ^4—to the C-19 androgens. The major Δ^5-androgens are dehydroepiandrosterone (DHEA) and Δ^5-androstenediol, also called dihydrotestosterone (DHT). The Δ^4-androgens are androstenedione (A'D) and testosterone (T) (Fig. 1).

Various sites on the C-19 androgen molecule determine androgenic potency and effect. They are C-17, C-3, and C-5. At the C-17 position, the conversion of the 17-ketogroup of A'D to the 17β-hydroxyl complex of T increases the androgen potency some sevenfold. DHEA is changed to the more potent A'D by the formation of a ketogroup at C-3. The introduction of a hydrogen atom in the α plane at C-5 increases the cytosol binding and therefore the potency of DHT over its precursor, T.

Androgens are distributed in the serum by several binding proteins that are important in androgen metabolism, as well as in the regulation of androgen effect.[25] They include albumin, cortisol-binding globulin, acid α_2-glycoprotein, and sex hormone–binding globulin (SHBG). Albumin has a much greater binding capacity than SHBG, but the affinity of T binding is approximately 100,000 times greater to SHBG than to albumin. SHBG binds the largest portion of plasma T and largely determines the amount of free or active T available to diffuse into the target cell from the intravascular space, eventually affecting androgen-sensitive tissues. SHBG is produced in the liver. Its synthesis is diminished by circulating androgens and by menopause, obesity, and hypothyroidism. The synthesis of SHBG is increased by circulating estrogen and hyperthyroidism.

The manifestation of androgen effect depends on both steroid production rate and tissue responsiveness. Male and female fetuses at 12 to 22 weeks' gestation have an equal potential to develop masculine sexual characteristics, based on tissue responsiveness and an equal ability to convert T to DHT (i.e., by means of 5α-reductase), the trophic hormone of the genital tubercle. The male fetus is thus differentiated from the female fetus by testicular production of T. In the absence of T or its inadequate receptor function, female genitalia develops, despite the chromosomal complement. The female fetus retains the ability to respond to androgen stimulation after birth. The skin, muscle, larynx, and urogenital system may be masculinized by supraphysiologic androgen levels, but complete phallic masculinization does not occur.

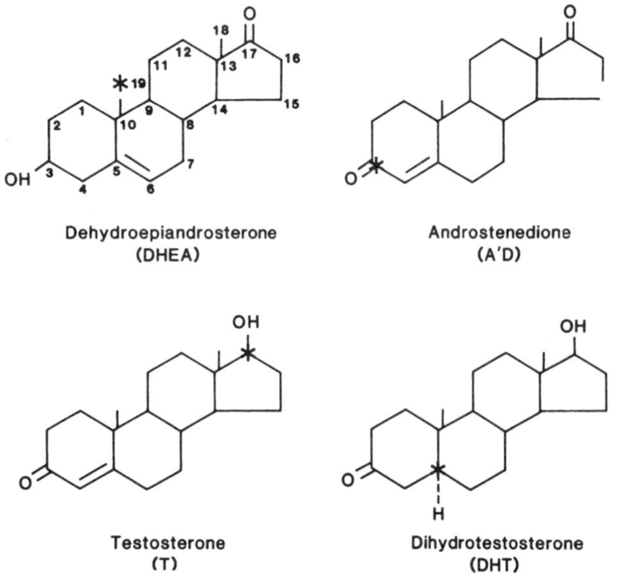

◊ HAIR PATTERNS

The hair follicles and sebaceous glands (i.e., pilosebaceous unit) are androgen-sensitive skin appendages. Hair follicles may produce vellus and terminal hair in humans. Vellus hair is light, finely textured, and short. Terminal hair is dark and coarse and may grow long. High levels of androgens, found normally in men and abnormally in women, stimulate terminal conversion of vellus hair in specified regions, including the face, sternum, back, and upper abdomen. Hair follicles in the axilla, lower pubic triangle, forearms, and legs are responsive to the lower androgen levels seen in normal women, as well as to the higher levels seen in the normal men. Sparse or absent hair growth is found in these areas in genetic males with complete androgen resistance (i.e., testicular feminization). Scalp hair ordinarily grows independently of a stimulatory androgen effect. In excess, however, androgens reverse the normal stimulation to terminal hair and convert the terminal scalp hair to vellus hair or the loss of hair in particular scalp regions (i.e., male-pattern baldness). Except in these relatively androgen-independent areas, hair follicles must be exposed to androgens for a prolonged period before terminal hair is produced. Conversely, terminal hair growth persists after the source of androgens is removed, albeit at a slower rate.

Hair growth is not a continuous process but rather cycles between three phases of hair follicle activity. The growth phase of the hair follicle is termed *anagen*, the resting phase *telogen*, and the intermediate phase (i.e., between resting and growth) *catagen* (Fig. 2). All follicles continually cycle through all three phases of activity; thus, there is a continual growth and shedding of hair. The length of time that a hair follicle spends in each phase varies with its anatomic location. The relatively short hair of the extremities, eyebrows, and eyelashes corresponds to a short anagen phase (2 to 4 months) and a longer telogen phase. Conversely, the long hair of the scalp has an extended anagen phase of 1 to 6 years with a short telogen phase. Androgens in responsive areas propel a hair follicle into the anagen phase and prolong the length of anagen time, resulting in excess terminal hair.[32]

During the anagen phase, there is downward proliferation of the basal epithelium of the hair shaft toward the bulb of the hair follicle in the dermis. Matrix cells then grow rapidly toward the skin surface, and the superficial matrix cells differentiate to form a keratinizing column. The bulb of the hair

FIG. 1. Major serum androgens. *Asterisks* indicate sites that affect androgen potency.

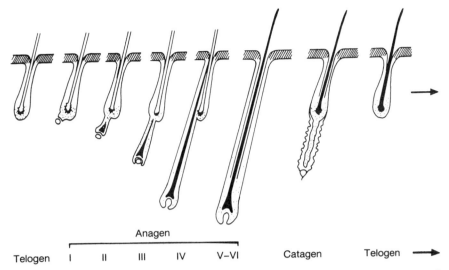

Anagen

Telogen | I | II | III | IV | V–VI | Catagen | Telogen ⟶

FIG. 2. Diagram of cyclic hair follicles, a club hair *(white)* in old telogen and early anagen *(I–IV)* follicles, and a new hair *(black)* in new anagen *(V–VI)* follicles. (From Uno H. *Seminars in reproductive endocrinology.* Vol.4. New York: Thieme,1986; with permission.)

follicle forms around the dermal papilla until the bulb sheds, marking involution (i.e., catagen). The follicle remains at this stage (telogen), if it is not stimulated to grow further. During the resting phase, the hair is loosely attached to the follicle and easily shed.

◊ SOURCES OF ANDROGENS AND THEIR METABOLISM

The principal androgens in women and men are DHT, T, A′D, DHEA, and DHEA sulfate (DHEAS). DHT is the most potent androgen, having about twice the biologic potency of T. Serum assays of DHT often do not reflect the clinical evidence of androgen excess.[48] DHT is cleared rapidly from the serum and is highly bound by SHBG. It is primarily derived from circulating A′D conversion in peripheral compartments (i.e., extrasplanchnic and nonglandular), the largest of which is the skin. There is no significant menstrual cycle or diurnal change in plasma DHT levels. Mauvais-Jarvis[44] demonstrated an elevated 5α-reductase activity in the skin of hirsute women compared with nonhirsute women, which also increases their DHT production. Lobo et al.[38] assayed the distal metabolites of DHT, finding 3α-androstenediol glucuronide (3α-diol G) to be elevated 10-fold in hirsute women compared to nonhirsute women with polycystic ovarian syndrome (PCOS). Significant elevations were also found in so-called idiopathic hirsutism (absent apparent pathologic cause of excess hair growth such as PCOS) (Fig. 3). Lobo et al.[38] reported a strong correlation between serum 3α-diol G and 5α-reductase activity in the skin. Subsequent studies analyzed in a review by Rittmaster[52] did not demonstrate the same magnitude of difference in 3α-diol G between hirsute and nonhirsute women. Furthermore, other studies have failed to demonstrate a decline in 3α-diol G levels with clinical improvement in hirsute women treated with gonadotropin-releasing hormone

analogs.[52] With few exceptions, serum levels of neither DHT nor 3α-diol G help appreciably in diagnosing or treating androgen excess states.

T is the second most potent androgen. About 1% of T circulates as free (i.e., unbound) T in normal women, whereas 3% is found unbound to SHBG in normal men.[58] Approximately 19% in both sexes is loosely bound to albumin. The direct ovarian contribution is between 5% and 20%, depending somewhat on the stage of the menstrual cycle. T has been used as an ovarian marker of androgen excess because of the relatively small direct contribution of adrenal secretion. More than one-half of T production is from the peripheral conversion of A′D to T, which primarily occurs in the liver, skin, fat, and skeletal muscles. Serum T levels show only slight diurnal variation, paralleling cortisol secretion. T and A′D are

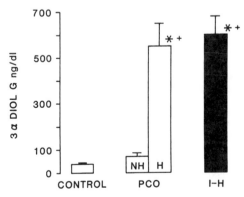

FIG. 3. Serum 3α-androstenediol glucuronide (3α-diol G) levels in controls, nonhirsute *(NH)*, and hirsute *(H)* women with polycystic ovarian syndrome *(PCO)*, and idiopathic hirsutism *(I-H)*. (From Lobo RA. Hirsutism. In: Sciarra JJ, Speroff L, Simpson JL, eds. *Gynecology and obstetrics*, vol 5. Philadelphia: JB Lippincott Co, 1988; with permission.)

reduced at the 5α-carbon to DHT and A'D, respectively. Both T and DHT are found in nanomolar concentrations in peripheral blood assays. Their primary metabolites, glucuronide and sulfa conjugates, are some 10 to 1000 times higher.

A'D is the obligate intermediate of estrone (E_1) but has the potential to be converted to T. It exhibits approximately 20% of the androgenic activity of T. The production rate of A'D is about equal from the ovary and the adrenal. About 10% of A'D is derived from the peripheral conversion of DHEA. A'D has a diurnal secretion that can vary as much as 50% and parallels cortical secretion from ACTH stimulation. It also changes to a smaller degree from the increased ovarian secretion at midcycle.

DHEA and DHEAS are weak androgens that may more accurately be termed *prehormones*, having less than 3% of the potency of T. Their androgen activity is essentially derived from their peripheral conversion into the more potent androgen forms, particularly at the level of the hair follicle.[39] Both DHEA and DHEAS are secreted directly and almost exclusively from the adrenal (85% and 95%, respectively), with only small contributions from the ovary. Serum DHEA levels, much more than DHEAS levels, vary with cortisol circadian rhythmicity.

◊ ANDROGEN EXCESS SYNDROME

The development of hirsutism and acne from androgen stimulation to the pilosebaceous unit is one of the earliest signs of hyperandrogenism. Approximately 90% of hirsute women have a production elevation in one or more of the androgens. Table 1 lists the various causes of hyperandrogenism.

TABLE 1. *Causes of hyperandrogenism*

Ovarian causes—functional
Polycystic ovarian syndrome
Hyperthecosis
Obesity, insulin resistance, and acanthosis nigricans

Neoplastic
Sertoli-Leydig cell tumor
Lipid tumor
Hilus cell tumor
Luteoma
Other

Adrenal causes—functional
Congenital adrenal hyperplasia
Acquired adrenal hyperplasia

Neoplastic
Adrenal tumor
Adrenal carcinoma
Cushing syndrome
(Cushing disease)

Mixed ovarian-adrenal causes
Other causes
Drug therapy
Excess peripheral androgen production
XY gonadal dysgenesis

Ovarian-related Causes of Androgen Excess

Polycystic Ovarian Syndrome

The most common cause of ovarian androgen excess and probably the most common cause of hirsutism in women is PCOS. Goldzieher and Axelrod[27] found a nearly 70% prevalence of hirsutism in women with PCOS. It is likely that PCOS is the end point in a spectrum of several physiologic abnormalities. The clinical manifestations, including hirsutism, anovulation, and infertility, are found in more than 50% of women with polycystic ovaries. Other symptoms found with varying frequency include obesity, virilism, and dysfunctional bleeding. Histologically, the classic ovarian finding in PCOS is multiple, small follicular cysts with poor granulosa cell development (Fig. 4). The follicle is surrounded by a thickened, luteinized theca. The biochemical parameters that define PCOS remain ill-defined. Patients with the syndrome often have modestly elevated T, DHEAS, and prolactin (PRL) levels.[4] They often demonstrate a reversal of the estradiol (E_2) to E_1 ratio, and frequently the luteinizing hormone (LH) to FSH ratio is 3:1 or greater.

Several theories have been advanced to explain the biochemical abnormalities found in PCOS in light of the unique anatomic and physiologic findings. LH is generally elevated in patients with PCOS and may reflect greater pulse frequency and pulse amplitude in response to gonadotropin-releasing hormone (Gn-RH) from the hypothalamus. Because Gn-RH is the principal stimulant to gonadotropin secretion, abnormalities in its control and secretion have been sought to explain PCOS. Unfortunately, Gn-RH is not easily or accurately assayed in peripheral samples and, when obtained, is of questionable relevance to hypothalamic events. The neurotransmitter dopamine inhibits hypothalamic Gn-RH secretion in animals. The results of several studies imply an abnormal dopamine–Gn-RH dissociation, resulting in elevated Gn-RH pulse amplitude and frequency. Central opioids also have an inhibitory control over Gn-RH secretion and modulate dopamine activity. Similarly, abnormal opioid tone has been suggested as the cause of anomalous Gn-RH secretion. Naloxone (Narcan) infusion studies indicate a normal, intact opioid response in PCOS but suggest a possible interactional abnormality between the opioid and dopaminergic pathways. Clearly, more information is needed before the cause of PCOS can be resolved. Nonetheless, the net result is an elevated LH level and a preferential inhibition of FSH. FSH may be affected directly by secretion of inhibin from the multiple follicular cysts of the ovary. The consequence of the abnormal gonadotropin (i.e., LH:FSH) ratio is an LH-induced excess of A'D and T from ovarian thecal and stromal cells. Without requisite FSH levels, the normal granulosa cell aromatization of A'D and T to E_2 in cyclic manner is reduced. Erickson et al.[19] reported a reduction of estrogen production in granulosa cells cultured from characteristically small polycysts found in PCOS. However, when FSH was added to these cultures *in vitro*, estrogen production was greatly increased. Ovarian androgens are peripherally converted to estrogens, which are chronically elevated in a

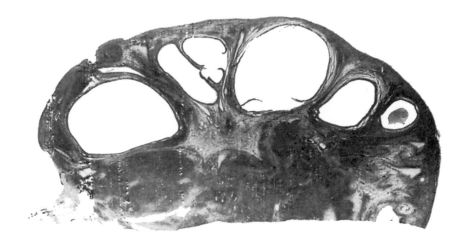

FIG. 4. Polycystic ovarian syndrome. This whole-mount view of a polycystic ovary reveals multiple follicular cysts below a thickened cortical stroma. The hilum of the ovary is prominent. The apparent thickened capsule is related to compression of the cortical stroma between the follicles and the overlying peritoneum (original magnification ×4). (Courtesy of E.J. Wilkinson, MD, Department of Pathology, University of Florida, Gainesville, FL.)

noncyclic manner in anovulatory patients with PCOS. The cycle is completed by the continued secretion of pituitary LH, sensitized by the elevated estrogen levels.

Hyperthecosis

Hyperthecosis shares many of the clinical features of PCOS but characteristically is associated with more severe hirsutism and often virilism. Histologically, this syndrome overlaps with PCOS to a large degree. Hyperthecotic ovaries, however, are found to have numerous islands of luteinized cells scattered throughout the stroma, often in proximity to the hilum (Fig. 5). Induction of ovulation in patients with hyperthecosis usually is extremely difficult because of elevated androgen levels, which are often as high as levels found in patients with androgen-secreting tumors. Therapy for these patients has often been relegated to wedge resection of the ovaries if fertility is to be preserved or bilateral oophorectomy if it is not.

Obesity, Insulin Resistance, and Acanthosis Nigricans

Obesity is associated with multiple general health problems and specific gynecologic abnormalities, including menstrual cycle irregularity, amenorrhea, and dysfunctional uterine bleeding. Although many obese women are eumenorrheic, the percentage of women with menstrual irregularity increases as weight increases above ideal body weight. Kaufman et al.[34] found elevated serum androgen and LH levels and reversal of the E_2 : E_1 ratio in obese adolescent girls. These findings, reminiscent of PCOS, are reversible with weight reduction.

Androgen levels are increased in obese women.[8] Both androgen production rates and clearance rates are increased. A reduction in SHBG associated with obesity increases the clearance of androgens but allows an elevation in free T levels. The degree of excess weight also correlates with the degree of extraglandular aromatization of androgens, primarily A'D, to estrogens. Elevated androgen levels, a high E_2 : E_1 ratio, and lower SHBG levels create a biochemical milieu that undoubtedly contributes to the PCOS state. More than

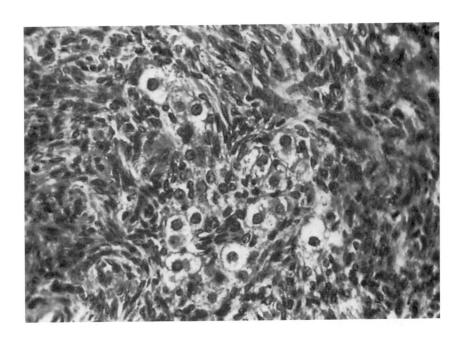

FIG. 5. Thecomatosis (hyperthecosis). This ovary was removed from a 310-lb anovulatory hirsute woman. The ovaries were slightly enlarged bilaterally. Ovarian stromal cells with prominent cytoplasm can be identified. The cytoplasmic contents are predominantly lipid, reflected here as a clear cytoplasm with no identifiable cytoplasmic features other than slight vacuole formation. The surrounding theca reveals its usual appearance (original magnification ×250). (Courtesy of E.J. Wilkinson, MD, Department of Pathology, University of Florida, Gainesville, FL.)

50% of patients with PCOS are obese. A reduction in weight can lower androgen levels, diminish hirsutism, and even restore ovulation in many women with PCOS.

Obesity, particularly when coupled with PCOS, has been associated with hyperinsulinemia, insulin resistance, and abnormal glucose tolerance testing. Hyperandrogenemia has in turn been associated with hyperinsulinemia and acanthosis nigricans.[6] Acanthosis nigricans is a hyperpigmentation of the skin generally found over the neck, in the axillae, in the vulva, and beneath the breasts. It has been used as a marker of insulin resistance, particularly in women with non-insulin-dependent diabetes mellitus. The relationship of insulin to androgen excess is becoming more evident.[17] Insulin belongs to a family of other insulin-like growth factors, particularly insulin-like growth factor 1 (IGF-1). IGF-1 increases thecal cell production of ovarian androgens. Because the receptors for insulin and IGF-1 are similar, insulin has been found to enhance T and A′D production *in vitro* from ovarian stromal and thecal cells. The observation that diminished insulin resistance and therefore lowered circulating insulin lower the level of androgens strengthens this insulin–androgen association. Insulin resistance in PCOS is most likely caused by a primary defect in insulin receptor mechanisms unique to this syndrome. It therefore appears to differ genotypically from other insulin-resistant states.

Obesity has been categorized as gynoid or android. Gynoid obesity describes fat distribution primarily in the gluteal and femoral region. The so-called pear-shaped morphotype is the obesity seen mainly in women. Android obesity describes fat distribution in the trunk and abdominal region. This apple-shaped morphotype is most often seen in men but confers greater cardiovascular risk in women found with this type of fat distribution. Kitabchi and Burrington[36] reported that women with abdominal obesity have significantly increased androgen levels, insulin resistance, and basal and glucose-challenged insulin production, compared to women with gluteal-femoral obesity. They were also found to have increased levels of cholesterol and LDL cholesterol and increased blood pressure.[18] It is recommended that in obese women with PCOS features weight control through diet and exercise and screening for dyslipidemia and glucose intolerance states be started soon after diagnosis.

Ovarian Neoplasms

Ovarian neoplasms that cause hyperandrogenism are rare. When found in patients in the reproductive-age group, they frequently present with amenorrhea and rapidly progressive hirsutism or virilism.

The most commonly found masculinizing tumors are the gonadal stromal group (Fig. 6). The Sertoli-Leydig cell tumor (arrhenoblastoma) is the most frequently found neoplasm of this group. It typically presents in women between 20 and 30 years of age, but there have been reports of it in a 2.5-year-old girl, as well as in a 70-year-old woman. Women who have such tumors generally report a cessation of menstrual periods and rapid hair growth. Tumors are characteristically unilateral and frequently palpable by pelvic examination; they also produce high amounts of T.[23] This is reflected in peripheral T serum concentrations often exceeding 200 ng/dl (i.e., approaching normal male levels). The hilus cell and mixed gonadal stromal (i.e., gyneandroblastoma) tumors are two other potentially masculinizing neoplasms derived from the gonadal stroma. The hilus cell and other lipid cell tumors often are usually nonpalpable, and patients with them may present with the development of hirsutism after menopause.

Other tumors may stimulate stromal activity and lead to a production of excess androgens. These include dysgerminoma, teratoma, Brenner tumor, serous cystadenoma, and Krukenberg tumor.[33] These tumors are typically associated with increased A′D production.

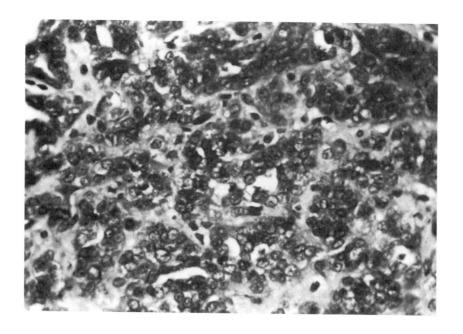

FIG. 6. Sertoli-Leydig cell tumor. The tubular structure of the Sertoli cells is evident. The nuclei of the epithelial cells lining these tubules are uniform and show minimal nuclear atypia. Between the tubules, stromal cells containing more prominent eosinophilic cytoplasm and larger nuclei can be seen, which represent the Leydig cells (original magnification ×250). (Courtesy of E.J. Wilkinson, MD, Department of Pathology, University of Florida, Gainesville, FL.)

Ovarian luteoma of pregnancy is a rare and potentially masculinizing tumor that may affect both the mother and the fetus.[24] It is a solid, frequently bilateral neoplasm that shares some histologic cellular features with theca-lutein cysts of pregnancy, which are always bilateral but not reported to cause masculinization. Virilism or hirsutism in pregnancy may occur with any of the tumors described.

Adrenal Causes of Androgen Excess

Congenital Adrenal Hyperplasia

The adrenal gland, alone or in combination with the ovary, has been implicated as the major source of hyperandrogenism in hirsute women in several studies. The most common congenital enzyme defect of the adrenal that causes androgen excess is 21-hydroxylase (21-OH) deficiency, producing congenital adrenal hyperplasia 21 (CAH-21, also designated CAH type III). This defect is usually manifested at birth by varying degrees of genital ambiguity and, more rarely, with severe salt loss resulting in hypotension and shock. Precocious masculinization and virilism may occur in affected and untreated male and female children. In addition to chronic glucocorticoid therapy for both girls and boys, severely affected girls may require reconstructive genital surgery.[2]

The CAH-21 defect results in the inability of the adrenal to produce sufficient quantities of glucocorticoids or mineralocorticoids. As a result, ACTH is increased and drives the overproduction of adrenal prehormones. Significant elevations of 17α-hydroxyprogesterone (17-OHP), a prehormone to cortisol and to the androgens, is found with CAH-21 (Fig. 7). 17-OHP levels are also diagnostically elevated in the amniotic fluid of affected fetuses and in the serum of affected neonates or children. CAH-21 is commonly associated with an increase in both DHEA and DHEAS.

11β-Hydroxylase (11β-OH) deficiency (CAH-11, CAH type IV) is the next most common congenital cause of androgen excess. As in CAH-21, the failure is found in the enzymatic conversion of cortisol precursors, which precludes adequate production of cortisol. ACTH is stimulated and drives the overproduction of glucocorticoid and mineralocorticoid prehormones, as well as androgens. 11-Desoxycorticosterone, a potent mineralocorticoid, is produced in excess and is frequently associated with salt retention and hypertension in neonates. The finding of an elevated serum 11-desoxycortisol level is diagnostic of CAH-11.

Reduction in levels of the 3β-hydroxysteroid dehydrogenase 4-5 isomerase enzyme (CAH-3 hsd, CAH type II)) results in diminished production of glucocorticoids, mineralocorticoids, and sex steroids. This rare defect leads to the clinical manifestations of salt wasting and inadequate masculinization in male neonates. Female children who survive childhood will not develop secondary sex characteristics because of deficient E_2 production but may present with hirsutism because of DHEA overproduction, which is undoubtedly converted to androgens in the skin.

Acquired Adrenal Hyperplasia

Nonclassic CAH (NC-CAH), also called late-onset, attenuated, or acquired CAH, refers to a functional derangement of the adrenal gland that produces an excess androgen effect that may be manifested before or after pubertal maturation rather than at childbirth or early in childhood.[22] These disorders are caused by incomplete deficiencies of 21-OH (NC-CAH-21), 3β-hydroxysteroid dehydrogenase (NC-CAH-3 hsd), and

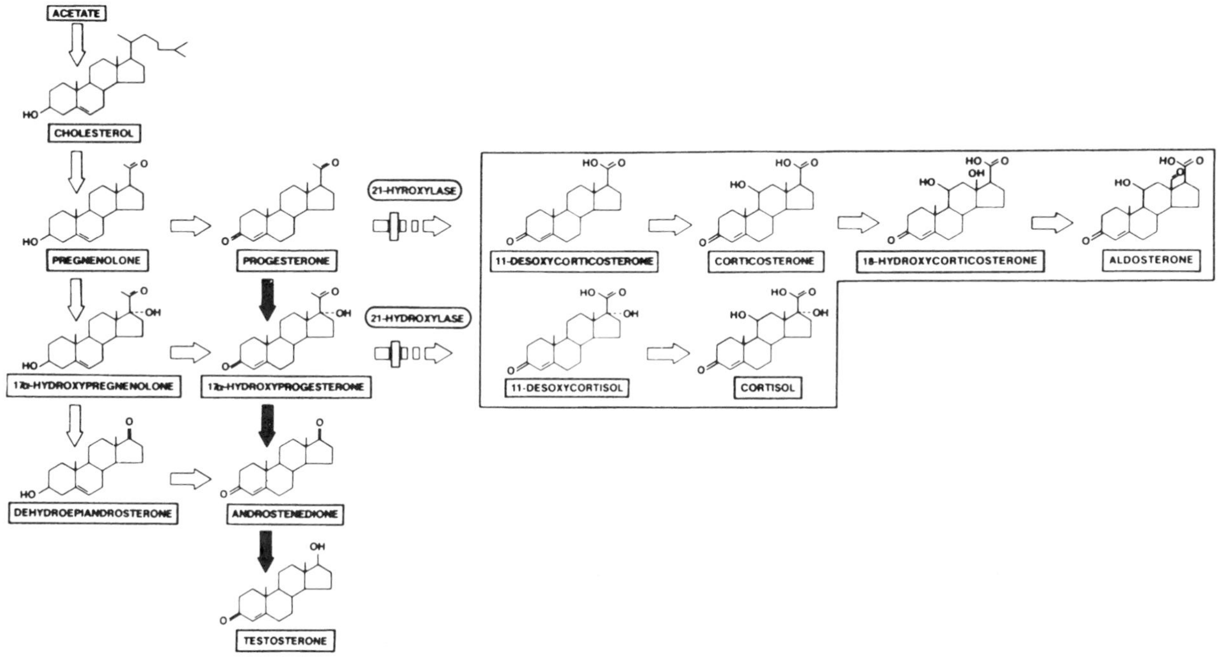

FIG. 7. Adrenal steroidogenesis: consequences of 21-hydroxylase deficiency. (From ref. 2, with permission.)

11β-OH (NC-CAH-11), listed in order of decreasing frequency in the population. NC-CAH-21 accounts for the vast majority of cases that present with peripubertal androgen excess.[37] The active gene coding for cytochrome P-450$_{C21}$OH enzyme is closely linked to the HLA-B and DR loci on the short arm of chromosome 6 (Fig. 8). A significant linkage disequilibrium has been demonstrated with HLA-Bw47 and DR7 in the classic defective disorder. The HLA-B14-DR1 allele has likewise been highly associated with NC-CAH-21 in DNA linkage studies. CAH-21 presenting in its classic or nonclassic form is an autosomal-recessive disease. Heterozygotes for CAH-21 (21-OH deficiency severe/21-OH normal) or NC-CAH-21 (21-OH deficiency mild/21-OH normal) do not manifest symptoms of masculinization. They do, however, differ biochemically from unaffected people and from homozygotes by having an intermediate production response of 17-OHP to synthetic ACTH stimulation.

Great phenotypic variability occurs in NC-CAH.[57] It is anticipated that a large genetic heterogenicity will be demonstrated. It is likely that there are three alleles for 21-OH deficiency: 21-OH normal, 21-OH mild, and 21-OH severe. A division based on HLA linkage and pedigree studies has been confirmed biochemically by Speiser and New.[57] Mild homozygotes (21-OH deficiency mild/21-OH deficiency mild) have a significantly diminished 17-OHP response to ACTH, compared with compound heterozygotes (21-OH deficiency severe/21-OH deficiency mild).

Various diagnostic tests have been used to define NC-CAH biochemically.[14] Basal levels of A'D, T, DHEA, or DHEAS are often but inconsistently elevated. Women with NC-CAH-21 are not easily differentiated from women with PCOS by clinical appearance or basal androgen levels. Basal or ACTH-stimulated 17-OHP levels obtained early in the morning are most consistently elevated in affected patients. A 17-OHP level greater than 300 ng/dl confirmed by an ACTH-stimulated level exceeding 800 ng/dl secures the diagnosis of NC-CAH.

In the absence of elevated serum androgen levels, particularly the more potent Δ^4-androgens, it is thought that the Δ^5-androgens and 17-OHP are converted in the peripheral tissues to more potent androgen forms.

NC-CAH-3 hsd and NC-CAH-11

NC-CAH-3 hsd has increasingly been recognized in association with peripubertal androgen excess. As with NC-CAH-21, the clinical features of NC-CAH-3 hsd are not distinctly different from those of PCOS, except that menstrual irregularity is not uniformly found. An incomplete deficiency in the microsomal 3β-hydroxysteroid dehydrogenase enzyme system in the ovary and adrenal gland allows excess production and secretion of 5β-steroids.[47] Diagnosis is made by basal and ACTH-stimulated elevations in 17-hydroxypregnenolone, DHEA, and DHEAS levels compared with those of the Δ^4-androgens 17-OHP, A'D, and T. NC-CAH-3 hsd does not have a HLA linkage, and the carrier status has not been identified.

NC-CAH-11 deficiency is an uncommon cause of androgen excess manifestations, although no reliable prevalence rates are available. The diagnosis should be considered, however, in hypertensive hirsute young women, particularly those with a positive family history. Biochemical abnormalities are similar to those for NC-CAH-21, but in addition levels of 11-desoxycortisol are elevated. No linkage association between CAH-11 and HLA genes has been demonstrated.

Adrenal Neoplastic Disorders

Cushing disease, the cause of 70% of hypercortisolism, is most often the result of an ACTH-secreting pituitary tumor. This tumor is associated with bilateral adrenal hyperplasia and cortisol elevation and may be associated with mild hirsutism and, rarely, virilization. Less frequent in occurrence (20%), Cushing syndrome is caused by a cortisol-secreting adenoma or carcinoma of the adrenal gland and is associated with a 20% incidence of virilism. The remaining causes of hypercortisolism are secondary to ectopically secreted sources of ACTH. The clinical signs and symptoms of Cushing syndrome include muscle weakness, ecchymosis, hypertension, abdominal striae, central obesity, osteoporosis, and hypokalemic alkalosis.

Severe hirsutism and virilism caused by adrenal sources may be seen in patients with androgen-secreting adrenal adenoma or carcinoma. Carcinoma and, rarely, adenoma produce combinations of Δ^4- and Δ^5-androgens, depending on the degree of tumor differentiation. A'D and T levels may be elevated in the absence of a significant DHEAS level. Generally, however, DHEAS levels in excess of 800 μg/dl are found in patients with adrenal neoplasms. Suppressive therapy with dexamethasone is usually not effective in these patients. Rarely, a pure T-producing tumor having the characteristics of an ovarian rest, including responsiveness to human chorionic gonadotropin (hCG), is found in the adrenal gland and manifests itself clinically with rapid virilism.

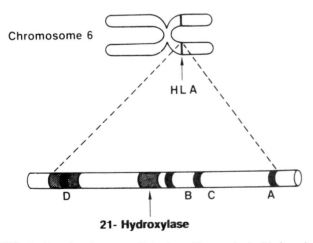

Chromosome 6

HLA

D   B C   A

21- Hydroxylase

FIG. 8. Nonclassic congenital adrenal hyperplasia 21. Localization of the 21-hydroxylase (cytochrome P-450$_{C21}$) gene within the HLA complex of human chromosome 6. (From ref. 2, with permission.)

Mixed Ovarian–Adrenal Hyperandrogenism

Excess androgen production by both the adrenal gland and the ovary has been found in several studies, based on adrenal and ovarian vein catheterization and dexamethasone suppression or hCG stimulation. Kirschner et al.[35] found that 30% of hirsute patients had both adrenal and ovarian sources of androgen excess. Abraham et al.[1] reported a 39% incidence. Adrenal androgens putatively affect the ovary either indirectly through estrogen conversion, thus increasing LH secretion and stimulation of ovarian androgens, or directly by inhibition of 3β-hydroxysteroid dehydrogenase and aromatase enzymes, causing inadequate follicular maturation and an elevated ratio of androgen to E_2 secretion by the ovary. Interpretation of the dexamethasone and hCG data must be guarded, however, because of the multiple glandular (e.g., pituitary, adrenal, ovary) effect of both hormones. Gn-RH agonists have successfully been used to anatomically isolate androgen production by suppressing ovarian secretion without apparent effect on the adrenal.

◊ CLINICAL EVALUATION

Endocrinologic evaluation is mandatory in girls presenting with prepubertal hirsutism and in any patient presenting with hirsutism of rapid onset or the onset of virilization at any age. The development of hirsutism in patients with associated menstrual abnormalities (i.e., in PCOS) may warrant evaluation to rule out a more serious process.

A thorough history should be obtained in evaluating hirsute patients, particularly the time of onset and velocity of hair growth[29] (Fig. 9). A history of rapid hair growth, often with virilism, suggests a neoplasm of adrenal or ovarian origin. Patients with features of PCOS, including chronic anovulation and hirsutism, usually note a gradual onset of excess hair growth that begins 2 to 3 years after the onset of menarche. Eumenorrheic women with androgen excess may have an adrenal source of hyperandrogenemia.

Patients presenting with primary amenorrhea and hirsutism should be evaluated with a leukocytic karyotype to exclude a Y-bearing dysgenetic gonad. Prepubertal girls presenting with hirsutism should be evaluated for CAH and adrenal or ovarian neoplasia. Finally, iatrogenic causes of excess hair growth should be sought. Danazol (Danocrine), frequently used in the treatment of endometriosis and benign cystic breast disease, may cause hirsutism and acne. Similarly, some of the 19-nortestosterone progestogens used in oral contraceptives have been reported to cause hirsutism and acne. Phenytoin sodium, penicillamine, minoxidil, and diazoxide may produce hypertrichosis, defined as an excess growth of nonsexual hair (i.e., vellus), which is also seen in patients with anorexia nervosa, dermatomyositis, and hypothyroidism.

The physical examination is used to quantify the signs of androgen excess. Hair morphology and distribution should be graded and photographed, if possible. Various scoring methods have been suggested in quantifying hirsutism. Perhaps the most functional and widely used is the Farriman-Galloway (F-G) scale, which semiquantitatively grades hair growth in 12 body areas (Fig. 10). The mean F-G score for normal women is 4 to 7. Individual area scores of 0 to 2 and a total F-G score of 8 are found in mild hirsutism. Women with mild hirsutism typically have fine, pigmented hair over the face (i.e., sideburns and chin but not a complete beard), chest, and lower abdomen. In moderate hirsutism, individual scores of 1 to 3 are found. These women have coarse, pigmented terminal hair over the extremities, face (but not a complete beard), chest, abdomen, and perineum. Severe hirsutism (i.e., scores of 3 to 4 and a total F-G of 16 or greater) is defined as coarse, pigmented hair over the whole beard area and thicker distribution over the rest of the androgen-sensitive areas. Evaluation of therapeutic efficacy in clinical drug trials has been made with reduction in hair shaft diameter.

Other indications of androgen excess, such as acne and signs of hypercortisolism (i.e., Cushing syndrome), should be carefully evaluated. Clitoromegaly is generally found with tumor levels of T. It has been useful to define clitoromegaly by measuring the clitoral area (i.e., multiplying the length times the width of the clitoris). A value greater than 35 mm^2 is indicative of abnormality. Others suggest the diagnosis can be made by clitoral width exceeding 1 cm. Abdominal and pelvic computed tomography (CT) or magnetic resonance (MR) imaging and pelvic ultrasound studies are used to investigate adrenal and ovarian neoplasms. A unilateral androgen-producing ovarian tumor can be palpated 60% to 80% of the time when present.

Laboratory Studies

Serum T, DHEAS, and PRL levels are obtained primarily as screening tests to rule out androgen-secreting neoplasms of the ovary and adrenal and PRL-secreting neoplasms of the pituitary. Secondarily, T and DHEAS levels often help define the source of androgen excess. Hirsute women with PCOS have high-normal to moderately elevated T levels (60 to 150 ng/dl). DHEAS is normal to slightly elevated (< 450 μg/dl). PRL may be elevated (> 30 ng/ml) in 10% to 30% of PCOS patients. An elevated T level, particularly greater than 150 ng/dl, warrants repeat sampling, which should be assayed at a reliable laboratory. Patients with ovarian tumors generally have T levels consistently greater than 200 ng/dl. Levels above this range are not necessarily diagnostic of ovarian neoplasia. Friedman et al.[23] found an ovarian neoplasm in only 2 of 11 women (i.e., without a palpable mass) explored at laparotomy with single T levels in excess of 200 ng/dl. Pelvic sonographic findings of bilateral ovarian enlargement and multiple ovarian cysts (Fig. 11) in the setting of elevated T levels suggest PCOS and probably warrant pursuing medical treatment rather than continuing diagnostic procedures (e.g., surgical exploration or venous catheterization). An elevated T level, a unilateral ovarian mass, and accelerating clinical signs of androgen excess warrant surgical exploration. If a small, nonpalpable ovarian tumor (e.g., hilus

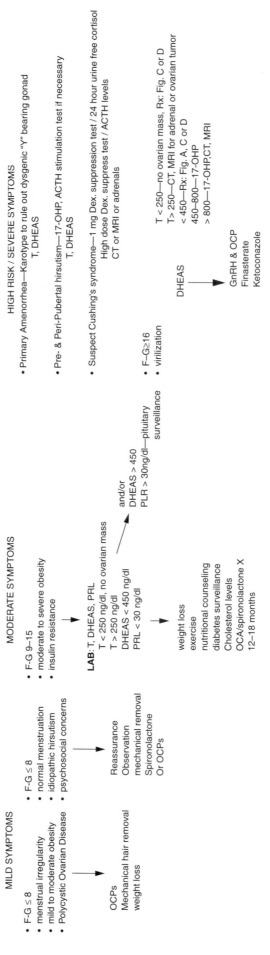

FIG. 9. Hirsutism workup.

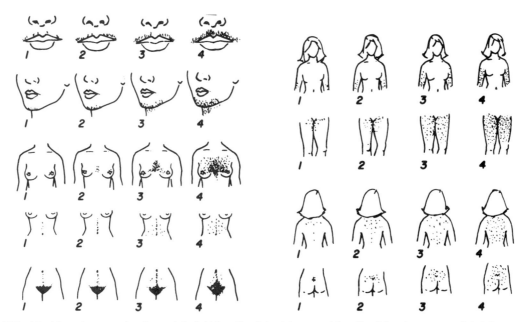

FIG. 10. Hirsutism scoring from 1 (mild hirsutism) to 4 (severe hirsutism) in nine areas. A total score exceeding 8 indicates hirsutism. (From ref. 29, with permission.)

cell tumor) is suspected in the setting of severe hirsutism or virilism, retrograde venous catheterization has been used to distinguish ovarian from adrenal sources. It is also helpful in lateralizing (i.e., right versus left) the involved side. Arterial or venous catheterization is technically difficult and carries a small but definite morbidity. It should be reserved for selected indications. MR imaging may be the most accurate means of tumor identification.

DHEAS elevations above 800 µg/dl are indicative of adrenal pathology. With elevated DHEAS levels, a family history of CAH, and perimenarcheal onset of severe hirsutism, basal and ACTH-stimulated 17-OHP levels should be obtained. If the rare conditions NC-CAH-3 hsd or NC-CAH-11 are suspected, the addition of A'D and Δ^5-androstenediol for $\Delta^5 : \Delta^4$ ratios in 3β-hydroxysteroid dehydrogenase deficiency and of 11-desoxycortisol in 11β-OH deficiency is needed. When adrenal neoplasms are suspected, imaging studies (MR imaging and CT) are the most accurate means of detecting adrenal tumors.

Elevated DHEAS and T levels may also be found in patients with Cushing disease or syndrome. If by history and examination hypercortisolism is suspected, a screening dexamethasone suppression test is performed.[16] Dexamethasone, 1 mg orally, is given at 11:00 p.m. A plasma cortisol level is obtained at 8:00 a.m. A cortisol level higher than 10 µg/dl is suggestive of Cushing disease or syndrome; values less than 6 µg/dl are normal. Elevated and consistently indeterminate levels may be further evaluated with 24-hour urinary levels of urinary free cortisol (upper limits of normal, 74 µg/24 hours) and 17-hydroxycorticosteroids (upper limits of normal, 8 mg/24 hours). These urinary levels are also used with both low-dose (0.5 mg orally every 6 hours for 2 days) and high-dose (2 mg every 6 hours for 2 days) dexamethasone suppression. Low-dose suppression of urinary free cortisol to less than 25 mg per 24 hours or 17-hydroxycorticosteroids to less than 3 mg per 24 hours rules out Cushing syndrome. Cortisol in Cushing disease may be suppressed with high-dose

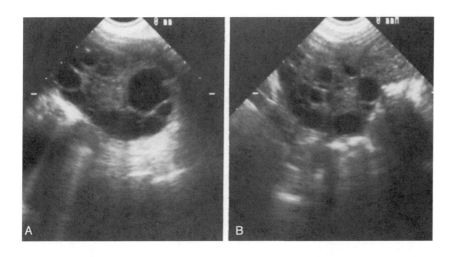

FIG. 11. Multiple small ovarian cysts demonstrated by vaginal sonography in a woman with polycystic ovarian syndrome and androgen excess. **A:** Right ovary. **B:** Left ovary.

dexamethasone, whereas patients with adrenal neoplasms or ectopic ACTH-secreting tumors (i.e., Cushing syndrome) generally do not suppress. Recently, the more accurate ACTH assays, catheterization studies of corticotropin-releasing factor (CRF), and liberalized use of adrenal CT and MR imaging have proved more reliable and sensitive in identifying the abnormalities that cause excess cortisol secretion.

Normal to slightly elevated levels of T and DHEAS are generally found in women with a slow progression of mild or moderate hirsutism. It is therefore uncertain whether any steroidal measurements are necessary. Treatment (as described below) is generally unaltered by T and DHEAS levels or ratios in nontumorous conditions. In these cases of idiopathic hirsutism, there are increases in peripheral conversion of circulating androgens to DHT. One might find mild elevations in circulating A′D or free (i.e., non–SHBG-bound) T. More specifically, however, 3α-diol G, a major metabolite of DHT, is elevated. The use of 3α-diol G has been largely limited to research protocols because of the difficult assay involved and the narrow indications for obtaining the levels.

PRL levels should be obtained when hirsutism is associated with menstrual irregularities because of the increased frequency of hyperprolactinemia. Of hyperprolactinemic women, 20% to 30% are reported to have elevated DHEAS levels but not elevated T or A′D levels.[11] PRL seems to have multiple androgen effects, including inhibition of SHBG levels and reduced 5α-reductase activity. Hyperprolactinemia-induced DHEAS elevation does not in and of itself cause hirsutism.

◊ TREATMENT

Treatment of hirsute women is based on the cause and source of androgen excess.[51] Surgical extirpation of an ovarian, adrenal, or pituitary tumor is required when these neoplasms are identified. A combination of glucocorticoid and mineralocorticoid is used to diminish the ACTH drive in CAH-21. This will lower the Δ5-androgens DHEA and DHEAS available for peripheral conversion.

Adrenal sources of androgen excess are best treated with a synthetic glucocorticoid such as dexamethasone, 0.25 to 0.5 mg at bedtime. Caution should be used in treating with dexamethasone, however, as chronically administered doses, particularly those over 0.5 mg per day, may result in cushingoid effects.[1] Conversely, serum monitoring of morning cortisol should be used to maintain the level of cortisol at 3 μg/dl or greater to avoid impairment of the pituitary–adrenal axis. Oral contraceptives and dexamethasone may also be effective when used together.

Oral Contraceptives

Oral contraceptives have been used as the first-line drug for mild forms of hirsutism. Oral contraceptives suppress pituitary secretion of LH and decrease ovarian production of A′D and T. The progesterone component may bind to glucocorticoid receptors and cause a reduction of adrenal androgen secretion. The estrogen component, through a direct effect on the liver, stimulates increased production of SHBG. Over the last several years, there has been little written about the exclusive use of oral contraceptives in treating hirsutism, particularly the severe forms. They have been used as an adjunct to more aggressive therapies, particularly when using Gn-RH agonists and antiandrogens. In combination with a Gn-RH agonist, oral contraceptives reduce the frequent side effects of hot flushes and vaginal dryness and may reduce other adverse reactions, including unfavorable changes in cholesterol and a reduction in bone density. Oral contraceptives are also useful in reducing the menstrual irregularities frequently seen with antiandrogens. The contraceptive effect is useful in preventing potential feminization of a male fetus if pregnancy occurred while antiandrogens were being used. Oral contraceptives may also lower adrenal androgen secretion, presumably by diminishing pituitary stimulation of the adrenal.

Ketoconazole

The antifungal agent ketoconazole (Nizoral) has been found to exert a blocking action on adrenal and gonadal steroidogenesis by inhibition of cytochrome P-450 enzymatic pathways that include androgen synthesis.[56] It has also been used in certain treatment protocols for prostate cancer, Cushing disease, precocious puberty, and adrenal cell adenoma or carcinoma. Hepatic damage has been reported, particularly with higher doses of ketoconazole.[3] The drug dosage is between 400 to 1200 mg per day. Generally, a lower dose is used over a period of 6 months. Prominent side effects include dry skin, nausea, fatigue, and hair loss. Because of its side effect profile, ketoconazole has not been used as extensively as other drug preparations.

Gn-RH Agonists

Gn-RH agonists are powerful suppressants of ovarian androgen secretion via pituitary suppression of gonadotropin secretion. Preparations are available for daily subcutaneous injection, nasal spray applied two to three times daily, monthly and thrice-monthly intramuscular depot administration, and subcutaneous pellet placement.[9] There is generally a decrease in ovarian T and A′D secretion after 1 to 2 months of therapy. Most side effects of Gn-RH agonists are secondary to the profound hypoestrogenemia produced.[42] These side effects include hot flushes, headaches, vaginal dryness, and mood swings. Prolonged treatment can also cause decreases in bone density. There appears to be no reduction in effectiveness by combining Gn-RH agonists with oral contraceptives, and in a double-blind, controlled trial, the combination was shown to improve the effectiveness of hair growth suppression.[5]

Antiandrogens

An antiandrogen effect is seen with a wide variety of drugs, caused by a competitive inhibition of the binding of T and DHT to androgen receptors.

Spironolactone

Spironolactone is a potassium-sparing diuretic that appears to inhibit hair growth by peripherally inhibiting 5α-reductase activity and binding competitively to the intracellular receptor for DHT.[41,46] Higher doses of spironolactone interfere with cytochrome P-450 activity, which may reduce the total amount of androgen synthesis and secretion.[54] Side effects of spironolactone include menstrual irregularity, as well as nausea and fatigue at with higher doses.[30] Because spironolactone is a potassium-sparing agent, women who are predisposed to hyperkalemia should be carefully monitored or should use an alternative drug.

Cyproterone Acetate

Cyproterone acetate is a potent progesterone that acts to inhibit pituitary gonadotropin secretion.[10,21] It is not yet available in the United States. It also competitively inhibits the binding of T and A′D to the androgen receptor. Cyproterone is stored in adipose tissue, where it is released relatively slowly. Because of its potent progestational effects, it is often given during the early part of a menstrual cycle (50 to 200 mg on days 1 to 10), with ethinyl estradiol added on days 5 to 25. In women using an oral contraceptive, cyproterone, 50 mg for 10 days, is well tolerated. In Europe, a low-dose combination pill containing 2 mg of cyproterone acetate and 50 mg of ethinyl estradiol is used on cycle days 5 to 25. Higher dosages of cyproterone, however, are more effective in reducing hirsutism.[28] Side effects from cyproterone include weight gain and edema. This is generally associated with a higher dose of cyproterone and is likely secondary to its weak glucocorticoid activity. There have also been reports of mild transient liver enzyme elevation and hepatitis. As with spironolactone, avoidance of pregnancy to protect against feminization of a male fetus is important.

Flutamide

Flutamide (Eulexin) is a pure nonsteroidal antiandrogen having no reported progestational, estrogenic, corticoid, or antigonadotropic activity.[13] In most studies, peripheral levels of T and free T are unchanged, although some have reported a possible modulation of androgen production. Flutamide has similar efficacy to spironolactone and cyproterone.[20] It has been used to treat prostate cancer in men. It is generally used in a dosage of 125 to 250 mg twice a day. The most common side effect is dry skin and increased appetite. The most worrisome concern is a potentially fatal drug-induced hepatitis that reportedly occurs in less than 0.5% of patients using this drug. Flutamide is also associated with feminization of male genitalia in the offspring of rats and should be considered to have the same possible effects in humans.

Finasteride

Finasteride (Proscar) has been used in the treatment of benign prostatic hypertrophy. It is generally regarded as a pure 5α-reductase inhibitor without other hormonal properties.[12] Serum levels of DHT and 3α-diol G are reduced by this drug after 3 months of treatment. Finasteride, 5 to 7.5 mg, is administered daily. Although doses up to 100 mg have been used in men without significant side effects, a smaller dose (1 mg) may be as effective as 5 mg in treating hirsutism. This hypothesis, however, has yet to be tested. There are no significant side effects reported for this medication, with the exception of an occasional report of mild headache and depression.[15] Finasteride may cause male genital feminization *in utero*. It may therefore be well suited to contracepting patients, those incapable of pregnancy, or postmenopausal hirsute women.

Mechanical Hair Removal

Mechanical hair removal, including shaving, plucking, depilatory creams, electrolysis, and waxing, may be very important adjuncts to medical therapy. Generally, it will take 3 to 6 months before any effect from medical therapy can be realized, and frequently this extends to more than a year of treatment. During this time, mechanical removal of hair (which has frequently not been emphasized by clinicians or taught to their patients) should be offered. It is a frequent misconception among patients that shaving increases the rate and density of hair growth. In combination with medical therapy, mechanical hair removal may increase patient compliance until hair growth stimulation is reduced. It may also be used following achievement of maximum effects of medical therapy. Chemical depilatories that dissolve hair by hydrolyzing the disulfite bonds may cause skin irritation and occasional dermatitis. Waxing or plucking may be beneficial for localized areas of hirsutism. Both can cause a folliculitis, and waxing is expensive and sometimes uncomfortable.[53]

Electrolysis is a commonly used therapy that attempts to destroy the hair follicle by electrolysis and thermolysis. Regrowth of hair is fairly common, however, with rates approaching 50%. Some patients have significant pain, scarring, and pigmentation problems following frequent visits for electrolysis therapy. Newer forms of epilation include laser therapy and light therapy (using selective wavelengths) that thermogenically destroy the hair and hair follicle. These methods may confer an advantage over electrolysis but have not been adequately studied at this time.

◊ EVALUATION OF MEDICAL THERAPY FOR HIRSUTISM

This section will evaluate studies that have been performed in the treatment of hirsutism from 1987 to 1997. It necessitates a fairly long introduction to the literature because of the unique nature of hirsutism. Hirsutism as treated by the clinician is almost always a cosmetic, if not a psychological, problem and not a disease state, the exceptions to this being the rare congenital or neoplastic conditions that have been described previously in this chapter. The evaluation of the literature in the treatment of hirsutism is difficult for a number of reasons. There is no recognized standard of treatment for evaluation. Farriman and Galloway's description in 1961 was originally developed as an epidemiologic tool. Studies have demonstrated both a large intra- and interobserver variability. Unfortunately, in most studies using the F-G grading score, a nonblinded observer was used.[7]

Quantitative measurements are more precise and reproducible. They include the measurement of the hair shaft diameter and the hair growth rate, which is determined by the weight of plucked or shaved hair. These quantitative measures were only reported in 25% of the studies presented here. The more objective quantitative methods themselves have lacked standardization in determining pharmacologic efficacy for treatment of hirsutism. Part of the problem lies in the considerable variation in the size of the hair shaft and in the distribution of hair in different body locations. The hair shafts themselves are oval in shape and difficult to measure uniformly. Shaving or plucking to determine hair weight is serially done in designated hirsute areas. This requires a tedious and labor-intensive measurement.

Many studies reported changes that occurred with baseline androgen levels, gonadotropins, SHBG, and a variety of other markers before and after treatment. These markers, while having academic interest, do not address the end point of treatment, which is the reduction of terminal hair density in androgen-sensitive areas. Very few studies report subjective evaluation by patients themselves. While improvement was difficult to standardize, some indication of it may be ascertained by reports of how frequently patients shaved or plucked their hair or had other therapy to treat hair growth.

Hirsutism Studies

Thirty-seven studies are evaluated here. Four studies use a double-blind, placebo-controlled methodology. The remainder are single-drug clinical trials or a randomization of two or more drugs or combinations of drugs. Semiquantitative or qualitative comparisons are reported as a baseline pretreatment measurement and are measured again at 6 months of therapy. The studies that did not report a 6-month evaluation could not be compared and thus were eliminated from review. However, the most beneficial effect of drug therapy may take up to 6 months, if not a year or more, to become apparent. There has been no attempt in this summary to distinguish the response in hirsute women with PCOS or from that of women with idiopathic hirsutism (IH). There was little if any difference in success rates between the two groups in any of the drug classifications reported.

Double-blind, Placebo-controlled Studies

There are four double-blind, placebo-controlled studies: one involving a Gn-RH agonist, one ketoconazole, and two spironolactone. Heiner et al.[31] randomized 64 women to one of four groups: (1) Gn-RH agonist nafarelin acetate (Synarel)

plus the oral contraceptive norethindrone and ethinyl estradiol (Norinyl 1 + 35), (2) Gn-RH agonist plus placebo, (3) oral contraceptive plus placebo, or (4) double placebo. They demonstrated a significant reducton in hair shaft diameter (21%) with the Gn-RH agonist plus oral contraceptive, but no reduction with the other treatment groups. There was also no significant change in the F-G scale between baseline and treated hirsutism scores in any of the groups.

Akaline[3] used ketoconazole in a randomized, placebo-controlled, double-blind crossover study involving 15 hirsute women. Nine were given ketoconazole, 600 mg per day, and six were given placebo. The F-G score was reduced at the end of 6 months by 41% in the treatment group and only 2% in the placebo group. Spironolactone was evaluated by Siegberg et al.[55] using a mixed PCOS/IH group and by McClellan et al.[45] using IH patients both in a double-blind, controlled study. Siegberg et al. showed no significant difference between the baseline and treated F-G scores, and McClellan et al. demonstrated no changes in hair shaft diameter or F-G hirsutism scores at the end of treatment.

Clinical Trials

Six classifications of drugs were evaluated from 31 studies. Several used a combination of quantitative (hair diameter/hair growth) and semiquantitative (F-G scores) systems. Results were presented as percentage changes from the baseline to the 6-month treatment evaluation in hair shaft diameter and/or hair growth or in F-G scores. There is considerable variation in the severity of hirsutism in the patients evaluated by these studies. There was also an apparent modification of the F-G scores, where some authors chose to eliminate evaluation of body areas that may not reflect androgen status (e.g., lower arm, lower leg, etc.). In summary, the studies showed that all the drugs evaluated have been effective in treating moderate to severe hirsutism.[7,26,49,50] There was no consistently superior drug demonstrated in the studies in which two or more drugs were evaluated head to head. In addition, in multiple randomizations, there was again no clear therapeutic advantage of one medication over another. The double-blind, randomized, controlled studies showed (somewhat predictably) less drug effectiveness than was demonstrated in the nonblinded, noncontrolled reports.

◊ CONCLUSION

There is no drug currently approved by the U.S. Food and Drug Administration for the treatment of hirsutism. In milder forms of hirsutism in women not satisfied cosmetically with mechanical removal, an oral contraceptive pill would seem to be the best first-line drug. Spironolactone and cyproterone[28] seem to be equivalent in effectiveness. Spironolactone seems to have less potential for side effects, and cyproterone is not available in the United States. In more severe forms of hirsutism, a Gn-RH agonist plus an oral contraceptive may be chosen over flutamide or ketoconazole, particularly when hepatic problems are a concern. Finasteride appears to have the least side effects of all and may be very effective in treating women with a low or no risk of pregnancy.

SUMMARY POINTS

◊ Hirsutism is the most common finding associated with androgen excess in women. If pathologic, it is often associated with menstrual dysfunction and infertility.

◊ DHT is biologically the most potent androgen in women, but serum levels often do not reflect elevations as the cause of clinical androgen excess.

◊ DHEA and DHEAS are weak androgens that serve as prehormones. They are almost exclusively produced in the adrenal glands.

◊ PCOS is the most common cause of androgen-related hirsutism, menstrual dysfunction, and infertility.

◊ The primary therapy of hirsutism is oral-contraceptive suppression, although ketoconazole, Gn-RH analogues (with or without "add back therapy"), and various antiandrogens have some utility.

◊ REFERENCES

1. Abraham GE, Maroulis GB, Buster JE, et al. Effect of dexamethasone on serum cortisol and androgen levels in hirsute patients. *Obstet Gynecol* 1976;47:395.
2. Adashi Eli Y, Levin PA. Pathophysiology and evaluation of adrenal hyperandrogenism. *Semin Reprod Endocrinol* 1986;4:155.
3. Akaline S. Effects of ketaconazole in hirsute women. *Acta Endocrinol* 1991;124:19–22.
4. Axelrod LR, Goldzieher JW. The polycystic ovary. III. Steroid biosynthesis in normal and polycystic ovarian tissue. *J Clin Endocrinol Metab* 1961;22:431.
5. Azziz R, Ochoa M, Bradley EL, et al. Leuprolide and estrogen. V. Oral contraceptive pills for the treatment of hirsutism: a prospective randomized study. *J Clin Endocrinol Metab* 1995;80:3406–3411.
6. Barbieri RL. Hyperandrogenism: new insights into etiology, diagnosis and therapy. *Curr Opin Obstet Gynecol* 1992;4:372.
7. Barth JH. How robust is the methodology for trials and therapy in hirsute women? *Clin Endocrinol* 1996;44:379.
8. Bates GW, Lucus JA. Hyperandrogenism and obesity. *Semin Reprod Endocrinol* 1986;4:189.
9. Bertoli A, Fusco A, Magnani A, et al. Efficacy of low-dose GnRH analogue (Buserellin) in the treatment of hirsutism. *Exp Clin Endocrinol* 1995;103:15.
10. Beslisle S, Love EJ. Clinical efficacy and safety of cyproterone acetate in severe hirsutism: results of 9 multicentered Canadian studies. *Fertil Steril* 1986;46:1015.
11. Carter JN, Tyson JE, Warne GL, et al. Adrenocortical function in hyperprolactinemic women. *J Clin Endocrinol Metab* 1997;45:973.
12. Castello R, Negri C, Tosi F, et al. Outcome of longterm treatment with the 5α-reductase inhibitor finasteride in idiopathic hirsutism: clinical and hormonal effects during a one-year course of therapy and one-year follow-up. *Fertil Steril* 1996;66:734.
13. Cesur V, Kamel N, Uysal AR, et al. The use of anti-androgen flutamide in the treatment of hirsutism. *Endocrine J* 1994;41:573.
14. Chetkowski RJ, DeFazio J, Shamonki I, et al. Incidence of late-onset congenital adrenal hyperplasia due to 21-hydroxylase deficiency among hirsute women. *J Clin Endocrinol Metab* 1984;58:595.
15. Ciotta L, Marietta E, Cianci A, et al. Clinical and endocrine effects of finasteride, a 5α-reductase inhibitor, in women with idiopathic hirsutism. *Fertil Steril* 1995;64:299.
16. Crapo L. Cushing's syndrome: a review of diagnostic tests. *Metabolism* 1979;28:955.
17. Dunaif A, Green G, Phelps RG, et al. Acanthosis nigricans, insulin action, and hyperandrogenism: clinical, histological, and biochemical findings. *J Clin Endocrinol Metab* 1991;73:590.
18. Dunaif A, Mandel J, Fluhr H, Dobrjansky A. The impact of obesity and chronic hyperinsulinemia on gonadotropic release and gonadal steroid secretion in the polycystic ovary syndrome. *J Clin Endocrinol Metab* 1988;66:131.
19. Erickson GF, Hsueh AJW, Quigley ME, et al. Functional studies of aromatase activity in human granulosa cells from normal and polycystic ovaries. *J Clin Endocrinol Metab* 1984;58:595.
20. Erenus M, Demicay Z, Gurbuz O, et al. Comparison of efficacy of spironolactone. V. Flutamide in the treatment of hirsutism. *Fertil Steril* 1996;61:613.
21. Erenus M, Durmusoglu F, Yucelten D, Pekin S, Gurbuz O. Comparison of spironolactone-oral contraceptive. V. Cyproterone acetate-estrogen regimens in the treatment of hirsutism. *Fertil Steril* 1996;66:216.
22. Feuillan P, Pang S, Schurmeyer T, et al. The hypothalamic-pituitary-adrenal axis in partial (late-onset) 21-hydroxylase deficiency. *J Clin Endocrinol Metab* 1988;67:154.
23. Friedman CI, Schmidt GE, Moon HK, Powel J. Serum testosterone concentrations in the evaluation of androgen-producing tumors. *Am J Obstet Gynecol* 1985;153:44.
24. Garcia-Bunuel R, Berek JS, Woodruff JD. Luteomas of pregnancy. *Obstet Gynecol* 1975;45:467.
25. Givens JR. Androgen metabolism. In Sciarra JJ, ed: *Gynecology and obstetrics.* Philadelphia: JB Lippincott Co, 1983:1.
26. Gokmen O, Senoz S, Gulekli B, Isik AZ. Comparison of four different treatment regimens in hirsutism related to polycystic ovary syndrome. *Gynecol Endocrinol* 1996;10:249.
27. Goldzieher JW, Axelrod LR. Clinical and biochemical features of polycystic ovarian disease. *Fertil Steril* 1963;14:631.
28. Hammerstein J, Meckies J, Leo-Rossberg I, et al. Use of cyproterone acetate (CPA) in the treatment of acne, hirsutism, and virilism. *J Steroid Biochem* 1975;6:827.
29. Hatch R, Rosenfield RL, Kim MH, Tredway D. Hirsutism: implications, etiology and management. *Am J Obstet Gynecol* 1981;140:815.
30. Helfer EL, Miller JL, Rose LI. Side-effects of spironolactone therapy in the hirsute woman. *J Clin Endocrinol Metab* 1988;66:208.
31. Heiner JS, Greendale GA, Karakami AK, et al. Comparison of a low-dose gonadotropin-releasing hormone agonist and a low-dose contraceptive given alone or together in the treatment of hirsutism. *J Clin Endocrinol Metab* 1995; 80:3412-3418.
32. Hideo U. Biology of hair growth. *Semin Reprod Endocrinol* 1986;4:131.
33. Ireland K, Woodruff JD. Masculinizing ovarian tumors. *Obstet Gynecol Surv* 1976;31:81.
34. Kaufman E, Mosman J, Sutton M, et al. Characterization of basal estrogen and androgen levels and gonadotropin release patterns in the obese adolescent female. *J Pediatr* 1981;96:990.
35. Kirschner MA, Zycher IR, Jesperson D. Idiopathic hirsutism—an ovarian abnormality. *N Engl J Med* 1976;294:637.
36. Kitabchi AE, Burrington CK. Body fat distribution and hyperandrogenicity and health risks. *Semin Reprod Endocrinol* 1994;12:6.
37. Lee PA, Gareis FJ. Evidence for partial 21-hydroxylase deficiency among heterozygote carriers of congenital adrenal hyperplasia. *J Clin Endocrinol Metab* 1975;41:415.
38. Lobo RA, Goebelsmann U, Horton R. Evidence for the importance of peripheral tissue events in the development of hirsutism in polycystic ovary syndrome. *J Clin Endocriol Metab* 1983;57:393.
39. Lobo RA, Wellington LP, Goebelsmann U. Serum levels of DHEAS in gynecologic endocrinopathy and infertility. *Obstet Gynecol* 1981;57:607.
40. London SN, Hammond CB. Hirsutism. *Postgrad Obstet Gynecol* 1983;3:1.
41. Loriaux DL. Spironolactone and endocrine dysfunction. *Ann Intern Med* 1976;85:630.

42. Marcos RN, Abdul-Malik ME, Shikroa E. Treatment of hirsutism with a gonadotropin-releasing hormone agonist and estrogen replacement therapy. *Fertil Steril* 1994;61:427.

43. Maroulis GB. Evaluation of hirsutism and hyperandrogenemia. *Fertil Steril* 1981;36:273.

44. Mauvais-Jarvis P. Regulation of androgen receptor and 5α-reductase in the skin of normal and hirsute women. *Postgrad Med J* 1989;65:459.

45. McClellan AR, Rentoul J, MacKie R, McInnes GT. Lack of spironolactone on hair shaft diameter in hirsute females. *Postgrad Med J* 1989; 65:459.

46. McMullen GR, Van Herle AJ. Hirsutism and the effectiveness of spironolactone in its management. *J Endocrinol Invest* 1993;16:925.

47. Medina M, Herrera J, Flores M, et al. Normal ovarian function in a mild form of late-onset 3-beta-hydroxy steroid dehydrogenase deficiency. *Fertil Steril* 1986;46:1021.

48. Meikle AW, Stringham JD, Wilson DE, Dolman LI. Plasma 5-alpha-reduced androgens in men and hirsute women: role of adrenals and gonads. *J Endocrinol Metab* 1979;48:969.

49. Moghtti T, Castello R, Magnani CM, et al. Clinical and hormonal effects of the 5α-reductase inhibitor finasteride in idiopathic hirsutism. *J Clin Endocrinol Metab* 1994;79:1115.

50. Muderis II, Kelestimur F, Bayman F, et al. The efficacy of 200 mg/day flutamide in the treatment of patients with hirsutism. *Fertil Steril* 1996; 66:220.

51. Rittmaster RS. Medical treatment of androgen-dependent hirsutism. *J Clin Endocrinol Metab* 1995;80:2559.

52. Rittmaster RS. Androgen conjugates as a major product of hyperandrogenism. *Semin Reprod Endocrinol* 1994;12:45.

53. Schriock EA, Schriock ED. Treatment of hirsutism. *Clin Obstet Gynecol* 1991;34:852.

54. Serafini P, Lobo RA. The effects of spironolactone on adrenal steroidogenesis in hirsute women. *Fertil Steril* 1985;44:595.

55. Siegberg R, Yolostalo P, Laatakainen T, Pelkonen R, Stenman U. Endocrine and clinical effects of spironolactone in female hyperandrogenism. *Arch Gynecol* 1987;240:67.

56. Sonino N, Scranoni C, Biason A, et al. Low-dose ketaconazole treatment in hirsute women. *J Endocrinol Invest* 1990;13:35.

57. Speiser PW, New MI. Genotype and hormonal phenotype in nonclassical 21-hydroxylase deficiency. *J Clin Endocrinol Metab* 1987; 64:86.

58. Wu CH. Plasma free and protein-bound testosterone in hirsutism. *Obstet Gynecol* 1982;60:188.

CHAPTER 40

The Breast

—— ◊ ——

James V. Fiorica

Breast cancer is quite likely the most feared disease by women in the United States at the current time. Its incidence continues to increase, with more than 180,000 new cases in 1997 and a corresponding reported mortality of 44,000 for 1997. In the United States, it is the leading cause of death from cancer in women between ages 30 and 54 years and represents 30% of the cancer incidence in women and 17% of total cancer deaths. The good news about breast cancer in 1997 is that the mortality in the United States is finally beginning to fall.

Obstetricians and gynecologists are commonly the primary care physicians for many women between 20 and 65 years of age. These physicians serve a key role in detecting breast abnormalities, as well as educating, screening, and counseling on all benign and malignant conditions. The American Board of Obstetricians and Gynecologists has made a curriculum for training residents and others in the behavioral, cognitive, and technical aspects of breast care. This chapter presents an overview of screening guidelines, common benign and malignant conditions of the breast, and the obstetrician/gynecologist's role as a clinician.

◊ DETECTION AND DIAGNOSIS

History and Physical Examination

A thorough initial history is critical and should be oriented toward risk factors for breast cancer (Table 1). The most recognized epidemiologic risk factors include previous breast cancer in the opposite breast or breast cancer in a first-degree relative. A family history of breast cancer increases the risk by two to three times to as high as nine times in cases of bilateral premenopausal breast cancer occurring in a first-degree relative. Nulliparous women, women whose menopause began after age 55, and women who had their first pregnancy after age 35 have a two to three times higher risk of breast cancer. Age is probably the most significant risk factor, because breast cancer risk increases with age throughout a woman's life. However, when risk factors are identified and analyzed either

alone or in combination, they explain only 21% of the breast cancer risk among women aged 55 to 84 years. Thus, from clinicians' point of view, all women are assumed to be at risk for breast cancer, particularly those older than 35 years. Breast cancer in the United States is more prevalent among women in the upper socioeconomic rather than the lower socioeconomic classes. In the past, whites have been reported to be more commonly affected than blacks, but this is true only among women older than 45 years. Mortality increases when urban as compared to rural areas are examined. Mortality is higher in the northeastern than in the southeastern United States, where it is lowest.

Several reproductive factors have been identified in association with increased risk of breast cancer, for example, the mother's age when the first child is born. If a woman is younger when the first birth occurs, it lowers her risk for breast cancer; it is not known why this association exists. In addition, several studies have indicated that lactation does decrease the risk for breast cancer, partly because it has been correlated with the number of full-term pregnancies and multiparity also appears to be protective. The effect of menopause has been examined as it relates to breast cancer, and late menopause poses a greater risk. If a woman has natural menopause at age 55 years or older, she is more likely to develop breast cancer; bilateral oophorectomy before natural menopause reduces the risk. If the ovaries are removed before age 35 years, there is a 70% reduction in the risk of breast cancer. These data suggest that the total number of years of menstrual activity is an associated factor.

The patient is the one who discovers most lumps. If a patient notices a breast lump, pertinent historical factors include the duration of the finding, the presence or absence of pain in relation to menses, and the presence or absence of dimpling of the skin. Pain is most common in cystic changes and is less common in carcinoma. If the pain is constant and only on one side in a postmenopausal patient who is not taking estrogen, more suspicion is appropriate. A premenstrual, tender thickening is more likely to be benign engorgement or fibrocystic

TABLE 1. *Risk factors for breast cancer*

Factor	Relative risk
Family history of breast cancer	
First-degree relative	1.8
Premenopausal first-degree relative	3.0
Postmenopausal first-degree relative	1.5
Premenopausal first-degree relative (bilateral breast cancer)	9.0
Postmenopausal first-degree relative (bilateral breast cancer)	4.0–5.4
Menstrual history (age in years)	
Menarche before age 12	1.7–3.4
Menarche after age 17	0.3
Menopause before age 45	0.5–0.7
Menopause from age 45–54	1.0
Menopause after age 55	1.5
Menopause after age 55 with >40 menstrual years	2.5–5.0
Oophorectomy before age 35	0.4
Anovulatory menstrual cycles	2.0–4.0
Pregnancy history	
Term pregnancy before age 20	0.4
First term pregnancy at age 20–34	1.0
First term pregnancy after age 35	1.5–4.0
Nulliparous patient	1.3–4.0
Noninvasive breast disease	
Atypical lobular hyperplasia	4.0
Lobular carcinoma *in situ*	7.2
Other neoplasms	
Contralateral breast cancer	2.0–10.0
Cancer of the major salivary gland	4.0
Cancer of the uterus	2.0

(From Marchant DJ. Risk factors. In: Marchant DJ., ed. *Breast disease.* Philadelphia: WB Saunders, 1997:119; with permission.)

changes rather than malignant disease. When the skin dimples, carcinoma is the likely underlying etiology. This dimpling is the result of the shortening of the Cooper ligaments. Nipple discharge must be evaluated; malignant discharges are usually unilateral, bloody, or spontaneous. When the patient is postmenopausal, nipple discharges should be carefully examined. A detailed history of prior surgery, infection, injury to the breast(s), or inappropriate lactation is pertinent.

There are numerous questions about when and how to perform a breast examination. The optimal time for performing one is right after menstruation and prior to ovulation. This avoids evaluating an engorged and tender breast and helps in performing an accurate evaluation. With the patient in the upright position, the breasts should be inspected for precancerous abnormalities including retraction, deviations, or inverted nipples, as well as for dermatologic disorders. They should also be examined with the patient's hands down at her side, then with her arms elevated, and finally with her arms tensing at her hips, contracting the pectoralis muscles (Fig. 1). Dermatologic disorders that could signal more serious conditions include edema, nevi, ulcers, or eczematoid reactions. If a scaly red eruption is noted around the areola, Paget disease should be suspected.

As the examination progresses, attention is directed toward the supraclavicular area and axilla. Digital palpation is performed beneath the lateral pectoralis muscles into the axilla itself. A clinically negative axilla contains metastatic lymph nodes in about 40% of breast cancer patients. Nonetheless, the axilla must be thoroughly examined.

The second phase of the breast examination is conducted with the patient in the supine position, and the examiner inspects the entire breast, chest wall, and axillae. It is important to instruct patients in the technique of breast self-examination. If physicians personally do the instruction, patients are much more likely to comply. Brochures are helpful but not nearly as effective as physician-directed discussion on breast self-examination. During this patient education, physicians have the opportunity to individualize the examination and reinforce what is normal versus abnormal to patients. Digital palpation is then carried out using the index and middle fingers and applying varying amounts of pressure with the flats or pads of the fingers. A thorough examination covers the entire breast and chest wall, first superficially at the skin and then intermediately within the breast stroma and subcutaneous tissue. Finally, the triple-touch technique is used deep against the chest wall. The entire breast must be examined systematically. The examination can be done in a clockwise direction or by rows (stripwise). It is important to carefully examine beneath the nipple–areolar complex and within the axilla. Half of breast cancers occur in the upper outer quadrant of the breast, 18% beneath the nipple–areola, and 15% in the upper inner quadrant.

If no lesions are noted on examination, it is critical to document negative findings, discuss cancer screening, and plan follow-up with the patient. A summary of pertinent negative findings might appear as follows: "No dominant masses, no retractions, no nipple discharge, or lymphadenopathy was noted in the sitting and supine positions." The date of the last mammogram should be recorded. Persistent risk factors are listed, as well as notation of what hormones were administered. Oral contraceptives should not be renewed without a documented annual breast examination. Hormones should not be renewed unless a breast examination and mammography are performed. These practices are good for patients and protect physicians, as a great deal of litigation results from failure to diagnose breast cancer. The Physician Insurers Association of America's breast cancer claims study, conducted in 1988, determined that 75% of successful malpractice lawsuits involved primary care physicians with practices in family medicine, internal medicine, or obstetrics and gynecology. It is important that the medical chart is carefully documented, as approximately one-third of the cases resulted from inadequate documentation.

Dominant Mass

During the breast examination, discovery of a lesion mandates determining whether or not it is cancerous. If a mass is palpated, the physician must determine whether the lesion is

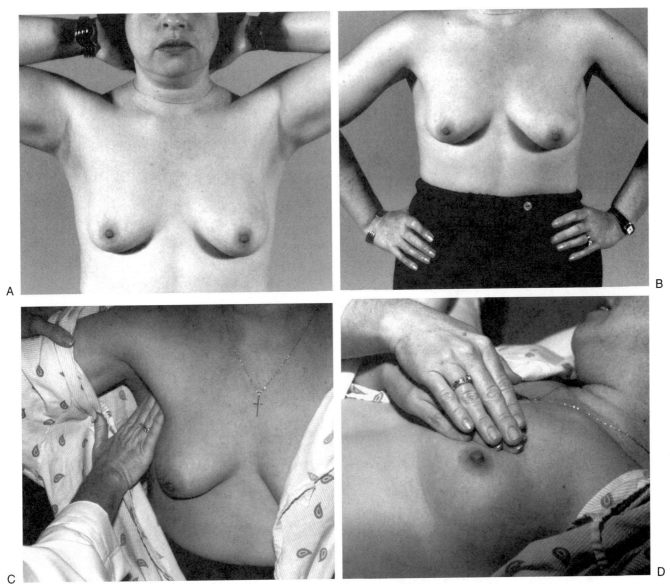

FIG. 1. Examination of the breast. **A:** The arms are extended above the head. Attention is directed to abnormal motion or skin retractions. Asymmetry, prominent veins, and skin changes may indicate cancer. **B:** Inward pressure on the hips tenses the pectoralis major muscle. Abnormal attachments to its overlying fascia and skin can produce retraction or dimpling of the skin. **C:** The axilla is best examined in the upright position. Proper placement of the examiner's hand and the arm is important to detect nodal enlargement. **D:** Thorough palpation of the entire breast for masses is performed with the patient in the supine position. This is the best opportunity to reinforce breast self-examination and individualize aspects of the breast examination.

a discrete three-dimensional mass rather than the thickening commonly noted when breasts have fibrocystic changes. Discrete masses are commonly referred to as dominant masses. Once a mass is identified, a diagnosis must be assigned and cancer ruled out.

The first step is to measure the size of the lesion. This can sometimes be done by compressing the lesion against the adjacent rib to stabilize it. The next step is to determine whether the lesion is solid or cystic. A simple cyst aspiration can be performed in the office. After the breast is prepped with an alcohol pad, a 23-gauge needle connected to a 10-ml syringe is placed directly into the mass while the opposite hand stabilizes it. Once the needle has passed through the skin, negative pressure is applied. If the mass is cystic, the fluid is completely evacuated, and the lesion should disappear completely. The suction is then taken off the syringe and the needle removed from the patient. The fluid is discarded if it is serous and nonbloody. The patient is instructed to return in 4 to 6 weeks for reexamination.

In a noncystic lesion, fine-needle aspiration (FNA) is done because the lesion is thought to be solid. Using the same technique described above, the needle, once placed in the mass, is moved back and forth eight to ten times while full suction is applied. The plunger of the syringe is then released, and the negative pressure normalized. The needle is withdrawn, and a smear is prepared for cytologic evaluation. Usually, two or three separate specimens are obtained from solid lesions to sample the mass adequately and increase cell collection. Cytologic preparation can be a monolayer smear, similar to a Papanicolaou test. However, the yield can be improved by lavaging the syringe in a specimen jar containing cytofixative, where a cell block is created for cytologic analysis (Fig. 2). The number of satisfactory collections by FNA sampling varies from 50% to 87%.

Physicians should *not* rely on negative FNA findings. The accepted standard of care is to excise all solid, three-dimensional masses unless a definite benign diagnosis can be made by FNA. An open biopsy is also required if a cystic lesion does not completely disappear on fluid aspiration, if bloody cyst fluid is obtained on aspiration, if a cyst recurs after one or two aspirations, if a solid dominant mass is not diagnosed as a fibroadenoma, or if the patient has bloody nipple discharge, nipple ulceration, or skin edema suspicious for carcinoma. The purpose of FNA is to determine whether or not a malignancy is present so that the patient may be counseled and triaged for immediate cancer treatment. If the lesion is cystic, FNA is therapeutic and diagnostic, with the patient's anxiety relieved. If the palpable mass is not a discrete dominant mass, the physician must determine whether or not the findings are consistent with fibrocystic changes versus asymmetric breast parenchyma that must be biopsied. In patients close to the start of menstruation, a repeat exami-

nation should be performed after the menstrual cycle. The sensitivity, specificity, positive predictive value, and negative predictive value of FNA are 82%, 97%, 95%, and 96%, respectively. A false-positive rate of 1.2% and a false-negative rate of 7.7% are generally seen. The differential diagnosis of a solid breast lesion includes the following:

◊ Inflammatory disorders: acute mastitis, plasma cell mastitis, subareolar abscess, and fat necrosis;
◊ Benign tumors: fibrocystic changes, lactating adenomas, intraductal papilloma, fibroadenoma, cystosarcoma phyllodes, adenoma of the nipple, and granular cell tumor;
◊ Malignant tumors: ductal carcinoma, lobular carcinoma, sarcomas and metastatic tumors.

Mammography

For several years, a debate has been ongoing as to the optimal age to start mammographic screening and the appropriate screening interval. In March 1997, the American Cancer Society (ACS) approved annual mammography for all asymptomatic women starting at age 40 years (Table 2). The justification for this was based on an ACS workshop reviewing old and new data on this controversial subject. Eight randomized clinical trials of mammography screening have been conducted. The most recent metaanalysis of these trials yielded an 18% mortality reduction (95% confidence interval [CI], 0.71 to 0.95) among screened women aged 40 to 49 years. Seven of the trials were population-based, and a metaanalysis of these

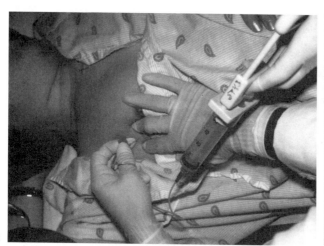

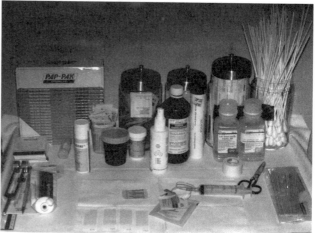

FIG. 2. A: After the mass is located and stabilized, the needle is inserted several times into it. **B:** The fine-needle aspirate is readied for processing on cytology slides. Note that the "tissue juice" remains in the needle and does not enter the syringe in the case of solid masses. **C:** When a cyst is encountered, the fluid is withdrawn into the syringe as the mass disappears with negative pressure.

TABLE 2. *American Cancer Society 1997 breast cancer screening guidelines*

Monthly breast self-examination for women aged 20 and older
Annual mammogram for women aged 40 and older
Breast clinical examination for women aged 20–40 every 3 years; every year for women older than 40

showed a 26% mortality reduction (95% CI, 0.63 to 0.88) in the same age group.

Two trials conducted in Sweden revealed a statistically significant reduction in mortality among women aged 40 to 49 years at randomization. The Gothenberg trial had 12 years of follow-up and showed a 44% reduction in mortality (95% CI, 0.32 to 0.98). The Malmo trial showed a 36% reduction in mortality (95% CI, 0.45 to 0.89). Relative mortality reductions appear later in women aged 40 to 49 years at randomization compared with women aged 50 years or older, according to these study results. This observation has raised questions about whether or not the benefit may be attributable to women randomized during their 40s who were diagnosed with breast cancer after age 50. It appears that the delayed appearance of a relative mortality reduction in younger women compared with older women is best explained by (1) small numbers of women in their 40s in the existing randomized trials, (2) a greater proportion of diagnosis of ductal carcinoma *in situ* in the group invited to screening (the greater lead time achieved from a diagnosis at this stage requires a longer period of follow-up), (3) lower incidence and mortality in women in their 40s, and (4) the observation that in most of the trials, screening intervals longer than 1 year were comparatively less effective in detecting more aggressive tumors at favorable stages.

Results from randomized trials and large community-based screening programs provided compelling evidence to support the existing ACS guidelines. Evaluation of interval cancers indicated that a greater proportion of breast cancers grow faster in younger women than in older women. Therefore, to achieve the maximal benefit from screening among women aged 40 to 49 years, it is important that the screening interval be the same in women younger and older than 50 years, that is, annual screening. Further, it is clear from the data presented that it is artificial to compare women aged 40 to 49 years with all women over the age of 50.

A standardized reporting system—the Breast Imaging Reporting and Data System (BI-RADS)—was developed in 1995 by the American College of Radiology (Table 3). In the past, a lack of uniformity in mammographic terminology and reporting often led to confusion as to the malignant nature of a lesion. Currently, BI-RADS employs a standardized lexicon to bring uniformity to the description of mammographic findings. The examination is categorized into one of five fixed assessment categories, and each of these categories is associated with one specific management recommendation.

Mammography should be performed before any open biopsy. A mammogram may better delineate the palpable lesion and identify other lesions in the same or opposite breast that may need treatment. Film screen mammography is the uniformly accepted radiologic screening test for breast cancer. In *diagnostic* mammography, breast x-ray images are obtained in patients with *breast symptoms*, *palpable masses,* or *a known history of mammographic abnormalities*. In these instances, the radiologist is present at the examination and can order additional films as necessary. In contrast, *screening* mammography is performed in asymptomatic patients, and a technician performs it without a radiologist necessarily being present. The radiologist reads the films later, thus potentially reducing the cost.

Mammographic abnormalities are grouped into three categories: densities, microcalcifications, and parenchymal asymmetry. The mammographic signs of early breast cancer are the following:

◊ Tumor mass, usually irregularly marginated or spiculated;
◊ Small, grouped (clustered) calcifications with or without a mass;
◊ Poorly defined, asymmetric breast density, especially if this developed since a prior examination;
◊ Distortion of the breast parenchymal architecture by scirrhous tumor.

Nonpalpable mammographic densities are handled in the same manner as their palpable counterparts. The densities are

TABLE 3. *Mammography final assessment categories*

Category	Assessment	Description	Recommendation
1	Negative	There is nothing to comment on	Routine screening
2	Benign finding	A negative mammogram, but the interpreter may wish to describe a finding	Routine screening
3	Probably benign finding	A very high probability of benignity	Short interval follow-up suggested to establish stability
4	Suspicious abnormality	Not characteristic, but a definite probability of malignancy	Biopsy should be considered
5	Highly suggestive of malignancy	A high probability of malignancy	Appropriate action should be taken.

(From American College of Radiology, 1995; with permission.)

either solid or cystic, new or old. Ultrasound examination can distinguish simple cysts, which are generally left alone unless a complex pattern is seen. Previous films can help differentiate old from new findings and determine whether or not a solid lesion is enlarging.

Microcalcifications may be scattered or clustered, coarse or fine, and new or old. Previous films and additional magnification views may be helpful. Typically, benign calcifications are normally more evenly scattered than clustered. Benign secretory calcifications are thick, smooth, or ring-like. Coarse calcifications within a well circumscribed density are characteristic of a fibroadenoma. There are many other benign types of calcifications, including ring calcifications of the skin, typical parallel linear vascular calcifications, and the layered appearance of "milk of calcium" in small cysts.

Possibly the most difficult radiologic abnormality one may encounter is parenchymal asymmetry. Previous breast films are important for comparison, and compression films of the breast should be ordered. The final recommendation as to whether or not a biopsy should be performed must made by a skilled breast radiologist. Certain types of cancer (e.g., lobular) can be concealed in an asymmetric parenchymal breast. Clinicians are more routinely using algorithms being developed at many breast centers to aid clinicians in the management of abnormal mammograms.

Breast Biopsy

It has been recommended that surgeons familiar with contemporary cancer treatment planning perform open biopsies when these are necessary. The American College of Obstetrics and Gynecology has stopped short of recommending that open biopsy may be performed by every obstetrician and gynecologist.

Once a lesion has been described as a mass and been measured or drawn, it must be analyzed to see whether it is benign or malignant. Initially, an attempt at FNA should be made. Many macrocysts, which are under a great deal of pressure, have all the characteristics of a solid mass by palpation. If the dominant mass is truly solid, a biopsy must be scheduled. Other indications for biopsy include the following:

◊ Marked erythema and edema suggestive of inflammatory carcinoma,
◊ Unilateral discharge in a postmenopausal patient,
◊ Serosanguineous or bloody nipple discharge,
◊ Persistent crusting of the nipple and, occasionally, ill-defined areas associated with suspicious mammographic findings.

It is prudent to schedule a biopsy as soon as possible. A biopsy can be performed on an outpatient basis under local anesthesia in the majority of patients.

Biopsy must be performed in an operating-room setting, where trained personnel familiar with the biopsy technique are present. It is important to choose the design and type of incision. A wide local excision may not be possible in cases in which the mass is located at some distance from the

nipple–areolar complex. The incision should be carefully chosen (Fig. 3). Despite an excellent cosmetic appearance, a circumareolar incision is normally not acceptable, except in the rare instances when the lesion is directly beneath the areolar complex. The incision should be marked with the patient sitting or standing, and then she is prepared and draped. Normally, local anesthesia is used. Fine instruments should be used. Cautery or fine suture ligatures control bleeding during the operative procedure. In most instances, an excisional biopsy is performed, and the entire lesion is removed. An incisional biopsy may be appropriate if a large lesion is discovered for which additional surgery is planned.

Once the lesion has been excised, fine ligatures are the preferred way to control bleeding. Bleeding points on the dense breast tissue itself are more easily controlled by cautery, but cautery should not be relied on to control bleeding from large vessels. The breast is then loosely reconstructed using fine suture material with a minimum number of sutures. It is not necessary to use a drain if the wound is dry. The skin is closed with either a subcuticular suture or fine vertical mattress sutures of nonabsorbable material. It is critical in the operation to place a pressure dressing secured with a large woven elastic bandage (e.g., Ace bandage). This dressing is left in place for 48 hours. Immobilization and application of pressure eliminate significant induration and hematoma formation. In 5 to 7 days, sutures are removed. If the lesion is malignant, treatment planning can be instituted.

As the biopsy often becomes part of the treatment, it must be meticulously planned and executed. Being appropriately skilled and knowledgeable prior to performing biopsies is imperative. Unfortunately, there are surgeons who are not aware of the requirements for conservative treatment of breast cancer. The incisions may be poorly chosen, and marked postbiopsy induration and hematoma can preclude additional wide local excision, resulting in unnecessary mastectomy. The pathologist has special responsibilities, which include carefully inking the margins of the excision. Sufficient tissue must be submitted for estrogen and progesterone analysis. It is critical to obtain free margins. If the lesion is not completely removed, reexcision or mastectomy will be required.

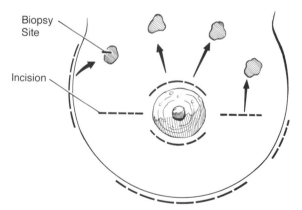

FIG. 3. Location of incisions for breast biopsy with good cosmetic result. (Modified from Keen G, et al. *Operative surgery and management.* New York: Macmillan, 1987.)

Needle localization biopsies have become an increasingly common surgical procedure. There are a number of lesions that are clinically not detectable. Localization of nonpalpable breast lesions is accomplished by insertion of a needle, usually containing an internal hook-wire, into the breast, and coordination of the topographic anatomy of the breast with mammographic images. The concept is to insert the needle into the breast so that the surgeon can make a small incision in the breast and follow the needle to the target. An x-ray image is taken to confirm the lesion is in the specimen after the specimen and needle are removed.

With advancements in mammographic technology, a histologic tissue diagnosis can be obtained with a stereotactic core needle biopsy (CNB), eliminating the need for a surgical biopsy. Many reports in the medical literature document the sensitivity and specificity of stereotactically guided CNB (sensitivity, 71% to 100%; specificity, 85% to 100%). The stereotactically guided nonsurgical core needle uses sophisticated radiographic equipment and an automated biopsy gun that cuts a core of tissue. Several cores can be taken from a nonpalpable mass or other suspicious areas within the breast without the need for a surgical incision. The advantages of this procedure include lower costs because operating-room charges are avoided. There is only a minimal scar, and there is no permanent effect on subsequent mammographic studies.

Discrepancies in the published results concerning CNB may be result of several factors, including basic definitions and methodology, case selection, gauge of the core biopsy needle used, and number of specimens obtained. In general, better results have been reported when 14-gauge needles are used rather than smaller-bore needles. Recent investigations showed that five specimens obtained with a 14-gauge needle achieve a 99% accuracy for masses; however, 10 or more stereotactically guided CNB specimens may be required for calcifications. Specimen radiography should be routinely performed on breast tissue obtained by stereotactically guided CNB to determine whether calcifications have indeed been obtained and to direct the pathologist's evaluation of the tissue specimens. One problem with this technique is that cancers may be missed during core-needle sampling, leading to a false-negative diagnosis. In one multiinstitutional study, 5.4% of women who were diagnosed with a benign lesion by stereotactically guided CNB were found to have carcinoma at follow-up. Proponents of stereotactically guided CNB have argued that although lesions are sometimes missed using this technique, up to 20% of nonpalpable lesions can also be missed at the time of image-directed excisional biopsy. However, radiologists and surgeons experienced in excisional biopsy guided by needle-wire localization have reported that only 0.2% to 0.3% of lesions are missed. Furthermore, radiography of the excised specimen identifies the "misses" immediately so that they can be managed appropriately. The actual false-negative rate for stereotactically guided CNB is not known, because most studies in the literature have not provided the rigorous long-term follow-up (at least 2 to 3 years) required to identify all false-negative diagnoses. Indications and relative contraindications for stereotactically guided CNB

TABLE 4. *Indications and relative contraindications for stereotactically guided core-needle biopsy*

Indications
A solid, nonpalpable mass associated with:
    Irregular shape
    Spiculated or ill-defined margins
    Microlobulations
    Suspicious calcifications
    Associated findings such as:
        Focal skin thickening
        Focal solitary dilated duct

Microcalcifications with the following features:
    Morphology: varying size or shape (pleomorphic), branching, or granular
    Distribution: clustered (grouped), linear, or regional

An area of suspicious architectural distortion in a known prior biopsy site that demonstrates a suspicious interval change since a prior mammogram

Asymmetry associated with suspicious calcifications, architectural distortion, a noncystic mass, a solitary dilated duct, or focal skin thickening

Solid, circumscribed mass that is dominant (usually >1 cm) or shows interval growth since a prior mammogram

Contraindications
Lesions in the benign or probably benign category such as:
    Masses that
        Are circumscribed, of low density, and <1 cm, unless changed since the prior mammogram
        Contain intralesional fat of a density that is pathognomonic for a lymph node, oil cyst, or hamartoma
        Are multiple, noncalcified, and circumscribed
    Microcalcifications that are
        Tiny, round or oval, uniform, and in localized cluster
        In a discrete cluster (or clusters) suggestive of milk of calcium, secretory disease, or sclerosing adenosis
        Diffuse, nonclustered, and suggestive of milk of calcium, secretory disease, or sclerosing adenosis

Unequivocal, palpable masses

(From Bassett et al., 1997, with permission.)

depend on practice variations and the experience of the physician performing the biopsy (Table 4).

A final method for locating masses is ultrasonography. Ultrasound equipment has improved to enable localizing and permitting a biopsy of nonpalpable masses. A skilled radiologist and a cooperative relationship between radiologist and surgeon are essential to properly prescribe the correct biopsy technique.

◊ BENIGN CONDITIONS

There is no lesion that is *obviously* benign. Some patients present with an irregular, tender dominant mass that may be related to trauma, but they cannot recall the actual incident. Others present with irregular, tender thickening in the upper outer quadrant of the breast. This is usually cyclic and often referred to as fibrocystic changes. A physician must first rule out breast cancer before assuming benignity (Fig. 4).

MANAGING BENIGN BREAST DISORDERS

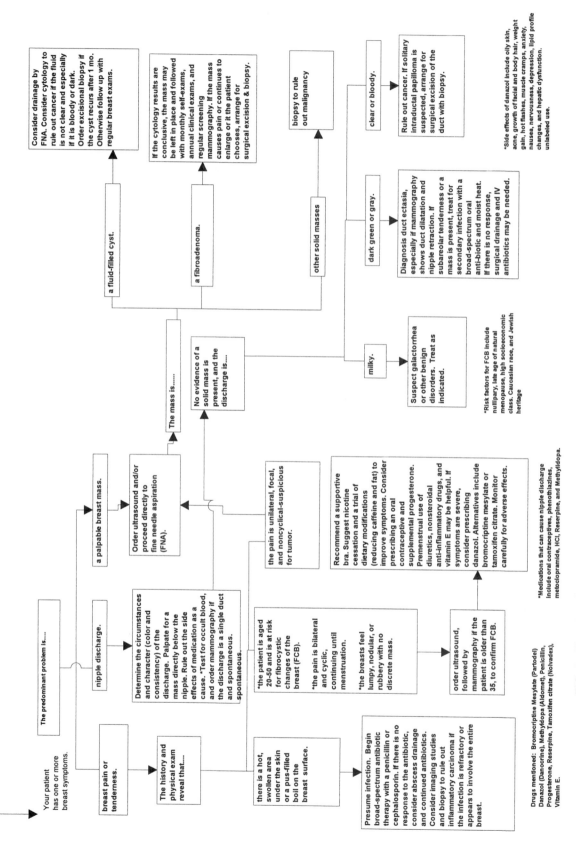

FIG. 4. Flowchart for managing benign breast disorders. (From Fiorica JV. Benign breast disorders: first rule out cancer. *Patient Care* Apr 15, 1997:144, 145; with permission.)

Fibrocystic Changes

The most common benign condition of the breast is fibrocystic change (FCC), an enhanced or exaggerated reaction by breast tissue in response to fluctuating levels of ovarian hormones. The incidence of FCC is greatest in women aged 20 to 50 years who are in their reproductive, premenopausal years. Pain (mastodynia) is the most common symptom of FCC. Because of fear of breast cancer, any discomfort in the anterior chest is usually perceived as breast pain. In addition to intrinsic breast disease, there are many causes of anterior chest pain: achalasia, cervical radiculitis, hiatal hernia, costochondritis (Tietze syndrome), neuralgia, cervical rib, cholelithiasis, coronary artery disease, myalgia, pleurisy, phantom pain, trauma, or herpes zoster. The pain from FCC is often bilateral and particularly noticeable during the premenstrual phase. The lumpiness (nodularity) may be unilateral or bilateral, localized or generalized. Occasionally, a spontaneous nipple discharge is present. Age, parity, genetic makeup, and lactational history may all have a bearing on FCC.

The pathogenesis is not precisely known, but it seems to be due to an imbalance in estrogen and progesterone levels. Epithelial and stromal changes may be induced by the cyclic changes of the breast tissue under the influence of hormones. Risk factors include nulliparity, late age of natural menopause, and high socioeconomic class.

Women with the highest risk for development of cancer—an 11-fold increased risk—had a positive family history for breast cancer and exhibited cellular atypia on biopsy. Unless proliferative changes with atypia are present, FCC is not a risk factor for cancer, and fortunately this is the case for the vast majority of women. FCC is histologic and can be divided into three prognostic categories: nonproliferative, proliferative changes with atypia, and proliferative changes without atypia. Of breast biopsies showing FCC, 70% are of nonproliferative lesions with no increased risk for cancer; of proliferative lesions (30%), 26% exhibit no cellular atypia and no apparent increased risk for breast cancer, while 4% show cellular atypia, which appears to have a fivefold increased risk for breast cancer.

Women who present with complaints of FCC should have a thorough breast examination. Most symptoms are treated by medical management, but a tissue biopsy is mandatory for a three-dimensional lump. Medical therapy for symptomatic FCC includes use of a support bra worn at all times to alleviate pain and heaviness. A diuretic, especially premenstrually, may transiently relieve discomfort. Studies have shown a correlation between the consumption of methylxanthines (e.g., caffeine) and tobacco and FCC. There was a 24% improvement in clinical symptoms by decreasing intake of methylxanthines and tobacco. Although this therapy has been refuted by some, discontinuing caffeine does no harm and may benefit symptomatic patients.

Oral contraceptives during the secretory phase of the menstrual cycle has had some effect on pain control. The preferred drug for the treatment of severe symptomatic FCC is danazol (Danocrine). A 3- to 6-month course of danazol, 100 to 400 mg per day, eliminates pain and nodularity in about 69% of women and reduces signs and symptoms in another 30%. This therapy may also focus attention on a dominant lump to be biopsied, reducing the need for additional biopsies as the other nodules respond to therapy. At the low doses recommended, side effects are minimal. Danazol's effects can last several months after discontinuation.

Fibroadenoma

Ultrasound and FNA can distinguish fibroadenomas from cysts. Fibroadenomas are benign breast masses that occur in as many as 10% of women. They are found in all age-groups but primarily during the 20s and early 30s; their incidence decreases with advancing age. Multiple fibroadenomas are found in 12% to 20% of cases and are frequently bilateral. These smooth, round, mobile lumps that can feel firm to rubbery are usually painless and tend to be discovered on breast examination. Cytologic examination of aspirate from a fibroadenoma reveals monolayers of benign ductal epithelial cells with dense stroma and abundant elongated nuclei. Where fibroadenomas are concerned, mammography is not helpful in definitively ruling out cancer. Fibroadenomas recur in about 20% of women. A clinically suspicious lesion should be evaluated by complete excision. When cytology provides a clear diagnosis of fibroadenoma, the mass can be left in place and followed with monthly breast self-examination, annual clinical breast examination, and regular screening mammography. Some fibroadenomas regress spontaneously, and they are not considered premalignant. Surgical excision and biopsy are often recommended when the following occur:

◊ The mass causes pain or continues to enlarge;
◊ The results of FNA are inconclusive or suspicious in any way;
◊ The patient needs further reassurance that biopsy can provide.

Other benign breast masses, such as tubular adenomas and hematomas, are often misidentified as fibroadenomas.

Nipple Discharge

A nipple discharge is a true drainage that is expelled directly from the mammary duct and appears on the surface of the nipple. The drainage may be milky, sticky, and consistent with galactorrhea. To be significant, nipple discharge should be persistent, true, spontaneous, and nonlactational. The cause of nonspontaneous discharge from multiple ducts of both breasts is generally pharmacologic or endocrinologic.

The most common of several causes of nipple discharge is mammary duct ectasia, which produces a multicolored (green, yellow, white, brown, gray, or reddish-brown) nipple discharge. The reddish-brown discharge is often mistaken for a bloody discharge. It is thought to be due to an increase in glandular secretions with the production of an irritating lipid fluid that can produce a nipple discharge. Mammary duct ectasia discharge occurs in middle-age women.

The next most common cause of a multicolored, sticky nipple discharge is nonpuerperal mastitis. The persistent type involves inflammation in deeper portions of the breast; the transient types are associated with periareolar inflammation. If the inflammation develops into an inflammatory mass, surgical excision and drainage are necessary. Medical management with local care, avoidance of all nipple manipulation, and nonsteroidal antiinflammatory agents, bromocriptine, and an antistaphylococcal antibiotic is often successful when infection is only suspected.

Intraductal papillomas are the most common cause of bloody nipple discharge. These bloody, persistent discharges warrant further investigation. The risk of cancer is increased when (1) discharge is unilateral from a single duct, (2) discharge occurs in a postmenopausal patient, or (3) a mass is present.

During the breast examination, physicians should look for an associated periareolar mass. The examination consists of gently and carefully palpating the subareolar region to identify the pressure point that produces the discharge. It is important to reproduce the discharge and demonstrate the breast quadrant from which it emanates. All significant nipple discharges warrant referral for tissue biopsy. Although a mass is usually present when the discharge is due to cancer, there is no palpable mass in 13% of cancers with nipple secretions. In addition, physicians should not rely solely on the cytology of the discharge, because there is an 18% false-negative rate and a 2.6% false-positive rate with standard cytology alone. Galactography (injecting radiopaque contrast into the discharging duct and then performing mammography) offers better visualization of small intraductal papillomas but cannot differentiate benign from malignant lesions. A surgical procedure is still necessary. Mammography has a 9.5% false-negative rate and a 1.6% false-positive rate for detecting cancer in patients with a nipple discharge.

A thorough initial history and physical examination should include whether the discharge is recurrent, spontaneous, or unilateral. If the drainage first appeared in the patient's bra or nightgown on awakening, this finding is more significant than discharge during a workout at the gym. It should be noted that postmenopausal discharges are always significant. Spontaneous bloody discharges occurring in the third trimester of pregnancy may be regarded as physiologic and do not require intervention, unless they persist for several months after delivery. Patients with such discharges should be aware of no contraindication to breast-feeding.

Pseudomasses in Adolescence

The risk of breast cancer in an adolescent is negligible. Adolescent breast development begins with formation of a breast bud. The appearance of a breast bud can cause alarm and suspicion of a breast mass. A unilateral lump can occur when one breast develops before the other. FNA or biopsy is not appropriate. Biopsy would only traumatize the young patient and potentially interfere with normal breast development. Ultrasound, only if it is necessary, can make the definitive assessment.

Mastitis

Mastitis is an infection and the most common benign breast problem during pregnancy and lactation. It can cause fever, pain, and swelling. The cause of the infection relates to retained breast milk that provides an ideal medium for bacterial growth. *Staphylococcus aureus* is the most likely causative organism, and antibiotic therapy involves a course of penicillin G or dicloxacillin sodium, 250 mg orally four times a day. Women with mastitis may continue to breast-feed. If the infection does not respond to treatment, an abscess might be present, requiring drainage with continued antibiotic therapy. In refractory cases in which the infection seems to involve the whole breast, it is necessary to rule out inflammatory carcinoma. Galactoceles are milk-filled cysts, probably caused by ductal obstruction. They can be tender and typically occur in the periphery of the breast. Galactoceles are not thought to be associated with a tendency to form breast cysts or with FCC. Aspiration of milk in the cyst, sometimes more than once, usually relieves the condition. Special attention must be paid to the skin and nipple–areolar complex. Persistent crusting of the nipples suggests Paget disease. A biopsy is required under such circumstances, as well as for new, unexplained nipple retractions.

Squamous metaplasia of the breast is a benign process and should not be confused with cancer. It is the most common form of nonpuerperal mastitis. Squamous metaplasia is the transformation of glandular or mucosal epithelium into stratified squamous epithelium. It may occur after trauma when fat necrosis may be thickening and erythema is present. Two types of metaplasia may occur in the breast: apocrine and squamous. It can mimic ductal ectasia or intraductal papillomas. Treatment is simple excision. If recurrent fistulous tracts occur, complete excision of the tract is recommended. The most important step in the differential diagnosis is to rule out an inflammatory cancer. This is done by a simple excisional biopsy of the breast, which constitutes treatment for squamous metaplasia.

◊ BREAST CARCINOMA

Staging

The diagnosis of breast cancer is made by surgical biopsy or radiologic core biopsy. Cytologic FNA in the office leads to a more rapid office diagnosis, allowing physicians to pursue better patient counseling before any surgery. Most cytologic diagnoses are confirmed histologically at the time of definitive surgery.

Staging of breast cancer is done using the tumor-node-metastasis (TNM) system. However, most physicians recognize that this system does not adequately segregate patients and select appropriate surgical treatments. Patients thought to have clinically negative nodes may have histologically positive nodes. It has been demonstrated that 25% of patients presumed to have clinically positive nodes are found to have negative nodes. In addition, it is difficult to accurately estimate tumor size. On palpation, a mass with surrounding inflammation and carcinoma *in situ* may represent an area not entirely composed of malignant cells. The staging must be recorded in hospital tumor registries, as mandated by the American College of Surgeons. Studies also show that 5% of patients have synchronous or multicentric disease, which underscores the need for mammography before cancer treatment.

There are two histologic categories of noninvasive breast cancer: ductal carcinoma *in situ* (DCIS) and lobular carcinoma *in situ* (LCIS); and two categories of invasive breast cancer: infiltrating ductal carcinoma and invasive lobular carcinoma. Statistically, 72% of breast cancers are infiltrating ductal carcinoma; infiltrating lobular tumors represent 10% to 15%. DCIS, LCIS, Paget disease, inflammatory carcinoma, and sarcomas account for the remaining cases.

The Breast Cancer Detection Demonstration Project (BCDDP) recently reported its 20-year follow-up data. Breast cancer screening has definitely resulted in an earlier diagnosis of breast cancer, thus opening the door to more breast-preserving surgical procedures. The BCDDP provided 5 years of screening with physical examination and two-view mammography for 280,000 volunteer women across the United States. Of the 4051 women diagnosed with breast cancer between 1973 and 1980, 2658 (66%) were alive. A high percentage of the tumors was detected by mammography alone, and 28.6% of all the cancers were smaller than 1.0 cm. The adjusted survival rate for the entire group was 80.5%. The observed survival rate was 61.7%. Prognostic indicators of survival were lymph node status and the size of the cancer at diagnosis. The study demonstrated adjusted survival rates of 85.5% among women with invasive cancer and negative lymph nodes and 90.2% for those with invasive cancer smaller than 1 cm.

Treatment Options

The most common treatment options for invasive breast cancer include a modified radical mastectomy or breast-conserving procedures that include a lumpectomy and axillary lymph node dissection with irradiation. Treatment planning for breast cancer includes a multidisciplinary approach. Although each patient should have a primary physician, treatment options require the expertise of not only a surgeon but also a radiotherapist and a medical oncologist. Some states mandate that physicians discuss alternative treatments with patients.

Once the clinical data are reviewed, it is now generally accepted that breast-conserving surgery and irradiation are a valid alternative to mastectomy (Table 5). A consensus development conference for the treatment of early-stage breast

TABLE 5. *Modern randomized trials comparing conservative surgery and radiation with mastectomy*

Trial	Points (n)	Survival at (yr)	Mastectomy (%)	Conservative surgery and radiation (%)
Milan	701	10	76	79
NSABP	1219	10	71	76
WHO	179	8	80	79
NCI	237	8	79	85
Denmark	859	6	82	79
EORTC	874	?	equal	

EORTC, European Organization for Research and Treatment of Cancer; NCI, National Cancer Institute; NSABP, National Surgical Adjuvant Breast Project; WHO, World Health Organization.
(From Wazer, 1997, with permission.)

cancer convened by the National Cancer Institute in June 1990 concluded that "breast conservation treatment is an appropriate method of primary therapy for the majority of women with Stage I and II breast cancer and is preferable because it provides equivalent survival to total mastectomy and axillary node dissection while preserving the breast." Complete removal of the breast with a modified radical mastectomy involves pectoralis major fascia and levels I and II axillary lymph nodes, with preservation of pectoralis muscles. A breast-conserving operation is a wide local excision and resection of the tumor with 1 or 2 cm of adjacent breast tissue. A quadrantectomy is resection of the tumor with the overlying skin and the involved quadrant of the breast. All these procedures are coupled with an axillary lymphatic dissection of levels I and II lymph nodes (removal of the axillary content from the tail of the breast to the latissimus dorsi, the axillary vein superiorly, and the lateral border of the pectoralis to beneath the pectoralis minor medially) (Fig. 5).

From the patient's standpoint, typically even a simple mastectomy is a radical procedure. This procedure implies that the entire breast is removed, including the nipple–areolar complex and the fascia over the pectoralis major muscle. A modified radical mastectomy is the preferred treatment in the following cases:

◊ Patients who have multifocal DCIS or LCIS,
◊ Patients who have tumor recurrence after partial mastectomy and have had axillary dissection or axillary radiation with or without breast irradiation,
◊ In selected patients for whom prophylactic removal of the opposite breast is recommended,
◊ Elderly patients or patients deemed poor operative risks who have no axillary adenopathy or evidence of distant disease,
◊ Patients with bulky or ulcerated lesions and distant metastases for whom local control will improve the quality of life.

Several factors influence the choice of surgical treatment, including size and location of the tumor and size of the breast. Poor candidates for breast preservation are women with large tumors, multifocal diffuse tumors, or small breasts. Age is not

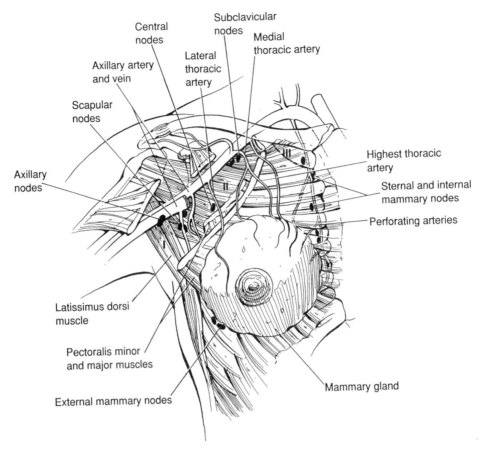

FIG. 5. Lymphatics and blood supply of the breast. Lymphatic drainage from the outer half of the breast goes first to the axillary nodes, shown here a levels I, II, and III. Medial lesions are more likely to metastasize first to the internal mammary chain. (From Rock JA, Thompson JD, eds. *TeLinde's Operative gynecology,* 8th ed. Philadelphia: Lippincott–Raven, 1997; with permission.)

a contraindication to breast preservation. Studies have indicated that even in the best performed subcutaneous mastectomy, breast tissue remains under the areola and is found in other locations in 80% of cases. Subcutaneous mastectomy is no longer recommended because it does not remove all breast tissue. If a truly prophylactic procedure is recommended, it seems reasonable to recommend a complete removal of breast tissue, although there are no studies indicating whether or not removal of 80% of the breast tissue would yield an equivalent reduction in risk. In addition to providing a less than satisfactory prophylactic operation, subcutaneous mastectomy yields variable cosmetic results. When breast cancer is detected early, breast preservation is an option for most patients. Breast-preservation surgery is generally coupled with adjuvant whole-breast radiation therapy when the patient's breast has healed.

Use of conservative surgery and radiotherapy requires consideration of the following criteria: (1) patient selection, (2) surgery of the primary tumor, (3) radiotherapy of the primary tumor, and (4) surgery of the axilla. Poor candidates for breast-conserving treatment include those who have widely separated primary tumors in the same breast, who have large tumors in a relatively small breast, or whose mammograms

reveal diffuse disease in many quadrants. The principal advantage of conservative treatment is cosmetic. There are no data indicating that the conservative approach provides improved survival, compared with radical or modified radical mastectomy. Thus, the major criterion for patient selection is the ability to adequately resect the primary tumor without cosmetic deformity. Patients with central lesions that involve the nipple–areolar complex can be successfully treated by resection of the nipple–areolar complex with careful attention to the final cosmetic result.

Adequate surgical resection implies grossly clear margins. The surgeon must appropriately mark the specimen for orientation by the pathologist. It is important to determine the distance from the tumor to the closest margin of resection. Tissue should be removed for estrogen and progesterone receptor studies without disturbing the evaluation of the resected margins. Microscopic involvement is best determined at the time of the evaluation of the permanent sections. Again, if the surgeon is to reexcise a lesion some weeks after the initial biopsy, it is essential that there be minimal induration and ecchymosis at the operative site; otherwise, it is impossible to define the lesion and provide a satisfactory cosmetic result.

Axillary lymphatic dissection is critical to determining the proper stage of the lymph nodes.

When breast conservation is chosen, the patient's radiotherapy is normally initiated as soon as the wounds are healed. It is generally agreed that the breast should be treated with 1.8 to 2.0 Gy per day for a total of 45 to 50 Gy. Doses in excess of 50 Gy result in fibrosis, retraction, and an unacceptable cosmetic result. For patients treated with wide local excision in whom the margins of resection are close on microscopic evaluation, an additional 10- to 15-Gy electron therapy to the operative area may be recommended.

There is no consensus concerning either the concomitant use of chemotherapy and radiotherapy or a sequence in administering adjuvant chemotherapy with radiotherapy. Such treatment must be decided after consultation with the radiation oncologist and the medical oncologist.

All patients should be presented with the option of breast reconstruction when a mastectomy is recommended. The reconstruction may be performed in conjunction with the primary surgery or delayed. Delay would mean waiting until completion of adjuvant chemotherapy and/or radiation therapy. Thoughts of disfigurement are ever present, and the physical and mental adjustments to the diagnosis of breast cancer and breast removal are an important part of the recovery process. Breast reconstruction is a vital aspect of that recovery process for some patients. The options for reconstruction include prosthetic augmentation with saline-filled implants or reconstruction with a myocutaneous flap, such as the rectus abdominis muscles. Decisions concerning reconstruction are made by the patient and her surgical team. Those decisions vary according to medical problems, prior surgery, and physique.

The role of axillary lymph node dissection in the conservative management of breast cancer is well established. The nodes serve as a guide for recommendations regarding systemic therapy. Surgeons no longer remove all three node levels, but customarily remove level I and a portion of level II lymph nodes. Axillary node dissections can be associated with chronic edema (5%), seromas (10%), paresthesias (3% to 4%), and pain.

Breast cancer specialists are considering lymphatic mapping and a sentinel node biopsy as an alternative to the standard dissection of levels I and II nodes. Such a procedure would further decrease complications while securing the same prognostic information. Patients undergo lymphoscintigraphy before surgery and are injected with a colloid tracer that identifies the lymphatic basins at risk for metastatic disease and the location of the sentinel node(s). Intraoperatively, radiocolloid is injected around the primary tumor and taken up by the lymphatic system. A hand-held gamma-detection probe that measures the radiolabeled colloid injected during lymphoscintigraphy is used intraoperatively to confirm the location of the sentinel node (Fig. 6). The procedure is especially effective because it allows the surgeon to give the pathologist only one or two sentinel lymph nodes. If these nodes are negative for malignancy, no further nodal dissec-

tion is necessary. If micrometastases are identified within the sentinel node or the sentinel node did not map, then the standard lymph node dissection is carried out. In the lymphatic mapping procedure, the sensitivity can be further increased with immunohistochemical staining, serial sectioning, and reverse transcriptase-polymerase chain reaction analysis of the sentinel node.

The Comprehensive Breast Program at the H. Lee Moffitt Cancer Center in Tampa, Florida, reported on 62 newly diagnosed breast cancer patients who underwent mapping. The sentinel node procedure was successful in 57 (92%) of the patients. Eighteen patients (29%) were found to have metastatic disease, and the sentinel node tested positive in all of them. There were no "skip" metastases, defined as a sentinel node that tested negative with a higher node that tested positive.

In Situ Carcinoma

Intraductal carcinoma *in situ* (DCIS) is breast cancer in which the cellular abnormalities are limited to the ductal epithelium and have not penetrated the base membrane. DCIS is not usually detected by palpation because the disease does not produce a definitive mass. It is classified into four histologic types based on architectural pattern: comedo, micropapillary, cribriform, or solid. Others have generalized the classification into comedo or noncomedo types. With the advent of screening mammography, the incidence of DCIS has increased to 20% of mammographically detected breast cancers. DCIS is generally believed to be a multicentric disease.

Mastectomy is the standard treatment for DCIS. There is approximately a 1% recurrence rate at 10 years, and the incidence of node positivity is less than 1%. The frequency of multicentricity is higher in the comedo than in the noncomedo types of DCIS. In cases of unifocal DCIS, breast preservation may be attempted. It is imperative that the surgical margins be clear, and radiation therapy is generally given to the residual breast tissue.

The National Surgical Adjuvant Breast Project (NSABP) B-17 protocol found a 5-year actuarial recurrence rate of 10% for lumpectomy with radiation compared to a rate of 21% with excision alone. The Breast Center in Van Nuys, California, is now further defining the risk of recurrence and the need for radiation or mastectomy. The Van Nuys Prognostic Index assigns lesions a score from 1 to 3 for each of three factors: tumor size, margin width, and pathologic classification (determined by nuclear grade and necrosis). In this manner, it may be possible to identify subgroups of patients who do not require irradiation. Although cure rates with mastectomy exceed 96%, breast preservation is frequently attempted to improve the cosmetic result. Since the incidence of nodal disease is low, patients with DCIS may wish to consider lymphatic mapping of the sentinel node to identify spread. Lymph node dissection in the majority of patients with DCIS is unnecessary.

An incidental finding in breast biopsies performed either because of a mammographic abnormality or a palpable mass is LCIS. It is very difficult to detect LCIS during a clinical

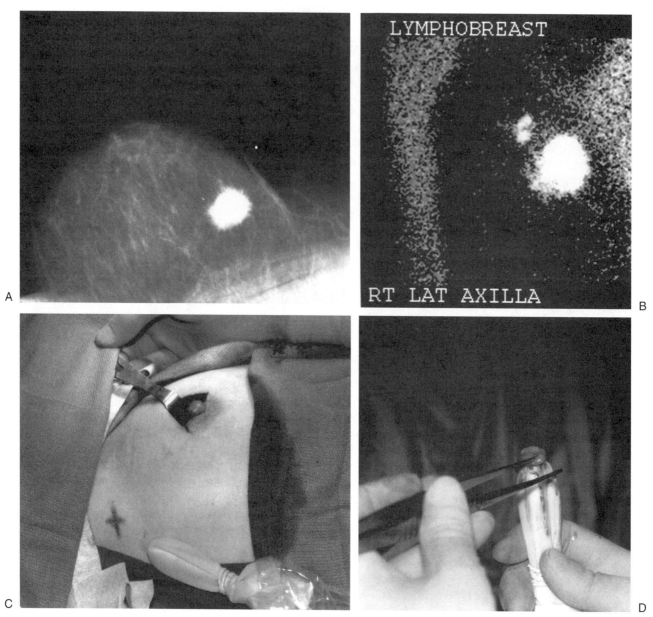

FIG. 6. A: Mammographic and palpable *(marker)* spiculated breast cancer. **B:** Lymphoscintigraphy. The larger white density corresponds to the breast cancer, while the smaller adjacent density represents the sentinel lymph node. **C:** The periareolar breast cancer has been excised, and the sentinel axillary lymph node marked *(X)* with the adjacent neoprobe. **D:** The isolated lymph node is excised and placed directly on the neoprobe to confirm uptake of the colloid tracer.

examination. There may be subtle breast thickening on palpation or subtle parenchymal thickening on mammographic screening. LCIS is found in 3% to 6% of breast biopsies. It is now accepted by most authorities as a genetic marker of predisposition for cancer. This cancer may be ductal, lobular, medullary, and so on and may affect *either* breast. A majority of surgeons concur that LCIS should be considered a risk factor only, such as a strong family history. Treatment for LCIS is wide local excisional biopsy alone. Patients with LCIS should receive the same careful breast cancer surveillance given patients with a strong family history of breast cancer.

Prognostic Factors

The primary prognostic factors used for metastatic disease are nodal status and tumor size. It is a proven fact that cancer screening has led to locating smaller tumors at the time of diagnosis. Women with tumors with a maximum size of 1 cm or less have a recurrence rate of less than 10%. With earlier diagnosis secondary to patient education and better mammography equipment, two-thirds of newly diagnosed breast cancers will have negative axillary nodes. Axillary lymph node status is the most important factor in the prognosis of patients with breast cancer. Patients with negative axillary nodes and tumors less than 2 cm have shown a recurrence rate of 11% compared to 22% for 2- to 3-cm tumors and 24% for tumors larger than 5 cm. Tumor size is independently important in predicting recurrence. The number of positive lymph nodes corresponds with the survival rate for patients. Tumor recurrences increase from 30% for patients with node-negative disease to 55% to 60% for patients with one to three lymph positive nodes and 85% to 90% for patients with four or more positive nodes. Gross nodal involvement is an adverse prognostic factor, compared to microscopic disease. Since recurrent disease will eventually develop in 25% to 30% of node-negative patients, who will die, other biologic prognostic factors are needed.

These factors include (1) estrogen receptor (ER) status, (2) vascular/lymphatic invasion, (3) tumor proliferation activity, (4) grade, and (5) histologic subtype. A high nuclear grade is associated with a high rate of relapse. Several well characterized histologic subtypes impact a favorable prognosis. These subtypes include tubular, colloid (mucinous), and papillary tumors. Invasive lobular and medullary lesions are intermediate, whereas signet-ring carcinoma and sarcomatoid carcinoma carry an unfavorable prognosis. It is standard practice to determine the presence of both estrogen and progesterone receptors at the time of diagnosis. ER-positive patients have an 8% to 10% better prognosis than ER-negative patients at 5 years. Peritumoral lymphatic and blood vessel invasion is an adverse prognostic factor independent of menopausal status and tumor size. The risk of recurrence is 4.7 times greater for patients with vascular/lymphatic invasion compared to those without it. Approximately 25% of all breast cancers and 15% of node-negative breast cancers show vascular/ lymphatic invasion.

Several investigational biologic markers are available for evaluating the risk of relapse. These include *erb B2 (NEU)* oncogene protein product, epidermal growth factor receptor, cathepsin D, quantification of microvessels, p53 expression, haptoglobin-related protein, heat shock protein, and PS2. Although these factors have predictive value, none meets the 90% specificity level for predicting the presence or absence of micrometastatic disease. Tumor proliferation activity can be assessed morphologically by mitotic counts or by simple immunohistochemical methods. Measurements of cellular proliferation in breast cancer specimens using a variety of techniques have shown a strong correlation with outcome. DNA flow cytometry provides an accurate and objective evaluation of cell cycle and is less laborious than thymidine-labeling index. The DNA content and S-phase fraction of the tumor are simultaneously measured. Tumors with a low S-phase fraction (less than 4.4% for diploid tumors and less than 7.0% for aneuploid tumors) had a better 5-year disease-free survival rate than patients with high S-phase fractions. Patients with a high S-phase fraction and micrometastatic disease are more likely to have recurrent disease.

Adjuvant Treatment

Several factors influence disease prognosis and the decision for recommending adjuvant therapy. These factors include tumor size, nodal status, histology, menopausal status or age, grade, ER status, slow or rapid progression, prior treatment, and evidence of metastatic disease. For half of patients, the decision regarding adjuvant therapy is straightforward. About 25% have small tumors (less than 1 cm) and favorable histologic types and should not be treated. Another 25% have large tumors, which are often associated with poor prognostic features, and most of these patients should be treated. The remaining 50% of candidates for adjuvant therapy have tumors of intermediate size. They constitute the group for which the above mentioned prognostic factors may be helpful.

Several studies have shown that mortality can be reduced by at least 20% in pre- and postmenopausal women with adjuvant therapy. In one study, adjuvant systemic chemotherapy decreased the odds of dying from breast cancer during the first 10 years following diagnosis by 25%. Adjuvant therapy in high-risk groups has shown a definite and sustained benefit in reducing both recurrence and mortality rates. Polychemotherapy improves outcomes for pre- and postmenopausal women, but this benefit appears to be greater in the menopausal group. In postmenopausal compared with premenopausal patients, there is greater improvement with tamoxifen citrate (Nolvadex), especially with ER-positive tumors. In some studies, chemotherapy has been shown to benefit postmenopausal patients. This is especially true in ER-negative patients at high risk of recurrence. A medical risk assessment is necessary for deciding which postmenopausal patient to treat with chemotherapy.

It is recommended that adjuvant chemotherapy be given to all premenopausal node-negative patients whose tumor is greater than 1 cm. Tamoxifen may help all postmenopausal node-positive and node-negative patients with tumors greater than 1 cm. If these patients are ER-negative, the risk–benefit analysis should guide whether or not chemotherapy is instituted. Adding tamoxifen to a chemotherapy regime is controversial. For postmenopausal patients, ER protein status becomes more important in the choice of therapy.

Several chemotherapy combinations are available. The following drugs and combinations have been used for therapy: cyclophosphamide, methotrexate, and fluorouracil (CMF), cyclophosphamide, doxorubicin (Adriamycin), and fluorouracil (CAF), or fluorouracil, doxorubicin, and cyclophosphamide (FAC). Another active drug in breast cancer is paclitaxel (Taxol), even in patients with prior doxorubicin exposure. Adjuvant tamoxifen reduces recurrence and mortality rates. However, tamoxifen carries some increased risk of endometrial cancer, which is a drawback.

Patients in the NSABP B-14 study were treated with tamoxifen, 20 mg per day, or placebo. When tamoxifen was given, there was an elevated risk of endometrial cancer developing in 2 in 1000. Tamoxifen-treated patients should have an annual gynecologic examination, and an evaluation should be performed in postmenopausal women with any vaginal bleeding. The role of intravaginal ultrasonography and random endometrial biopsies remains unclear and needs further study. If a typical hyperplasia of the endometrium develops, tamoxifen should be discontinued, or a hysterectomy should be considered.

Adjuvant radiotherapy to the axilla is generally recommended in patients who have more than three lymph nodes involved with tumor or have extracapsular lymph node spread. Patients with multiple abnormal lymph noes (10 or more) have a 70% risk of recurrence at 10 years and may wish to consider institutional protocols using high-dose therapy with bone marrow or peripheral blood stem cell support. The toxicity may be significant, including arm edema and fibrosis and limitation of range of motion. Axillary radiotherapy clearly controls regional disease, so patients should weigh the potential benefits with these risks.

Follow-up

Patients with a history of breast cancer need to be evaluated for both locoregional recurrence and a second breast cancer. Mammography must be routinely done on the unaffected breast once a year. If breast conservation is performed, it is recommended that cancer screening of the affected breast be performed every 6 months for the first 5 years. After that time, annual examinations including a history, physical examination, and mammography should provide sufficient surveillance. The risk of recurrence is 2% to 5% per year from years 2 to 6, dropping to 1% per year thereafter. Many tests, including tumor markers, computed tomography, are bone scans, are available to physicians and practitioners for follow-up evaluations. However, when intensive follow-up is compared with follow-up without these tests, there is no difference in survival rate.

Genetics/Family History

The area of genetics and family history is the new trend of the future. Genetic testing for inherited cancer susceptibility will play an increasingly important role in health care. When a patient is diagnosed with breast cancer, she reviews her family history. Other family members become concerned about the disease and ask about the contribution of a heritable predisposition. One must attempt to distinguish women carrying mutations in breast cancer susceptibility genes where the risk of disease is extremely high for other women in their families. The identification of new breast cancer susceptibility genes, *BRCA1* and *BRCA2,* has led to commercial availability of genetic testing for breast and ovarian cancer susceptibility. The clinical application of this information is not clear at this time.

The risk factors examined for determining the probability of an individual's carrying a *BRCA1* or *BRCA2* mutation include age at the time of diagnosis of breast or ovarian cancer, number and age at diagnosis of first- and second-degree rel-

atives with breast or ovarian cancer in the same parental lineage, the occurrence of any other associated tumors (e.g., prostate cancer) in the same lineage, and ethnicity. The best person to be tested is the family member with the cancer. A statement on genetic testing by the American Society of Clinical Oncology defined families with a high (greater than 10%) probability of a *BRCA1* mutation as follows:

◊ A family with two or more breast cancer cases and one or more cases of ovarian cancer diagnosed at any age,
◊ A family with three or more breast cancer cases diagnosed before age 50 years,
◊ Sister pairs with two breast cancers, two ovarian cancers, or a breast and an ovarian cancer, all diagnosed before age 50 years.

Genetic testing for inherited cancer susceptibility can affect an individual's personal, psychological, social, financial, and ethical well-being. The beneficial effects of this testing are not yet clear. Individuals considering genetic testing for inherited cancer susceptibility should receive appropriate education and pretest genetic counseling. Then, they can make an informed decision as to whether or not to proceed with testing. When the testing is complete, counseling and follow-up care must again be provided. Individuals considering genetic testing should be informed that there are currently no methods proven to reduce or prevent the risk of cancer in persons who harbor mutations.

Retrospective data in a recent abstract from the Mayo Clinic reported a 91% breast cancer reduction among the 2500 high-risk cases who underwent prophylactic surgery at the center. Prophylactic mastectomy is considered one option for some women with known genetic susceptibility to breast cancer. A total mastectomy is more effective than a subcutaneous mastectomy. From a population where 76 cancers were expected to occur, only nine were located. Future chemoprevention trials may hold potential promise in upcoming years. No data are yet available to quantify the risk reduction of breast cancer in women with *BRCA1* or *BRCA2* mutation.

Individuals who have negative genetic test results could still be at risk on the basis of age, environment, or other genetic factors or unknown mutations. They should be advised to continue annual cancer screening. Genetic susceptibility testing is a complex issue. Physicians should identify qualified professionals in their area who can provide genetic counseling and testing for patients who desire testing.

◊ CONCLUSION

Breast cancer can now be diagnosed at an early stage. The obstetrician-gynecologist is in the ideal situation to make an early diagnosis through patient education about proper screening techniques and through performance of a comprehensive breast examination. The American College of Obstetricians and Gynecologists (ACOG) has recommended breast cancer screening and adopted as goals the full education of obstetrician-gynecologists in the diagnosis and treatment of benign breast diseases and the reduction of mortality from breast cancer. To accomplish these goals, obstetrician/gynecologists must now recognize (1) that the breast examination, inspection, and palpation are integral parts of a complete examination, (2) that patients should be instructed in lifelong breast self-examinations, and (3) that screening mammography should be encouraged in all women.

The American Cancer Society now recommends annual mammography starting at age 40. Earlier screening should be performed in women who have first-degree relatives with breast cancer or who themselves had a prior breast cancer.

Women with breast symptoms should be evaluated. The first step in evaluation is distinguishing a dominant mass from FCC. If a mass is discrete and palpable, cyst aspiration should be performed to determine whether it is solid or cystic. Cancer must be ruled out in all solid masses. FNA can serve as an intermediate step in cancer diagnosis, but the majority of patients will require histologic tissue confirmation with a breast biopsy. The obstetrician-gynecologist should accept the responsibility for referring patients to a specialized physician, after carrying out the initial diagnostic steps. Diagnostic mammography and/or ultrasonography are warranted in symptomatic women. When a referral becomes necessary, ACOG emphasizes that the obstetrician-gynecologist should explain to patients the need for further care and provide the names of qualified physicians, as well as answering patient questions. The ACOG also encourages both clinical and basic research into the etiology, early diagnosis, and treatment of all breast diseases. This should be carried out through residency training programs and continuing medical education. Education should also concern early diagnosis and management options.

The majority of breast cancers are diagnosed at stages I and II due to improved screening modalities. Breast-preserving operations (lumpectomy with axillary lymph node dissection) have equivalent long-term survival rates to modified radical mastectomy. The National Institutes of Health recommends breast preservation as the preferred procedure, whenever possible. Radiotherapy to the breast is recommended when breast preservation is chosen.

Adjuvant chemotherapy or hormonal therapy has been shown to diminish recurrence rates and improve survival rates in patients with tumors larger than 1 cm or positive lymph nodes. Newer diagnostic techniques such as stereotactic CNB and lymphatic mapping of the sentinel node are being incorporated into medical practices. These procedures are designed to be less invasive while offering the same clinical information. At present, they require special expertise due to steep learning curves but are expected to be standard practices in the not too distant future.

Obstetrician-gynecologists are in a prime position to diagnose breast cancer. They should seize the opportunity to cure patients through early diagnosis. All are encouraged to do their part in breast cancer screening and treatment when warranted.

◊ RECOMMENDED READINGS

Albertini JJ, Lyman GH, Cox C, et al. Lymphatic mapping and sentinel node biopsy in the patient with breast cancer. *JAMA* 1996;276:1818–1822.

American College of Obstetricians and Gynecologists. *Non-malignant conditions of the breast. Technical Bulletin No. 156.* Washington, DC: American College of Obstetricians and Gynecologists, 1991.

American College of Obstetricians and Gynecologists. *Carcinoma of the breast. Technical bulletin no. 158.* Washington, DC: American College of Obstetricians and Gynecologists, 1991.

American College of Obstetricians and Gynecologists. *The role of the obstetrician-gynecologist in the diagnosis and treatment of breast disease. Committee opinion no. 186.* Washington, DC: American College of Obstetricians and Gynecologists, 1997.

American College of Radiology. *Breast imaging reporting and data system* (BI-RADS), 2nd ed. Reston, VA: American College of Radiology, 1995.

Andersson I. Results from the Malmo breast screening trial. Presented at the National Institutes of Health consensus development conference: breast cancer screening for women ages 40–49, Bethesda, MD, January 21–23, 1997.

Basset L, Winchester DP, Caplan RB, et al. Stereotactic core-needle biopsy of the breast: a report of the joint task force of the American College of Radiology, American College of Surgeons, and College of American Pathologists. *CA Cancer J Clin* 1997;47:171–190.

Berry DA, Parmigiani G, Sanchez J, et al. Probability of carrying a mutation of breast-ovarian cancer gene BRCA1 based on family history. *J Natl Cancer Inst* 1197;89:227–238.

Bjurstam N, Bjornel L, Duffy SW. The Gothenburg breast cancer screening trial: results from 11 years' follow-up. Presented at the National Institutes of Health consensus development conference: breast cancer screening for women ages 40–49, Bethesda, MD, January 21–23, 1997.

Consensus development conference on the treatment of early-stage breast cancer. *J Natl Cancer Inst Monogr* 1992;11:1.

Diamond TM, Sutphen R, Tabano M, Fiorica JV. Inherited susceptibility to breast and ovarian cancer. *Curr Opin Obstet Gynecol* 1998;10:3–8.

Donegan WL. Tumor-related prognostic factors for breast cancer. *CA Cancer J Clin* 1997;47:28–51.

Fisher B, Bauer M, Wickerham DL, et al. Relations of number of positive axillary nodes to the prognosis of patients with primary breast cancer: an NSABP update. *Cancer* 1983;52:1551–1557.

Fisher ER, Paleker A, Rockette H, et al. Pathologic findings from the National Surgical Adjuvant Breast Project (protocol no. 4) V. Significance of axillary nodal micro- and macrometastases. *Cancer* 1978;42:2032–2038.

Goldhirsch A, Wood WC, Senn H-J, et al. Meeting highlights: international consensus panel on treatment of primary breast cancer. *J Natl Cancer Inst* 1995;87:1141–1145.

Harmann L, Jenkins R, Scheid D, Tang P. Prophylactic mastectomy (PM): preliminary retrospective cohort analysis. *Proc Am Assoc Cancer Res* 1997;77:168(abst).

Henderson IC, Danner D. Legal pitfalls in the diagnosis and management of breast cancer. *Hematol Oncol Clin North Am* 1989;3:823–842.

Hendrick RE, Smith RA, Rutledge JH, et al. Benefit of screening mammography in women ages 40–49: a meta-analysis of new randomized controlled trial results. Presented at the National Institutes of Health consensus development conference: breast cancer screening for women ages 40–49, Bethesda, MD, January 21–23, 1997.

Lee NC. Results from the National Breast and Cervical Cancer Early Detection Program, 1991–1995. Presented at the National Institutes of Health consensus development conference: breast cancer screening for women ages 40–49, Bethesda, MD, January 21–23, 1997.

Leitch AM, Dodd GD, Costanza M, et al. American Cancer Society guidelines for the early detection of breast cancer: update 1997. *CA Cancer J Cin* 1997;47:150–153.

Linver MN. Mammography outcomes in a practice setting by age: prognostic factors, sensitivity, and positive biopsy rate. Presented at the National Institutes of Health consensus development conference: breast cancer screening for women ages 40–49, Bethesda, MD, January 21–23, 1997.

Marchant DJ. Invasive breast cancer: surgical treatment alternatives. In: Marchant DJ, ed. *Breast disease.* Philadelphia: WB Saunders, 1997:179–193.

McGuire WL, Clark GM. Prognostic factors and treatment decisions in axillary node-negative breast cancer. *N Engl J Med* 1992;326:1756–1761.

McKinnon WC, Baty BJ, Bennett RL, et al. Predisposition genetic testing for late-onset disorder in adults: a position paper of the National Society of Genetic Counselors. *JAMA* 1997;278:1217–1220.

Parker SL, Tong T, Bolden S, et al. Cancer statistics, 1997. *CA Cancer J Clin* 1997;47:5–27.

Recht A, Silen W, Schnitt SJ, et al. Time-course of local recurrence following conservative surgery and radiotherapy for early stage breast cancer. *Int J Radiat Oncol Biol Phys* 1988;15:255–261.

Report of the consensus development conference panel on breast cancer screening for women ages 40–49, January 21–23, 1997, Bethesda, MD. Bethesda, MD: National Institutes of Health, 1997.

Rosselli Del Turco M, Palli D, Cariddi A, et al. Intensive diagnostic follow-up after treatment of primary breast cancer. *JAMA* 1994;271:1593–1597.

Sickles EA. Screening outcomes: clinical experience with service screening using modern mammography. Presented at the National Institutes of Health consensus development conference: breast cancer screening for women ages 40–49, Bethesda, MD, January 21–23, 1997.

Silverstein MJ. Ductal Carcinoma *in situ* of the breast: the Van Nuys experience by treatment. *Breast J* 1997;3:232–237.

Smart CR, Byrne C, Smith RA, et al. Twenty-year follow-up of the breast cancer detection demonstration project. *CA Cancer J Clin* 1997;47:134–149.

Statement of the Amercian Society of Clincial Oncology: genetic testing for cancer susceptibility. *J Clin Oncol* 1988;14:1730–1738.

Swedish Cancer Society and Swedish National Board of Health and Welfare. Breast-cancer screening with mammography in women aged 40–49 years. *Int J Cancer* 1996;68:693–699.

Tabar L, Fagerberg G, Chen HH, et al. Tumour development, histology and grade of breast cancers: prognosis and progression. *Int J Cancer* 1996;66:413–419.

Wazer D. Radiation therapy in the management of early invasive breast cancer. In: Marchant DJ, ed. *Breast disease.* Philadelphia: WB Saunders,1997;195–201.

CHAPTER 41

Infertility and Assisted Reproduction

◇

Charles B. Hammond
Robert J. Stillman

Confusion exists regarding terms used in discussing human reproduction. Without clarity in such terms, it is very difficult for physicians and their patients to carefully evaluate alternatives in diagnosis and treatment of infertility problems. Many use the term *infertility* in various ways that often interfere with accurate communication. Table 1 provides definitions of terms used in discussions of human reproduction. In practice, a couple with relatively normal fertility will conceive within 1 year of regular coitus, if no contraception is used. No conception in 1 year of trying implies infertility, but if it is proven that conception is impossible, then the proper definition is *sterility*. Measures of probability of conception per cycle are one of the more meaningful ways to evaluate the reproductive performance of couples and advise them of the benefit of specific therapies; this is usually described as *cycle fecundity* or *fecundability*. Cycle fecundity, although a population-based measure, is the most useful single decision-making parameter in the care of infertile couples.

In the United States, about 2.5 million married couples are infertile.[14] The number of infertile couples and the overall incidence of infertility in the United States have not changed significantly in the past several decades. However, the number of physician office visits for infertility has dramatically risen in this interval. The likely factors in this increased demand for infertility services are numerous but seem to relate to increased problems resulting from delayed childbearing, expectations of the reproductive-age population, the decreased number of infants available for adoption, remarkable progress in available reproductive technologies, and increased social acceptability of being infertile and attempting to treat the problem. One measurable factor that clearly affects fertility is maternal age.[23,40] As shown in Figure 1, marital age-specific fertility rates in a series of historical populations in which contraception was not used show a dramatic decline after 35 years of age and are essentially nil for a number of years before the median age of menopause (i.e., 50 years). Much of this decline can be attrib-

uted to gradual alteration in ovulatory function; delay of childbearing also increases the risk of development of endometriosis and intercurrent injury, such as tubal occlusion and pelvic adhesions from pelvic inflammatory disease. None of these diagnostic categories is novel, but the relative incidences of various diagnoses may be quite different from those reported in previous decades because of the sociologic factors described.

◇ EVALUATION

The traditional approach to the diagnostic assessment of human infertility has been simply to follow the path of sperm up the genital tract to the point of fertilization and subsequent implantation. This conceptual approach suits our biologic understanding but is not representative of an efficient and practical diagnostic approach. As an alternative, infertility categories can be defined by diagnostic test groups. In this concept, there are three groups of factors:

◇ Male gamete factor,
◇ Female gamete factor,
◇ Female genital tract factors.

This simplified concept is compatible with the nature of the available diagnostic tests and is easy to explain to patients as their evaluation is undertaken.

◇ DIAGNOSIS AND TREATMENT

Male Gamete Factor

If the male partner produces no sperm, then azoospermia is the diagnosis, and the couple has sterility on the basis of male factor. Compromises of spermatogenesis that result in decreased number, motility, or fertilizing capability of spermatozoa are much harder to define. Many criteria have been applied to semen analysis results in an attempt to distinguish

TABLE 1. *Definitions of terms used in human fertility*

Term	Literal definition[a]	Practical definition
Fertile/fertility	Capable of conceiving and bearing young	Spontaneous conception in less than 1 year[b]; usually implies progression of pregnancy beyond the first trimester; may imply delivery of living infant
Sterile/sterility	Bearing no progeny	Incapable of conception
Infertile/infertility	Diminished or absent fertility; does not imply as irreversible a condition as sterility	No conception in 1 year or more[b]
Fecund/fecundity	Pronounced fertility; capability of repeated fecundation (impregnation)	Probability of achieving pregnancy each menstrual cycle[b]; also called cycle fecundity or fecundability
Prolific/prolificacy	Bearing many children	Number of fetuses or living infants per conception

[a] From *Stedman's Medical Dictionary,* 22nd ed. Baltimore: Williams & Wilkins, 1972.
[b] Assumes that the couple is not practicing contraception.

fertile from infertile men, but this effort has been frustrated by both the surprising fertility of some men with poor counts and the great variability in counts that is known to occur even in normal fertile men. Table 2 lists usual accepted standard semen analysis parameters. If a semen analysis falls below these measures of count and motility, then further evaluation of the male partner is appropriate, although some men in this category are fertile. Figure 2 shows an algorithmic approach to the evaluation of male infertility. A systemic evaluation is important but beyond the scope of this chapter. In brief, diagnoses resulting from such an evaluation range from normal findings on further seminal testing to a wide range of endocrine disorders, anatomic obstructions of the male system, and failure of the spermatogenic production constituents.[24,38,43] It is important to note, however, that with newer technologic advances in assisted reproduction (e.g., intracytoplasmic injection of sperm), pregnancy can now be accomplished where only a few years ago it was impossible because of very reduced sperm counts or other problems in sperm production. The incidence of ejaculatory dysfunction, including many forms of azoospermia, or sexual dysfunction in infertility populations is not well documented, but some

infertile couples benefit from urologic or psychiatric counseling services with a focus on sexual dysfunction problems.

Female Gamete Factor

The periodic shedding of an ovum is necessary for conception, and women who are physiologically anovulatory, such as prepubertal children, castrated women, and late postmenopausal women, are sterile. Infertility caused by an ovulatory problem in reproductive-age women is more difficult to define because all available measures in the clinical setting are indirect. In other words, the only absolute proof that ovulation has occurred is detection of a conception or observation of an egg outside the ovary. All other measures are indirect; these include menstrual rhythm, basal body temperature (BBT), changes in cervical mucus, systemic symptomatology, ovulation test kits, endometrial biopsy, serum progesterone levels, ultrasound monitoring of follicle growth and collapse, and oral and vaginal electrical resistance.[3] Therefore, all such tests of ovulation have some false-positive and some false-negative results. Consequently, the clinical significance of normal but rarely occurring ovulation (i.e., oligoovulation)

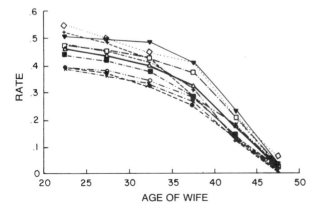

FIG. 1. Marital age-specific fertility rates of 10 historic populations. The common age pattern is shown (△–△). (From ref. 23; with permission.)

TABLE 2. *Standard semen analysis*

Parameter	Average values
Consistency	Fluid (after liquefaction)
Color	Opaque
Liquefaction time	≤20 min
pH	7.2–7.8
Volume	2–6 ml
Motility (grades 0–4)	≥50%
Count (millions/ml)	20–100
Viability (eosin)	≥50%
Morphology (cytology) cell types	≥60% normal oval
Cells (white blood cells, others)	None to occasional
Agglutination	None
Biochemical studies (e.g., fructose, prostaglandins, zinc) if desired	

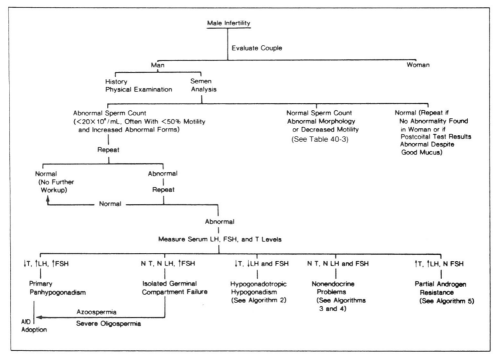

Algorithm 1.—Diagnostic evaluation of potentially infertile man. LH indicates luteinizing hormone; FSH, follicle-stimulating hormone; T, testosterone; N, normal; AID, artificial insemination donor.

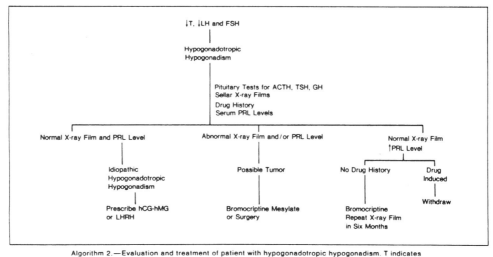

Algorithm 2.—Evaluation and treatment of patient with hypogonadotropic hypogonadism. T indicates testosterone; LH, luteinizing hormone; FSH, follicle-stimulating hormone; ACTH, adrenocorticotropic hormone; TSH, thyroid-stimulating hormone; GH, growth hormone; PRL, prolactin; hCG, human chorionic gonadotropin; hMG, menotropins (human menopausal gonadotropin); LHRH, gonadotropin releasing hormone (leuteinizing hormone-releasing hormone).

A

FIG. 2 A and **B.** Algorithms for the diagnosis and management of male infertility. (From ref. 38, with permission.)

and abnormal ovarian cycles (i.e., ovulatory dysfunction) remains a point of diagnostic contention among some infertility experts. Relatively subtle abnormalities of ovarian cycles can be practically grouped together, but there are definable subsets. Although it is not clear that detailed characterization of dysfunctional cycles is essential before the initiation of rational therapy, advances in the management of ovulatory dysfunction have probably been limited by inadequate scrutiny and subgrouping of study subjects. Numerous names given to abnormal ovarian cycles include anovulatory cycles, luteal-

phase deficiency, luteal-phase defect, short luteal phase, poor progesterone surge, luteinized unruptured follicle syndrome, and poor preovulatory follicular maturation. Although no broad-based prospective study of human populations will probably ever permit absolute characterization of the incidence and consequences of these entities, studies in animals such as rhesus monkeys and sheep strongly suggest that cycle fecundity is profoundly decreased in such abnormal cycles.

Thus, several diagnostic tests are available for assessing ovulatory function. A patient's history of menstrual interval is

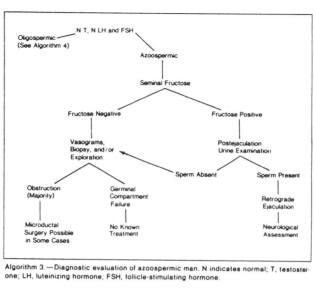

Algorithm 3.—Diagnostic evaluation of azoospermic man. N indicates normal; T, testosterone; LH, luteinizing hormone; FSH, follicle-stimulating hormone.

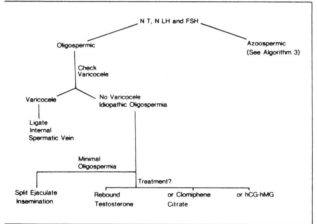

Algorithm 4.—Diagnostic evaluation of oligospermic man. N indicates normal; T, testosterone; LH, luteinizing hormone; FSH, follicle-stimulating hormone; hCG, human chorionic gonadotropin; hMG, menotropins (human menopausal gonadotropin).

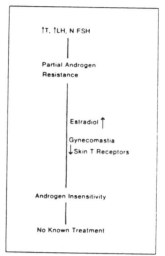

Algorithm 5.—Diagnostic evaluation of patient with partial androgen resistance. T indicates testosterone; LH, luteinizing hormone; FSH, follicle-stimulating hormone; N, normal.

B

FIG. 2. *Continued*

the defining parameter for distinguishing anovulation from normal or abnormal but cyclic ovarian function. Even if a patient is having relatively regular menses at a normal interval of 28 ± 2 days, additional tests are indicated to distinguish normal ovulatory function from abnormal cycles. The traditional BBT chart can be reassuring if measurements are normal, but it is difficult to interpret if it does not show a clear-cut stepwise shift of temperature at midcycle with an appropriate luteal interval of 12 ± 2 days. Figure 3 shows a normal biphasic BBT pattern for a group of presumably ovulatory subjects. In general, if a BBT chart looks normal, the clinician can be somewhat reassured, but confirmation of ovulatory status with additional testing (e.g., serum progesterone, endometrial biopsy) is usually appropriate. If the chart looks extremely abnormal or has a subtler change, such as a slow midcycle temperature rise or an apparently short luteal interval, then additional testing of ovulation is required to distinguish normal ovulatory function from ovulatory dysfunction.

Endometrial biopsy is commonly used to evaluate ovulatory dysfunction, and at the time of its initial validation, this technique was estimated to be about 80% accurate relative to menstrual interval, BBT charts, and progesterone levels. Direct measurement of serum progesterone levels also provides useful assessment of normality of ovarian cycles. A single midluteal progesterone level greater than 15 ng/ml is more than 80% accurate in distinguishing normal from abnormal cycles. Values between 10 and 15 ng/ml are often found in both normal and abnormal cycles, whereas values less than 10 ng/ml are rare in normal cycles, especially if samples are drawn during the morning hours and in the *mid*luteal interval. A powerful and persuasive assessment of ovarian function is the cycle profile. In this approach, detailed analysis of a cycle is generated by daily samples for a panel of reproductive hormones and by serial ultrasound scans to monitor follicle growth and subsequent collapse. Figure 4 shows such normal cycle profiles and represents the state-of-the-art characterization of

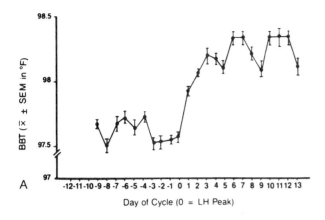

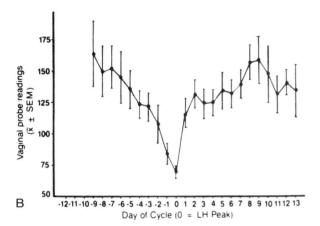

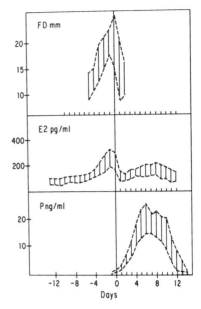

FIG. 4. Normal cycle profiles of follicular diameter *(FD)*, estradiol *(E₂)*, and progesterone *(P)* in 20 spontaneous ovulatory cycles. The 95% confidence intervals are shown. From the midluteal point onward, *n*=12 days since conception occurred in 8 of the 20 cycles. (From ref. 18, with permission.)

FIG. 3. Changes in *(A)* basal body temperature *(BBT)* and *(B)* vaginal electrical resistance during presumably normal ovulatory menstrual cycles. Note the coincidence of the luteinizing hormone *(LH)* surge with the distinct vaginal electrical resistance nadir. (From Albrecht BH, Fernando RS, Regas J, et al. A new method for predicting and confirming ovulation. *Fertil Steril* 1987;47:82; with permission.)

normal ovarian function. Such a detailed approach to cycle function is not a practical screening test; however, it does provide a potential standard with which other diagnostic tests can be compared. One such newer test is daily measurement of salivary and vaginal electrical resistance (see Fig. 3). Patients can easily take these readings and document characteristic resistance changes, which have greater than 80% correlation with more intensive cycle-monitoring schemes. Because these resistance changes precede ovulation in the cycle, such a self-administered test should be useful in timing such activities as coitus and insemination. Other, newer self-administered ovulation predictor tests depend on monoclonal antibodies to human luteinizing hormone (LH)[29] and immunosorbent colorimetric dipstick testing of urine samples. Semiquantitative color changes indicate recent occurrence of the LH surge and therefore would be expected to slightly anticipate the ovulatory event. These urine LH tests appear helpful in characterizing cycle events and improving the timing of intercourse because they predict ovulation in advance, compared to BBT

charts. Correlation of results obtained with LH kits from different manufacturers can be variable and accuracy estimates can vary.

Once anovulation or ovulatory dysfunction is diagnosed, some additional evaluation is necessary to distinguish certain endocrinopathies that commonly disrupt ovulatory function from primary ovulatory disorders. Many obvious systemic illnesses or metabolic or endocrine diseases can interfere with normal cyclicity, but only subtler hyperprolactinemia and hypothyroidism are commonly diagnosed during infertility evaluation.[18] Although a complete discussion of the evaluation and management of hyperprolactinemia and thyroid disorders is beyond the scope of this chapter, specific treatment of these entities often restores normal ovarian function.

Whether caused by pituitary adenoma or idiopathic excess, hyperprolactinemia commonly responds well to bromocriptine mesylate (Parlodel) or caberglide (Dostinex). These potent dopaminergic receptor agonists directly inhibit prolactin secretion from the anterior pituitary and are nearly universally effective in reducing prolactin secretion, whether or not an adenoma or microadenoma is present. Many patients with modest hyperprolactinemia have true amenorrhea, whereas others may simply have subnormal luteal-phase production of progesterone. When hyperprolactinemia is the cause of anovulation or ovulatory dysfunction, normalization of prolactin secretion with medical therapy can be expected to result in normal ovulatory function in most patients.

A related abnormality of hyperprolactinemia is primary hypothyroidism. When hypothyroidism is clinically apparent, there is no diagnostic difficulty. Some patients, however, present with a normal thyroid panel but an elevated thyroid-stimulating hormone (TSH) level, implying primary compensated (i.e., subclinical) hypothyroidism. Proper treatment of patients with mild elevations of TSH and prolactin is thyroid hormone replacement. The typical response is normalization of both TSH and prolactin levels, and restoration of normal ovarian cyclicity is common.

Three diagnostic categories of ovulatory dysfunction are independent of a prolactin- or thyroid-mediated mechanism. First, ovarian failure can occur at any age. Elevated gonadotropin levels are the findings of the usual diagnostic test. Treatment of infertility resulting from this cause requires modern reproductive technologies with donor eggs. Second, patients who have normal prolactin levels and no gonadotropin elevation but are relatively hypoestrogenic are usually described as having hypothalamic amenorrhea. Failure to bleed with a progestin challenge is the usual diagnostic hallmark of this group of hypogonadotropic hypogonadal patients. Truly specific therapy for this entity is available in the form of pulsatile administration of gonadotropin-releasing hormone (Gn-RH). This highly specific therapy for augmenting pituitary output of gonadotropins can be somewhat cumbersome but is successful, although pulsatile delivery (every 90 minutes) requires considerable logistical effort. Clomiphene citrate is occasionally useful, but human gonadotropin therapy is usually of aid.[42] Third, a wide range of ovulatory disturbances that occur in relatively well estrogenized patients is initially distinguished by withdrawal bleeding after progestin challenge. In general, the designation for all these estrogenized patients is polycystic ovarian syndrome, although there is a wide range of presentations from mild luteal dysfunction up to and including complete cyclicity and marked androgen excess. Many of these patients, especially those with milder disturbances, respond to clomiphene for ovulation induction. Figure 5 shows the hormone levels on a midluteal day in a patient who received clomiphene, 100 mg per day for 5 days, earlier in the cycle. The patient conceived a singleton gestation, and human chorionic gonadotropin (hCG) was first detectable in her serum on the day after the study sampling.

For patients who do not conceive after either specific, directed endocrine therapies or a trial of clomiphene, induction of ovulation with gonadotropins, such as human menopausal gonadotropins (hMG) or purified follicle-stimulating hormone (FSH) and hCG, is usually appropriate.[35,41] Administration of hMG typically begins between cycle days 2 and 5. Therapy is monitored with frequent estradiol assays and ovarian ultrasonic scans from about day 6 onward. Once one or more follicles exceed a diameter threshold (usually 18 mm), hCG is given for ovulatory release. Estradiol levels provide a measure of the functional state of all follicles within the ovary; thus, a low estradiol level with large follicles suggests relatively poor health, whereas a very high estradiol level implies a significant risk of hyperstimulation because of excessive recruitment of large numbers of small follicles.[13] An acceptable moderate response for an hMG-hCG cycle is shown in Figure 6.

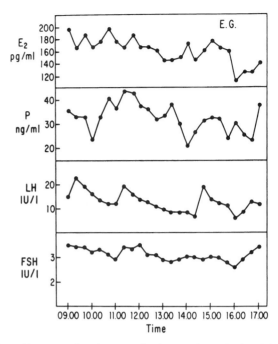

FIG. 5. Hormone levels on cycle day +9 from the luteinizing hormone *(LH)* surge in a patient given 15 μg of gonadotropin-releasing hormone subcutaneously every 90 minutes by pulsatile infusion pump for hypogonadotropic hypogonadism. *Arrows* indicate infusions. The patient did not conceive in this cycle but continued without interruption or change of dosage or infusion interval, and she conceived a singleton in the subsequent cycle (*E₂*, estradiol; *FSH*, follicle-stimulating hormone; *P*, progesterone). (From the Glasgow Royal Infirmary.)

Experience with hMG-hCG ovulation induction has shown that a significant number of failed cycles are caused by premature luteinization; that is, the LH surge, or at least a progressive rise in LH levels, may occur before follicle maturation is completed. Blockade of LH release with long-acting Gn-RH agonists that down-regulate the pituitary has been effective in preventing this premature luteinization phenomenon.[10] The hope that such agents would greatly reduce the risk of ovarian hyperstimulation has been only partially fulfilled.

Treatment of milder forms of ovulatory dysfunction, such as luteal-phase deficiency (i.e., luteal-phase defect), has often been undertaken by providing luteal-phase progesterone supplementation. This can be done with vaginal suppositories of 25 mg twice a day, and treatment of such luteal-phase abnormalities has typically been monitored by correction of endometrial biopsies from out of phase to in phase.[36] This treatment seems to have reasonable efficacy, which has been attributed to an endometrial action of the progesterone supplement. Studies have shown that in cycles in which the luteal progesterone production is subnormal, the LH secretory pattern is increased. Furthermore, administration of progesterone in the follicular phase reduces the LH secretory pulse pattern to that found in normal luteal phases. These observations certainly suggest that luteal-phase progesterone supplements may ac-

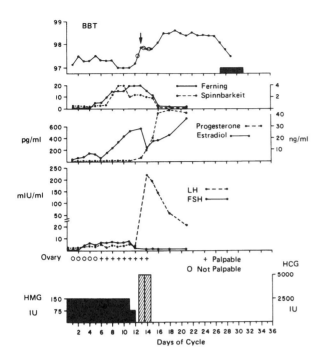

FIG. 6. Hormone levels on cycle day +8 from the luteinizing hormone *(LH)* surge in a patient given 100 mg of clomiphene citrate per day on cycle days 5 through 9 for polycystic ovarian disease–related anovulation. Although human chorionic gonadotropin was not detectable in these plasma samples, the patient did conceive a singleton in this cycle (*E₂*, estradiol; *FSH*, follicle-stimulating hormone; *P*, progesterone). (From the Glasgow Royal Infirmary.)

tually normalize function of the hypothalamic–pituitary axis as follicle recruitment is being initiated for the next cycle, rather than fixing an endometrial problem in the current treatment cycle.

Female Genital Tract Factors

Lower Genital Tract

Although it is obvious that complete or partial vaginal agenesis precludes conception, these types of defects are seldom found at the time of infertility evaluation. Virtually all these abnormalities are detected during the assessment of peripubertal symptoms such as amenorrhea and hematocolpos. Practically speaking, if coital frequency is at least two times per week and true intromission is occurring, then vaginal infertility factors do not exist.

Cervical factor infertility is often suggested by poor sperm motility or poor sperm survival in cervical mucus after intercourse 1 to 10 hours earlier. Cervical factor infertility as a single diagnosis seems to be relatively rare in practice, and it is easy to understand that cervical mucus may lack appropriate biophysical properties in women with hypoestrogenic states. There is little doubt that the most common cause of an abnormal postcoital test (PCT) is poor timing of the test within the cycle, with good cervical mucus occurring during the im-

mediate preovulatory interval (i.e., 1 to 3 days before ovulation). The easiest means to properly time a PCT is on the day following the change in an ovulation prediction kit. The second most common cause of a bad PCT is a male factor such as oligospermia. On the other hand, if the male partner has relative oligospermia but good PCT results can be obtained with the couple, then it is difficult to attribute the couple's infertility solely to lack of sperm in the female upper genital tract.

Other than the biophysical properties of cervical mucus that permit sperm penetration and survival, factors that might be injurious to sperm have also been identified or proposed. Antisperm antibodies have been detected in cervical mucus, and if one or more subsets of antibodies are directed toward critical surface components of spermatozoa, then an immune basis for infertility can be supposed. The difficulty is a technical limitation in distinguishing irrelevant antisperm antibodies from those that impede sperm migration or fertilization ability. Independent of immune-mediated mechanisms, an inflammatory process in the cervix, such as cervicitis, could be nonspecifically toxic to sperm or could alter the physicochemical properties of cervical mucus. Such a toxic mechanism for infertility can be readily imagined, but there seem to be few data to support this as an important infertility diagnosis.[9]

A common iatrogenic cause of hostile-appearing cervical mucus is the use of clomiphene for ovulation induction. Because clomiphene is an estrogen antagonist, estrogenic stimulation of cervical mucus production should be decreased. This virtually universal effect argues for the use of clomiphene relatively early in the cycle (i.e., days 3 to 7) rather than the more traditional use later in the follicular phase (i.e., days 5 to 9). There is certainly no pharmacologic justification for giving supplemental estrogens during clomiphene cycles because this amounts to giving exogenous agonist to compete with the administered antagonist, and if the early-follicular-phase administration of clomiphene has not engendered an adequate late-follicular-phase estradiol rise, then the dose was probably inadequate. Because there is a significant conception rate with clomiphene and because virtually all treated patients have some disturbance of cervical mucus production, it is difficult to conclude that the cervical mucus perturbation is of profound significance in clomiphene cycles.

No specific, directed therapy for cervical factor infertility exists short of intrauterine insemination (IUI) or the newer reproductive technologies that mechanically bypass the cervix. Therefore, a reasonable treatment strategy for a couple with cervical factor infertility would be an interval of prospective observation of 6 to 12 cycles with subsequent options, including first a series of washed IUIs, followed by a gamete intrafallopian transfer (GIFT) procedure or *in vitro* fertilization with embryo transfer (IVF-ET). Because the same sequence of treatment options applies for idiopathic infertility, there is a general trend sharply away from postcoital testing. If a specific, less invasive treatment is devised for the management of cervical factor infertility, then distinguishing between cervical factor infertility and idiopathic infertility will become clinically important rather than simply academically interesting.

Upper Genital Tract

Assessment of the upper female genital tract, including the uterus, fallopian tubes, and peritoneal cavity, is most efficiently accomplished by performance of a single combined procedure of laparoscopy, hysteroscopy, and hydrotubation. This outpatient surgical procedure does require an anesthetic but permits direct visualization of the endometrial cavity with concurrent inspection of the serosal surface of the uterus and adjacent structures, thereby enhancing the quality of the information obtained. Similarly, dye injection at the time of laparoscopy may detect tubal patency and permit direct inspection of the mobility and morphology of the fallopian tubes. The detection of endometriosis and pelvic adhesions requires inspection of the peritoneal cavity; these diagnoses cannot reliably be made without such direct inspection.[2]

Hysterosalpingography (HSG) or saline infusion sonogram (sonohysterogram) provides a useful adjunct in the assessment of the uterine cavity. HSG can also evaluate the fallopian tubes when hysteroscopy is not available or a confirmatory study of tubal patency is needed, especially if bilateral proximal tubal occlusion was believed to be present at laparoscopy and hydrotubation.

Intrauterine abnormalities can be found at hysteroscopy or HSG and at times on sonohysterogram, including retained intrauterine device, endometrial polyp, leiomyomata, intrauterine adhesions, and various developmental anomalies. On HSG, it may be difficult or impossible to distinguish a uterine septum (i.e., septate or subseptate) from a bicornuate or didelphic uterus. At combined hysteroscopy with laparoscopy, specific diagnosis can be immediately made, and if a septum is present, hysteroscopic resection can be performed at that time.

Occlusion of one or both fallopian tubes is most commonly detected at the time of dye injection, whether at laparoscopy or at HSG. Occlusion may be proximal or distal, or exist at a combination of those sites. If there is proximal tubal occlusion for which resection and end-to-end reanastamosis can be performed, then fertility rates can approach those of sterilization-reversal operations. If reimplantation is required, then the fertility prospects are poor, with no more than 10% of patients conceiving in the first 2 years after surgery. Distal tuboplasty of hydrosalpinges is commonly performed, and subsequent pregnancy rates vary widely. The biggest problem in estimating subsequent outcome is the inability to assess the functional integrity of the tubal mucosa. It is probably fair to advise patients that fimbrioplasties yield a 25% pregnancy rate in the first 2 years after surgery, but this outcome varies from individual to individual, depending on the degree of unmeasurable intraluminal injury.[34] Newer technologies, such as transcervical balloon tuboplasty,[8] have to date had variable success in aiding some of these therapies. Assisted reproductive technologies (ARTs) such as IVF provide a better opportunity for success than surgery in more severe tubal factor infertility.

Although laparoscopy may reveal pertinent observations, such as polycystic changes of the ovaries, the most significant diagnoses to be made are the presence and extent of pelvic adhesions and endometriosis. If pelvic adhesions are minimal but constrain tubal motility, then laparoscopic lysis of adhesions is a reasonable undertaking. Extensive adhesions would usually require laparotomy for lysis, with or without tuboplasties, and the results of such surgery are variable. Increasingly, newer barrier materials are available for use when adhesiolysis is extensive. If adhesions are extensive or if the patient has undergone prior procedures for lysis but has suffered reformation, then advancement to IVF would probably be the best strategy, if that is a financially available option for the patient. The selection of appropriate treatment—surgery or ART—is in transition. The choice often depends on the surgical skills of the operator, as well as the availability (affordability) and success of the newer technologies.[17]

Endometriosis is commonly found at laparoscopy in infertile couples either as the single detectable diagnosis or with other factors. In severe endometriosis, significant destruction of the ovaries and fallopian tubes and formation of extensive pelvic adhesions are associated with an exceedingly low cycle fecundity, which is only slightly higher than zero. All milder forms of endometriosis (i.e., minimal, mild, and moderate) seem to have a cycle fecundity that is one-half to one-fifth that of normal couples and is not graded in association with disease severity. This implies that the mechanism of infertility in milder forms of endometriosis may not be the same as that in severe disease. The best evidence is that endometriosis is associated with an intraperitoneal inflammatory process with elevated concentrations of chemical mediators of inflammation and an increased number of activated phagocytic cells. Either one or both of these aspects of an established inflammatory process could explain infertility in terms of decreased sperm survival and, possibly, injury of eggs or embryos.[25]

Treatment of endometriosis with medical therapies improves pelvic pain scores but does not clearly improve cycle fecundity. There is often a loss of four to six cycles of conceptive attempts with any of the medical regimens available (i.e., danazol [Danocrine], continuous progestin, continuous oral contraceptives, Gn-RH analogs), and this decreases the fecundity from time of diagnosis onward, even if there is an increase in fecundability in the first several cycles after therapy is completed. Laparoscopic ablation of endometriosis implants by either cautery or laser does not improve the long-term pregnancy achievement, and careful analysis of pregnancies that occur after such procedures suggests only a transient improvement in cycle fecundity in patients with moderate endometriosis. Major surgery is seldom indicated for milder stages of endometriosis for pregnancy but is appropriate when there is extensive endometriosis or consequential pelvic adhesions are present. Before conservative resection of endometriosis at laparotomy, it often is advisable to have the patient complete 3 to 6 months of medical suppressive therapy. Many small implants of endometriosis may disappear, and larger nodules (e.g., endometriomas within ovaries) will diminish in size and have much less associated induration. As a result, surgical planes are easier to develop, and operative technique is enhanced. If such medical or surgical therapies have been used or judged inappropriate, then the newer reproductive technologies are the appropriate next step, if financially possible. IUI in superovulation cycles, GIFT procedure, and IVF-ET all seem to be appropriate for patients with endometriosis that has been refractory to lesser therapies.[11,15]

Multifactorial Infertility

There is no reason to suppose that several infertility factors may not coexist in any couple, and the clinician and the couple must allow that the obvious factor is not the only problem. It is good practice to undertake the assessment of each couple in a systematic way and then proceed with less invasive or demanding therapies initially as therapeutic trials. Specifically,

male gamete factor can be evaluated by semen analysis and female gamete factor can be initially evaluated by a luteal-phase progesterone or endometrial biopsy, and a large fraction of diagnoses will be made (Table 3). It is then reasonable to proceed with a more detailed analysis of the male partner or complete the endocrine evaluation of the female partner with ovulatory dysfunction and to initiate a trial of therapy before proceeding with invasive assessment, such as laparoscopy and HSG. For example, if there appears to be ovulatory dysfunction and a trial of clomiphene is undertaken, four to eight cycles should be sufficient to determine whether or not this sole intervention has been effective. At this point, completion of the infertility survey is appropriate; this primarily means performance of laparoscopy, hysteroscopy, and hydrotubation.

If the patient's history or examination initially suggests a particular diagnosis such as female genital tract problems or

TABLE 3. *Infertility diagnoses, tests, and therapies*

Diagnosis	Incidence[a] (%)	Common tests	Diagnostic results	Initial therapy	Advanced therapies
Multifactorial	40	Complete survey[b]	See individual tests	Treat one or more specific factors	IUI, GIFT, IVF-ET
Endometriosis	17	Laparoscopy	Characteristic implants and adhesions	Prospective observation, suppression with medication or conservative resection at laparotomy	IUI, GIFT, IVF-ET
Male factor	12	Semen analysis	<20 million normal motile sperm per ejaculate	Prospective observation or donor insemination	IUI, GIFT, IVF-ET, ICSI
Ovulatory dysfunction	11	Midluteal serum progesterone; late-luteal endometrial biopsy	Progesterone <15 ng/ml is suspect; < 10/ml is abnormal. Biopsy lag ≥2 d	Directed therapies for endocrine diseases; otherwise, clomiphene	Human menopausal gonadotropin or gonadotropin-releasing hormone
Tubal factor/pelvic adhesions	8	Laparoscopy with hydrotubation; HSG	Tubal occlusion/presence of adhesions at laparoscopy. HSG does not show adhesions	Laser laparoscopy or lysis of adhesions and tuboplasties at laparotomy	IVF-ET
Cervical factor	1	Postcoital test	<5 motile sperm/hpf in late follicular phase mucus	Prospective observation	IUI, GIFT, IVF-ET
Uterine factor	1	Hysteroscopy; HSG	Septum, polyp, fibroid seen; HSG has a significant false-negative rate	Hysteroscopic resection	Metroplasty at laparotomy
Idiopathic	10	Complete survey	See individual tests	Prospective observation, empirical therapy: clomiphene or empirical antibiotics	IUI, GIFT, IVF-ET

GIFT, gamete intrafallopian transfer; hpf, high-power field; HSG, hysterosalpingography; ICSI, intracytoplasmic sperm injection; IUI, washed intrauterine insemination with husband's sperm, usually in superovulation cycles; IVF-ET, *in vitro* fertilization with embryo transfer.

[a] Approximate.

[b] Minimum of semen analysis, midluteal serum progesterone and laparoscopy or hysteroscopy with hydrotubation or hysterosalpingogram.

From Soper J. Clarke-Pearson D. Hughes C. Gynecologic surgery. In: Liechty RD, Soper Rt, eds. Fundamentals of surgery. 6th ed. St Louis: CV Mosby, 1989:526; with permission.

male gamete factor, then those specific areas should be pursued early in the assessment. For example, if the patient describes cyclic progressive dysmenorrhea, then it is appropriate as an early step to proceed with laparoscopy for evaluation of both her infertility and her pelvic pain syndrome.

Unexplained Infertility

The incidence of idiopathic (i.e., unexplained) infertility is relatively low. Estimates range from 5% to 20%, but the incidence seems to be inversely correlated with the severity of criteria used. If a couple has undergone a complete survey, which would include as a minimal assessment semen analysis, measurement of serum progesterone levels, laparoscopy, hysteroscopy, and chromoperturbation with or without a PCT, then idiopathic infertility can be tentatively diagnosed.

Treatment of multifactorial or idiopathic infertility usually comes down to empirical therapies that are either conservative or aggressive. The most conservative empirical therapy is prospective observation. This strategy of allowing conceptive attempts with no medical intervention for 6 to 12 months frequently makes practical sense and permits treatment-independent conceptions to occur. The next level of empirical therapies might include more precise timing of coital activity (e.g., by LH surge indicators or salivary and vaginal electrical resistance indicators) and the administration of clomiphene for six to eight cycles, or an empirical antibiotic, such as tetracycline, for the woman or couple to treat undetected genital tract pathogens. It seems inappropriate to extend such empiric therapies for longer than 6 to 12 months after the diagnosis of infertility has been made, even in younger patients. We would advise either more aggressive therapies or adoption at this time.

Additional aggressive empirical therapies include several technologic options. IVF-ET is effective when fallopian tubes are absent or occluded; it has also been used for various other diagnoses with apparent success. When the fallopian tubes are present and relatively normal, GIFT or superovulation with IUI can be used. These alternatives appear to be more effective treatment modalities for many couples in some of the various diagnostic subgroups. All these reproductive options require the use of ovulation-inducing drugs to increase the number of oocytes available. It remains to be seen whether these techniques actually increase the overall ultimate conception rate or simply compact several cycles of conceptive possibilities down into a single event. These advanced therapies are reviewed in greater detail later in this chapter.

◊ ASSISTED REPRODUCTIVE TECHNOLOGY

Stillman and colleagues coined the term "getting gametes together" to define the major goals of ARTs in the treatment of human infertility. For humans, ARTs began in the mid-1970s with experiments in oocyte retrieval, fertilization *in vitro* using improved culture media, and transfer of zygotes or preembryos into the uterus. Many cycles took place, most with-

out fertility drug use. Sophisticated technology was developed for monitoring the periovulatory phase of the cycle (e.g., estradiol and LH assays, ultrasound). These processes culminated in the birth of Louise Brown in 1978 through the pioneering work of Steptoe and Edwards.[37] Since the birth of this child, ARTs have flourished, being performed in hundreds of centers worldwide. Thousands of children have been born who, only a few years ago, could never have been born.[22] Unfortunately, there has occasionally been confusion about the success rates with various groups and techniques, making patient decisions difficult, and it seems that in some rare cases ethical practice may have been violated. Finally, due to the absence of health insurance or the vagaries of what such insurance provides, many patients are left without coverage or resources to pursue these expensive technologies. In some situations. patients may be forced to fall back on less expensive (or covered) approaches, such as attempts at reparative tubal surgery, when they are little indicated. It is hoped that the differences of science, technology, health insurance, and managed care will shortly come together to allow infertility care to pursue the therapy most likely to succeed rather than the one that is affordable.

ART is replete with many procedures, defined by a multiplicity of acronyms describing variations on the more standard theme of IVF. Figure 7 illustrates the steps in IVF. Table 4 presents some of the variations that can now be done with IVF using a husband's and/or wife's or donors' gametes and a wife or surrogate recipient. When one considers the addition of cryopreservation of gametes and embryos, the options are even further compounded. In addition to IVF, the various other technologies includw GIFT,[15] zygote intrafallopian transfer (ZIFT), tubal embryo transfer (TET), transuterine tubal insemination (TUTI), gamete manipulations, and intracytoplasmic sperm injection (ICSI). Each of these advances has consistently motivated advances in the clinical utility of these new reproductive technologies.

The information gained from ARTs and experience has increased understanding of the physiologic and pathophysiologic processes of ovarian function, ovarian reserve, sperm function, fertilization, culture and coculture systems, embryo development, implantation, and cryotherapeutics. These areas of progress in treating infertility also promise to improve diagnoses and therapies in many other fields. Examples of the research applications of ARTs to other fields include progress in contraception from the knowledge gained in fertilization processes, progress in genetic diagnoses and therapies gained from *in vitro* manipulation of preimplantation embryos, and progress in the use of gestational surrogacy to avoid fetal risk in a mother with prior Rh sensitization. The latter two conditions are also examples of the medically appropriate use of ARTs for couples without infertility problems.

ART programs continue to undergo innovation involving increased complexity and attempts at simplification. Practitioners are attempting to bring the technologies to many more couples seeking care and to improve the risk–benefit and cost–benefit ratios.

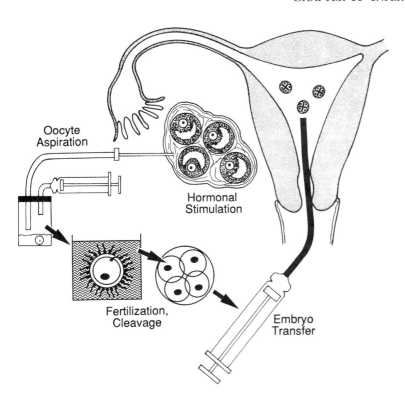

FIG. 7. Steps of *in vitro* fertilization (IVF) and embryo replacement are ovarian stimulation, monitoring, ultrasound or laparoscopy, oocyte retrieval, IVF, and uterine preembryo replacement.

In the following sections, we first explore the components of a typical ART protocol cycle and follow some of the increasingly dichotomous historical trends of increased complexity and simplification. We then review the means by which ARTs can optimize reproductive efficiency, including methods for evaluating and improving oocyte quality, spermatozoal quality, embryo quality, and implantation capacity.

Assisted Reproductive Technology Cycle Parameters

Patient Selection

Once reserved for patients with severe tubal factor infertility who had failed to conceive after pelvic surgeries, the indications for ARTs have expanded to include essentially all infertility patient categories. Once deemed only bypass procedures

TABLE 4. *Indications for gamete donors and embryo recipients using noncryopreserved embryos*

Source of sperm	Source of ova	Carrier	Couples' genes (%)	Indications
Husband[a]	Wife[a]	Wife	100	Female infertility (e.g., tubal, cervical, endometrial); immunologic infertility; infertility of unknown origin
Husband	Wife	Surrogate	100	Gestational surrogacy (i.e, "host uterus"); müllerian agenesis or duct malformation; wife with undesirable gestational environment (e.g., phenylketonuria, treatment with chemotherapy, irradiation, or surgery); high-risk pregnancy (e.g., diabetes, hypertension, postpartum psychosis, seizures, Eisenmenger complex)
Husband	Donor	Wife	50	Donor oocyte for wife without functioning or responding ovaries; wife is X-linked genetic disease carrier; autosomally failed fertilization with normal man
Donor	Wife	Wife	50	Absolute male infertility plus female infertility
Donor	Donor	Wife	0	Embryo adoption because of absolute male infertility and wife without ovaries or uterus
Husband	Donor	Surrogate	50	Surrogate motherhood (i.e., donor is the surrogate) because wife has no uterus or ovaries
Donor	Wife	Surrogate	50	Absolute male infertility and wife without uterus
Husband	Wife	Husband[b]	100	Reversal of childbearing roles; wife without uterus and no desire for surrogate

[a]The terms male partner and female partner may be substituted for husband and wife.
[b]It is theoretically possible for the husband to carry the fetus with hormone manipulation and peritoneal implantation.

for irreparable fallopian tubes, ARTs now bring multiple gametes into direct proximity to improve fecundity in diverse settings. Some investigators speculate on the possible extinction of the standard infertility workup, with the near-future offering some form of ART after a rudimentary evaluation of the uterus, day 3 FSH level, and semen parameters. Although this view of infertility therapy probably awaits further development of ART cycle success rates, the indications for the appropriate use of ARTs have broadened beyond the substitution of the test tube for the damaged fallopian tube.

Successful IVF with compromised semen parameters has led to the frequent use of IVF for patients in these circumstances. However, when normal male factor and tubal factor are present, ART may succeed with gamete transfers to the fallopian tube or its vicinity. This group may include patients with earlier stages of endometriosis and infertility of unknown origin, but some physicians still prefer the diagnostic capability of egg and sperm interaction by IVF rather than gamete transfers for even these disorders. The risk–benefit and cost–benefit analyses of which ART form to use, if any, must be calculated in each center, using its own statistics for comparing alternate therapies.

The indications for ARTs have expanded for the infertile population, and they have expanded beyond the usual definition of infertility to include perimenopausal and prematurely postmenopausal women with donor oocytes, gestational surrogates for women without a functional uterus, preimplantation genetics, and fetomaternal incompatibilities such as severe Rh sensitization or maternal chemotherapy. Expansion of the patient categories has altered patient selection for ARTs to those with or without gametes, with or without a uterus, and with or without infertility. Paradoxically, it has also made the field more complex by multiplying the means available to manage these groups, such as synchronized cycles for gestational surrogacy and embryo biopsy for preimplantation genetic analysis.

Ovarian Stimulation

ART began by using the natural cycle and retrieving the one dominant oocyte developed per menstrual cycle. When this technique showed minimal success because of variation in the ability to retrieve, fertilize, and culture a mature but unluteinized oocyte, ovarian stimulation was attempted with clomiphene and combinations of agents that included hMG. The most commonly employed method is pituitary downregulation with Gn-RH analogs, followed by high-dose gonadotropin stimulation. Innumerable variations on the basic theme exist, including additions of pure and recombinant FSH, growth hormone, and flareup with follicular Gn-RH analog (i.e., stimulating with Gn-RH analog in combination with high-dose gonadotropin stimulation).[5,6] The goal has been to "cheat" nature with the creation of numerous oocytes for manipulation for IVF and transfer or for IVF after GIFT.[5]

After appropriate ovarian stimulation has been achieved, the Gn-RH analog and gonadal stimulation are discontinued, and hCG is administered as the LH substitute to induce ovulation approximately 35 to 36 hours before planned retrieval to allow final maturation of the oocytes in vivo.[19]

Luteal support after aspirations of the oocytes, follicular fluid, and granulosa cells has used progesterone, divided doses of hCG, and no adjunctive support. Despite some studies demonstrating no statistically significant differences in pregnancy rates among the various luteal-support regimens, most groups use some therapy, and the most efficacious is probably hCG.

To contain costs, improve safety, and minimize the risk of multiple gestation, a simplified process of stimulation has been popularized with a back-to-the-basics version of minimal stimulation with clomiphene used during the natural cycle or retrieval and then culture of immature oocytes. ART cycle success rates usually correlate directly with the number of embryos developed for use in the cycle. Because these cycle designs expect the transfer of fewer preembryos than in gonadotropin-stimulated cycles, the decision for the patient is between the ease, expense, or risk of the procedure and the likelihood of pregnancy in an individual cycle.[8] Improving culture methods, including the use of coculture systems and the transfer of blastocyst-stage embryos, may improve implantation rates when fewer embryos are transferred.

Monitoring

Monitoring oocyte development has evolved from urine LH assays to rapid serum estradiol and daily transvaginal ultrasound evaluation of follicles. Ultrasound evaluation of the endometrial thickness and patterns has also been added. Before the use of Gn-RH analogs, serum or urine LH and serum progesterone also helped mark the course of oocyte development and minimize premature luteinization in the late follicular phases. With the use of Gn-RH analogs, the risk of unidentified and unwanted LH surges and premature luteinization are greatly reduced, and monitoring of preretrieval LH and progesterone is less important.

Gn-RH analogs are available today only as agonists. After initial stimulation, the Gn-RH agonist suppresses pituitary and ovarian function. This appears to allow some synchronization of oocyte development in response to subsequent gonadotropin stimulation, to ablate the LH surge to prevent spontaneous ovulation before oocyte retrieval, and to limit premature follicle luteinization because of increases in progesterone. The result has been a striking decrease in cycle cancellation rates and increases in oocyte yield per cycle, fertilization rates, number of embryos transferred, and cycle pregnancy rates.[5] Many practitioners have used the cycle control available with Gn-RH analogs (i.e., starting dates for gonadotropins, timing of the hCG ovulatory trigger) to orchestrate patient flow during an ART series. The need for the additional Gn-RH medication, which is administered subcutaneously or by nasal spray, and the increased amounts of gonadotropin usually required for adequate stimulation after Gn-RH suppression—and the costs of each—are generally outweighed by the benefits accrued. This cost–benefit ratio should improve with the marketing of pure Gn-RH antagonists.

Cycle monitoring has progressed toward cost control and simplification. In some standardized protocols, patients are given a set, unmodified medication regimen followed by little or no monitoring. Egg retrieval is preset for a specific day. Some of these protocols have achieved pregnancy rates similar to those of more interventionist programs. Satellite monitoring has also gained advocates, especially in rural areas. ART patients are monitored at a local center and then, according to standardized criteria, are sent to a centralized facility for oocyte retrieval and laboratory processing of the gametes and preembryos. This has obvious benefit for patients, and it limits the need for duplication of the more expensive laboratory facilities and personnel.

Oocyte Retrieval

Laparoscopy was the standard method of oocyte retrieval during the early stages of ART development. Through technologic advances in the mid-1980s, it became apparent that mature follicles 18 mm or larger were also amenable to aspiration under ultrasound guidance. The first such attempts used abdominal ultrasound transducers with and without abdominal fixed biopsy guides. This approach was followed by abdominal transducers with a free-hand transvaginal needle aspiration. The standard now is transvaginal aspiration with fixed needle guides on transvaginal ultrasound transducers (Fig. 8). Variations include periurethral, transvesical, and

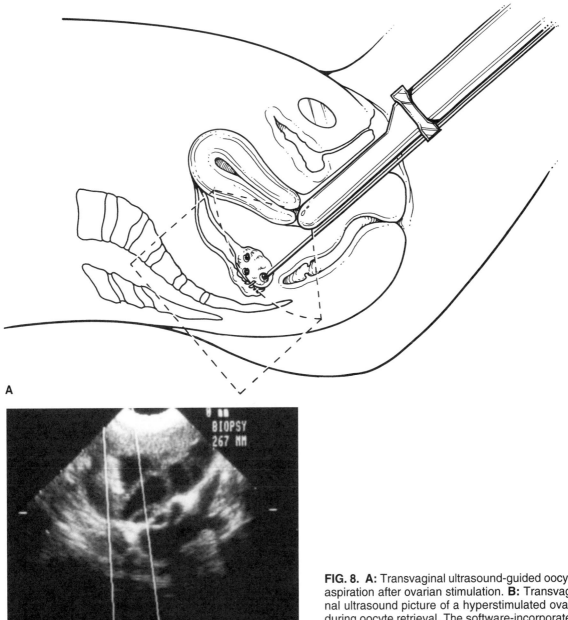

FIG. 8. A: Transvaginal ultrasound-guided oocyte aspiration after ovarian stimulation. **B:** Transvaginal ultrasound picture of a hyperstimulated ovary during oocyte retrieval. The software-incorporated biopsy guidelines and the bright-white echogenic needle within a follicle are visible.

transuterine techniques that are rarely used, compared with the transvaginal approach, although they are useful in certain clinical circumstances due to unusual anatomic locations of the ovaries.

A revival of laparoscopic oocyte retrieval had been initiated by some programs that have successfully combined oocyte retrieval with diagnostic infertility laparoscopy.[10] This approach combined diagnostic and therapeutic laparoscopy used for addressing infertility with early IVF or GIFT. In patients undergoing laparoscopy for assessment, prelaparoscopic ovarian stimulation and monitoring are performed. The timing of the laparoscopic procedure is dictated by the time of required oocyte retrial. If semen and tubal parameters are normal, GIFT may be performed. If either is not optimal or if diagnostic information about IVF is desired, IVF and uterine preembryo replacement are performed. Patients have the opportunity to conceive through the laparoscopic ART approach or, if unsuccessful, through the laparoscopic therapy that may have been employed in addressing the infertility.

Laboratory Culture Conditions

Laboratory techniques have evolved in complexity and sophistication, even as attempts have been made to simplify and standardize these methods. Sophistication has been increased with strict quality-control measures, the use of new culture media, and coculture technologies. Some attempts at simplification, such as intravaginal culture systems, have proven successful. Transport of gametes to centralized facilities for culturing and preembryo transfer after local oocyte retrieval has been introduced with some success.

Gamete and Embryo Replacement

Many types of gamete and embryo replacement techniques have been attempted. The standard approach is uterine preembryo replacement at the four- to eight-cell stage, usually after 48 to 72 hours in culture (Fig. 9). This approach attempts to replace the preembryos during the endometrial implantation window and limits the time in culture. The transcervical uterine preembryo replacement is performed earlier in endometrial development than the preembryo would usually enter the uterus from the fallopian tube. The longer the preembryo is kept in culture, the greater is the degree of endometrial and preembryo dysynchrony because the endometrium *in vivo* develops more rapidly than the *in vitro*–cultured preembryo.[16]

If early replacement is important to limit the time of preembryos in the artificial laboratory environment but falls too early in the optimal endometrial implantation window, better culture technologies or alternative replacement techniques are warranted. GIFT or ZIFT appears to satisfy both goals. ZIFT and GIFT were developed to simplify the process by avoiding the need for rigorous *in vitro* culture.

IVF, as noted, was initially used as a therapy for severe tubal factor infertility. Success expanded the indications for the procedure to include patients without tubal factors, and

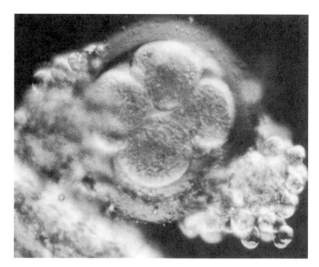

FIG. 9. Human four-cell embryo cultured for 48 hours after *in vitro* fertilization.

there were questions about whether clinical circumstances existed to avoid IVF, culture, and uterine preembryo replacement, especially if normal fallopian tubes existed, as in cases of infertility of unknown origin or minimal endometriosis. GIFT was an attempt to meet these needs. It is a simplification of the IVF culture technologies and avoids the rigorous laboratory conditioning by using the patient's tube as incubator instead of the laboratory's tube and incubator.[28]

ZIFT and TET were offshoots of GIFT technology. These methods overcame the failure of GIFT to confirm or influence fertilization, as in cases of infertility caused by male factors, and they decreased *in vitro* time requirements and allowed physiologic tubal preembryo development and timing of the transfer to the uterus by replacement in the fallopian tube. ZIFT and TET have their own problems. First, they require oocyte retrieval, some *in vitro* culture, and laparoscopic embryo transfer. Success with transtubal ZIFT or TET after transvaginal oocyte retrieval and *in vitro* culture has been disappointing.[30] Second, randomized studies do not show an improved pregnancy rate, even with laparoscopic ZIFT, compared with IVF and uterine preembryo transfer, despite the former method's placement of the preembryos into the tube. However, further work and refinement of these techniques, perhaps from transcervical tubal cannulation using linear everting catheters, should be encouraged.

The quest for simplification did not stop with ZIFT or GIFT. Several innovative attempts have been made to further simplify ARTs for patients with normal fallopian tubes. One involved peritoneal oocyte and sperm transfer (POST), which required ultrasound oocyte retrieval but not laparoscopic gamete transfer. The oocytes and sperm were placed into the cul-de-sac of Douglas for fallopian tube retrieval. Additional attempts to simplify the process maintained the controlled ovarian hyperstimulation regimes without oocyte retrieval. These have included direct intraperitoneal insemination (DIPI) and TUTI. With stepwise attempts at simplification of the original complex form of the IVF process using ovarian hyperstimulation and the development of multiple oocytes each month, the approach has evolved from IVF to GIFT to ZIFT or TET to POST and back to IVF.[23]

Reproductive Efficiency

ARTs are about enhancing reproductive efficiency, including oocyte, sperm, and embryo quality and implantation capacity. Representative examples of these are described in the following sections.

Oocyte Quality

Reproductive age adversely influences female fecundity and reproductive performance. The amount of hMG required for ovarian stimulation is greater, while the number of oocytes retrieved, the number of preembryos transferred, the pregnancy rate per cycle, and the ongoing pregnancy rate are all diminished in older women, especially those older than 40 years. Failed attempts at ART, defined by cycle cancellation and miscarriage rates, are also higher.[40] This basic defect related to maternal age is most vividly demonstrated in the remarkable success rates obtained using young donor oocytes in older women.[33] Donor oocytes are now regularly being used in women with poor ovarian reserve (as demonstrated by FSH values greater than 12 mIU/ml or estradiol greater than or equal to on cycle day 3 or on cycle day 10 after 5 days of clomiphene therapy).[39] Other categories of donor egg use include patients in whom the ovaries are anatomically inaccessible for retrieval, those who have experienced repeated failure of IVF due to lack of fertilization without male factor, those who have certain genetic disorders, and those who have suffered secondary ovarian failure as a result of gonadal dysgenesis, surgery, chemotherapy, or irradiation.

It is likely that some of the cohort of oocytes retrieved from natural or stimulated cycles may not be capable of being fertilized. Some may be immature, some postmature, and some may have abnormalities in the zona or in sperm binding. The appropriate maturational age is important for fertilizability. Newer technology is now allowing immature oocytes to be matured using special coculture techniques.

Finally, oocyte quality correlates with the likelihood of fertilization, with better preembryo development, and with a higher likelihood of implantation and pregnancy. Such oocyte quality can be assessed by various parameters from the spent culture medium (e.g., androgen–estrogen ratios). Chemotactic attraction of sperm to the oocyte is another active investigational area, as are other biochemical assessments and probes of oocyte health and maturity and our ability to influence oocyte quality.

Sperm Quality

One of the greatest advances in ARTs has been in the treatment of male factor infertility. Even the definitions of moderate and severe male factor infertility have dramatically changed. Various biochemical assays and bioassays have previously been used to evaluate sperm function, but generally they have been disappointing.[20] The results of IVF with human oocytes has aided the specificity of fertilization to be adequately proven. Although IVF-ET began as a therapy for tubal factor infertility, it rapidly became apparent that the concentration of spermatozoa needed for fertilization could be obtained from men having significantly compromised semen parameters. Now, even a very few sperm, even those with poor or no motility, can yield a pregnancy through micromanipulation techniques such as ICSI. Testicular biopsy, fine-needle aspiration, or epididymal sperm aspiration has made ICSI available and successful even for men with azoospermia. This exciting area is one of great interest to ART practitioners. Donor sperm may be used as a backup for all these techniques, particularly for those unsuccessful or not wishing to pursue these somewhat extraordinary measures.

Preembryo Quality

In an attempt to optimize reproductive efficiency in ARTs, preembryo quality can be assessed morphologically, biochemically, and chromosomally. Examples of how these criteria are used to measure preembryo health and quality and how these may be manipulated to optimize oocyte quality are discussed in the next sections. However, with the extensive and rapid advances in this field, these examples offer only a superficial view of what this science will bring in the future.

Morphologic Evaluation

Morphologic evaluation of preembryos is done in ART laboratories to decide which preembryos to transfer from the cohort produced by the fertilization of multiple oocytes obtained after controlled ovarian hyperstimulation. Preembryos are chosen for the greatest likelihood for implantation. The criteria used for these evaluations are qualitative and somewhat subjective. Cell number is a classic criteria; more rapid development usually correlates with higher preembryo implantation rates. The four- to eight-cell stage at 48 hours is used as a goal. Symmetry and roundness of the blastomeres and the lack of fragmentation or vacuoles are criteria used in this assessment by embryologists. Advances in semiquantitative and quantitative assessment beyond these morphologic assessments would be welcome.

Improvement in preembryo quality, as assessed by these morphologic criteria, can be obtained by strict laboratory quality-control conditions and carefully prepared culture media. Advances in coculture systems may bring about improvement in the percentage of blastomeres expanded, a decrease in the percentage of fragmentation, and an increase in blastomere adherence and zona thickness variation. These culture systems allow embryo culture to the blastocyst stage, at which the percentage of embryos that will implant is increased.

Embryo expansion and hatching out of the restricting zona pellucida are critical functions of the healthy preimplantation embryo. It has been suggested that hatching and implantation are more likely when early preembryos have significant variation in the thickness of the zona pellucida. A thickened zona or one without a thickness variation does not appear to implant with the same frequency. This has been one rationale for the therapeutic concept of assisted hatching.[6,7]

Biochemical Assessment

The preembryo *in vivo* is capable of significant active biochemical processes. If some of these can be assessed *in vitro*, the measurement of preembryo quality of health may be feasible. As it was used in assessing oocyte health, the spent culture media is also a method for biochemical evaluation of the preembryo. Correlation of culture media and embryo byproducts can be used to preselect healthy preembryos destined for implantation and determine those with lower potential for viability. The evaluation of substances synthesized by the preembryo in culture may lead to characterization and later synthesis of these chemicals. Such materials as oncofetal fibronectin, pregnancy-associated plasma protein A, and integrin molecules are all substances of diagnostic and therapeutic use in the assessment and therapy of the preembryo.

Chromosomal Evaluation

Micromanipulation is used in microsurgical fertilization and in assisted implantation through assisted hatching. The chromosomal evaluation of preembryo quality can also involve microsurgical manipulation by means of a blastomere biopsy for diagnosis. Dramatic advances in the field also promise realization of the potential for preembryo therapy. This growing field of preimplantation genetics is an excellent example of the use of ARTs for medical purposes other than treating infertility and of the use of molecular biology's newest tools such as the polymerase chain reaction and fluorescent *in situ* hybridization. The ability to use gene therapy by gene insertion has been performed in animals, as has cloning. Human trials will be a natural consequence of the work available in preimplantation genetics, although cloning has been likely relegated to major ethical decisions before its use is considered.

The uses of gene evaluation, diagnosis, and therapy employ ARTs for couples who may not otherwise be infertile. Patients with X-linked disorders have normal fertility, but circumstances dictated a technologic means by which to minimize or eliminate the ravages of the genetic disorder. The ethical and social implications of each of these scientific developments are impossible to ignore. Conservative, clear medical indications should exist before consideration is given to using embryo micromanipulation or ARTs. For example, the use of ART combined with blastomere biopsy to allow preembryo gender selection for social preference or other nonmedical indications should be condemned.

Implantation Capacity

Endometrial and maternal uterine receptivity play critical roles in implantation in cases of spontaneous and assisted conceptions.[2,4] Much clinical and basic research is being applied to ART implantation, because the implantation capacity is thought to be one of the rate-limiting factors in achieving pregnancy.

Hormonal Environment

Exceedingly high levels of estradiol, sometimes combined with the known adverse antiestrogenic consequences of clomiphene, may adversely influence the implantation capacity of the endometrium after controlled ovarian hyperstimulation. The artificial timing of preembryo transfer to the uterus may also play a role. The mechanism to overcome or overwhelm these implantation limitations has been to transfer multiple preembryos. This raises the ethical decision required in managing embryos that are created but not transferred (they are often dealt with by cryopreservation) and the risk of multiple pregnancies. The implantation rates in most successful IVF programs are 10% to 15% per preembryo. Higher rates are possible and have occasionally been achieved. The rate may be higher if the transfer of preembryos is made to artificial cycles using sequential estrogen and progesterone regimes synchronized to allow preembryo transfer during the implantation window. Implantation rates in donor oocyte programs, besides being significantly improved by the use of donor oocyte itself, have been further improved by artificial endometrial cycles that use Gn-RH down-regulation, if needed, and sequential estrogen and progesterone therapy. Evaluation of the endometrium during artificial cycles without transfer, combining endometrial biopsy or endometrial ultrasound evaluation of thickness and endometrial pattern, may allow assessment of endometrial implantation capacity.[1,32]

Another clinical direction designed to improve endometrial receptivity has been the use of natural IVF cycles. The apparent oxymoron of the term *natural* used with IVF brings us full circle to the original construct of Steptoe and Edwards, who initially retrieved a single dominant oocyte from an unstimulated but monitored cycle. The natural cycle theoretically provides a natural, unstimulated endometrial environment for implantation. Cost savings, simplicity for patients, and minimization of the risk of multiple pregnancy and the ethical concerns about extra embryos are also realized. Implantation rates of approximately 10% reported for these cycles do not seem to be a marked improvement over implantation rates in stimulated cycles. Randomized trials to determine whether the natural cycle or the artificial cycle provides an improved endometrial advantage are being initiated.[1,26,27] If cryopreservation technologies improve sufficiently, consideration of cryopreserving all preembryos from a stimulated cycle and delaying their transfer until later artificial or natural endometrial cycles (i.e., separate from the stimulated endometrium of the cycle of retrieval) may be warranted.[21] Maturation *in vitro* of immature oocytes retrieved without stimulation holds promise of greater success in unstimulated cycles than that achievable with a single oocyte.

One method to improve implantation in ARTs has been to place gametes or preembryos in a more physiologic environment for fertilization and early cell division: the fallopian tube. This placement helps ensure that preembryos are released from the fallopian tube into the uterus in the physiologic implantation window rather than one dictated by limitations of culture system and *in vitro* embryo and endometrial growth dysynchrony. GIFT allows fertilization in the fallopian tube, natural development of the preembryo, and its natural transfer into the uterus. Although implantation rates per embryo may be higher, the decrease in fertilization achieved with GIFT and the number of preembryos created minimize the reality of markedly improved pregnancy rates, especially compared with IVF in ART programs in which IVF pregnancy success rates are also high.[28,31]

Uterine Receptivity

The endometrial environment and implantation capacity may also be affected by the uterus itself. Significant synechiae, uterine malformations, *in utero* exposure to diethylstilbestrol, and persistent leiomyomata uteri may diminish implantation capacity and success of reproduction and of ART. These abnormalities, if amenable to therapy, should be treated prospectively before considering ARTs. However, if they are not amenable to therapy or if previous therapy has failed, gestational surrogacy may be entertained. The classic example of the use of gestational surrogacy is after hysterectomy without oophorectomy or for müllerian agenesis. In a patient previously considered sterile, normal ovaries with normal ovarian reserve reside, but with the gestational vessel absent. The transfer of *in vitro*–fertilized oocytes retrieved after ovarian stimulation from a woman with absent or diminished uterine capacity to a primed and synchronized host has proven quite successful.

Fetomaternal Incompatibility

Gestational surrogacy may be considered for an otherwise fertile woman who may be at medical risk if she is pregnant. Examples include severe hypertension, severe diabetes, and severe maternal cardiac disease. Surrogacy may also be the answer if the fetus may be at risk for being carried by his or her mother, as in cases of Rh sensitivity, maternal chemotherapy, or recurrent miscarriages. These may be grouped under the heading of fetomaternal incompatibility. The use of these technologies for other than a clear medical indication, such as women wishing to have a genetic child but not wanting to carry the gestation, has been raised and should be dismissed.

Embryo Signaling

The biochemical signals from the endometrium to the preembryo and from the preembryo to the endometrium that effect implantation are unknown. Numerous candidates for implantation signals are being studied, such as oncofetal fibronectin, the integrins, platelet-activating factor, and PAPP-A.[12] These substances may be assayed as measures of embryo health, but, more important, if characterized and synthesized, they may allow us to improve or alter implantation.

Goals of Reproductive Technology

Reproductive technology has developed with a speed and force unparalleled in medical progress. Basic science and clinical care have raced along with as much rapidity as the entrepreneurial interest in these areas. The social, ethical, and legal constructs lag far behind the scientific capabilities. Legitimate efforts in Australia, Europe, and the United States through the American Society for Reproductive Medicine (ASRM) to form the constructs for these developments are in need of constant updating. The National Board of Ethics in Reproduction, initially formed jointly by the American College of Obstetricians and Gynecologists and the ASRM, may fulfill some of this urgent need in the future.

Frozen embryo custody cases, spousal frozen semen custody cases, gestational surrogate visitation rights, death row inmates' procreative rights, paid oocyte donors, embryo biopsy, gender selection, cloning, and less than truthful advertising are examples of controversies raised worldwide by assisted reproduction. Through gestational surrogacy, we have changed the very definition of motherhood, for the first time separating the genetic mother from the birth mother. We have created technologies to allow grandmothers to carry their grandchildren for daughters without a uterus and allow menopausal women to bear children through donor oocytes.

These scientific achievements create wonderment and potential societal repercussions. Society looks to us for maintaining procreative rights within accepted societal frameworks. Regulating agencies, governments, insurance firms, and consumer groups have interfered and may continue to interfere with the scientific process. To minimize this, we must maximize introspection within the profession.

The medical goals should be to provide each couple with a legitimate medical need with the support by which they may choose from the technologies available the best means to fulfill the biologic desire to reproduce. We cannot abdicate our responsibilities to limit access to those presenting as patients—those with a known medical disorder; only in this way can we avoid social engineering and potential abuse of these technologies. Backlash would follow such misuses. Only with valid scientific investigation and conservative clinical use will society and law allow us to continue to provide these options to couples in need.

The techniques are evolving, and the discoveries continue. Micromanipulation, gene therapy, and improved knowledge of fertilization and implantation are the areas of greatest growth. It is up to us as health care providers to ensure these achievements are indeed medical and social progress.

SUMMARY POINTS

◊ Infertility is a common problem in the United States, occurring in approximately 15% of couples. For the majority, it is correctable using more routine treatment but also the new ARTs.

◊ Presently, the core infertility workup should include the following: seminalysis, documentation of ovulation, and testing of the anatomy and function of the female reproductive system (HSG, laparoscopy–hysteroscopy).

◊ Current therapies for infertility are in transition secondary not only to newer advances in ARTs but also to the vagaries of patient funding and/or the changing patterns of managed care in the United States.

◊ GIFT and gonadotropin superovulation plus IUI are two newer "intermediate level" ART procedures capable of enhancing conception rates in infertile patients with patent fallopian tubes (i.e., endometriosis, male factor infertility, unexplained infertility).

◊ Newer ART efforts, such as variants of more traditional IVF, allow dramatic improvement of management results in many previously untreatable categories (i.e., ICSI for couples with severe oligospermia).

◊ REFERENCES

1. Abyholm T, Tambo T, Dale PO, Magnus O. *In vivo* fertilization procedures in infertile women with patent fallopian tubes: a comparison of gamete intrafallopian transfer, combined intrauterine and intraperitoneal insemination, and controlled ovarian hyperstimulation alone. *J Assist Reprod Genet* 1992;9:19.
2. Adamson GD. Treatment of endometriosis-associated infertility. *Semin Reprod Endocrinol* 1997;15:263.
3. Al-Azzawi F. Hysteroscopy or ultrasound? *Curr Opin Obstet Gynecol* 1996;8:246.
4. Ben-Nun I, Jaffe R, Fejgin MD, Beyth Y. Therapeutic maturation of endometrium in *in vitro* fertilization and embryo transfer. *Fertil Steril* 1992;57:953.
5. Campbell KL. Methods of monitoring ovarian function and predicting ovulation: summary of a meeting. *Res Front Fertil Regul* 1985;3:1.
6. Cohen J. Assisted hatching of human embryos. *J In Vitro Fertil Embryo Transfer* 1991;8:179.
7. Cohen J, Alikani M, Malter HE, et al. Partial zona dissection or subzonal sperm insertion: microsurgical fertilization alternatives based on evaluation of sperm and embryo morphology. *Fertil Steril* 1991;56:696.
8. Confino E, Tur-Kaspa I, DeCherney A, et al. Transcervical balloon tuboplasty: a multicenter study. *JAMA* 1990;264:2079.
9. Coulam CB. Immunologic tests in the evaluation of reproductive disorders: a critical review. *Am J Obstet Gynecol* 1992;167:1844.
10. Dodson WC, Hughes CL, Whitesides DB, et al. The effect of leuprolide acetate on ovulation induction with human menopausal gonadotropins in polycystic ovary syndrome. *J Clin Endocrinol Metab* 1987;65:95.
11. Dodson WC, Whitesides DB, Hughes CL, et al. Superovulation with intrauterine insemination in the treatment of infertility: a possible alternative to gamete intrafallopian transfer and *in vitro* fertilization. *Fertil Steril* 1987;48:441.
12. Feinberg RR, Kliman HJ, Lockwood CJ. Rapid communication: is oncofetal fibronectin a trophoblast glue for human implantation? *Am J Pathol* 1991;138:3.
13. Frydman R, Forman R, Rainhorn JD, et al. A new approach to follicular stimulation for *in vitro* fertilization: programmed oocyte retrieval. *Fertil Steril* 1986;46:657.
14. Gray RH. Epidemiology of infertility. *Curr Opin Obstet Gynecol* 1990; 2:154.
15. Gindoff P, Hall J, Nelson L, Stillman R. Efficacy of assisted reproductive technology during diagnostic operative and non-operative infertility laparoscopy. *Obstet Gynecol* 1990;75:299.
16. Handyside AH, Pattinson JK, Renketh RJA, et al. Biopsy of human preimplantation embryos and sexing by DNA amplification. *Lancet* 1989;1:347.
17. Holst N, Maltau JM, Forsdahl F, Hansen LJ. Handling of tubal infertility after introduction of *in vitro* fertilization: changes and consequences. *Fertil Steril* 1991;55:140.
18. Hughes CL. Monitoring of ovulation in the assessment of reproductive hazards in the workplace. *Reprod Toxicol* 1988;2:163.
19. Licchiardi LF, Hung-Ching L, Rosenwaks Z. Day 3 estradiol serum concentrations as prognosticators of ovarian stimulation response and pregnancy outcome in patients undergoing *in vitro* fertilization. *Fertil Steril* 1995;64:991.
20. Liu DY, Baker HWG. Tests of human sperm function and fertilization *in vitro*. *Fertil Steril* 1992;58:465.
21. Mandelbaum J, Junca AM, Plachot P, et al. Human embryo cryopreservation, extrinsic and intrinsic parameters of success. *Hum Reprod* 1987;2:709.
22. Medical Research International. *In vitro* fertilization—embryo transfer (IVF-ET) in the United States: 1990 results from the IVF-ET registry. *Fertil Steril* 1992;57:15.
23. Menken J, Larsen U. Fertility rates and aging. In: Mastroianni L, Paulsen CA, eds. *Aging, reproduction and the climacteric*. New York: Plenum Publishing, 1986:147.
24. Morritz de Kretser D, Baker HWG. Human infertility: the male factor. In: Adashi EY, Rock JA, Rosenwaks Z, eds. *Reproductive endocrinology, surgery, and technology*. Philadelphia: Lippincott–Raven, 1996:2031.
25. Olive DL, Haney AF. Endometriosis-associated infertility: a critical review of therapeutic approaches. *Obstet Gynecol Surv* 1986;41:538.
26. Paulson RJ, Sauer MV, Francis MM, et al. *In vitro* fertilization in unstimulated cycles: a clinical trial using hCG for timing of follicle aspiration. *Obstet Gynecol* 1990;76:788.
27. Paulson RJ, Sauer M, Lobo R. Embryo implantation following human *in vitro* fertilization: importance of endometrial receptivity. *Fertil Steril* 1990;53:870.
28. Perone N. Gamete intrafalloipian transfer (GIFT): historic perspective. *J In Vitro Fertil Embryo Transfer* 1991;8:1.
29. Ralt D, Goldenberg M, Fetterold P, et al. Sperm attraction to a follicular factor(s) correlates with human egg fertilizability. *Proc Natl Acad Sci USA* 1991;88:2840–2844.
30. Risquez F, Mathieson J, Zorn J-R. Tubal cannulation via the cervix: a passing fancy—or here to stay? *J In Vitro Fertil Embryo Transfer* 1990; 7:301.
31. Robinson D, Syrop C, Hammitt D. After superovulation-intrauterine insemination fails: the prognosis for treatment by gamete intrafallopian transfer/pronuclear stage transfer. *Fertil Steril* 1992;57:606.
32. Sauer MV, Paulson RJ, Lobo RA. Reversing the natural decline in human fertility: an extended clinical trial of oocyte donation to women of advanced reproductive age. *JAMA* 1992;268:1275.
33. Sauer MV, Paulson RJ, Lobo RA. A preliminary report on oocyte donation extending reproductive potential to women over 40. *N Engl J Med* 1980;323:1157.
34. Schlaff WD, Hassiakos DK, Damewood MD, Rock JA. Neosalpingostomy for distal tubal obstruction: prognostic factors and impact of surgical technique. *Fertil Steril* 1990;54:984.
35. Simon A, Avidan B, Mordel N, et al. The value of menotropin treatment for unexplained infertility prior to an *in-vitro* fertilization attempt. *Hum Reprod* 1991;6:222.
36. Soules MR. Luteal phase deficiency: an underdiagnosed and overtreated reproductive endocrine disorder. *Obstet Gynecol Clin North Am* 1987; 14:865.
37. Steptoe PC, Edwards RG. Birth after implantation of a human embryo. *Lancet* 1978;2:336.
38. Swerdloff RS, Boyers SP. Evaluation of the male partner of an infertile couple. *JAMA* 1982;247:2418.
39. Toner JP, Philput CB, Jones GS, Muasher SJ. Basal follicle-stimulating hormone level is a better predictor of *in vitro* fertilization performance than age. *Fertil Steril* 1991;55:784.

40. Van Noord-Zaadstra BM, Looman CW, Alsbach H, Habbema JD, te Velde ER, Karbaat J. Delaying childbearing: effect of age on fecundity and outcome of pregnancy. *BMJ* 1991;302:1361.

41. Vlahos N, Garcia JE. New developments in gonadotropin therapy. *Postgrad Obstet Gynecol* 1997;17(24):1.

42. Wallach EE. Induction of ovulation: general concepts. In: Wallach EE, Zacur HA, eds. *Reproductive medicine and surgery*. St. Louis, MO: Mosby–Year Book, 1995:555.

43. Zinaman MJ, Sachs PC. Evaluation of male infertility. *Postgrad Obstet Gynecol* 1993;13(1):1.

CHAPTER 42

Endometriosis

— ◊ —

Robert S. Schenken

Endometriosis is characterized by the presence of endometrial glands and stroma outside the endometrial cavity and uterine musculature. The pelvis is the most common site of endometriosis, but endometriotic implants may occur nearly anywhere in the body. Although there are numerous theories to explain why women develop endometriosis, no one theory has been conclusively proven. Endometriosis is a common gynecologic problem in reproductive-age women who present with pelvic pain, dyspareunia, or infertility. The management of endometriosis is controversial, but recent randomized clinical studies have substantiated some therapeutic approaches.

◊ PATHOGENESIS

Several theories have been proposed to explain the histogenesis of endometriosis.[21] The *implantation* theory proposes that endometrial tissue desquamated during menstruation passes through the fallopian tubes, where it gains access to and implants on pelvic structures. The incidence of retrograde menstruation is similar in women with and without endometriosis. Thus, the development of endometriosis could depend on the quantity of endometrial tissue reaching the peritoneal cavity or the capacity of a woman's immune system to remove the refluxed menstrual debris.

The *direct transplantation* theory is the probable explanation for endometriosis that develops in episiotomy, cesarean section, and other scars following surgery. Endometriosis in locations outside the pelvis likely develops from dissemination of endometrial cells or tissue through lymphatics or blood vessels. The *coelomic metaplasia* theory proposes that the coelomic (peritoneal) cavity contains undifferentiated cells or cells capable of dedifferentiating into endometrial tissue. This theory is based on embryologic studies demonstrating that all pelvic organs, including the endometrium, are derived from the cells lining the coelomic cavity. The *induction* theory, an extension of the coelomic metaplasia theory, postulates that the refluxed endometrial debris releases a product that activates undifferentiated peritoneal cells to undergo metaplasia. There is no conclusive proof that peritoneum can undergo spontaneous or induced metaplasia.

Anatomic alternations of the pelvis that increase tubal reflux of menstrual endometrium may increase a woman's chance of developing endometriosis. The incidence of endometriosis is increased in young women with genital tract obstructions that prevent expulsion of menses into the vagina and increase the likelihood of tubal reflux.[15] Other studies have suggested that deficient cellular immunity results in an inability to recognize the presence of endometrial tissue in abnormal locations.[23] Decreased natural killer cell activity resulting in decreased cytotoxicity to autologous endometrium has been reported in women with endometriosis.[17] The presence of increased concentrations of leukocytes and their cytokine products in peritoneal fluid of women with endometriosis may play a role in the initiation and growth of the ectopic implants.[10] The immune system clearly has an important, albeit unclear, role in the pathogenesis of endometriosis.

The possibility of a familial tendency for endometriosis has been recognized for several decades. If a patient has endometriosis, a first-degree female relative has a 7% likelihood of being similarly affected.

◊ EPIDEMOLOGY

The true prevalence of endometriosis in the general population is not known. Estimates of its prevalence are based on visualization of the pelvic organs. Pelvic endometriosis is present in approximately 1% of women undergoing major surgery for all gynecologic indications, 6% to 43% of women undergoing sterilization, 12% to 32% when laparoscopy is performed to determine the cause of pelvic pain in reproductive-age women, and 21% to 48% of women undergoing laparoscopy for infertility.[20] Endometriosis is found in 50% of teenagers undergoing laparoscopy for evaluation of chronic pelvic pain or dysmenorrhea.[6]

The influence of age, socioeconomic status, and race on the prevalence of endometriosis remains controversial.[11] The age at time of diagnosis is commonly 25 to 35 years, and endometriosis is rarely diagnosed in postmenopausal women.[16] Many believe that endometriosis is more common in women of upper economic classes because they delay pregnancy, which is postulated to increase the risk of developing endometriosis. It is unknown whether this reflects a true increased incidence or results from greater access to medical care. Recent evidence indicates that blacks have a prevalence of endometriosis similar to that in whites when controlled for socioeconomic status.

◊ PATHOLOGY

The most common sites of endometriosis, in decreasing order of frequency, are the ovaries, anterior and posterior cul-de-sac, posterior broad ligaments, uterosacral ligaments, uterus, fallopian tubes, sigmoid colon, appendix, and round ligaments.[12] Other sites less commonly involved include the vagina, cervix, and rectovaginal septum. These lesions usually result from extension and invasion of posterior cul-de-sac implants. Uncommon locations include the inguinal canal, abdominal or perineal scars, ureters, urinary bladder, umbilicus, kidney, lung, liver, diaphragm, vertebrae, and extremities.

Macroscopic Appearance

Endometriotic implants have a variety of appearances. Superficial lesions on the ovarian or peritoneal surface are commonly reddish maculae or nodules similar in consistency to normal endometrium. These implants vary from 1 mm to several centimeters in size. Collection of hemosiderin results in yellow-brown or black discoloration ("powder-brown" lesions). Nonpigmented disease appears as whitish opacified peritoneum, translucent blebs, or pinkish polyploid implants. Scarring with retraction of adjacent peritoneum and peritoneal pockets may occur.

Endometriosis may also appear as a deeply infiltrative disease. Tumor-like masses form from invasion, and diffuse fibrosis usually develops in the posterior cul-de-sac, pelvic side wall, or posterior broad ligament and ovary. Lesions in the cul-de-sac may invade the rectovaginal septum. The rectosigmoid and small bowel may become adherent to these areas. Endometriotic foci on the ovarian surface may develop a fibrous enclosure and manifest cyst formation as a result of accumulation of fluid and blood. These endometriotic cysts ("endometriomas") vary from several millimeters to over 10 cm in size. Bleeding with menses gives the cyst a dark-red or bluish hemorrhagic color. The degradation of blood pigment over time resulted in thick, tarry contents, and hence the term "chocolate cysts." Occasionally, the contents changes to a yellow straw color or clear fluid. Filmy or dense fibroid adhesions from these cysts to the pelvic side wall and fallopian tubes are common and may obscure visualization of the cyst.

Microscopic Appearance

Endometriosis is histomorphologically similar to eutopic endometrium. The four major components of endometriotic implants are endometrial glands, endometrial stroma, fibrosis, and hemorrhage. The relative amount of each component is highly variable and dependent in part on the age and location of the lesions. Identifying the endometrial elements in individual implants requires an adequate tissue specimen, proper orientation, and often serial sections of the specimen.

The endometrial glands in ectopic implants lack uniform size and shape. The glands may show normal cyclic change with mitotic figures and pseudostratification in response to estrogen or vacuoles and intraluminal secretion in response to progesterone. The response to endogenous and exogenous hormones is inconsistent. This may imply differences in steroid hormone receptor content and function. When glands are responsive, the epithelium becomes attenuated, and hemorrhage ensues at the time of menstruation.

The stromal cell morphologies of ectopic and eutopic endometrium are similar. Small arterioles, similar to the spiral arterioles of normal endometrium, are usually present in implants. Interstitial hemorrhage with accumulation of blood products and hemosiderin-laden macrophages is a frequent finding.

Fibrosis may occur in older endometriotic implants. This is very common in the lining of endometriomas, where the only histologic finding may be fibroblast proliferation and hemosiderin pigment deposition.

◊ SYMPTOMS

The common signs and symptoms of endometriosis are pelvic pain, dysmenorrhea, dyspareunia, abnormal uterine bleeding, and infertility. The type and severity of symptoms are dependent on the extent of disease, the location, and the organs involved. Even limited amounts of disease may cause significant symptomatology.

Endometriosis is present in approximately one-third of patients with chronic pelvic pain. The pain may be described as crampy, dull, or sharp and usually increases around menses. The discomfort may be unilateral or bilateral, and many patients complain of rectal pressure or low backache. Acute abdominal pain may result because of hemorrhage secondary to a ruptured endometrioma.

Dysmenorrhea is a more frequent complaint than dyspareunia. There is some correlation between the extent of disease and the severity of pain. The morphologic appearance of an endometriotic implant appears to be unrelated to pain symptomatology. Dyspareunia is more common in women with invasive endometriotic nodules in the cul-de-sac, uterosacral ligaments, rectrovaginal septum, and vagina.

Abnormal uterine bleeding occurs in up to one-third of women with endometriosis and presents as oligomenorrhea, polymenorrhea, and midcycle or premenstrual spotting. The abnormal bleeding likely results from conditions associated with endometriosis: oligoanovulatory, luteinized unruptured

TABLE 1. *Proposed mediators and mechanisms of infertility*

Anatomic distortion and tubal obstruction
Anovulation, luteal phase defects, and hormonal abnormalities
Galactorrhea/hyperprolactemia
Autoimmunity
Peritoneal leukocytes and the peritoneal inflammatory response
Peritoneal fluid prostaglandins
Peritoneal fluid cytokines
Embryo implantation defect and spontaneous abortions

TABLE 2. *Clinical signs*

Localized tenderness in the cul-de-sac or uterosacral ligament
Palpable tender nodules in the cul-de-sac, uterosacral ligament, or rectovaginal septum
Pain with uterine movement
Tender, enlarged adnexal masses
Fixation of adnexa or uterus in retroverted position

follicles, luteal phase defects, and other pathology such as uterine fibroids.

Endometriosis involving the gastrointestinal or urinary tracts and extrapelvic sites presents with symptoms characteristic of the location of disease. Bladder involvement is associated with frequency and urgency. Invasion of the mucosa results in hematuria. Ureteral and rare cases of renal endometriosis occasionally present with flank pain or gross hematuria. Symptoms suggestive of gastrointestinal involvement include, in decreasing order of frequency, diarrhea, rectal bleeding, constipation, and dyschezia. All symptoms are usually exacerbated catamenially.

There are numerous case reports of extrapelvic endometriosis. Pulmonary endometriosis presents with catamenial hemoptysis and dyspnea. Cutaneous lesions present with catamenial bleeding, tenderness, and swelling.

It is estimated that 25% to 50% of infertile women have endometriosis, and 30% to 50% of women with endometriosis are infertile. Although the association of endometriosis and infertility is well recognized, the pathophysiological mechanisms are poorly understood. Endometriomas and endometriosis with adhesions distort pelvic anatomy and impair tubal ovum pickup, which is an acceptable explanation for infertility. In less severe cases, there are several theories to explain the observed subfecundity (Table 1).

Recent research to explain the subfertility has focused on peritoneal fluid leukocytes and their cytokine products. Studies have suggested that constituents in the peritoneal fluid inhibit sperm function, fertilization, embryonic development, and implantation. The clinical significance of these findings has not been established.

◊ DIAGNOSIS

Endometriosis is usually diagnosed in the third and fourth decades of life. It has not been found in prepubertal girls and is rarely diagnosed in postmenopausal women. Endometriosis should be suspected in any woman having the classic symptoms of pelvic pain, dysmenorrhea, dyspareunia, abnormal menstrual bleeding, and infertility. These symptoms are present in other gynecologic disorders. No one constellation of signs or symptoms is pathognomonic of endometriosis. Many women with endometriosis are completely asymp-

tomatic, and endometriosis should be considered in all reproductive-age women with infertility or an adnexal mass.

Physical findings in women with endometriosis are variable and dependent on the location and severity of disease (Table 2).[25] Frequently, there are no obvious findings on pelvic examination. When findings are present, the most common is tenderness when palpating the posterior fornix. Nodules of endometriosis on the uterosacral ligaments, enlarged ovaries as a result of endometriotic cysts, and a uterus fixed in the cul-de-sac by adhesions may be detected on pelvic exam. Uterosacral implants are best palpated on rectovaginal examination. On the other hand, many patients with these clinical findings on pelvic exam later turn out not to have endometriosis.

The optimal way to diagnose endometriosis is by direct visualization of the site of suspected involvement. Because endometriosis is located primarily in the pelvis, laparoscopy is the preferred technique to make an accurate diagnosis. A double-puncture technique is necessary to adequately view all structures that may contain implants. Peritoneal fluid should be aspirated to see the entire cul-de-sac. Adhesions should be lysed to view the entire surface of the ovaries and the fossa ovarica. These sites are commonly involved with endometriosis when the ovary is adherent to the pelvic side wall. Suspected endometriomas should be aspirated and resected to confirm the diagnosis. Biopsy and histologic study of any suspicious areas are helpful when the diagnosis is questionable.

Transvaginal ultrasound can be used to identify ovarian endometriomas, but it is of little utility to diagnose peritoneal implants. The use of other radiologic studies and blood tests to diagnose endometriosis is rarely required. Radioimmunoassay for the tumor marker CA-125 has been used, but the test is not sufficiently sensitive, and patients having conditions other than endometriosis may test positive.[22]

◊ CLASSIFICATION

A number of classifications have been developed for staging endometriosis. The most widely used classification system for endometriosis was introduced by the American Society for Reproductive Medicine (ASRM) in 1979 and revised in 1985 and in 1997.[3] This system assigns a point score for the size and location of endometriotic implants and associated adhesions. The new ASRM endometriosis classification for infertility includes the morphologic appearance of the implant. There is also a form published by the ASRM to assist in the management of endometriosis in the presence of pelvic pain.

Endometriosis is classified as minimal, mild, moderate, and severe. Mild disease is characterized by superficial implants less than 5 cm in aggregate scattered on the peritoneum and ovaries. Minimal or no adhesions are present. Moderate forms are characterized by multiple implants, both superficial and invasive. Peritubal and periovarian adhesions may be evident. Severe forms are characterized by multiple superficial and deep implants, including large ovarian endometriomas. Filmy and dense adhesions are usually present.

◊ TREATMENT

The treatment of endometriosis is dependent on (1) the severity of symptoms, (2) the extent of disease, (3) the location of disease, (4) the patient's desire for pregnancy, and (5) the age of the patient. Treatment options are presented in Table 3.

Expectant Management

Avoiding specific therapy is considered when patients have minimal or no symptoms and minimal or mild endometriosis. Patients in this category may benefit from cyclic oral contraceptives to retard progression of the disease and protect against unwanted pregnancy. Minor pain may be controlled by nonsteroidal antiinflammatory drugs and/or analgesics. Infertile women having limited disease may be observed without treatment.[2] However, one study suggests that surgical treatment of mild endometriosis results in higher pregnancy rates than expectant management.[13] If pregnancy occurs, regression or complete resolution of the disease is common. Perimenopausal women may be managed expectantly even when the disease is advanced because endometriotic implants usually regress in the absence of ovarian hormone production after menopause.

Medical Therapy

Endometriotic implant growth is highly dependent on ovarian steroids. Medical therapy attempts to "induce" pseudopregnancy or menopause, the two physiological states believed to inhibit or delay progression of endometriosis by

TABLE 3. *Treatment options*

Expectant management
Medical therapy
    Progestins
    Danazol
    GnRH analogs
Surgical therapy (laparoscopy or laparotomy)
    Conservative: retains uterus and ovarian tissue
    Definitive: removal of uterus and possibly ovaries
Combination therapy
    Preoperative medical therapy
    Postoperative medical therapy

interrupting cyclic ovarian hormone production. Progestins alone or in combination with estrogen hormonally mimic pregnancy. Danazol and gonadotropin-releasing hormone (GnRH) analogs induce a state of "pseudomenopause." Medical therapy has some advantages over surgery: (1) avoidance of the surgical risks of damaging pelvic organs and causing postoperative adhesions, and (2) treatment of implants that are not visible at surgery. Disadvantages of medical therapy are the associated side effects, high recurrence rates following discontinuation of treatment, lack of an effect on endometrioma and adhesions, and inability to conceive because of medically induced anovulation. Medical therapy has never been shown to enhance fertility (Fig. 1). Thus, it is not appropriate for women with advanced stages of endometriosis and adhesions or women desiring pregnancy. The most commonly used medications to treat endometriosis are continuous oral contraceptives, progestins, danazol, and GnRH analogs. They should be considered only after a definitive diagnosis of endometriosis has been made by direct visualization of the implants.

Progestins inhibit endometriotic tissue growth by a direct effect on the implants, causing initial decidualization and eventual pseudodecidual necrosis (CO) or atrophy (progestins). Progestins also inhibit pituitary gonadotropin secretion and ovarian hormone production. Treatment may consist of medroxyprogesterone acetate (10 mg three times a day) or norethindrone acetate (5 mg daily), usually continued for 6 months. Medroxyprogesterone may also be given as an injection (100 to 150 mg monthly).[14] Side effects include irregular menstrual bleeding, nausea, breast tenderness, fluid retention, and depression. The effectiveness of continuous oral contraceptives or progestins in eliminating implants and the risk of recurrent endometriosis following treatment are not precisely known. Over 80% of women have partial or complete pain relief. Pregnancy rates in patients with less severe stages of disease are equivalent to those following expectant management.

Danazol is the isoxazol derivative of 17α-ethinyltestosterone. Danazol has three mechanisms of action: (1) inhibition of pituitary gonadotropin secretion, (2) direct inhibition of endometriotic implant growth, and (3) direct inhibition of steroidogenic enzymes. Danazol is given orally in divided doses ranging from 400 to 800 mg daily, generally for 6 months. Most women taking danazol have side effects, but only a small percentage of patients discontinue the drug because of unwanted effects. Side effects, in decreasing order of frequency, include weight gain, muscle cramps, decreased breast size, acne, hirsutism, oily skin, decreased high-density lipoprotein levels, increased liver enzymes, hot flashes, mood changes, and depression. Danazol decreases the size of implants, especially in treating mild or moderate stages of disease. Endometriomas and adhesions do not respond well to danazol treatment. More than 80% of patients experience relief or improvement of pain symptoms within 2 months of treatment.[4] Pregnancy rates following treatment approximate 40% and are independent of the disease severity. Danazol is

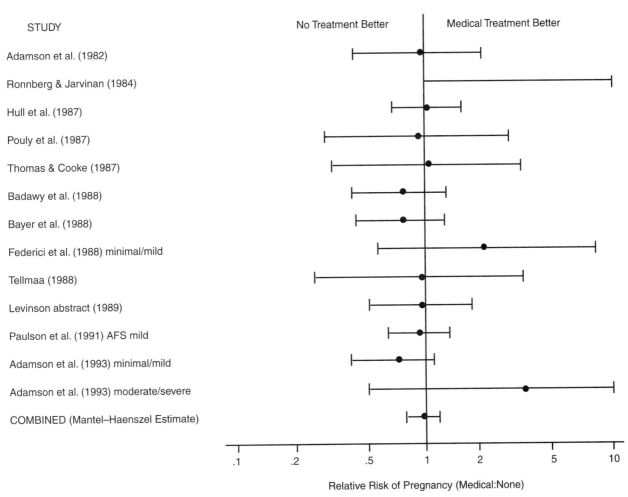

FIG. 1. Metaanalysis of studies comparing medical treatment with no treatment.

no more effective than expectant management for treating infertility.

The GnRH analogs profoundly suppress ovarian estrogen production by inhibiting pituitary gonadotropin secretion. These medications are administered by nasal spray or injections. The usual dose is 400 to 800 mg daily for nasal nafarelin, 3.6 mg for monthly subcutaneous goserelin, and 3.75 mg for monthly intramuscular leuprolide. Side effects of the hypoestrogenemia are common and include hot flashes, vaginal dryness, decreased libido, insomnia, breast tenderness, depression, headaches, and transient menstruation. In addition, GnRH analog treatment[4] for the recommended 6-month period decreases bone density and total body calcium, but most of the bone loss is reversible.[8] Hypoestrogenic side effects and bone loss may be prevented by add-back therapy with high-dose norethindrone (10 mg daily) or the daily combination of low-dose norethindrone (2.5 mg), sodium etidronate (400 mg), and calcium carbonate (500 mg).[24] The GnRH analogs effectively reduce the size of endometriotic implants, even with add-back therapy. Recurrence rate over 5 years ranges from 37% for patients with mild disease to 74% for severe disease.[26] The GnRH analogs are as affective as other

medical therapy in relieving pain symptoms, but they do not enhance fertility.[9]

Surgical Management

Surgery for endometriosis is considered conservative when the uterus and as much ovarian tissue as possible are preserved. Definitive surgery involves hysterectomy with or without removal of the fallopian tubes and ovaries.

Surgery is indicated when the symptoms are severe, incapacitating, or acute and when the disease is advanced. Surgery is preferred over medical therapy for advanced stages of disease with anatomic distortion of the pelvic organs, endometriotic cysts, or obstruction of the bowel or urinary tract. Women who are older than 35 years of age, infertile, or symptomatic following expectant or medical management should be treated surgically.

Laparoscopy is the preferred approach to perform conservative surgery.[7] Treatment of endometriosis is possible at the initial laparoscopy to diagnose the condition. This offers the advantage of ablating the implants and adhesions while avoiding possible progression of disease or symptoms and the expense and side effects of medical therapy. Disadvantages include possible damage to bowel and bladder, infection, and mechanical trauma that may result in adhesion formation.

Conservative surgery involves excision, fulguration, or laser ablation of endometriotic implants and removal of associated adhesions. The goal is to restore normal pelvic anatomy. Laparoscopic treatment offers advantages over laparotomy, including shorter hospitalization, anesthesia, and recuperation times. Laparotomy is advisable to deal with extensive adhesions or invasive endometriosis located near structures such as the uterine arteries, ureter, bladder, and bowel. Ancillary procedures include presacral neurectomy or uterosacral interruption of sensory nerves innervating the pelvis to relieve midline pelvic pain. Uterine suspension may be performed to avoid adhesion formation from the cul-de-sac to the posterior surface of the uterus, tubes, and ovaries.

Surgery effectively removes pathology and restores normal anatomy in most cases. The disease recurrence risk is estimated to be as much as 40% with 10 years of follow-up.[27]

Pain relief is achieved in 80% to 90% of patients. Presacral neurectomy provides additional pain relief, but its benefit is not lasting,[5] and bladder dysfunction occasionally occurs after the procedure. The chance for pregnancy following surgery is related to the stage of disease and presence of other infertility factors. Approximate pregnancy rates after surgery in patients with mild, moderate, and severe endometriosis are, respectively, 60%, 50%, and 40%.[1] Surgery is performed over expectant or medical management for infertile women with endometriosis (Fig. 2).

Definitive surgery for treatment of endometriosis is indicated when significant disease is present and future pregnancy is not desired, when incapacitating symptoms persist following medical therapy or conservative surgery, and when coexisting pelvic pathology requires hysterectomy. The decision to perform hysterectomy is dependent on the patient's interest in maintaining child-bearing potential. The ovaries may be conserved in younger women to avoid the need for estrogen replacement therapy. Removal of both ovaries is appropriate

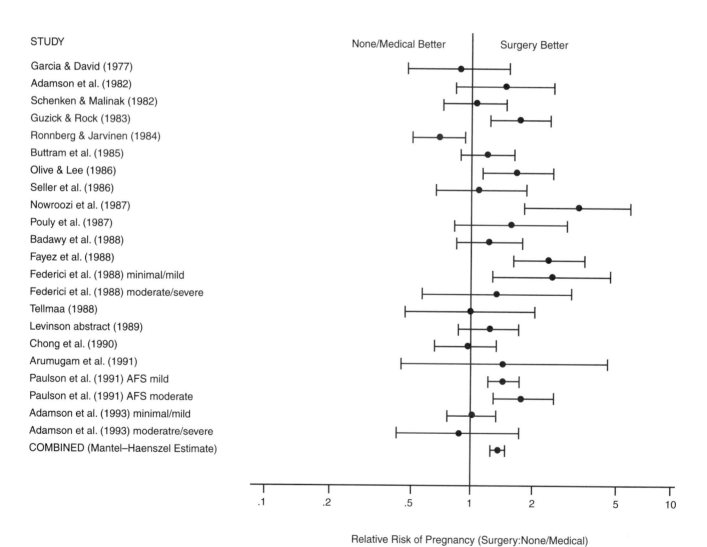

FIG. 2. Metaanalysis of studies comparing surgical treatment (operative laparoscopy or laparotomy) with nonsurgical treatment (medical treatment or no treatment).

when the ovaries are extensively damaged by endometriosis or when menopause is approaching. Endometriosis may recur even with castration.[19] Menopausal hormonal replacement is indicated when the ovaries are removed, even when surgery has not removed all endometriotic implants. The chance for symptomatic recurrence in these cases is small except when endometriosis involves the bowel.

Combination Medical/Surgical Therapy

Medical therapy is used before surgery to decrease the size of endometriotic implants and thus reduce the extent of surgery. In cases in which complete removal of implants is not possible or advisable, postoperative medical therapy is used to treat residual disease. Progestin, danazol, or GnRH analogs may be used in conjunction with conservative or definitive surgery. Preoperative medical therapy may decrease the amount of surgical dissection required to remove implants, but it does not prolong pain relief, increase pregnancy rates, or decrease recurrence rates.[18] Postoperative treatment with GnRH analogs will delay the recurrence of pelvic pain,[28] but there is no evidence to support its use in infertile patients.

SUMMARY POINTS

◊ The histogenesis of endometriosis is poorly understood, but emerging evidence supports the causative role of retrograde menstruation and implantation of endometrial tissue.

◊ Endometriosis is a common in women with pelvic pain or infertility.

◊ Laparoscopy is the optimal technique to diagnose pelvic endometriosis.

◊ In most cases, surgical therapy at the time of initial diagnosis effectively relieves pain and may enhance fertility.

◊ Alternatively, medical therapy with progestins, danazol, or GnRH analogs will ameliorate pelvic pain, but they do not enhance fertility.

◊ Endometriosis is a recurrent disease, and definitive treatment with removal of pelvic organs may be necessary.

◊ REFERENCES

1. Adamson GD, Hurd SJ, Pasta DJ, Rodriguez BD. Laparoscopic endometriosis treatment: Is it better? *Fertil Steril* 1992;59:35–44.
2. Adamson GD, Pasta DJ. Surgical treatment of endometriosis-associated infertility: Meta-analysis compared with survival analysis. *Am J Obstet Gynecol* 1994;171:1488.
3. American Society for Reproductive Medicine. Revised American Society for Reproductive Medicine classification of endometriosis. *Fertil Steril* 1997;67:817–821.
4. Barbieri RL, Evans S, Kistner RW. Danazol in the treatment of endometriosis: Analysis of 100 cases with a 4-year follow-up. *Fertil Steril* 1982;37:737.
5. Candiani GB, Fedele L, Vercellini P, et al. Presacral neurectomy for the treatment of pelvic pain associated with endometriosis: A controlled study. *Am J Obstet Gynecol* 1992;167:100.
6. Chatman DL, Ward AB. Endometriosis in adolescents. *J Reprod Med* 1982;27:156.
7. Crosignani PG, Vercellini P, Biffignandi F, et al. Laparoscopy versus laparotomy in conservative surgical treatment for severe endometriosis. *Fertil Steril* 1996;66:706.
8. Dawood MY, Ramos J, Khan-Dawood FS. Depot leuprolide acetate versus danazol for treatment of pelvic endometriosis: changes in vertebral bone mass and serum estradiol and calcitonin. *Fertil Steril* 1995;63:1177.
9. Dlugi AM, Miller JD, Knittle J, Lupron Study Group. Lupron depot (leuprolide acetate for depot suspension) in the treatment of endometriosis: a randomized, placebo-controlled, double-blind study. *Fertil Steril* 1990;54:419.
10. Dmowski WP, Gebel HM, Braun DP. The role of cell-mediated immunity in pathogenesis of endometriosis. *Acta Obstet Gynecol Scand [Suppl]* 1994;159:7.
11. Houston DE. Evidence for the risk of pelvic endometriosis by age, race, and socioeconomic status. *Epidemiol Rev* 1984;6:167.
12. Jenkins S, Olive DL, Haney AF. Endometriosis: Pathogenetic implications of the anatomic distribution. *Obstet Gynecol* 1986;67:335.
13. Macroux S, Haheux R, Berube S, et al. Laparoscopic surgery in infertile women with minimal or mild endometriosis. *N Engl J Med* 1997;337:217.
14. Olive DL. Medical treatment: alternatives to danazol. In: Schenken RS, ed. *Endometriosis: Contemporary concepts in clinical management.* Philadelphia: JB Lippincott, 1989;189.
15. Olive DL, Henderson DY. Endometriosis and mullerian anomalies. *Obstet Gynecol* 1987;69:412.
16. Olive DL, Schwartz LB. Endometriosis. *N Engl J Med* 1993;328:1759.
17. Oosterlynck DJ, Cornillie FJ, Waer M, et al. Women with endometriosis show a defect in natural killer activity resulting in a decreased cytotoxicity to autologous endometrium. *Fertil Steril* 1991;56:45.
18. Parazzini F, Fedele L, Busacca M, et al. Postsurgical medical treatment of advanced endometriosis: Results of a randomized clinical trial. *Am J Obstet Gynecol* 1994;171:1205.
19. Redwine DB. Endometriosis persisting after castration: clinical characteristics and results of surgical management. *Obstet Gynecol* 1994;83:405–413.
20. Sangi-Haghpeykar H, Poindexter AN. Epidemiology of endometriosis among parous women. *Obstet Gynecol* 1995;85:983.
21. Schenken RS. Pathogenesis. In: Schenken RS, ed. *Endometriosis: Contemporary concepts in clinical management.* Philadelphia: JB Lippincott, 1989:1.
22. Schenken RS, Vancaillie TG, Riehl RM, et al. New developments in diagnostic techniques. In: Chadha DR, Buttram VC Jr, eds. *Current concepts in endometriosis.* New York: Alan R. Liss, 1990:137.
23. Steele RW, Dmowski WP, Marmer DJ. Immunologic aspects of human endometriosis. *Am J Reprod Immunol* 1984;6:33.
24. Surrey ES, Voigt B, Fournet N, Judd HL. Prolonged gonadotropin-releasing hormone agonist treatment of symptomatic endometriosis: the role of cyclic sodium etidronate and low-dose norethindrone add-back therapy. *Fertil Steril* 1995;63:747–755.
25. Vercellini P, Trespidi L, De Giorgi O, et al. Endometriosis and pelvic pain: relation to disease stage and localization. *Fertil Steril* 1995;65:299.
26. Waller KG, Shaw RW. Gonadotropin-releasing hormone analogues for the treatment of endometriosis: long-term follow-up. *Fertil Steril* 1993;59:511.
27. Wheeler JM, Malinak LR. Recurrent endometriosis: incidence, management, and prognosis. *Am J Obstet Gynecol* 1983;146:247.
28. Winkel CA, Bray M. Treatment of women with endometriosis using excision alone, ablation alone, or ablation in combination with leuprolide acetate. *Am J Obstet Gynecol* (in press).

CHAPTER 43

Climacteric

———— ◊ ————

Charles B. Hammond

The population of the United States is aging. More than 50 million women have reached the climacteric, that phase of life for women that marks the transition from being able to reproduce to being nonreproductive. The most visible event in this transition is the cessation of physiologic uterine bleeding, referred to as the menopause. Although different, the terms *menopause* and *climacteric* are often used interchangeably.[2]

The approximate age of menopause for white women in the United States is 51 years; the mean life expectancy of these women is over 85 years. Most women in the United States will live more than one-third of their lives without significant estrogen production. The special health problems created by prolonged estrogen deprivation are just beginning to be appreciated.[69]

◊ HISTORY

Estrogen was chemically synthesized in the 1920s. Mazer and Israel first reported successful treatment of menopausal vasomotor symptoms with estrogen in 1935. Davies described improvement of atrophic vaginitis by treatment with estrogen. Albright and colleagues observed that estrogen had a beneficial effect on osteoporosis. These findings confirmed that estrogen was effective treatment for the menopausal syndrome. Initially, some gynecologists had reservations about using estrogen in menopausal women. In 1940, Emil Novak stated the following:

> There is perhaps no gynecologic disorder in which the indication for organotherapy (estrogen) is more rational than in the treatment of typical climacteric symptoms. . . . The question of the possible hazard of inciting malignancy in cancer-susceptible individuals cannot be described in the present state of our knowledge.

In 1966, Robert A. Wilson[79] in *Feminine Forever* referred to the menopause as a curable disease state. After this disclosure, estrogen sales increased approximately 400% between 1966 and 1975. In December 1975, two articles and an editorial were published, linking continuous estrogen replacement therapy (ERT) alone to an increased risk of endometrial cancer. Several other articles with similar conclusions soon appeared, and the use of estrogen dropped dramatically. In the late 1970s and early 1980s, a series of articles was published that clearly documented that the increased risk of endometrial cancer associated with continuous estrogen therapy could be largely negated by the regular addition of a potent synthetic progestin to the estrogen.

Attention has now turned to the apparent significant benefit of ERT on cardiovascular mortality, particularly coronary artery disease. Some still challenge these observations, based on what may be bias in selection. While it will be a number of years before several ongoing, large, randomized trials provide better answers, I believe that ERT/hormone replacement therapy (HRT) does significantly reduce cardiovascular disease in women. Data are rapidly being developed to demonstrate not only a reduction in cardiovascular disease by ERT/HRT but also a significant reduction in osteoporosis and related fractures. Additionally, newer data suggest that ERT/HRT may have a role in the reduction of certain types of urinary incontinence, in Alzheimer's disease, and in colon cancer. Perhaps, there may also be a role for estrogen in adult macular degeneration.

It thus appears that ERT/HRT can be of major benefit for the control of menopausal symptoms (e.g., hot flushes, vaginal atrophy) and can also retard the development of other major metabolic diseases of aging women. Of residual concern, however, is the potential impact of such treatment on the incidence of breast cancer, a concern fueled by several recent articles purporting a causal linkage but negated by many other reports not identifying such a concern.

In summary, the menopause (i.e., climacteric) continues to be a controversial epoch in women's lives. Many data now exist to support a major protective role for ERT/HRT, although several other concerns have not yet been fully answered. This chapter provides an overview of this important aspect of women's health.

◊ CAUSE OF MENOPAUSE

No single all-inclusive theory adequately explains the menopause. However, there is no doubt that the ovary is primary to it. The exhaustion of gonadotropin-responsive follicular units is responsible for the reduction of estrogen secretion and the cessation of menses. The average age of a woman at menopause, which has remained unchanged since the 6th century, is 51.4 years, with a standard deviation of 3.8 years. The age at which menopause occurs is unaffected by race, socioeconomic status, number of pregnancies, oral contraceptive use, education, physical characteristics, alcohol consumption, age of menarche, or date of last pregnancy. Only cigarette smoking, irradiation, and certain types of chemotherapy have conclusively been shown to moderately hasten follicular exhaustion.

◊ OVARY AND MENOPAUSE

The ovary develops on the medioventral border of the urogenital ridge, adjacent to the kidney and the primitive adrenal. Until 42 days' gestation, the gonads are indifferent; that is, on a morphologic basis, the ovary and testis are indistinguishable. This indifferent gonad is formed from a proliferation of the mesodermal coelomic epithelium, the mesenchymal cell mass on the urogenital ridge, and mesonephric elements. Additionally, the indifferent gonad contains large primordial germ cells that migrated from the yolk sac to the genital ridge during the fifth week of embryonic life. The 300 to 1300 primordial germ cells that have seeded the indifferent gonad will become either oogonia or spermatozoa. In females, they undergo mitosis to form oogonia. The oogonia replicate so that there are approximately 600,000 by 8 weeks' gestation and 6 to 7 million by 20 weeks' gestation.

Between 8 and 13 weeks' gestation, meiosis is initiated under the influence of a meiosis-inducing substance secreted by the rete ovarii. The initiation of meiosis converts the oogonia to primary oocytes, some of which become surrounded by precursors of granulosa cells, thus creating primordial follicles. Conversion of oogonia to primary oocytes and formation of primordial follicles are not completed until 6 months after birth. Primary oocytes that do not form primordial follicles degenerate. It has been estimated that of the 6 million oogonia present in the fetal ovaries at 20 weeks' gestation, only 700,000 to 2 million will form primordial follicles. Thus, human females has a variable but finite number of primordial follicles.

The primordial follicles present at birth are lost from the ovary by either ovulation or follicular atresia. Follicular atresia is the physiologic degeneration of the oocyte and its surrounding stroma. Atresia begins at 5 months of fetal life and continues until all follicles are exhausted. Atresia occurs continuously during the menstrual cycle and even during pregnancy. The factors determining whether a primordial follicle ovulates or undergoes atresia are unknown. The total number of oocytes at puberty and the efficiency of the atretic process may determine the age of menopause.

Some primordial follicles can still be found in the ovaries of postmenopausal women. This suggests that the more functionally normal follicles are depleted first. Thus, as a woman ages, she is left with more gonadotropin-resistant, less hormonally active follicles. This concept may help explain the signs and symptoms of the climacteric. As the number of quality follicular units declines, the ovary undergoes gross and microscopic changes. Ovarian weight declines from 14 g in the fourth decade to approximately 5 g postmenopausally. Microscopic examination of the postmenopausal ovary reveals the remaining primordial follicles undergoing follicular atresia. The ovarian stroma is also more prominent, with increased numbers of medullary stromal and interstitial cells.

◊ SYSTEMIC CHANGES WITH AGING

Senescence is the process or condition of aging. The term *disease* is defined as a morbid process with a characteristic train of symptoms. Senescence produces its own symptoms that in a young person would be considered a disease. Physicians have been unwilling to accept involution and the symptoms that aging produces as a natural and inevitable phase of life. Because the menopause is the most obvious sign of senescence in women, many signs and symptoms, as well as diseases, are incorrectly attributed to gonadal failure. Many organ systems are affected by the aging process independently of gonadal failure. Changes in some of the major organs are briefly outlined below and summarized in Table 1.[35]

Nervous System

Neural cells reach maturity and stop dividing in infancy. With normal aging, the brain loses 5% to 10% of its gross weight, and the total number of brain cells decreases 20% to 50%. Aging brain cells show a decline in functional ability. There is significant slowing in the transmission of impulses between neurons, but intraneuronal depolarization remains normal. Cerebral blood flow may decline 30% to 40% with age. This decrease does not correlate with alterations in cognitive function. All people show some deterioration in short-term memory with age, even in the absence of organic brain disease. Other changes include difficulties with thermoregulation, eyesight, hearing, smell, taste, and touch. The sense of taste shows a particularly dramatic decline with age. A 75-year-old person may have only 20% of a 20-year-old person's ability to taste.

Cardiovascular System

With regard to the cardiovascular system, it is often difficult to tell where normal aging ends and disease begins. Certain changes occur so frequently that they may be normal. Physical changes include hypertrophy of the myocardium and calcification of the heart valves. There is a decrease in maximal oxygen consumption that parallels a decrease in cardiac output. This decline is at the rate of 1% per year, starting in the third

TABLE 1. *Changes associated with aging*

Organ system	Clinical manifestation	Age-related change
Central nervous system	Postural hypotension Slowness of movement Decreased rate of learning	Diminished autonomic regulation Neuronal loss in nucleus basalis Diminished neuronal transmission rates
Cardiovascular system	Diminished cardiac reserve	Decreased myocardial cell number Calcification of heart valves
Gastrointestinal system	Dysphagia Constipation	Decreased esophageal motility Decreased intestinal motility
Immune system	Increased susceptibility to infections Impaired response to immunization	Diminished cellular immunity Diminished primary antibody response
Endocrine-metabolic	Relative glucose intolerance Relative hypothyroidism	B-cell degeneration Glandular fibrosis
Skin	Wrinkling Slow healing	Decreased elasticity Decreased cell replication

(Adapted from ref. 35.)

decade. The aging heart usually functions well for everyday activities but has significantly diminished reserves for stress.

Respiratory System

Some amount of emphysema is inevitable with advancing years. The alveolar septal membranes weaken and break down, leaving depleted alveoli. Normal aging also causes the collagen in septa to become rigid. This rigidity causes a restrictive limitation on pulmonary functions. There is a diminution in vital capacity and maximum breathing capacity and an increase in residual volume. In people 75 years of age, maximum inspiratory and expiratory pressures may have dropped 50% and voluntary ventilation 60%.

Urinary Tract

The aging kidney has a diminished ability to clear medications. This may be a reflection of the decrease in cardiac output, which decreases renal plasma flow. The kidney may also lose the ability to concentrate urine. On microscopic examination, the aging kidney will show evidence of interstitial fibrosis, tubular atrophy, and glomerular degeneration.

Gastrointestinal System

Few structural changes occur in the gastrointestinal tract, but digestive disorders are common among the elderly. There is age-related atrophy of the intestinal mucosa and marked reduction in gastric secretions. This results in an increased incidence of gallstones, gastrointestinal cancer, and diverticulosis with advancing age. Additionally, diminished integrity of the gastroesophageal sphincter leads to increased gastric reflux.

Immune System

The immune system shows a steady decline in function from adolescence to death. The reasons for this are unknown. Histologically, there is a reduction in the number of stem cells in the bone marrow, an increase in B cells in the spleen and lymph nodes, and a decrease in circulating lymphocytes. Functionally, there is a decrease in antibody response of B cells to antigens, an increase in autoantibodies, a decrease in proliferative responses of T cells and B cells, and changes in modulators to include B-cell suppression and helper T-cell formation.

Skin and Musculoskeletal System

The skin loses its subcutaneous fat and elasticity with age. Collagen is reduced. This results in skin that is easily traumatized and slow to heal. The increased incidence of arthritis in elderly people is partly due to degenerative changes in the articular surfaces and perichondrial margins of the joints.

Endocrine System

The pituitary loses 20% of its volume by the ninth decade of life but still maintains normal concentrations of growth hormone, adrenocorticotropic hormone, and thyroid-stimulating hormone. Anatomically, the thyroid gland undergoes progressive fibrosis with age. In people older than 50 years, concentrations of triiodothyronine are diminished by 25% to 40%. Still, elderly patients remain clinically euthyroid.

Beta-cell degeneration of the pancreas progresses with age. By age 65 years, 50% of patients have chemically abnormal responses to the glucose tolerance test. Frank diabetes is clinically evident in only 7%.

◊ REPRODUCTIVE ENDOCRINE CHANGES IN CLIMACTERIC WOMEN

Hypothalamus–Pituitary

Changes in the hypothalamic–pituitary–gonadal axis are responsible for the menstrual irregularity associated with the perimenopause. As women approach the age of menopause, their menstrual interval usually lengthens. The luteal phase remains 14 days, but the follicular phase often lengthens. The prolonged follicular phase is probably due to the diminished supply of gonadotropin-sensitive follicles. These gonadotropin-insensitive follicles take longer to produce preovulatory estrogen levels. When the preovulatory estrogen levels are not attained, an anovulatory cycle results. By measurement of luteinizing hormone (LH), follicle-stimulating hormone (FSH), estradiol, and progesterone levels during the menstrual cycles of women aged 46 to 56 years and of women aged 18 to 30 years, it has been shown that the older women had higher FSH levels, lower estradiol levels, and equivalent LH levels, compared with the younger women.

During the perimenopause, FSH values of 40 mIU/ml or more are often found. Values greater than 100 mIU/ml almost certainly indicate follicular exhaustion. FSH levels for the first time since puberty exceed LH levels. The maximal increase in LH and FSH levels occurs 2 to 3 years after menopause. Gonadotropin concentrations over the next five decades remain stable or decrease slightly. In contrast, surgical menopause results in rapid and dramatic changes in FSH and LH levels. Twenty days after oophorectomy, FSH values are greater than 70 mIU/ml, and LH values are greater than 50 mIU/ml. Maximum concentrations are reached by 45 days. ERT/HRT will significantly lower LH and FSH levels, but usually not to premenopause levels. The inability to reduce FSH and LH levels to normal values is explained by the loss of inhibin production from ovarian granulosa cells.

As peripheral gonadotropin levels rise, abnormal pulse patterns of LH are observed. Menopausal women have a pulse frequency of 10 to 20 minutes compared with a 90- to 120-minute pulse frequency in the early follicular phase of reproductive-age women. There also appears to be a loss of opioid inhibition of gonadotropin release in postmenopausal women. The physiologic significance of these changes remains unknown at this time.

Although there is no appropriately sensitive or specific assay for measuring circulating gonadotropin-releasing hormone (Gn-RH), the increased pulse frequency and amplitude of LH release are probably the result of increased Gn-RH release. The results of a few published reports on serum and urine Gn-RH levels in postmenopausal women indicate an overall increase. Administration of Gn-RH to a postmenopausal woman results in an LH and FSH response similar to that in a woman of reproductive age, although the response is greater in magnitude. This may be due to diminished circulating estradiol concentrations and therefore diminished negative feedback with Gn-RH.

Estrogen Production

The principal circulating estrogen in premenopausal women is estradiol-17β. Serum concentrations of estradiol-17β fluctuate in relation to maturation and involution of the ovarian follicle and the corpus luteum. Estradiol is produced either by direct ovarian secretion or by peripheral conversion of testosterone and estrone. The exact percentages of total estrogen production from each source vary with the phase of the menstrual cycle and age.[53] The adrenal gland has not been shown

to secrete estradiol directly in any significant quantities. During the reproductive years, 80 to 500 μg of estradiol are produced daily.[20]

Oophorectomy in premenopausal women reduces circulating estradiol concentrations from a mean of 120 pg/ml to 18 pg/ml. This suggests that 95% of circulating estradiol is derived from the ovary. Estradiol production in the ovary is achieved by the synergistic actions of the granulosa and theca cell components. According to the two-cell theory, the theca produces 19-carbon (C-19) steroids, which are converted to estrogens by the aromatase system in the granulosa. The granulosa cells are stimulated by FSH and estradiol, whereas the theca and stromal cells respond to LH. As follicular exhaustion occurs, estrogen concentrations gradually decrease. As time passes, fewer and fewer follicles remain, and estradiol concentrations approximate those of oophorectomized premenopausal women.

The predominant estrogen of the postmenopausal woman is estrone. The biologic potency of estrone is only one-third that of estradiol. Virtually no estrone is produced by the postmenopausal ovary or adrenal gland. Oophorectomy in postmenopausal women produces no discernible change in circulating estrone or estradiol levels. Most estrone is formed by the peripheral conversion of androstenedione by extraglandular aromatase. Aromatase has been identified in the liver, fat, and certain hypothalamic nuclei. The activity of extraglandular aromatase is age- and weight-dependent and increases twofold during the perimenopause. Production rates postmenopausally are 40 μg per day for estrone and 6 μg per day for estradiol, compared with 80 to 500 μg per day for estradiol and 80 to 300 μg per day for estrone in reproductive-age women.[25]

Essentially all estradiol in postmenopausal women can be accounted for by the conversion of estrone to estradiol. Even though testosterone production in postmenopausal women remains constant, only about 0.1% of testosterone is converted to estradiol.[30] Unlike premenopausal women, whose production rates of estrogens vary with the ovarian cycle, postmenopausal women have fairly constant circulating levels of estrone and estradiol. The concentration of estrone rises to four times that of estradiol after the menopause. Both estrone and estradiol are inactivated by the sulfotransferase enzyme system. Interestingly, estrone sulfate has an average concentration of 128 pg/ml, compared with only 35 pg/ml for estrone. The conjugated form may form a pool from which biologically active estrogens can be produced.

Androgen Production

In 1942, Fuller Albright suggested that there was an "adrenopause" as well as a menopause in women. He made this statement on the basis of a 20% and 40% decrease in dehydroepiandrosterone sulfate (DHEAS) levels and dehydroepiandrosterone (DHEA) levels, respectively, in postmenopausal women. ERT/HRT produces a twofold increase in DHEAS values. Therefore, the magnitude of the diminished concentrations of the two androgens is probably due to estrogen deprivation.

Serum cortisol concentrations remain unaffected by ERT/HRT. *In vitro* data suggest that estrogen is a noncompetitive inhibitor of 3β-hydroxysteroid dehydrogenase. A relative block at this site would augment DHEA and DHEAS production.

Androstenedione, the most extensively produced androgen in reproductive-age women, declines in the climacteric. Androstenedione production decreases from 1500 pg/ml to 800 pg/ml in postmenopausal women. Overall, the postmenopausal ovary contributes only 20% to the circulating androstenedione. Testosterone levels in postmenopausal women decline, but not to the same extent as those of estrogen. In premenopausal women, circulating testosterone is derived from three sources: the ovary (25%), the adrenal gland (25%), and extraglandular conversion from androstenedione (50%). The postmenopausal ovary produces a larger percentage of testosterone than does the premenopausal ovary, yielding about 50% of circulating concentrations (Fig. 1).[4]

◊ MENOPAUSAL SYNDROME

Many signs and symptoms attributable to aging have often been erroneously attributed to estrogen deprivation. For a symptom to have been caused by estrogen deprivation, it should occur in patients of any age after ovarian failure, whether natural or surgical, and must be relieved with the addition of estrogen. Signs and symptoms of the menopause can be classified as one of the following: definitely estrogen deficiency–related, probably estrogen deficiency–related, or possibly estrogen deficiency–related. Definite hormone-related symptoms are genitourinary atrophy, vasomotor instability, and osteoporosis. Probably hormone-related symptoms include atherosclerotic cardiovascular disease and psychosocial symptoms of insomnia, fatigue, and possibly depression.

Vasomotor Symptoms

Hot flashes are experienced by 75% to 85% of perimenopausal and postmenopausal women. Thirty-seven percent to 50% of premenopausal women after bilateral oophorectomy likewise develop hot flashes. Vasomotor symptoms are most common in the early menopause. Eighty percent of women who experience hot flashes have symptoms for more than 1 year, but somewhat less than 25% have symptoms for more than 5 years. The hot flash is described as a warmth that begins in the face, spreads to the chest, and is often accompanied by a visible red flush. The hot flash is episodic rather than continuous and is frequently associated with nausea, dizziness, headache, palpitations, diaphoresis, and night sweats.

Meldrum et al.[54] standardized a technique for measuring changes in skin temperature during hot flashes and noted a mean interval of 54 ± 10 minutes between hot flashes. These investigators also found that the subjective sensation of warmth precedes any changes in skin temperature and is over before the maximal peripheral change is measured. Therefore, the origin of hot flashes is not a peripheral disturbance. Several investigators have tried to correlate hot flashes with circulating levels of gonadotropins. There is no difference in the ratio of LH to FSH or total estrogens in patients with vasomotor symptoms compared with those without. Others also failed to identify any significant change in estrone or estradiol levels at the time of reported hot flashes. Interestingly, increases in DHEA, androstenedione, and cortisol were noted 10 to 20 minutes after observed hot flashes. The significance of these observations is unknown. Hot flashes do not occur in women with gonadal dysgenesis who have not been exposed to exogenous estrogen. A close temporal relationship between each hot flash and a pulse of LH has been observed. This suggests that either LH itself or factors that initiate the release of LH are responsible for hot flashes in patients with

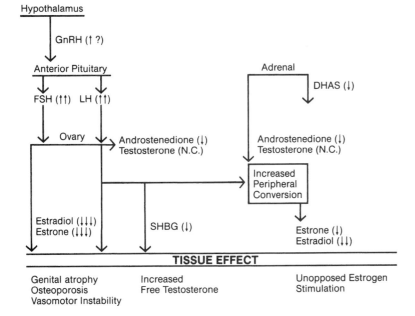

FIG. 1. Schematic diagram of hormonal changes after menopause. *Arrows* refer to direction of change in menopausal women (*DHAS*, dehydroepiandrosterone sulfate; *FSH*, follicle-stimulating hormone; *GnRH*, gonadotropin-releasing hormone; *LH*, luteinizing hormone; *N.C.*, no change). (Adapted from Hammond CB, Maxson WS. *Physiology of the menopause. Monograph in current concepts.* Kalamazoo, MI: Scope Publications, 1983.)

gonadal failure. Administration of exogenous LH, however, does not cause hot flashes. To determine which is responsible, investigators studied women with pituitary insufficiency and found both subjective and objective evidence of hot flashes. Thus, it seems that LH elevation per se is not responsible for hot flashes.

These studies suggest that hypothalamic factors that stimulate LH release are responsible for hot flashes. The hypothalamic centers that control thermoregulation are located in the preoptic and anterior hypothalamic nuclei. The four neurotransmitters active in these nuclei are Gn-RH, norepinephrine, dopamine, and β-endorphin, all of which affect gonadotropin secretion. Because dopamine and β-endorphin exert inhibitory influences on gonadotropin secretion, they probably do not play a role in hot flashes. Because norepinephrine stimulates gonadotropins, it is more likely to play a role. Given that hot flashes occur in patients with Kallmann syndrome after discontinuation of ERT/HRT, Gn-RH itself is probably not primal to the initiation of the hot flash. In ovariectomized rats, there is an increase in the concentration and turnover of hypothalamic norepinephrine. In humans, clonidine, an α-adrenergic agonist-antagonist, can be used to treat hot flashes fairly effectively. Therefore, one possible explanation of their origin is that gonadal failure may increase hypothalamic norepinephrine, which increases pulsatile Gn-RH and subsequently LH. The increase in norepinephrine results in activation of the autonomic nervous system that controls thermoregulation.

Experimental evidence suggests that estrogen deficiency is the primary abnormality affecting the hypothalamic neurons that produce hot flashes. Although serum concentrations of estrogen are similar in women with and without symptoms, there appears to be a difference between the groups in biologically available estrogen. Animal studies have shown that only estrogen not bound to sex hormone–binding globulin (SHBG) is available to be transported across the blood-brain barrier and into the brain tissue. Erlik and colleagues have been able to predict which women would have hot flashes on the basis of biologically available estradiol.[20,54]

Estrogen has traditionally been the drug of choice to relieve hot flashes.[54] However, a number of other drugs can effectively suppress them. These agents are particularly useful in women who have a contraindication to ERT/HRT. Medroxyprogesterone acetate, 10 mg or more orally daily or 100 mg injected monthly, can be effective. Phenobarbital/ergotamine tartrate/belladonna (Bellergal-S), an ergot alkaloid, has been found to be slightly effective in the treatment of hot flashes. Clonidine, 0.1 to 0.2 mg twice daily, is also effective. However, in nonhypertensive patients, side effects are common.

Genitourinary Atrophy

The vagina, vulva, urethra, and trigone of the bladder share embryonic proximity, and all contain large numbers of estrogen receptors. Therefore, genitourinary senescence is modified by the amount of circulating estrogen. Genitourinary tissues do not atrophy at the same rate. Atrophy begins in the premenopausal period and continues over many years. The vulva, although not derived from müllerian structures, undergoes accelerated atrophy with estrogen deprivation. Age alone causes thinning of the hair of the mons and shrinkage of the labia minora. The labia majora flatten as the subcutaneous fat and elasticity of the structures diminish.

The most common vulvar symptom of the menopause is pruritus. ERT/HRT is usually quite effective in relieving pruritus. However, vulvar dystrophies also present with pruritus vulvae. It is important to separate dystrophy from simple atrophy, because squamous cell carcinoma is present in 5% of vulvar dystrophies on initial examination and may develop in another 5% in the succeeding 3 to 5 years after diagnosis. Estrogen deprivation does not appear to be a primary causal factor in either vulvar dystrophy or carcinoma.

With estrogen loss, the vagina becomes pale and its epithelium thins, resulting in diminished distensibility and reduced secretion. The estrogen-deficient vagina is easily traumatized. Vaginal trauma may account for as much as 15% of all postmenopausal bleeding. The incidence of vaginitis increases during the postmenopausal years. Estrogen deficiency changes the vaginal pH from 3.5 to 4.5 to a pH of 6.0 to 8.0. The alkaline environment predisposes the vagina to colonization by a multitude of bacterial pathogens. Estrogen administered systemically or intravaginally reverses the thinning of the vaginal mucosa and lowers vaginal pH. Treatment must be continuous for 1 to 3 months. After the initial continuous therapy, only intermittent therapy is necessary to maintain the effect.

Postmenopausally, the three cervical lesions—erosion, ectropion, and ulcer—become more common. Endocervical glandular tissue becomes less active in the menopause and produces only scant mucin. This contributes to the overall vaginal dryness that is often a presenting complaint. The squamocolumnar junction and transformation zone migrate highly into the endocervical canal. This may pose a problem for accurate colposcopy if Papanicolaou smears show an abnormality.

The incidence of descensus of the uterus, cystocele, and rectocele is increased in the climacteric. However, there is only limited evidence to suggest that estrogen deprivation is the cause. Probably, the increase in incidence is due to estrogen loss coupled with age-related slowing of cell division and to a decrease in tissue elasticity. The urethra is also affected by estrogen loss. The distal urethra may become rigid and inelastic. This predisposes to the formation of ectropion (i.e., urethral caruncle), diverticula, and urethrocele. The most common problem in postmenopausal women related to urethral changes is the urethral syndrome. The urethral syndrome consists of burning, frequency, hesitancy, nocturia, and urgency. The diagnosis is made when these symptoms are associated with sterile urine cultures. This condition is treatable by estrogen therapy, urethrotomy, or urethral dilation. Despite the changes in the urethra and supporting pelvic fascia, there are few data to support a proven increase in the incidence of true stress urinary incontinence.

Bacteriuria is found in 7% to 10% of postmenopausal women, compared with 4% of premenopausal women. The higher incidence in postmenopausal women may be due to mucosal atrophy and increased vaginal contamination caused by the lowering of the external urethral orifice into the anterior vaginal canal. Estrogen therapy frequently improves urinary frequency, dysuria, nocturia, urgency, postvoid dribbling, and, to some extent, stress urinary incontinence. Additionally, estrogen causes proliferation of the vaginal epithelium and can provide relief from the symptoms of vaginitis and frictional dyspareunia.

Osteoporosis

Osteoporosis is a condition in which bone has lost sufficient mass to become predisposed to mechanical failure (i.e., fracture).[1] It is classified as either primary or secondary. Primary osteoporosis is often referred to as senile osteoporosis and usually affects women between the ages of 55 and 70 years. The most common sites of fracture are the vertebrae and the long bones of the arms and hips. Secondary osteoporosis is defined as pathologic fracture caused by a specific disease. Many diseases have been recognized as causing osteoporosis (Table 2).[34]

It is estimated that one in three women in the United States will develop some complication of osteoporosis postmenopausally. Postmenopausal osteoporosis is the cause of 1.3 million fractures each year.[47] Most of the 250,000 hip fractures that occur in people over age 45 years are due to primary osteoporosis. After hip fracture, approximately 15% of patients will die within 1 year, usually because of some complication related to prolonged immobilization. Perhaps equally as tragic is that 75% of hip fracture patients will lose their independence. About 25% of hip fracture patients will require prolonged skilled nursing care. Besides the human suffering caused by osteoporotic hip fractures, the economic impact of this disease is tremendous. Approximately $12 billion a year is spent treating complications of osteoporosis.[46–49]

Menopause and Bone Loss

In both sexes, maximal skeletal mass is attained by age 35 years. By age 50 years, both men and women have begun to experience a generalized loss of bone. Throughout, women have significantly less bone mineral content than men of similar age and race. After oophorectomy, bone loss averages 3.9% per year for the first 6 years after surgery and 1% per year thereafter. Overall bone loss after natural menopause averages 1% to 2% per year. By age 80 years, some untreated white women have lost 30% to 50% of their skeletal mass.[46]

A woman's genetic background, lifestyle, dietary habits, coexisting endocrine disease, and age of menopause are the major factors that determine whether or not she will develop osteoporosis. Bone density parallels skin pigmentation, with African-Americans having more bone mineral mass than whites. Women with a family history of osteoporosis are at increased risk.[12]

The value of exercise in the development and prevention of osteoporosis is poorly understood. Inactivity produces muscular and skeletal degeneration. Astronauts on long space missions who did not exercise showed a significant loss of bone mineral content. Exercise in outer space was found to prevent bone loss. Unfortunately, the type of exercise that will produce a positive bone balance has yet to be defined. However, some type of weightbearing exercise would appear to be the best. Cigarette smoking and caffeine and alcohol consumption are factors that may be associated with osteoporosis. Whether they are independent lifestyle risk factors or confounders has yet to be determined.[58]

Dietary habits determine whether enough calcium is present for effective bone formation. Heaney et al.[36] demonstrated that calcium intake in the United States is usually well below the level of calcium lost from the body. In average postmenopausal women, there is a negative calcium balance of 40 mg per day. It is recommended that postmenopausal women ingest a minimum of 1500 mg of calcium per day.[36]

Premature menopause is an extreme risk factor for osteoporosis. Data from the Mayo Clinic demonstrated that women who had undergone an oophorectomy approximately 20 years before (current mean age, 50 years) and postmenopausal controls who had reached natural menopause 20 years before (current mean age, 70 years) had similar bone mineral masses. Both groups showed approximately a 15% to 18% reduction in radial bone mass.[26]

Estrogen and Bone Mineral Metabolism

Bone is continuously being deposited and resorbed. Resorption and formation are coupled in time, degree, and quality. This continuous remodeling provides a mechanism for bone repair and for liberation of calcium from skeletal stores on demand.

Two cells, the osteoblast and the osteoclast, are responsible for bone remodeling. Bone resorption initiates the process. Osteoclasts, derived from bone marrow, attach to the bone and dissolve the mineral and organic matrix, thus creating a lacuna. Osteoclasts are then replaced by cells that resemble macrophages, and these cells digest any remaining organic matrix and elaborate a signal that recruits the osteoblasts. Osteoblasts that come from the bone marrow deposit an amorphous organic matrix called osteoid. The precipitation of calcium and phosphate to form hydroxyapatite results in hardening of the osteoid. A bone remodeling cycle takes approximately 100 days. On average, 1 to 2 mg (0.02% to 0.04%) of the skeleton is formed and resorbed daily.[26]

TABLE 2. *Differential diagnosis of osteoporosis*

Postmenopausal	Leukemia
Thyrotoxicosis	Alcoholism
Glucocorticoid excess	Long-term heparin therapy
Multiple myeloma	Immobilization
Hyperparathyroidism	

The bone remodeling process is controlled systemically by parathyroid hormone (PTH), vitamin D, and calcitonin. Local factors such as interleukin-1 also play a role in the remodeling process. Calcium plays a crucial role in the maintenance of skeletal integrity. Of the 1 to 2 kg of calcium in the body, 98% is contained in bone. PTH is the critical modulator of calcium balance. In response to hypocalcemia, PTH exerts the following effects:[15]

◊ Stimulation of renal mitochondrial α_1-hydroxylation, which converts 25-hydroxyvitamin D_3 to the biologically active form α_1-25-dihydroxyvitamin D_3,
◊ Direct action on bone, causing rapid release of calcium within several minutes,
◊ Reduction in renal calcium clearance rate with augmented tubular resorption of calcium after glomerular filtration.

Bone remodeling is a late effect that occurs several hours after PTH infusion, during which time osteoclasts increase in number and activity.

Vitamin D deficiency also causes substantial bone loss. Vitamin D is a hormone derived from 5,7-diene steroids. The parent compound is acquired from dietary sources or photobiosynthesis in the skin. Vitamin D exists in three forms with varying biologic activities: Vitamin D, the weakest form, is first hydroxylated in the liver to form 25-hydroxyvitamin D_3. The second hydroxylation to α_1-25-hydroxyvitamin D_3 occurs in the kidney and produces the most active form of vitamin D. The hydroxylase enzyme in the kidney is under the influence of PTH. α_1-25-Dihydroxyvitamin D_3 stimulates the absorption of both calcium and phosphorus from the intestinal lumen into the circulation. Long-term vitamin D deficiency reduces intestinal absorption of calcium, requiring the bone to be the main source of serum calcium.

Calcitonin, derived from the C cells of the thyroid gland, inhibits osteoclastic activity and lowers serum calcium. Estrogen, like calcitonin, opposes the resorptive action of PTH. Estrogen loss appears to make bone more sensitive to the effects of PTH. The increase in serum calcium that suppresses PTH release, and subsequently reduces α_1-25-dihydroxyvitamin D_3, lowers calcium absorption.

Because the body is deprived of its intestinal source of calcium, bone becomes the primary source of calcium. Some studies indicate that calcitonin production declines with estrogen deficiency. Several reports have definitely demonstrated that there are estrogen receptors within bone. Therefore, it is likely that estrogen, like calcitonin, modulates bone remodeling directly by either inhibiting osteoclast activity or stimulating osteoblast activity.[26]

Diagnosis

Symptomatic osteoporosis will develop in 30% to 35% of women. Because most women will not become symptomatic, some means to distinguish those who will fracture from those who will not becomes important. No method for measuring bone mineral mass can yet be endorsed as a routine part of the health care of postmenopausal women. Debates about bone mass measurement revolve around the technique, frequency of measurement, site of measurement, and cost effectiveness (Table 3).

Single-photon absorptiometry has been most widely used for obtaining accurate measurements (i.e., capability of measuring absolute amount of the substance of interest) with a good degree of precision (i.e., capability of repeating a measurement reliably). Single-photon scans accurately measure only peripheral bone, which is mostly cortical. Additionally, variable findings have been found in the mineral content of the axial skeleton, where osteoporosis strikes first, and of the appendicular skeleton. The accuracy of the technique is 4% to 5%. The peripheral skeleton changes less than 1% per year. Therefore, a patient would have to be followed for a minimum of 3 years before bone loss could be identified.

Dual-photon absorptiometry is a technique that allows bone mass measurements to be made in the lumbar vertebrae or in the femoral neck. Unfortunately, dual-photon absorptiometry takes 60 to 90 minutes for measurements in these areas. Accuracy and precision are 5% and 2%, respectively, but the cost of $100 to $200 per measurement limits its use as a screening tool. Computed tomography (CT) has the advantage of measuring trabecular bone exclusively. However, questions have been raised about its accuracy and precision. Dual-energy CT improves accuracy and precision but at the expense of increased radiation exposure. Radiation doses of 200 mrem have been quoted for this technique. Quantitative digital radiography now seems to be the most reproducible,

TABLE 3. *Techniques for measurement of bone mass*

Technique	Site	Precision error (%)	Exam time (min)	Dose of radiation (mrem)[a]	Approx. cost ($)
Radiographic absorptiometry	Hand	1–2	3–5	100	75–125
Dual-energy x-ray absorptiometry (DXA)[b]	Spine, wrist, hip, total body	0.5–2	1–7	1–3	125[c]
Ultrasound[d]	Os calcis	2–3	2–3	—	50–75

[a] One chest x-ray is 20 to 50 mrem, a full dental x-ray 300 mrem, and an abdominal CT 1 to 6 mrem.
[b] DXA or peripheral DXA techniques.
[c] Medicare reimbursement.
[d] Experimental.
(Adapted from ref. 57; courtesy of The Resource Group, New York, NY.)

accurate, and sensitive study available for determining bone density and has the added advantage of minimal radiation.

A group of biochemical markers of bone remodeling has been identified. It includes markers associated with bone formation—osteocalcin (bone Gla-protein) and bone-specific alkaline phosphatase—and with bone resorption—collagen cross-links, cross-linked N-telopeptides, and cross-linked C-telopeptides. These newer urinary tests may serve to predict bone loss, bone density, and fracture risk (hip). Current data suggest the specific ability of markers of bone resorption to predict the response of bone mineral density to ERT/HRT and to monitor its therapeutic effect. More study is needed to fully define the roles of these tests in women's health care.

Despite their limitations as screening tools, bone mineral mass assessments do have value in patients at high risk for osteoporosis. Bone mass measurements provide a quantitative value that can encourage modifications in lifestyle and diet, as well as in any distaste for taking estrogen replacement. It is important to remember that other entities besides aging can produce osteoporosis. In women with an extreme reduction of bone mineral mass quantitated by one of the methods mentioned, I recommend measurements of serum calcium, inorganic phosphate, creatinine, alkaline phosphatase, electrolytes, glucose, aspartate transaminase, bilirubin, albumin, and total protein; testing should also include serum protein electrophoresis, complete blood cell count with differential, routine urinalysis, and a 24-hour urine test for calcium and creatinine. In some patients, an iliac crest bone biopsy may be necessary to establish a definitive diagnosis.

Estrogen Therapy to Prevent Osteoporosis

Although the exact mechanism by which estrogen prevents bone loss is unknown, several large clinical studies have demonstrated a causal relationship between estrogen deprivation and accelerated bone loss. Though numerically small, a 10-year, double-blind, prospective study by Nachtigall et al.[56] showed a dramatic difference in bone mineral density between estrogen- and placebo-treated patients if estrogen was started within 3 years of the loss of ovarian function. More importantly, there was a significant difference in the number of fractures between estrogen- and placebo-treated patients. In the study, 7 of 62 placebo-treated patients had fractures.[56,57] This study, together with a large number of well designed controlled trials, as well as cohort and case–control trials (Fig. 2), cause me to believe there is good evidence to support the recommendation that estrogen can be used to reduce the risk of postmenopausal osteoporotic fractures. Many other studies have clearly shown a reduction in fractures with ERT/HRT.[47] (Strength of evidence: A.)

Cessation of ERT/HRT results in rapid and progressive loss of bone mineral content. Lindsay[46] reported a 2.5% per year average rate of loss of bone mineral content among women whose ERT/HRT had been stopped. This rate of bone loss is comparable to that during the first 2 years after bilateral oophorectomy. In Lindsay's study, 4 years after cessation of ERT/HRT, total bone mineral content in formerly treated patients was equivalent to that in women who had never received estrogen replacement.

Other work by Lindsay and colleagues has suggested that the earlier that ERT/HRT is started after menopause, the more protective is its effect on bone density. However, even if therapy is started at longer intervals after menopause, it seems to provide at least cessation of further loss[47] (Fig. 3). The role of estrogen in the treatment of established osteoporosis is less clear. Two large, uncontrolled studies suggested that estrogen reduces the rate of further fractures in patients who had at least one osteoporotic fracture at the start of treatment. These data suggest that estrogen may be useful in the treatment of established osteoporosis. (Strength of evidence: B—fair.) However, the doses used for treatment are higher than those used for prevention and may thus be associated with a greater likelihood of side effects. The dosage of estrogen necessary to prevent bone loss depends on its type and route of administration. A dose of 0.625 mg of conjugated estrogen per day, or its equivalent in other estrogen, provides adequate protection against the development of osteoporosis for most women.

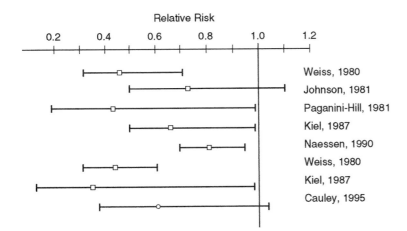

FIG. 2. Effect of hormone replacement therapy on hip fracture. (Adapted from ref. 26.)

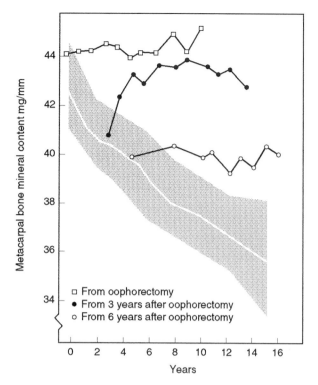

FIG. 3. Effect of delay of onset of estrogen replacement therapy on bone loss. (Adapted from ref. 46; courtesy of The Resource Group, New York, NY.)

Other Therapies for Osteoporosis

The second-generation bisphosphonate, alendronate sodium (Fosamax), has also been shown to significantly reduce the development of postmenopausal osteoporosis.[40] These data, based on both international and United States trials, show even some gain in bone density during alendronate therapy. (Strength of evidence: A—good.) Side effects of therapy include an erosive esophagitis, the incidence and severity of which can be greatly reduced if the patient remains upright during the first hour after taking the medication. This nonhormonal therapy seems quite useful in women not suitable for ERT/HRT or calcitonin. No data yet exist to demonstrate the efficacy of simultaneously taking several of these therapies.

Calcitonin has been approved for the prevention and treatment of osteoporosis. It is expensive but can now be administered by nasal spray. The most effective dose of calcitonin is 100 MRC units (100 medical research council units = 1 mg) at least three times per week. In smaller doses, calcitonin is relatively ineffective. Other therapies, such as coherence therapy and sodium fluoride, are still investigational.[47–49]

Atherosclerotic Cardiovascular Disease

Each year, more than 500,000 women in the United States die of cardiovascular disease, twice as many as those who die of cancer. The evidence that postmenopausal ERT/HRT lowers the relative risk for coronary heart disease becomes stronger with each passing year. Still, a few well performed studies show no or minimal protection. Until more data are available, cardiovascular disease prevention must be considered a possible benefit of ERT/HRT. (Strength of evidence: B—fair.)

Obstetrician-gynecologists are the primary care physicians for many American women. As such, they must assume responsibility for detecting patients who are at risk for coronary heart disease and for providing therapy to lower that risk. Risk factors for cardiovascular disease include chronologic age, early menopause, family history of cardiovascular disease, elevated cholesterol level, hypertension, diabetes mellitus, and cigarette smoking. Gynecologists can do nothing about a patient's chronologic age, age of menopause, or family history. However, they can help alter a patient's blood pressure, cigarette smoking, and total cholesterol level.[7] Hypertension is an independent risk factor for cardiovascular disease. Although 95% of cases of hypertension are idiopathic, high sodium intake, obesity, heavy drinking, and stress are probably involved. If nutritional and hygienic measures do not achieve the desired reduction in blood pressure, drug therapy is usually effective. Cigarette smoking contributes to cardiovascular disease in several ways. Possible mechanisms include the direct effect of nicotine on the sympathetic nervous system, desaturation of hemoglobin by carbon monoxide, and increased platelet adhesiveness. Physicians must encourage their patients to stop smoking at every encounter.

Elevation of total cholesterol level has been identified as a major risk factor for coronary heart disease. The Framingham Study clearly shows that the higher the level of total serum cholesterol is, the higher the rate of coronary heart disease.[11] For every 1% increase in the total serum cholesterol level, a corresponding 2% increase is observed in the incidence of coronary heart disease in both younger and older women. How lipids may affect cardiovascular disease requires a brief review of lipoprotein metabolism and a review of lipids in coronary heart disease.[50]

Lipoproteins are globular particles of high molecular weight that transport triglycerides and cholesterol esters through the plasma. Because triglycerides and cholesterol are not soluble in water, they must associate with these proteins for transport. Differences in density on centrifugation are used to classify lipoproteins. The density of the lipoprotein particle depends on the amount of cholesterol and triglyceride attached to the protein. Three major density classes have been identified: very-low-density lipoprotein (VLDL), low-density lipoprotein (LDL), and high-density lipoprotein (HDL).[73]

The liver actively secretes VLDL. VLDL is triglyceride-dominated but also contains cholesterol, phospholipids, and the apolipoproteins B-100, E, and C. In the fat, lipoprotein lipase converts the VLDL to intermediate-density lipoprotein (IDL). Apoproteins E and C are later cleaved, converting the IDL to LDL. LDL is cholesterol-rich and is the major transporter of cholesterol in normal individuals. Apoprotein B-100 is the signal for the uptake of LDL in many tissues. LDL cholesterol is critical for the formation of steroid hormones in the adrenal glands and ovaries. LDL and IDL are cleared by the liver. The liver contains specific receptors for IDL and LDL. If IDL and LDL are produced in excess of available receptors, the numbers of which are genetically determined, excess IDL and LDL will accumulate. Increased IDL and LDL causes cholesterol accumulation and ultimately leads to atherosclerosis.

The cholesterol released from the transformation of VLDL to IDL and of IDL to LDL is removed by the HDL fraction. HDL is structurally and physiologically distinct from LDL. HDL is derived from both the liver and the intestine. Several subtypes of HDL exist. Initially, HDL is secreted as a small, dense HDL_3 particle. After picking up cholesterol, HDL_3 particles are converted to HDL_2 particles. The uptake of cholesterol by HDL aids the liver in the removal of excess cholesterol from the circulation. In summary, the VLDL-IDL-LDL system promotes atherosclerosis, whereas the HDL_3-HDL_2 system promotes removal of cholesterol, preventing atherosclerosis.[9]

In addition to the important roles of blood pressure and lipids in regard to coronary artery disease, Wagoner et al.[77] contributed important information as to the effects of estrogens and progestins on "vasomotion," the dilating effects of various substances on the coronary vessels in monkeys. Now also demonstrated angiographically in humans as well, this is likely to be another important finding as more is learned about this number one cause of death in women.

At the time of the menopause, women experience a rapid increase in the incidence of clinical cardiovascular diseases. The possibility that estrogen deprivation may be related to this increase is suggested by what happens to women who have a premature surgical menopause. These patients have an increased relative risk of 2.2 for the development of cardiovascular disease. These patients' relative risk can be reduced to 1 if they take estrogen replacement after removal of the gonads.

The majority of studies to date have shown that postmenopausal ERT/HRT reduces the risk for development of cardiovascular disease (Fig. 4). (Strength of evidence: B—fair.) However, several investigators recently raised concerns that women who elect to take estrogen replacement are healthier than women who do not.[5,51] The authors suggested that unintended selection of more healthy women to treat with estrogen may, at least in part, explain these findings.

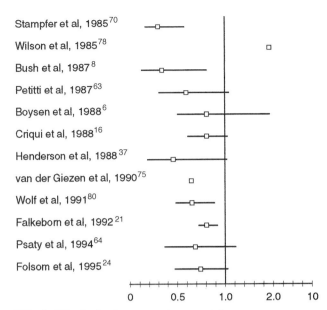

FIG. 4. Effect of estrogen replacement therapy on coronary artery events. (Adapted from ref. 9; courtesy of The Resource Group, New York, NY.)

Interestingly, several studies show that ERT/HRT provides secondary prevention for women who already have cardiovascular disease. They show that ERT/HRT use in women with established coronary artery disease reduces the risk of death and future events by 50% to 90%.[37,38,44] This degree of reduction in risk is marked, but it has also been observed following successful reduction of elevated cholesterol. (Strength of evidence: B—fair.) In similar fashion, Sullivan et al.[72] showed that ERT/HRT clearly improved 10-year survival, even in women in the most severe categories of coronary atherosclerosis (by angiogram). Figure 5 illustrates a summary of the arteriographic studies of ERT/HRT and coronary artery stenosis. (Strength of evidence: B—fair.)

Data from studies of the relationship of ERT/HRT and the risk of stroke are also suggestive, but do not prove, protection by such therapy (Fig. 6). These observational studies remain

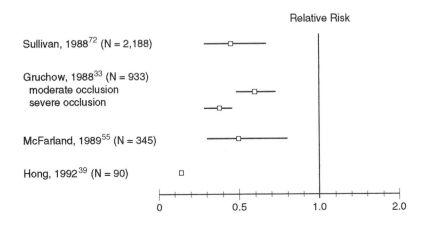

FIG. 5. Summary of angiographic studies of estrogen replacement therapy and coronary artery stenosis. (Adapted from ref. 12; courtesy of The Resource Group, New York, NY.)

Relative Risk

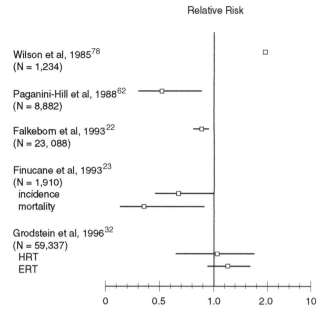

FIG. 6. Summary of observational studies of estrogen replacement therapy and risk of stroke. (Adapted from ref. 14; courtesy of The Resource Group, New York, NY.)

to be proven in well done randomized trials. (Strength of evidence: B—fair.)

It is important to know that better answers to these important questions may soon be available, as there are at least three major randomized, controlled trials under way. Until data from these trials are available, it is my belief that ERT/HRT is cardioprotective, may reduce the risk of stroke, and, unless contraindicated, should be a part of a healthy lifestyle that includes diet and weight restriction, smoking cessation, cholesterol lowering, blood pressure and diabetic control, exercise and low-dose aspirin.

Psychosocial Problems

Sigmund Freud characterized menopausal women as "quarrelsome and obstinate, petty and stingy, sadistic, and anal-neurotic." Wilson[79] echoed this sentiment by stating that "the menopausal syndrome is based on an erratic disorientation of the woman's entire frame of mind." However, there is little evidence that estrogen deprivation causes psychiatric disorders.

Insomnia and fatigue affect 30% to 40% of all postmenopausal women. These symptoms may be related to estrogen deficiency. There is a close temporal relationship between hot flashes and waking episodes. Therefore, many postmenopausal women suffer chronic sleep deprivation. Two double-blind studies showed that insomnia is increased in untreated postmenopausal women and is specifically reduced by estrogen.[65–67]

Estrogen may combat depression through its effects on catecholamine metabolism. Klaiber et al.[43] demonstrated increased plasma monoamine oxidase activity in patients being treated for depression who had been given large daily doses of conjugated

estrogen. Dopamine and serotonin metabolism may also be modified by estrogens. All of this may be why estrogen is effective in treating some depressive illnesses in menopause.

There is a prevalent notion that sexuality is not important in old age. However, in a study of sexual activity of single women between 50 and 69 years of age, both previously married subjects and subjects who had never been married clearly maintained sexual activity, including masturbation (59% and 44%, respectively), coitus (37% and 25%), and orgasmic dreams (35% and 52%). Masters and Johnson showed that postmenopausal women have a reduced vasocongestive increase in breast size during the excitement phase, decreased generalized myotonic contraction, limited sexual flush, diminished vaginal lubrication, and a less expansive vagina.

Estrogen deficiency has been suggested as a cause for this decreased sexual response and loss of libido. It is hypothesized that disinterest may occasionally be a consequence of dyspareunia from atrophic vaginal mucosa, introital stricture, and decreased vaginal distensibility. However, significant dyspareunia occurs in fewer than 8% of postmenopausal patients. Additionally, oophorectomy in premenopausal patients apparently does not affect libido. There is no direct evidence to support hormonal deprivation as a cause of diminished sexual response. Dean adequately summarized the postmenopausal sexual decline as being one of circumstance, not potential.

Colon Cancer

Cancer of the colon is the third most common malignancy and cause of death from cancer in women. The incidence of this disease rises after age 40 years and peaks between 60 and 75 years. It is more common in women than in men, although men have more rectal cancer than women. Preliminary studies have suggested that recent and long-term use of ERT/HRT was associated with a substantial decrease in the risk of fatal colon cancer (Fig. 7) (Strength of evidence: B—fair.)[10] This remains an exciting area for further investigation.

Alzheimer's Disease

Alzheimer's disease (AD) is a neurodegenerative process of the brain that causes slow, progressive loss of mental function. Forty percent of individuals over age 80 years are affected, and it is obvious that many millions of individuals are likely to be affected as the population ages. After age 70 years, age-adjusted prevalence of AD is greater in women than in men. A number of studies now suggest that the risk of AD is reduced in women taking estrogen replacement, depending on the dose used and the duration of use.[61] Figure 8 illustrates the five studies that consistently demonstrate a 50% to 60% reduction in the risk of AD in women who have taken estrogen replacement. (Strength of evidence: B—fair.)

Age-related Macular Degeneration

The leading cause of legal blindness in the United States is age-related macular degeneration (AMD). In the early stages

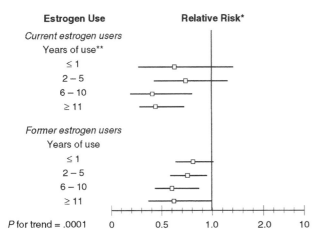

P for trend = .0001

*RR estimate adjusted for age and race
**Includes 50 non-case subjects with unclassified years of estrogen use.

FIG. 7. Estrogen and colon cancer: mortality by duration of use. (Adapted from ref. 67; courtesy of The Resource Group, New York, NY.)

of AMD, patients are usually asymptomatic; however, it can be found in 17% of the population 43 to 86 years old. The pathogenesis of AMD is unknown, and to date there are no effective therapies. Preliminary studies demonstrated that women with an early age at menopause had a significant increased risk of late AMD, compared to women with a later menopause. Several other case–control studies suggested that ERT/HRT reduces the risk of AMD. (Strength of evidence: B—fair.)

◊ RISKS OF ESTROGEN THERAPY

The benefits of ERT/HRT must be weighed against its potential risks. Definite risks of ERT/HRT are endometrial carcinoma and cholelithiasis. Possible risks are hypertension, glucose intolerance, breast cancer, and thrombophlebitis.

Definite Risks

Endometrial Carcinoma

The endometrium of both premenopausal and postmenopausal women can become hyperplastic when subjected to prolonged stimulation by estrogen in the absence of progesterone. One study observed 256 women with adenomatous hyperplasia of the endometrium and reported that 18.5% developed adenocarcinoma within a few years. Thirty percent of the women developed adenocarcinoma after 10 years of follow-up. Others followed 115 patients with either adenomatous hyperplasia or adenocarcinoma *in situ* without any therapy. Invasive carcinoma was detected in the study group within 2 years. By 8 years, invasive adenocarcinoma was found in 26.7% of those with adenomatous hyperplasia, 81.8% with atypical hyperplasia, and 100% with adenocarcinoma *in situ*. Thus, women with adenomatous hyperplasia can progress to invasive carcinoma at a rate that is dependent on their genetic predisposition and intensity of estrogen stimulation.

Numerous studies have documented that unopposed estrogen therapy will increase the relative risk for uterine cancer. In general, this augmented risk appears to be related to both the dosage and the duration of estrogen therapy. (Strength of evidence: A—good.)

The upsurge in the use of estrogen therapy between 1960 and 1970 was associated with an increased incidence of endometrial adenocarcinoma, but not of patient mortality. Patients on estrogen replacement tend to present early, and their lesions are minimally invasive and extremely well differentiated. The 5-year survival rate approaches 95% in women whose uterine cancer was diagnosed while they were taking estrogen replacement. Some have challenged this perception by suggesting that estrogen will increase the risk for both local and metastatic endometrial cancer. Their data suggested that women who have taken estrogen for 1 or more years remain at increased risk for endometrial carcinoma for as long as 10 years after they discontinue the medication.[60]

	Odds Ratio	95% CI	P Value for Trend Test
Estrogen dose*			
None	1.00	–	
≤ 0.625 mg	0.78	0.48 – 1.27	< .01
≥ 1.25 mg	0.54	0.32 – 0.92	
Estrogen duration			
None	1.00	–	
≤ 3 yrs	0.83	0.56 – 1.22	
4 – 14 yrs	0.50	0.31 – 0.81	< .001
≥ 15 yrs	0.44	0.26 – 0.75	

* AD – Alzheirmas diease
* Diagnosis inferred from death certificate; **Conjugated estrogens.

FIG. 8. Association of estrogen replacement therapy and Alzheimer's disease. (Adapted from ref. 74; courtesy of The Resource Group, New York, NY.)

The main reason for the development of uterine cancer when women are given unopposed estrogen seems to be the lack of progesterone. Progestational agents protect against endometrial carcinoma by inhibiting replenishment of estrogen receptor, creating a pseudodecidual endometrium, inducing the enzyme estradiol dehydrogenase, which converts estradiol to estrone, and causing endometrial shedding. Numerous studies have shown that adding cyclic progesterone to estrogen reduces the risk for endometrial carcinoma below the incidence of untreated controls.[27,28,34] (Strength of evidence: A—good.)

The duration of the progestin therapy is as important as the dose. Progestin therapy for only 5 to 7 days is usually insufficient to reverse most endometrial hyperplasias and thus prevent endometrial cancer. Giving a progestin for 10 to 14 days will reverse approximately 98% of all endometrial hyperplasia. Giving a progestin for 13 days each month will reduce the incidence of hyperplasia to almost zero. Full endometrial protection will never be achieved, however, because some areas of the endometrium may not contain progesterone receptors. It is important to remember that adequate progestin therapy is not a guarantee that endometrial carcinoma will never develop in a patient.

Cholelithiasis

Several studies have suggested a relative risk of 2.5 for gallbladder disease in postmenopausal women taking estrogen replacement. The annual incidence in women aged 45 to 49 years is 87 per 100,000 for those not on estrogen, compared with 218 per 100,000 for estrogen users. The exact mechanism for this increase is unknown, but estrogen-induced alterations in bile salts may favor stone formation.

Possible Risks

Breast Cancer

The potential role of estrogen in the generation of breast carcinoma comes primarily from the ability of estrogen to induce mammary tumors in mice. In humans, estrogen's role is far less clear. Few patients with metastatic breast carcinoma respond beneficially to oophorectomy. Breast cancer must be considered a multifactorial disorder in which genetic predisposition, endocrine milieu, and environmental toxins all play a part. However, fear of this disease remains a major concern for many women and is an important reason why many women do not to consider ERT/HRT.

Observational studies and one small prospective, controlled long-term trial have evaluated whether ERT/HRT is associated with the incidence of breast cancer (Fig. 9).[31,42] In addition, a series of metaanalyses has been published (Table 4).[3,14,19,68,71,76] Despite intense debate in both the lay and the medical press, whether or not ERT/HRT increases the risk for breast cancer and whether or not the known risk

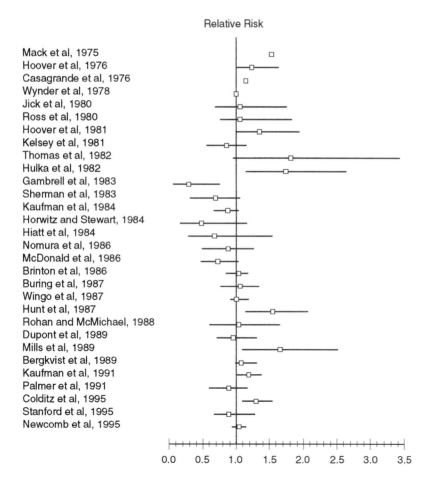

FIG. 9. Relative risk for breast cancer with estrogen replacement therapy. (Adapted from ref. 50; courtesy of The Resource Group, New York, NY.)

TABLE 4. *Metaanalyses of estrogen replacement therapy and relative risk for breast cancer*

Reference	RR	CI	Duration of ERT	Fam hx cancer
Armstrong (1988)[3]	1.01	(0.95−1.08)	NS	↑(1.25RR)
Steinberg et al., (1991)[70]	1.0	(0.96−1.20)	↑	↑(3.4RR)
Dupont and Page (1991)[18]	1.08	(0.96−1.20)	NS	
Silero-Arenas et al., (1992)[67]	1.06	(1.00−1.12)	↑	
Colditz et al., (1993)[13]	1.02	(0.93−1.02)	NS	NS

↑, increased; NS, not significant; RR, relative risk.
(Adapted from ref. 75; courtesy of The Resource Group, New York, NY.)

factors of family history or proliferative breast pathology by biopsy should serve as contraindications have not been clearly shown.[45] Until the long-term randomized trials previously mentioned are available, it is my opinion that if taking estrogen replacement increases the incidence of breast cancer at all, the increase must be very little. Any minimal increase, if present, would be greatly overshadowed by the other dramatic benefits of such treatment. (Strength of evidence: B—fair.)

Whether or not the addition of a progestin to ERT/HRT will lower the risk of breast cancer is controversial, at least. Most authors do not believe such protection occurs. However, three studies show a lower incidence of breast carcinoma in estrogen-plus-progestin users compared with untreated women. In the study by Nachtigall et al.,[56,57] there were four cases of breast cancer in 84 placebo users and none in 84 estrogen–progestin users. In the Wilford Hall studies of Gambrell,[27] estrogen–progestin users had an incidence of breast cancer of 66.8 per 100,000, compared with 343.5 per 100,000 in nonusers. There was a statistically significant difference between estrogen–progestin users and nonusers, but not between estrogen–progestin users and unopposed-estrogen users. When the estrogen–progestin group was compared with the National Cancer Institute data for 1980, it had a statistically significantly lower incidence of carcinoma. However, there was no statistically significant difference between the estrogen–progestin group and women taking unopposed estrogens. A West German study showed that breast carcinoma was significantly lower in estrogen–progestin users (109 per 100,000) than in either estrogen users or nonusers. Therefore, the value of progesterone with estrogen in the prevention of breast carcinoma remains controversial.

Although the results are inconclusive, it appears that the prognosis for breast cancer, like that for endometrial cancer, may be better for estrogen users than for nonusers. At Wilford Hall, from 1972 to 1981, 256 postmenopausal women developed breast cancer. Overall mortality was 30.5%. Mortality for estrogen users was 16%, compared with 35.8% for nonusers.[27,28] Other studies have shown similar results. Whether the improved survival rate resulted from increased surveillance or from the protective effect of the hormone remains open to speculation.

Thromboembolism

Older data from studies involving high-dose (greater than 50 µg), estrogen-containing oral contraceptives suggested a link with thromboembolism. Until recently, there had not been an association between postmenopausal ERT/HRT and *de novo* thromboembolic disease in women. Several studies now suggest a modest increased risk.[17,18,41] A report by Grodstein et al.[32] using primary pulmonary embolus (no identified antecedent cancer, trauma, surgery, or immobilization) as its end point demonstrated a relative risk of 2.1 (95% confidence interval, 1.2 to 3.8). By their calculations, this would be associated with 5 additional cases per 100,000 postmenopausal women aged 50 to 59 years that are attributable to ERT/HRT. Figure 10 illustrates the limited data existing on this point. (Strength of evidence: B—fair.)

Hypertension

The Royal College of General Practitioners' Study demonstrated a 2.5-fold increased risk for hypertension in high-dose oral contraceptive users. However, the relationship between ERT/HRT and the risk of hypertension is unresolved. Administration of 1.25 mg of a conjugated estrogen or 0.05 mg of ethinyl estradiol can raise renin substrate threefold. Percutaneous applications of estradiol do not seem to alter plasma renin. If an elevation of blood pressure occurs, most women return to pretreatment levels within a short time after discontinuing the estrogen. In general, hypertensive changes are seen less frequently during ERT/HRT than during oral contraceptive therapy. Still, blood pressure measurements should be routine for all postmenopausal women treated with estrogen replacement. There are no data to suggest that adding ERT/HRT to a patient with stable, fixed hypertension is in any way detrimental, and some data exist to suggest that it may even be beneficial.

Glucose Intolerance

Estrogen in doses for replacement therapy seldom precipitates frank diabetes. Estrogens exert a tropic effect on the pancreas and increase insulin secretion. Despite this insulinotropic

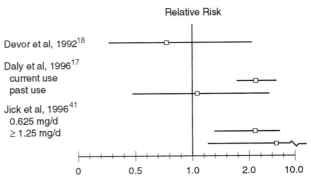

FIG. 10. Effect of estrogen replacement therapy on risk of deep venous thrombosis *(DVT)*. (Adapted from ref. 16; courtesy of The Resource Group, New York, NY.)

effect, many studies have demonstrated impaired glucose tolerance in women taking estrogen. These studies show a delay in glucose absorption and a postponement of peak plasma insulin after a glucose load. However, an equal number of studies has shown that estrogen does not produce any negative affect on glucose tolerance. In oral contraceptive agents, the progestational component may be the cause of impaired glucose tolerance. Diabetic control may be more difficult in the luteal phase. In high doses, exogenous progestins may increase plasma insulin to levels similar to those of late pregnancy. Use of cyclic progestin therapy is unlikely to have a significant impact on carbohydrate metabolism. In general, estrogen-plus-progestin therapy does not result in significant or prolonged abnormalities of carbohydrate metabolism, and diabetes is not an absolute contraindication to ERT/HRT.

◊ ESTROGEN PHARMACOLOGY

More than 90% of circulating estrogen is thought to be associated with a transport protein. Approximately 38% of estradiol is bound to SHBG, 60% is bound to albumin, and 2% to 3% is unbound or free in the circulation. SHBG is produced in the liver, with one binding site per molecule. Estradiol, testosterone, and 5α-dihydrotestosterone bind it competitively, with affinitive ratios of approximately 0.4:1:3. Albumin has a higher affinity for estrone, estrone sulfate, and estriol than for estradiol.

Free estrogen is the biologically active form of the hormone. The concentration of free hormone is a function of total hormone concentration, SHBG concentration, and metabolic clearance rate. The metabolic clearance rate of a given steroid is inversely proportional to the extent of protein binding. Therefore, SHBG plays a central role in the amount of free hormone presented to the tissues. Because the amount of free hormone to which the tissues are exposed can vary from tissue to tissue, it is difficult to construct potency tables. Several factors affect biologic potency comparisons:

◊ Assay system used,
◊ Route of administration,
◊ Dosage,
◊ Duration in assay system.

The potency of a particular estrogen will vary with the assay system used. For example, diethylstilbestrol (DES) is a potent estrogen if assessed by its ability to cornify the mouse vagina, but it is a weak estrogen if assessed by its ability to inhibit LH secretion. Potency estimates must consider duration of exposure as well as molar quantities. For example, estriol occupies the nucleus for only 1 to 4 hours and thus has a weak uterotropic effect in the rat bioassay. However, if estriol is infused or given by repetitive injection, a uterotropic effect similar to that of estradiol can be obtained.

Many estrogen preparations are available for clinical use. Comparison of the biologic potencies of the clinically available estrogen compounds in humans is difficult because there is no single, uniform bioassay for estrogen and variations in the dose, route, and frequency of administration can turn a weak estrogen into a potent one. Estrogen potency in humans is analyzed by changes in the maturation index, endometrial proliferation, and cervical mucus fern. Table 5 illustrates the dosages of estrogens that are in use and are comparable.

In the United States, conjugated equine estrogens are the most commonly prescribed estrogens for ERT/HRT (Table 6). These estrogens are obtained from the urine of pregnant mares and contain approximately 48% estrone sulfate, 20% equilin sulfate, 15% 17α-dihydroequilin sulfate, and smaller amounts of many other conjugated estrogens. The major circulating estrogen in women receiving conjugated estrogens is equilin. In humans, equilin is both potent and long-lasting. According to the mouse uterine weight bioassay, the relative potencies of DES, equilin sulfate, and estrone sulfate are 2.5, 2.0, and 0.4, respectively. There is no evidence that equilin has detrimental effects in humans other than those inherent in all estrogens. A report by investigators using pure equilin sulfate indicated that it is the main mediator of the plasma lipid change associated with oral conjugated equine estrogens. Gonadotropins can be partially suppressed by as little as 0.3 mg of conjugated equine estrogen. However, in postmenopausal women, 1.25 mg of conjugated equine estrogen given daily will not suppress LH and FSH to normal premenopausal levels. A possible explanation is that other substances such as inhibin are required for complete suppression. This points out the problem of trying to follow the adequacy of ERT/HRT by measuring FSH. The amount of FSH suppression will depend on the type of estrogen given, time since last dose, and dosage involved.

Estradiol, estrone, or estriol would be a reasonable choice for ERT/HRT. However, these estrogens are virtually insoluble in water and are rapidly metabolized by the gastrointestinal mucosa. Therefore, they must be esterified or given in a sulfated form for oral absorption. In the past, micronization (i.e., making the estradiol particles small enough to permit gastrointestinal absorption) has been the only way to give estradiol easily. Estrogens are well absorbed from mucosal membranes, particularly the vagina. Intravaginally administered estrogen can result in physiologic levels. Use of vaginal estrogen can cause endometrial stimulation, and all standard estrogen contraindications apply to intravaginal use. A transdermal method of delivering estradiol-17β has become available in the United States.[13] Two dose sizes, 0.05 mg and 0.1 mg, are available. A change of 40 to 80 pg/ml from baseline is achieved with transdermal estradiol. The patch is replaced every 3 days. There is fluctuation around the physiologic level in users of the patch, and an absolute steady state is not easily accomplished.

TABLE 5. *Relative potencies of estrogens*

Type of estrogen	Potency
Conjugated estrogens	0.625–1.25
Micronized estradiol	1–2
Transdermal estradiol	0.05–0.1
Esterified estrogens	0.9–1.50

TABLE 6. *Commonly used estrogens for replacement therapy*

Generic or chemical name	Commercial preparation	Doses available (mg)	Usual starting dose (mg)
Estradiol	Transdermal system: Climara, Estraderm, Vivelle	0.05; 0.1	0.05
	Cream, tablets: Estrace	1; 2	1
Conjugated Estrogens	Premarin	0.3; 0.625; 0.9; 1.25; 2; 5	0.625
Estropipate	Ogen	0.625; 1.25; 2.5; 5	1.25
Esterified Estrogens	Estratab, Menest	0.3; 0.625; 1.25; 2.5	0.625

(Adapted from ref. 51.)

Therefore, relatively physiologic levels of estrogens may be achieved with a variety of preparations given through various routes. With the exception of transdermal or intravaginal estradiol, estrone levels will exceed estradiol levels. The clinical significance of the reversal of the estrone-to-estradiol ratio is not known. There is no evidence that one form of estrogen is therapeutically superior to another or that one is more likely to cause major side effects than another if relative dose is considered. Equally important is that no one form of estrogen appears to be therapeutically superior in preventing the long-term consequences of estrogen deprivation.[29]

◊ PROGESTIN PHARMACOLOGY

Progesterone is secreted by the corpus luteum for approximately 14 days. It decreases the receptor content and mitotic activity of the endometrium, induces estradiol dehydrogenase (the main detoxifier of estradiol in the endometrium), and facilitates endometrial shedding. Thus, the addition of progesterone to ERT is a logical extension of the concept of physiologic hormone replacement.

Native progesterone is poorly absorbed through the gastric mucosa. Oral progestational activity is obtained by modifying progesterone at the C-17 position (17-acetoxyprogestins) or by removing C-19 from testosterone and placing an ethinyl group at C-17 (19-norprogestins). The most commonly used 17-acetoxyprogestin is medroxyprogesterone acetate, which, in addition to the 17-hydroxyl group, has an acetate group attached at C-6. The 19-norprogestins are norgestrel, norethindrone, and norethynodrel, and they are commonly used in birth control pills.

There is tremendous individual variation in absorption of the synthetic progestins. Therefore, it is difficult to construct potency ratios for the various progestins. Absorption of medroxyprogesterone acetate after a 10-mg oral dose causes a peak level in 1 to 4 hours with almost complete excretion by 24 hours. Administration of 1 mg of norethindrone produces peak concentrations in 1 to 3 hours with almost complete excretion in 24 hours. Thus, there is tremendous individual variation among patients because of differences in gastrointestinal absorption.

Oral administration of the 17-acetoxyprogestins or 19-norprogestins does not affect SHBG and has minimal effects on clotting proteins. Whether or not progestins affect glucose tolerance is debatable; there are many conflicting observations.

Interestingly, progestins appear to have a beneficial effect on bone mineral metabolism. Both 17-acetoxyprogestins and 19-norprogestins reduce calcium-to-creatinine ratios. Some studies suggested that estrogen plus progestin may actually increase bone mineral mass, rather than just stabilizing bone mass.

Micronized oral progesterone has been used in Europe. Given in divided doses, it can produce serum levels greater than 10 ng/ml and a secretory endometrium. Micronized progesterone is subject to first-pass hepatic effects. Characteristic of these changes is the rapid conversion of progesterone to desoxycorticosterone. This conversion is not encountered with parenteral administration, and its clinical relevance is unknown.

Native progesterone is well absorbed through mucous membranes and can be administered by suppositories. Mucosal administration (i.e., vaginally or rectally) results in levels of circulating progesterone that are higher than those with oral micronized administration.

All progestins affect lipid metabolism adversely. However, no investigations have been published that clearly demonstrate that such progestin-induced lipid changes translate to an increase in clinically defined cardiovascular disease. All progestins elevate LDL cholesterol levels, while lowering HDL cholesterol levels. The amount of androgenic activity possessed by a progestin correlates with its lipid effect. In general, the 19-norprogestins affect lipids more than the 21-acetoxyprogestins. Still, 10 mg of medroxyprogesterone acetate will clearly lower HDL levels. To date, oral micronized progesterone has been devoid of adverse lipid effects. Despite adverse effects, progestins must continue to be given to protect the endometrium from hyperplasia. Data from Padwick et al.[60] suggested that as little as 0.35 mg of norethindrone or 5 mg of medroxyprogesterone acetate, given for 14 days, will give adequate endometrial protection.

◊ MANAGEMENT OF ESTROGEN THERAPY IN MENOPAUSE

Before estrogen is prescribed, the physician and the patient must discuss the potential benefits of therapy versus its potential risks. If a patient has an absolute contraindication to estrogen, then the risk–benefit ratio is of concern. If a patient has a relative contraindication to ERT/HRT, then the reason for suggesting ERT/HRT should be carefully considered. The following are absolute contraindications to ERT/HRT:

◊ Known or suspected estrogen-dependent neoplasia,
◊ Undiagnosed genital bleeding,
◊ Active thrombophlebitis or thromboembolic disorder,
◊ Active liver disease,
◊ Known or suspected pregnancy.

ERT/HRT should be considered in all women who have symptoms related to estrogen deficiency (see "Menopausal Syndrome" above). All women who are at risk for the development of osteoporosis or who have a strong family history of cardiovascular disease should consider ERT/HRT.

If a decision has been made to prescribe ERT/HRT, the physician is left with three basic questions: which estrogen to prescribe, which dosage and route of administration to use, and how to monitor therapy.

No single estrogen or progestin has been shown to be clinically superior when equivalent doses are compared. The dosage and route of administration have undergone tremendous change since the early 1980s. In the United States, estrogen traditionally has been given in a cyclic manner. Estrogen has been administered for the first 25 days of the month, and the progestin has been added for the last 10 days, with a 5-day estrogen-free period. This regimen provides excellent protection against endometrial hyperplasia and carcinoma. Unfortunately, during estrogen-free days, many women experience a return of estrogen deficiency symptoms. Estrogen has been given continuously (i.e., 365 days a year) with a progestin added for the first 10 to 14 days of the month. Initial data indicate that this method is equally protective against the development of endometrial carcinoma. An additional benefit of prescribing estrogen in this manner is that the bleeding pattern gives some indication of the status of the endometrium. Padwick et al.[60] demonstrated that if a woman begins menstrual bleeding before the tenth day of the month, a proliferative endometrium is likely, and this group of patients needs a higher dose of progestin, as well as endometrial sampling. If a patient begins bleeding after the tenth of the month but before day 18, then there is full secretory transformation.

Many physicians are now using replacement regimens of continuous estrogen and continuous progestin to enhance compliance by reducing withdrawal bleeding. Data now exist to suggest that such regimens are protective against endometrial hyperplasia/neoplasia and that bleeding will cease entirely in up to 70% of such patients. However, a fairly common drawback has been irregular bleeding in the remaining group. The physician must then decide whether to sample the endometrium, stop treatment, or return to a cycling regimen. Dosages used for this include both conjugated estrogen, 0.625 mg or its equivalent among the other available estrogens (see Table 6), and medroxyprogesterone acetate, 2.5 mg or its equivalent, daily without interruption.[27]

The dose of estrogen should be the least that will control the symptoms but provide protection against osteoporosis. A dose of 0.625 mg of conjugated equine estrogen is known to prevent osteoporosis in most women. The physician cannot assume that an equivalent amount of a different estrogen will prevent bone loss. For optimal protection, the estrogen should be supplemented with 1500 mg of calcium daily and an exercise program. Because rapid bone loss follows discontinuation of estrogen therapy, estrogen therapy should be continued until the patient is in her 70s or beyond. Women who receive calcium supplementation initially should have periodic checks of serum calcium and phosphorus to detect otherwise asymptomatic hyperparathyroidism. The dose of progestin that will protect the endometrium as well as produce the least effect on lipids is unknown. However, norethindrone, 0.35 mg, or medroxyprogesterone acetate, 5 mg, given for 14 days of the month appears to be adequate to protect the endometrium. In general, I have not given estrogen to women who have had their uterus removed.

All patients on ERT/HRT should be seen at least yearly. At the time of the annual examination, a thorough medication review should be obtained, as well as nutritional information. As people age, their nutritional habits decline, and those who previously did not need calcium supplementation may require it. During the annual examination, it is necessary to screen patients for other carcinomas (Table 7). A breast and pelvic examination, a Papanicolaou test, and a fecal occult blood test are mandatory. It is not unreasonable to recommend that patients use a home stool guaiac kit (Hemoccult) at least four times during the year. Right-sided colon cancers bleed intermittently, and a single stool guaiac test may miss an early colon cancer. At the annual visit, the physician should also stress the need for mammography and should follow the National Institutes of Health's guidelines for lipid screening.[59,74]

If a patient develops abnormal uterine bleeding, then sampling of the endometrium is necessary. It is not recommended that routine, intense sampling be used in patients who either do not bleed or bleed only in the expected, postprogestin interval.

TABLE 7. *Cancer screening for the climacteric woman*

Type of cancer	Screening test
Laryngeal cancer	Examination with persistent hoarseness. Stop using tobacco products
Lung cancer	No screening available. Stop smoking
Breast cancer	Annual physician examination, monthly patient self-examination, mammography every 1 to 2 yrs
Skin cancer	Check skin; have any suspicious lesions removed
Colorectal cancer	Stool samples (2–3/yr) for occult blood
Vulvar cancer	Yearly pelvic examination; evaluation of persistent vulvar itching
Cervical cancer	Annual Pap smear
Endometrial cancer	Aggressive investigation of any abnormal vaginal bleeding
Ovarian cancer	Yearly pelvic examination

(Adapted from ref. 51.)

◊ PREMATURE OVARIAN FAILURE

Premature ovarian failure is defined as cessation of menstruation before age 40 years. The term was coined because initially it was thought that no follicles remained in the ovary, because most patients presented with FSH levels greater than 40 mIU/ml. However, these patients occasionally resumed cyclic menstruation or even became pregnant. Study of these patients and others revealed that premature ovarian failure is a heterogenous disorder with numerous causes.

The exact prevalence of premature ovarian failure is unknown. However, it has been estimated that of the 43 million women in the United States of reproductive age, 3% could have primary or secondary amenorrhea. Of these, 10% could have premature ovarian failure, thus giving a frequency of approximately 0.3% of the total reproductive-age population. Another study, examining the records of women in Rochester, Minnesota, calculated the frequency of premature ovarian failure at 0.9%.

The cause of premature ovarian failure may be broken down into five categories: genetic, autoimmune, metabolic, environmental, and surgical. Genetic disorders always involve some abnormality of the X chromosome. Two intact X chromosomes are necessary for the maintenance of intact follicles. Structural abnormalities of the X chromosome can lead to premature follicle loss. Premature ovarian failure has been reported in women who have abnormalities of both the short and long arm of the X chromosome. Many of the women who have deletions in the short or long arm will have reproduced, and there will be a familial occurrence.

Many autoimmune diseases have been associated with the development of premature ovarian failure. Usually, ovarian failure is associated with women who have polyglandular failure, including thyroiditis, hypoadrenalism, and hypoparathyroidism. Many investigators have detected antibodies to ovarian tissue in patients with premature ovarian failure. Still, the presence of circulating antibodies does not conclusively prove that these antibodies are the cause of ovarian failure.

Galactosemia is a deficiency of the enzyme galactose 1-phosphate uridyltransferase involved in galactose metabolism. It appears that high levels of galactose are toxic to oocytes. The exact reason for this is unclear.

Numerous environmental agents can cause oocyte toxicity, as well as destruction. Antineoplastic drugs, especially alkylating agents, induce amenorrhea in more than 50% of patients. The duration of the amenorrhea is related to the dose and patient age at the time of exposure. Younger women appear to be less affected than older women. Permanent ovarian failure can be caused by 800 cGy delivered over 3 days. Patients who receive treatment for Hodgkin disease typically receive 400 to 500 cGy over 4 to 6 weeks. One-half of these women will have permanent ovarian failure. In others, only temporary hypergonadotropic amenorrhea will occur. Unfortunately, individual sensitivity cannot be predicted before therapy.

Therapy for premature ovarian failure depends on a patient's desire for pregnancy. Some women, particularly if they have ovarian antibodies, may rebound after a prolonged course of combined estrogen and progestin. Other investigators have achieved pregnancy by pretreatment with estrogen followed by human menopausal gonadotropin. If a patient is not desirous of pregnancy, then ERT/HRT is indicated. If a patient present with primary amenorrhea, it is better to start with low-dose estrogen and increase gradually over time. This regimen allows completion of the arrested maturation of the secondary sex characteristics. This is particularly true of women who present with cytogenetic abnormalities such as Turner syndrome. This slow approach may allow some growth before the estrogen fuses the epiphyses.

◊ REFERENCES

1. Aitken JM, Hart DM, Lindsay R. Oestrogen replacement therapy for prevention of osteoporosis after oophorectomy. *BMJ* 1973;3:515.
2. Andrews WC. The transitional years and beyond. *Obstet Gynecol* 1995;85:1.
3. Armstrong BK. Oestrogen therapy after the menopause—boon or bane? *Med J Aust* 1988;148:213.
4. Bardin CW, Swerdloff RS, Santin RJ. Androgens: risks and benefits. *J Clin Endocrinol Metab* 1991;73:4.
5. Barrett-Connor E, Wingard DL, Criqui MH. Postmenopausal estrogen use and heart disease risk factors in the 1980's. *JAMA* 1989;261:2095.
6. Boysen G, Nyboe J, Appleyard M, Sorensen PS, Boas J, Somnier F. Stroke incidence and risk factors for stroke in Copenhagen, Denmark. *Stroke* 1988;19:1345.
7. Bush TL, Comstock CW. Smoking and cardiovascular mortality in women. *Am J Epidemiol* 1983;118:480.
8. Bush TL, Barrett-Connor E, Cowan LD, et al. Cardiovascular mortality and noncontraceptive use of estrogen in women: results from the Lipid Research Clinics Program Follow-up Study. *Circulation* 1987;75:1102.
9. Bush TL, Cowan LD, Barrett-Connor E, et al. Estrogen use and all-cause mortality: preliminary reports from Lipid Research Clinic's follow-up study. *JAMA* 1983;249:903.
10. Calle EE, Miracle-McMahil HL, Thun MJ, Heath CW Jr. Estrogen replacement therapy and risk of fatal colon cancer in a prospective cohort of postmenopausal women. *J Natl Cancer Inst* 1995;87:517.
11. Castell WP, Garrison RJ, Wilson PWF, et al. Incidence of coronary heart disease and lipoprotein cholesterol levels: the Framingham Study. *JAMA* 1986;256:2835.
12. Christianson C, Riis BT, Nilas L, et al. Uncoupling of bone formation and resorption by combined oestrogen and progestogen therapy in postmenopausal osteoporosis. *Lancet* 1985;2:800.
13. Cicinelli E, Ignarro LJ, Schonauer LM, Matteo MG, Galantino P, Balzano G. Effects of short-term transdermal estradiol administration on plasma levels of nitric oxide in postmenopausal women. *Fertil Steril* 1998;69:58.
14. Colditz GA, Egan KM, Stampfer MJ. Hormone replacement therapy and risk of breast cancer: results from epidemiologic studies. *Am J Obstet Gynecol* 1993;168:1473.
15. Cummings SR, Black DM, Nevitt MC, et al. Appendicular bone density and age predict hip fracture in women. The Study of Osteoporotic Fractures Research Group. *JAMA* 1990;263:665.
16. Criqui MH, Suarez L, Barrett-Connor E, McPhillips J, Wingard DL, Garland C. Postmenopausal estrogen use and mortality. *Am J Epidemiol* 1988;128:606.
17. Daley E, Vessey MP Hawkins MM, Carson JL, Gough P, Marsh S. Risk of venous thromboembolism in users of hormone replacement therapy. *Lancet* 1996;348:977.
18. Devor M, Barrett-Connor E, Renvall M, Feigel D Jr, Ramsdell J. Estrogen replacement therapy and the risk of venous thrombosis. *Am J Med* 1992;92:275.

19. Dupont WD, Page DL. Menopausal estrogen replacement therapy and breast cancer. *Arch Intern Med* 1991;151:67.
20. Erlik Y, Meldrum DR, Judd HL. Estrogen levels in postmenopausal women with hot flashes. *Obstet Gynecol* 1983;59:403.
21. Falkeborn M, Persson I, Adami HO, Bergstrom R, Eaker E, Lithell H. The risk of acute myocardial infarction after oestrogen and oestrogen-progestogen replacement. *Br J Obstet Gynaecol* 1992;99:821.
22. Falkeborn M, Persson I, Terent A, Adami HO, Lithell H, Bergstrom R. Hormone replacement therapy and the risk of stroke: follow-up of a population-based cohort in Sweden. *Arch Intern Med* 1993;153:1201.
23. Finucane FF, Madams JH, Bush TL, Wolf PH, Kleinman JC. Decreased risk of stroke among postmenopausal hormone users: results from a national cohort. *Arch Intern Med* 1993;153:73.
24. Folsom AR, Mink PJ, Sellers TA, Hong CP, Zheng W, Potter JD. Hormonal replacement therapy and morbidity and mortality in a prospective study of postmenopausal women. *Am J Public Health* 1995; 85:1128.
25. Fotherby K. Variability of pharmacokinetic parameters of contraceptive steroids. *J Steroid Biochem* 1983;19:817.
26. Gallagher JC. Estrogen: prevention and treatment of osteoporosis. In: Marcus R, ed. *Osteoporosis.* San Diego, CA: Academic Press, 1996.
27. Gambrell RD Jr. Role of hormones in the etiology and prevention of endometrial and breast cancer. *Acta Obstet Gynecol Scand* 1982;106 (suppl):37.
28. Gambrell RD, Babgnell CA, Greenblatt RB. Role of estrogens and progesterone in the etiology and prevention of endometrial cancer: a review. *Am J Obstet Gynecol* 1983;146:696.
29. Gelety TJ, Judd HL. Menopause: new indications and management strategies. *Curr Opin Obstet Gynecol* 1992;4:346.
30. Geola FL, Freeman AM, Tataryn IV, et al. Biological effects of various doses of conjugated equine estrogen in postmenopausal women. *J Clin Endocrinol Metab* 1980;51:620.
31. Gibbons WE. Evaluating studies linking hormone replacement therapy and breast cancer. *Contemp Obstet Gynecol* 1992;37:127.
32. Grodstein F, Stampfer MJ, Manson JE, et al. Postmenopausal estrogen and progestin use and the risk of cardiovascular disease. *N Engl J Med* 1996;335:453.
33. Gruchow HW, Anderson AJ, Barboriak JJ, Sobocinski KA. Postmenopausal use of estrogen and occlusion of coronary arteries. *Am J Heart* 1988;115:954.
34. Hammond CB, Jelovsek FR, Lee KL, et al. Effects of long-term estrogen replacement therapy. II. Neoplasia. *Am J Obstet Gynecol* 1979; 133:537.
35. Hazzard WR. The biology of aging. In: Brunwald E, Isselbacker KJ, Petersdorf RG, et al., eds. *Harrison's principles of internal medicine,* 11th ed. New York: McGraw-Hill, 1987.
36. Heaney RP, Recker RR, Soville PD. Menopausal changes in calcium balance performance. *J Lab Clin Med* 1978;92:953.
37. Henderson BE, Paganini-Hill A, Ross RK. Estrogen replacement therapy and protection from acute myocardial infarction. *Am J Obstet Gynecol* 1988;159:312.
38. Henderson BE, Ross RK, Lobo RA, et al. Re-evaluating the role of progestin therapy after the menopause. *Fertil Steril* 1988;49(suppl):95.
39. Hong NK, Romm PA, Reagan K, Green CE, Rackley CE. Effects of estrogen replacement therapy on serum lipid values and angiographically defined coronary artery disease in postmenopausal women. *Am J Cardiol* 1992;69:176.
40. Hosking D, Chilvers CE, Christiansen C, et al. Prevention of bone loss with alendronate in postmenopausal women under 60 years of age. *N Engl J Med* 1998;338:485.
41. Jick H, Derby LE, Myers MW, Vassilakis C, Newton KM. Risk of hospital admission for idiopathic venous thromboembolism among users of postmenopausal oestrogens. *Lancet* 1996;348:981.
42. Kaufman DW, Miller DR, Rosenberg L, et al. Noncontraceptive estrogen use and the risk of breast cancer. *JAMA* 1984;252:63.
43. Klaiber EL, Broverman DM, Vogel W, Kobayashi Y. The use of steroid hormones in depression. In: *Psychotropic actions of hormones: proceedings of the first world congress in biologic psychiatry, Buenos Aires, Argentina.* New York: Spectrum, 1974.
44. Krauss RM. Lipids and lipoproteins in postmenopausal women. *Postgrad Med* Sept 14, 1987:56.
45. Lauritzen C, Meier F. Risks of endometrial and mammary cancer morbidity and mortality in long-term estrogen treatment. In: van Herendael HB, Riphagen FE, Goessens L, et al., eds. *The climacteric—an update.* Lancaster, England: MTP Press, 1984.
46. Lindsay R. The menopause: sex steroids and osteoporosis. *Clin Obstet Gynecol* 1987;30:847.
47. Lindsay R, Hart DM, Clark DM. The minimum effective dose of estrogen for prevention of postmenopausal bone loss. *Obstet Gynecol* 1984; 63:759.
48. Lindsay R, Hart DM, Forrest C, Baird C. Prevention of spinal osteoporosis in oophorectomized women. *Lancet* 1980;2:1151.
49. Lindsay R, MacLean A, Kraszowski A, et al. Bone response to termination of oestrogen treatment. *Lancet* 1978;1:1325.
50. Lipid Research Clinics Program. The Lipid Research Clinics Coronary Primary Prevention Trial Results. II. The relationship of reduction in incidence of coronary heart disease to cholesterol lowering. *JAMA* 1984; 251:365.
51. Lobo RA, Speroff L. International consensus conference on postmenopausal hormone therapy and the cardiovascular system. *Fertil Steril* 1994;62(suppl 2):176S.
52. London SN, Chihal HJ. *Menopause: clinical concepts.* Durant, OK: Essential Medical Information Systems, 1989.
53. Longcope C. Metabolic clearance and blood production rates of estrogens in postmenopausal women. *Am J Obstet Gynecol* 1971;111:778.
54. Meldrum RD, Erlik Y, Lu JKH, Judd HL. Objectively recorded hot flashes in patients with pituitary insufficiency. *J Clin Endocrinol Metab* 1981;52:684.
55. McFarland KF, Boniface ME, Hornung CA, Earnhardt W, Humphries JO. Risk factors and noncontraceptive estrogen use in women with and without coronary disease. *Am J Heart* 1989;117:1209.
56. Nachtigall LE, Nachtigall RH, Nachtigall RD, Beckerman EM. Estrogen replacement therapy: a 10-year prospective study in the relationship to osteoporosis. *Obstet Gynecol* 1979;53:277.
57. Nachtigall LE, Nachtigall RH, Nachtigall RB, et al. Estrogen replacement. II. A prospective study in the relationship to carcinoma and cardiovascular and metabolic problems. *Obstet Gynecol* 1979;54:74.
58. Notelovitz M. Osteoporosis: screening, prevention and management. *Fertil Steril* 1993;59:707.
59. Ottosson UB, Johansson BG, von Schoultz B. Subfractions of high-density lipoprotein cholesterol during estrogen replacement therapy: a comparison between progestogens and natural progesterone. *Am J Obstet Gynecol* 1985;151:746.
60. Padwick ML, Pryse-Davies J, Whitehead MI. A simple method for determining the optimal dosage of progestin in postmenopausal women receiving estrogens. *N Engl J Med* 1986;315:930.
61. Paganini-Hill A, Henderson VW. Estrogen replacement therapy and risk of Alzheimer's disease. *Arch Intern Med* 1996;156:2213.
62. Paganini-Hill A, Ross RK, Henderson BE. Postmenopausal oestrogen treatment and stroke: a prospective study. *BMJ* 1988;297:519.
63. Petitti DB, Perlman JA, Sidney S. Noncontraceptive estrogens and mortality: long-term follow-up of women in the Walnut Creek Study. *Obstet Gynecol* 1987;70:292.
64. Psaty BM, Heckbert SR, Atkins D, Lemaitre R, Koepsell TD, Wahl PW. The risk of myocardial infarction associated with the progestins in postmenopausal women. *Arch Intern Med* 1994;154:1333.
65. Sherwin BB. The impact of different doses of estrogen and progestin on mood and sexual behavior in postmenopausal women. *J Clin Endocrinol Metab* 1991;72:336.
66. Sherwin BB, Gelfand MM. The role of androgen in the maintenance of sexual functioning in oophorectomized women. *Psychosom Med* 1987;49:397.
67. Sherwin BB, Karper D. Estrogen and memory in postmenopausal women with Alzheimer's disease. Presented at the third annual meeting of the North American Menopause Society, Cleveland, Ohio, September 7, 1992.
68. Silero-Arenas M, Delgado-Rodriguez M, Rodrigues-Canteras R, Bueno-Cavanillas A, Galvez-Vargas R. Menopausal hormone replacement therapy and breast cancer: a meta-analysis. *Obstet Gynecol* 1992; 79:286.
69. Speroff L. The menopause, a signal for the future. In: Lobo RA, ed. *Treatment of the postmenopausal woman: basic and clinical aspects.* New York: Raven Press, 1994:1.
70. Stampfer MJ, Willett WC, Colditz GA, Rosner B, Speizer FE, Hennekens CH. A prospective study of postmenopausal estrogen therapy and coronary heart disease. *N Engl J Med* 1985;313:1044.
71. Steinberg KK, Thacker SB, Smith SJ, et al. A meta-analysis of the effect of estrogen replacement therapy on the risk of breast cancer. *JAMA* 1991;265:1985.

72. Sullivan JM, Vander Zwaag R, Lemp CF, Hughes JP, Maddock V, Kroetz FW. Postmenopausal estrogen use and coronary atherosclerosis. *Ann Intern Med* 1988;108:358.

73. Tepper R, Goldberger S, May JY, Luz IJ, Beyth Y. Hormonal replacement therapy in postmenopausal women and cardiovascular disease: an overview. *Obstet Gynecol Surv* 1992;47:426.

74. Timmons MC, Hammond CB. *Osteoporosis. ACOG technical bulletin no. 167.* Washington, DC: American College of Obstetricians and Gynecologists, 1992.

75. van der Giezen AM, Shopman Geurts van Kessel JG, Schouten EG, Slotboom BJ, Kok FJ, Collete HJ. Systolic blood pressure and cardiovascular mortality among 13,740 Dutch women. *Prev Med* 1990;19:456.

76. Vassilopoulou-Sellin R. Estrogen replacement therapy in women at increased risk for breast cancer. *Breast Cancer Res Treat* 1993;28:167.

77. Wagner JD, Clarkson TB, St Clair RW, Schwenke DC, Shively CA, Adams MR. Estrogen and progesterone replacement therapy reduces low-density lipoprotein accumulation in the coronary arteries of surgically postmenopausal cynomolgus monkeys. *J Clin Invest* 1991; 88:1995.

78. Wilson PWF, Garrison RJ, Castelli WP. Postmenopausal estrogen use, cigarette smoking, and cardiovascular morbidity in women over 50: the Framingham Study. *N Engl J Med* 1985;313:1038.

79. Wilson RA. *Feminine forever.* New York: Mayflower-Dell, 1966.

80. Wolf PH, Madans JH, Finucane FF, Higgins M, Kleinman JC. Reduction of cardiovascular disease-related mortality among postmenopausal women who use hormones: evidence from a national cohort. *Am J Obstet Gynecol* 1991;164:489.

CHAPTER 44

Perioperative Care

———— ◇ ————

Philip J. Di Saia
Joan L. Walker
Michael A. Gold

The ultimate goal of perioperative patient management is an uncomplicated recovery after surgery. Most patients present to the operating room expecting this outcome. Good surgeons are secure in the knowledge that they have taken appropriate precautions to reduce the risk of a complication's occurring. They also are aware that no surgery is without risk and that many intraoperative and postoperative complications are not preventable. This discrepancy in expectation can be the source of much dissatisfaction for both patients and physicians if it is not recognized from the beginning. Thorough preoperative patient education and counseling can assist in improving patient understanding of the nature of the procedure and the risks and benefits involved. Careful preoperative evaluation, including patient history, physical examination, and laboratory and radiographic studies, will aid in risk assessment and identify comorbid conditions that can be medically optimized prior to surgery. Similarly, physician knowledge regarding potential postoperative complications allows the institution of prophylactic measures preoperatively. With this accomplished, the successful surgeon can proceed to the operating room, confident that his or her patient has a realistic understanding of the risks and benefits of the procedure and that appropriate precautions have been undertaken to ensure the best outcome possible.

◇ PREOPERATIVE PREPARATION

General Considerations

Surgery is anxiety-provoking for everyone. Preoperative concerns develop regarding alterations in body image, lifestyle, social situation, and postoperative pain. Because of the very nature of the organs involved in obstetric and gynecologic surgery, concerns about reproductive capacity, continuation of sexual function, or alterations in bowel or bladder function or physical appearance may be foremost in a patient's mind.

No surgeon can guarantee a desired outcome, but a patient must be assured that her wishes will be respected and carry equal weight to that of the physician's professional judgment. In ethical principles, this is described as balancing patient autonomy with physician beneficence, as balancing the right of self-determination on the part of a patient with the physician's obligation to promote the patient's medical well-being. A frank discussion addressing these issues preoperatively, involving a patient's family members if desired, can often prevent dissatisfaction with surgical outcomes if they differ from those desired by the patient or physician. Finally, the nature of the discussion, as well as the scope of the counseling given a patient, should be incorporated into the medical record.

Operative Permit/Informed Consent

After discussing the potential risks and benefits of a proposed procedure, the physician is obligated to have the patient sign an operative permit, thus obtaining informed consent. Although this is usually required by both legal and hospital policies, the primary directive for obtaining informed consent comes from an ethical obligation. According to the American College of Obstetricians and Gynecologists, "informed consent is an expression of respect for the patient as a person," encompassing both patient autonomy and physician beneficence. In the process, the patient demonstrates an understanding of her physician's description of the operative procedure, what benefits she might expect, and what untoward events or complications might reasonably occur. She should be given a realistic appraisal of the possible positive results to be obtained from the operative procedure, along with the most frequent complications. A similar process should be undertaken for the transfusion of blood and blood products. The patient should be educated by the physician as to the potential risks and benefits of transfusion prior to signing a transfusion consent form stating acceptance or refusal of blood and blood products.

The physician must use some discretion when discussing potential rare and catastrophic complications, however, as this may only cause undue patient anxiety. The most difficult of these catastrophic complications is likely to be the potential mortality of any operation. The informed consent process is a means of educating the patient and should serve as a way of relieving patient anxiety. She should come away from it with the outlook that the operative procedure is a way of potentially treating an existing problem, not of creating new ones. Thus, the medical team must carefully balance the process of informed consent against a possible loss of hope on the part of the patient. Data from the Centers for Disease Control and Prevention, for instance, have helped establish the overall mortality associated with hysterectomy in the United States. Wingo et al. (1985) documented an overall mortality of 12 per 10,000 hysterectomy procedures. The death rate was higher in women who were pregnant (29 per 10,000 patients) and in women with cancer (38 per 10,000 patients), whereas the death rate was only 6 per 10,000 hysterectomies performed for benign disease. Data such as these may be helpful in creating the proper perspective in discussions of informed consent when a hysterectomy is required. Finally, a summary of this discussion should be documented by a written progress note in the patient's chart.

History and Physical Examination

It has been estimated that 70% of the useful diagnostic information in the preparation of a surgical patient comes from the history, 20% from the physical examination, and only 10% from the special laboratory tests that are ordered. The challenge is to obtain all the information that the patient is able to give. This includes a thorough history of the present illness in addition to gynecologic, medical, and surgical histories and a complete review of systems. Information about cigarette, alcohol, and drug use is also obtained. Concise recording of the entire history on a standardized form will be useful for review later, and ample room should be available in the chart for the recording of details that do not fit into the form. Patients appreciate a physician's sympathetic attitude and seemingly unhurried willingness to listen to the account of their illness. The physician–patient relationship is formed during this initial interview process and is essential in creating a sense of confidence in the physician on the part of patients.

Information obtained from the patient's history will also help to define the patient's operative risk. The typical healthy, ambulatory woman with a localized gynecologic complaint is an excellent operative candidate. Not all patients are without comorbidities, however, and questioning a patient about her exercise tolerance can reveal important information about any cardiopulmonary compromise that might exist. A healthy person has unlimited tolerance for walking on level ground, whereas older or overweight women may only be able to ambulate if they walk at a slow and leisurely pace. Special preoperative testing such as cardiac and pulmonary function tests are warranted if a patient describes a specific quantified limitation to her ambulation, such as if she states that she must stop and rest after walking only a few blocks.

After gathering the patient's history, the physician next performs a complete physical examination. The information gathered from the patient's history will help direct the physician's attention to potential abnormalities. Frequently, however, signs develop independently of symptoms, and a systematic method of conducting the physical examination will yield the most information. A search for unexpected disease is a priority, with special attention paid to the pulmonary and cardiac assessments. This will help determine whether special preoperative studies or medical consultations are necessary. The pelvic examination should be performed last, both to ensure that the physician's attention is not diverted from the overall assessment and to aid in the preservation of the patient's comfort. The examination should be explained to the patient before it is executed to further assist with patient comfort. All information obtained during this evaluation should be documented clearly and will assist the physician in formulating a diagnosis, defining operative risk, and preventing postoperative complications.

Laboratory Studies

Preoperative laboratory evaluations are coming under increasing scrutiny as physicians, patients, and insurers strive for cost containment. Laboratory studies and diagnostic procedures therefore should be limited to those that are appropriate to the findings elicited during the history and physical examination. In addition to these "case-specific" studies, all women scheduled for elective gynecologic procedures should have a preoperative Papanicolaou test (Pap smear) within the 12 months preceding surgery, a pregnancy test if they are of reproductive age, and a hematocrit. Other studies, such as creatinine and electrolytes, coagulation studies, electrocardiogram (ECG), and chest radiographs, should be based on evaluation of the patient, her age, and the consultant's recommendations. Most anesthesia departments have adopted the guidelines suggested by Roizen (1994) (Table 1). Patients with medical illnesses such as cardiac or pulmonary disease or endocrine disorders need to be in optimal control before surgery. Their medical therapies should be reevaluated, special testing performed, and medical consultation obtained to ensure that the best preoperative condition is achieved and that the operative risk is minimized.

All women should be carefully questioned about their smoking history and exercise tolerance, as even young smokers can have significant pulmonary abnormalities. Patients with known chronic obstructive pulmonary disease as a result of long-term smoking are at significantly increased risk of complications secondary to general anesthesia and abdominal surgery. Preoperative evaluation will often include pulmonary function testing and an arterial blood gas measurement. Clinically important decreases in serum carbon monoxide levels and improvement in spirometry values are known to occur

TABLE 1. *Guidelines for preoperative testing*

Condition	CBC with Plt*	Chem-7	LFTIs	Coags	Chest x-ray	ECG
Age <65	X	—	—	—		
≥65	X	X	—	—	X	X
Cardiovascular disease	X	—	—	—	X	X
Pulmonary disease	X	—	—	—	X	X
Hepatic disease	X	—	X	X	—	X
Renal disease	X	X	—	—	—	—
Diabetes mellitus	X	X	—	—	—	—
Smoking	X	—	—	—	—	—
Bleeding disorders	X	—	—	X	X	—

*Complete blood count with platelet.
(Adapted from Roizen, 1994.)

with several days of smoking cessation, so it is vitally important that all smokers be requested to stop smoking at least 1 week preoperatively.

Patients undergoing preoperative evaluation for a pelvic or adnexal mass represent another special group of patients. The indiscriminate use of barium enema examination, intravenous pyelography (IVP), and computed tomography (CT) in these patients should be discouraged. Ultrasonography should be performed to assess the mass with particular attention to wall thickness, inner wall structure, echogenicity, and the presence or absence of septations. These findings can help differentiate benign from malignant masses. The most dependable value of ultrasound is its negative predictive value for malignancy in the case of a simple ovarian cyst. The addition of a CA 125 assay is of little benefit in the premenopausal population, since such common medical problems as endometriosis, pregnancy, pelvic inflammatory disease, menses, and leiomyomata can lead to elevations in this tumor marker. In a postmenopausal patient, however, an elevated CA 125 has a positive predictive value of 80% to 98% and, when combined with ultrasonography, can significantly improve the sensitivity and positive and negative predictive values of this test. A normal CA 125 value does not rule out malignancy, however, as early-stage disease and nonserous ovarian adenocarcinoma may not be associated with elevated values. Surgical evaluation therefore is recommended for all postmenopausal patients with an adnexal mass and all other patients suspected of having an ovarian malignancy. Preoperative consultation with a gynecologic oncologist will ensure that proper staging and optimal surgical resection of ovarian malignancies will occur.

Other preoperative findings can alert the physician to the possibility of a diagnosis other than an ovarian malignancy and require specific studies for their evaluation. A patient with gastrointestinal symptoms, age greater than 50 years, blood in the stool, or a left-sided pelvic mass suggestive of diverticulitis requires barium enema examination and/or sigmoidoscopy preoperatively. Urinary tract evaluation is generally necessary only if a patient has a fixed, solid pelvic mass suggestive of malignancy, a pelvic kidney, or unexplained renal insufficiency. For patients with diabetes or poor renal function, IVP should only be performed if absolutely necessarily. Noninvasive renal ultrasound can be substituted in

these patients, especially if hydronephrosis is suspected. Finally, the finding of unexplained hematuria, confirmed by a catheterized urinalysis, requires cystoscopic evaluation. Obviously, no study should be performed if the results are not going to be utilized preoperatively in the management of patients. Surgeons therefore must ensure that all preoperative studies are reviewed and abnormal findings appropriately evaluated before the patient arrives in the operating room.

◊ DETERMINING SURGICAL RISKS

Most surgical procedures are reasonably well standardized, and it is usually possible for the surgeon to make a good statistical estimate of how a proposed surgical procedure will affect the course of a specific problem. Considerable variability exists in the individual aspects of a patient's health, however, and this can significantly affect the overall risk assessment. A thorough preoperative evaluation, including patient history, physical examination, and laboratory assessment, is essential to the accurate calculation of the risk of operative morbidity and mortality.

Operative Mortality

The most common causes of operative mortality are pulmonary embolus, heart disease, myocardial infarction, and infection. Preoperative prediction of those at risk for these life-threatening complications allows the institution of preventive measures. One of the most widely used predictors of surgical risk is the American Society of Anesthesiologists (ASA) physical status classification system (Table 2). Based on a patient's comorbid conditions, this system has demonstrated an excellent correlation between preoperative physical status and operative mortality (Table 3). Emergency surgery constitutes a special risk factor and doubles the perioperative mortality risk for classes I, II, and III.

Thromboembolism is one of the most common complications in gynecology, being responsible for 40% of all deaths following gynecologic surgery. Because all patients undergoing major gynecologic procedures are at risk for this potentially fatal complication, the preoperative institution of prophylactic measures is vital. Risk factors associated with an increase in risk for perioperative myocardial infarction

TABLE 2. *American Society of Anesthesiologists'*
physical status classification

Class	Description
I	Normal, healthy patient
II	Mild systemic disease—no functional limitation
III	Severe systemic disease—functional limitations but not life-threatening
IV	Incapacitating systemic disease—life-threatening
V	Moribund with life expectancy 24 h without surgery
Emergency (E)	Emergency surgery—the suffix *E* is added to denote the poorer status of any patient in one of these five categories who is operated on as an emergency

(Adapted from Schneider, 1983.)

have been described by Goldman et al. (1977,1979) and include age greater than 70 years, myocardial infarction in the previous 6 months, S_3 gallop, jugular venous distention, rhythm other than sinus, premature atrial contractions on the last preoperative ECG, more than five premature ventricular contractions per minute, and emergency surgery. Based on the number of risk factors present, patients are assigned to a cardiac class that is associated with a well defined risk of perioperative cardiac morbidity and mortality (Table 4).

Noncardiac causes of postoperative death are rare. Life-threatening infection is very uncommon following gynecologic surgery. Women at risk are those who have a ruptured tuboovarian abscess, an unrecognized bowel complication, gynecologic cancer, or immunosuppression. Finally, anesthesia itself is a rare cause of operative mortality. Approximately 1 death per 10,000 procedures is directly related to anesthesia, and another 4 deaths per 10,000 procedures are anesthesia-related. Appropriate prophylactic measures should be undertaken to reduce the risk of these complications occurring, and patients should be counseled preoperatively regarding them.

Emergency Surgery

The preoperative evaluation of a patient may be abbreviated at times but should never be omitted, even if the procedure is emergent. Obstetrics and gynecology patients are at increased risk of requiring emergency surgery, which can double the op-

TABLE 3. *American Society of Anesthesiologists'*
physical status classification and overall death rate

Physical status	Number	Deaths	Mortality rate (%)
I	50,703	43	0.08
II	12,601	34	0.27
III	3626	66	1.82
IV	850	66	7.76
V	608	57	9.38

(Adapted from Vacanti et al., 1970.)

TABLE 4. *Goldman cardiac risk class and overall*
morbidity and mortality

Class	No or only minor complications[a]	Life-threatening complications[b]	Cardiac deaths[c]
I	532 (99)	4 (0.7)	1 (0.2)
II	295 (93)	16 (5)	5 (2)
III	112 (86)	15 (11)	3 (2)
IV	4 (22)	4 (22)	10 (56)

[a]$n=943$
[b]$n=39$
[c]$n=19$
[d]Numbers in parenthesis indicate % within each class.
n=number of patients incidence
(Adapted from Goldman et al., 1977.)

erative mortality even without significant blood loss. The incidence of ectopic pregnancy is rapidly increasing, for instance, and these patients often present to the emergency department in a hypovolemic state with a hemoperitoneum. Unfortunately, there is often little time for preoperative stabilization. Immediate transfer to the operating room with intravenous colloid and blood and blood product administration can be life-saving. Hemodynamic stability then can be achieved through surgical intervention. Vomiting due to a full stomach is another complication of emergency surgery. A pregnant woman is considered to have a full stomach for 8 to 12 hours after she has eaten, placing her at risk for aspiration pneumonia. Even in situations requiring emergent surgery such as these, the surgeon should make every effort to quickly take a focused history, examine the patient, determine her operative risk, inform her of the nature of the proposed procedure, and receive her consent.

◊ IMMEDIATE PERIOPERATIVE MANAGEMENT

Blood Availability and Transfusion

Before any operative procedure that carries the risk of significant blood loss, a sample of the patient's blood should be made available in the blood bank for a type and screen. This will ensure that blood will be available within 30 minutes if the need arises. For procedures associated with minimal blood loss, such as tubal ligation, dilation and curettage, laparoscopy, and hysteroscopy, no preoperative specimen is necessary.

Because the use of blood components is not without risks, careful assessment of the benefit-to-risk ratio must be made prior to transfusion. As described above, patients should be counseled and consent received prior to all transfusions, unless the situation is emergent and the patient unable to give consent. Documented risks of transfusion include allergic reactions consisting of fevers, chills, and urticaria in 1 to 2 per 100 units, hemolytic transfusion reactions in 1 in 6000 units, and fatal hemolytic transfusion reactions in 1 in 100,000 units. Current infectious risks in the United States include transmission of human immunodeficiency virus in an estimated 1 in 493,000 units, hepatitis B virus in 1 in 63,000 units, and hepatitis C virus in 1 in 103,000 units. Overall, the estimated risk of viral transmission from a blood transfusion is 1 in 34,000 units.

In an attempt to decrease the risks associated with transfusion, many have advocated the use of preoperatively donated autologous blood. Because the shelf life of stored blood is now approximately 45 days, patients scheduling elective procedures may schedule their surgery sufficiently far in advance to permit correction of donation-associated anemia with iron supplementation. Recently, however, recommendations against the routine use of preoperative autologous blood donation prior to abdominal hysterectomies were made by the National Heart, Lung, and Blood Institute. In support of this recommendation, Kanter et al. (1996) demonstrated an increase in the overall incidence of posthysterectomy transfusion from 0.8% in women not donating blood to 9.9% in women who donated preoperatively. This increase in transfusion rate is concerning because, despite precautions to prevent the administration of an incorrect unit of blood, estimates suggest that clerical error is responsible for autologous blood being administered to the incorrect patient in 1 30,000 to 50,000 transfusions.

Currently, the use of blood and blood products in the perioperative period appears to be on the decline. Because cardiac output does not appear to increase significantly in otherwise healthy humans until the hemoglobin levels fall below 7 g/dl, a National Institutes of Health consensus panel recently recommended that unless patients are unstable or symptomatic, transfusions above this value may not be necessary. Although this may serve as a general guideline for the use of red cell transfusions, no single hemoglobin concentration should ever "replace good clinical judgment as the basis for decision making regarding perioperative transfusion" (National Institutes of Health, 1988). Thus, before any operative procedure, patients should be counseled as to the risk of significant blood loss requiring transfusion, and preparations should be made to ensure that blood is available if needed.

Preoperative Admission

Outpatient surgery and same-day admission have almost completely replaced preoperative admission for gynecologic procedures. Occasionally, however, a patient will require preoperative admission due to concurrent medical conditions. In general, any patient with severe systemic disease classified as ASA class III or higher (see Table 2) warrants admission prior to surgery. This decision is often best made in conjunction with the anesthesiologist and other physicians involved in the patient's care.

Thromboembolism

Venous thromboembolism is a significant cause of postoperative morbidity and mortality. The overall incidence of thromboembolic disease in the postoperative period for gynecologic patients is approximately 25% and for gynecologic oncology patients 40%. Current methods of prophylaxis are directed at modifying the identifiable risk factors for thromboembolic disease. Virchow's triad remains valid in defining the most important of these: hypercoagulability, venous stasis, and vessel injury. Other associated risk factors include advanced age, prior venous thromboembolism, malignancy, abdominal or pelvic surgery, obesity, congestive heart failure, stroke, and high-dose estrogen use. Two methods of prophylaxis currently in use are low-dose unfractionated heparin and low-molecular-weight heparin. These agents each lower the risk of thromboembolism to between 3% and 9% but are associated with a 3% to 6% incidence of postoperative bleeding complications, including wound hematomas, and an increase in operative blood loss. Sequential pneumatic compression stockings and elastic stockings are directed toward prevention of venous stasis. A metaanalysis of studies involving the use of sequential compression stockings in moderate-risk surgery (abdominal, gynecologic, and neurosurgery) demonstrated a 68% risk reduction compared to controls. In contrast, the benefit derived from simple elastic stockings has not been well demonstrated, and these may actually increase the incidence of postoperative thromboembolism if they do not fit properly. Obviously, the more immobile a patient is, the greater the risk of venous stasis will be, as well as the subsequent risk for development of deep vein thrombosis. Thus, early ambulation and leg exercises while in bed should be encouraged for all postoperative patients in addition to the use of any mechanical or pharmacologic measures.

Bowel Preparation

Preoperative cleansing of the bowel has several benefits for patients undergoing intraabdominal procedures including laparoscopy. It appears to lessen the severity of postoperative ileus, facilitates operative manipulation of the colon, and decreases aerobic and anaerobic bacterial counts. Patients should be restricted to clear liquids for 1 to 2 days before surgery to decrease the number of enemas required to cleanse the bowel in the immediate preoperative period and to minimize the probability of dehydration. When surgery on the gastrointestinal tract is anticipated or a gynecologic malignancy is suspected, a more thorough cleansing is in order. A nonabsorbable antibiotic, such as erythromycin and neomycin base, 500 mg of each orally every 6 hours for 48 hours prior to surgery, has been recommended, but its advantages are controversial. A more rapid yet effective method is to restrict patients to clear liquids for 1 to 2 days, followed by the administration of 4 liters of GoLYTELY (polyethylene glycol 3350 and electrolytes for oral solution) or 1 to 2 bottles of magnesium citrate on the day before surgery. If colorectal surgery then becomes necessary, a protective diverting colostomy might be avoided, and the incidence of postoperative complications such as abscess formation and anastomotic disruption will be decreased.

Preoperative Cleansing

Overall, 60% to 80% of all postoperative infections are incisional, and much attention has been paid to preoperative cleansing in an attempt to reduce this by decreasing bacterial flora. Methods of skin preparation vary from hospital to hospital but routinely consist of a combination of scrubbing, painting, and spraying the operative site with an antimicrobial preparation. Studies suggest that after mechanical cleansing of obvious dirt, grime, and dried blood, all techniques of antimicrobial application are equivalent in preventing postoperative infection as long as the antimicrobial preparation is in contact with the skin for at least 2 minutes. Vaginal preparation with antiseptic solutions has never been tested in well controlled trials, and its use has been essentially intuitive. The primary reason for removal of hair from the operative site is to aid in the reapproximation of the wound. Shaving the patient in advance of a surgical procedure causes small cuts in which infections can develop and actually increases the risk of postoperative wound infection. Clipping the hair with an electric razor appears to be the best technique when hair removal is absolutely necessary.

Prophylactic Antibiotics

Much like perioperative skin cleansing, prophylactic antibiotics are used primarily to decrease the incidence of postoperative surgical site infection. For both vaginal and abdominal hysterectomies, which are considered "clean-contaminated" procedures due to entry into the vagina, the routine use of prophylactic antibiotics is recommended. A metaanalysis of antibiotic prophylaxis in abdominal hysterectomies clearly demonstrated the benefit of antibiotic prophylaxis with a variety of antibiotics (Mittendorf et al., 1993) (Fig. 1). Adnexal surgery, on the other hand, is considered a "clean" procedure, and unless there is evidence of a prior pelvic infection or vaginal contamination, prophylactic antibiotics are not recommended. Many surgeons order antibiotics for their patients undergoing infertility procedures, however, because the consequences of postoperative infection are devastating. The drug of choice for prophylaxis varies from institution to institution, depending on individual hospital costs and antimicrobial

Study		Year	# Pts
1.	Allen	1972	168
2.	Ohm	1975	93
3.	Mathews	1977	59
4.	Jennings	1978	102
5.	Holman	1978	80
6.	Roberts	1978	47
7.	Appelbaum	1978	104
8.	Grossman-cef	1979	163
9.	Grossman-pen	1979	160
10.	Adno	1979	37
11.	Polk	1980	429
12.	Itskovitz	1980	69
13.	Stage	1982	110
14.	Duff	1982	91
15.	Walker	1982	88
16.	Vincelette	1982	106
17.	Gall-cefop	1983	39
18.	Gall-cefam	1983	36
19.	Hemsell	1983	100
20.	Kauppila	1983	112
21.	Houang-sul	1983	100
22.	Houang-met	1984	107
23.	Gonen-cef-3	1985	116
24.	Gonan-cef-6	1985	143
25.	Crosthwaite	1985	67
26.	Evaldson	1986	98
27.	Hakim-cef	1986	105
28.	Hakim-mez	1986	107
29.	Davey-mez	1988	203
30.	Davey-cephr	1988	199
31.	Munck	1989	166
Overall			3604

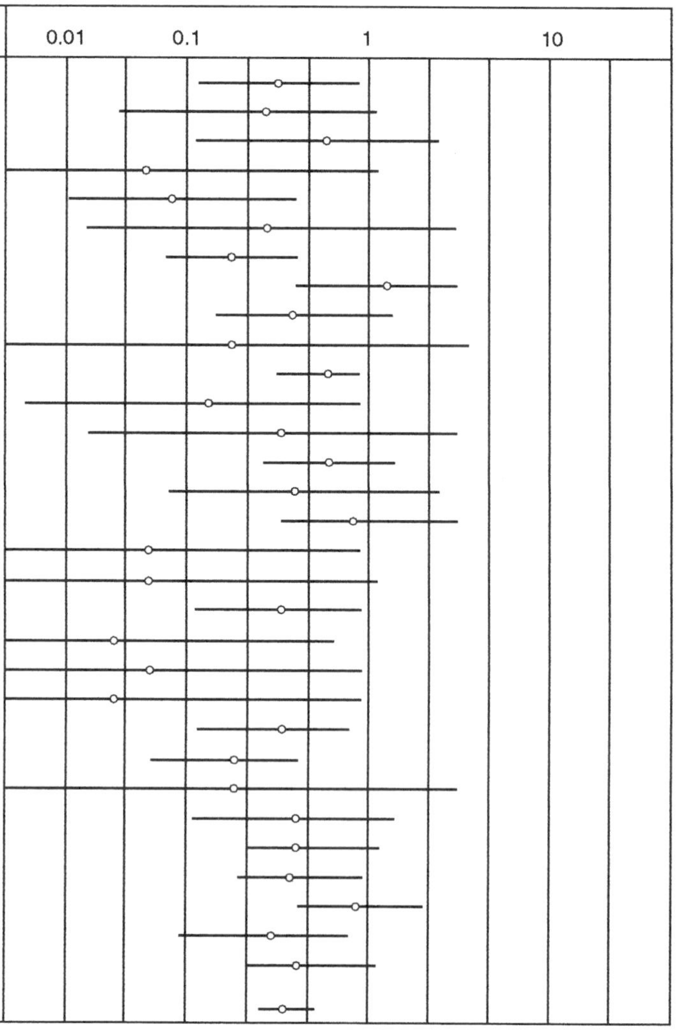

Adapted from Mittendorf R[6]

FIG. 1. Prehysterectomy antibiotic prophylaxis studies. (Adapted from Mittendorf et al., 1993.)

sensitivities. In general, a single dose of a penicillin or a first-, second-, or third-generation cephalosporin prior to the induction of anesthesia will be adequate prophylaxis, although some evidence exists that continuation of an antibiotic for the first 24 hours postoperatively is beneficial. We recommend the use of cefotetan disodium (Cefotan) because of its excellent broad-spectrum coverage and 12-hour dosing. For patients with a β-lactam allergy, doxycycline, clindamycin, or metronidazole are all effective as prophylactic agents.

Patients with indwelling implanted devices such as orthopedic, cardiac, or vascular prostheses may require special broad-spectrum antibiotic coverage, such as with ampicillin and gentamicin, before and again 8 and 16 hours after surgery to prevent the spread of infection to these devices. Similarly, broad-spectrum coverage may be necessary for women at risk for bacterial endocarditis secondary to valvular heart disease or congenital cardiac anomalies. The American Heart Association's most recent recommendations consider prophylaxis optional for vaginal hysterectomies and vaginal deliveries, unless they are complicated by suspected bacteremia. Prophylaxis is not recommended for cesarean section, uterine dilation and curettage, therapeutic abortion, sterilization procedures, or the insertion or removal of intrauterine devices, unless the tissues involved are known to be infected. When deemed necessary, prophylaxis is usually accomplished with ampicillin, 2 g, and gentamicin, 1.5 mg/kg (not to exceed 120 mg), administered intravenously 30 minutes prior to the procedure, followed by ampicillin, 1 g, 6 hours later. Vancomycin, 1 g, should be substituted for penicillin-allergic patients and does not need to be repeated postoperatively.

Two known causes of posthysterectomy wound infection deserve special mention. Soper et al. (1990) demonstrated a relationship between bacterial vaginosis and trichomonal vaginitis and both cuff cellulitis and cuff abscess. Indeed, the presence of these conditions increased the risk of posthysterectomy infection threefold. In women with bacterial vaginosis, there appears to be a 1000-fold increase in anaerobic bacterial concentration in the vagina, causing increased contamination and potential infection. Based on these data, it is recommended that women be examined for both of these infections before a proposed hysterectomy and treatment be undertaken prior to surgery. Both conditions can be easily treated with metronidazole, 500 mg twice daily for 7 days.

Hydration and Medication

To minimize the risk of vomiting and intraoperative aspiration, patients are routinely required not to take anything by mouth for 8 to 12 hours before surgery. In certain situations, such as treatment of elderly patients or following a mechanical bowel preparation, this may have a negative impact on the patient's level of hydration. This is particularly true for patients who are on the operative schedule late in the day or whose surgery may have been intentionally or unintentionally delayed. In such instances, intravenous fluids should be administered during the period of delay prevent the consequences of dehydration. In patients with extremely tenuous fluid balance, such as those with aortic stenosis, severe pulmonary hypertension, or the very elderly, adequate hydration may require preoperative admission on the day before surgery.

In addition to causing potential problems with hydration, prohibiting oral intake on the morning of surgery can be difficult for patients required to take oral medications. In general, patients should take their medications on the morning of surgery with a small sip of water. Exceptions to this rule include patients taking monoamine oxidase inhibitors, which alter intrinsic catecholamine uptake and thus influence myocardial excitability; tricyclic antidepressants, which may have a chronotropic and arrhythmogenic influence in association with some anesthetic agents; and aspirin, whose antiplatelet effect remains for the life of the platelet (approximately 10 days). These medications should be stopped 1 to 2 weeks prior to surgery, if at all possible.

For patients with hypertension, good blood pressure control on the day of surgery is essential for optimizing surgical outcome. Chronic hypertensive patients with diastolic blood pressures maintained below 120 mm Hg can usually undergo elective surgery without increased risk, but inadequately controlled pressures above this are dangerous and can result in cancellation of surgery. It is therefore essential that these patients continue their antihypertensive medications throughout the entire preoperative period. In particular, beta-blockers, nitrates, calcium channel blockers, and α_2-adrenergic stimulants should be continued, as their abrupt withdrawal can result in rebound hypertension. If a patient is to remain without oral intake for any length of time postoperatively, intravenous or transdermal formulations of these agents should be continued.

Patients with endocrine disorders are also required to continue their medications in the preoperative period. It is recommended that insulin-dependent diabetic patients take one-half of their usual daily dose of NPH insulin on the morning of surgery after which intravenous supplementation can be administered intraoperatively, if indicated. Oral hypoglycemic agents, on the other hand, should be discontinued 1 to 3 days prior to surgery, depending on the half-life of the medication. Finally, patients taking chronic adrenal corticosteroids require perioperative coverage for the stress of surgery. This usually consists of supplemental doses of hydrocortisone, 100 mg, on the evening before surgery, at the beginning of surgery, and every 8 hours thereafter until there is minimal stress. No tapering is necessary if the duration of therapy is just several days.

Positioning the Patient

Patient positioning on the operating table must always be done with care. A balance must be found between obtaining adequate exposure for the surgeons and providing for a noncompromising position for an anesthetized patient. Many patients complain postoperatively of pressure pain that undoubtedly resulted from uncomfortable positioning during anesthesia. Indeed, peripheral nerve palsies can actually result when the extremities are placed in extremes of position and may range from minor self-limiting injury to permanent loss of function. In addition, the incidence of postoperative thrombosis in peripheral veins is often related to pressure on major veins due to incorrect intraoperative patient positioning. The extremities should therefore always be properly padded and persistent pressure on any body part by either a surgeon or an instrument should be avoided at all times.

The sciatic nerve can be injured during pelvic surgery by excess abduction and hyperflexion of the thigh against the abdomen in the exaggerated dorsal lithotomy position. Temporary footdrop is the most common result, although motor and/or sensory loss to the posterior lateral lower leg and foot can also result. Peroneal nerve injury commonly results from external rotation of the leg against the operative stirrup causing pressure on the fibular head. This can lead to difficulty with ambulation secondary to footdrop and inability to abduct or evert the foot. The femoral nerve is vulnerable to injury by excessive lateral traction, most commonly in association with a low transverse or Pfannenstiel incision and self-retaining retractors. Direct pressure of the retractor blade on the nerve itself and compression of both the psoas muscle and the femoral nerve against the lateral pelvic side wall are thought to be the most common etiologies. Prevention entails the use of the shortest retractor blades possible, appropriate padding, and examination of the operative field to ensure that the retractor blade is not pressing on the psoas muscle. Inadvertent injury will result in numbness to the anterior portion of the thigh and/or difficulty with leg flexion or knee extension. Finally, injury to the obturator nerve, which results in sensory loss to the medial aspect of the thigh and difficulty in adduction, may occur during a retropubic urethropexy but is more commonly associated with radical pelvic surgery and deep pelvic lymph node dissection.

◊ IMMEDIATE POSTOPERATIVE CARE

The most critical period in any postoperative course occurs within the first 72 to 96 hours after surgery. It is during this period that the patient's physiologic reserve must be accurately assessed. Precise evaluation of the cardiovascular, urinary, and respiratory systems will provide essential information about a patient's postoperative condition. Control of these three organ systems results in the accurate management of a patient's physiologic response to the gynecologic surgery. The surgeon must diligently evaluate the patient daily for evidence of surgical complications, the most serious of which is postoperative bleeding. Alterations in the patient's vital signs and urine output are often the first symptoms of a potentially life-threatening hemorrhage. Early recognition can significantly reduce the morbidity and mortality associated with this. Prophylactic measures aimed at the prevention of all postoperative complications are instituted or continued throughout the immediate postoperative period, and all untoward events and appropriate therapy

given should be clearly documented in progress notes in the patient's chart.

Pain Control

The surgeon must make arrangements for adequate pain relief in the postoperative period. In addition to providing for the subjective comfort of patients, effective pain control allows them to take deep breaths, cough, and ambulate more easily, decreasing their risk of postoperative complications. Pain control is usually initiated in the recovery room with intravenous administration of a narcotic such as morphine. This route of analgesia may be continued once patients are in their room, or it may be converted to intramuscular or oral dosing, depending on patients' anticipated bowel function. Patient-controlled analgesia pumps that can combine a steady infusion of morphine with an as-needed, patient-controlled bolus are extremely effective and actually decrease the amount of narcotic used. The addition to a systemic opioid of an antihistamine, such as hydroxyzine, or a nonsteroidal antiinflammatory drug is well documented to have an additive or synergistic effect. This not only improves analgesia, but it also results in an opioid-sparing effect and may contribute to a reduction in the nausea, vomiting, and postoperative ileus associated with narcotic use. Finally, continuous postoperative epidural analgesia employing a combination of a local anesthetic and an opioid is being more commonly used following major abdominal and pelvic surgeries. It too provides excellent pain relief, while decreasing the incidence of side effects associated with systemic narcotics.

Examinations

In addition to providing an opportunity to communicate the findings and results of surgery to patients, the postoperative examinations function as a survey for complications. Routine assessment should include the following:

◊ Neck veins to assess volume status;
◊ Heart for abnormal rhythm, murmur, or rub;
◊ Lungs for signs of atelectasis, pulmonary edema, or pneumonia;
◊ Abdomen for bowel activity and signs of distention;
◊ Extremities for edema, cellulitis at intravenous sites, and deep vein thrombosis.

Special attention is given to examining the wound for erythema, induration, tenderness, or drainage. A progress note should be entered into the chart to reflect these examinations.

Fluids

Fluid management is one of the most basic and essential concepts in postoperative care. Type and duration of the procedure, estimated blood loss, intraoperative fluid replacement, and comorbid conditions must all be taken into consideration before intravenous fluids are ordered. Postoperative examination of a patient's lungs, neck veins, heart, abdomen, and extremities provides an estimate of volume status and will further assist in choosing an intravenous rate of replacement. Isotonic solutions such as 5% dextrose in Ringer's lactate are usually used until spontaneous diuresis begins. Once vital signs and urine output have demonstrated adequate and stable volume status, the isotonic solution may be replaced with a hypotonic solution such as 5% dextrose in one-half normal saline.

Poor urine output may indicate postoperative bleeding, third spacing, or heart failure. If a urethral catheter is in place, it should be checked and irrigated to ensure that it is functioning properly. If the patient is without a catheter, one should be inserted to accurately measure urine output. Urinary retention is a common postoperative problem that is easily diagnosed by catheter placement. When the catheter appears to be working well but the patient remains oliguric, evaluation of cardiac status, intravascular volume, and renal status should be undertaken. A hematocrit should be obtained to investigate for possible postoperative hemorrhage. If the cardiac and pulmonary excesses are normal, a fluid challenge with 250 to 500 ml of normal saline solution should be administered. Immediate operative intervention is usually indicated for patients with falling hematocrits who demonstrate tachycardia, hypotension, and abdominal distention. For patients with a suspected intraabdominal hematoma who demonstrate normal vital signs and appear stable, treatment of oliguria with intravenous fluids and observation is appropriate. Evaluation of urine sodium, creatinine, and osmolality also can be helpful in the assessment of oliguria when urine output seems inappropriate for a patient's apparent volume status. This is only useful, however, if the patient has not received any diuretics in the preceding 24 hours.

Fluid management in the postoperative period in patients with cardiovascular compromise is more difficult. This often necessitates monitoring of central venous pressure, which may be done in consultation with a skilled internist or other appropriate specialist, if necessary. Cancer patients with ascites are another group for whom postoperative fluid management can often be difficult. They generally third-space fluid postoperatively, resulting in intravascular volume depletion, oliguria, and an increased hematocrit.

Bowel Function

Because dysfunction of the gastrointestinal tract is common following abdominopelvic surgery, most physicians will restrict their patients' oral intake following surgery until there is evidence of return of bowel function. The presence of normal bowel sounds without nausea or evidence of abdominal distention usually means that patients can tolerate a clear liquid diet. A regular diet is usually withheld until patients can tolerate liquids. Patients undergoing vaginal or laparoscopic surgery, surgery of short duration, or surgery involving minimal bowel manipulation generally recover bowel function quickly. Conversely, patients undergoing radical procedures requiring prolonged operative time and extensive bowel ma-

nipulation tend to experience prolonged postoperative bowel dysfunction.

When abdominal distention and discomfort are present postoperatively, the physician must determine whether they are the result of a slow return of normal bowel peristalsis or represent a more serious condition such as a postoperative bowel obstruction. Abdominal distention without bowel sounds is the hallmark of a paralytic ileus (Table 5). It may often be treated by bowel rest and patient ambulation, but occasionally requires nasogastric suctioning. When abdominal distention is accompanied by an unexpected amount of pain, nausea, and vomiting, the diagnosis of a bowel obstruction must be considered. Abdominal radiography in the supine and upright positions will help with the diagnosis. Complete small bowel obstruction may result in ischemia of the bowel wall secondary to distention and usually demands immediate surgical intervention to prevent bowel perforation. A partial obstruction will often resolve spontaneously if bowel edema is diminished through bowel rest and nasogastric suctioning. The diagnosis of a complete obstruction may remain elusive and may require administration of barium or meglumine diatrizoate (Gastrografin) into the nasogastric tube to document obstruction.

Fever

Fever, defined as two temperature elevations of 38.0°C (100.4°F) or greater observed at least 6 hours apart, is a common problem in postoperative patients. Overall, an estimated 28% to 45% of patients undergoing abdominal or pelvic surgery will experience a fever, and an infectious etiology will be identified in approximately 36% of these. It is not surprising, however, that the frequency of an identifiable infectious etiology increases with the degree of temperature elevation. In one study, only 19.4% of patients with fevers less than 38.5°C (101.3°F) had a demonstrable source, whereas 45.2% of patients with fevers of 38.5°C or higher were found to have an infectious etiology. It is the physician's responsibility to evaluate patients' vital signs, urine output, physical examination, and available laboratory and imaging studies to determine whether fever represents a self-limited episode or an infection that could become life-threatening if not treated appropriately. Ordering of laboratory studies such as a complete blood cell count, urinalysis and culture, chest

TABLE 5. *Clinical manifestations of ileus versus partial small bowel obstruction*

Ileus	Obstruction
Pain from distention	Pain from cramps
Absent bowel sounds	Peristaltic rushes
Distention	Distention
Vomiting	Vomiting
Onset usually within 72 h	Onset usually 5–7 d postoperatively
X-ray gas pattern with large and small bowel gas	Small bowel gas in loops with air-fluid levels

radiograph, and blood cultures should be guided by patients' symptoms and signs identified on physical examination.

During the first 24 hours after surgery, the most likely causes of fever are nonspecific, and an infectious etiology is rarely identified. Physical examination will often demonstrate atelectasis, with decreased expansion of the lungs and inspiratory crackles that clear with cough. Aggressive use of incentive spirometry, deep breathing, coughing, and early ambulation will help resolve atelectasis. Recently, however, Engoren demonstrated a lack of association between the incidence of radiographically diagnosed atelectasis and postoperative fever. Therefore, possible sources of postoperative infection should be considered in every febrile patient. The most common sites of infection in the postoperative period are urinary tract, lower respiratory tract, and wound. Urinary tract infections are common, occurring in as many as 40% of all women postoperatively, but do not generally cause high fevers, unless there is obstruction or pyelonephritis. A urinalysis and subsequent culture is helpful in making the diagnosis, and, if costovertebral angle tenderness is present, a renal ultrasound is indicated to look for hydronephrosis secondary to a ureteral injury. Early postoperative fever found in association with pulmonary findings on examination is suggestive of pneumonia. Pulmonary infiltration seen on a chest radiograph is diagnostic, and sputum should be collected for microbiologic examination.

Vaginal cuff cellulitis after hysterectomy is usually a diagnosis of exclusion. A vaginal examination should be performed if fever develops 48 to 72 hours after surgery and no other source of infection is identified. In most cases, no pelvic mass will be identified, but tenderness will be noted. Antibiotic therapy should treat Enterobacteriaceae and anaerobes generally found in the vaginal flora. If a patient does not improve in 24 hours, enterococcus coverage should be added. In other cases, purulent drainage or a mass will be found at the vaginal cuff. This indicates a cuff abscess and warrants drainage and broad-spectrum antibiotic coverage. If this can not be accomplished by simple opening of the vaginal incision or if the patient remains febrile despite appropriate antibiotics, a pelvic ultrasound or CT scan and placement of a pelvic drain may be necessary.

When fever presumed to be secondary to a vaginal cuff cellulitis does not respond to antibiotics, septic pelvic thrombophlebitis should be considered. This is treated by the initiation of heparin anticoagulation to achieve a partial thromboplastin time of approximately two times control. Although thrombi in the ovarian veins occasionally can be found by radiologic studies, such studies are not necessary, and the diagnosis is confirmed when the patient has resolution of her fever 24 to 48 hours after the initiation of heparin.

Finally, surgical wound infection is a common cause of a fever arising late in the postoperative course. Careful examination of the wound for erythema and induration may reveal a cellulitis with underlying seroma or abscess. Opening of the wound followed by drainage and irrigation is warranted. If a marked cellulitis is present, initial therapy with parenteral antibiotics may be indicated, followed by an oral antibiotic, such as cephalexin or dicloxacillin, 250 to 500 mg four times a day. Dressing changes should be performed two to three times a day until the wound appears healthy, clean, and pink with granulation tissue, at which time the edges may be reapproximated with adhesive tape or sutures to diminish the width of the scar.

Pulmonary Complications

Some degree of postoperative pulmonary dysfunction occurs in all patients who receive general anesthesia and is the result of atelectasis—the collapse of the peripheral small airways of the lung with loss of lung volume and difficulty in clearing secretions. Preoperative pulmonary compromise is well known to exacerbate this complication and increase a patient's risk for pneumonia and hypoxemia. Patients at risk may benefit from preoperative instruction in incentive spirometry and coughing techniques, as well as from early ambulation postoperatively. Known risk factors include advanced age, history of smoking, obesity, prolonged hospitalization, preexisting pulmonary disease such as asthma and chronic obstructive pulmonary disease, prolonged anesthesia, and ASA class III or higher.

Prevention remains the key to the treatment of atelectasis. Patients at risk should be identified and counseled on the importance of postoperative incentive spirometry, deep breathing, and coughing despite the discomfort of an abdominal incision. Aerosolized bronchodilator treatments and chest physiotherapy may be employed in the most severe patients, and, as described earlier, preoperative admission may be beneficial. Patients at risk for hypoxemia should be monitored with bedside pulse oximeters or arterial blood gas measurements, and supplemental oxygen can be administered, if needed to maintain oxygen saturation above 90%. If pneumonia is diagnosed on the basis of a persistent fever in association with findings on physical examination or chest radiograph, aggressive respiratory toilet should be continued in addition to the initiation of broad-spectrum antibiotics.

Possibly the most devastating pulmonary complication that can occur postoperatively is pulmonary embolism. As discussed previously, even with aggressive prophylactic measures, thromboembolic disease will complicate between 3% and 9% of all major abdominopelvic surgeries, and pulmonary embolism will be the result in approximately 10% of these patients. The sudden onset of chest pain, dyspnea, tachypnea, and tachycardia heralds a pulmonary embolus, although the majority of patients present with only a few subtle or ambiguous symptoms. In fact, more than 70% of patients who die of a pulmonary embolus are not suspected of having one before their death. The national collaborative Prospective Investigation of Pulmonary Embolism Diagnosis (PIOPED) examined patient history and physical examination, chest radiograph, ECG, and arterial blood gas analysis to assess their utility in the diagnosis of pulmonary thromboembolism. Unfortunately, such significant inadequacies of both sensitivity and specificity were found for each of these noninvasive tests alone or in combination that they were determined to be insufficient to diagnose pulmonary embolism. They remain important diagnostic tools as part of the clinical assessment, however, and should still be performed before more expensive and invasive testing is ordered. The PIOPED trial also evaluated pulmonary ventilation and perfusion scans. Nearly all patients found to have pulmonary embolism had an abnormal scan (high, intermediate, or low probability), but so did most patients who did not have a pulmonary embolus (sensitivity, 98%; specificity, 10%). The predictive values of both the high- and low-probability lung scans were markedly improved, however, when combined with good clinical judgment. The gold standard remains pulmonary arteriography, resulting in an unchallenged diagnosis in 96% of patients. The invasive nature of arteriography also makes it the most morbid, however, with a major nonfatal complication rate of 1%, and a minor complication rate of 5%. The conclusion

drawn from the PIOPED trial was that "the risks of pulmonary angiography were sufficiently low to justify it as a diagnostic tool in the appropriate clinical setting [but] good clinical judgment is probably the most important consideration in the assessment of risk" (Stein et al., 1992). An algorithm for the evaluation of ventilation scintigraphy results is presented in Figure 2 and demonstrates the importance of clinical suspicion. If the diagnosis is made, heparin therapy is instituted and maintained until therapeutic levels of warfarin are achieved. Warfarin should be started on the first or second day of heparinization and continued for at least 3 months, with therapy aimed at prolonging the prothrombin time to an international normalized ratio of 2.0 to 3.0.

There are many other causes of chest discomfort and hypoxemia, and the most serious deserve consideration. If myocardial ischemia is responsible for the discomfort, changes may be seen on the ECG. Serial evaluation of cardiac isoenzymes, such as CPK, lactate dehydrogenase, and troponin,

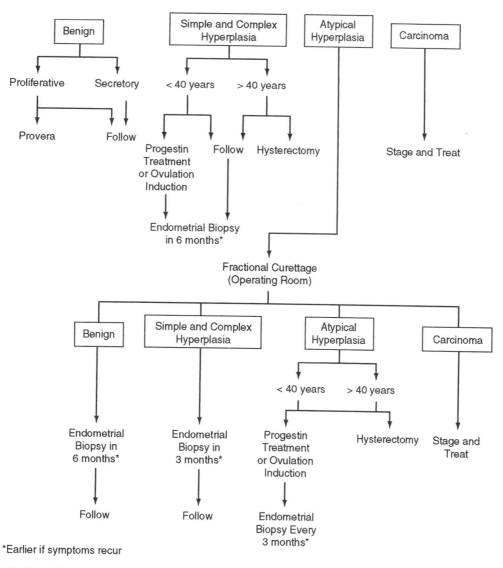

FIG. 2. Algorithm for assessment ventilation—perfusion scan results. (Adapted from Rosenow, 1995.)

can further assist with the diagnosis. Similarly, pneumonia, pneumothorax, pulmonary edema, and pericardial tamponade can be diagnosed on a chest radiograph. It is prudent in such cases to reevaluate the need for more aggressive nursing care and monitoring of patients and to decide whether or not transfer to an intensive care setting is required.

Wound Complications

Wound dehiscence is defined as a disruption of any of the layers of the surgical incision. Superficial wound disruption involving only the skin and subcutaneous tissue is fairly common and occurs in approximately 2% to 5% of gynecologic laparotomies. Classically, however, dehiscence has been used to describe separation of the skin, subcutaneous tissue, and fascia while the peritoneum remains intact. This usually occurs between postoperative days 5 and 10 and occurs in approximately 0.5% to 2.0% of gynecologic laparotomies. Evisceration, defined as the breakdown of all layers of the abdominal incision with protrusion of intraabdominal contents through the incision, is extremely rare.

The most common cause of wound dehiscence and evisceration is a concomitant wound infection. Prevention of wound infection, as previously described, is the hallmark of preventing wound complications. Other predisposing factors include a previous history of a wound infection, obesity, diabetes, chronic obstructive pulmonary disease, steroid therapy, malnutrition, peritonitis, intraabdominal malignancy, ascites, and previous irradiation therapy to the abdomen and pelvis. Closure with a Smead-Jones technique results in a marked reduction in the rate of dehiscence and is recommended for all high-risk patients. This employs a far-far/near-near suturing technique in which only the anterior fascia is included in the near-near bite (Fig. 3). There appears to be little benefit to interrupted primary closure of the anterior abdominal wall over continuous closure, and continuous closure is significantly faster. Use of polyglycolic acid–type sutures helps further reduce the incidence of these complications. Catgut sutures such as plain and chromic should never be used for fascial closure because of their relatively short half-lives. Further, because they are degraded by leukocyte-released proteolytic enzymes, a superficial wound infection may result in a fascial dehiscence.

Two patient populations that deserve special mention are obese patients and patients with a contaminated wound. Superficial wound separation occurs in as many as 30% of obese patients who undergo abdominal surgeries. Closure of the subcutaneous adipose tissue has been shown to significantly reduce this complication. Despite anecdotal evidence to the contrary, however, no definitive reduction in the rate of wound separation has been seen with the use of subcutaneous closed-drainage systems. Closure of the contaminated wound has traditionally been by delayed primary closure or by secondary intention. With the advent of modern broad-spectrum intravenous antibiotics, primary closure of the contaminated wound has become a safe and accepted practice.

The spontaneous passage of serosanguineous fluid from the abdominal incision is a classic sign of an impending wound disruption. When this occurs, the wound should be carefully probed at the bed side with a sterile cotton swab. A few staples or sutures can often be removed to determine the presence and extent of a fascial defect. Small, superficial defects can be treated by simple cleaning of the wound and allowing healing by secondary intention. Fascial defects of 1 to 2 cm without evidence of bowel herniation can be closed at the bed side or left intact, and the overlying skin closed secondarily. Patients with large defects and evisceration should be taken to the operating room, where foreign material, sutures, clots, and necrotic debris can be removed prior to wound closure. This can be performed with interrupted Smead-Jones or retention-type sutures. Prophylactic antibiotics should be administered in the event of reoperation for a wound disruption.

Urinary Tract Complications

Urologic injuries and complications are uncommon in gynecologic surgery, occurring in approximately 0.5% of benign

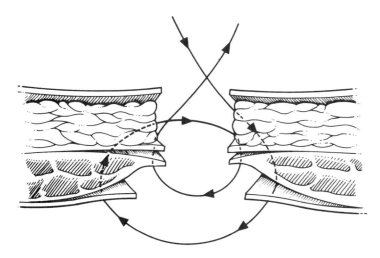

FIG. 3. Modified Smead-Jones abdominal wall closure.

gynecologic procedures and 2.0% of urogynecologic procedures. The physician must thoroughly understand the signs and symptoms of these disorders, however, because early recognition is important for successful correction without long-term morbidity. Ideally, good surgical technique will either prevent these problems or identify them intraoperatively. Whenever there is cause for concern, intraoperative evaluation and consultation, if necessary, are preferable to observation.

The most common urologic complaint following obstetric and gynecologic procedures is urinary retention, which occurs in approximately 10% to 15% of cases. Finding more than 100 ml of urine by catheterization is diagnostic of this problem. In addition to the inability to void, urinary retention can present as overflow incontinence and is diagnosed in a similar manner. This problem most commonly occurs after radical pelvic surgery or urinary incontinence procedures, but it can occur in association with almost any obstetric or gynecologic procedure. Intermittent catheterization is the treatment of choice.

Ureteral injury is another complication of obstetric and gynecologic surgery, and its incidence varies from procedure to procedure. For radical hysterectomy, the incidence is approximately 1% to 2%, for abdominal hysterectomies 0.5 to 1%, and for vaginal hysterectomies and adnexal procedures 0.1%. If ureteral obstruction is bilateral, this injury will present with anuria and rising blood urea nitrogen and creatinine levels. More commonly, however, the injury is unilateral and is either asymptomatic or presents with only mild flank pain and ileus. An ultrasound showing hydronephrosis may be helpful in the diagnosis, but an IVP showing obstruction or spillage of contrast into the peritoneal cavity is diagnostic of a ureteral injury.

Postoperative leakage of clear fluid from the vagina is the dreaded sign of a urinary fistula. Localization of the fistula site can be accomplished at the bed side with indigo carmine dye studies. A Foley catheter is first placed in the bladder, and 300 ml of water and dye are instilled in a retrograde fashion. The vagina is observed for leaking, and if none is seen, a tampon is then inserted into the vagina, and the patient asked to ambulate. The tampon is then inspected for dye staining. When positive results are found, a vesicovaginal fistula is diagnosed. A negative result suggests that the urine leak originates higher in the urinary tract. An ampule of dye is then injected intravenously. Within a few minutes, the dye will begin to color the urine blue, and if the dye is observed in the vagina, a ureterovaginal fistula is identified.

The treatment of a fistula depends on the site. A small vesicovaginal fistula may heal spontaneously if the bladder is allowed to drain by means of a catheter. Bladder fistulas greater than 1 cm in size usually require operative repair performed either immediately after diagnosis if the tissue appears clean and healthy or 2 to 3 months later if time is needed for inflammation and edema to resolve. A ureterovaginal fistula may be secondary to ligation and obstruction of the ureter, a crush injury, or ureteral devascularization. Cystoscopy and retrograde pyelography will identify which ureter is involved

and whether or not there is an associated obstruction or the fistula is compound. Attempted retrograde stenting of the involved ureter can also be performed at this time. If retrograde stent placement is unsuccessful, percutaneous nephrostomy tube placement and subsequent antegrade stenting may be successful and result in spontaneous healing within 14 to 21 days. If this does not occur, reimplantation of the ureter into the bladder will be necessary.

◊ POSTOPERATIVE COUNSELING AND DISCHARGE

In the postoperative period, patients should receive a careful explanation of the surgical procedures performed, the intraoperative findings, and the results of the pathologic evaluation of removed tissues, when available. All intra- and postoperative complications should be discussed along with their necessary management. It is essential to the physician–patient relationship that the surgeon allow adequate time for queries from patients and their family. Sometimes written as well as oral explanations are helpful. Diagrams may be especially valuable because they can be studied by patients and their family after the physician has left. Staging of patients with gynecologic malignancies or endometriosis, follow-up planning, and proposed treatments should all be discussed in the immediate postoperative period to allow patients time to consider the treatment options prior to their first return appointment. On discharge, oral and written instructions regarding postoperative home care should be given to patients. Appropriate instructions for contacting the physician both during and after office hours, as well as needed prescriptions for the immediate postoperative period, are also essential. As with all other types of perioperative counseling described in this chapter, documentation of all discussions should be entered into patients' permanent medical records.

◊ RECOMMENDED READINGS

Allen JR, Hightower AW, Martin SM, Dixon RE. Secular trends in nosocomial infections: 1970–1979. *Am J Med* 1981;70:389.

American Board of Anesthesiology. New classification of physical status. *Anesthesiology* 1963; 24:111.

American College of Obstetricians and Gynecologists. *Antibiotics and gynecologic infections. ACOG educational bulletin no. 237.* Washington, DC: ACOG, 1997.

American College of Obstetricians and Gynecologists. *Ethical dimensions of informed consent. ACOG committee opinion no. 108.* Washington, DC: ACOG, 1992.

Dajani AS, Taubert KA, Wilson W, et al. Prevention of bacterial endocarditis: recommendations by the American Heart Association. *JAMA* 1997; 277:1794.

Garner JS. CDC guidelines for the prevention and control of nosocomial infections: guidelines for prevention of surgical wound infections, 1985. *Am J Infect Control* 1986;14:71.

Goldhaber SZ, Savage DD, Garrison RJ, et al. Risk factors for pulmonary embolism: the Framingham Study. *Am J Med* 1983;74:1023.

Goldman L, Caldera DL. Risks of general anesthesia and elective operation in the hypertensive patient. *Anesthesiology* 1979;50:285.

Goldman L, Caldera DL, Nussbaum SR, et al. Multifactorial index of cardiac risk in noncardiac surgical procedures. *N Engl J Med* 1977;297:848.

Haley RW, Hooten TM, Culver DH, et al. Nosocomial infections in U.S. hospitals, 1975–1976: estimated frequency by selected characteristics of patients. *Am J Med* 1981;70:947.

Jeffcoate TNA, Tindall VR. Venous thrombosis and embolism in obstetrics and gynecology. *Aust N Z J Obstet Gynaecol* 1965;5:119.

Kaiser AB. Antimicrobial prophylaxis in surgery. *N Engl J Med* 1986; 315:1129.

Kanter MH, van Maanen D, Anders KA, Castro F, Mya WW, Clark K. Preoperative autologous blood donations before elective hysterectomy. *JAMA* 1996;276:798.

Lunn JN, Hunter AR, Scott DB. Anaesthesia-related surgical mortality. *Anaesthesia* 1983;38:1090.

Mittendorf R, Aronson MP, Berry RE, et al. Avoiding serious infections associated with abdominal hysterectomy: a meta-analysis of antibiotic prophylaxis. *Am J Obstet Gynecol* 1993;169:1119.

National Institutes of Health. *Perioperative red cell transfusion. National Institutes of Health Consensus Development Conference Statement.* Bethesda, MD: US Department of Health and Human Services, 1988:1–19.

Roizen MF. Preoperative evaluation. In: Miller RD, ed. *Anesthesia*, 4th ed. New York: Churchill Livingstone, 1994:872.

Rosenow EC III. Venous pulmonary thromboembolism: an algorithmic approach to diagnosis and management. *Mayo Clin Proc* 1995;70:45.

Schneider AJL. Assessment of risk factors and surgical outcome. *Surg Clin North Am* 1983;63:1113.

Schreiber GB, Busch MP, Kleinman SH, Korelitz JJ. The risk of transfusion-transmitted viral infections. *N Engl J Med* 1996;334:1685.

Soper DE, Bump RC, Hurt WG. Bacterial vaginosis and trichomoniasis vaginitis are risk factors for cuff cellulitis after abdominal hysterectomy. *Am J Obstet Gynecol* 1990;163:1016.

Stein PD, Athanasoulis C, Alavi A, et al. Complication and validity of pulmonary angiography in acute pulmonary embolism. *Circulation* 1992; 85:462.

Vacanti CJ, Van Houten RJ, Hill RC. A statistical analysis of the relationship of physical status to postoperative mortality in 58,388 cases. *Anesth Analg* 1970;49:564.

Wells PS, Lensing AWA, Hirsh J. Graduated compression stockings in the prevention of postoperative venous thromboembolism: a meta-analysis. *Arch Intern Med* 1994;154:67.

Wingo PA, Huezo CM, Rubin GL, Ory HW, Peterson HB. The mortality risk associated with hysterectomy. *Am J Obstet Gynecol* 1985;152:803.

CHAPTER 45

Pelvic Organ Prolapse

◇

John O. L. DeLancey

Management of pelvic organ prolapse is one of the most unique aspects of obstetrics and gynecology. It has helped define our specialty and continues to lie in the exclusive province of the obstetrician-gynecologist. Although often discussed as a purely mechanical phenomenon, prolapse is associated with significant functional problems. Stress urinary incontinence, micturitional difficulties, and problems with defecation are all associated with prolapse. These functional derangements are not simply results of altered support of the bladder and rectum but have to do with the innervation and musculature of the urinary and intestinal tracts as well. This chapter reviews the structural and functional aspects of prolapse necessary to understand and manage these conditions.

◇ PELVIC FLOOR AND THE NATURE OF GENITAL PROLAPSE

The pelvis lies at the bottom of the abdominopelvic cavity, and the pelvic floor closes the canal within the bony pelvis (Fig. 1). The pelvic floor forms a supportive layer that prevents the abdominal and pelvic organs from falling through the opening within the pelvic bones. Its structural role can best be appreciated by considering a surgeon's hand placed through a transabdominal incision that pushes caudally on the pelvic organs. All of the structures that prevent this hand from passing through the pelvic canal constitute the pelvic floor. In addition to this supportive role, the pelvic floor must provide for conception and parturition, while also controlling storage and evacuation of urine and feces. To understand the pelvic floor and genital prolapse, it is necessary to understand the mechanical strategies that evolution has put in place to prevent downward descent of the pelvic organs, as well as the process by which genital prolapse occurs. As Victory Bonney[1] pointed out, the phenomenon of prolapse is similar to the maneuver that a scrub nurse uses to evert the in-turned finger of a surgical glove (Fig. 2). Compressing the air within the glove drives the invaginated finger outward in much the same way that increases in intraabdominal pressure force the

vagina and the uterus to prolapse downward. It is not the weight of the uterus that is important in the development of prolapse, but rather the forces placed on the pelvic floor by increases in intraabdominal pressure.

There are two mechanical principles that explain how the pelvic floor prevents prolapse (see Fig. 2). First, the uterus and vagina are attached to the walls of the pelvis by a series of ligaments and fascial structures that suspend the organs from the pelvic side walls. Second, the levator ani muscles constrict the lumina of these organs closed, forming an occlusive layer on which the pelvic organs may rest. It is a combination of these two factors—suspension of the genital tract by the ligaments and fasciae and closure of the pelvic floor by the levator ani—that holds the vagina over the levator ani muscles and forms a flap-valve closure. This flap-valve mechanism is instrumental in keeping the posterior cul-de-sac closed and preventing the development of an enterocele.

◇ EPIDEMIOLOGY OF SURGICALLY MANAGED PELVIC ORGAN PROLAPSE AND URINARY INCONTINENCE

Olsen et al.[2] recently reported the prevalence of surgery for pelvic organ prolapse and urinary incontinence within a defined population. They studied 149,554 women over 25 years of age who were members of the Kaiser Permanente Northwest Health Maintenance Organization. During 1995, 384 women were identified who had surgical treatment for either pelvic organ prolapse, urinary incontinence, or both these problems. A woman's lifetime risk for needing a single operation by age 80 years was 11.1%. Among this group of women, there was great variety in types and sizes of prolapse (Table 1), and the overall incidence of surgery increased with age (Fig. 3). This was primarily due to the increase in surgery for prolapse. Reoperation was remarkably common, with 29.2% of patients requiring a second operation.

These data show the remarkable frequency with which women require surgery for incontinence and prolapse but

713

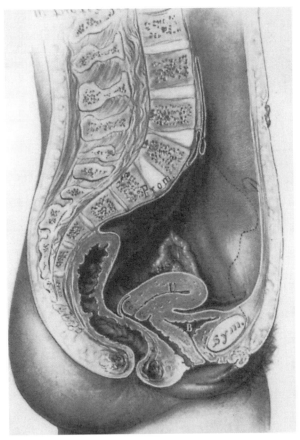

FIG. 1. Sagittal section of the abdomen and pelvis shows the relation of the pelvic floor to the abdominal cavity. (From Kelly HA. *Gynecology.* Baltimore: Appleton and Co, 1928:64; with permission.)

probably underestimate the prevalence of these problems within the population. One would expect that many women who have prolapse and incontinence choose not to have surgery, so these data represent only those women operated on. Therefore, serious consideration needs to be given these conditions.

Effects of Vaginal Delivery on Pelvic Organ Prolapse

Although it is commonly accepted that vaginal delivery increases the likelihood that pelvic organ prolapse will develop, the magnitude of this effect has not been precisely quantified. Some idea of the effect of parity on increasing incidence of organ prolapse can be gleaned from a study in Scandinavia performed by Timonen et al.[3] They compared information concerning parity in 1422 patients operated on in their hospital between 1955 and 1965 for prolapse with national parity data in Finland; these data are displayed in Figure 4. Only 4% of women with prolapse are nulliparous, while among the Finnish population 13.3% of women are nulliparous. In addition, they evaluated the size of the largest infant delivered by women in whom prolapse subsequently developed (Fig. 5) and compared that with birthweight information for Finland ($n=52,955$) during the same period (1957 to 1958). These data lend some sense of the degree to which vaginal birth influences pelvic organ prolapse.

◊ BASIC ANATOMY AND PATHOPHYSIOLOGY OF THE PELVIC FLOOR

Viscerofascial Layer

The topmost layer of the pelvic floor is a combination of the pelvic viscera and their connections to the pelvic walls and

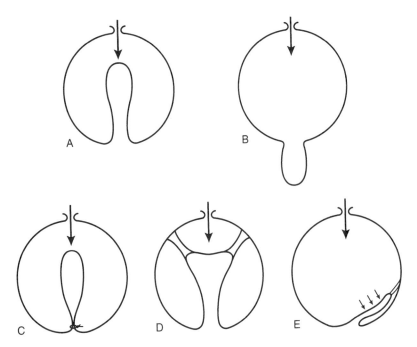

FIG. 2. A: Diagrammatic representation of the vagina within the abdomen shows how increases in abdominal pressure *(arrow)* force the vagina to prolapse downward. **B:** This prolapse may be prevented by **(C)** constricting the lower portion of the vagina, **(D)** suspending the vagina from the pelvic walls, and **(E)** forming a flap-valve closure, wherein the vagina is pinned against surrounding structures.

TABLE 1. *Preoperative prolapse severity according to operative site*

	Anterior compartment [n (%)]	Posterior compartment [n (%)]	Apex [n (%)]	Worst grade [n (%)]
No prolapse	36 (9.4%)	61 (15.9%)	80 (20.8%)	14 (3.6%)
Grade 1	81 (21.1%)	73 (19.0%)	20 (5.2%)	54 (14.1%)
Grade 2	124 (32.3%)	92 (24.0%)	63 (16.4%)	173 (45.1%)
Grade 3	41 (10.7%)	21 (5.5%)	26 (6.8%)	61 (15.9%)
Not assigned	34 (8.9%)	25 (6.5%)	27 (7.0%)	59 (15.4%)
Not documented	68 (17.7%)	112 (29.2%)	168 (43.8%)	23 (6.0%)

n=384.
(From ref. 2; with permission.)

will be referred to as the viscerofascial layer. Although it is common to speak of the fasciae and ligaments alone as separate from the pelvic organs, unless these fibrous structures have something to attach to (e.g., the pelvic organs), they have no structural integrity.

The uterus and vagina are attached to the pelvic walls by the fibrous tissue referred to as the endopelvic fascia. It forms a sheet-like mesentery that is continuous from the uterine artery to the point at which the vagina fuses with the levator ani muscles and passes through the urogenital hiatus. Those tissues that connect the uterus are called the parametria, and those that attach to the vagina are the paracolpia. Although they are given regional names, they are one continuous mass. The parametria comprise the cardinal and uterosacral ligaments.[4,5] These are two different elements of the same tissue (Fig. 6). The uterosacral ligaments are the visible and palpable medial margin of the cardinal–uterosacral ligament complex. As is true of the remainder of the parametria, they contain smooth muscle, nerves, and blood vessels and are not the same type of tissue seen in the "fascia" of the rectus abdominus muscle, which is dense regular connective tissue.

Opposite the external cervical os, the sheet of tissue that attaches the genital tract to the pelvic wall arbitrarily changes name from the parametrium to the paracolpium.[6] The paracolpium has two portions (Fig. 7). The upper portion (i.e., level I) consists of a relatively long sheet of tissue that sus-

pends the vagina by attaching it to the pelvic wall in an area similar to that of the cardinal–uterosacral ligament complex. It is this portion that prevents the vagina from prolapsing after the uterus has been removed.

In the midportion of the vagina, the paracolpium attaches the vagina laterally and more directly to the pelvic walls (i.e., level II). This stretches the vagina transversely between these two lateral attachments (Fig. 7B). This arrangement has functional significance. The structural layer that supports the bladder (i.e., pubocervical fascia) is composed of the anterior vaginal wall and its attachment through the endopelvic fascia to the pelvic wall. It is not a separate layer from the vagina. Similarly, the posterior vaginal wall and endopelvic fascia (i.e., rectovaginal fascia) form the restraining layer that prevents the rectum from protruding forward. In the distal vagina (i.e., level III), the vaginal wall is directly attached to surrounding structures without any intervening paracolpium.

The support that lies under the urethra has special importance for urinary incontinence. The endopelvic fascia in this region is better developed than it is tougher in the vagina in the area under the bladder, thereby providing better support for the vesical neck than for the bladder. This layer of suburethral endopelvic fascia attaches laterally to the arcus tendineus fasciae pelvis and also to the medial border of the levator ani muscles. Loss of this normal support of the urethra at the vesical neck is responsible for stress incontinence of urine.

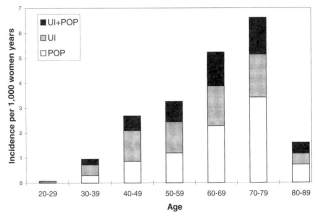

FIG. 3. Age-specific incidence of surgery for pelvic organ prolapse and/or urinary incontinence. (Adapted from ref. 2; with permission.)

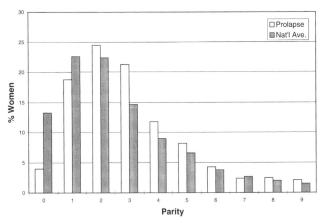

FIG. 4. Parity information for women operated on for pelvic organ prolapse compared with national average. (From ref. 3; with permission.)

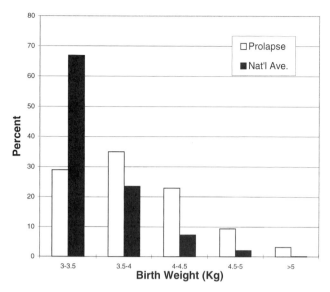

FIG. 5. Birthweight of largest infant delivered vaginally to women with pelvic organ prolapse and normative birthweight data for Finland. (From ref. 3; with permission.)

Levator Ani Muscles

Below the uterus, vagina, bladder, and rectum lie the levator ani muscles (Fig. 6B). The medial portion of the levator ani muscles has frequently been called the pubococcygeus but is more appropriately called the puborectalis or pubovisceral muscle because it extends from the pubic bone and attaches to the vagina and rectum, with only a few insignificant fibers ending in the coccyx. This strong, robust striated muscle starts on the inner surface of the pubic bone near the midline and passes behind the rectum to return to the pubic bone on the other side. The lateral walls of the vagina are attached to this muscle, which then inserts into the rectum, as well as passing around its dorsal surface in a sling-like loop. The normal resting tone of this muscle[7] squeezes the rectum, vagina, and urethra closed by compressing them against the pubic bone. Lateral to this is the flat, sheet-like iliococcygeus muscle that forms a horizontal shelf on which the upper pelvic organs rest.

Interaction between the Muscles and Fasciae

The interaction between the pelvic floor muscles and ligaments is critical to proper function. As long as the pelvic floor

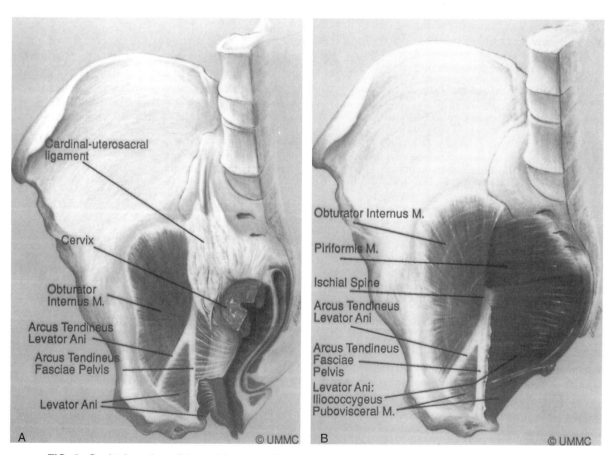

FIG. 6. Sagittal section of the pelvis shows the support structures of the genital tract. **A:** The bladder, urethra, and uterine corpus (above the cervix) have been removed. **B:** All of the pelvic organs have been removed to show the levator ani muscles.

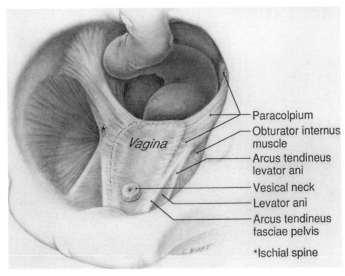

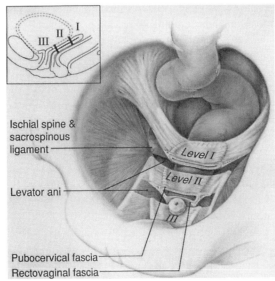

A

B

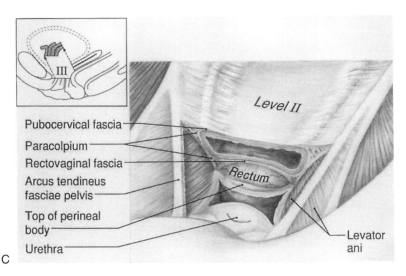

C

FIG. 7. Support structures of the vagina after hysterectomy. The bladder has been removed to expose the vagina. **A:** The paracolpium. **B:** The different levels of support structures. **C:** The details of the pubocervical and rectovaginal fasciae after a wedge of vagina and urethra has been removed **(inset).** (From ref. 6; with permission.)

musculature functions normally, the pelvic floor is closed, and the ligaments and fasciae are under no tension. They simply act to stabilize the organs in their position above the levator ani muscles. When the pelvic floor muscles relax or are damaged, the pelvic floor opens and the vagina lies between the high intraabdominal pressure and low atmospheric pressure where it must be held in place by the ligaments. Although the ligaments can sustain these loads for short periods of time, if the pelvic floor muscles do not close the pelvic floor, then the connective tissue will become damaged and eventually fail to hold the vagina in place.

◊ ISSUES RELATING TO INCONTINENCE

The mechanisms of urinary and fecal incontinence are more difficult to explain than the mechanical basis of genital tract support, and they are not entirely understood. As is true for genital prolapse, urinary continence depends on both support of the urethra and its ability to remain closed as a result of its innate constriction. Normal support of the urethra allows it to

be compressed closed by increases in abdominal pressure (i.e., pressure transmission). Although support of the urethra and pressure transmission are important for stress urinary continence, they are not the only factors involved. Stress incontinence may occur in women with normal urethral support in the lumen of the vesical neck and urethra but with inadequate constriction by the muscles within the walls. This is especially true when the α-adrenergically innervated smooth muscle of the vesical neck does not function normally and the vesical neck is open; this is referred to as type III incontinence to differentiate it from types I and II incontinence, which involve different degrees of support loss.[8] When the proximal urethra is patent at rest, urine already lies below the area where pressure transmission has its effect and therefore bypasses this mechanism of continence.

The support of the urethra is not due exclusively to fascial structures; active muscle contraction plays an important role in urethral support.[9] In addition, the musculature of the urethra contracts during a cough and increases urethral closure. Therefore, neuromuscular mechanisms play an important role in the pathophysiology of stress incontinence and must be considered in understanding this group of diseases.[10]

◊ CAUSES OF PELVIC FLOOR DAMAGE

Several factors influence the development of genital prolapse and urinary incontinence (Table 2). The inherent strength of the muscles and connective tissue of an individual, damage to these structures that occurs with birth, the rate at which they deteriorate with age, and the loads that they are subjected to during life—all play a role in the development of genital prolapse and incontinence. Understanding the interplay between these various factors is critical to appreciating the pathophysiology of genital prolapse.

Although it is obvious that the native strength of the levator ani muscles and endopelvic fascia plays an important role in prolapse, the changes that vaginal birth causes in the pelvic floor deserve specific examination. Distention of the vagina during vaginal birth is usually blamed for prolapse, and yet the cervix undergoes a much greater degree of dilation during parturition but recovers so sufficiently that forceful dilation is needed at the time of dilation and curettage later in life. Damage to the levator ani muscles and their innervation is common during vaginal birth,[11] and loss of the muscle's ability to support the pelvic organs and unload the ligaments may be partially responsible for the breakage and elongation of the ligaments later in life.

Certainly, some damage to the connective tissue of the parametria and paracolpia occurs during childbirth and can also contribute to subsequent prolapse. Although usually thought of as stretching, prolapse also includes instances in which the connective tissue supports rupture.[12] This acute injury mechanism is much more likely than stretching, because it is usually rupture that occurs with overload of other ligaments in the body (e.g., knee). Chronic injury through attenuation of the endopelvic fascia with age also contributes and explains why prolapse presents many years after childbirth. Failure of connective tissue to heal the many minor injuries that occur from day to day may also play a role. Age and chronic disease may cause weakening of the tissues, and heavy lifting or chronic coughing may cause progressive damage. This wear and tear on the connective tissues depends on the

TABLE 2. *Factors involved in pelvic organ prolapse*

Inborn strength of connective tissue and muscle
Loss of connective tissue strength
   Damage at childbirth
   Deterioration with age
   Poor collagen repair
Loss of levator function
   Neuromuscular damage during childbirth
   Metabolic diseases that affect muscle function
Increased loads on the supportive system
   Prolonged lifting
   Chronic coughing from chronic pulmonary disease
Disturbance of the balance of the structural parts
   Alteration of vaginal axis by urethral suspension
   Failure to reattach the cardinal ligaments at hysterectomy

magnitude of the stresses placed on them, as well as how well damage is repaired by the body.

◊ DIAGNOSIS AND CLASSIFICATION

Determining the type and severity of prolapse present in any given patient is a skill that should be acquired through practice and careful observation. Characterizing the degree of support loss as normal or abnormal depends on comparisons with the findings in normal multiparous women in the examiner's experience. It is therefore helpful to perform the same examination on a sufficient number of asymptomatic patients without prolapse to become familiar with the range of normal support. In performing an examination to determine the type and severity of prolapse, the practitioner has two important points to consider:

◊ Examination must be made with the patient straining forcefully enough that the prolapse is at its greatest.
◊ The examiner must examine each different element of support independently.

If a patient is not able to strain sufficiently in the lithotomy position so that the prolapse is at its largest, examination in the standing position may be necessary. This is a critical point because it is only when the prolapse can be seen in its fullest extent that all of its various elements can be assessed. If the entire extent of the prolapse is not observed, some element may be overlooked. For example, a large cystocele may be seen initially when the patient strains. It may only be with continued effort by the patient that the enterocele and prolapse of the vaginal apex that are present can be demonstrated. To make sure all aspects of the prolapse can be evaluated, the patient should be asked how large her prolapse is at its largest, and the physician should persist in the examination until that size is achieved. Once the prolapse is visible, the elements of the vagina and pelvic organs that have prolapsed can be evaluated. The examination should then focus on what specific defects in support are present and how severe the prolapse is, and there should be some evaluation of the cause of the prolapse. Once the prolapse is maximally developed, the physician should begin by identifying how much the anterior wall, cervix, and posterior wall have prolapsed downward. The anterior and posterior walls should be examined separately by retracting the opposite wall with the posterior half of a vaginal speculum. This is important because a large cystocele, for example, may hold a potential rectocele in place and therefore hide it. If this is not recognized preoperatively, the rectocele may not be repaired and will become symptomatic postoperatively.

◊ EVALUATING INDIVIDUAL ELEMENTS OF SUPPORT

Anterior Vaginal Wall

Examination of the anterior vaginal wall should establish the status of urethral support, as well as bladder support. The urethra is fused with the lower 3 to 4 cm of the vaginal wall,[13] and abnormal support in this region is properly referred to as a urethrocele (Fig. 8). Defective support of the upper portion of the vagina is called a cystocele because the bladder lies adjacent to this portion of the vaginal wall (Fig. 9). The urethrovesical crease, normally visible on examination, forms the line of demarcation between these two areas of support (Fig. 10). When support of the entire anterior wall is defective, the term *cystourethrocele* is used.

The anterior vaginal wall should be above the hymenal ring during straining. Descent of the lower anterior vaginal wall to the level of the hymenal ring during straining is characteristic of a urethrocele and is often seen in patients with stress urinary incontinence. This is due to loss of urethral support and corresponds to the loss of the posterior urethrovesical angle on radiographic studies of patients with stress incontinence. The lower anterior vaginal wall is mobile in all women and may move significantly in continent multiparas. Therefore, motion of this region does not establish stress incontinence but rather indicates the degree to which the support of the urethra has failed. Descent below the hymenal ring is definitely abnormal and indicates the presence of a cystourethrocele whether or not stress incontinence is present.

The anterior vaginal wall above the urethrovesical crease usually lies in a flat plane at about a 45-degree angle from the horizontal (Fig. 2). Descent below the level of the hymenal ring is significant. This descent can be caused by one of three entities:

◊ Separation of the paravaginal attachment of the pubocervical fascia from the white line,

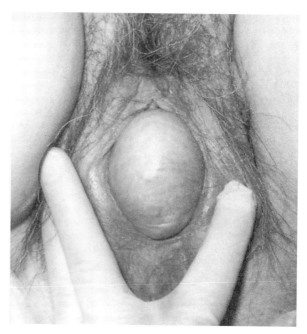

FIG. 9. Distention cystourethrocele caused by midline failure of the pubocervical fascia. (Copyright © DeLancey, 1993.)

◊ Loss of the vagina's attachment to the cervix,
◊ Tearing in the pubocervical fascia that results in herniation of the bladder through this layer.

Uterus and Vaginal Apex

The vagina and cervix are fused with one another, and prolapse of the uterine cervix is invariably associated with prolapse of

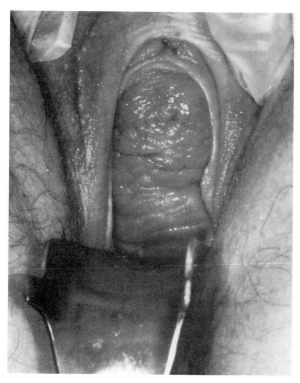

FIG. 8. Displacement cystourethrocele with intact rugal folds caused by lateral detachment of the pubocervical fascia. (Copyright © DeLancey, 1993.)

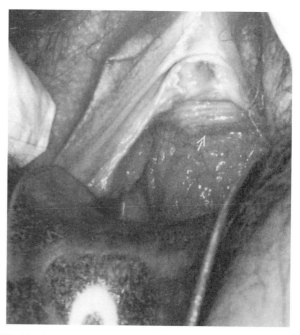

FIG. 10. Angulation in the anterior vaginal wall, called the urethrovesical crease *(arrow)*, indicates the location of the urethrovesical junction. (Copyright © DeLancey, 1993.)

the upper vagina as well. When the uterus descends below its normal level, the term *uterovaginal prolapse* is appropriate, although uterine prolapse is also commonly used. In patients in whom the uterus was previously removed, descent of the vaginal apex below its normal position in the pelvis is referred to as prolapse of the vaginal apex, and when the vagina turns entirely inside out, the term *vaginal eversion* is used.

The location of the cervix is customarily used to gauge the severity of uterine prolapse (Fig. 11). Its position relative to the hymenal ring should be noted while the prolapse is at its greatest. If the cervix is not visible because of the presence of a cystocele or rectocele, then its location may be palpated while having the patient strain. When the cervix descends to within 1 cm of the hymenal ring, there is a significant loss of support. In instances in which the uterus is not necessarily going to be removed, the normality of uterine support should be tested before it is assumed that the uterus is well supported. This can be done by grasping the cervix with a tenaculum or ring forceps and applying traction until it stops descending.[14] Occult prolapse in which the cervix comes below the hymenal ring can be detected in this way.

In addition to determining how far the cervix descends, its length should be measured. Cervical elongation is frequent in individuals with prolapse, and the uterine corpus may often lie in its normal location. Awareness of the presence of cervical elongation preoperatively will allow the surgeon to proceed expeditiously with the hysterectomy, rather than hoping with every pedicle that the uterine arteries will soon appear.

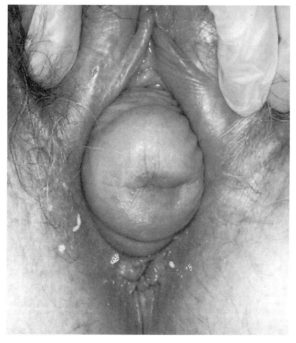

FIG. 11. Uterine prolapse with the cervix extending 3 cm below the hymen. (Copyright © DeLancey, 1993.)

Posterior Vaginal Wall

The posterior vaginal wall is the site of both rectoceles and enteroceles. Evaluation and correction of these two problems challenge even the most experienced gynecologic surgeon, and they are probably the most difficult to understand of all pelvic support defects. Because dyspareunia can follow repair,[15,16] correction of asymptomatic posterior wall defects is not without risk. On the other hand, having a rectocele or enterocele develop after vaginal hysterectomy and anterior colporrhaphy is an undesirable outcome, and careful consideration of the support of the posterior vaginal wall is important.

Three questions should be asked by the physician when examining the posterior wall:

◊ Is it normally supported?
◊ If not, is it a true rectocele or a pseudorectocele?
◊ Is an enterocele present?

A rectocele is present when the anterior rectal wall and overlying vagina protrude below the hymenal ring. An enterocele exists when the cul-de-sac becomes distended with the intestine and bulges the posterior vaginal wall outward. There are also occasions in which the posterior wall appears to bulge into the vagina, not because of poor support of the rectal wall but because of a deficiency in the perineal body. This has been referred to by Nichols and Randall[17] as a pseudorectocele and can be easily differentiated from a true rectocele because the anterior rectal wall contour is normal on rectal examination.

Enterocele

There is always a cul-de-sac between the upper vagina and the rectum. This allows a culdocentesis to be performed and a colpotomy to be made through the posterior vaginal wall at the beginning of a vaginal hysterectomy. This peritoneal pouch extends 3 to 4 cm beyond the junction of the vagina and cervix.[18] Therefore, the absence of an enterocele in normal women must be explained by factors that keep the cul-de-sac closed rather than by the absence of a peritoneal space between the upper vagina and rectum. It is the suspension of the upper vagina near the sacrum in a position where it may rest over the rectum and intact levator plate that keeps this space closed.

There are two types of enteroceles: pulsion enterocele and traction enterocele. A pulsion enterocele exists when the cul-de-sac is distended with and presents as a bulging mass that is inflated by increases in abdominal pressure. This may occur with either the vaginal apex or uterus well suspended, in which case the cervix or vaginal apex is at a normal level and the enterocele dissects between the vagina and the rectum. When an enterocele is also associated with prolapse of the uterus or vaginal apex, then the prolapse and enterocele occur together.

A traction enterocele represents a situation in which prolapse of the uterus pulls the cul-de-sac peritoneum down with it but there is no bulging or distention of the cul-de-sac when abdominal pressure rises. This condition is usually found at the time of vaginal hysterectomy when the cervix has prolapsed. It represents a potential enterocele rather than an actual enterocele because there is no bulging mass separate from the uterus.

Unlike uterine prolapse, which is obvious because of the protrusion of the easily recognized uterine cervix, enteroceles and rectoceles are rarely self-evident on examination. Therefore, the key to detecting an enterocele lies in actively looking for it whenever a patient who has prolapse is examined. Detection of an enterocele is best performed in the awake, straining patient by noting a mass of small intestine between the rectum and vagina; it may not be suspected in a supine individual at rest.

Anatomically, an enterocele extends from the apex of the vagina downward, whereas a rectocele typically begins in the lower portion of the vagina. An enterocele is sometimes evident as a bulge that overrides the more caudal rectocele (Fig. 12). Careful inspection of the posterior vaginal wall with a speculum retracting the anterior wall can sometimes suggest that an enterocele is present. The key to detecting a pulsion enterocele lies in palpating the small bowel between the vagina and rectum during rectovaginal examination with the patient straining so that the prolapse is protruding. To do this, an index finger is placed in the rectum and a thumb is placed in the vagina. Then, with the patient straining, the rectovaginal space may be palpated to detect the bulge of the enterocele and the presence of small bowel, omentum, or large bowel in this region.

Rectocele

The hallmark of a typical rectocele is the formation of a pocket that allows the anterior rectal wall to balloon downward through the introitus. When a rectal examination is performed

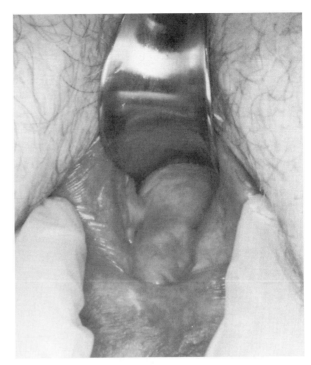

FIG. 12. "Double hump" sign of an enterocele overriding a rectocele. (Copyright © DeLancey, 1993.)

with the prolapse fully developed, a rectocele exists if there is an extension of the rectal lumen below the axis of the anus (Fig. 13). This not only provides the diagnosis but also illustrates the mechanism by which rectoceles create their symptoms. As long as the anterior rectal wall has a smooth contour

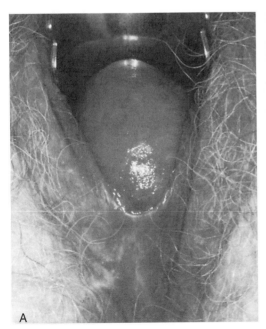

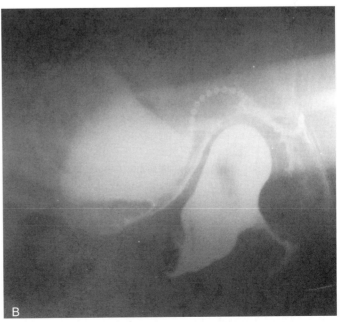

FIG. 13. A: Pelvic examination shows a rectocele. B: Lateral bead chain cystourethrogram with the patient supine and with contrast in the vagina and rectum shows a protruding rectocele. (Copyright © DeLancey, 1993.)

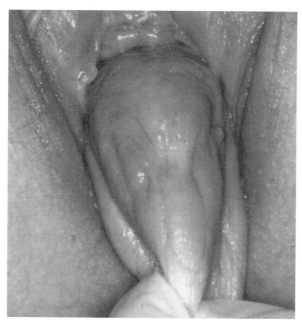

FIG. 14. Eversion of the vagina after hysterectomy. Note that the vaginal apex, indicated by the puckered scar where the cervix had been removed, lies below the hymenal ring. (Copyright © DeLancey, 1993.)

and no sacculation, even though it may be more mobile than normal, stool will pass out through the anus. However, when a pocket develops as the patient strains, stool becomes trapped in it, and difficulty with evacuation can occur.

Prolapse Subsequent to Hysterectomy

Special consideration should be given to patients who have prolapse after hysterectomy to assess whether or not prolapse of the vaginal apex is present. When the uterus is *in situ,* the cervix calls attention to the fact that the cervix and upper vagina are poorly supported. In instances of posthysterectomy vaginal prolapse, descent of the vaginal apex is more easily missed. If it is overlooked and an anteroposterior colporrhaphy is not accompanied by suspension of the vaginal apex, the colporrhaphy will fail to cure the apical prolapse, and the problem is not corrected. Examination of patients who have previously had a hysterectomy should include a specific effort to determine the location of the vaginal apex when the prolapse is at its largest. The apex is identified by the scar that exists where the cervix was removed (Fig. 14). Vaginal prolapse is present when the vaginal apex lies below the level of the hymenal ring.[19] If the apex descends to within the lower one-third of the vagina with straining, a significant deficit in support of the apex is present, and the vagina should be resuspended during repair.

◊ PELVIC ORGAN PROLAPSE CLASSIFICATION

Several classification systems have been used to describe the size and type of pelvic organ prolapse present in an individ-

ual woman. Because many of these systems use similar words to indicate different degrees of prolapse, confusion has arisen concerning the size of prolapse present. For example, grade 2 uterine prolapse in some systems indicates that the cervix descends halfway between its normal position and the introitus. While in other classifications, grade 2 can mean that half of the uterus is outside the introitus. Recently, a system that standardizes terminology has been proposed.[20] This standardized terminology provides a system that can unambiguously describe the type of prolapse present, as well as quantifying the degree of prolapse in each area. Although this standardized system seems somewhat cumbersome when described in writing, in actual practice it is quite simple. The following section first considers the measurements that describe the type and size of prolapse present and then discusses the measurements concerned with the changes in the urogenital hiatus in the levator ani muscles through which the prolapse descends.

Measurements Describing Prolapse Type and Size

To describe the nature of a woman's prolapse, it is necessary to

◊ Document what part or parts of the genital tract have prolapsed,
◊ Indicate how far down each part of the vaginal wall or cervix has descended.

Prolapse description must include a consideration of anterior vaginal wall descent, posterior wall descent, and uterine descent (or prolapse of the vaginal apex after hysterectomy). Furthermore, because different parts of the anterior wall might suffer support damage, the system provides for determining the status of each level of vaginal support. For example, the distal anterior vaginal wall adjacent to the urethra may be well supported, while the portion of the vagina under the bladder may prolapse. This system addresses the need to have individual assessments of different parts of the vaginal wall.

Three levels of vaginal support must be assessed, corresponding to the different anatomic regions of vaginal support:

◊ Level I: support of the vaginal apex and uterus,
◊ Level II: support of the bladder and rectum,
◊ Level III: support of the the urethra and perineal body.

In levels II and III, the anterior and posterior vaginal wall are considered separately, while in level I the cervix (or vaginal apex) and posterior fornix must be assessed.

To understand the classification system, refer to Figure 15. The size and type of prolapse present is measured by determining the location of a series of points on the anterior and posterior vaginal walls relative to the hymenal ring. Points at each of the three levels are measured. It should be noted that this descriptive scheme does not distinguish between rectocele and enterocele but simply provides a way to quantify the

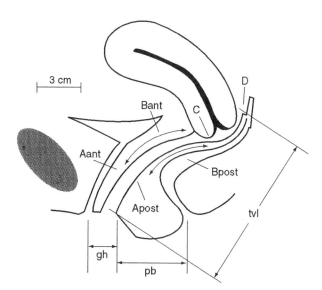

FIG. 15. Six sites (points A_{ant}, B_{ant}, C, D, B_{post}, and A_{post}), genital hiatus *(gh)*, perineal body *(pb)*, and total vaginal length *(tvl)* used for pelvic organ support quantitation. (Adapted from ref. 20.)

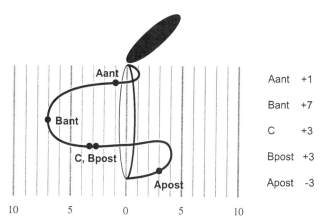

FIG. 16. Diagram of prolapse sites. (From ref. 21; with permission.)

amount of vaginal wall descent in each specific area. Additional examination and written comments concerning these important differences should be made.

To measure the lower third of vaginal support (level III), the location of a pair of points lying 3 cm above the hymenal ring is assessed. In this level, these are called points A. Anteriorly, this corresponds to the approximate location of the urethrovesical junction, and this measurement assesses urethral descent (A_{ant}). Posteriorly, this region is normally occupied by the tissues of the perineal body (A_{post}). By definition, the highest position of either point A_{ant} or A_{post} is 3 cm above the hymen, and the lowest position is 3 cm below the hymen.

To assess midvaginal support (level II), the most dependent part of the vaginal wall above point A_{ant} is used. This point is called B_{ant} on the anterior wall and B_{post} on the posterior wall. This is therefore not a fixed point along the surface of the vagina, but rather it is marked at whatever location is the most caudal portion of that vaginal segment at maximum prolapse protrusion. In a normally supported vagina, this will be the same as point A_{ant}, whereas in a woman with procidentia it will be the same as point C. The same is true for the posterior vaginal wall at point B_{post}. Point C corresponds to the most distal portion of the uterine cervix or of the hysterectomy scar in the vagina in those patients who have previously had the uterus removed. Point D denotes the posterior fornix (that point at which the posterior vaginal wall changes direction). In addition to the positions of these points, the total length of the vagina is noted. Once these data have been gathered, a simple line diagram can be constructed by plotting these points relative to the hymen to provide a graphical representation of the prolapse (Fig. 16).[21]

So far, each element of the prolapse has been considered separately. It is also possible to give an overall description to the size of the prolapse by looking at the most dependent part of the protruding vagina or uterus. In this way, different stages—stage 0 through stage IV—can be defined; a description of these is shown in Table 3.

Pelvic Floor Measurements

In normal women, the levator ani muscles close the pelvic floor. In women with pelvic organ prolapse, the urogenital hiatus within the levator ani muscles is the opening through which the vagina prolapses. This hiatus is enlarged in women with pelvic organ prolapse.[22] The size of the urogenital hiatus and thickness of the perineal body can easily be measured to describe the changes that have occurred in the pelvic floor. The anteroposterior diameter of the genital hiatus extends

TABLE 3. *Stages of pelvic organ prolapse based on measurement of specific sites*

Stage 0	No prolapse is demonstrated. Points A_{ant}, A_{post}, B_a, and B_p are all at -3 cm and either point C or D is between $-$ total vaginal length (TVL) cm and $-(TVL-2)$ cm (i.e., the quantitation value for point C or D is $\le -[TVL-2]$ cm)
Stage I	The criteria for stage 0 are not met, but the most distal portion of the prolapse is >1 cm above the level of the hymen (i.e., its quantitation value is <-1 cm)
Stage II	The most distal portion of the prolapse is between 1 cm above and 1 cm below the plane of the hymenal ring (i.e., its quantitation value is ≥ -1 cm but $\le +1$ cm)
Stage III	The most distal portion of the prolapse is >1 cm below the plane of the hymen but protrudes no farther than 2 cm less than the TVL in centimeters (i.e., its quantitation value is $>+1$ cm but $<+[TVL-2]$ cm)
Stage IV	Essentially, complete eversion of the total length of the lower genital tract is demonstrated. The distal portion of the prolapse protrudes to at least (TVL-2) cm (i.e., its quantitation value is $\ge +[TVL-2]$ cm)

from the arch of the pubic bone to the front of the perineal body, while the thickness of the perineal body is measured from the anterior margin of the perineal body to the center of the anal verge. The urogenital hiatus is held closed by the constant activity of the levator ani muscles, and the diameter of this opening enlarges in many women with prolapse.

This classification system is detailed and specific. It requires careful examination and assessment. Although it seems at first quite detailed, it is simply the quantitative documentation of the individual defects present that experienced surgeons have always found necessary to assess. Some clinicians will not find it expedient to measure each of these sites, but intelligent, detailed analysis of each site of support is important to properly plan any repair for pelvic organ prolapse.

◊ SYMPTOMS

All types of prolapse have several symptoms in common. Once the vagina prolapses below the introitus, it becomes the structural layer between the high pressures in the intra-abdominal space and the relatively low atmospheric pressure. The downward force that this pressure differential creates puts tension on the fasciae and ligaments that support the vagina and uterus. This results in a dragging sensation where the tissues connect to the pelvic wall, usually identified by patients as occurring in the groin, and in sacral backache caused by traction on the uterosacral ligaments. This type of discomfort resolves when the patient lies down and the downward pressure is reduced. In addition, exposure of the moist vaginal walls leads to a sensation of perineal wetness that may be confused with urinary incontinence, and it can also give rise to ulceration of the vaginal wall. Most patients also have an underlying sense of insecurity that is difficult for them to describe and is often expressed as a feeling that "something is just not right." Although this is difficult for patients to put into words, it causes them significant distress and should not be ignored.

Symptoms of Anterior Wall Prolapse

The symptoms of cystourethrocele are varied,[23] and the two primary ones are paradoxical. On the one hand, loss of support of the urethra and the lower vaginal wall is associated with stress urinary incontinence, whereas loss of support of the upper anterior vaginal wall and bladder base can cause difficulty in emptying the bladder. This inability to completely empty the bladder is probably related to voiding by the Valsalva maneuver. If there is a detrusor contraction, then there should be no reason for a woman with a cystocele not to empty her bladder, and many women with a significant cystocele have a normal postvoid residual urine volume. When a woman strains to void, however, the cystocele simply gets bigger, and no impulse is provided for urine to flow through the urethra.

In addition to these functional symptoms, many patients with a cystourethrocele complain of urinary urgency and fre-

quency. This probably arises from stretching of the bladder base that accompanies its prolapse through the vaginal introitus; it is often less pronounced at night when patients are supine.

Patients have a varying amount of support loss under the urethra or bladder, and symptoms vary along the spectrum from incontinence to urinary retention. As is true for other forms of prolapse, it is important to correlate a patient's symptoms with the physical findings, so these problems can be addressed.

Symptoms Associated with Prolapse of the Uterus, Prolapse of the Vaginal Apex, or Enterocele

Few specific symptoms are related to prolapse of the uterus, prolapse of the vaginal apex, or enterocele. Patients with these conditions usually complain of the generalized symptoms of prolapse mentioned above. Some have urgency and frequency, probably related to pressure of the prolapse on the bladder base, but this is variable. In addition, patients with large, thin enteroceles occasionally have a sense of impending rupture. Although this is an uncommon problem, it should not be overlooked.

Symptoms of Rectocele

The cardinal symptom of a rectocele is difficulty in emptying the rectum.[10] As a woman bears down to evacuate the rectum, stool is pushed into the rectocele, and the harder she strains, the bigger the rectocele becomes. Because constipation is common in older women, it is important to differentiate between infrequent bowel movements due to poor colonic motility or inadequate dietary fiber and difficulty due to a rectocele. Many women have found that if they press between the vagina and rectum to elevate the rectocele, this maneuver helps with defecation. This finding supports the fact that the rectocele is the source of the problem.

◊ WHO SHOULD BE TREATED SURGICALLY

A decision about when an operation for prolapse should be performed is based on each individual woman's situation. It depends on the size of the prolapse, the presence or absence of symptoms, and whether or not physiologic complications have arisen because a prolapse is present.

When the prolapse lies at or above the level of the hymenal ring, surgery should be performed only if definite symptoms are present and can be reliably attributed to the prolapse. Examples of this are a patient with a cystourethrocele at the level of the hymen who has significant stress incontinence, or a woman with the cervix in the lower one-third of the vagina who has the characteristic dragging discomfort of a prolapse that resolves when she lies down or puts a supportive pessary in place. Another example is a patient with a small rectocele in whom a definite pocket can be detected on rectal examination and elevation of the perineum relieves problems with defecation.

It is unusual for women in whom the uterus has not yet descended to the level of the hymenal ring to have symptoms caused by descent of the uterus. Symptoms of pressure, back pain, or feelings that something is coming out should be studied to confirm that they are related to the prolapse and not to other factors, before a decision to operate is made. If the symptoms go away when a pessary is placed or a patient notices prompt relief when she lies down, this helps to confirm the fact that the prolapse is the source of the symptoms. A woman with low back pain whose discomfort persists after she is supine is more likely to have arthritic or musculoskeletal pain than pain caused by uterine prolapse, and the results of surgery are likely to disappoint her.

In patients whose prolapse descends several centimeters below the hymenal ring, symptoms are usually present, and surgery will relieve these patients of this distress. Some women with a large prolapse will deny any symptoms because they do not wish to undergo surgery or because they simply are not troubled by the presence of the prolapse. Their wishes should be respected. On the other hand, potential problems from the prolapse should be considered and discussed frankly, so that possible complications from the prolapse are taken into account.

Specific problems that indicate that a prolapse should be repaired, despite its lack of symptoms, include the presence of recurrent urinary tract infections associated with an increased postvoid residual urine volume. Ureteral dilatation caused by the prolapse, which leads to an impairment of renal function, occurs in some patients with large prolapses and should be considered an indication for repair. An intravenous pyelogram (IVP) and renal function testing can detect these abnormalities and indicate the need for treatment. The IVP should include films made with the patient standing and the prolapse present, because the supine position may mask the presence of significant dilatation.

◊ SURGICAL PROCEDURES

Vaginal Hysterectomy and Anteroposterior Colporrhaphy

Vaginal hysterectomy and appropriate anteroposterior colporrhaphy is the operation most often performed for the treatment of uterovaginal prolapse. Because simple removal of the uterus does nothing to correct the prolapse of the vaginal walls that accompanies descent of the cervix, it is necessary to consider how an operation works to properly cure these conditions.

Basic Principles Underlying the Surgical Repair of Prolapse

Removal of the uterus does not improve support of the genital tract. It is the way in which a surgeon resuspends the vagina and repairs other defects in pelvic organ support when performing a vaginal hysterectomy and anteroposterior repair that determines the success of surgery for prolapse. Once the

uterus has been removed, the vaginal apex should be attached to a point of fixation that is higher in the pelvis than the vagina to elevate it to a normal position. During the vaginal hysterectomy, the cardinal and uterosacral ligaments can be shortened and used to resuspend the vagina. In addition, techniques such as McCall cul-de-plasty anchor a suture to a point on the uterosacral ligaments higher than the preoperative position of the vagina and use this suture to pull the vaginal apex to a point higher in the pelvis. It is the elevation of the vagina rather than removal of the uterus that is critical.

Preoperative Considerations

In addition to the usual thorough history, physical examination, and other medical measures necessary prior to any major operation, preoperative preparation for vaginal hysterectomy should include a pelvic examination, Pap smear, and urinalysis. Special care should be taken, as previously described, to determine the exact type and degree of prolapse present and to detect any potential ovarian malignancy. A Fleet enema the night before surgery empties the rectum in the event that a rectal examination is required during surgery and provides more room posteriorly, improving exposure. Patients should receive a prophylactic antibiotic to minimize the risk of postoperative infections (cefazolin sodium, 500 mg intramuscularly or intravenously, on call to the operating room is appropriate).[24] If abnormal uterine bleeding was present, the endometrium should have been sampled preoperatively. Finally, special consideration should be given to assessing whether or not concomitant cystocele, stress incontinence, enterocele, or rectocele is present.

Before the hysterectomy is begun, the bladder is drained, and a sterile preparation performed. An indwelling catheter is usually not placed at this point to allow the bladder to accumulate enough urine so that an inadvertent cystotomy may easily be recognized. Care should be taken in positioning and draping the patient to avoid compression of the femoral or peroneal nerve, but there should be adequate access to the operative site. An examination should be performed under anesthesia to once again assess whether or not any abnormalities are present that would make vaginal hysterectomy impossible and would indicate a switch to an abdominal approach.

Technique of Vaginal Hysterectomy

The elements of vaginal hysterectomy in the United States are derived from the operation described by Heaney[25,26] (Fig. 17). It is begun by making a circumscribing incision through the vaginal wall at the cervicovaginal junction (Fig. 17A). Anteriorly, the incision is placed at the lower edge of the bladder to allow entry into the vesicovaginal space. The lower edge of the bladder can be palpated against the cervix to determine where this incision should be made. In addition, the junction of the vaginal rugae and the smooth mucosa of the cervix can be used as a landmark to identify the proper site of incision. Some operators inject saline into the tissues

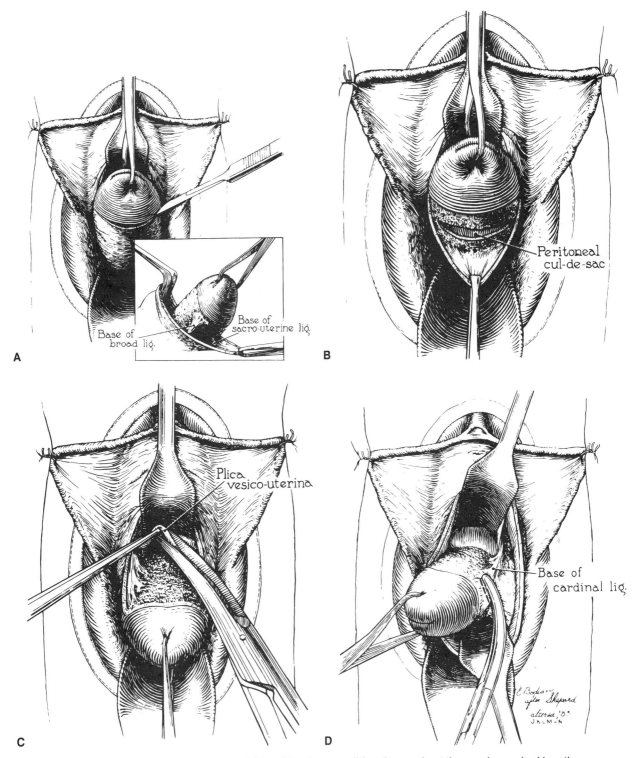

A

Base of broad lig.

Base of sacro-uterine lig.

B

Peritoneal cul-de-sac

C

Plica vesico-uterina

D

Base of cardinal lig.

FIG. 17. A: Vaginal hysterectomy is initiated by circumscribing the cervix at the cervicovaginal junction. **B:** The posterior cul-de-sac is opened. **C:** The peritoneum of the anterior cul-de-sac is incised. **D:** The base of the uterosacral and cardinal ligament is usually clamped in two bites. **E:** The upper cardinal ligament is clamped prior to its transection. **F:** The uterine fundus is delivered, and the connections between the adnexal structures and uterine corpus are clamped. **G:** Ligaments and vaginal cuff as they appear after hysterectomy. The posterior cuff is whip-stitched **(inset). H:** Technique for resuspension of the vaginal cuff and obliteration of the cul-de-sac: *1,* placement of suture through exteriorized ligaments and vaginal wall; *2,* reefing sutures placed in peritoneum; *3,* modified internal McCall suture; *4,* high purse-string suture to close the cul-de-sac. (From Mattingly RF, Thompson JD, eds. *TeLinde's operative gynecology,* 6th ed. Philadelphia: JB Lippincott Co, 1985:554; with permission.)

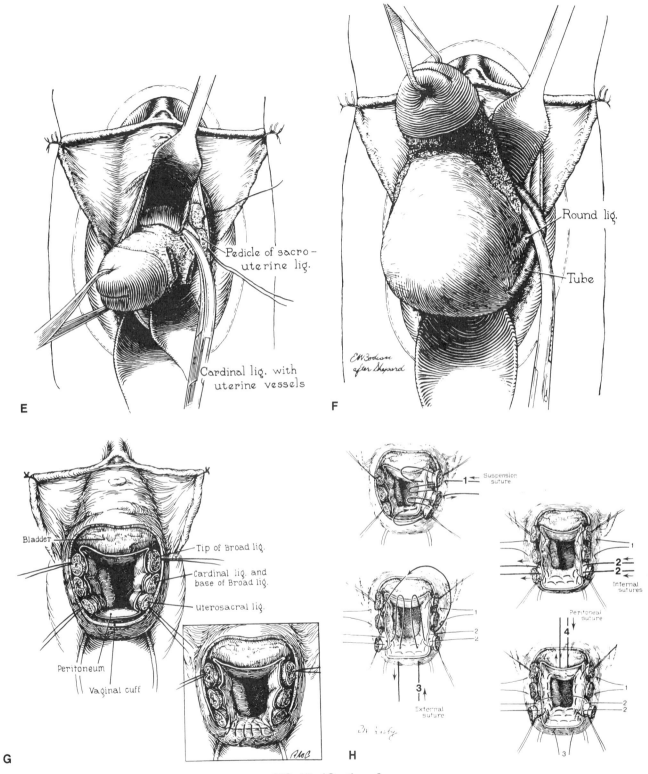

FIG. 17. (*Continued*)

around the cervix to facilitate dissection, but this should not contain a vasoconstrictor because use of these substances increases the incidence of postoperative pelvic infection.[27]

The incision should be made through the full thickness of the vaginal wall. This can be determined by placing a retrac-tor anteriorly while pulling forcefully on the cervix so that the vaginal wall is placed under tension. Once the vagina has been transected, it separates, exposing the underlying cleav-age plane. On the posterior aspect of the cervix, this exposes the area of the cul-de-sac. Blunt dissection here frees the peritoneum, which can then be grasped and entered (Fig. 17B). Care should be taken not to dissect the peritoneum off the uterus because that makes entry more difficult. Once the cul-de-sac incision has been extended laterally as far as the medial margins of the uterosacral ligaments, it can be sutured to the posterior vaginal cuff to minimize bleeding. At this point, it is appropriate to palpate the adnexal structures through the colpotomy to detect unsuspected tumors and also to make a final decision concerning the feasibility of the vaginal approach if any doubt had existed. This is an easy time to acquire this valuable information, and if unsuspected disease is found, an abdominal approach can be taken.

Next, the long blade of an Auvrard retractor is placed into the cul-de-sac, and attention is turned to entering the anterior cul-de-sac. Dissection along the vesicocervical plane is best performed by lifting the fascia anteriorly while cutting with Mayo scissors placed tip down on the cervix. This avoids the problems with dissecting into the cervix that sometimes occur when a knife is used, because the scissors held in this orientation will not cut into the dense fibrous tissue of the cervix. Once the cleavage plane of the vesicocervical space is reached, gentle dissection with a gloved finger is all that is needed to elevate the bladder off of the cervix. If the bladder pillars are prominent, they can be clamped next to the cervix, transected, and ligated to provide better lateral exposure. The location of the peritoneum may be detected by moving a finger from side to side and feeling the way in which the two slippery mesothelial surfaces slide on one anther. The peritoneum can then be lifted up, transilluminated, and incised (Fig. 17C). After the incision is extended laterally, a suture is placed in its vesical edge and held with a hemostat to facilitate its identification at the time of reperitonealization.

Once the cul-de-sacs have been entered, the ureter should be palpated to determine its position prior to shortening and transecting the cardinal ligaments. This is a critical step, because only if the ligaments are shortened will the vagina be held at a level higher than that of the prolapsed cervix. A retractor is placed in the lateral fornix of the vagina and a finger in the anterior cul-de-sac. Because the ureter must pass under the uterine artery and end in the bladder anterior to the examining finger, it can be palpated against the retractor blade. The characteristic snap of the ureter permits its identification, and it can be followed for some distance by moving the retractor and examining finger anteriorly and posteriorly.

After the ureter is identified here, the uterosacral and cardinal ligaments are shortened by clamping them at a safe distance from the ureter, somewhat lateral to the cervix (Fig. 17D,E). After the ligaments are cut and suture-ligated, the sutures are left long and marked for use in resuspending the vagina at the end of the procedure. The uterine arteries are similarly clamped, transected, and suture-ligated, but they are not tagged to avoid dislodging the suture from this vascular pedicle.

At this point, the corpus of the uterus is usually brought through the posterior colpotomy by pulling on it with a tenaculum to expose the connections between the adnexal structures and the uterus (Fig. 17F). When this is not possible because of

a small vagina or large uterus, the uterus can be divided along its sagittal plane, and one-half can be pushed up into the peritoneal cavity. A long tenaculum is left attached to the elevated half of the uterus to allow its later retrieval, while the contralateral adnexal pedicles are dealt with. Clamps are placed across the adnexal structures, with care taken not to include bowel or adjacent structures, and the pedicles are transected.

Next, consideration should be given to removal of the ovaries.[28] If the ovaries are to be removed, the mesovarium or infundibulopelvic ligament is clamped, the ovary is removed with or without the fallopian tube, and the remaining pedicle is suture-ligated.

Management of the Cul-de-Sac and Suspension of the Vaginal Apex

Once the uterus has been removed, the anterior colporrhaphy has been completed, and the ligaments have been prepared by shortening them, the reconstructive phase of the operation begins. These steps use the ligaments that were tagged during the hysterectomy (Fig. 17G). The goals are to close the peritoneum and suspend the vaginal apex while also correcting any existing enlargement of the cul-de-sac. The cul-de-sac peritoneum is attached to the uterus. Whenever the uterus prolapses, it pulls the cul-de-sac peritoneum with it. If this extension is not distended with bowel, it is referred to as a traction enterocele, and when the cul-de-sac is not only elongated but also distended with bowel, it is referred to as a pulsion enterocele, a true enterocele.

When little prolapse has been present (i.e., the cervix does not extend below the hymenal ring), simple closure of the cul-de-sac and attachment of the ligaments to the vaginal cuff suffice. A Foley catheter is usually placed at this time to drain the bladder. This brings the anterior peritoneum closer to the surgeon and thereby facilitates its closure.

Closure of the vaginal cuff should accomplish two things: resuspension of the vaginal apex and closure of the cul-de-sac (Fig. 17H). A suture is placed through the vaginal cuff and through the ends of the suspensory ligaments to reattach them to the vagina. Next, the cul-de-sac may be reefed and a suture placed through the uterosacral ligaments to bring them to the midline. Finally, the peritoneum is closed with a purse-string suture of 0-silk placed at the highest level possible, beginning on the vesical peritoneum. A finger is placed in the peritoneum while this suture is tied to avoid trapping intraabdominal contents in the suture, and it is removed as the suture is snugged down.

Anterior Colporrhaphy

After the uterus has been removed and before the ligaments are reattached to the vaginal cuff, an anterior colporrhaphy is performed in patients with cystocele (Fig. 18). Scissors are used to undermine the mucosa of the anterior vaginal wall as far as the midurethra, and this is incised (Fig. 18A). The vaginal fascia is then mobilized widely from the vaginal mucosa

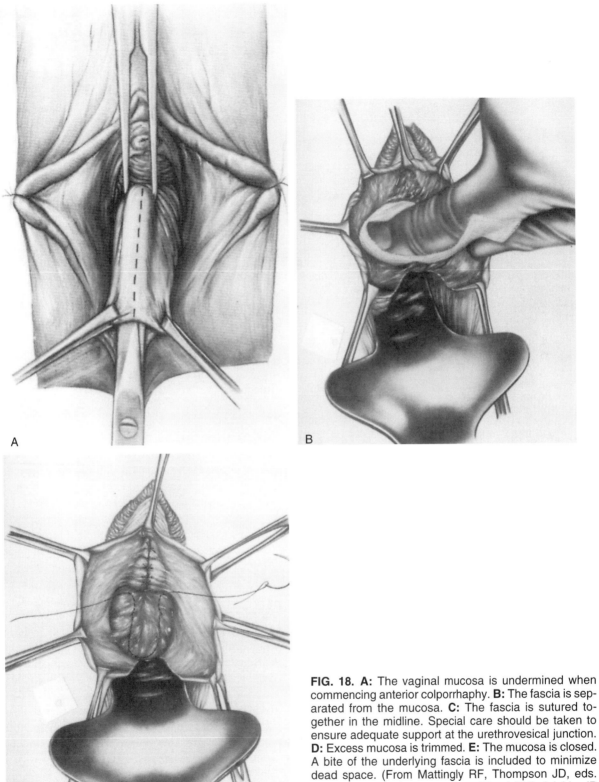

FIG. 18. A: The vaginal mucosa is undermined when commencing anterior colporrhaphy. **B:** The fascia is separated from the mucosa. **C:** The fascia is sutured together in the midline. Special care should be taken to ensure adequate support at the urethrovesical junction. **D:** Excess mucosa is trimmed. **E:** The mucosa is closed. A bite of the underlying fascia is included to minimize dead space. (From Mattingly RF, Thompson JD, eds. *TeLinde's operative gynecology*, 6th ed. Philadelphia: JB Lippincott Co, 1985:612; with permission.)

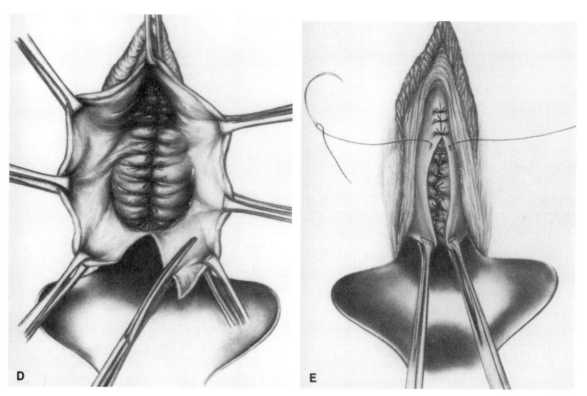

FIG. 18. (*Continued*)

with use of a combination of sharp and blunt dissection until the superior lateral sulcus of the vagina is reached (Fig. 18B). Care should be taken to remain superficial in this dissection to avoid transecting the fascia that is to be plicated in the midline. Special attention should be given to adequately developing the fascia that lies under the urethrovesical junction, because this is critical to improving urethral support. Once mobilization has been accomplished, a series of plication sutures are taken in the fascia, just medial to the junction of the anterior and lateral vaginal walls (Fig. 18C).

Plication of the suburethral fascia deserves special attention. Once the first suburethral suture has been placed and tied, it pulls some of the more lateral fascia into view, and this offers an opportunity to place a second suture in this same region and improve the elevation that was possible with the first suture. Once the remainder of the fascia has been closed, the cranial edge of the fascia at the vaginal apex should be tagged so that it may be included in the sutures that reattach it to the cardinal and uterosacral ligaments, because these will help elevate the upper margin of the fascia and pull it higher in the pelvis. An appropriate amount of vaginal mucosa is then trimmed (Fig. 18D), and the mucosa is closed with running or interrupted sutures (Fig. 18E).

Posterior Colpoperineorrhaphy

Next, any rectocele that is present must be corrected. Although often undertaken at the end of a tiring operation, this repair requires the most skill and judgment of all phases of surgery for prolapse. Overcorrection of the posterior wall may leave the patient unable to have satisfying intercourse, yet a failure to reinforce the supportive position of the posterior vaginal wall may increase the likelihood that prolapse will recur. The goal of this portion of the operation is to reinforce the rectovaginal septum and to return the size of the introitus to normal.

The posterior colporrhaphy is begun by determining the size that the introitus should be at the end of the procedure. This is done by estimating the amount of vaginal mucosa that must be removed to return the introitus to a normal diameter. Allis forceps are placed to grasp a solid bite of tissue at the hymenal ring bilaterally at the margins of the mucosa that is to be excised. These forceps are then approximated in the midline to bring the soon-to-be-united parts of the introitus together. This allows a preview of the degree to which the introitus will be narrowed. Adjustments may then be made in the placement of the forceps to obtain an optimal result before an irrevocable incision is made into the perineum. Patients with a normal introitus who have a rectocele above this level need not have any tissue excised, and a vertical incision can be made in the introitus.

After the skin of the introitus is incised, the mucosa is undermined (Fig. 19A). The vagina and perineal body are fused, so dissection in the 3 cm inside the hymenal ring must be done sharply. If the rectovaginal septum is thin, placing a finger in the rectum to guide dissection will minimize the likelihood of proctotomy.

The rectovaginal space begins at the top of the perineal body and lies between the rectovaginal fascia and the rec-

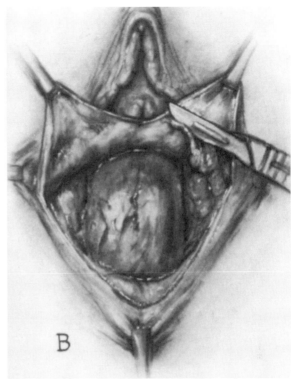

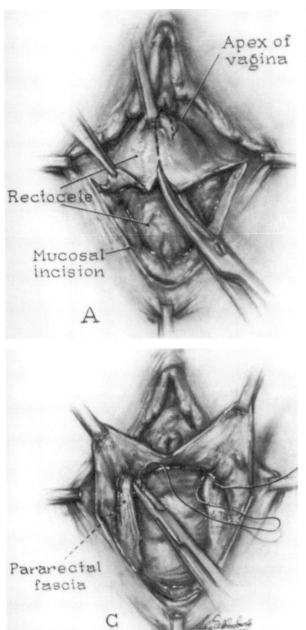

FIG. 19. A: To begin posterior colporrhaphy, a transverse incision is made in the perineal body, and a vertical incision is extended toward the vaginal apex. B: The perirectal fascia is mobilized from the mucosa. C: The perirectal fascia is sutured, beginning above the site of the rectocele. D: The inner surface of the levator ani muscles are approximated in the perineal body, and redundant mucosa is excised. E: The mucosa and perineal skin are closed. (From Mattingly RF, Thompson JD, eds. *TeLinde's operative gynecology*, 6th ed. Philadelphia: JB Lippincott Co, 1985:578; with permission.)

tum. It is a loose areolar plane and dissects easily. Once it is entered, it should be developed laterally (Fig. 19B) until the inferior lateral sulcus of the vagina has been reached and the inner surfaces of the levator ani muscles can be felt. The upper limit of the dissection depends on the location of the rectocele and should extend at least to a point several centimeters above the upper limit of the bulge. When a posterior repair is used in a patient who previously had a hysterectomy, the upper vaginal dissection should include a search for an enterocele.

Once the rectovaginal space has been adequately developed, the repair may begin. With a finger depressing the rectum, the connective tissue lateral to the rectum is grasped with

a needle and elevated, and the needle is retrieved (Fig. 19C). A similar bite of the endopelvic fascia on the contralateral side is then taken. Successive sutures are then placed from that point to the introitus. After this is complete, it is prudent to make sure that no ridge has formed. If it has, the offending suture should be removed and replaced to avoid distortion. After this first layer has been placed, the space between the levator ani muscles may be narrowed by suturing their fascial covering, and the perineal body can be reconstructed (Fig. 19D). This requires a second layer of sutures in the distal 3 cm of the vagina. After these sutures are placed, usually one final stitch may be placed at the level of the hymenal ring to establish the triangular nature of the perineal body when seen

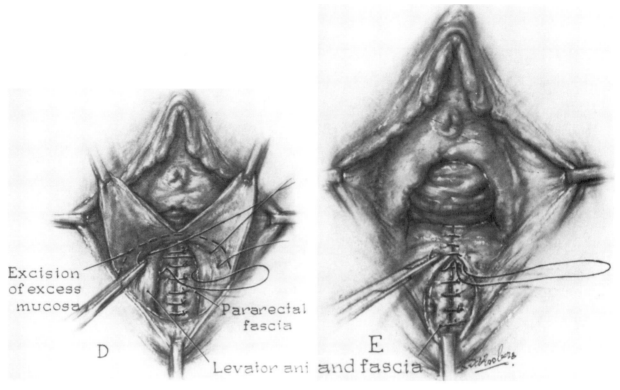

FIG. 19. (*Continued*)

in sagittal section. Finally, an appropriate amount of vaginal mucosa is trimmed, and the vaginal edges are reapproximated with interrupted or running absorbable sutures (Fig. 19E).

When the operation is complete, the adequacy of the vagina for intercourse should be assessed. Despite precautions to avoid stenosis of the vagina, it is sometimes noted after the repair is complete. If so, relaxing incisions may be made in the vaginal wall to relieve the stricture, or part of the repair may be taken down and resutured. Time rarely improves a bad initial repair, and correction in the operating room is far superior to taking the patient back to the operating room later for revision of the vagina.

Le Fort Partial Colpocleisis

In elderly patients with prolapse who will no longer be engaging in intercourse, a colpocleisis may be used to cure the prolapse. This operation carries less operative and postoperative morbidity and may be performed under local anesthesia in the rare patient whose medical condition puts her at too great a risk to have a regional anesthetic. It consists of denuding a rectangle of vagina anteriorly and posteriorly and sewing these together (Fig. 20). This prevents the uterus and vagina from prolapsing downward. An adjunctive high perineorrhaphy at the time of the colpocleisis forms a shelf for the repair to rest on so as to lessen the likelihood of prolapse reoccurring. Channels are left below the cervix and lateral to the closure to provide egress of cervical secretions and blood, should postmenopausal bleeding occur. Because the uterus is not removed and access to the cervix is blocked, care should

be exercised in the preoperative evaluation to make sure that endometrial carcinoma is not present or likely to develop.

Stress incontinence may follow colpocleisis if there is poor urethral support associated with the prolapse. In this instance, steps should be taken during the operation to improve this situation. Preoperatively, occult stress incontinence may be detected by examining the patient with a full bladder and having her cough with the prolapse reduced. If stress incontinence is elicited, steps must be taken to improve urethral support by plicating the endopelvic fascia under the urethra or using a needle bladder neck suspension.

Vaginal Repair of the Posthysterectomy Enterocele

The description earlier in this chapter concerning care of an enterocele and the cul-de-sac involves management of an enterocele encountered with the uterus *in situ* during vaginal hysterectomy. Because enterocele after hysterectomy is a significant problem in its own right,[29] it will be considered separately here. Certain special features of enterocele, such as its occurrence after high retropubic urethral suspension,[30] warrant its special consideration. Repair of an enterocele should not only obliterate the cul-de-sac but also pull the vagina over the rectum by shortening the ligamentous suspension of the vagina so that the normal closure of this space may be maintained. In addition, if the vaginal wall has been stretched because of its protrusion below the pelvic floor, the excess vaginal wall must be excised. Although transabdominal enterocele repairs (e.g., Moschcowitz, Halban) are useful as prophylaxis at the time of abdominal repair, an enterocele that presents

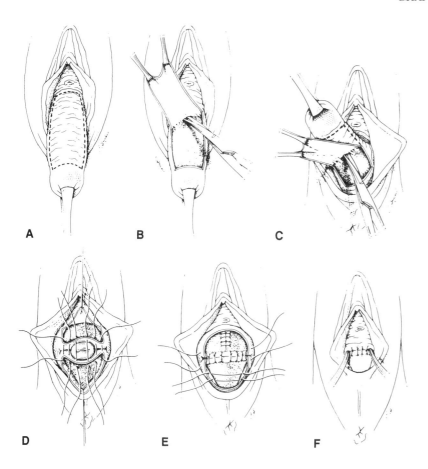

FIG. 20. A–C: In Le Fort colpocleisis, rectangles of vaginal mucosa are removed from the anterior and posterior vaginal walls. **D,E:** The denuded areas are then sutured together, leaving **(F)** channels on each side open. (From Mattingly RF, Thompson JD, eds. *TeLinde's operative gynecology*, 6th ed. Philadelphia: JB Lippincott Co, 1985:562; with permission.)

after hysterectomy can almost always be repaired vaginally. This is the preferred method because it avoids the morbidity of an abdominal incision and is much easier to perform.

The vaginal wall is opened over the enterocele sac. If a concomitant rectocele is present, this may be done by extending the incision made for the posterior repair up to the apex of the vagina. If a pure enterocele is present, the incision is made directly over the enterocele. In instances where the prolapsed vaginal wall has become stretched, a diamond-shaped incision may be made to excise the excess vaginal skin (Fig. 21A). Once identified, the peritoneum is separated from the vaginal wall (Fig. 21B). Once this has been done, the excess peritoneum is excised. Next, the remnants of the uterosacral ligaments are brought together under the peritoneum and attached to the vaginal apex to improve its support (Fig. 21C). At that point, any excess vaginal wall is trimmed, a posterior repair performed if needed, and the vaginal incision closed. Most enterocele repairs should be accompanied by a posterior colpoperineorrhaphy.

Posthysterectomy Prolapse

Prolapse subsequent to hysterectomy deserves special consideration. One-third to one-half of women will have had a hysterectomy by the age of 65, so prolapse in older women will often occur in the absence of a uterus. Although it might appear that these individuals would have only a cystocele or rectocele, because there could be no uterine pro-

lapse, prolapse of the vaginal apex is often present and must be recognized; otherwise, repair of a cystocele or a rectocele in the presence of prolapse of the vaginal apex is doomed to failure.

When the apex of the vagina, marked by the scar at the former location of the cervix, prolapses downward below the hymenal ring, vaginal prolapse is present. This is usually accompanied by an enterocele and is often seen in combination with a cystocele or a rectocele. To cure these patients, the apex of the vagina must be returned to and held in its normal position in the pelvis, and the cystocele or rectocele must be repaired. This may be accomplished by suturing the vaginal apex to the sacrospinous ligament[19,31] (Fig. 22A) or to the sacrum using an interposing graft in an operation known as abdominal sacral colpopexy[32] (Fig. 22B). Each of these operations is accompanied by repair of the enterocele and whatever other prolapse must be addressed. In women who are no longer interested in preserving coital function, a complete colpocleisis obliterates the vagina and prevents prolapse from occurring, and this provides an easy, safe, and effective technique to relieve the symptoms of prolapse.

Paravaginal Repair

When a cystourethrocele persists or returns soon after anterior colporrhaphy, this often means that the loss of anterior vaginal wall support is due to a paravaginal separation of the pubocervical fascia from its normal lateral attachment to the

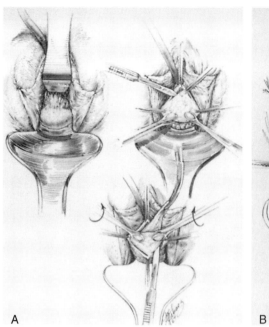

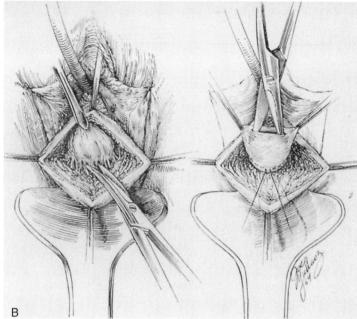

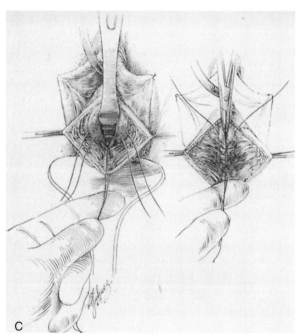

FIG. 21. A: The enterocele is exposed, and a diamond-shaped piece of vaginal wall is excised to reduce the size of the stretched upper vagina. **B:** The peritoneum is dissected from the surrounding structures, and it is dosed with a purse-string suture. **C:** The uterosacral ligaments are defined by creating opposing traction with a retractor and suture to complete repair, after which the vaginal wall is closed. (From ref. 35; with permission.)

arcus tendineus rather than to a midline defect in the fascia. In this instance, repeating the anterior colporrhaphy will not be effective, and repair of the separation will be required. Although the paravaginal repair is usually described as an operation to treat stress incontinence associated with cystourethrocele,[33] it is also helpful in treating cystourethrocele in the absence of stress urinary incontinence, especially when an anterior colporrhaphy has failed. This retropubic operation reattaches the lateral margin of the pubocervical fascia to the pelvic side wall along a line from the undersurface of the pubic symphysis to the ischial spine, along the line of the arcus tendineus. This reestablishes the normal lateral attachments of the pubocervical fascia and therefore prevents downward displacement of the bladder. It has not yet been established as a necessary procedure in the primary treatment of cystourethrocele without stress incontinence, but in instances of recurrent cystocele after anterior repair, simply repeating an operation that has not helped the patient is not desirable.

Conservative Measures

Vaginal pessaries are perhaps the oldest effective treatment for prolapse.[34] Named after an oval stone (i.e., a pessos) used in certain Greek games, innumerable natural and man-made materials have been used to make pessaries. These ob-

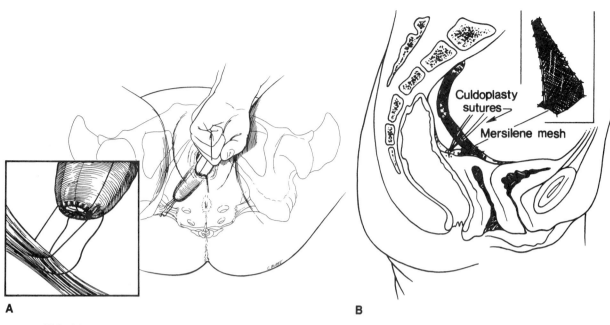

FIG. 22. A: The vagina is fixed to the sacrospinous ligament. (From ref. 19, with permission.) **B:** The vaginal apex is attached to the sacrum with an intervening graft. (From ref. 36; with permission.)

jects are placed in the vagina. Because they are larger than the introitus, they are retained in the vagina above the pelvic floor musculature and thereby prevent the somewhat smaller uterine cervix from passing through the opening. When the pelvic muscles are relatively normal, these devices work well. When the pelvic floor opening is enlarged because of damage to the levator ani, a pessary may not be able to be retained.

There are countless varieties of pessaries. The ones most commonly used for prolapse are the doughnut-shaped pessaries, either permanently inflated or inflatable. The largest pessary that the vagina will accommodate without undue pressure on the vaginal walls is inserted. Often, patients can be taught how to place and remove them. Having the patient remove the pessary at night minimizes the discharge inevitably associated with its use. Adjunctive treatment with topical or systemic estrogen helps the vaginal mucosa tolerate the foreign body. Because pessaries may erode and cause ulceration, they should be checked periodically, and if an ulcer is developing, the pessary should be discontinued or a smaller one fitted, and the ulcer should be monitored until it heals.[35,36]

◊ REFERENCES

1. Bonney V. The principles that should underlie all operations for prolapse. *J Obstet Gynecol Br Emp* 1934;41:669.
2. Olsen AL, Smith VJ, Bergstrom JO, Colling JC, Clark AL. Epidemiology of surgically managed pelvic organ prolapse and urinary incontinence. *Obstet Gynecol* 1997;89:501.
3. Timonen S, Nuoranne E, Meyer B. Genital prolapse: etiological factors. *Ann Chir Gynaecol Fenn* 1968;57:363.
4. Range RL, Woodburne RT. The gross and microscopic anatomy of the transverse cervical ligaments. *Am J Obstet Gynecol* 1964;90:460.
5. Campbell RM. The anatomy and histology of the sacrouterine ligaments. *Am J Obstet Gynecol* 1950;59:1.
6. DeLancey JOL. Anatomic aspects of vaginal eversion after hysterectomy. *Am J Obstet Gynecol* 1992;166:1717.
7. Parks AG, Porter NH, Melzak J. Experimental study of the reflex mechanism controlling muscles of the pelvic floor. *Dis Colon Rectum* 1962;5:407.
8. McGuire EJ. Urodynamic findings in patients after failure of stress incontinence operations. *Prog Clin Biol Res* 1981;78:351.
9. DeLancey JOL. Structural aspects of the extrinsic continence mechanism. *Obstet Gynecol* 1988;72:296.
10. Smith ARB, Hosker GL, Warrell DW. The role of pudendal nerve damage in the aetiology of genuine stress incontinence in women. *Br J Obstet Gynaecol* 1989;96:29.
11. Allen RE, Hosker GL, Smith ARB, Warrell DW. Pelvic floor damage and childbirth: a neurophysiological study. *Br J Obstet Gynaecol* 1990;97:770.
12. Richardson AC, Lyons JB, Williams NL. A new look at pelvic relaxation. *Am J Obstet Gynecol* 1976;126:568.
13. Krantz KE. The anatomy of the urethra and anterior vaginal wall. *Am J Obstet Gynecol* 1951;62:374.
14. Bartscht KD, DeLancey JOL. A technique to study cervical descent. *Obstet Gynecol* 1988;72:940.
15. Jeffcoate TNA. Posterior colporrhaphy. *Am J Obstet Gynecol* 1959;77:490.
16. Arnold MW, Stewart WR, Aguillar PS. Rectocele repair: four years' experience. *Dis Colon Rectum* 1990;33:684.
17. Nichols DH, Randall CL. *Vaginal surgery*, 2nd ed. Baltimore: Williams & Wilkins, 1983.
18. Kuhn RJP, Hollyock VE. Observations on the anatomy of the rectovaginal pouch and septum. *Obstet Gynecol* 1982;59:445.
19. Morley GW, DeLancey JOL. Sacrospinous ligament fixation for eversion of the vagina. *Am J Obstet Gynecol* 1988;158:872.
20. Bump RC, Mattiasson A, Bo K, et al. The standardization of terminology of female pelvic organ prolapse and pelvic floor dysfunction. *Am J Obstet Gynecol* 1996;175:10.
21. Viereck V, Peschers U, Singer M, Schuessler B. Metrische Quantifizierung des weiblichen Genitalprolapses: eine sinnvolle Neuerung in der Prolapsdiagnostik? *Geburtshilfe Frauenheilk* 1997;57:177.
22. DeLancey JOL, Hurd WW. Size of the urogenital hiatus in the levator ani muscles in normal women and women with pelvic organ prolapse. *Obstet Gynecol* 1998;91:364.

23. Gardy M, Kosminski M, McGuire EJ, Elkins TE, DeLancey JOL. Stress incontinence and cystoceles. *J Urol* 1991;145:1211.

24. Hemsell DL, Johnson ER, Hemsell PG, Nobles BJ, Heard MC. Cefazolin for hysterectomy prophylaxis. *Obstet Gynecol* 1990;76:603.

25. Heaney NS. Report of 565 vaginal hysterectomies performed for benign pelvic disease. *Am J Obstet Gynecol* 1934;28:751.

26. Heaney NS. Vaginal hysterectomy: its indications and technique. *Am J Surg* 1940;48:284.

27. England GT, Randall HW, Graves WL. Impairment of tissue defenses by vasoconstrictors in vaginal hysterectomies. *Obstet Gynecol* 1983;61:271.

28. Sheth SS. The place of oophorectomy at vaginal hysterectomy. *Br J Obstet Gynaecol* 1991;98:662.

29. Symmonds RE, Williams TJ, Lee RA, Webb MJ. Post-hysterectomy enterocele and vaginal vault prolapse. *Am J Obstet Gynecol* 1981;140:852.

30. Burch JC. Cooper's ligament urethroversical suspension for stress incontinence. *Am J Obstet Gynecol* 1968;100:764.

31. Nichols DH. Sacrospinous fixation for massive eversion of the vagina. *Am J Obstet Gynecol* 1982;142:901.

32. Addison WA, Livengood CH, Sutton GP, Parker RT. Abdominal sacral colpopexy with Mersilene mesh in the retroperitoneal position in the management of posthysterectomy vaginal vault prolapse and enterocele. *Am J Obstet Gynecol* 1985;153:140.

33. Richardson AC, Edmonds PB, Williams NL. Treatment of stress urinary incontinence due to paravaginal fascial defect. *Obstet Gynecol* 1981; 57:357.

34. Emge LA, Durfee RB. Pelvic organ prolapse: four thousand years of treatment. *Clin Obstet Gynecol* 1966;9:997.

35. Segala CJ. New technique for the repair of vaginal vault prolapse following hysterectomy. *Int Surg* 1969;51:36.

36. Addison WA, Timmons MC, Wall LL, Livengood CH. Failed abdominal sacral colpopexy: observations and recommendations. *Obstet Gynecol* 1989;74:480.

CHAPTER 46

Endoscopic Surgery

———— ◇ ————

Howard T. Sharp

Gynecologic endoscopy involves the use of a small telescope to view the peritoneal cavity (laparoscopy) and endometrial cavity (hysteroscopy). These techniques have evolved from being used primarily for diagnostic purposes into sophisticated systems for performing major surgery. The goal of endoscopic surgery is to provide excellent patient outcomes with reduced hospital stay, quicker recovery time, and lower cost. This concept has led to the descriptive term "minimally invasive surgery." Though clear benefit has been shown with some endoscopic procedures, data are still lacking in other areas in terms of cost effectiveness and long-term outcomes.

◇ LAPAROSCOPY

To perform safe and effective laparoscopy, the surgeon should be adequately trained in laparoscopic surgical techniques, including knowledge and experience with laparoscopic instrumentation for proper tissue manipulation and an understanding of the energy sources for dividing tissue and achieving hemostasis.

Instrumentation for Operative Laparoscopy

Because of the many specialized instruments needed for operative laparoscopy, a basic laparoscopy tray with a relatively small number of commonly used laparoscopic and nonlaparoscopic instruments is useful to avoid confusion. The basic laparoscopic components consist of a laparoscope, insufflation unit, video unit, light source, trocars, and laparoscopic forceps, scissors, needle drivers, irrigator-aspirator, staplers, vascular clips, and uterine manipulator. Nonlaparoscopic instruments include those used for making trocar incisions (scalpel), aiding with the specimen removal (Kocher clamps), and closing trocar incisions ("S" retractors, needle driver, scissors). Less commonly used instruments should be kept in a designated area where they are accessible. This instrumentation should be managed by a dedicated operating room team.

Laparoscopes

The laparoscope is a 2- to 11-mm rigid telescope containing fiberoptic light bundles, which transmit light from a light source to the peritoneal cavity (Fig. 1). It may have an operative channel through which instruments may be passed, such as a laser fiber for tissue cutting or desiccation or bipolar forceps for tubal cautery.

Insufflation Unit

The insufflation unit provides delivery of CO_2 for creation of a phisoperitoneum for optimal visualization. As carbon dioxide flows into the peritoneal cavity, parameters may be set to control the flow rate and pressure.

Video Unit

Though a video unit is not absolutely necessary to perform laparoscopy, it allows the surgeon to stand upright instead of bending over to look through the laparoscope. Additionally, it allows the assistant and other operating room personnel to see the operating field. The video camera attaches to the eyepiece of the laparoscope and is equipped with a focus or autofocus mechanism to adjust for various focal lengths. The image captured by the camera is transmitted and processed by a video recorder and is displayed on a video monitor.

Light Source

A light source is necessary to transmit light into the peritoneal cavity. A xenon light source is commonly used and is considered a "cool" light source. This is not to say that the end of the light cord can not be very hot but merely that the light is transmitted through fiberoptic cables. The end of the light cord should not be allowed to come in contact with the surgical drapes or the patient because of the potential to cause skin burns.

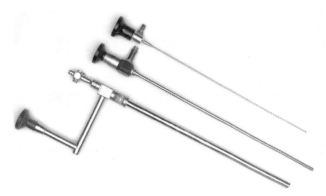

FIG. 1. Three different size of endoscopes used in laparoscopy: 2 mm **(top)**, 5 mm **(middle)**, and 10 mm **(bottom)**. The 10-mm laparoscope has an operating channel and an offset eyepiece.

Trocars

Trocars may be made of steel and be reusable or may be plastic disposable models (Fig. 2). The more frequently used trocars are between 2 and 12 mm. Trocars typically have an inner sharp trocar and an outer sheath. The trocar tip may be conical, pyramidal, or may consist of a more complicated retracting razor blade as in the disposable trocars.

Operating Instruments

There are several types of tissue graspers available. Graspers with atraumatic ends may be used on delicate structures such as bowel and fallopian tubes, whereas traumatic graspers are

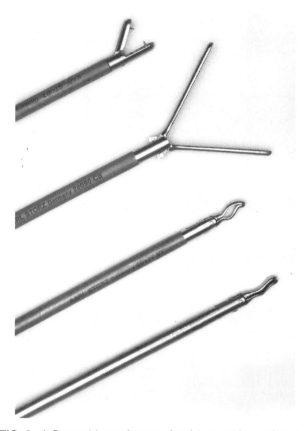

FIG. 3. A Semm biopsy forceps **(top)** is used for performing tissue biopsy and delicate dissection. The bowel grasper **(second from top)** is used to grasp bowel atraumatically. The fallopian tube forceps **(second from bottom)** is used for atraumatic handling of the fallopian tube, and the atraumatic grasp **(bottom)** is used to atraumatically handle a variety of tissues (Karl Storz, Culver City, CA).

typically used for tissue removal and biopsy (Fig. 3). Endoscopic scissors may be used to cut mechanically as well as electrosurgically (Fig. 4). Needle drivers and knot pushers are available for intracorporeal and extracorporeal suturing.

Irrigator-Aspirator

Fluid may be pumped into or aspirated from the pelvis with an irrigator-aspirator. These systems range from a simple cannula with an attached syringe to highly efficient motorized systems for rapid, high-pressure fluid flow.

Staplers

In 1990, a laparoscopic stapling device called the Endo-GIA (gastrointestinal anastamosis) was introduced for securing and dividing tissue (Fig. 5). When the jaws of the instrument are closed over tissue and the grip is squeezed, six staggered rows of staples 3 cm in length are placed, and a knife blade simultaneously divides the tissue leaving three rows of staples on each side of the incision.

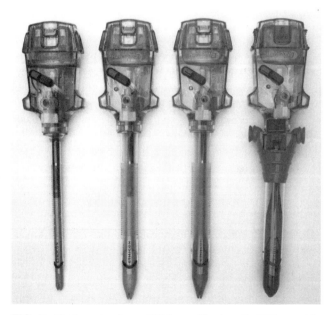

FIG. 2. Various trochars (Ethicon, Cincinnati, OH) used in laparoscopy: 5, 11, and 12 mm trochars and a 12-mm trochar used for open laparoscopy **(from left to right).**

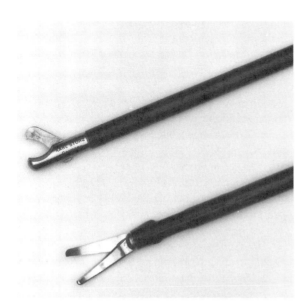

FIG. 4. Reusable endoscopic scissors (Karl Storz, Culver City, CA) may be used **(top)** as well as disposable scissors (Ethicon, Cincinnati, OH) **(bottom)**.

Vascular Clips

Endoscopic vascular clips may be used to achieve hemostasis of bleeding vessels (Fig. 5). These offer the advantage of being used near vital structures where the use of cautery would otherwise result in lateral thermal damage. They are particularly useful on oozing endo-GIA pedicles.

Uterine Manipulators

There are a number of uterine manipulators that may be placed within the uterus or cervix to gain better access to the pelvis by uterine manipulation anteriorly, posteriorly, or laterally. Many of these also offer the ability to perform chromotubation for documentation of fallopian tube patency.

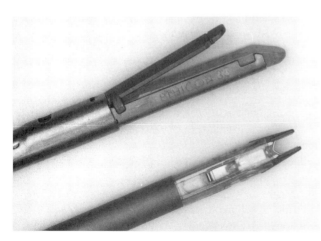

FIG. 5. The Endo-GIA for securing and dividing tissue is shown on **top**, and the Endoclip for achieving hemostasis is shown **below** (Ethicon, Cincinnati, OH).

Laparoscopic Energy Sources

The term "pelviscopy" was originally coined to refer the use of mechanical energy such as suture ligation for securing large tissue pedicles and obtaining hemostasis while completely avoiding the use of electrical energy. This was prompted in part by a number of severe electrical injuries that occurred in patients undergoing monopolar electrosurgical tubal sterilization. With improved technology, a number of energy modalities are available for use in endoscopic surgery.

Endomechanical Energy

The simplest laparoscopic ligature to apply is the Roeder loop, which was modified by Semm for laparoscopic use. This is available as a pretied slip knot on a push rod that is used to push a suture loop around a tissue pedicle for hemostasis (Fig. 6). Laparoscopic suturing can be used to close raw peritoneal surfaces, repair uterine incisions from myomectomy, repair damaged bowel or bladder, secure tissue pedicles at laparoscopic hysterectomy, and perform retropubic urethropexy.

Laparoscopic knots may be tied outside (extracorporeal) or within the body (intracorporeal). Extracorporeal knots may consist of multiple and single-pass knots. Multiple-pass knots are sliding square knots pushed through a trocar sleeve to the target by multiple passes of a knot pusher, which serves as the surgeon's finger. Single-pass knots are slip knots that are tied similarly to the Roeder and Fisherman's knot and then pushed through the trocar sleeve to the tissue by the single pass of a knot pusher. Intracorporeal knots are tied within the abdomen by looping the suture material around the laparoscopic needle holders using the same technique as an "instrument tie." In general, the strongest laparoscopic knots are the intracorpreal flat square knot and extracorporeal sliding square knot with multiple throws.[1] The only single-throw slip knots with knot

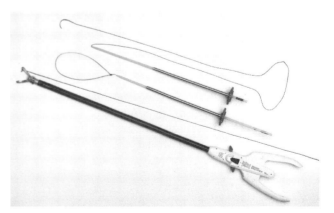

FIG. 6. The Surgiwhip **(top)** is used as a pretied method of performing extracorporeal suturing. The Endoloop **(middle)** is used to secure a tissue pedicle when no suturing is needed. The Endostitch **(bottom)** is used for suturing tissue by using a toggle switch, which obviates the need for manipulating a needle (United States Surgical Corp., Norwalk, CT).

strength similar to these knots are the 4-S knot and the Fisherman's knot.[2] These stronger knots are recommended in cases where continued tissue tension will be required, as in laparoscopic retropubic urethropexy.

Laparoscopic suturing requires considerable practice to confidently load the needle into the needle driver and place sutures accurately. To this end, the endostitch (U.S. Surgical Corp., Norwalk, CT) was developed wherein the needle is preloaded and the suture is passed through tissue up to 2 cm thick by closing a handle and a toggle switch. The endostitch is a 10-mm instrument with jaws measuring 4 mm wide and 2 cm long (Fig. 6).

Electrosurgery

Electrosurgical energy can be used to cut, desiccate, and fulgurate tissue. Many of the risks of monopolar electrical current have been eliminated by technological advances such as the isolated electrosurgical unit and return electrode monitoring (quality contact monitoring). However, the surgeon should be aware of other phenomena such as direct and capacitive coupling as well as lateral thermal conduction away from the site of the active electrode.

Capacitive coupling may allow 5% to 40% of the current flowing through an insulated conductor to be transferred or "coupled" into another conductor. The insulated active electrode of a unipolar instrument passed down the operating channel of a laparoscope can transfer up to 40% of its current into the laparoscope and cause tissue in contact with the laparoscope to sustain electrical injury. This risk can be minimized by using a metallic (conductive) trocar sleeve to provide a low-power-density pathway through the abdominal wall so that electricity may reach the return electrode without causing damage. The greatest risk of generating capacitive coupling occurs when "hybrid" trocars are used (metallic cannulas with plastic abdominal wall grips).

Bipolar forceps operate by conducting current between the jaws of the forceps, which serve as both an active and a return electrode. Hence, coupling accidents are virtually eliminated. However, lateral thermal tissue damage occurs in the tissue adjacent to the electrode. In the case of suspected small bowel injury, minilaparotomy with resection of the bowel segment in question should be considered. Because electrical damage always extends past the limits of the obvious lesion, these injuries must be resected, never oversewn. Additionally, staple lines should not be electrocoagulated because the tissue may shrink, which could result in bleeding, and the staples may conduct electricity to unrecognized pathways, causing tissue damage.

Laser

The term "laser" is an acronym for *light amplification by spontaneous emission of radiation.* Surgical lasers available for gynecologic use include CO_2, argon, potassium-titanyl-phosphate (KTP), and neodymium:yttrium-aluminum-garnet (Nd-YAG). These have the ability to vaporize, cut, and, to varying degrees, coagulate tissue. There is no need to worry about alternate ground site burns, direct or capacitive coupling, or current division and the path of least resistance, as is the case with electrosurgery.

There are advantages and disadvantages to the use of each wavelength. The CO_2 laser produces excellent vaporization of tissue and little residual thermal damage. Irrigation fluid also serves as an excellent backstop for CO_2 laser energy. For surgeons who prefer to cut tissue by contact, fiberoptic lasers can be used, such as the Nd-YAG coaxial fiber equipped with an artificial sapphire tip. Raw Nd-YAG laser energy delivered through a quartz fiber has the ability to penetrate tissue for up to 4 mm, which must be considered when working near the ureter and bowel. However, the sapphire tip limits the egress of laser energy, and tissue damage when cutting with the sapphire is usually less than 1 mm. The use of laser has diminished in recent years, mostly because of its higher cost and the improved safety of other energy sources.

Harmonic Scalpel

The harmonic scalpel (Ethicon Inc., Cincinnati, OH) uses vibration at the rate of 55,000 cycles per second as an energy source to break hydrogen bonds in tissue, resulting in cutting or coaptation of vessels. The harmonic scalpel is available as a 5- or 10-mm rounded "scalpel" or as a 10-mm "shear." This modality may result in less lateral thermal spread of energy, and there is no risk of electrical injury.

Positioning the Patient for Laparoscopic Surgery

The patient should be placed on the operating table with the buttocks at or slightly over the table's edge to allow placement and use of an intrauterine manipulator. The patient's thighs should be in the same plane as the abdomen rather than the dorsal lithotomy position, to allow freedom of motion for laparoscopic instrumentation. Stirrups should have ample padding to support the lower legs without creating any pressure points. It is preferable to use a stirrup that can be elevated without undraping the patient so that the lithotomy position can be used for easier vaginal access (O.R. Direct, Acton, MA, and Allen Medical Systems, Garfield Hills, OH).

Entering the Abdominal Cavity

The abdominal cavity may be initially entered at the umbilicus by Veress needle (Fig. 7), direct trocar insertion, or by open laparoscopy. The first two procedures are blind insertion techniques, whereas open laparoscopy is performed by making an incision approximately the size of the trocar and entering the abdominal cavity directly using a scalpel. This is often used if subumbilical adhesions are known or suspected.

When the Veress needle is to be used, an initial skin incision is made at the umbilicus. The umbilicus should be elevated, and the knife blade held parallel to the long axis of the patient, to avoid incising the great vessels inadvertently.

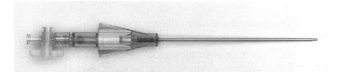

FIG. 7. Veress needle (Ethicon, Cincinnati, OH).

Having the anesthesiologist decompress the stomach with a nasogastric tube will decrease the risk of accidentally inserting the Veress needle or trocar into an overdistended stomach. The patient's abdomen should be completely relaxed to allow adequate elevation for Veress needle or trocar insertion. The patient should also be positioned flat on the table because if Trendelenburg positioning is used initially, the needle may be directed closer to the great vessels rather than the pelvic cavity. In the thin patient, the needle or trocar should be directed at a 45° angle from vertical to avoid the great vessels. In the obese patient, the aorta is typically above the level of the umbilicus, and therefore, the Veress needle or trocar may be inserted directly vertically, 90° to the long axis of the patient, as long as the abdominal wall has been elevated adequately.[3] If the Veress needle is inserted correctly into the abdominal cavity rather than the preperitoneal space, lifting up on the anterior abdominal wall should produce a negative pressure reading on the insufflator. When low-flow insufflation is performed (flow rate approximately 1 liter/min), the intraabdominal pressure should be less than 8 mm Hg. If the "intraabdominal" pressure reading is higher than 8 mm Hg, the probability of extraperitoneal insufflation is high, and the approach should be reassessed.

Alternative sites for insufflation may also be utilized. These include left anterior axillary line of the left upper quadrant, posterior cul-de-sac, superior aspect of the umbilicus, and midway between the umbilicus and symphysis pubis.

Secondary Trocar Placement

One or two secondary ports are usually adequate for most laparoscopic procedures. These may be placed lateral to the inferior epigastric artery or in the midline above the bladder. The size and number of trocars will depend on the procedure and equipment to be used. A 2- to 5-mm trocar may be used for diagnostic laparoscopy to maneuver pelvic organs for adequate visualization. Most instruments will fit through a 5-mm port. In the case of advanced operative laparoscopy, if an Endo-GIA is to be used, a 12-mm trocar must be placed. Insertion of a 22-gauge needle through the anterior abdominal wall at the intended site of the trocar can assist in determining a safe path away from the inferior epigastric artery. Secondary trocars should be inserted in a controlled fashion, under direct vision.

Tissue Removal

Small tissue fragments may be removed through 5-mm trocar sleeves, whereas large, dense specimens such as myomas can be time consuming to remove. Fluid-filled specimens such as ovarian cysts may be placed in a plastic specimen removal bag and drained while in the bag to avoid spillage (Endocatch, U.S. Surgical Corp., Norwalk, CT, and Endopouch II, Ethicon Inc, Cincinnati, OH) (Fig. 8). The cul-de-sac offers a large site for specimen removal. Posterior colpotomy may be performed vaginally or laparoscopically. If the laparoscopic approach is performed, a lubricated sponge stick is placed in the posterior fornix for cul-de-sac elevation, and an incision is made between the uterosacral ligaments into the vagina on top of the sponge by using laser, unipolar scissors, or harmonic scalpel. Alternatively, morcellation may be performed with a hand-held morcellator or an electromechanical morcellator (Karl Storz, Culver City, CA). In general, morcellation should not be performed with unipolar cautery if the specimen has been disconnected from the pelvis because the specimen is "grounded" only when it touches other tissue.

Laparoscopic Management of the Adnexal Mass

The role of laparoscopy in the evaluation and treatment of the adnexal mass remains controversial. The problem lies in determining preoperatively which masses are most likely to be benign, recognizing and treating malignancy intraoperatively, and knowing the effect of intraoperative spill of malignant tumor on prognosis. The preoperative evaluation of the adnexal mass cannot guarantee the exclusion of malignancy. However, in the vast majority of cases, strong suspicion should exist if the proper workup has been completed. If malignancy is found, the surgeon should be ready to perform the proper surgical staging procedures.

The effect of intraoperative rupture of ovarian neoplasms on prognosis is an unsettled issue. In 1973, Webb et al. reported a poorer prognosis after tumor spill.[4] However, with the use of multivariate analysis, newer data do not confirm this finding. Dembo et al. studied 519 patients with stage I epithelial ovarian cancer and found that the only factors influencing relapse rate were tumor grade, the presence of

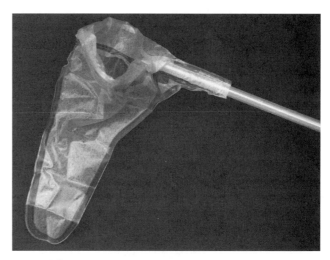

FIG. 8. Endopouch II (Ethicon, Cincinnati, OH).

dense adhesions, and large-volume ascites.[5] Intraoperative rupture was not found to have a negative prognostic effect. Sainz de la Cuesta et al. reported a poorer prognosis in patients with intraoperative rupture but acknowledged that the difference in survival did not reach statistical significance.[6]

When laparoscopy is performed for evaluation of an adnexal mass, peritoneal washings should be obtained with the use of an irrigator-aspirator. The pelvis and upper abdomen should be inspected for any sign of metastasis, and both ovaries should be examined for surface abnormalities. The goal of laparoscopy is to rule out cancer and treat benign adnexal pathology in an appropriate manner. Immediate laparotomy is indicated if cancer is encountered. If there is no obvious sign of malignancy on inspection, a tissue diagnosis is still necessary to rule out cancer. A frozen section should be sent on any specimen that is not clearly benign on gross inspection.

Technique of Salpingo-oophorectomy

Techniques for adnexal removal include the use of loop ligatures, sutures, bipolar and unipolar electrocautery, and staples. The ureter should be identified, and this is usually easily accomplished by looking near the bifurcation of the common iliac artery. If it can not be visualized directly, it may be dissected out, or a ureteral stent may be placed cystoscopically. Whether the infundibulopelvic ligament is taken with bipolar electrocautery or a stapler, it should be put on stretch in order to move it away from the ureter and pelvic side wall. If a stapling device is used, one or two applications will carry the dissection to the suspensory ligament of the ovary, and a single endo-GIA or coagulation with the bipolar forceps will suffice to complete the operation.

Ovarian Cyst Aspiration with Cystectomy

Ovarian cyst aspiration with subsequent cystectomy has been performed successfully in postmenopausal patients with low-risk preoperative findings. However, salpingo-oophorectomy may be a better procedure in this population. Because ovarian function has ceased, malignancy must be excluded. In the reproductive-aged patient, ovarian cystectomy is usually preferred to preserve ovarian function. Most benign ovarian cysts are relatively easy to remove from surrounding normal ovarian tissue having a good plane of cleavage.

Very large cysts may be difficult to remove laparoscopically, and as size increases above 10 cm, the operator must carefully consider the advisability of laparoscopy. To perform cyst aspiration and subsequent ovarian cystectomy, the ovary should be mobile. If the cyst is to be aspirated first, a 20-gauge spinal needle may be passed through the abdominal wall, or a 5-mm needle cannula may be used through a laparoscopic port. After aspiration, an incision is made over the cyst down to its capsule. The edges of the cyst wall and ovary are grasped with stout grasping forceps. Traction and countertraction are used to separate the ovarian cyst from the ovary. The specimen is then removed by one of the methods

outlined in the section on tissue removal. If there is reasonable coaptation of the raw ovarian surfaces, no suturing is necessary. If there is gross discrepancy, and in the operator's opinion the ovary must be repaired, 6-0 absorbable suture may be used to join stroma together. Avoiding cortical suturing may decrease the likelihood of adhesion formation.

Laparoscopically Assisted Vaginal Hysterectomy

The laparoscopically assisted vaginal hysterectomy (LAVH) is intended to convert an abdominal hysterectomy into a vaginal procedure, thus offering the advantage of a less invasive approach in a patient who would otherwise be a candidate for abdominal hysterectomy. The need to perform additional surgery in the abdominal cavity such as adhesiolysis, removal of endometriosis, or evaluation and removal of an adnexal mass are some of the reasons to perform LAVH. Although removal of the ovaries can usually be performed vaginally, the use of the laparoscope may be helpful in some cases. If vaginal hysterectomy can be performed in the absence of an indication for abdominal hysterectomy, this is the route of choice with no laparoscopic assistance. In a randomized trial, Summitt et al. demonstrated that LAVH provides no benefit over vaginal hysterectomy in terms of recovery and is significantly more expensive.[7] Vaginal hysterectomy and LAVH are associated with a shorter recovery time than is abdominal hysterectomy.[8] Though studies have shown benefits in terms of quicker discharge from the hospital and time to recover with LAVH compared with abdominal hysterectomy, in-hospital charges associated with LAVH usually result in higher total costs, mostly because of additional expensive instrumentation.[9]

There are several variations in the LAVH technique. These range from simply inspecting the peritoneal cavity and then performing a vaginal hysterectomy to performing a total laparoscopic hysterectomy without a vaginal approach. Most commonly, the laparoscope is used to assist removing the adnexa or disconnecting the upper portion of the uterus to the level just above or below the uterine artery.

When endo-GIA staples are used, two 12-mm lateral ports are placed in addition to the umbilical port. If the ovaries are to be removed, the ureter is first identified retroperitoneally, or it may be dissected out. The endo-GIA is then placed across the infundibulopelvic ligament. Both sides of the endo-GIA should be inspected before the staple is "fired" to be sure there are no vital structures involved. Additional endo-GIA loads may be used until the level of the uterine artery is reached. Avoiding the uterine artery is advised because the endo-GIA is 1 cm wide. In some cases this is the approximate distance from the uterine artery to the ureter, and the endo-GIA staple line is not always hemostatic and may require addition of vascular clips near the ureter. The bladder peritoneum may be taken down with laparoscopic scissors. The patient's position then is changed to the dorsal lithotomy position for the vaginal portion. At the end of the procedure, the pelvic cavity should be inspected to ensure hemostasis. Last, the 12-mm lateral ports are closed at the level of the fascia to avoid hernia complications.

Pelvic Pain and the Role of Laparoscopy

Pelvic pain is the most commonly reported indication for laparoscopy. Pent found pathology in only 53% of chronic pelvic pain patients, and Lundberg et al. found pathology 60% of the time.[10,11] In a 1993 review, Howard examined the role of laparoscopy in the diagnosis and treatment of chronic pelvic pain. He found that in spite of its frequent use, fewer than 50% of patients improved after laparoscopy.[12] Clearly, the laparoscope has not solved the problem of diagnosing and treating chronic pelvic pain.

Endometriosis

Although endometriosis has been described as blue-black "powder burn" spots, it also may appear as black, white, red, yellow-brown, and clear lesions.[13] To optimally visualize these lesions, two or more abdominal ports should be used along with Trendelenburg positioning and a uterine manipulator. If atypical or subtle lesions are the only evidence of endometriosis, a biopsy should be considered for microscopic verification.

Is the laparoscopy superior to laparotomy in the conservative treatment of severe endometriosis? In a review of 14 studies using conservative surgery for severe endometriosis by laparotomy and 15 studies of laparoscopic surgery (Table 1), it was concluded that "there are still not sufficient data to compare, reliably, the results of laparotomy and laparoscopy in terms of morbidity, pregnancy rates, pain relief, and recurrence."[14] The laparoscopic treatment of severe endometriosis should not be taken lightly. Resection of infiltrating cul-de-sac endometriosis has been reported but should be reserved for the expert endoscopic surgeon.

Laparoscopic Denervation Procedures

A report by Tjaden et al. is often cited as evidence of the efficacy of presacral neurectomy.[23] These authors reported that midline pain was relieved in four patients randomized to undergo laparotomy with excision of endometriosis and presacral neurectomy, whereas none of the four patients who received resection of endometriosis alone obtained relief. Unfortunately, the study was stopped at that point by the Institutional Review Board, who declared that these preliminary findings

TABLE 1. *Conservative surgery versus expectant management in endometriosis[a]*

	Odds ratio (95% CI)
All patients	2.2 (1.2, 4.0)
Mild endometriosis	0.4 (0.1, 1.6)
Moderate endometriosis	3.9 (1.6, 9.4)
Severe endometriosis	27.9 (1.6, 497)

[a]Adapted from Olive and Lee, Analysis of sequential treatment protocols for endometriosis-associated infertility. *Am J Obstet Gynecol* 1986; 154:613–619.

rendered it unethical to refuse patients the benefits of presacral neurectomy. Eleven of 13 subsequent nonrandomized patients who underwent presacral neurectomy experienced relief. None of the nine patients without presacral neurectomy obtained relief. Case series have been reported with success rates ranging from 70% to 97%.[15,16] Few randomized prospective trials have been reported.[17] A report of 71 patients by Candiani et al. demonstrated a marked reduction in the midline component of menstrual pain but no statistically significant difference in the frequency or severity of dysmenorrhea, pelvic pain, or dyspareunia.[18] Laparoscopic presacral neurectomy should be performed by surgeons who have received training in advanced operative laparoscopy and have familiarity with this procedure. This denervation procedure should be reserved for the patient with significant midline dysmenorrhea refractory to an adequate trial of conservative management.

Observational studies of laparoscopic uterosacral nerve ablation (LUNA) performed at the time of laparoscopic treatment of endometriosis show success rates similar to that of patients undergoing treatment of endometriosis alone, with 72% to 92% experiencing relief from dysmenorrhea.[19,20] The LUNA procedure seems to yield only partial and temporary relief of pelvic pain and is associated with serious complications; therefore, it is not recommended except in extraordinary circumstances.

Tubal Sterilization

Several methods for laparoscopic tubal sterilization have been designed for specific tubal segments. Knowledge of these techniques and their intended tubal segments is critical, as higher failure rates are associated with deviation from standard techniques.[21] Most electrocautery sterilizations performed today use bipolar rather than unipolar instruments (Fig. 9). The key concepts with bipolar electocautery include the use of matching electrosurgical components, grasping a midtubal segment within the concave portion of the cautery forceps so that the duck-billed tongs cauterize the vascular supply through the mesosalpinx, coagulating with 25 watts in three contiguous areas (at least 3 cm) until an ammeter confirms the cessation of current flow, avoidance of the cornual region (more vascular with a greater potential to form a fistula), and avoiding contact with any other tissues.

The spring-loaded plastic Hulka-Clemens clip should be applied at a 90° angle to the isthmic portion of the fallopian tube, 2 to 3 cm distal to the uterotubal junction, perpendicular

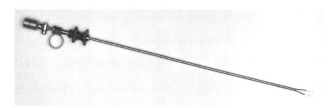

FIG. 9. Kleppinger bipolar forceps.

to the tube. After the clip is placed, the tube should be examined to ensure that the entire tube has been covered. If the clip has not been placed properly, a second clip may be placed. With recent FDA approval, a second clip composed of titanium lined with silicone rubber (called the Filshie clip, Avalon Medical Corp., Williston, VT) is now available. The Filshie clip is placed at a right angle to the proximal isthmus of the tube, within 2 to 3 cm of the cornu. The lead portion of the applicator should be visualized through the mesosalpinx to confirm that the tube is completely covered. These methods offer the advantage of less destruction of the tube in patients seeking tubal anastamosis.

The fallope ring is placed on the ampullary portion of the fallopian tube. The tube is grasped and drawn into the applicator cylinder. The applicator should be moved toward the tube to reduce any tension, which may result in bleeding. After application of the tubal ring, the banded loop of tube should be 1 to 2 cm and have two complete tubal lumens within it.

The U.S. Collaborative Review of Sterilization (CREST) study, a prospective cohort study performed at nine medical centers that reported on 10,685 women followed for 8 to 14 years, found that the failure rates of many methods of tubal sterilization were higher than expected. The study showed that within 5 years of sterilization, 1% of women will become pregnant. The cumulative 10-year probability of pregnancy was lowest after unipolar coagulation and postpartum partial salpingectomy. The highest 10-year failure rate was reported with the Hulka-Clemmens clip (36.5 per 1000 procedures).

Ectopic Pregnancy

Though the laparoscopic management of ectopic pregnancy has been studied more than other laparoscopic procedures, most of the favorable evidence to support the laparoscopic management of ectopic pregnancy comes from cohort, case-control, and descriptional studies. One RCT with 60 patients (30 in each group) comparing laparotomy to laparoscopy demonstrated a shorter stay and quicker recovery rate in the laparoscopically treated group.[22] However, to demonstrate a 50% decrease in morbidity ($p < 0.05$) and an 80% power, 948 patients would be needed.[23]

Technique of Linear Salpingectomy for Ectopic Pregnancy

To minimize bleeding, 5 ml of a dilute vasopressin solution (20 U in 100 cc saline) may be injected into the mesosalpinx below the ectopic pregnancy and over the antimesenteric surface of the tube with a 21-gauge spinal needle or a laparoscopic needle. A 1- to 2-cm linear incision is then made with a microelectrode or laser over the antimesenteric surface of the thinnest segment of the bulging tube. The fallopian tube is best accessed by holding it with gentle traction with an atraumatic forceps through the ipsilateral port while the incision is made through the contralateral port. The ectopic products usually easily dislodge with hydrodissection or may be teased out with laparoscopic forceps. If bleeding persists at the im-

plantation site, it is gently cauterized with a microbipolar forceps, needle electrode, or defocused laser beam.

Laparoscopic Myomectomy

Laparoscopic myomectomy is considered one of the more difficult laparoscopic surgeries because it requires expert skill to adequately suture the resultant uterine defect. There is no absolute size contraindication to the laparoscopic approach, as the procedure is highly operator dependent. Large pedunculated fibroids (8 to 10 cm) are fairly simple to remove but may take considerable time to morcellate manually. On the other hand, large intramural fibroids may take 4 hours to remove even by "expert" laparoscopic surgeons.[34] Most reports of laparoscopic myomectomy are limited to case series without comparison to open procedures.[24,25] Furthermore, these series do not distinguish between the treatment of simple subserous pedunculated fibroids and large intramural fibroids, which can be quite tedious to remove. Stringer and colleagues recently retrospectively compared their experience with open myomectomy (1983 to 1995, $n = 49$) to laparoscopic myomectomy (1993 to 1995, $n = 49$).[26] The mean operating room time was significantly higher with the laparoscopic approach; however, mean number of hospital days, mean blood loss, and postoperative complications were significantly lower in the laparoscopic group. There was no statistical difference in cost. The uterine size in the open group was 12 to 14 weeks, versus 9 to 11 weeks in the laparoscopic group, which may account for some bias toward the laparoscopic group. To date, there are not sufficient data regarding the long-term effects of these repairs on future pregnancy.

Laparoscopic Colposuspension

To date, most data regarding the efficacy and safety of laparoscopic urethropexy comes from case series with limited follow-up. No 5-year follow-up data exist to compare this technique with traditional open methods. In 1993, Liu reported the results of 58 cases of a laparoscopic modification of the Burch urethropexy.[27] His success rate was 95% at 6- to 22-month follow-up. The mean operating time was 73 minutes (excluding other concomitant laparoscopic and vaginal procedures) with an estimated blood loss of 50 cc. The mean hospital stay was 1.2 days, and two patients experienced bladder injury (8.5%). Three patients were diagnosed as having postoperative detrusor instability and responded favorably to medical management. Liu updated his series in 1994 to include a total of 132 patients, with 127 patients satisfied with the surgery (96%).[28] At the time of data collection (August 1993), 55 patients had been followed for 1 to 2 years, but only 10 patients had been followed for more than 2 years. These data suggest that in the hands of an experienced laparoscopic surgeon, the short-term clinical results of the laparoscopic Burch procedure are quite good.

Polascik et al. reported a case-control study of 22 patients who underwent either laparoscopic ($n = 12$) or traditional Burch urethropexy ($n = 10$).[29] In the laparoscopic group,

10 women (83%) were successfully treated for stress incontinence at a mean follow-up of 20.8 months. Of the 10 women in the open group, only seven were cured (70%) with a mean follow-up of 35.6 months. The laparoscopic route took on average 1.5 hours longer to perform ($p < 0.01$) but required less postoperative analgesia ($p < 0.01$) and had significantly reduced hospital stays (1.9 versus 4.9 days). Though these results appear encouraging for the laparoscopic Burch procedure, the mean follow-up between the two groups was quite dissimilar, and the sample size too small, to draw firm conclusions in terms of efficacy.

Burton presented data at the International Continence Society in 1994, from a randomized clinical trial of 60 women, comparing these two techniques.[30] The mean number of leaks in 24 hours was two in the open group and six in the laparoscopic group ($p < 0.05$). There is currently at least one multicenter randomized clinical trial ongoing to better compare these two methods.

Office Laparoscopy and Microlaparoscopy

Office laparoscopy refers to the use of laparoscopy in a non-hospital environment, using conscious sedation (intravenous sedation) and local anesthesia without the assistance of an anesthesiologist. Microlaparoscopy refers to the use of 2- or 3-mm instrumentation but may be performed using conscious sedation or general anesthesia. Local anesthesia and conscious sedation have long been used to perform tubal ligation. The use of microlaparoscopic instrumentation has assisted in performing laparoscopy under conscious sedation in an office setting for pain mapping in chronic pelvic pain patients.[31] Pain mapping may be useful in patients with chronic pelvic pain of uncertain etiology, as this enables the patient to participate in the evaluation of the pelvis while searching for a painful focus. Because this is a relatively new procedure, the effects of pain mapping have not been evaluated in terms of long-term outcomes.

◊ HYSTEROSCOPY

Hysteroscopy was first performed by Pantaleoni in 1869 using an adaptation of a cystoscope. As lenses and light sources evolved, the hysteroscope was used to visualize the endometrial cavity and the tubal ostia. With further technologic advances, the hysteroscope is now used to resect submucous myomas, remove uterine septae and synechiae, perform sterilization, canalize and visualize fallopian tubes, and ablate the endometrium in cases of dysfunctional uterine bleeding. Hysteroscopy is now routinely performed concomitantly with uterine dilation and curettage to avoid performing a "blind procedure."

Instrumentation

Rigid and flexible hysteroscopes were developed based on cystoscopes and gastrointestinal endoscopes. Depending on whether they are used for diagnostic or operative purposes,

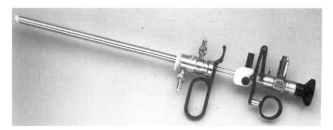

FIG. 10. The operative hysteroscope (courtesy of Karl Storz).

the outer diameter may range from 2 to 10 mm. Diagnostic rigid hysteroscopes are composed primarily of two pieces, the telescope and the outer sheath. The rigid hysteroscopic telescope is available with viewing angles that range from 0° to 70°. The outer sheath is used to instill a distending medium. The operative hysteroscope consists of three pieces: the telescope, the working element, and the outer sheath (Fig. 10). The working element has the capability to house a rollerball, loop, or vaporizing electrode (Fig. 11). These may be powered by electricity and are considered monopolar instruments. Nd:YAG, argon, and KTP lasers also may be passed through the operative channel. In addition, other instruments (such as graspers and scissors, which do not require electricity) may also be passed down an operative channel. A light source also is needed and video monitoring is available. Separate channels for fluid inflow and outflow are available so the fluid can be continuously exchanged for better visualization.

In contrast to the multisheathed rigid hysteroscope, the flexible hysteroscope consists of a single steerable unit. Its distal tip may be deflected 130° to 160°. The outer diameter usually ranges from 3.5 mm to 5 mm, and a 1-mm channel is used to instill a distending medium.

Distending Media

The use of a distending medium transforms the uterine cavity from a potential space into a cavity offering a panoramic

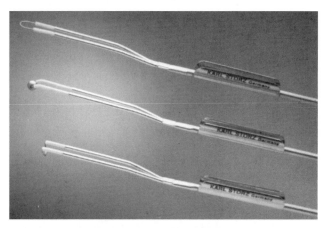

FIG. 11. The straight loop electrode **(top)** is used for division of uterine septae and adhesions; the rollerball **(middle)** is used for endometrial ablation; and the bent loop **(bottom)** is used for myoma and endometrial resection (courtesy of Karl Storz).

view of the endometrium. Several media are available, depending on surgeon preference and the operative setting. For office-based diagnostic hysteroscopy, usually of short duration, carbon dioxide, normal saline, or Ringer's lactate is typically used. Nonelectrolyte solutions must be used for most operative cases performed in the operating room.

Gas

Carbon dioxide offers the advantage of creating less mess with no fluid to collect. It provides excellent visualization and safety. It is important that a hysteroscopic rather than a laparoscopic insufflator be used, with a pressure set point of 100 mm Hg and a flow rate of less than 100 cc/min to avoid the complication of carbon dioxide embolus. The disadvantages of carbon dioxide include the accumulation of gas bubbles and bleeding, which may impair visualization. Also, CO_2 is not compatible with use of the Nd:YAG laser.

Low-Viscosity Electrolyte Solutions

Normal saline and Ringer's lactate commonly are used for diagnostic purposes. They offer the advantage of being relatively inexpensive and readily available. However, because they contain electrolytes, they should not be used in conjunction with a monopolar electrode. Recently, a system has been developed to use electricity with normal saline by having an attachable sheath that acts as a return electrode (ERA resectoscopic sheath, Conceptus, San Carlos, CA). This was developed in hopes of decreasing the risk of hyponatremia.

Low-Viscosity Nonelectrolyte Solutions

The most commonly used nonelectrolyte solutions are 1.5% glycine and 3% sorbitol. These offer the ability to use electricity safely. However, because they are hypotonic solutions, they pose the risk of causing hyponatremia. They readily mix with blood, which may make visualization difficult in the face of bleeding. In addition, when absorbed into the circulation, glycine is metabolized into ammonia and eventually to urea. Patients with impaired liver function may be at risk for ammonia intoxication, and patients with renal impairment may be at risk for urea toxicity. The most common problem is pulmonary edema.

High-Viscosity Solution

Hyskon (32% dextran 70 in dextrose) is a nonelectrolyte solution that does not mix with blood, thereby offering excellent visual quality and the ability to use electricity. The disadvantages with this medium are that it can be messy and may add to clean-up time. If the hysteroscope is not adequately cleaned, the instrument port may become clogged as the hyskon hardens. Intravascular absorption of hyskon can lead to serious hyponatremia complications, as it is a significant plasma expander. The osmotic properties of hyskon will expand plasma

with a ratio of 1:8. Hyskon also affects platelets, factor VII, and fibrinogen and may mimic von Willebrand's disease in rare circumstances. Rare but significant anaphyactoid reactions have also been reported. Operative procedures should be performed using between 100 and 500 ml to avoid fluid overload.

Diagnostic Hysteroscopy

Cervical dilation is rarely necessary when a small diagnostic hysteroscope is used. Before insertion, a bimanual exam should be performed to assess the axis of the cervix and the uterus to avoid perforation. The anterior lip of the cervix is grasped with a single-toothed tenaculum to straighten the cervical canal. As the hysteroscope is inserted through the cervical os, the angle of the telescope should be taken into account; if a foreoblique view is used, the view will be somewhat forward. As the hysteroscope is advanced under direct visualization, the endocervical canal is assessed. As the endometrial cavity becomes distended, a panoramic view of the endometrial cavity should be obtained. Any specific areas of abnormality within the endometrial cavity should be investigated, and the tubal ostia should also be evaluated. The entire examination need not take more than a few minutes.

Operative Hysteroscopy

Operative hysteroscopy is performed in the face of a known abnormality and usually requires cervical dilation to allow the passage of a larger hysteroscope, typically with an 8-mm outer diameter. The use of preoperative passive cervical dilators such as laminaria tents is helpful in preparing the cervix and may reduce the risk of uterine perforation. A medium should be selected that is compatible with the surgical equipment to be used. Fluid input and output must be monitored to avoid inadvertent fluid overload syndrome. Three-liter bags are often used in operative hysteroscopy, which may contain variable amounts of fluid, making calculation of input and output difficult if a visual system is used to estimate input and output. Systems are now available to determine fluid balance on a second-to-second basis based on fluid weight with significant accuracy (Flo-Stat Fluid Management System, FemRx, Sunnyvale, CA).

Leiomyomata

Patients with symptomatic submucous leiomyomata are often candidates for hysteroscopic resection. The use of a GnRH agonist for 2 months preoperatively may be useful in allowing time to raise the patient's hematocrit and may reduce the mean volume of the uterus by 30% to 50%.[32] The loop electrode is commonly used to shave the myoma flush with the endometrium. Cutting or coagulating current of 100 to 120 watts may be used. The loop should be advanced to the cephalad aspect of the myoma, and resection is carried out by pulling the loop toward the operator. In the case of pedunculated fibroids, the stalk should not be cut until the end of the procedure, as this anchors the specimen to the uterine wall, making resection easier. As several pieces of myoma collect and obscure visualization, the hysteroscope may be withdrawn, and polyp forceps may be used to remove myoma sections. Recently, the VaporTrode (Circon ACMI, Santa Barbara, CA) has been designed to vaporize myomas and thus eliminate the need to remove myoma chips. The VaporTrode uses 160 to 200 watts of pure cutting current. Because of the rare malignant tumor, it is recommended to resect a portion of the tumor to send for histologic confirmation. It is too soon to know how this new technology will compare to resection techniques.

Septate Uterus

There are no clear-cut or universal criteria for metroplasty. In general, this is performed when a patient has a history of adverse pregnancy outcomes thought to be attributed to the uterine septum. Indications may include repeated first-trimester losses, second-trimester loss, or history of premature births. For the treatment of the septate uterus, hysteroscopic septum resection can be performed with excellent results with fewer complications and for less cost than traditional abdominal approaches.[33–35]

Scheduling the surgery during the early follicular phase will aid in visualization because of relative thinning of the endometrial lining. Prophylactic antibiotics are recommended by some authors. The straight loop rather than the 90° loop is preferable for septum resection. If the loop electrode is to be used, a nonelectrolyte solution must be used (sorbitol or glycine). As the electrode is passed through the septum, it should be aimed at the center of the septum so that the tissue will retract and become flush with the endometrial cavity. Laparoscopic visualization should be performed simultaneously to avoid uterine perforation. In a series of 91 patients undergoing hysteroscopic metroplasty for a history of one or more miscarriages or late second-trimester losses, an 85% live birth rate was obtained.[36] Some surgeons administer estrogen after septum resection to build up the endometrial lining over the resected areas in hope of avoiding intrauterine adhesions. One prospective, randomized, blinded study showed no benefit to estrogen use after septum resection.[37]

Dysfunctional Uterine Bleeding: Endometrial Ablation/Resection

The Nd:YAG laser initially was used to ablate the endometrium. Subsequently, electrosurgical methods have been employed, including rollerball and rollerbarrel ablation and loop resection of the endometrium. The preoperative use of a GnRH agonist has been shown to increase the success rate after endometrial ablation or resection. In a large multicenter randomized, placebo-controlled, double-blind study comparing GnRH agonist to placebo before endometrial ablation, Donnez et al. found a 40% amenorrhea rate at 2 years using GnRH agonist versus a 26% amenorrhea rate with placebo.[38]

Overall, amenorrhea rates after endometrial ablation range from 25% to 60%, with a trend toward higher rates in patients followed for a shorter interval.[39–42] In the short term, endometrial ablation appears to offer an economic advantage over hysterectomy for menorrhagia;[43] however, in one study, 34% of women underwent hysterectomy within 5 years of endometrial ablation.[44] Satisfaction with the procedure approaches 90% in most series.

Endometrial resection is performed with a loop electrode using 100 watts of cutting current to resect the endometrium in contiguous 4-mm strips starting anteriorly and proceeding in a 360° fashion. If endometrial ablation with the rollerball is to be used, care should be taken to avoid ablating the endocervical tissue to avoid iatrogenic cervical stenosis. This may be avoided by first cauterizing a 360° rim around the border of the endocervix and the endometrial cavity to mark the limits of the ablation. The fundus and anterior wall are ablated first, and then the lateral and posterior walls. The cornu are ablated last, as this area is the area most likely to result in perforation and would result in halting the procedure. The rollerball should be gently pressed against the cornual regions to avoid perforation. Complications occur in approximately 12% of cases and include fluid overload syndrome and uterine perforation. Rarely, a missed endometrial cancer or pregnancy complicates this procedure.[45–47]

◊ CONCLUSION

Though a variety of new laparoscopic and hysteroscopic procedures are being performed, few have been studied extensively in properly designed randomized clinical trials (RCT). Randomization is the only known method of effectively controlling selection bias, but there are several problems with this approach that are difficult to overcome. Randomized clinical trials may not be representative because patients who volunteer seek randomization to the often "expert" surgeons who participate in surgical RCTs. It also is sometimes difficult to recruit a sufficient number of patients so that a RCT will have a sample size large enough to provide adequate statistical power. Well-designed case-control studies and cohort studies may be a more realistic way to study these surgical procedures.

◊ REFERENCES

1. Dorsey JH, Sharp HT, Chovan JD, Holtz PM. Laparoscopic knot strength: a comparison with conventional knots. *Obstet Gynecol* 1995; 86:536–540.
2. Sharp HT, Dorsey JH, Chovan JD, Holtz PM. The effect of knot geometry on the strength of laparoscopic slip knots. *Obstet Gynecol* 1996;88:408–411.
3. Hurd WW, Bude RO, DeLancey JOL, Pearl ML. The relationship of the umbilicus to the aortic bifurcation: implications for laparoscopic technique. *Obstet Gynecol [Suppl]* 1992;80:48.
4. Webb MJ, Decker DG, Mussey E, et al. Factors influencing survival in stage I ovarian cancer. *Am J Obstet Gynecol* 1973;116:222–228.
5. Dembo A, Davy M, Stenwig A, et al. Prognostic factors in patients with stage I epithelial ovarian cancer. *Obstet Gynecol* 1990;75:263–273.

6. Sainz de la Cuesta R, Goff BA, Fuller AF, et al. Prognostic importance of intraoperative rupture of malignant ovarian epithelial neoplasms. *Obstet Gynecol* 1994;84:1–7.

7. Summitt RL, Stovall TG, Lipscomb GH, Ling FW. Randomized comparison of laparoscopic-assisted vaginal hysterectomy with standard hysterectomy in an outpatient setting. *Obstet Gynecol* 1992;80:895.

8. Doucette RC, Scott JR. Comparison of laparoscopically assisted vaginal hysterectomy with abdominal and vaginal hysterectomy. *J Reprod Med* 1996;41:1–6.

9. Dorsey JH, Holtz PM, Griffiths RI, McGrath MM, Steinberg EP. Costs and charges associated with three alternate techniques of hysterectomy. *N Engl J Med* 1996;335:476–482.

10. Pent D. Laparoscopy. Its role in private practice. *Am J Obstet Gynecol* 1972;113:459–468.

11. Lundberg WI, Wall JE, Mathers JE. Laparoscopy in the evaluation of pelvic pain. *Obstet Gynecol* 1973;42:872–876.

12. Howard FM. The role of laparoscopy in chronic pelvic pain: promise and pitfalls. *Obstet Gynecol Surv* 1993;48:357–387.

13. Stripling MC, Martin DC, Chatman DL, et al. Subtle appearance of pelvic endometriosis. *Fertil Steril* 1988;49:427–431.

14. Candiani GB, Vercellini P, Fedele L, et al. Conservative surgical treatment for severe endometriosis in infertile women: Are we making progress? *Obstet Gynecol Surv* 1991;46:490–498.

15. Garcia CR, David SS. Pelvic endometriosis: infertility and pelvic pain. *Am J Obstet Gynecol* 1977;129:740–747.

16. Polan ML, DeCherney A. Presacral neurectomy for pelvic pain in infertility. *Fertil Steril* 1980;34:557–560.

17. Tjaden B, Schlaff WS, Kimball A, et al. The efficacy of presacral neurectomy for the relief of midline dysmenorrhea. *Obstet Gynecol* 1990;76:89–91.

18. Candiani GB, Fedele L, Vercelli P, et al. Presacral neurectomy for the treatment of pelvic pain associated with endometriosis: A contolled study. *Am J Obstet Gynecol* 1992;167:100–103.

19. Sutton C, Hill D. Laser laparoscopy in the treatment of endometriosis. *Br J Obstet Gynaecol* 1990;97:181–185.

20. Perez JJ. Laparoscopic presacral neurectomy. *J Reprod Med* 1990;35:625–630.

21. Stovall TG, Ling FW, O'Kelley KR, et al. Gross and histologic examination of tubal ligation failures in a residency program. *Obstet Gynecol* 1990;76:461–465.

22. Vermesh M, Silva PD, Rosen GF, Stein AL, Fossum GT, Sauer MV. Management of unruptured ectopic gestation by linear salpingostomy: a prospective trial of laparoscopy versus laparotomy. *Obstet Gynecol* 1989;73:400–404.

23. Grimes DA. Frontiers of operative laparoscopy: A review and critique of the evidence. *Am J Obstet Gynecol* 1992;166:1062–1071.

24. Nezhat C, Nezhat F, Silfen SL, et al. Laparoscopic myomectomy. *Int J Fertil* 1991;36:275–280.

25. Dubussion JB, Lecuru F, Foulot H, et al. Myomectomy by laparoscopy: A review of 43 cases. *Fertil Steril* 1991;56:827–830.

26. Stringer NH, Walker JC, Meyer PM. Comparison of 49 laparoscopic myomectomies with 49 open myomectomies. *J Am Assoc Gynecol Laparosc* 1997;4:457–464.

27. Liu CY. Laparoscopic retropubic colposuspension (Burch procedure). A review of 58 cases. *J Reprod Med* 1993;38:526–530.

28. Liu CY. Laparoscopic treatment for genuine urinary stress incontinence. *Bailliere's Clin Obstet Gynecol* 1994;8:789–798.

29. Polascik TJ, Moore RG, Rosenberg MT, Kavoussi LR. Comparison of laparoscopic and open retropubic urethropexy for treatment of stress urinary incontinence. *Urology* 1995;45:647–652.

30. Burton G. *A randomized comparison of laparoscopic and open colposuspension.* Abstract presented at the International Continence Society, Prague, Czech Republic, 1994.

31. Palter SF, Olive DL. Office microlaparoscopy under local anesthesia for chronic pelvic pain. *J Am Assoc Gynecol Laparosc* 1996;3:359–364.

32. Crosignani PG, Vercellini P, Meschia M, Oldani S, Bramante T. GnRH agonists before surgery for uterine myomas. A review. *J Reprod Med* 1996;41:415–421.

33. DeCherney AH, Russell JB, Graebe RA, et al. Resectoscopic management of Mullerian fusion defects. *Fertil Steril* 1986;45:726–728.

34. Hassiakos DJ, Zourlas PA. Transcervical division of the uterine septum. *Obstet Gynecol Surv* 1990;45:165–173.

35. Daly DC, Maier D, Soto-Albors C. Hysteroscopic metroplasty: Six years' experience. *Obstet Gynecol* 1989;73:201–205.

36. March CM, Israel R. Hysteroscopic management of recurrent abortion caused by septate uterus. *Am J Obstet Gynecol* 1987;156:834.

37. Dabirashrafi H, Mohammad K, Moghadami-Tabrizi N, Zandinejad K, Moghadami-Tabrizi M. Is estrogen necessary after hysteroscopic incision of the uterine septum? *J Am Assoc Gynecol Laparosc* 1996;3:623–625.

38. Donnez J, Vilos G, Gannon MJ, Stampe-Sorensen S, Klinte I, Miller RM. Groerelin acetate (Zoladex) plus endometrial ablation for dysfunctional uterine bleeding: a large randomized, double-blind study. *Fertil Steril* 1997;68:29–36.

39. Vilos GA, Vilos EC, King JH. Experience with 800 endometrial ablations. *J Am Assoc Gynecol Laparosc* 1996;4:33–38.

40. Bae IH, Pagedas AC, Barr CA, Alexander C, Bae DS. Retrospective analysis of 305 consecutive cases of endometrial ablation and partial endomyometrial resection. *J Am Assoc Gynecol Laparosc* 1996;3:549–554.

41. Chullapram T, Song JY, Fraser IS. Medium-term follow-up of women with menorrhagia treated with rollerball endometrial ablation. *Obstet Gynecol* 1996;88:71–76.

42. Baggish MS, Sze EH. Endometrial ablation: a series of 568 patients treated over an 11-year period. *Am J Obstet Gynecol* 1996;174:908–913.

43. Vilos GA, Pispidikis JT, Botz CK. Economic evaluation of hysteroscopic endometrial ablation versus vaginal hysterectomy for menorrhagia. *Obstet Gynecol* 1996;88:241–245.

44. Unger JB, Meeks GR. Hysterectomy after endometrial ablation. *Am J Obstet Gynecol* 1996;175:1436–1437.

45. Scottish Hysteroscopy Audit Group. A Scottish audit of hysteroscopic surgery for menorrhagia: complications and follow-up. *Br J Obstet Gynaecol* 1995;102:249–254.

46. McLucas B. Pregnancy after endometrial ablation. A case report. *J Reprod Med* 1995;40:237–239.

47. Horowitz IR, Copas PR, Aaronoff M, Spann CO, McQuire WP. Endometrial adenocarcinoma following endometrial ablation for postmenopausal bleeding. *Gynecol Oncol* 1995;56:460–463.

CHAPTER 47

Urogynecology

——— ◊ ———

Janine K. Jensen
Donald R. Ostergard

Although the evaluation and treatment of problems of the lower urinary tract have been the province of gynecologists since the first fistula was repaired by Sims in 1846, the field of urogynecology is a relative newcomer to obstetrics and gynecology. One of the early developers in the field was Howard Kelly, known for his vaginal approach to the treatment of stress incontinence, the account of which was published in 1914. During the ensuing years, the approach to disorders of the lower urinary tract was largely clinical, with diagnosis and therapy based almost exclusively on history and physical examination.

Since the late 1970s, a new approach to the entire field has developed, and urogynecology has come of age. Treatment of patients with lower urinary tract symptoms is based on history, physical examination, and objective evaluation with sophisticated endoscopic and urodynamic equipment, enabling the treating physician to develop a rational approach to patient management, particularly for patients who are incontinent or who have other lower urinary tract disorders. This chapter acquaints the student of gynecology with the basic fundamentals of urogynecology needed to develop a rational treatment plan for women with lower urinary tract complaints.

◊ NORMAL LOWER URINARY TRACT

Embryology

An understanding of embryologic events clarifies some aspects of therapy for women with lower urinary tract disorders. In the approximately 4-mm-long embryo, the cloaca exists as a blind pouch (Fig. 1). The cloacal membrane then forms between the exterior of the embryo and the cloaca. Eventually, the cloaca is divided by the urorectal fold into the anterior urogenital sinus and the posterior rectum (Fig. 2). These structures are of endodermal origin. The urogenital sinus is subsequently partitioned into an anterior vesicourethral canal, which ultimately forms the bladder and the upper urethra, and the pelvic portion, which forms the main part of the urethra, including the periurethral glands and the lower one-fifth of the vagina. This development is complete by the fourth month of gestation.

Understanding the nature of the close embryologic development of the urethra and vagina is important in managing estrogen-deficient conditions of the lower urinary tract. Because the vagina and the urethra are derived from estrogen-sensitive structures, the replacement of estrogen can be important in managing lower urinary tract estrogen deficiencies that occur during menopause.

Chronic inflammation of the periurethral glands is important in the genesis of the urethral syndrome and probably important in the development of urethral diverticula. The largest of these periurethral glands are the Skene ducts, which have their orifices at approximately the 4-o'clock and 8-o'clock positions at the external urethral meatus and may be involved in gonorrheal infection. Many small periurethral glands enter the urethra throughout its length, and if they are obstructed, debris can accumulate within the lumina of these glands, resulting in a sterile, inflammatory reaction that generates the lower urinary tract symptoms characteristic of the urethral syndrome. If the orifice of one of these ducts remains plugged for a long time, a urethral diverticulum may develop. Urethral diverticula may also develop congenitally.

The posterior urethral and trigonal musculatures have the same embryologic origin and are continuous (Fig. 3). Similarly, the anterior urethral musculature is continuous with the anterior bladder musculature. This association is important from the standpoint of opening of the urethra during the development of a vesical contraction at the initiation of micturition. The continuous nature of these fibers causes funneling of the upper urethra and the subsequent opening of the urethra during micturition. The bladder has many levels of decussating muscle fibers but does not have distinct layers. The interdigitation of these fibers is important in the genesis of an orderly, propagated vesical contraction.

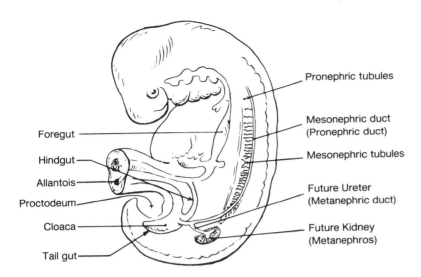

FIG. 1. The 4-mm embryo, in which the cloaca exists as a blind pouch. (From Ostergard DR. Embryology and anatomy of the female bladder and urethra. In: Ostergard DR, ed. *Gynecologic urology and urodynamics: theory and practice*, 2nd ed. Baltimore: Williams & Wilkins, 1985:4; with permission.)

Anatomy

The urethra and the bladder are intimately related to the lower reproductive tract. The urethra adheres closely to the anterior vaginal wall, and no surgical planes exist in this area. A plane may be artificially developed between the urethra and the anterior vaginal wall during dissection of this area, particularly in treating cystocele and stress incontinence.

The urethrovesical junction (UVJ) is normally maintained in a high retropubic position at the level of the junction of the lower and middle thirds of the symphysis pubis. This support is maintained to some degree by the pubourethral ligaments, the endopelvic fascia, and the urogenital diaphragm, which support the urethra, the UVJ, and the base of the bladder. The endopelvic fascia is attached laterally to the arcus tendineus fasciae pelvis, a band of fibers that runs on the inner surface of pelvis, originating approximately 1 cm inferior to the pubic tubercle and ending at the ischial spine. Failure of these supports, with resultant prolapse of the UVJ, is a major factor in the genesis of stress incontinence. All primary surgical procedures for stress incontinence are designed to resuspend the prolapsed UVJ.

Anteriorly, the urethra and anterior bladder wall are exposed to the retropubic space; this space exists between the posterior symphysis pubis and these structures. It is a poten-tial space that is developed during retropubic surgical treatment of stress incontinence (Fig. 4). In this area, several structures are identifiable that are important during surgery, including the Cooper ligament, extending laterally from the pubic tubercle, and the vaginal wall and surrounding adventitia. Between the vaginal wall and the pelvic side wall, most patients have an abundance of fat that must be removed during the surgical procedure. Veins arise in the obturator fossa and extend up to the external iliac vein, crossing over the superior part of the Cooper ligament. They are usually buried within a fat pad and must be avoided during surgical procedures in this area. The applications of these anatomic markers in the treatment of stress incontinence are discussed more thoroughly in the evaluation and treatment sections of this chapter.

Neurology

The neurologic control of the lower urinary tract is unique in that the bladder is the only smooth muscle organ that is under voluntary control. All humans are born incontinent and must learn to control the lower urinary tract to allow socially acceptable micturition habits.

The parasympathetic nervous system stimulates vesical contraction and inhibits urethral muscle activity. It originates from spinal cord segments S-2 through S-4, with long pregan-

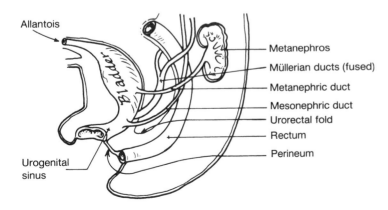

FIG. 2. The cloacal division. The urorectal fold divides the cloaca into the anterior urogenital sinus and the posterior rectum. (From Ostergard DR. Embryology and anatomy of the female bladder and urethra. In: Ostergard DR, ed. *Gynecologic urology and urodynamics: theory and practice*, 2nd ed. Baltimore: Williams & Wilkins, 1985:5; with permission.)

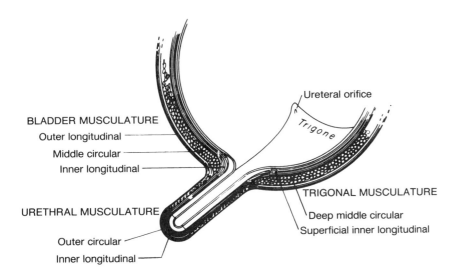

BLADDER MUSCULATURE
Outer longitudinal
Middle circular
Inner longitudinal

Ureteral orifice

Trigone

TRIGONAL MUSCULATURE

Deep middle circular
Superficial inner longitudinal

URETHRAL MUSCULATURE
Outer circular
Inner longitudinal

FIG. 3. The muscular layers of the urethra, bladder, and trigone. Notice the continuation of the deep trigonal musculature with the urethral musculature and the continuation of the anterior bladder musculature with the urethral musculature. (From Ostergard DR. Embryology and anatomy of the female bladder and urethra. In: Ostergard DR, ed. *Gynecologic urology and urodynamics: theory and practice*, 2nd ed. Baltimore: Williams & Wilkins, 1985:7; with permission.)

glionic fibers coursing through the pelvic nerve to the ganglion within the wall of the end organ. Its postganglionic fibers are short. Acetylcholine is thought to be the major neurotransmitter, but evidence suggests that there are also nonacetylcholine substances that mediate detrusor neurologic responses.

The sympathetic nervous system originates from spinal segments T-10 through T-12 down to the L-2 segment. The ganglion is somewhat distant from the end organ, with a short preganglionic fiber and a long postganglionic fiber. The sympathetic nervous system is divided into alpha and beta components. The bladder is primarily a β-adrenergic organ, and the urethra is primarily an α-adrenergic organ,

with high concentrations of their respective receptors. This difference is important in the treatment of various lower urinary tract disorders because α-adrenergic stimulation causes contraction of the urethra but not contraction of the bladder; the β-adrenergic component has the opposite effect.

It is helpful to conceptualize the volitional control of the lower urinary tract in terms of four loops or circuits that are involved in neurologic control of micturition:

◊ *Loop I*, the cerebral–brain stem loop originates in the frontal lobes and terminates in the brain stem (Fig. 5). This loop coordinates the voluntary control of

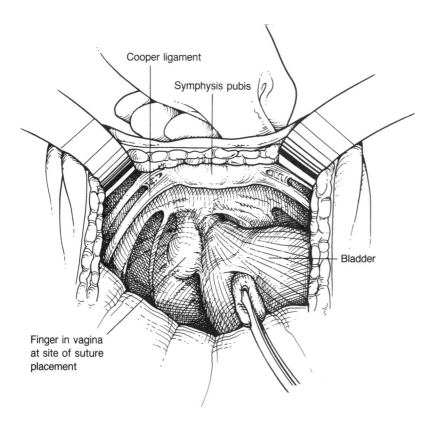

Cooper ligament
Symphysis pubis

Bladder

Finger in vagina at site of suture placement

FIG. 4. This surgeon's view of the retropubic space demonstrates the Cooper ligaments, the pelvic floor, and movement of the bladder away from the site where sutures will be placed. (Adapted from Burch JC. Cooper's ligament urethrovesical suspension for stress incontinence. *Am J Obstet Gynecol* 1968;100:764.)

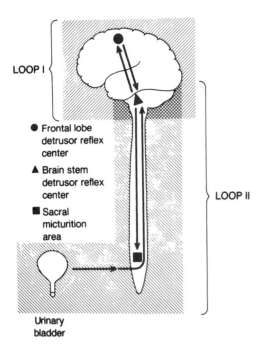

FIG. 5. Neurologic loops I and II. Loop I originates in the cerebrum and terminates in the brain stem. Loop II originates in the brain stem and terminates in the sacral micturition area. (From Ostergard DR. Neurologic control of micturation and integral voiding relfexes. In: Ostergard DR, ed. *Gynecologic urology and urodynamics: theory and practice*, 2nd ed. Baltimore: Williams & Wilkins, 1985:30; with permission.)

micturition. Because this is a central nervous system loop, it is affected by cerebrovascular accidents, tumors, and other central nervous system disorders.

◊ *Loop II* originates in the brain stem and terminates in the sacral micturition area of the sacral spinal cord (see Fig. 5). This loop provides the neurologic stimulus for a detrusor contraction of sufficient duration to empty the bladder completely. Because it is an upper motor neuron loop, diseases of the spinal cord, such as multiple sclerosis and tumors, can affect its function. Its afferent arm originates in the bladder, bypasses the sacral micturition area without synapsing, and terminates in the brain stem.

◊ *Loop III* connects the bladder with the sacral micturition area of the spinal cord and the striated component of the urethral sphincter (Fig. 6). Loop III coordinates vesical contraction and urethral sphincter relaxation during voiding.

◊ *Loop IV* originates in the frontal lobe and terminates in the sacral micturition area (Fig. 7). It controls voluntary activity of the urethral sphincter.

Although neurologic control of the lower urinary tract can be categorized by these four loops, the functions of each loop is not independent. Integration is required for coordinated bladder filling, storage, and evacuation. Many disorders of bladder function, including overflow incontinence and detrusor hyperflexia, are a result of neurologic insult. Detrusor

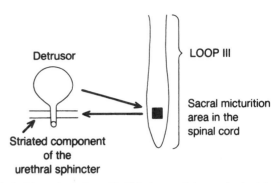

FIG. 6. Neurologic loop III. This loop originates in the bladder with synapses in the sacral micturition area of the cord and terminates in the striated component of the urethral sphincter. (From Ostergard DR. Neurological control of micturation and integral voiding reflexes. In: Ostergard DR, ed. *Gynecologic urology and urodynamics: theory and practice*, 2nd ed. Baltimore: Williams & Wilkins, 1985:31; with permission.)

instability, the majority of cases being idiopathic, may actually represent cortical atrophy or subtle breaks in the nervous system pathways. Stress urinary incontinence has traditionally been approached as a condition related to poor anatomic support of the UVJ, although it may be a disease of the nervous system with denervation of the pelvic floor rather than a disorder of the anatomic associations of the UVJ.

Pharmacology

Neurologic control of the lower urinary tract is based on the appropriate functioning of the sympathetic and parasympathetic nervous systems. The bladder is stimulated by cholin-

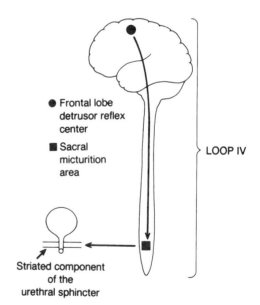

FIG. 7. Neurologic loop IV. This loop originates in the cerebral cortex and terminates in the sacral micturition area. (From Ostergard DR. Neurological control of micturation and integral voiding reflexes. In: Ostergard DR, ed. *Gynecologic urology and urodynamics: theory and practice*, 2nd ed. Baltimore: Williams & Wilkins, 1985:32; with permission.)

ergic activity and relaxed by anticholinergic activity. In certain disease states, it is necessary to relax the detrusor so that it does not contract spontaneously, if contraction and subsequent evacuation of the bladder are undesirable. If the bladder is overactive, a variety of medications can be used, including dicyclomine, flavoxate (Urispas), imipramine, oxybutynin chloride (Ditropan), and propantheline bromide (see "Detrusor Instability," below). Occasionally, it is also necessary to increase the muscular tone of the bladder, for which cholinergic medications are used. The major cholinergic medication is bethanechol chloride, used for conditions in which the bladder is relatively acontractile.

For some diseases of the urethra, it is occasionally necessary to relax this organ if urethral spasm is caused by overactivity of the urethral smooth muscle or skeletal muscle. Many experts in the field do not consider overactivity of smooth muscle to be the cause of this condition and therefore rarely use smooth muscle relaxants. The spasm is probably a result of overactivity of skeletal muscle, which usually is treated with skeletal muscle relaxants, such as diazepam. Much more important are patients who have a relaxed urethral sphincter and associated stress urinary incontinence. These patients frequently benefit from the use of α-adrenergic-stimulating agents, the most important of which phenylpropanolamine. Imipramine may be used for a combination of stress incontinence and unstable bladder.

Because the urethra, the base of the bladder, and the vagina have similar embryologic origins, an important pharmacologic consideration is the use of estrogen for treating several diseases of the lower urinary tract. When inspection of the vagina reveals hypoestrogenism, the lack of estrogen usually also affects the urethra and the base of the bladder. In the absence of contraindications, an oral estrogen or topical estrogen cream should be used. The latter provides a much better local effect and is useful in the management of a variety of lower urinary tract conditions.

◊ EVALUATION OF THE LOWER URINARY TRACT

Triage of Patients with Lower Urinary Tract Symptoms

History alone does not provide an accurate basis for treating lower urinary tract conditions, in particular urinary incontinence, although it can direct the appropriate sequence for evaluation.[15] The physical examination may reveal specific conditions that can be treated, and the results can guide further diagnostic evaluation. Diagnostic evaluation is divided into a series of steps, each of which is completed before advancing to the next (Table 1). Many of the diagnoses mentioned in the evaluation process are discussed in later sections of the chapter.

Step 1: Urinalysis and Culture

Cystitis may be responsible for many symptoms referable to the lower urinary tract, including incontinence. The initial

TABLE 1. *Evaluation of lower urinary tract*

Step 1: Urinalysis and culture
Step 2: Office evaluation, including history and physical examination, neurologic screen, urolog summary, uroflowmetry, residual urine, Q-tip test, urethral calibration
Step 3: Dynamic cystourethroscopy, stress test, screening cystometrography
Step 4: Multichannel urodynamic assessment, including urethral closure pressure profiles, rest and stress; voiding mechanism; electromyography

infection must be treated before continuing the evaluation. If the patient's symptoms persist despite adequate therapy, the evaluation proceeds to the next step.

Step 2: Office Evaluation

Step 2 includes the medical history, physical examination, urolog, uroflowmetry, residual urine determination, Q-tip test, and urethral calibration.

The medical history may reveal congenital defects, psychiatric problems, or medication use. Congenital defects require appropriate evaluation, including radiographic procedures and endoscopy. Psychiatric problems may require consultation, evaluation, and treatment before further management of incontinence. Medications known to affect the lower urinary tract may require alterations of dosage or substitution with other types of medication to minimize urinary tract side affects. Physical examination may reveal abnormal neurologic findings, hypoestrogenism, fistula, urethral diverticulum, or genital prolapse. Postmenopausal patients should be treated with vaginal estrogen before continuing the evaluation. The patient with abnormal neurologic findings requires neurologic consultation and appropriate management.

A fistula or a urethral diverticulum necessitates further evaluation by endoscopy and radiographic methods. Residual urine is considered abnormal if the amount is greater than 100 ml. The cause must be investigated and treatment introduced. Therapy may consist of double-voiding techniques or intermittent self-catheterization if the patient has symptoms, particularly recurrent urinary tract infections. Abnormal uroflowmetry results necessitate evaluation to rule out the possibility of detrusor-sphincter dyssynergia (i.e., obstructed voiding), urethral syndrome, and other local abnormalities of the lower urinary tract.

The urolog is a 24-hour voiding diary. Knowledge of a patient's maximal daily fluid intake and urine output may uncover significant medical conditions, including diabetes mellitus, diabetes insipidus, and psychogenic polydipsia.

The Q-tip test is used to assess possible hypermobility of the urethra. This test is important in planning surgery for stress incontinence, as a well supported UVJ (negative Q-tip test) responds poorly to standard urethropexy procedures. Urethral calibration determines urethral size and the potential need for dilation if the urethra is too small to admit the endoscopic instruments to be used in the next step.

Step 3: Dynamic Cystourethroscopy, Stress Test, and Screening Cystometry

Urethroscopic examination may reveal features compatible with the urethral syndrome. If a urethral diverticulum is detected, further evaluation is required by urethral pressure profilometry and radiography. Lesions of the bladder wall detected at cystoscopy, such as interstitial cystitis, necessitate further evaluation. The stress test is used to observe urinary loss associated with straining or coughing, and it is performed in the standing position with a full bladder. A positive stress test confirms the sign of stress incontinence. If stress loss is seen in the lithotomy position especially with a relatively empty bladder, intrinsic damage of the urethral sphincter is possible. Screening cystometry is used to rule out detrusor instability. Occasionally, the cystometrogram (CMG) or residual urine determination detects a hypotonic bladder. The physician must then rule out diabetes, hypothyroidism, postoperative conditions, and postherpetic infections.

Step 4: Multichannel Urodynamic Assessment

This examination is reserved for patients who are not diagnosed by the initial three steps of the evaluation, including most patients referred to a tertiary care center. Approximately 10% of patients presenting with urinary tract complaints are unable to be treated before the multichannel urodynamic assessment. Patients who have continuing symptoms of incontinence after the first three steps of investigation or who have urethral diverticula must undergo urodynamic assessment. This tool is used for presurgical assessment of patients with a mixed pattern of urge and stress incontinence and patients with stress incontinence to rule out low urethral pressure, which is an indicator of intrinsic urethral sphincter damage. Patients at higher risk for low urethral pressures include those with recurrent urinary incontinence, those over age 50 years, and those with a history of radical pelvic surgery or radiation therapy.

Urodynamic assessment is performed using microtransducer catheters that measure pressure in the urethra, bladder, and vagina simultaneously. Instantaneous subtraction of bladder pressure from urethral pressure provides the urethral closure pressure, and subtraction of vaginal pressure from bladder pressure indicates the pressure resulting from intrinsic activity of the bladder musculature. Electromyography of the pelvic floor is also useful (Fig. 8). Additional uses of this technique are described later.

Multichannel CMG detects detrusor instability and is useful in patients with combined genuine stress incontinence and detrusor instability to assess the degree of severity of each condition. Patients who have genuine stress incontinence may be managed by a program of medical intervention; those who have an anatomic defect may go on to operative intervention. Urodynamic assessment with urethral closure pressure profilometry is useful in diagnosing patients with urethral diverticulum to determine the location of peak urethral pressure in relation to the diverticulum. For patients with genuine stress

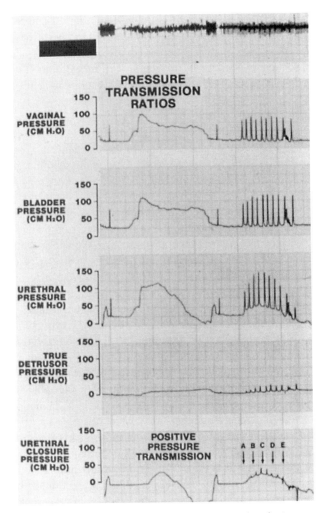

FIG. 8. Multichannel urodynamic assessment by electromyography. True detrusor pressure is bladder pressure minus vaginal (intraabdominal) pressure. The urethral closure pressure is the urethral pressure minus bladder pressure. Pressure transmission to the urethra is equal to or greater than that to the bladder, as evidenced by positive pressure transmission at *B, C,* and *D.* The electromyographic study shows a quiet tracing with increased activity during coughing.

incontinence but no demonstrable anatomic defect, a stress urethral closure pressure profile and Valsalva leak-point pressure measurement are indicated to assess the function of the urethra. Patients who have low urethral closure pressure (< 20 cm H_2O) or low Valsalva leak-point pressures (< 65 cm H_2O) are considered to have intrinsic sphincter deficiency and are managed in a different fashion than from those with genuine stress urinary incontinence.

Patients' voiding mechanism is also measured during urodynamic testing. If flow is obstructed, patients may require dilation or medication. The voiding mechanism may help to detect patients who will have difficulty voiding postoperatively.

With a systematic evaluation, patients may be selected for treatment at any step in the triage. If symptoms persist or reappear, further evaluation is indicated in the sequence presented (see Table 1).

History and Physical Examination

The urogynecologic history is facilitated by a questionnaire sent to patients before their scheduled appointment. Patients also complete a urolog, which is a 24-hour summary of voiding times and amounts, episodes of leakage, and fluid intake. This record serves as a clinical CMG and can guide the evaluation and management strategies. The history encompasses the chief complaints and details about the current illness, past medical and surgical history, and a list of medications used. Specific questions regarding urinary function define the specific problem, its degree of severity, aggravating or relieving factors, and past treatment (Table 2).

The physical examination concentrates on the genital and lower urinary tract. The neurologic evaluation of lower urinary tract function includes lower-limb sensory examination, reflex testing, and estimation of motor strength. With patients in the lithotomy position, the bulbocavernosus reflex is elicited by stroking lateral to the labia minora with the end of a Q-tip and observing the anal reflex contraction. The clitoral reflex is elicited by gently tapping the clitoris with the Q-tip while watching for anal contraction. The vulva is examined for signs of chronic irritation or localized inflammation.

A speculum examination is performed, the vagina is assessed for an estrogen effect, and a Papanicolaou smear may be taken. A Sims speculum or the posterior blade of a Graves speculum is used to depress the posterior vaginal wall during observation for anterior relaxation or uterine prolapse while the patient strains and coughs vigorously. Urine loss is occasionally seen at this time in patients with severe incontinence, even when the bladder is almost empty. This may indicate intrinsic damage to the urethral sphincter. The urethra is palpated to check for tenderness and urethral diverticulum, to assess tissue mobility, and to detect fibrosis around the UVJ. The speculum blade is reversed to retract the anterior vaginal wall, and the posterior wall is inspected during straining and coughing for evidence of enterocele, rectocele, and vaginal vault prolapse. A rectal examination is performed to evaluate rectal tone, to help in identifying an enterocele, and to assess the pelvis. The vaginal cuff is observed with straining to help detect vault pro-

lapse. The urethra and hymenal ring are examined for possible fusion, which may be a cause of recurrent urinary tract infections. The examination should be repeated in the standing position to assess the severity of pelvic floor relaxation.

The sequence of tests depends on whether or not patients come to the office with a full bladder. The examiner should complete a stress test, uroflowmetry, residual urine determination, collection of urine for culture if needed, Q-tip test, and, in some cases, a screening cystometry (i.e., eyeball urodynamics). If a patient has arrived with a relatively full bladder, a stress test can be performed. She is asked to cough vigorously while in the lithotomy position, and if no loss is observed, the test is repeated in the standing position. This test can demonstrate urine loss and clinically confirm a patient's complaint of stress incontinence. An empty supine stress test can be performed if a patient has already voided. The presence or absence urine loss observed in the supine position with Valsalva or cough can be used in a low-prevalence population to screen for intrinsic sphincter deficiency, virtually excluding this diagnosis if the test is negative.[19]

Patients should complete a uroflow test, and the amount of urine is measured. If the volume is less than 300 ml, a negative stress test result requires repeat testing with a full bladder. After the patient has emptied the bladder, the amount of postvoid residual urine is determined. The urine is sent for culture, if needed, or a microscopic examination can be done. While the straight catheter is in position, a screening cystometry can be performed by attaching a catheter syringe to the catheter and filling the bladder in 50-ml increments. The bladder capacity can be determined (normal, 350 to 500 ml), and if bladder activity (i.e., detrusor contraction) occurs, the fluid column in the syringe begins to rise, or fluid loss may occur around the catheter. After the bladder has been filled, the stress test or uroflowmetry can be performed, if not completed previously.

The Q-tip test is performed with patients in the lithotomy position. A cotton-tipped sterile applicator, well lubricated with lidocaine 2% (Xylocaine) jelly, is placed directly into the bladder and then gently pulled back against the UVJ. The angle made by the Q-tip with the horizontal is measured with a goniometer equipped with a level in the resting and straining positions (Fig. 9). The patient should be asked to strain and then relax, and she should then cough vigorously three to four times while the maximal deflection of the Q-tip from the horizontal is measured. Urethral hypermobility exists when the upward deflection during straining is greater than 30 degrees from the horizontal. This test reflects the anatomic support of the UVJ and is not diagnostic for the condition of genuine stress incontinence. The test should be used only to determine if a bladder neck suspension procedure would be helpful in patients with genuine stress incontinence.

TABLE 2. *Questions to ask patients with urinary incontinence*

Do you lose urine in spurts during coughing, lifting, or aerobic activity?

Is the urge to void ever strong enough that you would leak if you do not reach the bathroom in time?

Have you leaked urine because you could not reach the bathroom in time?

How frequently do you urinate during the day?

How many times do you get up from sleep to urinate?

Have you wet the bed in the past year?

When you are passing urine, can you stop the flow?

Do you wear protection (pads) to protect your clothing from the loss of urine?

How severe a problem do you consider your urinary leakage to be?

Do you leak urine during intercourse?

Uroflowmetry

Uroflowmetry is a measure of urine volume voided during the interval required to complete the voiding episode.[1] Normally,

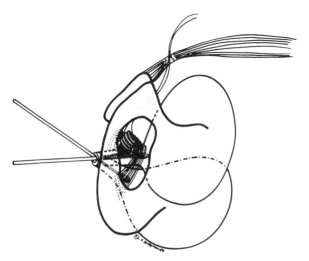

FIG. 9. Q-tip test. At rest, the Q-tip is in a horizontal position, but with straining and coughing, it shows a positive deflection because of inadequate support at the urethrovesical junction.

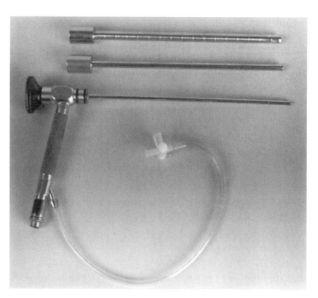

FIG. 10. Urethroscope with a 0-degree lens, sheaths, and a port for saline solution infusion.

200 ml of urine can be voided within 20 seconds at a maximum flow rate of 20 ml per second and with residual urine of less than 50 ml. The measurement is most simply performed using a stopwatch and a beaker in which to collect the urine; a reliable patient can do this in privacy. The more complex measurement is called electronic uroflowmetry, in which a pressure-sensitive electronic device directly records the flow time, volume voided, peak flow, time to peak flow, and average flow. Residual urine is immediately measured after voiding, and a sample is sent for culture. A voided volume of less than 150 ml is considered insufficient for accurate results.

The major abnormalities detected are prolonged voiding time and elevated residual urine. After surgical procedures for incontinence, both conditions can be aggravated. Other conditions associated with abnormal uroflowmetry results include recurrent cystitis associated with high residual urine, and detrusor-sphincter dyssynergia in which voiding is obstructed and residual urine is increased. Uroflowmetry is also performed with microtransducer catheters that measure intravesical, intraurethral, and intraabdominal pressures (i.e., instrumented uroflow). This determines patients' voiding mechanism and whether or not detrusor contraction or urethral relaxation occurs.

Cystourethroscopy

Urethroscopy is the examination of the urethra with a 0-degree lens to obtain a straight-on, wide-angle view (Fig. 10). The bladder base and trigone can be observed, but the entire bladder cannot be fully inspected. Cystoscopy is the systematic examination of the bladder using a 30- or 70-degree lens. The urethra cannot be adequately examined with these lenses.

Urethroscopy is performed with patients in the lithotomy position after the urethra is cleaned. Topical lidocaine is not used because it irritates the urethral mucosa and obscures

observation. Carbon dioxide, sterile water, or preferably a saline solution may be used as the infusing medium. With flow turned on, the urethroscope is inserted into the urethra and gradually passed to the UVJ. The mucosa should be pink, urethral glands may be seen, and vascular pulsations are frequently observed in the midurethra. The trigone is observed by angling the instrument downward and slightly laterally just inside the UVJ. Each ureteral orifice should be seen to open during contraction of the ureter. The instrument is withdrawn to the UVJ, and bladder filling proceeds. The patient is asked to hold her urine, squeeze her rectum, strain down, and cough while the bladder is being filled and again when it is full. The UVJ should close with these maneuvers and should gradually close with filling.

When the bladder has reached maximal fullness, the patient is asked to void while the examiner observes the UVJ open and whether or not the urethra funnels if the patient is able to void. She is asked to inhibit voiding and should be able to do so. With the examiner's finger in the vagina, the urethroscope is slowly withdrawn while palpation of the urethra is performed through the anterior vaginal wall. There should be no fixation of tissues or fibrosis, and there should be little or no debris exuding from the periurethral glands or other orifices.

Cystoscopy is performed by insertion of the lubricated cystoscope through the urethral meatus into the bladder. The air bubbles are observed at the 12-o'clock position for orientation. The instrument is then gradually withdrawn, while the areas corresponding to each hour of the clock are observed. Reinsertion to the bladder dome is performed under direct vision after each segment of the bladder is viewed. The trigone is observed last by rotating the instrument upside down. The mucosa should appear smooth and mildly pink. The vascular pattern is prominent but regular, and the trigone is somewhat reddened with a granular pattern.

TABLE 3. *Indications for urethroscopy and cystoscopy*

Condition	Urethroscopy	Cystoscopy
Incontinence	+	+
Recurrent urinary tract infection	+	+
Irritative urinary symptoms	+	+
Diverticulum (urethral or bladder)	+	+
Hematuria	+	+
Fistula	+	+
Interstitial cystitis		+
Intraoperative findings	+	+
Cervical cancer		+

+, indication.

The purposes of urethroscopy are to observe for diverticula, evidence of chronic urethritis, dynamic function of the UVJ, and ureteral function. Cystoscopy is performed to examine the ureters and to rule out foreign body, tumor, infection, and inflammation of the bladder wall. Both examinations give an indication of bladder capacity and, when performed together, are complementary in assessing the anatomic aspects of the urethra and bladder (Table 3).

Cystometry

Cystometry is the pressure–volume relation observed during bladder filling.[1] The CMG test uses carbon dioxide, water, saline solution, or induced diuresis as a filling medium. Pressure is measured by a catheter attached to a vertical fluid column, a pressure transducer, a microtip, or a fiberoptic sensor. The test should be performed in a full sitting or standing position. The patient's bladder is gradually filled with fluid, and the pressure inside the bladder is recorded continuously at filling increments of 50 to 100 ml. A second catheter provides a measure of intraabdominal pressure; this is subtracted from bladder pressure to get true detrusor pressure. Cystometry is indicated to rule out detrusor instability in incontinent patients. Specific indications include patients with symptomatic urinary frequency, urgency, urge incontinence, nocturnal enuresis, and sudden episodes of urine loss. All patients who undergo incontinence surgery should have a preoperative CMG.

During normal filling with carbon dioxide or water, the patient's first sensation of filling is with 50 ml of gas or up to 100 ml of water. A sensation of fullness is experienced with 100 ml of gas and 250 to 350 ml of water. The maximum capacities are 200 to 250 ml of gas and 350 to 550 ml of water. A positive test result is recorded when uninhibited detrusor contractions are observed during bladder filling. The test is more sensitive when performed with the patient standing and with the provocative stimulation of coughing, heel bouncing, or the presence of running water.

The simplest cystometer unit consists of a Foley catheter, three-way stopcock, tubing taped vertically along a 100-cm measuring stick on an intravenous pole, and tubing leading to an infusing medium. The patient is standing, and the zero mark on the measuring stick is placed at the level of the patient's upper symphysis pubis. Fifty milliliters of water or saline solution is infused, and the stopcock switched to measure the height of the water column, which usually is 10 to 15 ml of water and represents intraabdominal pressure. Additional increments of fluid are infused, and repeated pressure measurements are taken until a satisfactory test has been performed and the patient can tolerate no further filling (Fig. 11).

This technique and single-channel pressure recordings with a pressure transducer, microtip, or fiberoptic transducer also do not measure intraabdominal pressure, and false elevations of pressure may be observed from Valsalva activity. During a bladder pressure rise, the patient is asked to inspire to

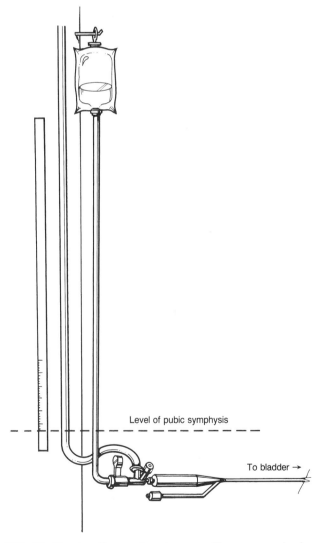

FIG. 11. Simple office cystometrogram. The zero mark of a meter stick is aligned with the upper margin of the patient's symphysis pubis, and a Foley catheter is in place for infusion of fluid. (Adapted from the American College of Obstetricians and Gynecologists, Bent AE, ed. *Urogynecologic evaluation, endoscopy, and urodynamic testing in the symptomatic female.* Washington, DC: ACOG Audiovisual Library, 1990.)

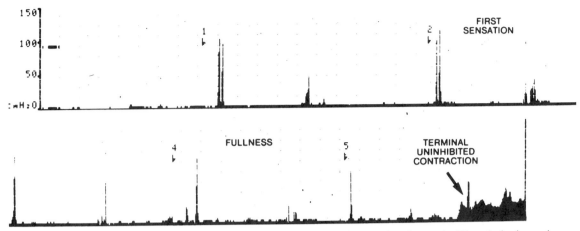

FIG. 12. Single-channel cystometrogram. A pressure rise is observed at the end of the study *(arrow)*, suggesting detrusor instability. The patient's abdomen is palpated to ensure that she is not straining or holding her breath. (From Bent AE. Evaluation of urinary incontinence. In: Hurt WG, ed. *Urogynecologic surgery.* Gaithersburg, MD: Aspen Publishers, 1992:39; with permission.)

remove the effect of raised intraabdominal pressure (Fig. 12). True detrusor pressure readings using intravesical and intraabdominal pressure measurements, performed in the standing position, provide the most sophisticated approach for these measurements. If a detrusor contraction occurs, it is important to determine whether or not the patient can inhibit it.

Urethral Pressure Profiles

Cystourethroscopy assesses the anatomic integrity of the urethra and bladder, and urethral pressure profilometry assesses the function of the urethra. The urethral pressure profile is a record of the pressure along the urethral lumen as a dual-sensor, pressure-sensitive catheter is withdrawn from the bladder through the urethra. The test should be performed in a full sitting or standing position with a full bladder. The urethral pressure is a measure of the urethral wall pressure or the pressure needed to bring the urethral walls together and hold them together against the force of urine in the bladder. Urethral pressure originates from several sources, including urethral smooth muscle, striated muscle of the external sphincter, elastic fibers in the urethral wall, the submucosal vascular plexus, and intraabdominal pressure transmitted to the urethra.

The urethral closure pressure is the pressure in the urethra in excess of the simultaneously measured bladder pressure.[1] Intravesical pressure depends on the amount of fluid in the bladder, detrusor muscle tone, elastic components of the bladder wall, and transmitted intraabdominal pressure. The functional urethral length is a measure of the length of the urethra over which the urethral pressure exceeds the bladder pressure (Fig. 13).

The urodynamic technique recommended for measuring urethral pressure profiles uses microtip transducer catheters attached to a recording device that measures simultaneous urethral and bladder pressure and prints out subtracted (i.e., closure) pressure at the same time (see Fig. 8). It cannot be performed with a single-sensor catheter, since a bladder contraction stimulated by the catheter movement may not be detected. Urethral pressure reflexively decreases during a bladder contraction. The double-transducer catheter is placed into the bladder and withdrawn by a pulley mechanism such that the urethral pressure is measured from the UVJ to the urethral meatus, while the intravesical pressure is constantly measured by a transducer on the end of the catheter. A normal patient has a urethral closure pressure in the range of 40 to 60 cm H_2O and a functional urethral length of 2.5 to 3.5 cm (Fig. 14). A patient with genuine stress incontinence has diminished closure pressure and a urethral functional length that tends to decrease during bladder filling and assuming an upright position. Measurement of these parameters is particularly useful for the evaluation of urinary stress incontinence.

Many investigators recommend urethral pressure profilometry for all patients with stress incontinence. Urethral closure pressure profiles are necessary in patients who have previous failed surgery, continuous incontinence, clinically severe stress incontinence, stress incontinence after age 50 years, genital prolapse with or without incontinence, symptoms without demonstrable urine loss, or actual or suspected urethral diverticula. Pressure profiles are also used to help identify cases of combined genuine stress incontinence and detrusor instability. A subtype of genuine stress incontinence associated with low urethral closure pressure (i.e., intrinsic sphincter deficiency) is associated with failure of standard repairs for stress incontinence. Suspicion of low urethral closure pressure is another reason to obtain urethral closure pressure profiles.

A specific diagnosis of genuine stress incontinence is made after the use of resting and dynamic urethral pressure profilometry. The cough or stress profile provides this dynamic assessment of urethral competency. During coughing, when bladder pressure is greater than the simultaneously measured urethral pressure, the urethral closure pressure is 0. This is called pressure equalization; it establishes the diagnosis of

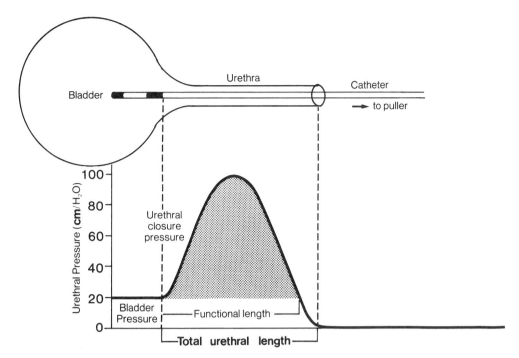

FIG. 13. Urethral closure pressure profile. A dual-sensor catheter is slowly withdrawn from the bladder. The distal sensor measures the bladder pressure constantly, while the proximal sensor measures the urethral pressure. The urethral closure pressure and functional urethral length are shown in the shaded portion of the graph. (From the American College of Obstetricians and Gynecologists, Bent AE, ed. *Urogynecologic evaluation, endoscopy, and urodynamic testing in the symptomatic female.* Washington, DC: ACOG Audiovisual Library, 1990; with permission.)

genuine stress incontinence when it occurs in the absence of detrusor activity (Fig. 15). Urethral and bladder pressures must be measured simultaneously to ensure detection of a detrusor contraction.

An important subcategory of patients are those with severe pelvic relaxation. These patients may initially have very high urethral closure pressures due to a urethral kinking effect due

to the prolapse. After the anatomic defect is reduced by insertion of a pessary, the stress urethral closure pressure profile often demonstrates pressure equalization and indicates a latent or potential genuine stress incontinence that must be corrected during surgery for the prolapse (Fig. 16).

Valsalva Leak-point Pressure

Valsalva leak-point pressure is a recently described test that determines the absolute ability of the urethra to resist expulsive forces transmitted to the bladder as a result of increased intraabdominal pressure.[23] Valsalva leak-point pressure was originally described as a test performed during videourodynamics, equivalent to the lowest intravesical pressure that causes urine to enter the urethra when the patient is asked to valsalva or cough. During multichannel urodynamic evaluation, the Valsalva leak-point pressure corresponds to the lowest intravesical pressure that causes urine leakage from the urethral meatus (Fig. 17). The patient should have a bladder volume of at least 150 ml when performing this test. A Valsalva leak-point pressure less than 65 cm H_2O is considered diagnostic of intrinsic sphincter deficiency, although there remains controversy regarding the test's ability to diagnose intrinsic sphincter deficiency, a poorly defined entity. Furthermore, the test has not yet been standardized in regard to patient positioning, catheter size, bladder fullness, or the effect of significant genital prolapse.

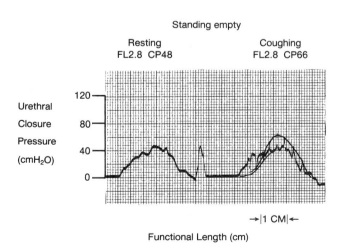

FIG. 14. Normal resting urethral closure pressure profile. During coughing or straining, the pressure may increase, indicating a normal continence mechanism and a competent bladder neck.

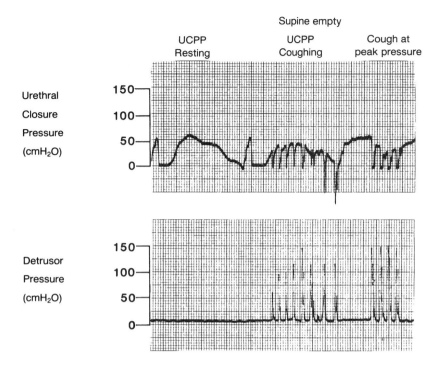

FIG. 15. Genuine stress incontinence. Although the resting profile in this patient appears normal, there is pressure equalization during coughing, while the detrusor pressure remains low.

Radiographic Examination

Several radiographic techniques are used in urogynecology. Plain x-ray films of the pelvis may be required for patients with detrusor instability in whom a neurologic deficit is expected. A congenital abnormality of the sacrum, such as spina bifida occulta or sacral agenesis, may be found. Acquired conditions include spondylolisthesis and intervertebral disc disease.

Intravenous pyelography (IVP) is indicated preoperatively for difficult pelvic surgical procedures and incontinence operations, especially those involving fistula or suspected congenital abnormalities, such as an ectopic ureter. Postoperatively, IVP is used in patients who have unexplained fever or unilateral flank pain suggesting a possible ureteral obstruction.

A voiding cystogram is an x-ray examination of the bladder during voiding. It is useful in determining whether or not vesicoureteral reflux or vesical diverticula are present, and in some cases it may be useful in assessing vesicovaginal fistulas or urethral diverticula.

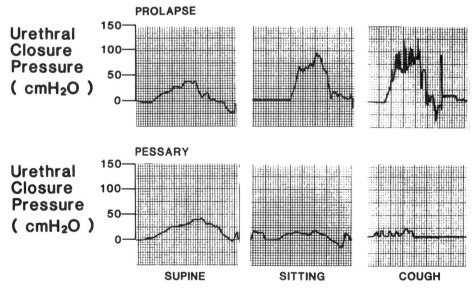

FIG. 16. Effect of pessary placement on urethral closure pressure in a patient with a severe cystocele. (From Richardson DA, Bent AE, Ostergard DR. The effect of uterovaginal prolapse on urethrovesical pressure dynamics. *Am J Obstet Gynecol* 1983;146:902; with permission.)

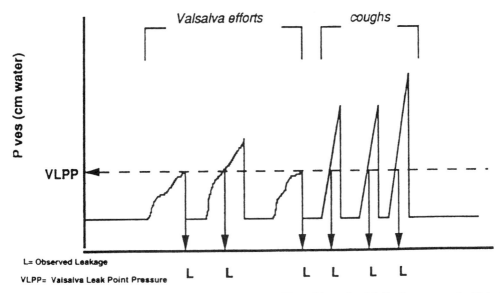

FIG. 17. Performance of a Valsalva leak-point pressure. (From Montella JM. Performance of a Valsalva leak-point pressure. *Am Urogynecol Soc Q Rep* 1994;12:3; with permission.)

A stress cystogram may be used to evaluate the anatomy of the UVJ before incontinence surgery and postoperatively; a chain cystogram is still performed in many centers. This test provides information on the shape, resting position, mobility, and position of the UVJ relative to the rest of the bladder. The posterior urethrovesical angle and angle of inclination are not important in the evaluation of incontinent patients. For this technique, radiopaque dye is placed into the bladder until subjective fullness, and barium paste is used to outline the bladder

base and UVJ. An 8-French (8-Fr) (2.6-mm) pediatric feeding tube or barium paste outlines the urethra. X-ray films and video recordings are taken in the anteroposterior and lateral projections with the patient at rest and while straining. In normal patients, the UVJ is opposite the lower one-third of the posterior aspect of the symphysis pubis, there is no funneling of the proximal urethra, the UVJ descends less than 15 mm during staining compared with the resting position, and the most dependent part of the bladder is not the bladder neck (Fig. 18).

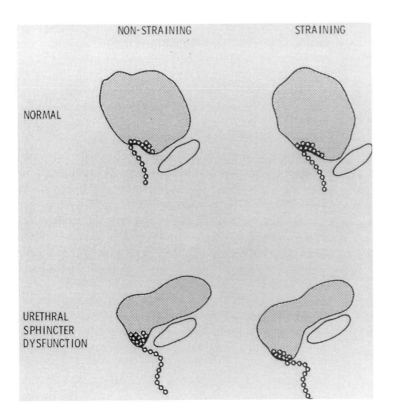

FIG. 18. Bead-chain cystourethrography in a normal patient and in a patient with urethral sphincter dysfunction. (From Hodgkinson CP. Metallic bead chain urethrocystography in preoperative and postoperative evaluation of gynecologic urologic problems. *Clin Obstet Gynecol* 1978;21:725; with permission.)

Videocystourethrography combines a micturating cystogram and fluoroscopic view of the UVJ with simultaneous recordings of intravesical, intraurethral, and intraabdominal pressures and urinary flow rates.

A Tratner catheter study is performed if urethral diverticulum is suspected. A triple-lumen Tratner or Davis catheter is placed into the bladder and maintained in position by inflation of the proximal balloon with 20 ml of air. The distal balloon at the perineum is inflated with 50 ml of air, which maintains this balloon snugly against the urethral meatus. The third channel is used to infuse contrast material by positive pressure into the urethra to outline the diverticulum (Fig. 19).

Ultrasound examination is used in some centers to assess the urethra and bladder base. Ultrasound is useful in cases of genuine stress incontinence, in which mobility of the UVJ may be measured during stress. The UVJ should not move more than 15 mm from a resting to a straining position. Investigators are also putting together ultrasound visualization of the lower urinary tract in conjunction with multichannel urodynamic testing. This combination appears promising, offering simultaneous visual and electronic assessment of

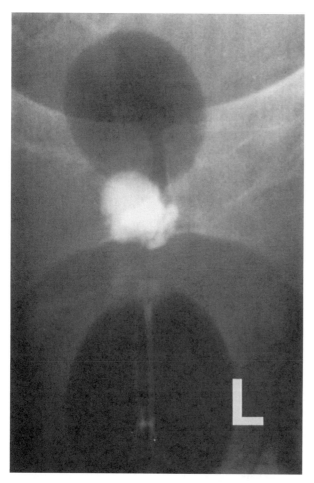

FIG. 19. Urethral diverticulum. The dark circular outlines indicate the proximal and distal air-filled balloons of the Tratner catheter. Contrast material reveals the urethral diverticulum (*L*, left).

function of the lower urinary tract and pelvic floor, similar to videourodynamics, without exposure to radiation or contrast materials.

◊ TREATMENT OF LOWER URINARY TRACT DISORDERS

Urethral Syndrome

The urethral syndrome is a chronic symptom complex consisting of irritative lower urinary tract complaints in the absence of a positive urine culture. Patients complain mostly of dysuria, frequency, and urgency, but they may also experience lower abdominal pressure, dyspareunia, and postvoid fullness. Another commonly used term for this condition is sensory urgency.

Estimates of the frequency of this diagnosis in a premenopausal population or in the general geriatric population have ranged from 5% to 15%. Although several diagnoses may coexist, the usual patient with urethral syndrome has had the condition for several months, has been treated numerous times for supposed cystitis or bladder infections with various responses, is frequently still on antibiotics, is perimenopausal or between 20 and 35 years of age, and complains persistently of frequency and urgency but seldom of incontinence.

The causes of the urethral syndrome include periurethral gland inflammation secondary to infection, trauma, or blocked gland ducts that create a chronic inflammatory response in the urethral mucosa and submucosal tissues. Hypoestrogenism in the perimenopausal or postmenopausal patient creates an atrophic urothelium in the urethra and trigone that is susceptible to chronic inflammation and irritation. The distal urethra is chronically colonized with bacteria, and although urine culture results may be negative, infective foci in the urethra may predispose to symptoms. Functional obstruction may occur as a result of spasticity of smooth muscle in the urethral wall or overactivity of the striated sphincter at midurethra. Recurring traumatic causes include diaphragm use, tampons or other vaginal inserts, and intercourse. Chemical sources include perfumed sanitary napkins, sprays, douches, and topical preparations. Less frequent causes include psychogenic, neurologic, allergic, and anatomic variants, such as urethrohymenal fusion. Excess ingestion of coffee and other caffeine-containing liquids may also aggravate symptoms.

The diagnosis is suggested by a history of chronic or recurrent symptoms associated with a negative urine culture result. There are no specific findings that determine the diagnosis. Vaginitis, vulvitis, acute urethritis, and other local pathologic conditions must be excluded by physical examination and appropriate laboratory testing. Evaluation also includes a residual urine determination, urethral calibration, and a urolog summary. Endoscopy is ideally performed before treatment intervention. Urethroscopy can exclude urethral diverticula, but the finding of acute urethral inflammation with redness and exudate does not necessarily correlate with the presence or severity of urethral syndrome. Cystoscopy can exclude bladder lesions. Urodynamic studies including CMG, urethral closure pressure profiles, and voiding mechanisms may be required to rule out other diagnoses in difficult or resistant cases.

The differential diagnosis includes acute urethritis, urinary tract infection, interstitial cystitis, hypotonic bladder with high residual urine, detrusor instability, urethral diverticulum, vaginal infection, acute and chronic vulvitis, atrophic vaginitis, urethral caruncle, lower urinary tract neoplasm, and severe pelvic relaxation.

The many treatments available indicate the complexity of the condition, and no one therapy suffices for all cases. The initial approach is to supply estrogen to perimenopausal and postmenopausal patients, using one-fourth to one-third of an applicator of a vaginal estrogen cream at bedtime nightly for 2 weeks and then two to three times each week.[13] After 3 months, the dose may be reduced to once or twice per week. In premenopausal patients for whom the main symptoms are urgency and frequency, initial therapy may consist of behavior modification. Patients are asked to keep a 2- or 3-day urolog, while noting the occurrence of their most annoying symptoms. Voiding intervals are established that allow patients to empty the bladder before the onset of symptoms. Intervals of voiding are gradually increased, and patients are encouraged to resist voiding before the assigned time interval. Given the diagnosis of a disorder, patients are encouraged during follow-up visits to alter their behavior to overcome the symptoms. This type of sensate defocus can be effective if other pathology is excluded and patients realize that they can modify the symptoms. Sometimes, patients do well when referred to a somatic symptoms clinic, where a multidisciplinary approach is used for diagnosis and management. Amitriptyline, 25 to 75 mg one to two times a day, may also assist patients in defocusing their attention to symptoms from the urethral area.

A second line of therapy, more frequently used if there is dysuria or pyuria, is chronic antibacterial therapy with nitrofurantoin, 50 mg per day, or trimethoprim/sulfamethoxazole (TMP/SMX), 400 mg/80 mg per day, for 3 to 6 months. Doxycycline, 100 mg twice daily for 2 to 4 weeks, can be used if hard-to-diagnose chlamydial, ureaplasmal, or mycoplasmal urethritis is considered in the differential diagnosis.

Urethral dilation, formerly used as initial therapy for premenopausal patients and with estrogen for older patients, is used less often as first-line treatment. Although there are no studies to indicate permanent adverse effects from urethral dilation, it is viewed by many as an invasive form of therapy, in which the beneficial effects may possibly be more related to the contact with the therapist and a positive reinforcement of active treatment for a prolonged, disabling condition. Urethral dilators or sounds from 24-Fr (8 mm) to 38-Fr (12.5 mm) are used in most cases, although a set with sizes from 12-Fr (4 mm) to 26-Fr (8.6 mm) should be available for patients with meatal stenosis. The urethra is cleaned and copious lidocaine jelly is injected into the urethral lumen and applied to the dilators, which are gently passed serially through the urethra, while the urethra is thoroughly massaged through the anterior vaginal wall to promote drainage of chronically obstructed periurethral glands. Patients usually tolerate the discomfort well, although a pillar block using 5 ml of lidocaine 1% may be administered submucosally at the 2-o'clock and 10-o'clock positions at the cervicovaginal junction or at the 4-o'clock and 8-o'clock positions at the UVJ if the uterus has been surgically removed. Treatments are repeated at 2- to 3-week intervals for two or three dilations. The response rate is 60% to 80% for these methods.

Patients for whom urethral dilation fails, especially those with dysuria or localized pain, may be treated by periurethral steroid injection, which is effective for 60% to 80% of patients. Functional obstruction from urethral spasm may be treated with a combination of diazepam, 2 mg two to four times daily, and prazosin, 1 to 2 mg two to three times daily. Selected patients benefit from urethroplasty, which is performed as an outpatient surgical procedure. Scar tissue in the urethrovaginal septum is incised or excised, with a cure rate in the range of 60% to 80%.

The frustration in treating urethral syndrome is that relapses frequently occur after therapeutic interventions. Physicians must provide periodic assessment, reevaluation for relapses, and encouragement to patients. Treatment, if not cure, is available for this annoying condition. Patients whose symptoms are understood and not passed off lightly will be forever grateful for planned therapeutic intervention.

Fistula

A fistula is an abnormal passageway between two body areas (e.g., cavities) normally separated by a tissue barrier. In urogynecology, fistulas are usually ureterovaginal, vesicovaginal, or urethrovaginal, although rare types, such as vesicouterine fistula, do exist. Patients complain of a constant urinary drainage that begins several days after hysterectomy, other pelvic surgery, or obstetric delivery.

Fistulas are uncommon, although postobstetric fistulas occur commonly in women in underdeveloped countries. In developed countries, hysterectomy is the most common cause. A ureterovaginal fistula may follow radical hysterectomy. Vaginal hysterectomy is less commonly associated with this fistula, although it occurs when the uterosacral-cardinal pedicle and uterine vessels are clamped without adequate mobilization of the bladder. A vesicovaginal fistula occurs after vaginal cuff closure if the bladder flap was not adequately mobilized from the anterior vaginal wall. Urethrovaginal fistula usually follows diverticulum repair, trauma, or other anterior vaginal surgery. The incidence of posthysterectomy fistula is less than 1%, but in some series urethrovaginal fistula may occur in as many as 5% to 10% of patients after diverticulum repair. A congenitally ectopic ureter may empty anywhere along the lower genital tract, including the bladder, vagina, or urethra. Other forms of congenital fistula are obvious at birth. Factors that promote poor healing and possible fistula formation include prior radiation therapy, impaired vascular supply, and general debilitation. Most other causes of incontinence are not preceded by surgery, and few patients have continuous incontinence. Severe genuine stress incontinence or detrusor instability requires diagnostic exclusion.

The physical examination after hysterectomy may reveal a vesicovaginal fistula with urine escaping just anterior to the healed vaginal cuff. If a suspected defect is not seen, the first diagnostic test is to instill methylene blue into the bladder, place a tampon into the vagina, and have the patient walk around. Blue dye on the superior aspect of the tampon indicates a vesicovaginal fistula. On cystoscopy, a posthysterectomy vesicovaginal fistula is usually found located above the trigone between the ureters.

If a ureterovaginal fistula is suspected and the methylene blue test result is negative, indigo carmine is injected intravenously or phenazopyridine given orally, a fresh tampon is placed into the vagina, and the patient again walks around the room. Dye on the superior aspect of the tampon suggests a ureterovaginal fistula. Confirmatory tests include endoscopy and IVP.

If the diagnosis is still uncertain, water is placed into the vagina with the patient in the knee-chest position. While the vaginal cuff site is viewed with a urethroscope, carbon dioxide is infused into the bladder through a catheter. Bubbles of carbon dioxide should be seen escaping through the vaginal site of the vesicovaginal fistula. A urethrovaginal fistula may be seen on direct inspection or by passing a catheter through the urethra into the bladder and palpating along the catheter. If this approach is unsuccessful, urethroscopy is performed. Seldom is urethrography required for documentation of this type of fistula.

A ureterovaginal fistula requires an abdominal approach to dissect and isolate the segment of involved ureter, followed by implantation directly into the bladder. In less favorable instances in which the site of the defect is more proximal, ureteroureteric anastomosis or a Boari flap and psoas hitch may be required. In acute cases, edema and hemorrhage can obscure tissue planes. Some fistulas occur after obstruction and decreased vascularity, which may cause renal impairment on the affected side.

A vesicovaginal fistula that follows hysterectomy should initially be placed at rest by insertion of a suprapubic catheter and observation at 2-week intervals for as long as 6 weeks. Spontaneous healing occurs in 20% of these patients, and even large defects become much smaller. If healing is complete, surgical repair may not be required. However, if a defect persists, the Latzko technique may be necessary. At this point, the tissues have minimal or no infectious or inflammatory residual. A pediatric Foley catheter is placed through the vaginal defect, if possible, and traction sutures are placed outside the fistula margins. The vaginal mucosa is injected with a vasoconstrictor agent, and the vaginal epithelium is removed to form a horizontal oval with 2-cm margins around the defect. The tissue is closed in three or more layers with polyglycolic acid sutures, with the last layer through the vaginal epithelium. In this manner, the vaginal tissue is invaginated into the bladder defect to form the new bladder wall. A suprapubic catheter is placed for 7 to 14 days.

Traditional fistula closure is performed by mobilization of tissues around the fistula, excision of the fistula tract, and closure without tension. The Latzko technique allows early closure of the defect and does not necessitate extensive mobilization or excision of the fistulous tract. It also involves less dissection with less risk for hematoma formation. Abdominal fistula repair is reserved for a large fistula that involves portions of a ureter, for repeated failure after the vaginal approach, and for operations after devitalizing procedures such as radiation therapy. An omental patch is mobilized and sutured between the vagina and the bladder wall; this approach usually allows a greater than 90% complete healing of the defect.

A urethrovaginal fistula is closed by dissection, tissue mobilization, and suturing of the defect without tension over a urethral catheter. A Martius fat pad is developed and sutured between the urethra and vaginal epithelium. Most of these repairs carry a success rate of approximately 80% to 90%. Fistula repair requires clean tissues, good hemostasis, closure without tension, and postoperative bladder drainage.

Diverticula

A urethral diverticulum is an outpouching of tissue from the lumen of the urethra that forms a sac-like structure, usually arising from a blocked periurethral gland duct. Many urethral diverticula are asymptomatic, but frequently symptoms include recurrent urinary tract infections, dysuria, frequency, urgency, postvoid urinary incontinence, and pain over the urethra during intercourse.

The incidence of urethral diverticulum is difficult to evaluate but is less than 1%. Although some diverticula are congenital, most form secondarily to periurethral gland duct blockage with subsequent gland enlargement and then reopening of a small channel into the urethra. Urethral diverticulum should be ruled out as a cause for many other lower urinary tract diagnoses, especially for urethral syndrome, recurrent urinary tract infection of unknown cause, and benign periurethrovaginal cysts.

The classic clinical finding is a suburethral, tender swelling that exudes pus from the urethral meatus on manual compression. Urethroscopy using carbon dioxide or saline solution is used to see the diverticular opening and observe pus or urine escaping from the diverticular orifice. Frequently, more than one diverticulum exists. Positive-pressure urethrography is performed using a Tratner or Davis catheter, as described previously (see Fig. 19). An approximate location of the diverticulum is obtained. This is physiologically confirmed by urethral closure pressure profilometry, which localizes the diverticulum as proximal or distal to the peak urethral closure pressure (Fig. 20).

Some diverticula are totally asymptomatic with negative urine culture results, and these require no treatment. Acute

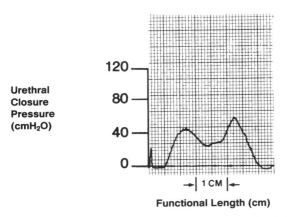

FIG. 20. Urethral diverticulum. The drop in the urethral closure pressure indicates the location of a diverticulum in relation to the peak pressure. Because the diverticular opening is proximal to the area of maximal urethral closing pressure, a Spence procedure should not be performed in this patient.

inflammation of a diverticulum has been treated with aspiration of the pus within the gland and urethral dilation and massage. In general, one of two surgical methods is used. If the diverticular opening is distal to maximal urethral closure pressure, a Spence procedure is performed. Scissors are placed with one blade in the urethra up to the diverticulum and the other blade into the vagina. The scissors are closed to divide the urethrovaginal septum, and a running locked suture is used to provide hemostasis. No hospitalization or catheter is required. Cure rates are more than 90%, and there are few complications. If the diverticulum is proximal to peak urethral closure pressure, direct dissection is carried out until the diverticulum can be excised, with care taken to save enough of its wall to aid in transverse closure of the urethral defect without tension over the catheter. A three-layer closure is performed to provide adequate protection during healing. Surgical success is high, but there is a 20% complication rate, including stricture and fistula.

Lower Urinary Tract Infection

Lower urinary tract infection is generally defined as a bacterial inflammation of urothelium in the bladder or urethra characterized by irritative urinary tract symptoms. For the bladder, a growth of 10^5 colonies/ml from a midstream urine culture on two occasions or 1000 colonies/ml on a catheterized specimen is considered significant growth.[8]

The traditional symptoms of a lower urinary tract infection (i.e., cystitis) are urinary frequency, dysuria, and urgency. Less common symptoms include suprapubic pain and hematuria. The infection may be asymptomatic. Asymptomatic bacteriuria (i.e., significant growth of bacteria without symptoms) occurs in 1% of preschool-age children, 5% of reproductive-age women, and 10% of postmenopausal women. Many women have had at least one bladder infection, and 20% may have more than one infection in a lifetime.

There are two other classifications of urinary tract infections. Unresolved bacteriuria during therapy means persistent infection despite antibiotic therapy. Recurrent bacteriuria refers to reinfection immediately after treatment of the original infection. There are numerous pathways for infection in the lower urinary tract. The outer one-third of the urethra is always colonized with bowel flora, and the short length of the female urethra predisposes to bladder colonization. Intercourse and use of diaphragms cause minor trauma to the urethra and help move organisms into the bladder, hence the term "honeymoon" cystitis.

Atrophic vaginitis secondary to estrogen deficiency allows pathogenic bacteria to grow more readily in the vagina, and atrophic urothelium predisposes to decreased urethral resistance. Infrequent voiders are subject to bladder wall ischemia, and infrequent bladder emptying allows the bacterial inoculum within the bladder to multiply to the point of causing infection. Altered bladder mucosal elements prevent the normal destruction of bacteria in the bladder, while infected calculi continually shower the urinary tract with bacteria. Patients with diabetes mellitus have poor resistance to recurrent infection, and increased urine glucose may provide a rich medium for bacterial proliferation. Structural disorders, such as urethrohymenal fusion, vesicoureteral reflux, and congenital anatomic defects of the urinary tract, lead to infections and recurrent infections.

The infecting organism is *Escherichia coli* in 80% of cases; less commonly found organisms include *Staphylococcus saprophyticus*, *Klebsiella*, and *Enterobacter aerogenes*. *Proteus* organisms revealed by culture suggest the presence of struvite stones. *Pseudomonas* organisms are uncommon but occur with prolonged catheterization, repeated treatment for other pathogens, and nosocomial infections.

The differential diagnosis includes acute urethritis, urethral syndrome, pyelonephritis, urethral diverticulum, and interstitial cystitis. An initial urinary tract infection is frequently diagnosed by one midstream urine culture showing more than 100,000 organisms/ml in a pure growth. The confidence level is only 85%, even with two such cultures, but patients are usually treated based on the characteristic symptoms and a single positive culture result. A presumptive diagnosis in a symptomatic patient may also be made, before the culture results are received, by a urinalysis that reveals bacteria, erythrocytes, or a positive nitrite chemistry test result. Recurrent or persistent cases should have catheterized urine sent for culture and sensitivity.

Physicians should confirm urinary pathogens before treatment. Many patients have been inadequately or inappropriately treated on the basis of symptoms alone. Other than upper respiratory tract viral infections, urethral syndrome prompts the administration of more unnecessary antibiotics than most other conditions. Patients who do not have resolution of an infection, those with a *Proteus* infection, and those with frequent recurrent infections require repeat urine culture and sensitivity tests, intravenous urography or renal ultrasonography, and endoscopy.

An isolated infection in an acutely symptomatic patient who cannot wait for a confirmatory culture and sensitivity report may be treated with one of several regimens: (1) TMP/SMX, three double-strength tablets, or ampicillin, 3 g orally, in one dose; (2) TMP/SMX, one double-strength tablet twice daily for 5 days, or ampicillin, 250 mg four times daily for 5 days; (3) nitrofurantoin, 100 mg four times daily for 4 days and then 50 mg four times daily for 4 days; (4) sulfisoxazole (Gantrisin), 500 mg per day for 7 days; and (5) (uncommon) gentamicin, 80 mg intramuscularly in one dose. Advantages to shorter courses of therapy include increased compliance, fewer side effects, and decreased cost. Three-day antibiotic regimes appear to be optimal, with equivalent efficacy rates to most 7-day regimes.[14] Single-dose therapy should only be used in patients who experience isolated urinary tract infections and are considered to be at low risk for relapse because single-dose therapy has a significantly higher treatment failure rate, compared to longer antibiotic regimens. Single-dose or short-course therapy should not be prescribed to the elderly, patients with a past history of recurrent, chronic or persistent infections, or patients who are diabetic or pregnant or have a renal tract abnormality. Too many patients are treated with ampicillin, to which many strains of *E. coli* are now resistant. Tetracyclines have no place in therapy for most urinary tract infections, and cephalosporins are effective but expensive.

Resistant or recurrent infections demand repeat culture and sensitivity testing and other appropriate evaluation. Depending on the sensitivities, the usual antibiotics used are TMP/SMX or a cephalosporin. The fluoroquinolones have a good spectrum of activity even against organisms such as *Proteus* species, some *Klebsiella* strains, and *Pseudomonas* species. Intramuscular therapy or intravenous therapy on an inpatient or outpatient basis is seldom required.

Patients who have recurrent urinary tract infections with common pathogens three or more times in a year should be placed on postcoital prophylaxis or continuous prophylaxis for 3 to 6 months. Nitrofurantoin, 50 mg daily at suppertime for 6 months, or TMP/SMX, one regular-strength tablet, is recommended. Postcoital prophylaxis is best used in patients who can clearly associate their urinary tract infections with intercourse. Nitrofurantoin has only a 2% incidence of resistant strains developing during prophylaxis, and the medication is not absorbed into the gastrointestinal tract. Its minor alterations in bowel or vaginal flora do not produce resistant strains. However, a rare idiosyncratic reaction causing pulmonary fibrosis prohibits its long-term administration. TMP/SMX has a 9% incidence of resistant strains developing.

During pregnancy, certain antibiotics with known or unknown effects should be avoided. These include tetracyclines and sulfa drugs in the last months of pregnancy. The usual recommendation is nitrofurantoin, ampicillin, or a cephalosporin.

Adjunctive therapy for urinary tract infection includes hydration to allow flushing of the bladder and a urinary analgesic such as phenazopyridine. Perineal hygiene and adequate bladder emptying, especially after intercourse, are necessary to prevent recurrences.

Interstitial Cystitis

Interstitial cystitis is a chronic inflammation of all layers of the bladder wall. Patients present with incapacitating suprapubic pain and urgency with bladder filling and with urinary frequency and nocturia to keep the bladder empty. Infrequently does incontinence pose a problem.

The incidence of interstitial cystitis is 1 in 350 persons, with women affected ten times more often than men. The disorder predominantly affects those between 40 and 60 years of age, although it is found in women of all ages. Although many theories have been proposed, the cause of interstitial cystitis remains unexplained. No specific pathogen has been found to date, and pathologic diagnosis is inconsistent. There is some evidence to support an autoimmune or an allergic process. Current investigation also suggests the possible alteration in the surface layer of glycosaminoglycans allowing noxious agents in the urine to contact the bladder mucosa. At various times, tissue examination reveals epithelial denudation, subepithelial edema and capillary dilatation, and edema and inflammation of the muscularis. These pathologic tissue findings are nonspecific and do not allow a diagnosis based on bladder biopsy.

The diagnosis is based on clinical symptoms in association with specific cystoscopic findings. The classic Hunner ulcers appear as a pale mucosa with linear scars that split on bladder distention to form zigzag bleeding fissures. Less severe findings in persons with a normal or reduced bladder capacity include discrete generalized submucosal hemorrhages. When suspicion is strong enough but the usual findings are not seen during cystoscopy under local anesthesia, patients must undergo cystoscopy under general anesthesia. Urodynamics may show decreased accommodation during cystometry (Fig. 21). Carcinoma *in situ* of the bladder must be differentiated by bladder biopsies. Other diagnoses are rare but include tuberculosis, schistosomiasis, and radiation cystitis.

Traditional therapy frequently occurs during diagnosis under general anesthesia when the bladder is overdistended with fluid. This is thought to impair neural pathways and detrusor muscle stretch receptors, resulting in increased bladder capacity that may last for 3 to 6 months. Therapeutic prolonged bladder distention is performed under epidural blockade as well. Instillation of dimethyl sulfoxide 50% (DMSO) or a 1:2000 silver nitrate solution at 1- to 2-week intervals provides relief for 60% to 80% of patients after 3 to 6 weeks. Steroids, heparin, diphenhydramine, lidocaine, and sodium bicarbonate have been combined with DMSO for instillation and may improve the response rates. Some patients respond to transcutaneous electrical nerve stimulation therapy or amitriptyline, 75 mg at bedtime. There are ongoing studies evaluating the efficacy of Elmiron as an instillation and an oral agent. Heparin has also been used in a subcutaneous injection two or three times per week, during which time the patient must be followed for bleeding diathesis. Other substances under investigation include cimetidine, hyaluronic acid, hydroxyzine, nifedipine, and BCG vaccine.[22]

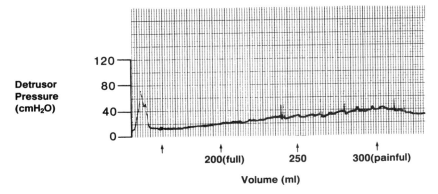

Impaired Bladder Compliance

FIG. 21. Interstitial cystitis. During bladder filling, the patient experiences pain and a feeling of fullness, which occur well before the normal expected bladder capacity of 400 to 500 ml. The detrusor pressure rises rapidly because of impaired bladder wall compliance.

Dietary therapy, with avoidance of irritative food substances, can ameliorate symptoms. Specific substances that commonly aggravate the bladder include caffeine, alcohol, chocolate, and spicy or acidic foods. Patients are also assisted in dealing with their chronic condition by self-help groups, regular exercise, and stress reduction techniques.

If the described measures fail, the next step may be neodymium : yttrium-aluminum-garnet (Nd:YAG) laser therapy for the bladder mucosal lining, which benefits some patients. Although relapses may occur, retreatment can be carried out. Surgical procedures are reserved for the most resistant conditions and include selective sacral neurectomy, inferior hypogastric nerve resection, cystoplasty, cystolysis, and bladder augmentation procedures. Many patients who suffer severe disability may be significantly improved by noninvasive techniques and function adequately in their environment.

Detrusor Instability

Detrusor instability or unstable bladder is the occurrence of involuntary, uninhibited bladder contractions that are usually associated with urine loss or urinary urgency. The main complaints of patients with detrusor instability are frequency, urgency, nocturia, and sudden urine loss with or without urgency. Patients usually state that episodes of incontinence occur with little warning and frequently cause soaking of the clothing. Some patients wear protection at all times, and some have nocturnal enuresis.

All infants have unstable bladders, and toilet training involves the training of neural pathways and reflexes that allow the bladder to store urine and permit urine emptying in a controlled manner at appropriate intervals. Approximately 5% of premenopausal patients have detrusor instability; this number increases steadily with aging up to 15% to 20% in the ambulatory adult female population and even higher among the institutionalized elderly.

The main causes of detrusor instability are idiopathic, cerebrovascular insufficiency, outflow obstruction, local irritation or infection, and psychosomatic or psychogenic conditions. If upper motor neuron disease exists, the disorder is called detrusor hyperreflexia. "Neurogenic bladder" is a term that should be avoided. In the elderly population, most cases are caused by cerebrovascular insufficiency with ischemic interruption of essential neural pathways. Premenopausal patients usually do not have a specific cause identified and constitute most of the idiopathic group. Outflow obstruction in women may be related to postsurgical events, typically overcorrection of UVJ support, or to learned patterns of functional obstruction. Local irritants include foreign bodies, renal calculus, and trauma. Psychogenic causes may be uncovered after other possibilities are excluded. Few conditions cause the inconvenience and social interruption that these patients experience.

The differential diagnosis includes severe genuine stress incontinence, fistula, interstitial cystitis, severe urinary tract infection, and severe urethral syndrome. In addition to history, the analysis of a 24-hour voiding diary can alert physicians to the possibility of detrusor instability. A urine culture is obtained to rule out cystitis. The diagnosis is made by CMG, preferably performed in the standing position with the provocative measures of cough, heel bounce, and the sound of running water. Uninhibited involuntary detrusor contractions during controlled bladder filling establish the diagnosis (Fig. 22).

Treatment measures include behavioral therapy, biofeedback, functional electrical stimulation, medications, surgery, psychological counseling, and an indwelling catheter. Behavioral therapy is a bladder-retraining program to allow patients to regain cortical control over detrusor activity. Toilet training in infants involves learned cortical inhibition of reflex bladder emptying. Through operant learning, the developing child learns to inhibit detrusor contractions and to contract or relax the urethral striated muscle. Idiopathic detrusor instability develops when a person loses this control in the absence of a diagnosed neurologic deficit. Patients are assigned a voiding interval that is compatible with their current voiding pattern according to their urolog and are asked to void regularly, whether or not they have a desire; urges to void at other times are ignored. The patient must adhere to this schedule during waking hours. The voiding interval is increased weekly or every 2 weeks until a satisfactory interval is achieved. The success rate is 60% to 80% and depends on weekly or biweekly contact with the therapist.

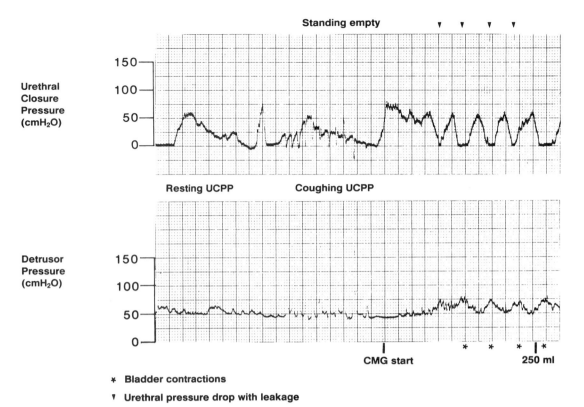

* **Bladder contractions**
▼ **Urethral pressure drop with leakage**

FIG. 22. Detrusor instability. This patient has pressure equalization with coughing. During bladder filling, regular bladder contractions occur with coincident urethral relaxation, followed by urinary leakage. The patient cannot inhibit the activity of an unstable bladder.

Biofeedback is a type of bladder training performed in a laboratory setting by inserting a pressure recording line into the bladder and providing the patient with a visual and an auditory signal when bladder pressure increases with filling. Patients attempt to retrain themselves by muscle-relaxing exercises to reduce pen deflection on the screen and reduce the noise signal. Weekly sessions are followed by practice at home to decrease undesired voiding urges. The success rate for this therapy has been 50%, but the method is therapist-intensive.

Functional electrical stimulation uses a vaginal probe connected to a battery-generated intermittent electrical impulse, which stimulates and reorganizes neural impulses to the detrusor muscle. Sessions are performed at home for 15 minutes twice daily over a 6- to 12-week period; 60% of patients report improvement or cure. Treatment can also be carried out in the office setting weekly using acute maximal electrical stimulation for 6 to 10 weeks.

Medications to control detrusor instability are anticholinergic or antispasmodic preparations. These include oxybutynin, 5 mg two to four times per day; dicyclomine, 10 to 20 mg two to four times per day; flavoxate, 200 mg two to four times per day; and imipramine, 25 to 75 mg once or twice daily. Patients with neurologic deficits may do poorly with behavioral therapy, but if it is combined with medication, they can frequently adhere to the scheduled voiding intervals. Drug therapy alone has a response rate of 60%.

Surgical measures are reserved for severely affected patients in good medical health who have not responded to conservative measures. Procedures include partial denervation of the hypogastric nerve plexus, implantation of sacral root–stimulating electrodes, cryoneurolysis of sacral nerve roots, transection of the bladder neck, and, in some cases, urinary diversion.

Some patients require psychological counseling and, through therapy, may uncover unsuspected triggers for loss of urinary control. Other patients may be better able to cope with their problem without achieving a complete cure. Occasionally, elderly institutionalized patients who have not been controlled by fluid restriction, caffeine reduction, regular toileting at 2-hour intervals, and frequent pad changing may be controlled by continuous bladder drainage.

Patients may not be completely cured by one or a combination of treatments, but the approach is one of genuine concern in understanding the problem associated with an acceptable plan of therapy that can at least provide a satisfactory level of functioning. Reassessment should be ongoing, and other problems should be managed concurrently to reduce adverse influences.

Stress Incontinence

Genuine stress incontinence is the socially unacceptable, involuntary loss of urine associated with increased intra-abdominal pressure in the absence of detrusor activity. Stress incontinence is a symptom that describes loss of urine during physical exertion (e.g., cough, aerobics, lifting, running). It is also a sign elicited by physicians that denotes loss of urine from the urethra associated with sudden cough or strain.

The incidence of genuine stress incontinence is less than 10% among reproductive-age women but may approach 10% to 20% among postmenopausal patients. Factors that promote the development of stress incontinence include congenital defects in structure or tissue, trauma secondary to childbearing, aging (including estrogen deficiency), obesity, chronic coughing, and iatrogenic causes. Pelvic floor denervation secondary to childbirth and aging are the primary causes.

The pathophysiology of stress incontinence includes defects in one or more of three continence-maintaining mechanisms. First, the internal urethral sphincteric mechanism consists of the urethral epithelial lining, submucosal elastic and connective tissues, submucosal venous plexus, and urethral smooth musculature. This sphincter maintains a resistance to urine passage from the bladder by coaptation of mucosal surfaces, compressibility of elastic tissues, and urethral muscular tonicity. Second, the striated muscle component of the external urethral sphincter has fast-twitch fibers that respond immediately to increased intraabdominal pressure and slow-twitch fibers that help maintain chronic tone. Specific exercises may strengthen this muscle. Third, fascial and muscular supports maintain the proximal urethra in its normal intraabdominal location such that increased intraabdominal pressure may be transmitted equally to the bladder and urethra and ensure continence during physical exertion.

Causative factors affect one or more of the components that maintain continence. Iatrogenic causes include local vaginal surgery and surgeries that destroy and scar components of the internal urethral mechanism. Other surgeries or repairs may alter support structures at the UVJ. In procidentia or severe cystocele, correcting the defect may cause stress incontinence.

The differential diagnosis includes detrusor instability, urethral diverticulum, ectopic ureter, fistula, and overflow incontinence. Diagnostic techniques include detailed history and physical examination to rule out other local defects. Residual urine determination, urine culture, Q-tip test, and demonstration of urine loss with stress are part of these simpler measures. Detrusor instability must be excluded by history, urolog analysis, and a standing CMG. In patients younger than 50 years, urethral closure pressure profiles are not required, but they are suggested if surgery is contemplated. Urethral closure pressure profilometry is recommended for patients older than 50 years or those with severe or continued incontinence, prior failed retropubic surgery, stress incontinence not demonstrable in the laboratory, or no anatomic defect. The examiner must rule out intrinsic sphincter deficiency, which may predispose to the failure of standard surgical procedures. Intrinsic sphincter deficiency is diagnosed by demonstration of a poorly functioning urethra. Contributing factors include low urethral closure pressure, bladder neck immobility, scarred vaginal tissue, prior failed surgery, and prior pelvic irradiation. Proximal urethral function and bladder neck mobility may be observed fluoroscopically or during urethroscopy, ultrasound, or videocystourethrography.

Medical Treatment of Stress Incontinence

Treatment of stress incontinence may be directed toward the three components that normally maintain continence during the course of increased intraabdominal pressure. Topical estrogen therapy improves urothelium, submucosal vascularity, and submucosal elastic tissues. Postmenopausal patients with mild stress incontinence may have complete relief after using one-fourth to one-third of an applicator of a vaginal estrogen cream three times a week for 6 to 12 weeks. α-Adrenergic stimulators, such as phenylpropanolamine, 25 to 150 mg per day, or imipramine, 25 to 150 mg per day, increase the tone of smooth muscle and may improve mild to moderate stress incontinence.

Pelvic floor exercises, with or without the aid of a perineometer or biofeedback, and functional electrical stimulation are designed to improve the voluntary external urethral sphincter by contracting the pubococcygeus muscle.[6] Patients must be instructed to perform the exercise correctly. During the hold or squeeze command, the exercise should compress a vaginal finger or a perineometer without an increase in intraabdominal pressure. Pelvic floor muscles are contracted maximally for 10 to 12 seconds and released for 15 seconds. Fifteen repetitions are performed one to three times daily. A therapist is required for proper instruction and follow-up to achieve maximal benefit (Table 4).[7] Functional electrical stimulation is delivered through a vaginal probe for 15 minutes twice daily. Improvement occurs in 40% to 50% of patients with either treatment protocol and is usually seen within 6 weeks of initiating therapy.

Surgical measures are intended to resupport the UVJ in its normal intraabdominal position to allow equal transmission of increased intraabdominal pressure to the bladder and the proximal urethra. The primary surgical approach is reserved for failures of medical therapy.

Surgical Treatment of Stress Incontinence

Many surgical procedures have been advocated for the treatment of genuine stress incontinence, ranging from a simple bladder neck elevation procedure performed entirely vaginally to an abdominal approach with the procedure accomplished entirely through the retropubic space. In recent years, laparoscopic procedures for bladder neck suspension have been developed. Various combinations of procedures have been reported, including the use of artificial materials to support

---

TABLE 4. *Basics of pelvic floor muscle training*

Repetition: graded activity to a desired maximum
Regular program: every other day or three times each week for 3 to 6 mo
Maximum intensity: squeeze pelvic floor muscles for 12 sec and relax for 15 sec (i.e., use resistance training)
Maintenance program: 15 repetitions performed one to three times each day
Follow-up: written record and weekly or biweekly visits to a therapist, who evaluates success

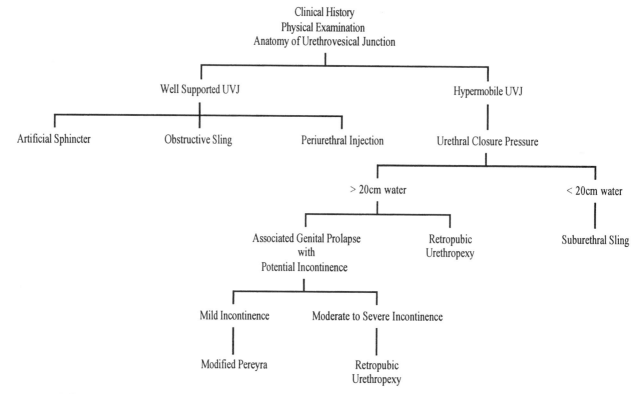

FIG. 23. Objective selection of surgical procedures for genuine stress incontinence. This schema can assist in selecting the appropriate surgical procedure for stress incontinence based on urethral pressure and the presence or absence of hypermobility of the urethrovesical junction.

the UVJ. Artificial sphincters may provide continence by entirely mechanical means. Given the variety of procedures available to the practicing gynecologist to treat genuine stress incontinence, selection of the appropriate procedure for each individual patient is important to ensure operative success and patient satisfaction (Fig. 23). The following discussion reviews the more commonly employed surgical procedures for genuine stress incontinence, and their relative merits.

Vaginal Approach

Anterior vaginal repair was originally described by Howard Kelly in 1914. This approach begins with a dissection of the anterior vaginal wall, separating the vaginal wall from the bladder and the proximal urethra (Fig. 24). Plication sutures are placed at the base of the UVJ, and an attempt is made to support the UVJ by pushing it upward with these plication sutures. This procedure is gradually being abandoned by gynecologic surgeons, because it does not provide long-term results that are as good as a retropubic urethropexy or suburethral sling procedure.

A review of the medical literature demonstrates successful outcomes in most series of only 50% to 60% at 2 years after surgery. Few studies compared this approach with other techniques in a systematic, prospective manner. One study found that the objective cure rate as determined by postoperative urodynamic studies was 73% if the abdominal route was chosen

and only 40% if the vaginal route was chosen.[4] Most urogynecologists do not choose a primary vaginal approach of the anterior repair type for treatment of genuine stress incontinence.

Retropubic Urethropexy

When a patient's urethral closure pressure is greater than 20 cm H_2O and an anatomic defect of the UVJ of greater than 30 degrees can be demonstrated with a Q-tip test, the retropubic approach is chosen. The retropubic approach provides the greatest chance of success in a consistent manner in these patients.

The surgical procedure begins with a standard entry into the retropubic space through a vertical lower abdominal incision or a Pfannenstiel incision. The muscle bellies are split in the midline, and the retropubic space is entered. The operating surgeon must visualize the entire paravaginal retropubic space to approach the vaginal wall and the site of suture placement in a safe manner. Using a retractor, the surgeon moves the bladder superiorly and views the retropubic space. Traction on the previously placed Foley catheter demonstrates the location of the balloon at the UVJ. This is an important anatomic landmark, because dissection above the level of the UVJ will injure the bladder or the ureters.

The operating surgeon places two fingers of the nondominant hand into the vagina to elevate the vaginal wall. This vaginal wall is cleared of all overlying fatty tissue, and the

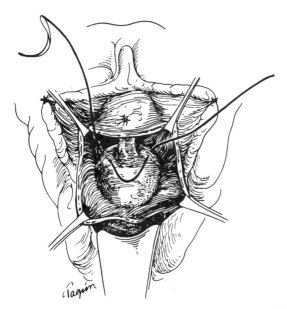

FIG. 24. Classic anterior vaginal repair. After dissection of the anterior vaginal wall from the paravesical adventitia, plication sutures are placed under the urethrovesical junction in an attempt to elevate it. (From Green TH Jr. Urinary stress incontinence, differential diagnosis, pathophysiology, and management. *Am J Obstet Gynecol* 1975;122:368; with permission.)

bladder is moved away from this area superiorly. The operating surgeon must avoid the large venous plexus that is usually in this area. The base of the bladder is marked by a large vein coursing along its lower border. This is commonly injured during this dissection, and care must be taken to adequately control any bleeding that may ensue. After the bladder has been mobilized, the shiny vaginal wall can be seen; it is unmistakable and cannot be confused with the muscular tissue of the bladder wall.

There are two major retropubic urethropexy procedures: the Burch operation and the Marshall-Marchetti-Krantz operation.

In the Burch retropubic urethropexy procedure, the surgeon further identifies the entire paravaginal space and removes all fat from a site approximately 2 cm lateral to the urethra, where the sutures will be placed, down the vaginal wall to the pelvic floor and up the pelvic side wall. All this fatty tissue must be removed to allow adequate adherence of the vaginal wall to the pelvic side wall. After this has been accomplished, suture material of a permanent type is used, such as Gore-Tex, Tycron, or Ethibond. A figure-of-eight suture is placed at the level of the UVJ 2 cm lateral to the midline, followed by a second suture placed more inferiorly to the first approximately 2 cm lateral to the urethra (Fig. 25). After the sutures are in place, the procedure is repeated on the opposite side.

The Cooper ligament is a firm, fibrous band on the pelvic side wall into which the sutures will be anchored. It is frequently necessary to clear the ligament of fatty tissue for some distance to expose enough of it to allow adequate placement of sutures through it. Of concern at this point is the aberrant obturator vein, which arises in the obturator fossa and empties into the external iliac vein. Although this vessel is called aberrant, it is constantly present and is usually hidden in fatty tissue at the upper extent of the dissection along the Cooper ligament. With this vessel retracted, the sutures are placed through the Cooper ligament, taking care to stagger their placement so that they are not exactly parallel to the Cooper ligament fibers.

After all eight strands have been placed through the ligament bilaterally, an assistant places two fingers in the vagina and holds the urethra in a horizontal position. The surgeon then ties the lower sutures, maintaining this horizontal position, and does not bring the vaginal wall any higher than the assistant's fingers indicate. The upper sutures are then tied in a similar manner. Even though this may leave a space between the Cooper ligament and the vaginal wall, this is of no concern, because the vaginal wall and the pelvic side wall must eventually fuse to provide for the permanence of the operation. This fusion takes place during the 3 months after

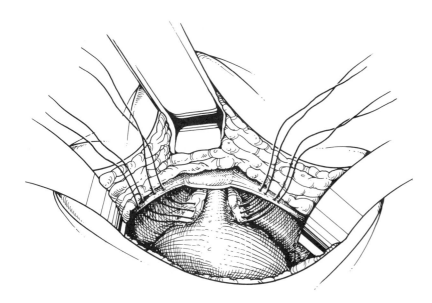

FIG. 25. Burch retropubic urethropexy. Sutures are placed lateral to the urethrovesical junction and lateral to the midurethra and brought to the Cooper ligament bilaterally. (Adapted from Tanagho EA. Colpocystourethropexy: the way we do it. *J Urol* 1976;116:751.)

surgery. During that period, patients must remain relatively inactive to allow the fusion to occur. Fusion gives permanence to the procedure. The sutures must be considered as temporary struts in this area to hold the vaginal wall and the pelvic side wall in contact long enough for fusion to occur. The simultaneous performance of a hysterectomy does not improve the results of incontinence surgery.

The Marshall-Marchetti-Krantz urethropexy procedure is similar to the Burch, except that the sutures that are placed periurethrally in the vaginal wall and are brought anteriorly and anchored in the periosteum of the symphysis pubis. Usually, absorbable sutures such as Dexon or Vicryl are used. This procedure has a 5% incidence of osteitis pubis secondary to this location for suture placement and a lower success rate than the Burch procedure.

At the termination of either procedure, it is important to determine that no damage or compromise has occurred to the ureters. Their function is checked bilaterally by the insertion of a cystoscope into the bladder transurethrally or by the use of suprapubic cystoscopy. The examiner should view both ureters and determine that they are functioning properly and that no damage has occurred to them. This is best assessed following the administration of intravenous indigo carmine, with visualization of free efflux of blue-stained urine from the ureteral orifices bilaterally. At the same time, the interior of the bladder is evaluated to be sure that no suture material is within the bladder, indicating inadvertent perforation of the bladder during placement of the sutures. The suprapubic catheter is then inserted through the incision used for suprapubic cystoscopy.

Postoperative management is similar to that for other abdominal surgical procedures. It is usually possible to allow patients to have oral intake soon after the operation, because the peritoneal cavity was not entered. The bladder is drained continuously for the first 1 or 2 postoperative days, and then the suprapubic catheter is occluded and patients are asked to indicate when they feel that the bladder is full. They are then allowed to void, and the amount of urine remaining inside the bladder is measured by the nursing personnel. The measurement of this residual urine is an important determination, and the suprapubic catheter should be left in place until patients are able to void adequately with small amounts of residual urine (< 100 ml or < 25% of the total volume in the bladder) consistently for 48 hours. It may take a few weeks or, rarely, months for patients to be able to void adequately.

Complications include those common to any surgical procedure, especially infection and bleeding. Urethral, ureteral, and vesical injury may occur during the procedure, and patients must be evaluated for these problems before leaving the operating room. A major complication is obstructive voiding postoperatively, and if it is persistent, it can be managed by intermittent self-catheterization. A long-term complication is the development of an enterocele. Approximately 10% of patients develop enteroceles after this type of surgical procedure. However, only 1% develop enteroceles that are symp-

tomatic. It is unnecessary to open the peritoneal cavity in 100 patients to prevent one symptomatic enterocele. Postoperatively, patients are observed for this problem, and it is managed if it occurs.

Success rates for the retropubic urethropexy range from 80% to 90% after 1 year in studies reporting objective preoperative and postoperative urodynamic assessments. Success rates are considerably better if patients with low urethral pressures are given a suburethral sling procedure.[22] In primary cases with normal urethral pressures, the objective success rate is approximately 90% after 1 year of observation.

The laparoscopic approach to retropubic urethropexy has been described utilizing multiple different techniques, including the use of mesh and staples or laparoscopic suturing, to give support to the proximal urethra. Subjective success rates of these procedures have been reported in short-term studies to be above 90%. Unfortunately, very few studies have included objective preoperative and postoperative urodynamic testing and clear-cut objective criteria of cure. Although equivalent success rates would theoretically be expected whether the Burch or Marshall-Marchetti-Krantz procedure was performed in an identical fashion through an open or laparoscopic approach, these data are not presently available.

Paravaginal repair has also recently been touted as another retropubic procedure to be used for the correction of genuine stress incontinence. The abdominal paravaginal repair was first used by Burch in his initial attempts to surgically support the UVJ. Due to poor results, Burch modified his procedure, elevating the sutures from the endopelvic fascia to the Cooper ligament rather than the arcus tendineus fasciae pelvis (ATFP). Paravaginal repair was reintroduced by Richardson as a procedure to correct paravaginal (lateral) defects in anterior vaginal wall support. Although others have suggested that the procedure may also be used as an antiincontinence surgery, closer examination of the procedure performed indicates that the investigators combined Burch stitches to the Cooper ligament with paravaginal stitches to the ATFP. The only randomized, prospective study comparing the Burch procedure to a pure paravaginal repair, with pre- and postoperative objective follow-up, indicates that the paravaginal repair yields inferior cure rates (75% versus 100%) in treating genuine stress incontinence.[10] The paravaginal repair should be considered as procedure for correcting anterior lateral vaginal wall defects and not as an antiincontinence procedure.

Combined Retropubic and Vaginal Approaches

The combined vaginal-retropubic approach was first popularized by Pereyra in 1956. His approach was to open the anterior vaginal wall in a manner similar to that of the anterior vaginal repair and to place a bifid needle blindly through the retropubic space to perforate the periurethral tissue. Two sutures were brought back up through to the retropubic space, after having been placed around the paraurethral tissue and vaginal wall. This approach has been modified by several investigators, including Stamey and Pereyra himself, to make it less blind and therefore much more useful.[16]

The surgical technique for the modified Pereyra procedure uses an anterior vaginal wall incision in a manner similar to that used for the traditional anterior vaginal repair. The vaginal mucosa is dissected from the underlying pubovesical tissue and the bladder. The retropubic space is entered bluntly precisely at the point where the endopelvic fascia attaches to the descending pubic ramus to avoid trauma to the large venous plexus situated more medially, just adjacent to the urethra.

A permanent suture of 0 nylon, Prolene, or Gore-Tex is used in a continuous helical manner along the endopelvic fascia, taking three to five bites of the needle (Fig. 26), and this is repeated on the opposite side. A small transverse suprapubic incision is made to the level of the anterior rectus fascia, and a ligature carrier is passed through the rectus fascia and guided through the retropubic space into the vaginal surgical site by the surgeon's index finger (Fig. 27). The sutures are withdrawn to the anterior abdominal wall with the use of the ligature carrier. Intraoperative transurethral cystoscopy is performed to confirm that no sutures are located inside the bladder.

The anterior vaginal wall is closed before tying the Pereyra sutures, because it may be difficult to close the anterior vaginal wall after the sutures have been tied. The suspension sutures are tied, using deflection of a Q-tip in the urethra to −10 degrees from the horizontal as a guide to tightness. A urethroscope may also be inserted into the urethra to be sure that there is complete closure of the UVJ. The sutures should

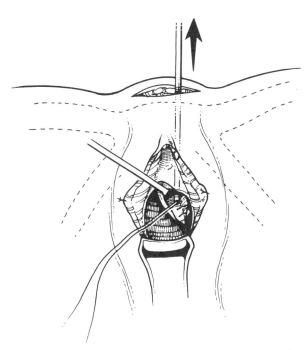

FIG. 27. Modified Pereyra procedure. The ligature carrier is used to withdraw the ends of the sutures to the anterior abdominal wall. (Adapted from Cutner LP, Ostergard DR. Modified Pereyra procedure: vaginal approach to retropubic urethropexy. In: Ostergard DR, ed. *Gynecologic urology and urodynamics: theory and practice*, 2nd ed. Baltimore: Williams & Wilkins, 1985:531.)

be tied to the rectus fascia, as well to each other across the midline.

The Raz procedure differs from the Pereyra procedure in two ways. The first is that the incision made along the anterior vaginal wall, and the second involves the placement of the anchoring sutures. In opening the anterior vaginal wall, an inverted-U incision is made rather than a vertical midline incision. Placement of the anchoring sutures includes not only the endopelvic fascia but also the full thickness of the anterior vaginal wall.

In the Stamey procedure, the endopelvic fascia is not perforated from below, and there is no dissection of the retropubic space. Sutures are brought to the anterior abdominal wall by the placement of needles through the retropubic space, through the endopelvic fascia, to the vaginal incision. This procedure is repeated with penetration of the endopelvic fascia in a different location. A bolster is placed on the exposed suture (Fig. 28). Because bladder perforation is a common hazard, cystoscopy is used to detect intravesical sutures.

Newly reported bone anchor procedures utilize intravesical sutures to attach the sutures anteriorly to the pubic bone. Due to the incidence of osteomyelitis associated with these procedures, they must be used cautiously.

The complications of combined vaginal-retropubic procedures include possible injury to the bladder, urethra, and ureters, which must be determined at the time of the surgical procedure. Infection and hemorrhage may occur. A suprapubic catheter is inserted for postoperative bladder drainage, and the complications discussed previously for obstructed

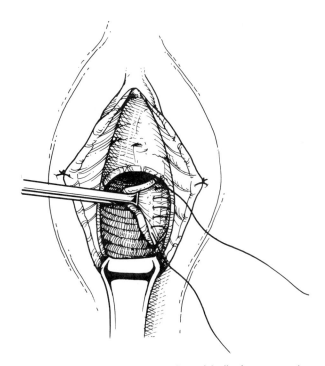

FIG. 26. Modified Pereyra procedure. A helical permanent suture is placed on the paravaginal fascia. (Adapted from Cutner LP, Ostergard DR. Modified Pereyra procedure: vaginal approach to retropubic urethropexy. In: Ostergard DR, ed. *Gynecologic urology and urodynamics: theory and practice*, 2nd ed. Baltimore: Williams & Wilkins, 1985:533.)

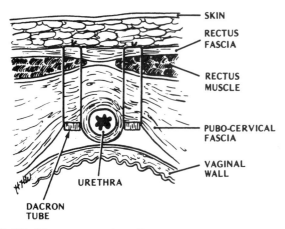

FIG. 28. Stamey procedure. Buttresses are used under the urogenital diaphragm to protect the fascia after elevation with the sutures attached to the anterior rectus fascia. (From Stamey TA. Endoscopic suspension of the vesical neck for urinary incontinence in females: report on 203 consecutive patients. *Ann Surg* 1980;192:465; with permission.)

used, the material is cut approximately 22 cm long with a 3-cm wide suburethral segment and 1-cm arms. The sling itself is sutured such that two-thirds of the 3-cm-wide sling are under the urethra and one-third is under the trigone (Fig. 29).

A short suprapubic incision is made to the level of the anterior rectus fascia. A stab wound is made through the rectus fascia 2.5 cm lateral to the midline just above the symphysis. A uterine packing forceps is passed through this incision down into the vagina, guided by the surgeon's index finger. The arm of the sling is grasped and withdrawn up to the anterior rectus fascia. The procedure is repeated on the opposite side. At this point, a cystoscope is introduced into the bladder to ascertain whether or not perforation of the bladder has occurred and ureteral function remains normal. A Q-tip is then placed in the urethra, and the sling is drawn upward so that the Q-tip makes a 0- to +10-degree angle with the horizontal. A urethroscope may be introduced into the urethra to ascertain that the UVJ is closed.

voiding postoperatively are identical. Rarely must a patient self-catheterize to empty the bladder for the long term. Cure rates have recently been reported to be equivalent to those for anterior vaginal repair, and therefore the place of these operations is in question.

Suburethral Sling Procedures

The suburethral sling procedure was first described by Giordano in 1907 and underwent modification by Goebell, Frankenheim, and Stoeckel. The procedure was used primarily for patients who had had multiple procedures and were thought to face failure if adequate support was not given to the UVJ. Renewed interest has occurred because the suburethral sling procedure has been more effective than retropubic urethropexy in patients whose urethral closure pressure is less than 20 cm H_2O. Sling procedures are used in primary and secondary cases for support of the UVJ. Suburethral sling procedures may use autologous materials or foreign materials to support the UVJ. Autologous materials such as fascia lata may be obtained from the leg, or rectus fascia from the anterior abdominal wall has also been used. Synthetic materials, such as Marlex, Mersilene, and Vicryl meshes and Gore-Tex patches, have been used for suburethral slings with success. Recently, allograft fascia has been used with similar success rates to those of other sling materials.

The surgical technique begins with opening of the anterior vaginal wall in a manner similar to that used for a traditional anterior vaginal repair. The retropubic space is entered in a manner identical to that performed in the Pereyra procedure. A subvesical and suburethral plication of perivesical adventitia is performed to provide thicker tissue between the urethra, trigone, and bladder and the material to be used for the sling. Sling material is harvested from the fascia lata or the rectus muscle. If Gore-Tex, Marlex, Mersilene, or Vicryl mesh is

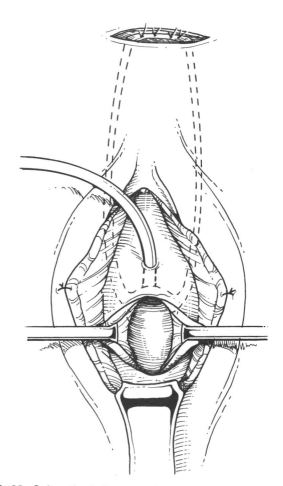

FIG. 29. Suburethral sling procedure. After dissection of the anterior vaginal wall, the sling is anchored underneath the urethrovesical junction, and the arms are brought to the anterior rectus fascia, where they are similarly anchored. (Adapted from Horbach N, Blanco J, Ostergard DR, et al. A suburethral sling procedure with polytetrafluoroethylene for the therapy of genuine stress incontinence in patients with low urethral closure pressure. *Obstet Gynecol* 1988;71:648.)

The anterior vaginal wall is approximated. The sling is sutured first to the rectus fascia and then to itself to provide secure placement of the sling material. The anterior abdominal wall incision is closed, and a suprapubic catheter is inserted.

Postoperatively, the suprapubic catheter is managed in a manner identical to that for retropubic urethropexy. The median time to removal of the catheter is 28 days, and patients must be warned in advance that they will have the catheter in place for a prolonged period. Ten percent of patients may eventually need to do intermittent self-catheterization. Most patients accept this, because it is preferable to having continued urine loss.

Complications of the suburethral sling procedure include the possibility of erosion of the sling material into the vagina or the anterior abdominal wall with sinus tract formation. Occasionally, slings must be removed because of this problem. Slings may also be removed from patients who develop marked obstruction and who do not want to use self-catheterization on a permanent basis. The elevation of the UVJ is usually permanent by this point, and recurrent incontinence does not usually result after a sling is removed. Success rates of 80% to 90% for the sling procedure have been reported.

Artificial Urinary Sphincters

Some patients have undergone multiple surgical procedures for persistent stress incontinence but have adequately positioned vesical necks. This group of patients responds best to the placement of an artificial urinary sphincter.[17] The artificial urinary sphincter was slow to gain widespread acceptance in female patients because of the difficulty of placement of the cuff around the vesical neck and the reluctance of surgeons to adequately expose the UVJ using a vaginal approach. The vaginal approach allows plication of perivesical adventitia underneath the vesical neck and urethra to provide a greater tissue gradient between the sphincter and the urinary tract.

The artificial sphincter has three components: a pressure-regulating balloon, a control pump, and a cuff (Fig. 30). The cuff is placed around the proximal urethra. The control pump is surgically implanted in the major labium, and the pressure-regulating balloon is located in the retropubic space. The surgical procedure is performed entirely in the retropubic space in a combined vaginal-abdominal approach or in a totally vaginal approach.

The totally retropubic approach is the traditional approach, but it does not allow suburethral plication or the possible enhancement of vascularity by the introduction a bulbocavernosus fat pad graft. Erosion into the urinary tract is a common problem. The retropubic space is entered in the manner identical to that for retropubic urethropexy, and the proximal urethra is identified. A right-angle scissors is used to dissect between the urethra and the anterior vaginal wall. After an adequate tunnel has been dissected, the artificial sphincter cuff is brought through the defect to surround the urethra. The

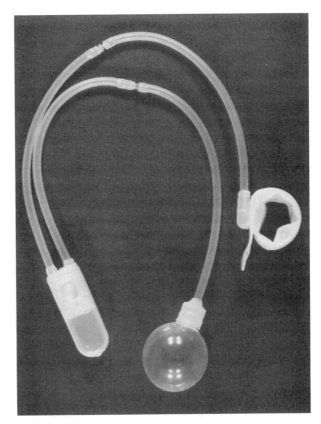

FIG. 30. Artificial urinary sphincter. The reservoir bulb (left) is connected to the poppet valve, which is connected to the cuff that is placed around the proximal urethra. (Model AS 800: courtesy of American Medical Systems, Minneapolis, MN.)

pressure-regulating balloon is placed in the retropubic space, and the control pump is located in the major labium.

Infection is not an inevitable result when the vagina is entered during this procedure, and this approach facilitates placement of the sphincter in a secure position. The total vaginal approach to the placement of the sphincter begins with incision in the anterior vaginal wall and entry into the retropubic space after the bladder and its fascia are separated from the vaginal mucosa in a manner identical to that of a modified Pereyra procedure or suburethral sling procedure. A tunnel is created into the major labium for placement of the pump. The pressure-regulating balloon is placed into the retropubic space, and the cuff is implanted around the proximal urethra after suburethral plication has been performed. Depending on the surgeon's clinical impression of the degree of vascularity under the urethra, it may be appropriate to bring a Martius fat pad graft into the area to increase vascularity and decrease the likelihood of infection. The surgical procedure is terminated by closing the anterior vaginal wall.

Postoperative care is similar to that for any vaginal or retropubic surgical approach. The artificial urinary sphincter is not activated until approximately 6 weeks have passed. The occluding cuff will not be inflated until after that time to enable adequate healing in the cuff placement area. When the pump is to be activated, a small valve called a poppet valve is located in the control pump, which allows activation of the system. When the patient feels bladder fullness, she manipulates the control pump of the activated system so that the fluid is transferred from the vaginal cuff to the reservoir. The fluid stays in the reservoir for approximately 1 minute, and then the cuff gradually begins to refill to provide urethral occlusion.

The artificial urinary sphincter is an alternative to previous surgical approaches of all types. It offers the greatest advantage for patients whose vesical neck is adequately supported but who still have urinary stress incontinence.

Periurethral injection

Several different substances have been injected submucosally at the UVJ to act a bulking agent to increase outflow resistance to prevent urine leakage. The substances can be injected via a transurethral mucosal route or a periurethral submucosal route. The procedure can be performed in an outpatient facility or in the office. This type of therapy is designed to treat patients who have intrinsic sphincter deficiency, specifically those with a well supported UVJ, and who would otherwise be candidates for artificial sphincters.

To date, silicone, Teflon, autologous fat, and bovine collagen have been used for periurethral injection. Each material has its merits and unique problems. Silicone and Teflon have been noted to migrate in the body and incite significant granulomatous reactions. Autologous fat harvested from the anterior abdominal wall has a limited length of efficacy due to rapid reabsorption of the transplanted tissue. Collagen has been available since 1995 and has largely replaced the other substances.[2]

Contigen is sterile, purified, bovine dermal type I collagen that is cross-linked with glutaraldehyde; as a substance, it is biocompatible and biodegradable. Acute bladder infection and known hypersensitivity to bovine collagen are contraindications to this form of treatment, whereas the presence of detrusor instability is a relative contraindication. Pretreatment skin testing is mandatory to identify patients with preexisting hypersensitivity to bovine collagen. Periurethral injection of collagen is not a one-time event, potentially requiring several injection procedures to obtain continence and intermittent reinjection over time to maintain continence. Success rates in one study of 148 patients followed for over 2 years were 55 (37%) dry, 57 (39%) improved, and 36 (24%) not improved.

Selecting the Appropriate Surgical Procedure for Genuine Stress Incontinence

Selection of a surgical procedure for a given patient has until recently been based on the operating surgeon's impression of the clinical complaints and the physical examination findings. The surgeon was aided by clinical evidence of urethral fibrosis interfering with normal urethral function. This is commonly associated with prior urethral surgery and can be demonstrated in its end stage as a functionless tube on urethroscopic evaluation. Objective urodynamic assessment of the patient and subsequent correlation of clinical surgical results allow the selection of a surgical procedure for a given patient based on urodynamically defined parameters (see Fig. 23). The most important considerations are the amount of urethral closure pressure available in the patient's urethra to prevent urine leakage and the degree of UVJ support. Urodynamic studies provide this information.

If a patient's urethral pressure has been considered normal (greater than 20 cm H_2O), a retropubic urethropexy of the Burch type is preferred for management of this patient's stress incontinence. If the urethral pressure is less than 20 cm H_2O, a suburethral sling procedure should be considered.[23] In both circumstances, it is assumed that inadequate support of the UVJ is present, as indicated by a Q-tip test that is greater than 30 degrees from the horizontal during straining. If the UVJ is well supported, as indicated by a Q-tip deflection on straining of less than 30 degrees from the horizontal, the patient is less likely to respond to either of the aforementioned procedures, and other surgical means may be indicated for treatment. Options for treatment of intrinsic sphincter deficiency, those with a low-pressure urethra and a well supported bladder neck, include an artificial sphincter, periurethral injection, or an obstructive sling. With the latter choice, the patient needs to be informed of the extremely high probability that lifelong self-catheterization may be required to empty the bladder.

There has been much discussion regarding the different procedures used to treat genuine stress incontinence in regard to efficacy and long-term success. Unfortunately, most studies in the literature have lacked objective pre- and postoperative assessment and therefore an objective measurement of cure. Table 5 presents the studies that have included objective pre- and postoperative urodynamic testing and highlights the handful of studies that have been prospective, randomized, controlled trials.[3–5,9–12,20,25,26] As previously mentioned, it is very evident that the anterior repair should not be considered an antiincontinence procedure, given the reported dismal long-term success rates compared to other surgical options.

An ongoing controversy has been the place of the combined vaginal-retropubic approach (needle procedures) in treating female stress urinary incontinence.[16] Although short-term studies have shown a cure rate of greater than 85% with the needle procedures, studies with objective measures of cure have shown an increased failure rate that increases with time following the procedure. This trend has been apparent in the gynecologic and the urologic literature.[3–5,12,18] In a comparison of the needle procedures to the retropubic procedures, the latter come out on top, with consistent long-term success rates over 80%, compared to 43% at 5 years for the needle procedures.

Due to this low long-term success rate, the combined vaginal-retropubic approach is not recommended for pri-

TABLE 5. *Urinary incontinence procedures: objective cure rates*

Trial	Length follow-up	Anterior repair (%)	Needle procedure (%)	Burch (%)	MMK (%)	Paravaginal (%)	Suburethral sling (%)
Henriksson and Ulmsten (1978)[a]	4–6 mo	—	—	—	100	—	100
Stanton and Cardozo (1979)[a]	6 mo	36	—	84	—	—	—
Milani (1985)[a]	22–73 mo	—	—	79	71	—	—
van Geelen (1986)	1–2 yr	44.6	—	84	—	—	—
Hilton (1989)[a]	2 yr	—	80	—	—	—	90
Bhatia and Bergman (1989)	1 yr	—	85	98	—	—	—
Bergman et al. (1989)[a]	1 yr	65	72	91	—	—	—
Bergman and Elia (1994)[a]	5 yr	37	43	82	—	—	—
Colombo et al. (1994)[a]	2–7 yr	—	—	80	65	—	—
Colombo and Milani (1996)[a]	2 yr	—	—	100	—	61	—

[a]MMK, Prospective, randomized, controlled clinical trial.

mary treatment of genuine stress incontinence. The vaginal-retropubic approaches are primarily relied on in cases of severe genital prolapse, in which repair of the genital prolapse would result in stress incontinence. This condition has been labeled potential incontinence and has been found in 60% to 80% of patients with severe vaginal vault inversion or with severe uterine prolapse. It is accepted medical practice to support the UVJ when other surgical procedures are being done to correct severe uterovaginal prolapse. The potential incontinence can be demonstrated in the urodynamic laboratory during multichannel urodynamic studies using a pessary to simulate the effects of the surgical procedure. Alternatively, a simple office demonstration of stress incontinence with the bladder full and the prolapse replaced by a pessary or a Sims speculum is sufficient to indicate that such an elevation of the UVJ is appropriate. Even in this scenario, the vaginal-retropubic procedures should be reserved for patients with mild potential incontinence and should not be used in those whose major complaint is symptomatic urinary incontinence or moderate to severe amounts of potential incontinence. Patients who have significant potential stress incontinence with reduction of their uterovaginal prolapse are best treated by a retropubic procedure, which offers them the best success rate over time. In this situation, the vaginal correction of pelvic relaxation is performed first, followed by the abdominal incision and retropubic procedure to give support to the UVJ.

◊ Selection of the appropriate surgical procedure for the correction of genuine stress incontinence should be based on urethral function and the presence or absence of UVJ hypermobility.

◊ Retropubic urethropexy procedures, specifically the modified Burch procedure, offers the best long-term support of the UVJ and cure of incontinence.

◊ Intrinsic sphincter deficiency should be considered in patients with severe leakage with minimal activity or those with recurrent incontinence, a history of radical pelvic surgery, or radiation, Options for therapy include periurethral injection of bulking agents or artificial sphincter in patients with a well supported UVJ, or a suburethral sling when UVJ hypermobility is present.

◊ Detrusor instability should be looked for in every patient with urinary incontinence, most importantly prior to any surgical antiincontinence procedure. It is best treated with anticholinergic medication or bladder retraining.

SUMMARY POINTS

◊ Diagnosis of lower urinary tract conditions, particularly urinary incontinence, can not be made based on symptoms alone. A systematic urodynamic evaluation of urethral and bladder function and structure is necessary and may include endoscopy, radiographic studies, and/or multichannel urodynamics.

◊ Anterior colporrhaphy is not considered a procedure for urinary incontinence.

◊ REFERENCES

1. Abrams P, Blaivas JG, Stanton SL, et al. The standardization of terminology of lower urinary tract function recommended by the International Continence Society. *Int Urogynecol J* 1990;1:45–52.
2. Appell RA. Collagen injection therapy for urinary incontinence. *Urol Clin North Am* 1994;21:177–182.
3. Bergman A, Elia G. Three surgical procedures for genuine stress incontinence: five-year follow-up of a prospective randomized study. *Am J Obstet Gynecol* 1995;173:66–71.
4. Bergman A, Ballard CA, Koonings PP. Comparison of three different surgical procedures for genuine stress incontinence: prospective randomized study. *Am J Obstet Gynecol* 1989;160:1102–1106.
5. Bhatia NN, Bergman A. Modified Burch versus Pereyra retropubic urethropexy for stress urinary incontinence. *Obstet Gynecol* 1985;66:255–261.
6. Bø K. Pelvic floor muscle exercise for the treatment of stress urinary incontinence: an exercise physiology perspective. *Int Urogynecol J* 1995;6:282–291.
7. Bump RC, Hurt WG, Fantl JA, Wyman JF. Assessment of Kegel pelvic muscle exercise performance after brief verbal instruction. *Am J Obstet Gynecol* 1991;165:322–327.

8. Childs S. Current diagnosis and treatment of urinary tract infections. *Urology* 1992;40:295–301.

9. Colombo M, Milani R, Vitobello D, Maggioni A. A randomized comparison of Burch colposuspension and abdominal paravaginal defect repair for female stress incontinence. *Am J Obstet Gynecol* 1996;175:78–84.

10. Colombo M, Scalambrino S, Maggioni A, et al. Burch colposuspension versus modified Marshall-Marchetti-Krantz urethropexy for primary genuine stress urinary incontinence: a prospective, randomized clinical trial. *Am J Obstet Gynecol* 1994;171:1573–1579.

11. Henriksson L, Ulmsten U. A urodynamic evaluation of the effects of the abdominal urethrocystopexy and vaginal sling urethroplasty in women with stress incontinence. *Am J Obstet Gynecol* 1978;131:77–82.

12. Hilton P. A clinical and urodynamic study comparing the Stamey bladder neck suspension and suburethral sling procedures in the treatment of genuine stress incontinence. *Br J Obstet Gynaecol* 1989;96:213–220.

13. Ishigooka M, Hashimoto T, Tomaru M, et al. Effect of hormone replacement therapy in postmenopausal women with chronic irritative voiding symptoms. *IntUrogynecol J* 1994;5:208–211.

14. Hooten TM, Winter C, Tiu F, Stamm WE. Randomized comparative trial and cost analysis of 3-day antimicrobial regimens for treatment of acute cystitis in women. *JAMA* 1995;273:41–45.

15. Jensen JK, Nielsen FR, Ostergard DR. The role of patient history in the diagnosis of urinary incontinence. *Obstet Gynecol* 1994;83:904–910.

16. Karram MM, Bhatia NN. Transvaginal needle bladder neck suspension procedures for stress urinary incontinence: a comprehensive review. *Obstet Gynecol* 1989;73:906–914.

17. Kreder KJ, Nygaard IE. Treatment of stress urinary incontinence with artificial urinary sphincter. *Int Urogynecol J* 1994;5:168–173.

18. Leach GE, Dmochowski RR, Appell RA, et al. Female stress urinary incontinence clinical guidelines panel summary report on surgical management of female stress urinary incontinence. *J Urol* 1997;158:875–880.

19. Lobel RW, Sand PK. The empty supine stress test as a predictor of intrinsic urethral sphincter dysfunction. *Obstet Gynecol* 1996;88;128–132.

20. Milani R, Maggioni A, Colombo M, et al. Burch colposuspension versus modified Marshall-Marchetti-Krantz for stress incontinence. *Neurourol Urodyn* 1991;9:454–455.

21. Milani R, Scalambrino S, Quadri G, Algeri M, Marchesin R. Marshall-Marchetti-Krantz procedure and Burch colposuspension in the surgical treatment of female urinary incontinence. *Br J Obstet Gynaecol* 1985;92:1050–1053.

22. Morales A, Emerson L, Curtis Nickel J. Treatment of refractory interstitial cystitis. *Int Urogynecol J* 1996;7:215–220.

23. Sand PK, Bowen LW, Panganiban R, et al. The low pressure urethra as a factor in failed retropubic urethropexy. *Obstet Gynecol* 1987;69:399–402.

24. Stanton SL, Cardozo LD. A comparison of vaginal and suprapubic surgery in the correction of incontinence due to urethral sphincter incompetence. *Br J Urol* 1979;51:497–499.

25. Swift SE. Intrinsic urethral sphincteric deficiency. In: Ostergard DR, Bent AE, eds. *Urogynecology and urodynamics: theory and practice*, 4th ed. Baltimore: Williams & Wilkins, 1996:151–163.

26. Van Geelen JM, Theeuwes AGM, Eskes TKAB, Martin CB. The clinical and urodynamic effects of anterior vaginal repair and Burch colposuspension. *Am J Obstet Gynecol* 1988;159:137–144.

CHAPTER 48

Vulvar and Vaginal Disease

$\Diamond$

Philip J. Di Saia

◊ BENIGN LESIONS OF THE VULVA

The vulvar skin is of ectodermal origin; it is subject to diseases that are common to the skin elsewhere and to infectious processes that are more or less specific to the genital area.

Benign lesions of the vulva may be classified as follows:

Inflammatory lesions
    Common dermatitides
        Reactive (not allergic)
        Intertrigo (i.e., seborrheic dermatitis)
        Psoriasis
        Candidiasis
        Tinea (various types)
        Vestibular (major and minor) gland infections
    Viral diseases
        Herpes simplex
        Condyloma acuminatum
        Molluscum contagiosum
    Ulcerative lesions
        Venereal (e.g., syphilis, lymphogranuloma, chlamydial infection) and granuloma inguinale (i.e., *Calymmatobacterium granulomatis*)
        Behçet disease
        Crohn disease
        Nonspecific (e.g., hidradenitis, ecthyma, folliculitis, factitious, decubitus) lesions
Traumatic lesions
    Hematomas
    Lacerations
White lesions, excluding neoplasms
    Absence of pigment
        Leukoderma or vitiligo
    Hyperkeratotic
        Inflammatory lesions
        Benign neoplasms
    Vulvar dystrophies
        Hyperplastic dystrophy without atypia
        Hyperplastic dystrophy with atypia

Lichen sclerosus
        Mixed dystrophy (i.e., lichen sclerosus with foci of epithelial hyperplasia) without atypia
        Mixed dystrophy with atypia
Benign neoplasms
    Solid tumors: granular cell myoblastoma, lipoma, fibroma, hemangioma, hidradenoma, nevus, condyloma, acrochordon (i.e., fibroepithelial polyp), endometrioma, pyogenic granuloma
    Cystic lesions: inclusion, Bartholin duct, mucous, canal of Nuck (i.e., hydrocele).

Because cancer of the vulva may be associated with ulcerative, erythematous, proliferative, or hyperkeratotic lesions, biopsies must be used freely if malignancy is to be diagnosed in its early or preinvasive stages. The instruments shown in Fig. 1 are used for single or multiple biopsy of all suspicious or controversial lesions to prove the true histologic nature of the disease. The physician can expect no concomitant spread of malignancy from the procedure, and the patient can be afforded an accurate evaluation and therapy.

The use of 1% toluidine blue as a local nuclear stain may assist in selecting sites for biopsy, but this technique is cumbersome. The value of careful inspection of the vulva with a good light during a routine gynecologic examination cannot be overstated. Identification of atypical areas on the vulva can be greatly enhanced with the use of 5% acetic acid, as is customary before colposcopic examination of the cervix; 3% acetic acid is customarily used on vaginal and cervical epithelium. I have not used the colposcope routinely for magnification when inspecting the vulva; I instead use a large magnifying lens. The field of vision with the colposcope is quite narrow and reduces the speed at which the inspection can take place. The application of toluidine blue and acetic acid leads to some false-positive and false-negative results, and liberal use of biopsy should be encouraged because a histologic examination is often essential for proper diagnosis. The presentation of vulva intraepithelial neoplasia can be subtle.

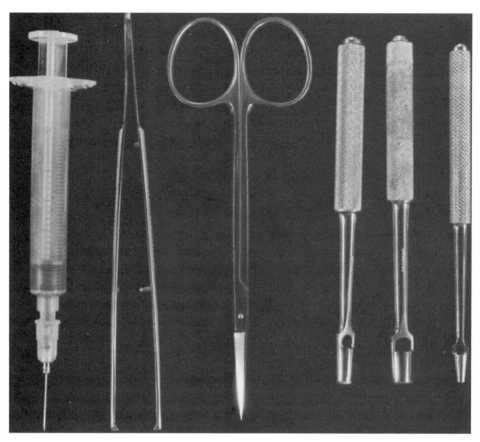

FIG. 1. Instruments used for biopsy of the vulva **(left)** and three types of Keyes dermatologic punches **(right)**.

To avoid delay, the physician must exercise a high degree of suspicion.

Inflammatory Lesions of the Vulva

The most common benign affliction of the female external genitalia is contact dermatitis, formerly called eczema or eczematoid dermatitis. Most dermatoses are caused by local irritants, such as tight underclothing that retains moisture, aerosol sprays, bubble bath and bath oils, colored toilet paper, detergents used in washing underclothing, perfumed soaps and powders, and a variety of other agents to which the vulva is commonly exposed. The treatment is to eliminate the irritant and apply local fluorinated hydrocortisones, which are extremely powerful and should be used sparingly in strengths of 0.025% to 0.1%. The fluorinated hydrocortisones should be used only for symptomatic relief because prolonged usage has been reported to produce systemic reaction or local fibrosis.

Intertrigo and seborrheic dermatitis are commonly seen in the diabetic patient. The elimination of moisture by the use of cornstarch and the topical use of fluorinated hydrocortisone creams or lotions for the pruritus are the appropriate approaches to the acute problem. The classic agents used for dandruff elsewhere may be applied to the vulva, but elimination of moisture and local irritants and the use of antipruritic

agents are usually sufficient. The chronic hyperkeratotic alterations are the group of white lesions, which are discussed later in this chapter (see White Lesions).

Psoriasis is usually multifocal. The classic picture on extragenital skin is characterized by silver scales and associated redness with linear excoriation. On the moist vulva, psoriasis appears as an erythematous patch without scales. The entire patient should be examined, not just the vulvar area, if the appropriate diagnosis is to be made.

Candidiasis of the vulva is commonly associated with a vaginal infection (see Chapter 37). Diabetes is often accompanied by such lesions.

Tinea cruris is usually sharply marginated, affects the adjacent skin surfaces, and is often found elsewhere on the body. Accentuation of the skin markings occurs in the more chronic situations. Clotrimazole (Lotrimin, Mycelex) is most commonly used in the treatment of such lesions. Tolnaftate (Tinactin) and ketoconazole (Nizoral) are also effective.

Infection in the major vestibular (Bartholin) gland is well known, and if an abscess develops, it should be incised.

Minor vestibular glands are superficial and lie just external to the hymenal ring. Inflammation of these glands gives rise to a condition called vestibular adenitis. The diagnostic criteria for vestibular adenitis are severe pain on vestibular touch or attempted vaginal entry, tenderness to pressure localized within the vulvar vestibule, and physical signs limited to vestibular erythema. Many patients have suffered for years as it progresses to a point where coitus is impossible. Patients also complain of burning pain on wearing tight pants or on insertion of a tampon. Inspection of the vestibule reveals foci of erythema within the hymenal sulcus. When these areas are pressed with a cotton-tipped applicator, a burning pain is described that is most pronounced on the lower half of the vestibule. Treatment has been varied and often disappointing. Submucosal injection of interferon to the vestibule several times each week for 4 weeks has proven effective. Topical therapy using steroids or antibiotics has not been successful. Surgical excision of the vestibule with accompanying glands has given pain relief in 60% to 80% of afflicted patients.

Ulcerative Lesions

Among the conditions causing ulcerative lesions, Crohn disease is especially important. Approximately 25% of patients with classic enteritis also have draining sinuses, fistulous tracts in the perineum, or fissuring at the outlet and edema. Unless this relationship is appreciated, inappropriate therapy may be instituted. Simple incision and drainage of the sinuses may lead to rectovaginal fistula or breakdown of the perineum. Prednisone is the classic treatment, usually in doses of approximately 40 mg/day. The addition of metronidazole (1000 to 1500 mg/day) to the therapeutic regimen has made it possible to reduce the dosage of cortisone. Treatment with corticosteroids should be continued indefinitely. Metronidazole should be continued if surgery is contemplated.

Behçet disease, which is probably an autoimmune disease, is characterized by ulcerations on the vulva and adjacent perineum that are associated with similar lesions on the buccal mucous membrane. The third member of this triple symptom syndrome, iritis, is not commonly recognized. Iritis is the most serious manifestation of all because it may progress to fatal neurologic disease. The fundamental treatment is prednisone (40 mg/day), the dosage of which is reduced if possible at the end of 1 month. There are many theories about the origin of this disease, and many therapies have been instituted. Spontaneous regressions and recurrences are common and constitute a major difficulty in the management of this disease.

White Lesions

Vitiligo is common on the vulva, often appears at the time of puberty, and is seldom symptomatic (Fig. 2). Associated depigmented areas are often found elsewhere on the body. When symptoms arise in this context, they usually are related to a superimposed dermatitis. Although there is often a family history, the cause is unknown. Vitiligo may appear at any time after middle age and anywhere on the body (Fig. 3). The melanocytes are apparently intact but do not deposit melanin in the affected epidermal areas. Vitiligo should not be misconstrued as a manifestation of systemic disease. It is purely a cosmetic defect, particularly disfiguring in blacks.

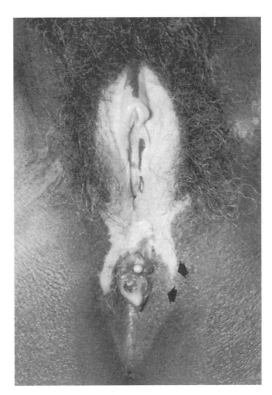

FIG. 2. Vitiligo with differential pigmentation on the labia minora and prepuce. The patient had perianal pruritus, and small areas of depigmentation caused by chronic dermatitis (i.e., vitiligo) are apparent *(arrows).*

Hyperkeratotic lesions may be recognized in a variety of circumstances. Increased deposition of keratin (i.e., hyperkeratosis) is a protective phenomenon seen particularly on traumatized skin and may be associated with any irritation, from chronic inflammatory disease to carcinoma. The white or grayish-white appearance of the skin in such situations is caused by the absorption of moisture by the keratin.

Intertrigo, probably the most frequent dermatitis in which hyperkeratosis develops on the vulva, is found most commonly in the interlabial and crural folds and is extremely difficult to combat, particularly in the obese, diabetic woman, in whom it is commonly found. Seborrhea (i.e., seborrheic dermatitis) is a corollary of intertrigo and is often found in the moist atmosphere of the vulva. Chronic dermatitis results from a variety of locally irritative conditions and similarly produces a thick, protective layer of keratin. The acuminate wart in its initial state is brown or reddish brown and microscopically shows superficial parakeratosis, but in its later stages, it is characterized by the development of hyperkeratosis. The chronic irritative lesion, regardless of cause, may eventually produce the superficially protective keratin coat.

Dystrophy refers to a disorder resulting from abnormal nutrition. The term has been applied to lesions that are characterized by a keratin layer of varying thickness, which accounts for a white or grayish-white color; an abnormal thinning or thickening of the epithelial layer; an underlying chronic inflammatory infiltrate; and the various degrees of

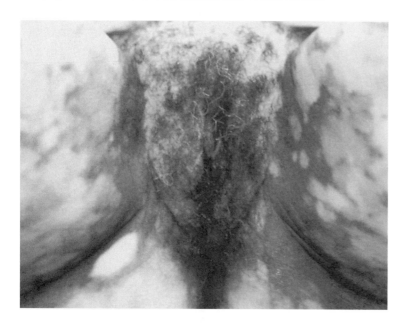

FIG. 3. Vitiligo in an African-American patient. (This figure is printed in color as Plate 14.)

change in the subepithelial connective tissue. The latter may be related to nutritional deficiencies, as evidenced by the vascular patterns. These dystrophies are the most common lesions. They were previously diagnosed as leukoplakia, and in current terminology, the word dystrophy is reserved for hyperkeratosis and lichen sclerosis with or without atypia.

Leukoplakia means a white patch, and it is a term that at one time or the other has been applied to almost every white lesion on the vulva. It is highly nonspecific and should be eliminated from the terminology of vulvar disease. A variety of other terms demand careful evaluation and modifications. Kraurosis is a clinical designation meaning shrinkage. The microscopic correlate classically is lichen sclerosus. The term kraurosis vulvae should be eliminated in favor of more specific clinical and histopathologic interpretations.

Lichen sclerosus (Fig. 4) has been recognized on the vulva in all age groups (Fig. 5). Girls in the first decade of life have been afflicted with this nonspecific, patchy, white alteration of the labial skin (Fig. 6). Most of these young patients im-

prove at the time of menstruation, but the lesion may occur throughout the menstrual years, usually beginning as small, bluish-white papules with eventual coalescence into white plaques. In its initial phases, lichen sclerosus is asymptomatic and demands no therapy. It assumes major significance in the postmenopausal patient, in whom it is commonly associated with severe and recalcitrant pruritus, shrinkage of the vulvar skin, and introital stenosis.

In the prepubertal patient, relief of symptoms is most important. Local corticosteroids are usually effective. Testosterone is not recommended for these patients, but 2% progesterone cream has been used for symptomatic relief. It is in the postmenopausal patient that long-term treatment with topical testosterone is sometimes effective. Clitoral enlargement and increased libido are associated with the use of testosterone in approximately 20% of patients. Recent literature suggests better results in the treatment of lichen sclerosus of the vulva utilizing topical corticosteroids at moderate to high strengths. Clobetasol propionate is a very potent corticosteroid and has

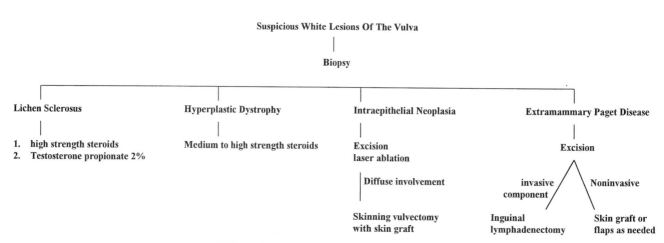

FIG. 4. Suspicious white lesions of the vulva.

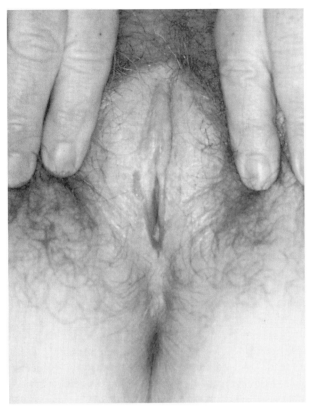

FIG. 5. Lichen sclerosus with an area of excoriation involves the labia minora and majora. (This figure is printed in color as Plate 15.)

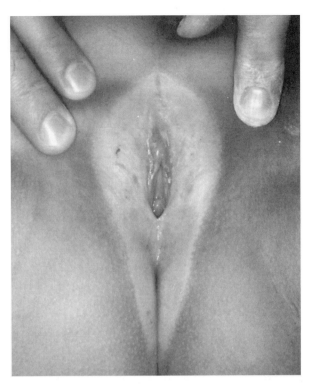

FIG. 6. Lichen sclerosus involving the vulva and perianal area in a 5-year-old girl. (This figure is printed in color as Plate 16.)

been reported effective in controlling clinical and histologic signs of lichen sclerosus after 3 months of therapy. It appears to be far more effective than testosterone. Clobetasol propionate is usually applied topically at a strength of 0.025% once a day 5 days a week for at least a year. The epidermal effects are reduction of hyperkeratosis and thickening of the epithe-

lium as a result of an increase in the number of mitoses of the keratinocytes.

The microscopic picture of lichen sclerosus is characterized by moderate hyperkeratosis, a thinning of the epithelium with loss of the rete pegs, underlying collagenization, and inflammatory infiltrate (Fig. 7). The later stages of lichen sclerosus are commonly associated with dyspareunia caused by constriction of the outlet and fissure formation at the fourchette. The terms primary senile atrophy and atrophic

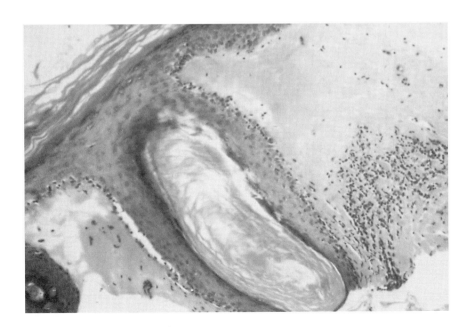

FIG. 7. Classic microscopic appearance of lichen sclerosus. Thin epithelium with underlying collagenation, inflammatory infiltrate, and follicular plugging.

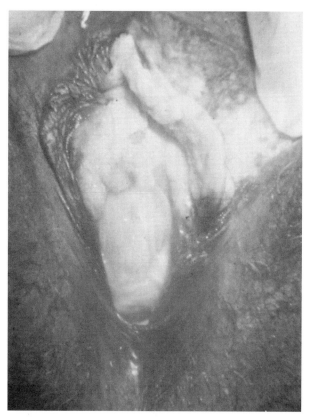

FIG. 8. Thick, white hyperkeratotic changes are characteristic of hypertrophic dystrophy. Biopsies should be used liberally for these patients to rule out malignancy. (This figure is printed in color as Plate 17.)

vulvitis should be eliminated as diagnoses because most of these lesions are variations of lichen sclerosus.

Hyperplastic dystrophy is characterized by gross lesions that are white or grayish white and may be diffuse or focal. The patches are firm and often cartilaginous on palpation (Fig. 8). They simulate the appearance of the lesions previ-

ously diagnosed as leukoplakia. Histologically, the keratin layer is usually thicker than that seen with lichen sclerosus, and the epithelium is more proliferative, with elongated and often blunted rete pegs. In typical hyperplasia, there is an increase in the cellular elements of the epithelium but no abnormality of maturation. Underlying chronic inflammatory infiltrates vary in degree. Many of these alterations are caused by chronic dermatitis, and treatment should be symptomatic. Biopsy must be used freely to eliminate the possible coexistence of cellular atypia.

Local fluorinated hydrocortisone is the best of the antipruritic agents. Occasionally, very hypertrophic and often atypically pigmented areas may not respond to local or systemic hydrocortisones, but the subcutaneous injection of such preparations may be dramatically effective. Small areas of 2 to 3 cm may be injected with 2 to 3 ml of fluorinated hydrocortisone, such as triamcinolone (Kenalog), producing dramatic results in eliminating the symptoms and restoring the normal coloration. Local measures to eliminate irritation are similar to those described previously, and regardless of the pathology, all patients should be instructed to observe these rules. Infrequently, these conditions are solitary and can be locally excised. However, the existence of multicentric foci must be eliminated by thorough investigation of the adjacent tissue. Diagnosis must be confirmed in all cases by biopsy. Multiple specimens are necessary in most instances because various patterns often coexist.

Atypical hyperplastic dystrophy is usually a white lesion, but red or pigmented lesions may show similar alterations. The latter do not simulate the epithelial changes described for cervical neoplasia. Atypical maturation and intraepithelial pearl formation are the hallmarks of atypical hyperplastic dystrophy and often occur adjacent to invasive vulvar cancer (Fig. 9). Histologic abnormalities may be associated with severe viral disease, such as human papillomavirus (HPV) infection and herpetic lesions. These undoubtedly account for the reversible atypias that have been described.

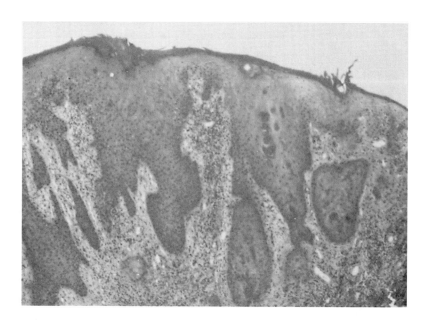

FIG. 9. Atypical hyperplastic dystrophy.

Mixed dystrophy is a combination of lichen sclerotic changes and hyperplasia. Biopsy is important in identifying the malignant potential of the lesions and must be used liberally. Colposcopy and cytology have not been helpful in differentiating the degrees of cellular atypia. Biopsy is simple and essentially painless if the area is infiltrated with a local anesthetic agent and the Keyes dermatologic punch is used to remove the tissue (see Fig. 1).

The basic treatment of all irritative lesions of the vulva must begin with a positive diagnosis; biopsy is imperative. Assuming that no major atypia is discovered, the next step is to eliminate the irritation. It seems probable that the chronic alterations associated with scratching may be important in the genesis of neoplasia. The treatment includes the use of topical fluorinated hydrocortisones to control the symptoms and reduce the local inflammatory reaction, the use of estrogen intravaginally in the postmenopausal patient, the treatment of any associated intravaginal infection, and the elimination of local irritants.

Solid Tumors

Most benign solid tumors (e.g., lipoma, fibroma) occur only rarely on the vulva, and because they are similar to such lesions elsewhere, they need no special discussion here.

All varieties of vascular tumors on the external genitalia have been described, but the congenital variety deserves special attention. Appearing in the infant at 2 to 3 months of age, it produces remarkable distortion of the vulva but generally needs and should receive no therapy unless excessive bleeding occurs because these lesions disappear spontaneously. In the adult, small, elevated, hemorrhagic nodes are often mistaken for hemangiomas but are tiny varicosities that may produce an occasional episode of irregular bleeding. Varicosities may attain great size, and a varicocele, similar to that in men, can develop on the vulva. These lesions usually are unilateral and are much less common than those that develop as the result of obstruction in the vessels of the spermatic cord.

The hidradenoma is a rare lesion that, because of its intricate adenomatous pattern, has been confused with malignancy. Malignant alterations are extremely uncommon, and the lesion, rarely more than 1 cm in its largest dimension, can be treated by local excision (Fig. 10).

A variety of pigmented lesions are seen on the vulva. An irritative focus of chronic dermatitis may be pigmented, as may carcinoma *in situ* and the spreading melanoma. Biopsy is imperative to evaluate the histopathology of such lesions. More than 50% of melanomas arise from preexisting nevi.

Nevi are classified as intradermal, junctional, and compound lesions. The malignant potential of the intradermal lesion is essentially nil. Junctional and compound nevi occur frequently and should be removed for accurate diagnosis. The junctional nevus is the one most likely to become malignant, although compound nevi also have malignant potential. Malignancy cannot be ruled out without excision and careful histopathologic study. The risk factors for melanoma are given in Table 1. Ominous patterns, such as atypical melanocyte hyperplasia (i.e., melanoma *in situ*), cannot be grossly differentiated from benign pigmented lesions.

A variety of papillary lesions can occur on the vulva. The common acuminate wart, which is of viral origin, constitutes a recurring therapeutic problem and is thought by some to be a precursor of malignancy. HPV particles have been identified in anogenital warts by electron microscopy (Fig. 11).

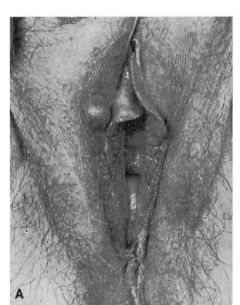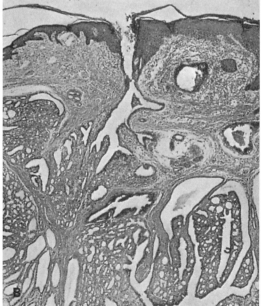

FIG. 10. (A) Hidradenoma on the right inner labium majus. A rectocele is also visible inside the introitus. **(B)** Photomicrograph of hidradenoma of vulva. (From Novak ER, Woodruff JD. *Gynecologic and obstetric pathology.* Philadelphia: WB Saunders, 1962; with permission.)

TABLE 1. *Risks for developing melanoma*

Family history of melanoma in blood relatives
Poor or no tanning ability, often with a history of sunburn in adolescence
Unusual moles with any of the following characteristics:
  Dark (i.e., blue-black) color
  Speckled or splotchy color pattern
  Jagged or fuzzy border
Recent change in size, shape, or color of a mole
Any mole larger than a dime

After inoculation, HPV preferentially infects the epithelial basal cell layer of the skin and mucous membranes, producing cellular proliferation. Viral replication is confined to the nucleus of the squamous epithelium, but a latent viral genome may also be present in the normal-appearing surfaces with no active virus replication. This characteristic of viral latency may explain the high rate of clinical relapse after ablative therapy of individual warts.

As stated above, genital HPV infection has been associated with neoplasia. Although cause and effect have not been firmly established, almost 85% of malignant and premalignant cervical and vulvar lesions contain HPV DNA, HPV structural antigens, or both. The association with malignancy is greatest with HPV types 16 and 18 and less with types 6 and 11.

The natural history of HPV-induced warts is not fully understood. Exophytic anogenital warts often resolve spontaneously, giving rise over the centuries to faith in folk remedies. However, in view of the sexual transmission of HPV and the suspected malignant potential of certain HPV types, many believe that all anogenital warts should be treated if possible. The traditional initial therapy is to destroy individual lesions by cytotoxic agents or ablation. These approaches are often limited because many lesions are not visible or accessible. The response to cytotoxic treatment may be incomplete, and recurrences are common.

Cytotoxic agents used in the treatment of anogenital warts include podophyllin, trichloroacetic acid (TCA), and 5-fluorouracil (5-FU) cream. Podophyllin, which has cytodestructive and antimitotic properties, was the most widely used cytotoxic agent. Many investigators now prefer TCA applied as often as three times weekly to visible lesions. Both TCA and podophyllin must be applied carefully to avoid contact with normal tissue and reduce the risk of systemic toxicity and tissue destruction. The antimetabolite cream 5-FU (1%) is less destructive to normal tissue than podophyllin and TCA, but it is more difficult to apply effectively to the vulva; 5-FU may be more effective as a prophylactic agent after ablative therapy.

Vulvar warts may also be ablated by using liquid nitrogen, electrocauterization, or surgical excision. Ablation with carbon dioxide laser techniques has been popular, especially if the area of involvement is less than one-third of the vulva. If large areas of the vulva must be ablated, considerable postoperative pain may necessitate a staging procedure when laser is the treatment of choice. Intradermal interferon is a possible therapeutic option, and preliminary results are encouraging, especially for small numbers of lesions.

The fibroepithelial polyp, also called an acrochordon, is common in all areas subjected to irritation, and it needs no treatment other than accurate diagnosis.

Of special interest to pathologists and clinicians is the granular cell myoblastoma. This benign lesion arising from the nerve sheath is associated with extensive, overlying pseudo-epitheliomatous hyperplasia, often misdiagnosed as carcinoma *in situ* or early invasive cancer. Careful investigation of the underlying tissue is important to make an accurate evaluation and institute the appropriate therapy. The finding of large cells with prominent eosinophilic granules makes the accurate diagnosis. The myoblastoma is not a well-localized tumor and is subject to local recurrences, but malignant myoblastomas are uncommon. Although multicentric foci arising in diverse areas in the body are not infrequent, they should not be interpreted as metastases.

Vulvar endometriosis is uncommon and occurs most frequently in areas subjected to trauma. The incision or excision of the chronically infected Bartholin gland seems to be an ideal precursory event for the development of these lesions. Episiotomy sites are common foci for implantation of the stimulus, leading to the development of endometriosis. The

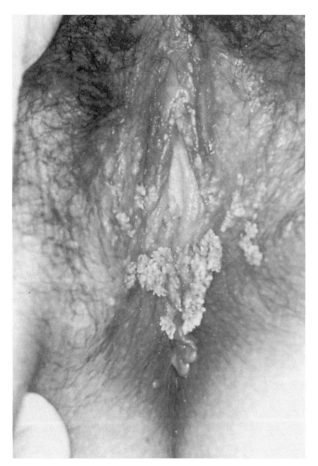

FIG. 11. Clusters of typical condylomata of the vulva. (This figure is printed in color as Plate 18.)

characteristic feature is cyclic swelling and pain. These lesions also develop in the inguinal canal and adjacent mons.

Cystic Lesions

The sebaceous cyst, more accurately called an epidermal inclusion, is the most common cystic lesion of the vulva. Although most lesions result from occlusion of a sebaceous gland on the labia minora or labia majora, microscopically they are epidermal inclusion cysts, and in the chronic, quiescent state, they are lined by stratified epithelium. Before the development of such lesions, the swelling contains only sebaceous material and is not a true cyst. These lesions need no treatment unless they become infected, at which time simple incision and drainage are usually sufficient. If they are recurrently infected, excision may be done, but recurrences are common.

Cystic dilation of the main Bartholin duct (Fig. 12) may be caused by chronic inflammatory reactions with scarring and occlusion or by trauma from lacerations or incisions in the area. Most are asymptomatic, and therapy is unnecessary. If symptomatic, marsupialization with the use of the indwelling Word catheter requires only local anesthesia and can be carried out as an office procedure. Excision is necessary only if marsupialization is unsuccessful in controlling the infection or if the diagnosis of malignancy is entertained. Whenever an enlargement of the Bartholin gland occurs in a postmenopausal patient, malignancy must be ruled out. All or part of the cyst or mass must be removed for histologic review.

Dysontogenetic (i.e., mucous) cysts are found at the introitus and adjacent labia minora. These cysts contain mucoid material and possibly represent the residua of incomplete separation of the cloaca by the urorectal folds; they represent dilations in rectal-like tissue. They may originate by occlusion of the minor vestibular glands that ring the outlet at the introitus. Regardless of origin, these lesions are benign.

Cysts that appear high in the labium majus (i.e., hydrocele of the canal of Nuck) correspond to the hydrocele in men. Because the round ligament has an investment of peritoneum, the latter may be occluded in the inguinal canal and allow the accumulation of fluid along the round ligament as it inserts into the labium majus. It is important to discover the origin of such lesions because simple incision and drainage leads to prompt recurrence. Furthermore, such lesions may be associated with inguinal hernias, and any portion of bowel that is present in the sac must be removed.

◊ BENIGN LESIONS OF THE VAGINA

Benign lesions of the vagina include inflammatory reactions (see Chapter 37), leukoplakia (i.e., hyperkeratosis resulting

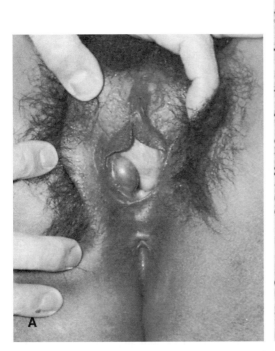
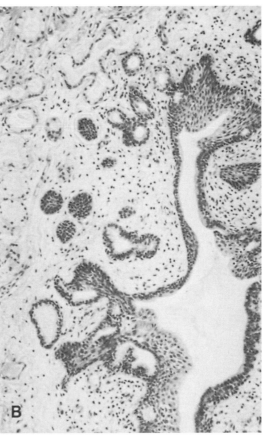

FIG. 12. (A) Bartholin duct cyst projecting into the introitus. **(B)** Various epithelia in the Bartholin gland, primarily transitional in the center with mucus-secreting acini.

from chronic irritation such as that associated with total prolapse of the uterus), cystic lesions, and solid tumors.

Cystic Lesions

Benign cystic lesions of the vagina are inclusion cysts, Gartner duct cysts, endometriosis, adenosis, and vaginitis emphysematosa.

The inclusion cyst is extremely common and occurs most frequently near the outlet at the site of previous lacerations or episiotomy scar. It seldom attains sufficient size to become symptomatic, and an associated inflammatory reaction is uncommon. Excision or incision and drainage are rarely necessary. The cyst is filled with desquamated cellular material from the stratified squamous epithelial lining.

The Gartner (i.e., mesonephric) duct may be the origin of multiple tiny cystic dilations or rarely of a large solitary cyst. The former are palpable only as fine elevations on the mucosal surface in the vaginal fornices or along the course of the mesonephric duct. They are common and rarely symptomatic. The latter may develop in the midline of the anterior vault and simulate a cystocele. Recognition of the nature of the lesion is important in determining therapy. Removal is usually not needed unless the lesions cause symptoms. Although no harm is done if the cyst is inadvertently opened during removal, the surgeon may be dismayed if he erroneously believes that he has incised the bladder. Malignancy rarely develops in these mesonephric remnants, although the mesonephroma described 40 or 50 years ago probably represents such a lesion.

Endometriosis usually develops as a penetration of cul-de-sac disease. It appears in the posterior fornix of the vagina, where it is characterized grossly by a bluish discoloration produced by the old blood. If penetration is incomplete, the associated nodular induration extending from the uterosacral ligaments into the vagina may simulate cancer. To rule out cancer, the vaginal lesion should be biopsied to establish the diagnosis. Nevertheless, because most of the vagina is of paramesonephric origin, endometriosis could arise in sites other than the cul-de-sac. If the lesion is asymptomatic and is the only abnormality present, no therapy other than accurate evaluation is indicated. Otherwise, appropriate medicinal or surgical therapy for endometriosis should be instituted.

Adenosis varies in gross appearance from diffuse granular thickening to an irregular, rugose, mucoid lesion. The frequency of adenosis is difficult to assess, but Sandberg suggests that more than 40% of all women have the subepithelial adenomatous structures. Any area of the vagina may be involved, but most commonly, it is the anterior or posterior wall of the upper half of the vault. Probably arising from aberrant ectopic and cervical-type glands (Fig. 13), the lesion is seldom symptomatic, and therapy is unnecessary. Interest in adenosis vaginae has increased with the appearance of these adenomatous elements in the vaginas of young women whose mothers had received diethylstilbestrol (DES) during pregnancy. The physician may be alerted to this group of lesions by the occasional presence of a transverse septum in the upper third of the vagina or the more frequent occurrence of a collar-like structure around the cervix (Fig. 14).

As of 1992, 587 cases of clear-cell-type vaginal adenocarcinoma of the vagina and cervix had been reported to the Registry for Research on Hormonal Transplacental Carcinogenesis. In approximately two-thirds of these cases, a suspicious history of maternal ingestion of some type of hormone has been elicited. Such neoplasms develop most commonly

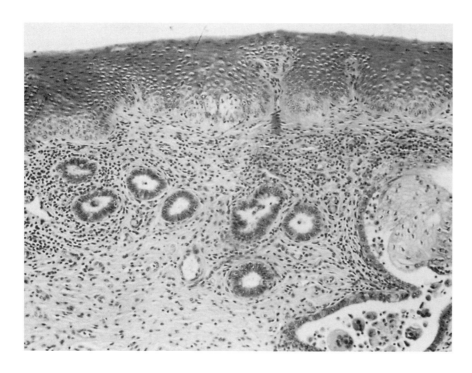

FIG. 13. Vaginal adenosis, showing surface-stratified epithelium with underlying glands, one of which contains metaplastic epithelium.

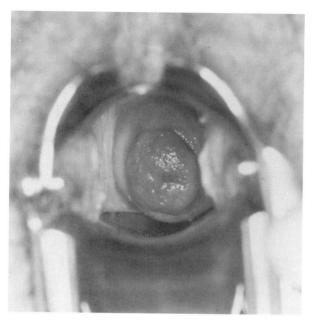

FIG. 14. The cervix of a 20-year-old diethylstilbestrol-exposed offspring demonstrates a complete cervical collar and polypoid structure of the central portion of the cervix. The anterior position is more prominent, giving rise to a partial deformity known as cockscomb. (This figure is printed in color as Plate 19.)

in the menarcheal years, but the lesions have been reported in a 7-year-old child, although the number of occurrences in those younger than 14 years of age is extremely small. The peak risk period for exposed women in the United States is between the ages of 15 and 22 years; the oldest patient was 42 years of age at diagnosis. Of importance is the magnitude of this at-risk population, which now must approximate more than 1 million young women. Methods of investigation of this special group have challenged the profession. The basic question is whether the young women at risk will develop mesonephroid carcinoma of the vagina, and the answer is yes for less than 0.1% of this group. The follow-up of the patient at risk should consist of careful palpation of the tissue with inspection and cytopathologic evaluation. Colposcopy has not been helpful in identifying the early adenocarcinoma. Most cases of clear-cell or mesonephroid carcinoma are found during the first study. However, at least four cases have been discovered in the follow-up study of initially benign adenosis; one of these was a multifocal lesion. Fortunately, the incidence of these rare vaginal malignancies has been declining over the last several years. In at least 25% of the cases of vaginal adenosis, there is no definable history of the maternal ingestion of DES or other hormones. Common to most sites of adenosis is active metaplasia similar to that which occurs at the squamocolumnar junction.

Of concern in the future may be the development of epidermoid neoplasia at the many squamocolumnar junctions produced by the change in the embryology of the area. Stafl, in his colposcopic studies, commented on this variety of histologic alteration. Nevertheless, there is no evidence that mul-

tiple squamocolumnar junctions place the patient at greater risk for the development of invasive neoplasia than does one. This is true despite the fact that Robboy has shown in cohort studies an increased incidence of intraepithelial neoplasia of the cervix and vagina in patients suspected of intrauterine DES exposure. Stafl reported that benign adenosis can be demonstrated colposcopically in up to 90% of the young women at risk, but the incidence of such alterations depends largely on the stage of the pregnancy at which therapy was instituted. For example, if treatment was begun before week 10 of gestation, adenosis occurs in approximately 90% of the female progeny. Conversely, if medication was instituted after week 16 of gestation, the risk factor is no greater than that for the female population at large. Microscopic examination of the adenomatous lesion reveals that the epithelia characteristic of the paramesonephric system (i.e., mucinous, endometrioid, endosalpingeal) may be found in many cases, but the mucinous or endocervical variety is the most common.

Another cystic lesion that is seldom diagnosed is vaginitis emphysematosa. Characterized by widespread submucosal cyst formation, this uncommon lesion is found in the pregnant woman or in the severely decompensated cardiac patient. The blebs are filled with carbon dioxide, and definitive infecting agents have not been recovered from the contents. Therapy should be directed toward the associated vaginitis, commonly found to be trichomonal in the pregnant woman. Complications have not been reported. Microscopically, the linings of the cavities are characterized by irregular, reactive giant cells (Fig. 15).

Solid Tumors

Benign solid tumors of the vagina include fibromyoma, polyps, papilloma, and condyloma.

Fibroma (i.e., fibromyoma), a rare solid tumor, may arise *de novo* from the connective tissue and smooth muscle elements of the vaginal wall. However, many of these lesions are intraligamentary uterine fibromyomas that have become divorced from the fundus and have dissected into the paravaginal area. These lesions, whether primary or secondary, are seldom symptomatic, and the incidence of sarcomatous change is negligible. Of major concern is the overdiagnosis of benign leiomyoma and polyps. Because of edema and degenerative changes, these lesions may be misconstrued as stromal malignancies. Excision usually is a minor procedure, but the uterine vessels or the ureter may be encountered if dissection is extensive. If any question exists about the nature of the tumor, excision must be performed because the treatment of vaginal malignancies is complicated by the necessity for radical surgery or technically difficult irradiation. Local excision is often followed by recurrence despite benign histology, probably because of incomplete excision.

True papillary tumors other than condylomata acuminata are rare. Most of these lesions are fibroepithelial tags. Although vaginal polyps are uncommon, they do occur and have been classically misinterpreted as sarcoma botryoides

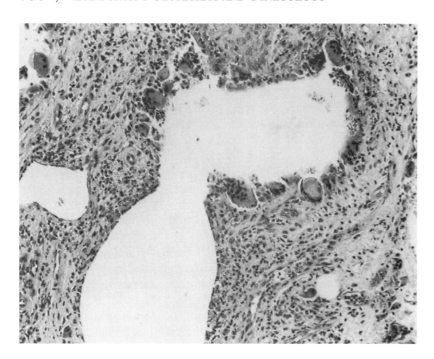

FIG. 15. Microscopic appearance of vaginitis emphysematosa. Cystic spaces are lined by giant cells.

because of the edematous nature of the lesion. A diagnosis of sarcoma botryoides is made on the basis of the histologic features. Although the polyp may recur, malignancy has not been reported in the follow-up of these patients.

Condylomata acuminata are common in the vagina and are often associated with condylomatosis of the vulva. The urethra, cervix, and perianal areas are also frequently involved. These lesions may become florid, particularly during pregnancy, where they can present major complications because of associated vascularity, edema, and an inflammatory reaction. One customary treatment, podophyllin, should not be used during pregnancy. The trauma of delivery may result in vaginal laceration and extensive bleeding. Nevertheless, because the acuminate wart is of viral origin, these lesion may spontaneously regress after delivery, especially with the institution of good local hygiene and the elimination of associated infection. Infrequently, laryngeal papillomas in the newborn have been associated with vaginal condylomatosis in the mother. Although these laryngeal lesions are benign, they do present problems in the care of the neonate. Cesarean delivery is often recommended for extensive vulvovaginal condylomatosis, not because of the possibility of infection of the newborn but because of the bleeding that may accompany the trauma of vaginal delivery.

In the nonpuerperal state, general cleanliness usually results in reduction in the size of the lesion. Podophyllin should be used sparingly in the vagina because local reactions may be severe. Anaphylactic shock has been reported as a complication of the injudicious use of this cauterizing solution. Local application to the individual lesion followed by vaginal douche within 2 hours of the application has seldom resulted in any unfavorable reaction. Although the small individual warts may be treated in this way, extensive involvement of

the vagina may require excision under general anesthesia. In resistant cases, 5-FU (Efudex) is often effective.

Caution should be exercised when using 5-FU cream in the vagina. Bedtime application is advised, with white petroleum jelly applied to the introitus and vulva for protection of those areas in case of extravasation during sleep. A tampon at the introitus also helps to prevent nighttime extravasation. The cream should be evacuated from the vagina each morning utilizing a warm water douche. Nightly applications for 5 consecutive days usually gives therapeutic results, but at least two 5-day treatments are necessary to give optimal results. For a few patients, it is necessary to continue with maintenance therapy in the form of weekly applications of the 5-FU cream to the vagina for several months to achieve a clinically free state.

Laser vaporization of lesions in the vagina is effective, but it must be done under general or regional anesthesia. As in all instances in which laser vaporization is used, at least 5 mm of normal surrounding epithelium or mucosa must be destroyed to achieve eradication of most virus particles. The depth of laser vaporization should not exceed 1 to 2 mm of normal mucosa beneath the lesion to avoid impaired healing and serious problems with scarring and stenosis of the vaginal wall. This technique is not applicable to patients who have diffuse involvement of the vaginal mucosa. In such patients, 5-FU cream appears to be the most effective therapy.

◊ MALIGNANT TUMORS OF THE VULVA

Vulvar anaplasia constitutes 3% to 4% of all primary malignancies of the genital tract. Despite the availability of these lesions for early investigation, there often is a longer interval between the appearance of symptoms and the establishment of diagnosis of carcinoma of the vulva than for any other primary malignancy of the female genitalia. Much of this delay may result from the reluctance of the elderly patient to seek medical advice, but the 30% to 35% of cases in which the physician is at fault may be related to the commonplace nature of the initial symptom: pruritus. Too often, local treatment is suggested over the telephone before a thorough study has been carried out.

The dystrophies may demonstrate a variety of histologic alterations, which are described as typical or atypical hyperplasias. Atypia and dysplasia are also used to describe atypical hyperplasia. In many series, these lesions are found because of the preexistence of cervical neoplasia (i.e., multifocal disease).

Vulvar malignancies may be classified as follows:

Primary malignancy
    Vulvar intraepithelial neoplasia (VIN)
        VIN I (mild dysplasia)—formerly mild atypia
        VIN II (moderate dysplasia)—formerly moderate atypia
        VIN III (severe dysplasia, CIS)—formerly severe atypia
        Squamous cell carcinoma *in situ*
    Paget disease
    Invasive cancer
        Squamous cell lesions (e.g., well differentiated)
        Basal cell carcinoma (histologic variations)
        Bartholin gland lesions
        Squamous cell lesions
        Transitional cell lesions
        Cribriform (i.e., adenocystic) lesions
        Verrucous carcinoma: locally invasive but not metastasizing; the histology is identifiable, and the treatment is wide excision; recurrences are common and often locally destructive
    Other malignancies, including melanotic and amelanotic melanoma, sarcoma, lymphoma, embryonal rhabdomyosarcoma, and breast cancer
Secondary malignancy.

Carcinoma *in Situ*

Carcinoma *in situ* occurs at any age, but it is more common during the third and fourth decades of life. Although a common presenting complaint is pruritus, the lesion may present as a lump or may be relatively asymptomatic. The gross appearance varies greatly. The classic (formerly referred to as bowenoid) lesion is scaly and characterized by a red background dotted with white hyperkeratotic islands (Fig. 16). Other lesions are almost entirely white or red (formerly referred to as erythroplasia of Queyrat) or a combination of these patterns (Fig. 17). Others are irregularly pigmented, with a diffuse but hazy background of hyperkeratosis (Fig. 18). These variable and bizarre patterns demand that all lesions be biopsied to determine their true nature. The increased frequency with which multiple areas of anaplastic change are found in the lower genital canal and perianal areas is note-

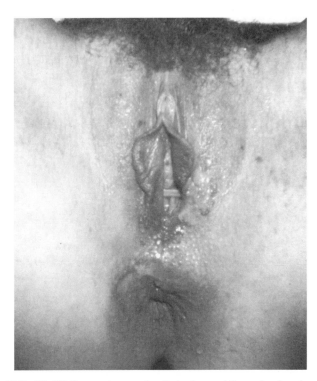

FIG. 16. White carcinoma *in situ* lesions of the vulva involve the left lower labium majus.

worthy. Such alterations demand thorough study of the entire region, initially and at follow-up examinations. Microscopic sections demonstrate variations in atypical cellular maturation (Figs. 19 and 20) in one and the same lesion, justifying the term carcinoma *in situ* in preference to a specific designation such as Bowen disease.

Of major interest are the variations in the histologic patterns adjacent to invasive cancer and those described as marked atypical hyperplasia or carcinoma *in situ*. It is possible that viral disease may produce histologic patterns that are indistinguishable from those of carcinoma *in situ*, representing the cases of reversible atypia.

If multiple foci of malignancy are carefully excluded by diligent inspection with magnification of skin moistened with 5% acetic acid followed by directed biopsies, wide local excision of the focal lesion is the acceptable treatment. Although vulvectomy has been a proposed therapy, more conservative approaches are indicated in most patients. Careful follow-up is essential because simple excision does not remove the precipitating agent, and the potential for recurrence always exists, regardless of whether the surgery is radical or simple. The use of topical chemotherapeutic agents (e.g., 5-FU cream) has not been successful in the hands of most clinicians, primarily because of the magnitude of local vulvar irritation that it is necessary to achieve for therapeutic results in most patients.

Surgical excision has been the mainstay of therapy. An important advantage is that excision allows complete histologic assessment, and lesions with microinvasive foci can be identified. As stated above, most localized lesions are managed

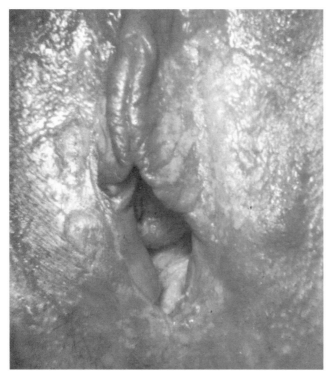

FIG. 17. Carcinoma *in situ* of the vulva presenting as multifocal red lesions.

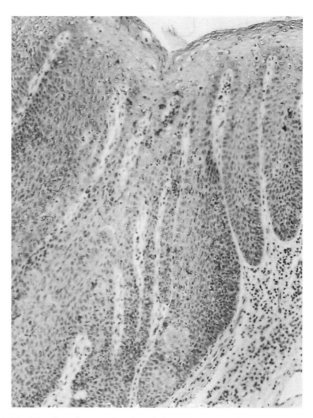

FIG. 19. Carcinoma *in situ* of the vulva showing intraepithelial pearl formation and individual cell anaplasia.

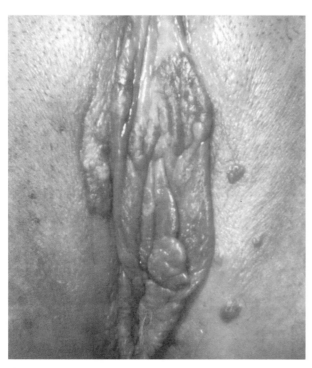

FIG. 18. Carcinoma *in situ* of the vulva presenting as irregularly pigmented lesions.

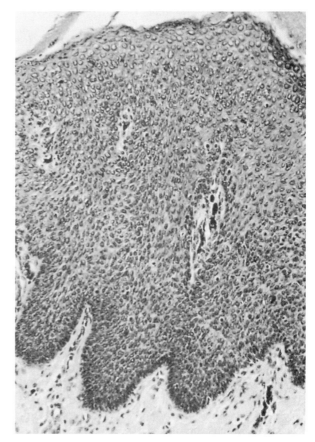

FIG. 20. Another pattern of intraepithelial vulvar carcinoma characterized by an increase in basal and parabasal cells.

effectively by wide local excision (i.e., disease-free border of at least 5 mm) with end-to-end approximation of the defect. Laser vaporization of these focal areas of involvement after multiple biopsies have ruled out invasive foci is also appropriate. With multicentric lesions, the problem becomes more complex. Laser vaporization over more than 30% to 40% of the vulva can result in intolerable postoperative discomfort. Many surgeons have used split-thickness skin grafts to replace the excised and involved vulvar skin. This skinning vulvectomy and skin graft procedure was introduced by Rutledge and Sinclair in 1968[9] (Fig. 21). Its purpose is to replace the skin at risk at the vulvar site with ectopic dermis from a donor site. The procedure was modified by Di Saia so that the clitoris can be preserved and any lesions on the glans clitoris are scraped off with a scalpel blade or superficially vaporized

with a laser; the epithelium of the glans regenerates without loss of sensation. Some reports have questioned this approach on the grounds that, at least in cases of vulvar dystrophy, the donated skin might be susceptible to a similar dystrophic process. However, neoplastic lesions have developed within the skin graft only rarely, and most recurrences have been outside the grafted area, on preserved skin.

Paget Disease

Like its counterpart on the breast, vulvar Paget disease (Fig. 22) is characterized grossly by a fiery red background mottled with white hyperkeratotic islands and, in this respect, resembles carcinoma *in situ*. Unlike the mammary lesion, which is usually associated with an underlying malignancy,

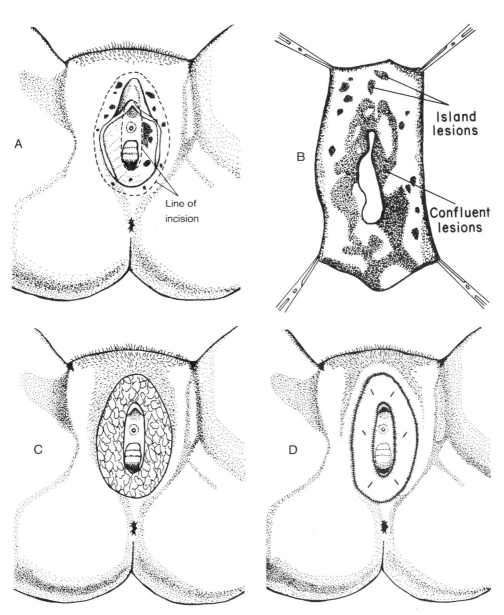

FIG. 21. Skinning vulvectomy and skin graft. **(A)** Excise all areas of involvement *en bloc*. **(B)** Lesions may be isolated or confluent. **(C)** Preserve all subcutaneous tissue as the graft bed. **(D)** Suture graft to graft bed. (From ref. 3.)

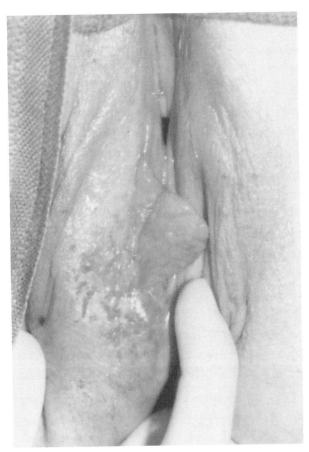

FIG. 22. Paget disease of the vulva presenting as a red background with mottled, white, hyperkeratotic islands. (This figure is printed in color as Plate 20.)

Microscopically, the characteristic large, pale cells of apocrine origin are found initially in the basal layer but eventually involve the entire surface epithelium and that of the underlying appendages (Fig. 23). The positive reaction of the cells to mucicarmine stain serves to differentiate the lesion from carcinoma *in situ* and melanoma.

Wide and deep excision of the involved skin is required to determine the extent of involvement of the underlying tissues. If invasive disease is recognized in the removed specimen, inguinal and femoral lymph node dissection is indicated. Because of the frequency of recurrence, careful follow-up is mandatory. Irradiation has been of little value for treating local or metastatic disease. The association with Paget disease of the breast has been recorded in several studies, and although they are uncommon, a thorough study of every patient should be made to rule out a mammary lesion. A similar statement is appropriate for malignant squamous lesions of the genital tract and anus as well as lesions of the lower colon, which have been reported to occur in patients with Paget disease.

Bergen and Di Saia described a series of patients with extramammary Paget disease of the vulva who were treated with wide local excision and split-thickness skin grafting. In their experience, extramammary Paget disease was most often intraepithelial, and patients with an underlying malignancy invariably had a palpable mass. Patients with disease limited to the epithelium can be identified and offered a more conservative approach than vulvectomy. This conservative approach requires careful margin checks at surgery to ensure optimal eradication of the lesion (Fig. 24). Recurrences are not infrequent, even with negative margins, but usually respond to local therapy. The subcutaneous tissue must be carefully inspected to avoid overlooking a small underlying invasive malignancy that may modify the surgeon's approach. The occurrence of this disease in sexually active middle-aged women has prompted the serious consideration of this less radical approach in an effort to preserve body image and sexual function.

the vulvar disease is solely intraepithelial in over 90% of patients. Nevertheless, the tendency to recur locally makes the neoplasm a constant threat. In addition to this threat, rare cases of malignancy have been reported to follow the initial intraepithelial lesion.

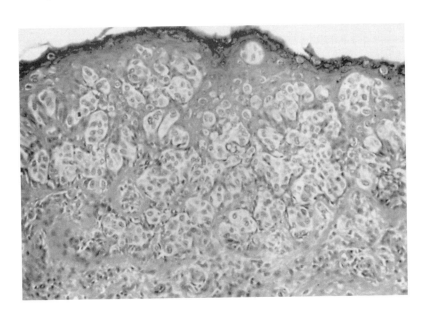

FIG. 23. Histology of Paget disease of the vulva. The large, pale cells of apocrine origin eventually involve the entire surface epithelium and underlying appendages. (This figure is printed in color as Plate 21.)

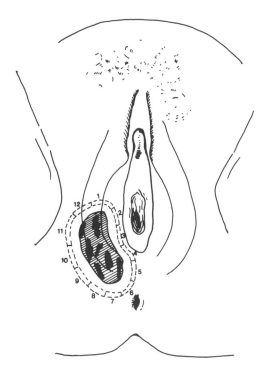

FIG. 24. A 2-cm margin is circumscribed around the gross Paget lesion, and another 5-mm strip is marked for excision. The perimeter is divided into 12 segments for identifying the frozen sections.

Invasive Carcinoma

The common vulvar malignancy is a skin cancer and should be classified as squamous cell, not epidermoid, carcinoma (Figs. 25, 26, and 27). Approximately 65% to 70% are ma-ture, pearl-forming tumors, and the remainder are poorly differentiated or a mixture of patterns. There is no difference in survival between these histologic variants. The average age of patients with vulvar cancer is 60 to 65 years. Approximately 10% of these malignancies are found in the third and fourth decades of life.

The primary symptom is pruritus, especially if the preceding disease is of the dystrophic type, but many patients have noticed a lump or local irritation for many years. Patients with chronic granulomatous disease or a long-standing benign tumor that has undergone malignant alteration usually complain of a mass, local discomfort, and bleeding. Diagnosis is made on examination of the biopsy material. Diagnostic problems lie in differentiating benign proliferating tumors and chronic granulomatous disease from their malignant counterparts.

Other Primary Malignancies

The vulva is the site of origin of approximately 2% to 3% of malignant melanomas in women. Because the spreading and the nodular varieties are difficult to differentiate from many of the benign pigmented lesions (Fig. 28), biopsy should be used freely. Early diagnosis is essential. Survival is directly related to the depth of invasion, which is categorized by the five Clark levels. Levels 1 and 2 (i.e., involvement of the intrapapillary ridges) are associated with essentially 100% 5-year survival; conversely, the salvage in level 5 tumors (i.e., involvement of the subcutaneous fat) is an unimpressive 0% to 20%.

Surgery is the treatment of choice, and irradiation and chemotherapy have added little to the salvage rate. Current

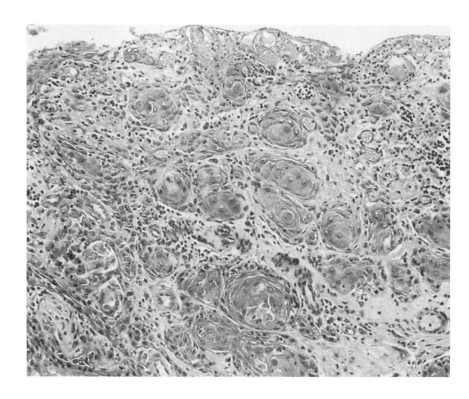

FIG. 25. Invasive cancer characterized by pearl formation without overlying full-thickness epithelial changes.

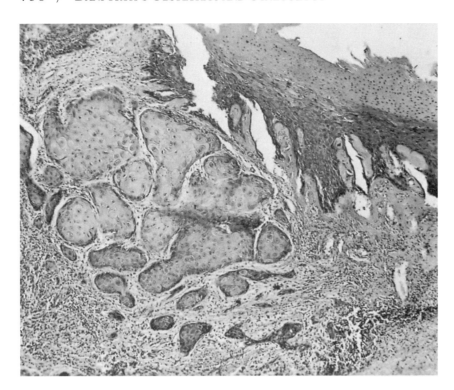

FIG. 26. Invasive carcinoma **(left)** with atypical maturation of invasive epithelium. Abnormal changes **(right)** are characterized by parakeratosis and irregular rete pegs with collagenation (i.e., leukoplakia).

thought suggests that there is no need for radical surgery in patients with involvement of only the epithelium and the rete ridge. Breslow has suggested depth measurement as a more accurate determinant of prognosis. For lesions that are less than 0.75 mm (i.e., Clark level 1), the 5-year survival rate is 100%; only rare patients with lesions extending from 0.75 to 1.5 mm (i.e., Clark levels 1 and 2) are found to have nodal involvement (Fig. 29). Therapy for these early lesions

is limited to wide local excision with no lymph node dissection.

Procrastination in treatment most often results from misdiagnosis or lack of follow-up after a suspicious area is biopsied. Biopsy is the method of diagnosis, and there is no validity in the opinion that every such lesion must be completely excised because of the danger of spread induced by biopsy. There is no evidence that the prognosis is worse for patients who are diagnosed during pregnancy or for individuals who choose to become pregnant subsequent to diagnosis and treatment of melanoma.

Rare cases of various sarcomas, including neurofibrosarcoma, leiomyosarcoma, and fibrosarcoma, have been reported arising primarily in the external genitalia. Surgery is the treatment of choice, although triple chemotherapy has been suggested by some researchers.

Lymphoma and embryonal rhabdomyosarcomas have been reported on the external genitalia. These cases classically arise in young people, and genital lymphoma often is the superficial demonstration of an underlying lesion.

Secondary Malignancies

Most secondary malignancies arise in the adjacent area and affect the vulva by direct extension; malignancies of the cervix, vagina, and rectum are common offenders. Adenocarcinoma of the endometrium and choriocarcinoma show a predilection for metastasizing to the external genitalia, and the diagnosis of trophoblastic malignancy sometimes is first made on examination of biopsy material from the vulvar metastasis. Extension from the cervix, vagina, or rectum may occur.

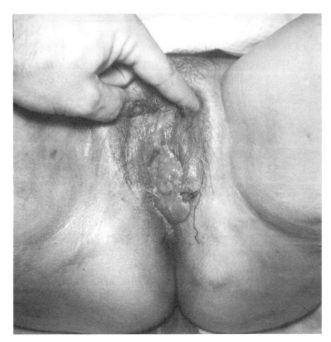

FIG. 27. Squamous cell cancer of the vulva.

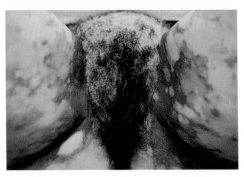

PLATE 14. Vitiligo in an African-American patient. (This plate is printed in black and white as Figure 48-3.)

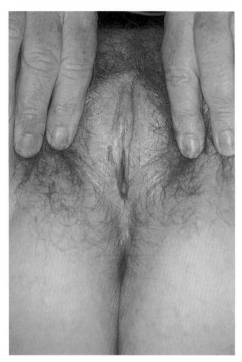

PLATE 15. Lichen sclerosus with an area of excoriation involves the labia minora and majora. (This plate is printed in black and white as Figure 48-5.)

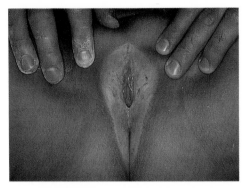

PLATE 16. Lichen sclerosus involving the vulva and perianal area in a 5-year-old girl. (This plate is printed in black and white as Figure 48-6.)

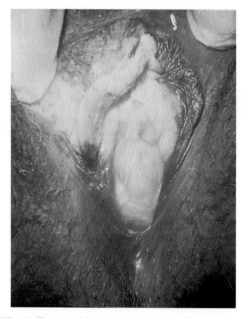

PLATE 17. Thick, white hyperkeratotic changes are characteristic of hypertrophic dystrophy. Biopsies should be used liberally for these patients to rule out malignancy. (This plate is printed in black and white as Figure 48-8.)

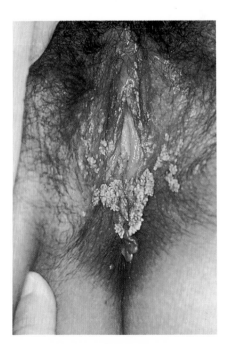

PLATE 18. Clusters of typical condylomata of the vulva. (This plate is printed in black and white as Figure 48-11.)

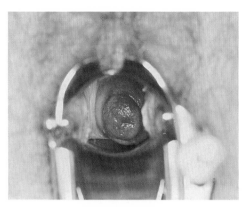

PLATE 19. The cervix of a 20-year-old diethylstilbestrol-exposed offspring demonstrates a complete cervical collar and polypoid structure of the central portion of the cervix. The anterior position is more prominent, giving rise to a partial deformity known as cockscomb. (This plate is printed in black and white as Figure 48-14.)

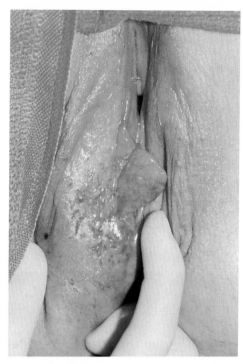

PLATE 20. Paget disease of the vulva presenting as a red background with mottled, white, hyperkeratotic islands. (This plate is printed in black and white as Figure 48-22.)

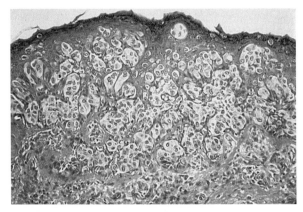

PLATE 21. Histology of Paget disease of the vulva. The large, pale cells of apocrine origin eventually involve the entire surface epithelium and underlying appendages. (This plate is printed in black and white as Figure 48-23.)

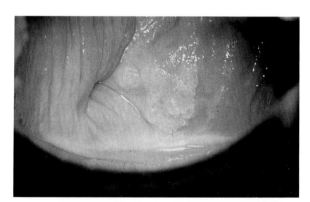

PLATE 22. Carcinoma *in situ* of the vaginal cuff after a hysterectomy for grade 3 cervical intraepithelial neoplasia. (Adapted from Cabanas RM. An approach to the treatment of penile carcinoma. *Cancer* 1997;39:456.) (This plate is printed in black and white as Figure 48-34.)

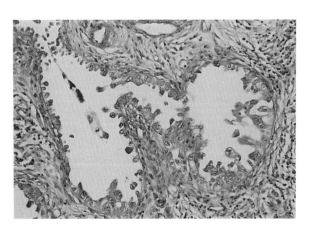

PLATE 23. Mesonephroid clear cell carcinoma was found in the vagina of an 18-year-old patient. High-power view reveals a hobnail pattern. (This plate is printed in black and white as Figure 48-36.)

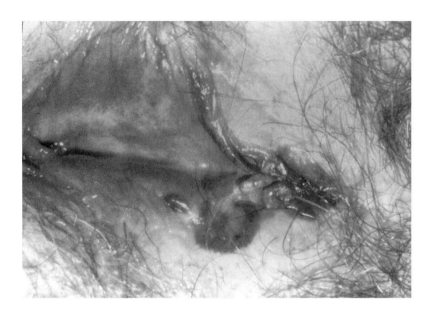

FIG. 28. Malignant melanoma of the clitoris.

Classification and Staging

The Fédération Internationale de Gynécologie et Obstetrique (FIGO) accepted in 1989 the classification of vulvar cancer. The TNM portion of the classification (i.e., tumor, nodes, metastases) is cumbersome and would be wisely eliminated. The final grouping of the FIGO classification, clinical staging, seems sufficient (Table 2).

Treatment

Treatment is fundamentally surgical, with removal of the vulva and the superficial and deep inguinal femoral nodes. The amount of normal skin and subcutaneous tissue routinely removed at the time of vulvectomy has gradually decreased over the past four decades, especially in the areas of the mons pubis and the groins.

The lymphatic drainage of the vulva is shown in Fig. 30. It has been suggested that there is cross-lymphatic circulation, and a bilateral lymphadenectomy should be carried out in most cases. Nevertheless, most studies suggest that unilateral lesions do not have contralateral nodal metastases if the ipsilateral nodes are not involved. In specific cases, unilateral node sampling may eliminate the need for the more extensive operation, which carries a predictably high postoperative morbidity. Extraperitoneal pelvic lymph node dissection is unwarranted today. Its place may be taken by pelvic irradiation if the superficial nodes are positive. An 85% to 90% sal-

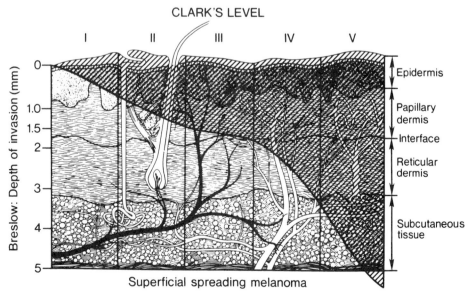

FIG. 29. Comparison of Clark and Breslow classifications. (From Prolog Unit #4, 1985. Courtesy of the American College of Obstetricians and Gynecologists.)

TABLE 2. *Fédération Internationale Gynecologie et Obstetrique clinical staging of invasive carcinoma of the vulva*

Stage 0	Carcinoma *in situ,* intraepithelial carcinoma
Stage I	Tumor confined to the vulva or perineum, ≤2 cm in greatest dimension, no nodal metastasis
Stage II	Tumor confined to the vulva or perineum, >2 cm in greatest dimension, no nodal metastasis
Stage III	Tumor of any size with (1) Adjacent spread to the lower urethra, the vagina, or the anus, or (2) Unilateral regional lymph node metastasis
Stage IVA	Tumor invades any of the following: upper urethra, bladder mucosa, rectal mucosa, pelvic bone, or bilateral regional node metastasis
Stage IVB	Any distant metastasis, including pelvic lymph nodes

vage may be expected if nodes are uninvolved, but even with metastasis to these regional sentinels, 5-year survival rates approximate 40%.

The incidence of positive inguinal and pelvic nodes varies considerably in the literature, but most investigators quote an incidence of roughly 40% for groin and pelvic node involvement and an overall 5% to 10% for pelvic node involvement alone. Some have quoted a 20% incidence of lymph node involvement if there is a stage I, T1 lesion (<2 cm in diameter). In T2 lesions (>2 cm in diameter but limited to the vulva), the incidence of lymph node involvement in some studies doubles to 40%. The rate of recurrence not only is dependent on the presence or absence of groin node metastases but also varies widely as a function of the number of nodes involved. Patients with only one or two small nodal metastases have an excellent outlook for survival (Table 3). Patients with positive inguinal nodes are given a course of radiation therapy to include the pelvic nodes. The practice of dissecting the pelvic nodes if the inguinal nodes are positive has been abandoned in the United States following the Gynecologic Oncology report of a randomized study of radiation therapy versus pelvic lymphadenectomy for patients with positive inguinal–femoral nodes.[6] Survival was improved in the group that received radical radiation therapy; more importantly, the incidence of complications was less in the group treated with radiation only. Pelvic irradiation can be limited to those patients with two or more positive inguinal–femoral nodes because these seem to be the only patients at a high risk for spread to the pelvic nodes.[5]

There is a lack of unanimity concerning the correct surgical approach to the patient with very early or macroscopic invasive carcinoma of the vulva. The morbidity associated with radical vulvectomy to body image and sexual function makes the issue worthy of serious consideration. In 1979, Di Saia

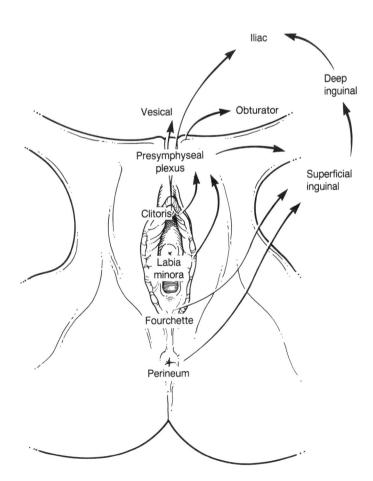

FIG. 30. Lymphatic spread of carcinoma of the vulva. (Adapted from ref. 8.)

TABLE 3. *Squamous cell cancer of vulva: Recurrence rate as a function of the number of positive groin node metastases*

		No. of recurrences (%)	
Study	n	≤ 2 nodes	≥ 3 nodes
Hoffman et al. (1985)	48	5/29 (17%)	14/19 (74%)
Hacker et al. (1984)	31	0/22 (0%)	4/9 (44%)
Curry et al. (1980)	30	7/21 (33%)	6/9 (67%)
Total	109	12/72 (17%)	24/37 (65%)

et al. published an alternative approach to early disease that stressed preservation of vulvar tissue, apparently without sacrificing curability.[4] This approach used all of the superficial inguinal nodes as sentinel nodes in the treatment planning when the central lesion was less than 1 cm in diameter and focal invasion was limited to 5 mm or less in depth. Patients with negative sentinel nodes in the inguinal area were candidates for wide local excision with or without skin grafting at the operative site. Berman et al.[1] reported on an additional group of patients using the Di Saia method but accepting lesions up to 2 cm in size with similar results. It is important to stress that all oblique and vertical nodes of the groin must be removed and declared negative to avoid subsequent groin recurrences. By these criteria, it appears that this approach is safe for treating early disease (Figs. 31 through 33).

Verrucous carcinoma is unique. Despite the massive local tumor, metastases to the regional nodes do not occur, and lymphadenectomy is unnecessary. Radiation therapy is contraindicated. Local recurrences are common and should be managed surgically.

Basal cell carcinoma constitutes less than 5% of all vulvar cancers. Like its counterpart on the skin elsewhere, it is a locally invasive but rarely metastasizing lesion. Wide local excision is the treatment of choice for these tumors.

Although the Bartholin gland is an uncommon site for primary malignancy, the tumors arising in the gland present a wide variety of patterns. The common squamous cell cancer develops at the orifice of the duct and represents a variant of primary vulvar carcinoma; it should not be classified as a Bartholin gland tumor. The transitional cell type arises from the characteristic urogenital epithelium of the duct. The true Bartholin gland cancer is a mucoid, cribriform adenocarcinoma that develops from the acini of the gland (i.e., adenoid cystic tumor). This variety deserves special mention because it is classically slow growing, indolent, and locally invasive, but late metastases occasionally appear in the lungs. The last type usually presents as an indurated mass in the deep recesses of the perineum, and the former types grossly simulate the common vulvar malignancies. Wide local excision is the treatment for the adenoid cystic lesion, but local recurrences are common.

◊ MALIGNANT TUMORS OF THE VAGINA

Primary malignancy arising in the vagina constitutes 2% to 4% of all anaplastic disease that arises *de novo* in the genital canal.

Vaginal malignancies may be classified as follows:

Primary malignancy
    Carcinoma
        Epidermoid carcinoma
        In situ (i.e., dysplasia)
        Invasive
        Adenocarcinoma
        Clear cell (i. e., mesonephroid carcinoma arising in adenosis)
        Adenocarcinoma in endometriosis

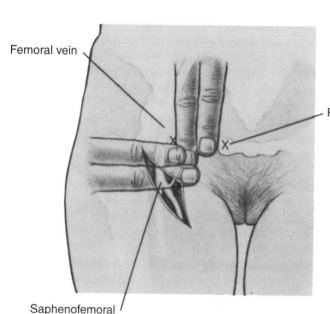

Femoral vein

Pubic tubercle

Saphenofemoral junction

FIG. 31. An incision can be made so that superficial inguinal nodes can be easily removed. (From ref. 2; with permission.)

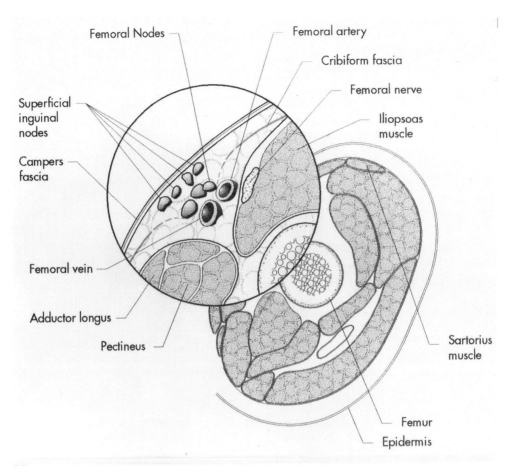

FIG. 32. Many inguinal nodes are located between the Camper fascia and the cribriform fascia, as noted on cross section through femoral triangle. Additional nodes are clustered in the foramen ovalis, in part protruding from beneath the plane of the cribriform fascia. (From ref. 2; with permission.)

Sarcoma
    Sarcoma botryoides
    Fibrosarcoma and leiomyosarcoma
    Rhabdomyosarcoma and lymphoma
Melanoma
Secondary malignancy, arising from primary lesion in cervix, endometrium, ovary, bowel, vulva, or urinary tract.

The FIGO staging system is used for describing primary carcinoma of the vagina:

Stage 0: Carcinoma *in situ*
Stage I: Carcinoma limited to vaginal wall
Stage II: Carcinoma involving subvaginal tissues but not extending to pelvic side wall
Stage III: Carcinoma extending to pelvic side wall
Stage IV: Carcinoma extending beyond true pelvis or involving mucosa of bladder or rectum (extension by bullous edema *per se* does not permit stage IV classification).

In Situ Epidermoid Carcinoma

In situ carcinoma of the vagina has been described as occurring in three situations: with other, similar lesions in the lower genital canal (i.e., possible regional response to a carcinogen); as residua after incomplete surgery for carcinoma *in situ* of the cervix (Fig. 34); and after irradiation for invasive carcinoma of the cervix. Preinvasive changes may be grossly evident before the development of invasive disease, but such lesions are in the minority. Although asymptomatic, these lesions can be recognized early if routine cytology is performed on all patients and if the possibilities of multicentric foci of original and postirradiation neoplasia are kept in mind.

Local excision of the involved area has been the mainstay of therapy. In many instances, a single isolated lesion can be removed easily in the office with biopsy forceps. If larger areas are involved, a partial vaginectomy may be necessary. The use of diluted solution of phenylephrine (Neo-Synephrine), which is injected submucosally at the time of surgery, facilitates the partial vaginectomy. Laser vaporization of involved areas to a depth of 1 to 2 mm is an alternative approach.

As with intraepithelial neoplasia of the cervix, outpatient modalities of therapy have been investigated for vaginal intraepithelial neoplasia (VAIN). The topical application of 5-FU cream has been advocated by many investigators. The technique of application of 5-FU cream to the vagina for

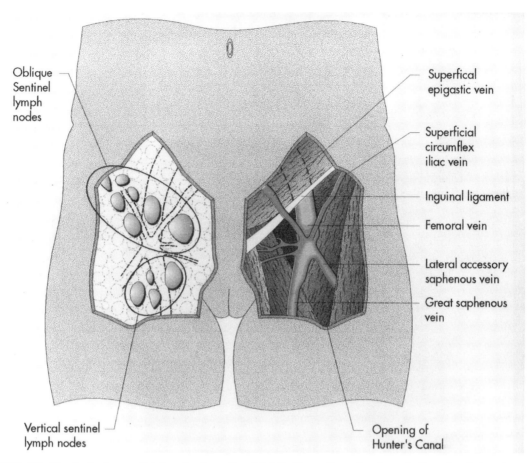

FIG. 33. The limit of superficial node dissection **(right)**. Dissection after the cribriform fascia has been removed **(left)**. The **right side** demonstrates the two groups of lymph nodes making up the "sentinel" nodes. The **left side** notes the limits of the dissection with the cribriform fascia removed. The triangle that is dissected in a full inguinal lymphadenotomy is clearly identified on the patient's left side. The inguinal ligament forms the base of the triangle, and the opening of Hunter's canal becomes the apex. The triangle is bound laterally by the sartorius muscle and medially by the adductor muscles and fascia. (From ref. 2; with permission.)

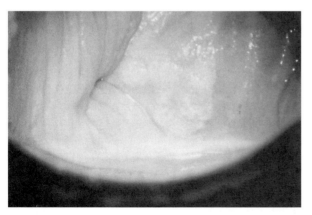

FIG. 34. Carcinoma *in situ* of the vaginal cuff after a hysterectomy for grade 3 cervical intraepithelial neoplasia. (This figure is printed in color as Plate 22.)

VAIN is identical to that described previously in this chapter for HPV lesions of the vagina (see Solid Tumors).

Some centers have advocated surface irradiation for VAIN, using an intravaginal applicator that delivers 5000 to 10,000 cGy to the vaginal mucosa, but most experience with this method of therapy has been discouraging, with a high recurrence rate and marked vaginal stenosis, making follow-up and further therapy extremely difficult. Total vaginectomy with vaginal reconstruction using a split-thickness skin graft is another option, but this should be reserved for the patient who has failed more conservative approaches.

Invasive Epidermoid Carcinoma

Invasive epidermoid carcinoma is the most common invasive neoplasm of the vagina. Approximately two-thirds of all patients are older than 50 years of age. The most common symptom is a bloody vaginal discharge, and in some series, total vaginal prolapse has been an associated finding. In the more extensive cases, urgency and pain on urination and defecation occur. The diagnosis is confirmed by biopsy.

Radiation therapy is still the most widely accepted primary treatment for invasive cancer of the vagina. External irradiation is usually followed by some type of brachytherapy, usually in the form of interstitial therapy, primarily using the isotope iridium. Interstitial therapy allows for a volume implant and more effective isodose curves than surface irradiation from an intravaginal application. The complications of radiation therapy, particularly vesicovaginal and rectovaginal fistulas, are more common than in the treatment of cervical cancer. Nonetheless, survival rates for vaginal cancer patients have improved to a point where the pessimism of the past should be abandoned. In a 1988 report by Perez et al., the actuarial disease-free 5-year survival rate for stage I was 75%; for stage IIA, 55%; for stage IIB, 43%; for stage III, 32%; and for stage IV, 10%.[7]

When invasive carcinoma involves the lower third of the vagina, the potential for inguinal lymph node involvement is similar to that of cancer of the vulva (Fig. 35). If inguinal nodes are involved with a lower vaginal lesion, management is usually the same as that for cancer of the vulva: radical surgery. If the lesion is in the upper vagina, the lymphatic spread pattern is similar to that of carcinoma of the cervix. Exenterative procedures should be reserved for patients who fail irradiation therapy, even in cases with involvement of the rectum, bladder, and urethra. Combinations of irradiation therapy and surgery may result in preservation of one or more of these pelvic organs.

More than 80% of the patients with recurrent disease have a pelvic recurrence that is clinically evident, and most recurrences develop within 2 years of primary therapy. Distant sites of involvement occur later and are much less frequent. Recurrent or persistent vaginal cancer requires ultraradical surgery of an exenterative type. Chemotherapy for recurrent squamous cell carcinoma of the vagina has been relatively ineffective, but cisplatin appears to be an active agent.

Adenocarcinoma

Primary adenocarcinoma is rare. In the last four decades, interest has been focused on one variety of adenocarcinoma that presumably arises in adenosis and develops most commonly in young women (i.e., 7 to 35 years of age) whose mothers may have received nonsteroidal estrogen therapy during pregnancy. These malignancies are difficult to diagnose in the early stages because of the infrequency with which the cells are shed from the deeper glandular elements. Colposcopy has not been able to identify the early malignant alterations in a potential group of 1 to 2 million exposed women. In view of the rarity of malignant change in such cases (i.e., 500 to 600 cases from a countrywide survey reside in the registry), it seems that the wisest approach to the patient at risk is careful observance with routine examina-

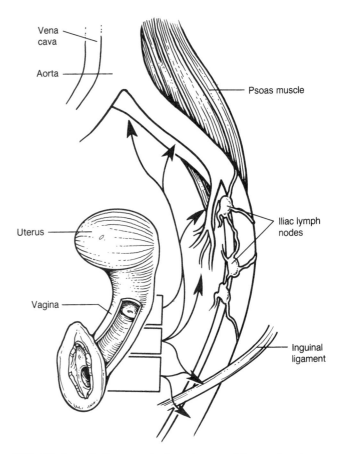

FIG. 35. Lymphatic spread of carcinoma of the vagina. Lymphatic channels from the lower one-third of the vagina drain into femoral and external iliac nodes (1). Channels from the middle one-third of the vagina drain into the hypogastric nodes (2). Channels from the upper one-third of the vagina drain into the common iliac, presacral, and hypogastric nodes (3). (Adapted from ref. 8.)

tions and multiple cytologic and colposcopic studies (Fig. 36; see Fig. 13).

If the malignancy arises in the upper half of the vagina in a young patient, the treatment most commonly prescribed is radical hysterectomy. This requires removal of the upper vagina, uterus, and pelvic lymph nodes, leaving the patient sterile. Fortunately, most patients present as stage I or IIA, when such therapy is reasonable. If there is extension of the disease to the bladder or rectum, or if the lower half of the vagina is involved, radiation therapy should be used as the primary approach. Radiation therapy has been used in some centers for most patients with good results reported. The overall 5-year survival rates are approximately 75%, with a high preponderance of patients presenting with stage I or IIA lesions. A few patients with very early lesions have been treated with investigative approaches that preserve childbearing capacity.

Sarcoma Botryoides

Although rare, sarcoma botryoides can be aggressive. This grape-like polypoid lesion arises from the lower end of the Müllerian tubercle. The initial symptom, a bloody vaginal dis-

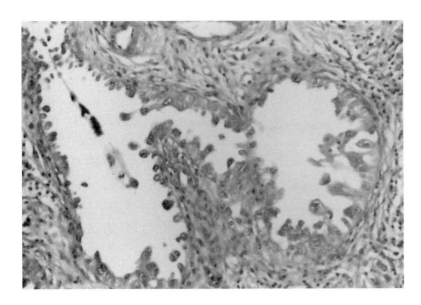

FIG. 36. Mesonephroid clear cell carcinoma was found in the vagina of an 18-year-old patient. High-power view reveals a hobnail pattern. (This figure is printed in color as Plate 23.)

charge, occurs in the first decade of life; two cases have been reported in newborns. The gross appearance is almost unmistakable, with grape-like clusters protruding from the introitus, although foreign bodies and acuminate warts may simulate the botryoid sarcoma. The microscopic picture is characterized by edematous blebs lined by a thin, stratified epithelium. The

loose stroma gives the false impression of benignity, but the elongated, malignant mesodermal elements that surround the rhabdomyoblast can be discerned by careful study.

Improvements in therapy were first reported with the use of exenterative surgery (Fig. 37), a loathsome procedure in these young children. Since the early 1970s, similar improved

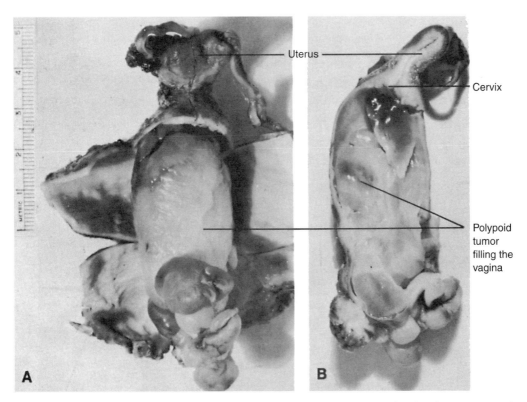

FIG. 37. Sarcoma botryoides, juvenile form. **(A)** Gross surgical specimen of lesion from a 16-month-old infant. The tumor arose in the vagina and invaded the pelvic tissues. The vagina has been split posteriorly to show the uterus and tumor. The patient was not given roentgenotherapy but was treated with aminopterin, a folic acid antagonist. She was alive and well 8 years later. **(B)** Midsagittal section of the specimen shown in **A**. Notice the lack of involvement of the uterus. (AFIP 218754-693 and 218754-694; specimen courtesy of Dr. Sidney Farber; from Hertig AT, Gore H. *Tumors of the female sex organs. Part 2. Tumors of the vulva, vagina and uterus.* Washington, DC: Armed Forces Institute of Pathology, 1960.)

results have been achieved with a combination of chemotherapy, irradiation, and less radical surgery. Few patients become candidates for exenteration, and most lesions can be controlled with a combination of therapies.

Other Primary Malignancies

Fibrosarcomas and leiomyosarcomas are rare primary malignancies of the vagina, as is malignant melanoma, although all such lesions have been reported. Prognosis depends on the extent of the lesion at the time of initial therapy. Most of the fibrosarcomas and leiomyosarcomas in young people are locally aggressive and recurring, but they seldom metastasize. The converse is true for the older patient.

Primary endodermal sinus tumors have been reported as primary lesions in the vagina. Fewer than 20 cases have been reported. The vagina actually represents an area close to the terminal portion of the line in the embryo, and it should not be surprising to see germ cell tumors in this area. It is important to detect them because triple chemotherapy has been effective in controlling these tumors in the ovary and should be instituted for similar lesions in the vagina. Surgery, as performed for sarcoma botryoides, is not the treatment of choice, and irradiation has been unsatisfactory for the similar lesion in the ovary.

Secondary Malignancy

Although primary neoplasia of the vagina is uncommon, secondary involvement by malignancies arising in the adjacent area is not. Direct extension from the cervix, rectum, or ovary may be found in the areas adjacent to the primary tumor. Metastases from endometrial cancer appear in the subepithelial lymphatics. Uterine choriocarcinoma may involve the vagina as a metastatic or locally invasive lesion.

◊ REFERENCES

1. Berman ML, Soper JT, Creasman WT, et al. Conservative surgical management of superficially invasive stage I vulvar carcinoma. *Gynecol Oncol* 1989;35:352.
2. Cabanas RM. An approach to the treatment of penile carcinoma. *Cancer* 1997;39:456.
3. Di Saia PJ, Creasman WT. *Clinical gynecologic oncology, 54th ed.* St Louis: CV Mosby, 1997.
4. Di Saia PJ, Creasman WT, Rich WM. Alternate approach to early cancer of the vulva. *Am J Obstet Gynecol* 1979;133:825.
5. Hoffman JS, Kumar NB, Morley GW. Prognostic significance of groin lymph node metastasis in squamous carcinoma of the vulvar. *Obstet Gynecol* 1985;66:402.
6. Homesley HD, Bundy BN, Sedlis A, Adcock L. Radiation therapy versus pelvic node dissection for carcinoma of the vulva with positive groin nodes. *Obstet Gynecol* 1986;68:733.
7. Perez CA, Camel HM, Galaktos AE, et al. Definitive radiation in the carcinoma of the vagina: long-term evaluation of results. *Int J Radiat Oncol Biol Phys* 1988;15:1283.
8. Plentl AA, Friedman EA. Lymphatic spread of carcinoma of the vulva. In: *Lymphatic system of the female genitalia.* Philadelphia: WB Saunders, 1971.
9. Rutledge FW, Sinclair M. Treatment of intraepithelial carcinoma of the vulva by skin excision and graft. *Am J Obstet Gynecol* 1968;102:806.

◊ RECOMMENDED READINGS

Anderson BL, Hacker NF. Psychosexual adjustment after vulvar surgery. *Obstet Gynecol* 1983;62:457.
Anderson WA, Franguemont DW, Williams J. Vulvar squamous cell carcinoma and papillomaviruses: two separate entities? *Am J Obstet Gynecol* 1991;165:329.
Andreasson B, Nyboe J. Value of prognostic parameters in squamous cell carcinoma of the vulva. *Gynecol Oncol* 1985;22:341.
Bergen S, Di Saia PJ. Conservative management of extramammary Paget's disease of the vulva. *Gynecol Oncol* 1989;33:151.
Borgno G, Micheletti L, Barbero M, et al. Topographic distribution of groin lymph nodes. *J Reprod Med* 1990;49:279.
Breslow A. Thickness, cross-sectional areas and depth of invasions in the prognosis of cutaneous melanoma. *Am Surg* 1970;172:902.
Burke TW, Stringer CA, Gershenson DM, et al. Radical wide excision and selective inguinal node dissection for squamous cell carcinoma of the vulva. *Gynecol Oncol* 1990;38:328.
Buscema J, Woodruff JD, Parmley TH, et al. Carcinoma *in situ* of the vulva. *Obstet Gynecol* 1980;55:225.
Clark WH Jr, From L, Bernardino EA, et al. The histogenesis and biologic behaviour of primary human malignant melanomas of the skin. *Cancer Res* 1969;29:705.
Curry SL, Wharton JT, Rutledge F. Positive lymph nodes in vulvar squamous carcinoma. *Gynecol Oncol* 1980;9:63.
Di Saia PJ, Rich WM. Surgical approach to multifocal carcinoma *in situ* of the vulva. *Am J Obstet Gynecol* 1981;140:136.
Eddy GL, Marks RD Jr, Miller C III, et al. Primary invasive vaginal carcinoma. *Am J Obstet Gynecol* 1991;165:292.
Hacker NF, Berek JS, Lagasse LD, et al. Individualization of treatment for stage I squamous cell carcinoma of the vulva. *Obstet Gynecol* 1984;63:155.
Hacker NF, Berek JS, Lagasse LD, et al. Management of regional lymph nodes and their prognostic influence in vulvar cancer. *Obstet Gynecol* 1984;63:155.
Helm CW, Hatch K, Austin JM, et al. A matched comparison of single and triple incision techniques for the surgical treatment of carcinoma of the vulva. *Gynecol Oncol* 1992;46:150.
Hoffman MS, Roberts WS, Finan MA, et al. A comparative study of radical vulvectomy and modified radical vulvectomy for the treatment of invasive squamous cell carcinoma of the vulva. *Gynecol Oncol* 1992;45:192.
Homesley HD, Bundy BN, Sedlis A, et al. Prognostic factors for groin node metastasis in squamous cell carcinoma of the vulva (A Gynecologic Oncology Group Study). *Gynecol Oncol* 1993;49:279.
Iversen T, Aas M. The lymph drainage from the vulva. *Gynecol Oncol* 1983;16:179.
Kaufman RH, Friedrich EG, Gardner HL. *Benign lesions of the vulva and vagina.* Chicago: Yearbook Publishers, 1989.
Mann MS, Kaufman RH, Brown D Jr, et al. Vulvar vestibulitis: significant clinical variables and treatment outcome. *Obstet Gynecol* 1992;79:122.
Perez CA, Camel HM. Long-term follow-up in radiation therapy of carcinoma of the vagina. *Cancer* 1982;49:1308.
Robboy SJ, Noller KL, O'Brien P, et al. Increased incidence of cervical and vaginal dysplasia in 3980 diethylstilbestrol-exposed young women. *JAMA* 1984;252:2979.
Sandberg EC. Benign cervical and vaginal changes associated with exposure to stilbestrol *in utero. Am J Obstet Gynecol* 1976;125:777.
Stafl A, Mettingly RF, Faley DV, et al. Clinical diagnosis of vaginal adenosis. *Obstet Gynecol* 1974;43:118.
Thomas GM, Dembo AJ, Bryson SC, et al. Changing concepts in the management of vulvar cancer. *Gynecol Oncol* 1991;42:9.
Trimble EL, Rubinstein LV, Menck HR, et al. Vaginal clear cell adenocarcinoma in the United States. *Gynecol Oncol* 1996;61:113.
Virgili A, Corazza M, Bianchi A, et al. Open study of topical 0.025% tretinoin in the treatment of vulvar lichen sclerosus. *J Reprod Med* 1995;40:614.

CHAPTER 49

Disorders of the Uterine Cervix

———— ◊ ————

Robert E. Bristow
Beth Y. Karlan

◊ BENIGN LESIONS

Anatomy and Physiology of the Cervix

Normal Findings

The cervix (Latin for neck) is a narrow, cylindrical segment of the uterus; it enters the vagina through the anterior vaginal wall and in most instances lies at right angles to it. In the average patient, the cervix is 2 to 4 cm long and is contiguous with the inferior aspect of the uterine corpus. The point of juncture is known as the isthmus; this area is marked by a slight constriction of the lumen. Anteriorly, the cervix is separated from the bladder by fatty tissue and is connected laterally to the broad ligament and parametria, through which it obtains its blood supply from the uterine artery. The cul-de-sac of Douglas lies immediately posterior to the cervix. The ureters are intimately associated with the cervix as they course inferomedially through the pelvis (Fig. 1). As they cross beneath the uterine artery, the ureters are approximately 1.0 to 1.5cm lateral to the uterine cervix.

The lower intravaginal portion of the cervix is a free segment that projects through the vault of the vagina and is covered with mucous membrane. The cervix opens into the vaginal cavity through the external os. The cervical canal extends from the anatomic external os through the internal os, where it joins the uterine cavity (see Fig. 1). In the internal os, there is a histologic transition from endocervical to endometrial glands. The portio vaginalis cervicis, also called the intravaginal portion of the cervix or ectocervix, is covered with stratified squamous epithelium that is essentially identical with the epithelium of the vagina. The endocervical mucosa is arranged in branching folds or crypts (i.e., plicae palmatae) and is lined by cylindrical epithelium. The stroma of the cervix is composed of connective tissue with stratified muscle fibers and elastic tissue. The elastic tissue is primarily found around the walls of the larger blood vessels.

Cervical mucus is produced by the secretory cells of the endocervical glands. The cervical canal contains approximately 100 crypts, often referred to as glands. The secretory cells in these crypts secrete mucus into the lumen of the endocervical canal. Under normal conditions, the mucus undergoes quantitative and qualitative changes, depending on the hormonal predominances in the different phases of the menstrual cycle. The cervix also undergoes anatomic changes during the menstrual cycle. The external os progressively widens during the proliferative phase, reaching maximal width just before ovulation occurs. At the time of maximal widening, cervical mucus usually exudes from the external os. After ovulation, the cervical os returns to a small diameter and the profuse, clear mucus becomes scant and viscid.

Abnormal Findings

Stenosis

Congenital stenosis of the endocervical canal is an uncommon finding occasionally encountered in the diagnostic evaluation of an infertile couple. The diagnosis is made by exclusion and is heralded by failure in attempts to pass a small catheter or probe into the endocervical canal. Stenosis of the cervix may follow chronic cervical infection, treatment of endocervicitis, cauterization of the cervix, cryosurgery or laser surgery of the cervix, radiation therapy, or senile atrophy. All of these factors must be excluded when a diagnosis of congenital stenosis is made.

Stenosis is usually asymptomatic, but it may cause abnormal genital bleeding, dysmenorrhea, and infertility. Stenosis can occur following diagnostic or therapeutic conization of the cervix by both cold knife and loop electrosurgical excision procedure techniques. For this reason, cervical patency should be ensured by sounding the cervical canal at postoperative examinations. If stenosis is complete or near complete, the accumulation of cervical or uterine secretions may

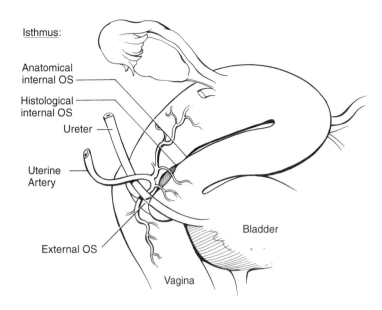

Isthmus:

Anatomical internal OS

Histological internal OS

Ureter

Uterine Artery

External OS

Vagina

Bladder

FIG. 1. Anatomy of the cervix.

cause distention of the uterus with blood (hematometra), fluid (hydrometra), or inflammatory exudate (pyometra). These conditions, which produce a distended, fluid-filled endometrial cavity, can be confused with adnexal masses of ovarian origin. They may be asymptomatic for prolonged periods and, on bimanual examination, often appear to be cystic. The diagnosis can often be confirmed by passing a small uterine sound or probe through the area of cervical stenosis into the fluid-filled endometrial cavity. Some patients must be treated with endocervical dilation and maintenance of a patent endocervical canal with an indwelling drain.

Polyps

Cervical polyps vary in length from a few millimeters to 3 cm. They are pedunculated, roughly pear-shaped, soft, smooth, and red or purple (Fig. 2). The pedicle almost always arises from the cervical canal, but occasionally it arises from the external surface of the cervix. In most cases, only a single polyp is present, but two or three may be found at the same time. When excised completely, polyps seldom recur after removal.

Microscopically, polyps are found to be a hyperplastic condition of the endocervical epithelium. They usually have a large number of blood vessels, especially near the surface. Associated inflammation and edema contribute to the size of the polyp. The chief symptoms of polyps are menorrhagia and leukorrhea, but women with cervical polyps are often asymptomatic. The polyp is often felt during bimanual examination, but in some patients it may not be evident until a speculum examination is performed. It is difficult to prevent the formation of polyps because their exact cause is unknown.

The treatment of cervical polyps is usually simple. A pedunculated polyp can often be avulsed hemostatically by grasping the polyp with a clamp and twisting repeatedly about the stalk. If the polyp is large, a clamp can be applied approximately 0.5 cm above the origin of the pedicle. A surgical ligature should be tied between the clamp and the cervix, and then the clamp can be removed. The polyp can be excised by cutting along the line of crush, or it can be allowed to remain

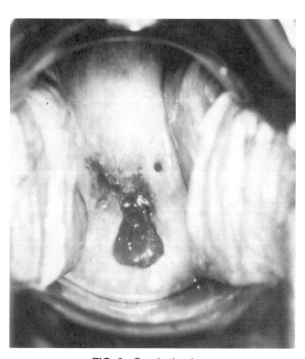

FIG. 2. Cervical polyp.

in situ, in which case it will undergo infarction and slough. All tissue removed should be sent for pathologic review because a malignancy can arise in these benign-appearing structures.

Hyperplasia and Metaplasia

Microglandular hyperplasia is a benign condition usually associated with the use of oral contraceptives or occasionally with pregnancy; it is rarely observed in their absence. Grossly, the lesion is soft, granular, tan-yellow, and usually flat. Microscopic examination demonstrates many small, closely packed glands devoid of intervening stroma. Microglandular hyperplasia is of considerable importance because it can often be misinterpreted as being a well differentiated adenocarcinoma by an inexperienced pathologist. The lesion is generally reversed when oral contraceptives are discontinued.

Metaplasia is defined as the replacement of one type of mature tissue by another equally mature type of tissue. In the cervix, squamous metaplasia is the replacement of the mucin-producing columnar epithelium by stratified squamous epithelium. The progression of squamous transformation of the endocervical ectropion is primarily dependent on local (vaginal) environmental factors, with the initial stimulus being the low (acid) pH of the vagina after puberty. Trauma, chronic irritation, or cervical infection also play a role in the development and maturation of the transformation zone by stimulating repair and remodeling.

One mechanism by which glandular cervical epithelium is replaced consists of direct ingrowth from the native portio squamous epithelium bordering the columnar epithelium, frequently referred to as squamous epithelialization. In this process, tongues of native squamous epithelium on the portio grow beneath the adjacent columnar epithelium and expand between the mucinous epithelium and its basement membrane. As the squamous cells expand and mature, the endocervical cells are gradually displaced upward, degenerate, and are eventually sloughed. In a typical area of epidermalization, the squamous epithelium differs from the normal tissue in that normal maturation and keratinization are absent, the cell layers are not apparent, and there may be a certain amount of epithelial architectural disorganization. The proximal or cranial edge of this process of epidermalization as it abuts the endocervical glands is the transformation zone, where active physiologic metaplasia takes place.

The second mechanism involved in replacement of columnar epithelium by a squamous epithelium, and the function of the transformation zone, is squamous metaplasia. Progressive growth and stratification of subcolumnar reserve cells is followed by differentiation into immature squamous cells. Immature squamous metaplasia is distinguished from its mature counterpart by a lack of surface maturation, and it is characteristically sharply demarcated from the native portio epithelium. As a result, the uninitiated observer may mistake immature squamous metaplasia for a preinvasive cervical lesion.

Eventually, the ectocervix is covered by a protective surface of mature squamous epithelium.

Inflammatory Lesions

Inflammation of the cervix is so prevalent that a physician must search long and hard to find a specimen without some indication of acute or chronic cervicitis. The cervix is constantly exposed to trauma during life processes (e.g., childbirth, coitus). The abundant mucus secretion of the endocervical glands, in conjunction with the bacterial flora of the vagina that bathes the cervix, creates an environment that is conducive to infection. In most women, cervicitis is a microscopic finding of no clinical consequence, and only a few patients are symptomatic and require treatment.

Acute Cervicitis

Acute cervicitis is most frequently associated with infection by either *Neisseria gonorrhoeae* or *Chlamydia trachomatis.* While both gonococcal and chlamydial infections can involve the endocervical glands, *N. gonorrhoeae* may also involve the glands of the urethra, the Skene glands, and the Bartholin gland. Other organisms, such as streptococci, staphylococci, enterococci, and *Gardnerella vaginalis,* may also infect the cervix and cause acute cervicitis.

Although the inflammatory process is usually confined to the endocervical glands, the squamous epithelium of the portio may become involved, a process called acute exocervicitis. The extent of endocervical involvement compared with exocervical involvement appears to have some relation to the infectious agent involved. Gonococcal and chlamydial infections are largely confined to the epithelial lining and ducts of the racemose endocervical glands located deep in the cervical stroma. Streptococcal and staphylococcal organisms tend to penetrate more deeply into the cervical wall and involve the gland acini themselves. This pathogenesis explains the manner in which streptococcal infections reach the lymphatic channels of the cervix and produce a pelvic cellulitis. Undoubtedly, this is the pathway of infection in septic abortions. Gonorrhea usually spreads along contiguous mucous membrane surfaces as a superficial infection.

The cervix and the rest of the vaginal canal are often red, swollen, and edematous, and a purulent discharge may exude from the cervical canal. The primary symptom of acute cervicitis is leukorrhea. The type of discharge varies considerably but may be purulent and profuse, particularly if the cause is gonorrhea. Other symptoms include backache, a bearing-down feeling in the pelvis, dull pain in the lower part of the abdomen, and urinary disturbances, especially frequency and urgency. Some women complain of painful intercourse. There is little in the way of a systemic reaction. There may be a slight elevation of body temperature, but most of the symptoms are concentrated in the genitalia. In many instances, the only symptom is profuse leukorrhea.

Tests for both gonorrhea (culture on Thayer-Martin media) and chlamydiosis, such as cell culture, enzyme-linked immunosorbent assay, or direct fluorescent antibody, should be performed. The microbial etiology of endocervicitis is unknown in approximately 50% of cases in which gonococci or chlamydiae are not detected. The treatment of acute cervicitis is limitation of pelvic activity and appropriate antibiotic therapy (Table 1).

Chronic Cervicitis

Between 90% and 95% of parous women have some evidence of chronic cervicitis, but this is usually minimal, asymptomatic, and not clinically apparent. The cervix that harbors chronic infection does not offer any consistent picture that may be regarded as characteristic. The most common clinical manifestation is cervical erosion. Erosion indicates the presence, around the cervical os, of a zone of infected tissue that has a granular, inflamed appearance. It implies the loss of superficial layers of the stratified squamous epithelium of the cervix (Fig. 3) and overgrowth of infected endocervical tissues. There is usually a yellow, mucopurulent discharge that on culture yields organisms such as *Escherichia coli* and *Enterobacter aerogenes*.

Chronic cervicitis can be associated with formation of a cervical ulcer, a lesion in which the full thickness of the cervical epithelium is lost and the underlying stroma is exposed and involved in the infection. A predisposing cause of erosion and cervical ulcer is a condition known as ectropion, in which there has been a laceration or dilatation of the external os, usually during previous childbirth, that leaves a considerable area of the endocervix exposed to the acid pH and bacterial flora of the vagina. Chronic cervicitis may appear as reddish granulation tissue raised above the surrounding surface, giving the impression of being papillary.

The inflammatory process stimulates a reparative attempt in the form of an upward growth of squamous epithelium, causing some of the ducts of the endocervical glands to be pinched off. Retention of mucus and other fluid within these glands results in the formation of nabothian cysts—endocer-

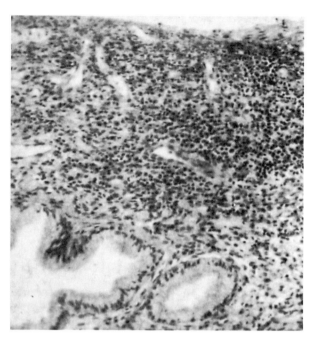

FIG. 3. In cervical erosion associated with chronic cervicitis, the surface squamous epithelium is absent, and the stroma is densely infiltrated with inflammatory cells.

vical glands filled with infected secretions whose ducts have become occluded secondary to inflammation and reparative processes. They may be single or multiple, and vary considerably in size. On drainage, they usually emit a clear mucus, but drainage sometimes reveals a mucopurulent material, signaling a recent infection.

The symptoms of chronic cervicitis are vaginal discharge that is usually yellowish white, thick, and tenacious and postcoital or postdouche spotting or bleeding. The endocervical epithelium is often swollen, edematous, and exposed; it is readily traumatized, with the result that patients frequently present with slight, irregular, intermenstrual bleeding. This can mimic the condition that often heralds a cervical polyp. Backache is a common complaint in patients who have chronic cervicitis. Other patients with chronic cervicitis complain of urgency and frequency of urination. Cystoscopic examination of these patients reveals an acute or chronic trigonitis of the bladder. It has been postulated that the trigonitis is secondary to spread of the infection from the cervix to the trigone by way of the lymphatic pathways to the floor of the bladder. This is the probable explanation of the condition known as "honeymoon bladder", in which excessive stimulation and trauma to the cervix results in a low-grade inflammatory process in the cervix that manifests itself as trigonitis. This condition has traditionally responded well to sexual abstinence, which undoubtedly results in avoidance of trauma to the cervix and decreased inflammation of the cervix and trigone.

The most important consideration in the diagnosis of chronic cervicitis is the exclusion of a malignant process. Before treatment is begun, a careful examination of the cervix, preferably with a colposcope, should be carried out. A Papanicolaou

---

TABLE 1. *Treatment regimens for gonococcal and chlamydial endocervicitis*

Gonococcal endocervicitis
Ceftriaxone sodium (Rocephin), 125 mg IM (single dose), or
Ofloxacin (Floxin), 400 mg PO (single dose), or
Cefixime (Suprax), 400 mg PO (single dose), or
Ciprofloxacin (Cipro), 500 mg PO (single dose)

Chlamydial endocervicitis
Doxycycline, 100 mg PO b.i.d. for 7 d, or
Azithromycin (Zithromax), 1 g PO (single dose), or
Ofloxacin, 300 mg PO b.i.d. for 7 d, or
Erythromycin base, 500 mg PO q.i.d. for 7 d, or
Erythromycin ethylsuccinate, 800 mg PO q.i.d. for 7 d

(From Centers for Disease Control and Prevention. *MMWR* 1993;42:51–57; with permission.)

test (Pap smear) should be performed, and any areas that appear suspicious should undergo biopsy. The final reports on cytologic smears and tissue biopsies should be acquired before treatment is instituted.

Treatment of chronic cervicitis and endocervicitis, erosions, and nabothian cysts is preventive and curative. Antibiotic therapy should be directed toward specific pathogens isolated on cervical culture. Prevention of recurrent infections of the cervix, such as gonorrhea, eliminates a large portion of cases, as does optimal obstetric care. Prophylactic measures during labor, such as awaiting spontaneous complete dilatation of the cervix before delivery is attempted and immediate repair of all cervical lacerations, decrease the incidence of ectropion, erosion, cervical ulcers, and chronic cervicitis. With appropriate antibiotic therapy, ablative treatment of chronic cervicitis has become primarily of historical interest only.

Cervical Tuberculosis

Cervical tuberculosis represents a small fraction of congenital tuberculosis, estimated to occur in only 1% of cases. Although older literature contains some correlations between cervical tuberculosis and epidermoid carcinoma of the cervix, no clear causative relation has been firmly established. On clinical inspection, the cervix is often found to be markedly irregular and sometimes ulcerated, a condition that can easily give the appearance of a malignant tumor. The diagnosis is easily made by performing a biopsy. The typical microscopic lesions are usually found; these include the tuberculous granuloma with epithelioid cells surrounded by lymphocytes and Langhans giant cells with little central cavitation.

Cervical Syphilis

Cervical chancre is caused by *Treponema pallidum* and is the second most common site after vulvar localization. This lesion is often confused with a simple cervical erosion. The chancre usually presents as an ulcer with an indurated base and elevated borders surrounded by a zone of edema or as a simple, nonindurated erosion covered by a gray, membranous exudate. It is painless and often accompanied by only a slight amount of serosanguineous discharge. It is particularly obvious during pregnancy because its indurated aspect contrasts sharply with the soft consistency of the cervix. A nontreponemal rapid plasma reagin test or VDRL test and a confirmatory treponemal test—fluorescent treponemal antibody absorption or microhemagglutinin *Treponema pallidum*—should be used to presumptively diagnose syphilis. Darkfield microscopic investigation may also be useful for diagnosis. The differential diagnosis includes granuloma inguinale, acute gonorrhea, chancroid, and carcinoma.

Herpetic Lesions

Human herpesvirus (HHV) 2, which is closely related to herpes labialis (i.e., herpes simplex virus type 1), can cause a lesion of the cervix that is similar to the vulvar lesion called herpes progenitalis (Fig. 4). The occurrence of these lesions on the cervix is considered to be a result of venereal transmission. The characteristic appearance on the cervix is similar to that on the vulva, with groups of multiple vesicles surrounded by a diffuse area of inflammation and edema. Occasionally, they are associated with a burning sensation in the vaginal area, but this is difficult to analyze, because they are often associated with vulvar lesions. These lesions may appear as multiple, small, superficial ulcers with or without vesicles. With the initial herpes infection, there may be a prodromal period of several days with constitutional symptoms, such as fever, malaise, and headache. Cervical and vaginal lesions are usually associated with leukorrhea, occasional abnormal spotting, vaginal pain, and dyspareunia. The differential diagnosis includes other venereal diseases such as syphilis, tuberculosis, condylomata, and chancre.

An initial episode of genital herpes can be treated with acyclovir (Zovirax), 200 mg orally five times daily for 7 to 10 days. Although this treatment regimen provides partial control of the symptoms and signs of clinical herpetic infection, it neither eradicates latent virus nor affects subsequent risk, frequency, or severity of recurrences after the drug is discontinued. Suppressive therapy (acyclovir, 400 mg orally twice daily) reduces the frequency of HHV recurrences by at least 75% among patients with six or more yearly recurrences of genital herpes.

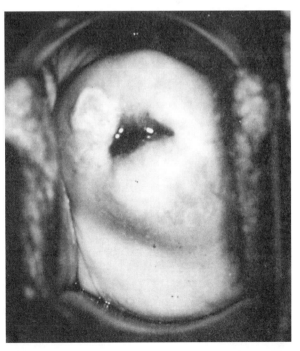

FIG. 4. Herpetic ulcer on the portio of the cervix. (From Di Saia PJ. The cervix. In: Romney S, Quilligan E, eds. *Gynecology and obstetrics.* New York: McGraw-Hill, 1981; with permission.)

Condylomata Acuminata

Condylomata acuminata are frequently multifocal warty growths caused by the human papillomavirus (HPV), usually types 6 and 11 (Fig. 5). The cervix is less frequently involved in these infections than either the vulva or vagina. As with other genital tract condylomata, pregnancy is likely to amplify the number of lesions. Very large growths are sometimes mistaken for carcinoma. A small biopsy is usually obtained for verification before medical therapy is begun. A satisfactory response can be obtained with podophyllin, which is contraindicated during pregnancy, or trichloroacetic acid. Lesions may also be destroyed by laser ablation, cryotherapy, electrodesiccation, or cautery. Immune therapy with intralesional or systemic interferon injections may be useful in some cases. There have also been some reports of successful use of 5-fluorouracil cream in the upper vagina. With most therapies, recurrence is common, since the virus is often incompletely eradicated.

Noninflammatory Benign Lesions

Leiomyomas

Tumors composed principally of smooth muscle fibers are common in the uterus, but the cervix is seldom their primary

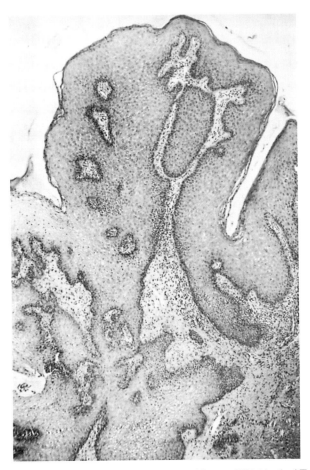

FIG. 5. Papillary condylomata. (From Kistner RW, Hertig AT. Papillomas of the uterine cervix: their malignant potentiality.

site. Radman observed three cervical leiomyomas in a series of 1068 patients who were admitted to the hospital for definitive therapy. These tumors caused an irregular enlargement of the cervix and sometimes led to ulceration of the mucous membrane. Any leiomyomas of the body of the uterus may secondarily involve the cervix by extension or by prolapse into the cervical canal. Myomas commonly present by aborting through the cervical canal, a process accompanied by uterine contractions and a considerable amount of discomfort. If the diagnosis is to be made by biopsy, the specimen must be of sufficient depth to reveal the characteristic microscopic pattern. Biopsies that go no more deeply than the mucosa cannot produce a definitive diagnosis.

Hemangioma

Hemangiomas are composed of small vascular channels with narrow lumina (capillary hemangiomas) or of distended, closely grouped vessels (cavernous hemangiomas). When the lesions are within the mucous membranes of the cervix, they appear as pink or red ill-defined areas. These lesions are usually asymptomatic but can cause hemorrhage and are commonly confused with endometriosis. Although biopsy is often associated with heavy bleeding, it is usually the only method of establishing the diagnosis.

Neurofibromas and hemangioendotheliomas have also been found in the cervix. These rare tumors are a curiosity and have no clinical significance, because they are usually asymptomatic. Treatment of all these lesions is necessary only if symptoms are annoying or if the lesions are a possible cause of infertility.

Endometriosis

Superficial endometriosis may readily be identified by examination. The lesion usually presents as a slightly raised, red area that does not fade when pressure is applied. Occasionally, there is a bluish discoloration with the erythema. However, visible lesions such as these are a rare finding, because endometriosis is usually found in the substance of the cervix and only rarely on the surface. In a high percentage of patients, it is associated with adenomyosis of the uterus and pelvic endometriosis. The treatment follows the same outline as for pelvic endometriosis.

Vestigial Mesonephric Structures and Adenosis

The adult cervix often harbors remnants of the mesonephric or wolffian ducts in the midlateral aspects of the connective tissue body. A specimen of cervical conization is likely to contain the lateral area of the cervix, where these structures occur; and in searching for other disease in the specimen, the physician is likely to find wolffian ductal remnants. They may present in a cystic or adenomatous form; rarely, an adenocarcinoma may arise from vestigial mesonephric remnants.

The term *adenosis* is used to describe another adenomatous retention, in which there are many more gland-like spaces due to failure of involution and persistence of a fetal duct. However, the neoplastic organization that could be described as an adenoma is absent. A considerable amount of evidence suggests that adenosis is of müllerian, not wolffian, duct origin. The adenocarcinoma that may arise from these remnants is the clear-cell variety, and it has been associated with maternal ingestion of diethylstilbestrol (DES) during the first and second trimesters of pregnancy.

Diethylstilbestrol-related Cervical Changes

Between 50% and 60% of DES-exposed female offspring have various degrees of anomalous cervical changes. DES-associated changes have been classified as

◊ Circular sulcus,
◊ Recessed ring surrounding the external os,
◊ Portio vaginalis completely covered by columnar epithelium,
◊ Endocervical gland hypertrophy with pseudopolyp formation,
◊ Anterior cervical lip protuberance (i.e., cock's comb).

All these changes can be associated with various degrees of vaginal stenosis and adenosis. It has been reported that DES-exposed women have an incidence of cervical and vaginal intraepithelial neoplasia twice that of unexposed women. Even in the absence of adenosis, these patients should have yearly surveillance with Pap smears taken from both the cervix and the upper vagina. While annual colposcopy is unnecessary, any Pap smear abnormality should be evaluated by an experienced colposcopist. If extensive adenosis is present, patients should have semiannual cervicovaginal cytology (every 6 months), and colposcopy should be performed at 2-year intervals. Cervical changes associated with DES exposure have been linked to cervical incompetence in pregnancy and to reduced fertility (e.g., spontaneous abortions, ectopic pregnancy).

Leukoplakia

Cervical leukoplakia is a term sometimes used to describe hyperkeratosis or parakeratosis; it can be found in up to 8% of women undergoing routine Pap smear screening. Both hyperkeratosis and parakeratosis can be recognized with the naked eye and have the gross appearance of a thickened white epithelium in either a focal or diffuse pattern. The etiologic and histogenic mechanisms of cervical hyperkeratosis are poorly understood. Most patients with diffuse hyperkeratosis have a prolapsed uterus. Focal areas of hyperkeratosis are sometimes associated with a local chronic irritation. These leukoplakia plaques are usually irregular, angular, and slightly raised from the surface. They are often loosely attached at the base, and vigorous wiping or scraping catches part or all of the white material. Although there is neither morphologic nor clinical evidence that hyperkeratosis or parakeratosis represents precursor lesions to cervical neoplasia, both can occur in association with squamous intraepithelial lesions (SIL; cervical intraepithelial neoplasia) and invasive cervical cancer. Recent evidence indicates that fewer that 4% of women with hyperkeratosis or parakeratosis without nuclear atypia on an otherwise negative Pap smear have SIL and that in all instances the SIL has been low-grade. While routine colposcopy of such women is unnecessary, all grossly visible white plaques on the portio vaginalis or vaginal epithelium should be biopsied, as hyperkeratosis may occasionally overlie an invasive carcinoma.

Cervical Pregnancy

Cervical pregnancy occurs in only 1 of 10,000 pregnancies. Implantation must occur below the internal os of the cervix. The space available for the developing pregnancy is obviously limited, resulting in the most frequent symptom of brisk, painless bleeding. Examination reveals a large, bulky, soft cervix with a small fundus protruding from above, resembling a subserous myoma. The appearance of the cervix is often confused with a malignancy because of the friable tissue within the canal. Ultrasonography is helpful in establishing the diagnosis. A cervical pregnancy rarely achieves viability, and the potential for life-threatening hemorrhage from the cervix always exists. Early recognition with evacuation is recommended, and a hysterectomy is usually necessary if bleeding from the cervix cannot be controlled. Investigations of the use of methotrexate therapy for this problem (as in tubal ectopic pregnancies) have been promising. Caution is required when patients with suspected cervical pregnancy are examined in the office because hemorrhage often follows digital manipulation of the canal. Maternal mortality rates as high as 5% have been reported.

The unique accessibility of the uterine cervix to direct physical examination, cytologic testing, and histologic study has facilitated the intensive investigation of incipient uterine neoplasia and revealed much about the histogenesis of cervical cancer. Although this knowledge is incomplete, we know that most cervical tumors have a gradual rather than explosive onset and that their precursors may exist in a reversible form that is present for several years prior to invasive tumor development. The wide use of cervical neoplasia detection techniques in asymptomatic women has undoubtedly contributed to the declining incidence of invasive cervical cancer observed in the past 30 years. This large screening window, coupled with effective preinvasive testing measures, has convinced many gynecologists that eradication of cervical cancer will be possible in the foreseeable future. Achieving this goal is primarily limited only by accessibility and utilization of cervical cancer screening resources.

Epidemiology

In the United States, cancer of the uterine cervix is the sixth most common solid cancer in women after carcinoma of the breast, lung, colorectum, endometrium, and ovary. The American Cancer Society (ACS) estimates that in 1998 there will be 14,500 new cases of invasive carcinoma of the cervix in the United States, over 50,000 cases of carcinoma *in situ*, and 4800 deaths from the disease. The mean age of diagnosis for cervical cancer is 52.2 years, and the distribution of cases is bimodal with peaks at 35 to 39 years and 60 to 64 years. Worldwide, cervical cancer continues to be a leading cause of death due to cancer among women, with approximately 500,000 cases occurring annually. Lifetime risks for cervical cancer show significant geographic variation, ranging from 0.4% in Israel to 5.3% in Cali, Colombia, where cervical cancer is the most common malignancy in women.

Risk Factors

Race

Although the incidence of cervical cancer in the United States has declined significantly over the past 50 years, the rates among African-Americans remain about twice as high as those among whites. The incidence is also approximately two times higher for Latino-Americans and even higher for Native Americans, while most Asian-American groups experience rates similar to whites. These differences are at least partially accounted for by the strong inverse association between cervical cancer incidence and socioeconomic factors. When socioeconomic differences are controlled for, the excess risk of cervical cancer among African-Americans is substantially reduced, from over 70% to less than 30%. Racial differences are also apparent in survival, with 59% of African-Americans with cervical cancer surviving 5 years, compared to 67% of whites with the disease.

Sexual and Reproductive Factors

First intercourse before 16 years of age is associated with a twofold increased risk of cervical cancer compared with that for women whose first intercourse occurred after age 20 years. Cervical cancer risk is also directly proportional to the number of lifetime sexual partners. Although difficult to separate epidemiologically, there is evidence to indicate that both early age at first coitus and the number of lifetime sexual partners have independent effects on cervical cancer risk. Increasing parity also appears to be a separate risk factor for cervical cancer, even after controlling for socioeconomic and reproductive characteristics. There is little evidence to support an association between age of menarche, age at menopause, or character of menses with carcinoma of the cervix.

Smoking

Cigarette smoking has emerged as an important etiologic factor in squamous cell carcinoma of the cervix. The increased risk for smokers is approximately twofold, with the highest risk observed for long-term or high-intensity smokers. Proposed mechanisms include genotoxic or immunosuppressive effects of smoke-derived nicotine and cotinine, which can be detected in high levels in the cervical mucus of smokers.

Contraceptive Use

Numerous confounding factors—time interval since last cervical smear, sexual behavior, and role of the male partner, among them—complicate the interpretation of the data on oral contraceptive use and cervical cancer. After controlling for these and other variables, it appears that long-term oral contraceptive users (5 years or more) have about a twofold increased risk of cervical cancer, compared to nonusers. Use of barrier methods of contraception, especially those that combine both mechanical and chemical protection, have been shown to lower the risk of cervical cancer, presumably because of reduced exposure to infectious agents.

Male Partner Contribution

Husbands of women with cervical cancer have been more likely to report a history of venereal infections, early sexual experiences, affairs during marriage, visits to prostitutes, and significantly more sexual partners, compared to control husbands. While it is possible that men may carry and transmit a causative agent(s), evidence for this hypothesis has been difficult to demonstrate.

Immunosuppression

Cell-mediated immunity appears to be a factor in the development of cervical cancer. Immunocompromised women (e.g., from renal transplantation or human immunodeficiency virus [HIV] infection) may not only be at higher risk for the disease but also demonstrate more rapid progression from preinvasive to invasive lesions and an accelerated course once invasive disease has been diagnosed.

Screening

Cytologic evaluation of cells obtained from the cervix and vagina was first proposed by Papanicolaou and Traut in the 1940s as a method for detecting cervical cancer and its precursors. Since that time, cervical cytology has proved to be the most efficacious and cost-effective method for cancer screening. By increasing detection of preinvasive and early invasive disease, cervical cancer screening with the Pap smear has decreased both the incidence and mortality from cervical cancer (Fig. 6). Nowhere in the world have the incidence and death rates of cervical cancer decreased without an active Pap smear screening program. A single negative Pap smear may decrease the risk for cervical cancer by 45%, and nine negative smears during a lifetime decreases the risk by as much as 99%. Eddy (1990), using a mathematical model, indicated that in women 35 to 64 years of age, screening intervals of 10, 5, and 3 years would reduce the incidence of invasive cervical cancer by 64%, 84%, and 91%, respectively.

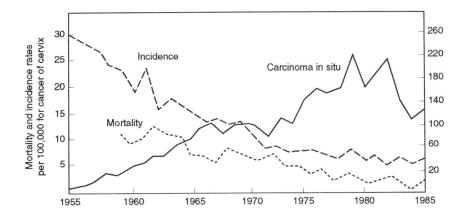

FIG. 6. The incidence of clinical invasive squamous cell carcinoma (SCC) of the cervix, squamous carcinoma *in situ* 1955 to 1985, and mortality from SCC of the cervix 1958 to 1985 in British Columbia, Canada (age-standardized rates per 100,000 women over age 20 years). (From Anderson et al., 1998; with permission.)

Despite the recognized benefits of cytologic screening, substantial subgroups of women in the United States have not been screened or are not screened at regular intervals. One-half of women with newly diagnosed invasive cervical carcinoma have never had a Pap smear, and another 10% have not had a smear in the 5 years preceding diagnosis. Unscreened populations include older women, the uninsured, ethnic minorities, and women of lower socioeconomic status, particularly those in rural areas.

The current Pap smear recommendations from the ACS and the American College of Obstetrics and Gynecology are that all women who are or have been sexually active or have reached the age of 18 years have an annual Pap smear and pelvic examination. After a woman has had three or more consecutive satisfactory normal annual examinations, the Pap smear may be performed less frequently in a low-risk woman, at her physician's discretion. Women with one or more risk factors for cervical cancer (e.g., HIV or human papillomavirus [HPV] infection, history of preinvasive cervical disease, high-risk sexual behavior) should continue to be screened annually. Women over age 65 years should continue to be screened, as 25% of all cases of cervical cancer and 41% of deaths from the disease occur in women in this age group.

Role of Human Papillomavirus

During the past decade, epidemiologic evidence has accumulated, implicating infection with HPV as a likely etiologic agent in cervical squamous cell carcinoma. All known types of HPV have a similar structural and genomic organization. They are nonenveloped virions with a double-stranded circular DNA genome of 7800 to 7900 base pairs and an icosahedral capsid. HPV DNA is present in virtually all cases (93%) of cervical cancer and its precursor lesions. While HPV infection is thought to be a component of neoplastic transformation, it is unlikely to be entirely sufficient in and of itself.

HPVs colonize mucosal or cutaneous epithelium and induce hyperproliferation, resulting in the formation of warts at the site of infection. Based on differences in DNA sequencing, over 70 different types of HPV have been identified, 23 of which are known to infect the anogenital tract. Low oncogenic

risk–type viruses include types 6, 11, 42, 43, and 44 and are associated with condyloma acuminatum and some cases of low-grade squamous intraepithelial lesions, but rarely with invasive cancer. High oncogenic risk–type viruses include types 16, 18, 31, 45, and 56 and are commonly detected in women with high-grade squamous intraepithelial lesions (HGSIL) and invasive cancer. HPV types 33, 35, 39, 51, and 52 can be considered as being of intermediate oncogenic risk, as they are associated with HGSIL but are uncommonly detected in invasive carcinomas.

Following acute HPV infection, three clinical sequelae are possible:

1. Latent viral infection occurs when the HPV genome becomes stabilized as a nonintegrated episome and remains in the host cell without clinical or morphologic changes in the squamous epithelium. Clinically, patients may display no gross or morphologic evidence of infection but still harbor virus as demonstrated by DNA detection techniques.
2. Active infection, manifested by proliferation of squamous epithelium into benign tumors (warts), is present when HPV undergoes vegetative replication.
3. Highly oncogenic HPV viruses associated with high-grade lesions can become integrated into the host genome, interrupting control of proliferation by certain oncoproteins.

Initiation of cervical dysplasia and carcinoma may involve interactions between HPV and specific genes that regulate cell growth. The E6 and E7 open reading frames of the HPV genome are particularly important in the immortalization and transformation of infected cells. In HPV types 16 and 18, the protein products synthesized from the E6 and E7 open reading frames can bind to the gene products of the p53 and retinoblastoma (Rb) tumor suppressor genes, respectively. Viral integration results in the overexpression of the E6 and E7 viral protein products with increased binding and inactivation of their respective tumor suppressor proteins. Removal of these two inhibitory influences on cellular proliferation is thought to provide HPV-infected cells with a growth advantage, ultimately leading to neoplastic transformation.

◊ PREINVASIVE CERVICAL NEOPLASIA

Definitions and Terminology

It is estimated that over 1 million women in the United States are diagnosed annually with cervical intraepithelial neoplasia (CIN) by means of a Pap smear. The concept of CIN was introduced in 1968, when Richart indicated that all dysplasias have the potential for progression to invasive cancer. It is now recognized that most early CIN lesions will regress spontaneously if untreated; nevertheless, CIN refers to a lesion that may progress to invasive carcinoma. This term is equivalent to the term *dysplasia*. The significant features included in the criteria for the diagnosis of intraepithelial neoplasia are cellular immaturity, cellular disorganization, nuclear abnormalities, and increased mitotic activity. The extent of these cytologic and histologic disturbances identify the degree of neoplasia. If mitoses and immature cells are present only in the lower one-third of the epithelium, the lesion is designated as CIN 1. Dysplasia involving of the middle third, upper third, or full thickness is diagnosed as CIN 2, CIN 3, or carcinoma *in situ* (CIS), respectively (Figs. 7 to 10).

CIN is a disturbance of growth, and the cellular changes are predominantly in the nuclei. Nuclear pleomorphism and hyperchromatism are characteristic. Multinucleation and abundant, abnormal mitosis are common, with the degree of abnormality corresponding to the grade of dysplasia. In addition to the changes in individual cells, there are changes in the relations of cells to one another. For example, the basal layer shows a disturbance in polarity, with cells growing haphazardly in every direction instead of conforming to the normal palisade arrangement.

The terminology used to classify preinvasive lesions of the cervix has changed many times over the last 50 years and continues to do so. A standardized method of reporting cytologic findings was needed to facilitate uniformity of diagnosis and treatment, peer review, and quality assurance. In 1989, a National Cancer Institute (NCI) workshop held in

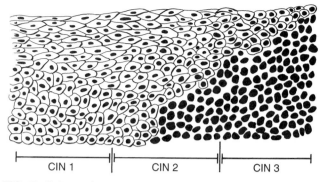

FIG. 7. Schematic representation of the different grades of cervical intraepithelial neoplasia (CIN). In CIN 1, dysplastic cells are limited to the lower one-third of the epithelium. In CIN 2 and CIN 3, dysplastic cells are located in the middle and upper thirds of the epithelium, respectively.

Bethesda, Maryland, resulted in the development of the Bethesda System for cytologic reporting. This system was subsequently revised in 1991 (Table 2). The major features of the Bethesda system are that it requires:

◊ An estimate of the adequacy of the specimen for diagnostic evaluation;

◊ General categorization of the specimen as either being within normal limits, showing benign cellular changes related to inflammation, or showing an epithelial abnormality;

◊ Descriptive diagnosis that includes evidence of infection, inflammation, and reactive changes;

◊ Description of epithelial cell abnormalities.

In the Bethesda System, potentially premalignant squamous lesions fall into three categories:

◊ Atypical squamous cells of undetermined significance (ASCUS),

◊ Low-grade squamous intraepithelial lesions (LGSIL),

◊ High-grade squamous intraepithelial lesions (HGSIL).

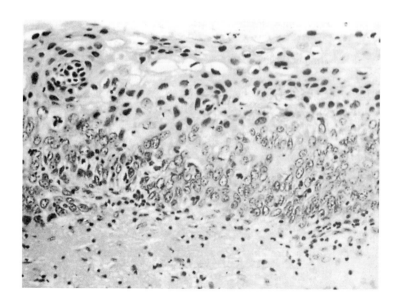

FIG. 8. Microscopic view of cervical intraepithelial neoplasia 2 showing hyperchromatism and pleomorphism of the nuclei in the upper one-half of the epithelial layer and evidence of an increased growth rate in the basal one-half. (From McKay DG, Terjanian B, Poschyachinda D, Younge PA, Hertig AT. Clinical and pathological significance of anaplasia (atypical hyperplasia) of the cervix uteri. *Obstet Gynecol* 1959;13:2; with permission.)

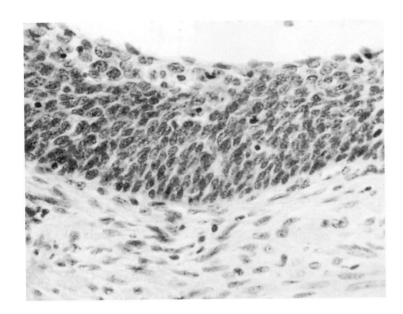

FIG. 9. Carcinoma *in situ* of the cervix showing spindle-shaped epithelial cells approaching the surface of the epithelial layer. (From McKay DG, Terjanian B, Poschyachinda D, Younge PA, Hertig AT. Clinical and pathological significance of anaplasia (atypical hyperplasia) of the cervix uteri. *Obstet Gynecol* 1959;13:2; with permission.)

LGSIL include CIN 1 (mild dysplasia) and cellular changes indicative of HPV infection, termed koilocytotic atypia. Cytologic changes consistent with CIN 2 and CIN 3 (moderate dysplasia, severe dysplasia, and CIS) are combined within the category of HGSIL (Fig. 11). This dichotomy of LGSIL and HGSIL has served to simplify the triage and clinical treatment protocols for these conditions.

Abnormal cells that do not fulfill the criteria for either LGSIL or HGSIL are described as ASCUS. This category includes many of the minor abnormalities that in the past were termed *atypical*. The undetermined significance phraseology reflects the uncertain relation of these cells to subsequent development of cervical cancer, HPV infection, or other conditions. The ASCUS category does not include benign, reac-

tive, or reparative changes that should be coded as normal in the Bethesda System. Similarly, the ASCUS category does not include condylomatous or koilocytotic atypia, which are now categorized as LGSIL. Using standardized diagnostic criteria, the rate of ASCUS Pap smears should be no more than 3% to 5% of all smears.

Natural History of Preinvasive Lesions of the Cervix

The behavior of squamous intraepithelial neoplasia has been extensively studied. In a comprehensive review, Oster (1993) found that for CIN 1 lesions the approximate likelihood of spontaneous regression is 60%, persistence 30%, progression to CIN 3 10%, and progression to invasive carcinoma 1%. Approximately one-third of high-grade lesions will spontaneously regress, while the majority of these lesions will persist or progress. The risk of CIN 3 progressing to invasive carcinoma was found to be at least 12% (Table 3). The transit time between different grades of SIL has been difficult to evaluate, primarily because most studies have used cervical biopsies to document cytologic abnormalities histologically and such biopsies may remove small precursor lesions in their entirety. In a large prospective study, Richart and Barron (1969) followed 557 patients using only cytology and colposcopy. Using life-table analysis, the mean transit time to CIS from very mild dysplasia was 85 months, from mild dysplasia 58 months, from moderate dysplasia 38 months, and from severe dysplasia only 12 months.

Diagnosis and Management

Current management of SIL of the cervix depends on a combination of cytology, colposcopic findings, and results of directed biopsy, as outlined in Figure 12. In general, all patients with a cytologic diagnosis of HGSIL should be evaluated colposcopically. Management of patients with LGSIL and ASCUS

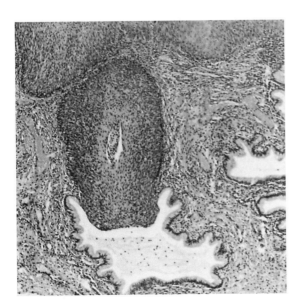

FIG. 10. Carcinoma *in situ* of the cervix with involvement of an endocervical gland.

TABLE 2. *The 1991 Bethesda system*

Adequacy of the specimen
Satisfactory for evaluation
Satisfactory for evaluation but limited by (specify reason)
Unsatisfactory for evaluation (specify reason)

General categorization
Within normal limits
Benign cellular changes (see descriptive diagnosis)
Epithelial cell abnormality (see descriptive diagnosis)

Descriptive diagnosis
Benign cellular changes
  Infection
    Trichomonas vaginalis
    Fungal organisms morphologically consistent
      with *Candida* sp.
    Predominance of coccobacilli consistent with shift in
      vaginal flora
    Bacteria morphologically consistent with *Actinomyces* sp.
    Cellular changes associated with herpes simplex virus
    Other
  Reactive cellular changes associated with
    Inflammation (includes typical repair)
    Atrophy with inflammation ("atrophic vaginitis")
    Radiation
    Intrauterine contraceptive device (IUD)
    Other
Epithelial cell abnormalities
  Squamous cell
    Atypical squamous cells of undetermined
      significance (qualify)
    Low-grade squamous intraepithelial lesion (LGSIL),
      encompassing human papilloma virus infection, mild
      dysplasia, CIN 1
    High-grade squamous intraepithelial lesion (HGSIL),
      encompassing moderate and severe dysplasia,
      CIN 2, CIN 3, and CIS
    Squamous cell carcinoma
  Glandular cell
    Endometrial cells, cytologically benign, in a
      postmenopausal woman
    Atypical glandular cells of undetermined significance
      (qualify)
    Endocervical adenocarcinma
    Endometrial adenocarcinoma
    Extrauterine adenocarcinoma
    Adenocarcinoma, not otherwise specified
  Other malignant neoplasms (specify)

CIN, cervical intraepithelial neoplasia; CIS, carcinoma *in situ.*

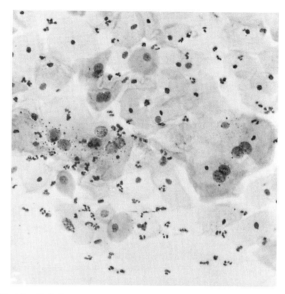

FIG. 11. Exfoliated cells on a Pap smear from a cervical intra-epithelial neoplasia. The neoplastic cells are binucleate, and the nuclei are considerably larger than those of the surrounding normal squamous cells. (From Takeuchi A, McKay DG. The area of the cervix involved by carcinoma in situ and anaplasia (atypical hyperplasia). *Obstet Gynecol* 1960; 15: 134; with permission.)

estrogen cream, respectively, may be useful prior to repeating cytology.

Colposcopy should generally be performed when a woman with an abnormal Pap smear has a significant chance of having SIL, a glandular lesion, or cancer. Colposcopic examination of the cervix is limited to the portio and outer third of the endocervical canal. Endocervical lesions are not adequately evaluated by colposcopy. The entire transformation zone and lesion, if present, must be visualized for the colposcopic examination to be considered satisfactory. Under colposcopic guidance, areas with the most pronounced epithelial and vascular abnormalities are sampled using a small punch biopsy instrument. A basic principle of colposcopic examination is that unless a SIL is visualized in its entirety during the examination, invasive cancer has not been ruled out and a cone biopsy is indicated, regardless of the grade of SIL.

Endocervical curettage (ECC) is performed to evaluate lesion distribution within the endocervical canal. When no exocervical lesion can be visualized or the squamocolumnar

on cytology is less well defined and should be individualized. In patients with LGSIL on Pap smear and high-risk factors for SIL (i.e., previous abnormal pap smear, history of HPV, smoker, immunocompromised, or multiple sexual partners), immediate colposcopic referral is prudent. However, in the absence of high-risk factors, patients with an initial LGSIL may be managed conservatively with a repeat Pap smear in 4 to 6 months. If the abnormality persists, then colposcopy should be performed. An ASCUS Pap smear can be triaged similarly, based on risk factors. In the presence of inflammation or postmenopausal atrophy, a trial of antibiotic treatment or vaginal

TABLE 3. *Natural history of cervical intraepithelial neoplasia (CIN)*

	Regress (%)	Persist (%)	Progress to CIS (%)	Progress to ICC (%)
CIN 1	57	32	11	1
CIN 2	43	35	22	5
CIN 3	32	56	—	12

CIS, carcinoma *in situ;* ICC, invasive cervical carcinoma. (From Oster, 1993; with permission.)

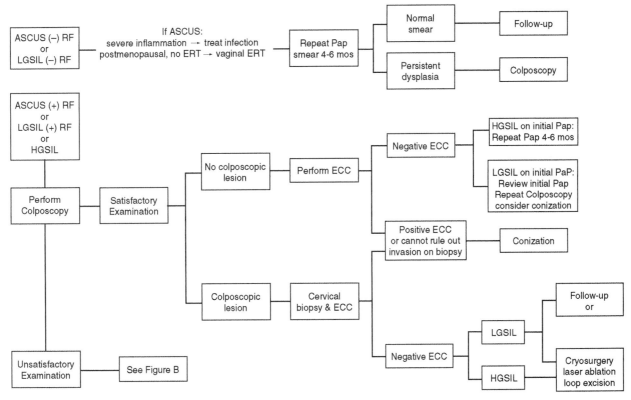

RF = Risk Factors: initial Pap suggestive of SIL or cancer, previous abnormal Pap smear,
A HIV infection, history of HPV infection, high risk sexual behavior.

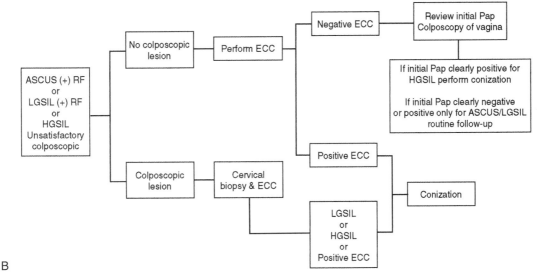

FIG. 12. Suggested protocol for the management of an abnormal Pap smear. **A:** Evaluation and treatment of squamous intraepithelial lesions (SIL) of the cervix when colposcopy is satisfactory. **B:** Evaluation and treatment of SIL of the cervix when colposcopy is unsatisfactory.

junction is within the endocervical canal, ECC is particularly useful to enhance the diagnostic accuracy of the colposcopic examination.

Cervical conization can be both a diagnostic and therapeutic procedure. Diagnostic indications for cervical conization are shown in Table 4. A cervical conization specimen represents a conically shaped section of cervix that varies in size according to the distribution of the lesion. For example, a broad, shallow conization is performed for a predominantly exocervical lesion, while a narrow, deep conization is appropriate for a predominantly endocervical lesion (Fig. 13).

The primary objectives in managing SIL are to (1) exclude the presence of invasive cancer, (2) determine the extent and distribution of noninvasive lesions, and (3) provide appropriate

TABLE 4. *Indications for conization of the cervix*

Abnormal cytology with unsatisfactory colposcopy
  (squamocolumnar junction not seen)
Limits of the lesion cannot be visualized colposcopically
Positive endocervical curettage
Lack of correlation between cytology, biopsy, and
  colposcopic findings
Microinvasive carcinoma on biopsy or colposcopy
  suspicious for carcinoma
Adenocarcinoma *in situ* on biopsy or endocervical curettage

therapeutic management based on lesion size, distribution, and grade.

Treatment Methods

Cryosurgery is frequently used to treat cervical SIL limited to the portio. Cryodestruction of cervical tissue is caused by freezing tissue below −20°C to −30°C, crystallizing the intracellular water and resulting in cell lysis. The margins of the iceball should extend at least 5 mm beyond the limits of the lesion. The failure rate or incidence of residual dysplasia (5% to 10%) and the long-term recurrence rate (1 in 1000 women per year after successful cryotherapy) are no greater than those following therapeutic conization. Cure rates are not affected by the grade of lesion treated; however, larger lesion size and the presence of endocervical gland involvement are associated with higher failure rates. Optimal candidates for cryotherapy should have a small ectocervical lesion, a negative ECC, and no endocervical gland involvement on biopsy.

The carbon dioxide (CO_2) laser is another treatment modality used for noninvasive lesions of the cervix. The laser's energy is absorbed by the intracellular and extracellular water in tissues, elevating tissue temperatures above 100°C. The tissue "boils" and the exploded cells are vaporized. The cervical tissue should be ablated to a depth of 7 mm, which is the location of the deepest endocervical gland. The failure and recurrence rates following CO_2 laser treatment are similar to those of cryotherapy.

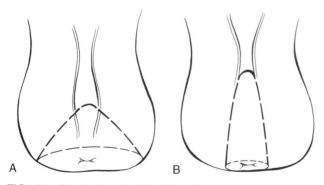

FIG. 13. Cervical conization. The shape of the conization specimen should be tailored to the size and distribution of the cervical lesion. **A:** Predominantly exocervical lesions are treated with a broad, shallow conization. **B:** Predominantly endocervical lesions are treated with a narrow, deep conization.

Recently, the loop electrosurgical excision procedure (LEEP) has become a valuable tool for both the diagnosis and treatment of SIL. The effect of electricity on the cervical tissue is dependent on the power (watts), concentration of electrons (wire size), and water content of the tissue. Thermal damage can be avoided by using a small diameter wire loop (0.5 mm) and relatively high power (35 to 55 W on cutting current). The cutting effect is produced by a steam envelope developing at the interface between the wire loop and the water-laden tissue. LEEP has the advantage over ablative techniques of providing a tissue sample for histologic analysis. Complications following LEEP are usually minimal and compare favorably with those following laser ablation and conization. Cervical stenosis occurs in approximately 1% of patients.

Screening/Triage Adjuncts

Advances in molecular biology have made testing for the presence of HPV DNA in cervical specimens increasingly accurate and available. Commonly used methods include the hybrid capture system, polymerase chain reaction–based tests, and *in situ* hybridization. Use of HPV testing for primary screening may have clinical utility in developing countries or underserved populations but is not yet applicable to populations with successful cytologic screening programs already in place. In selected settings, HPV testing may also be useful as a secondary triage tool for women with minimally abnormal Pap smears (ASCUS, LGSIL), although the precise role of this technology is yet to be determined. Automated computer-assisted Pap smear screening techniques are increasingly being used for cytologic quality assurance and may ultimately reduce the number of false-negative smears.

Glandular Abnormalities

The Bethesda System specifies a category for glandular abnormalities that includes atypical glandular cells of undetermined significance (AGCUS). Atypical endocervical cells are important because of their associated high risk for significant cervical disease. In a recent series, Zweizig et al. (1997) reported on 85 women with AGCUS Pap smears who underwent histologic assessment of the lower genital tract. Clinically significant pathology was detected in 48% of patients; diagnoses included invasive cervical adenocarcinoma (3.5%), cervical adenocarcinoma *in situ* (1.1%), squamous intraepithelial neoplasia (21.2%), endometrial adenocarcinoma (5.9%), endometrial hyperplasia (11.8%), and ovarian cancer (1.1%). Endometrial lesions were significantly more common in older women. It appears that the presence of AGCUS on cervical cytology is a marker for significant gynecologic neoplasia and should be evaluated with colposcopically directed biopsies, ECC, and, in older women, endometrial biopsy.

In adenocarcinoma *in situ* (AIS), endocervical glandular cells are replaced by tall columnar cells with nuclear stratification, hyperchromatism, irregularity, and increased mitotic activity (Fig. 14). About 50% of women with AIS also have

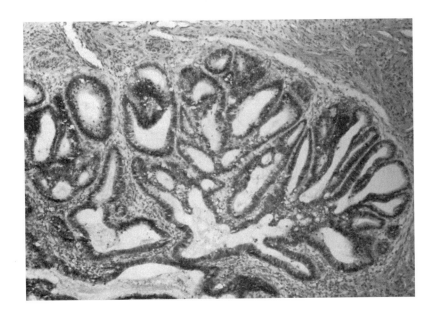

FIG. 14. Cervical adenocarcinoma *in situ* showing tall columnar cells with nuclear stratification, hyperchromatism, and irregularity.

squamous CIN. Obtaining endocervical specimens with the cytobrush may improve detection of AIS; however, if the focus of AIS is small, even cervical biopsy and ECC may be negative. In such cases, a more comprehensive survey of the cervix is necessary, usually in the form of conization. This type of evaluation also allows exclusion of a coexisting adenocarcinoma.

A point of major concern regarding AIS is that these lesions are frequently multifocal, so that conization margins are not useful in predicting the presence of residual disease. Poyner et al. (1995) reported a series of 28 patients with AIS in which 4 of 10 patients with negative conization margins had residual AIS in hysterectomy or repeat conization specimens. Of the eight patients with positive margins who underwent repeat conization or hysterectomy, three had residual AIS, and one patient had adenocarcinoma. Of the 15 patients managed conservatively with repeat conization of the cervix and close follow-up, seven (47%) had a recurrent glandular lesion detected after the conization, including invasive adenocarcinoma in two women. AIS must be considered a precursor of invasive cervical adenocarcinoma. The entire endocervical canal is at risk, and the accuracy of detection with cytology or ECC has not been determined. Some believe that any patient with a positive conization margin should undergo at least repeat conization. If fertility is undesired, a hysterectomy should be performed because of the risk of recurrence, even in the presence of negative margins.

◊ INVASIVE CERVICAL CARCINOMA

Clinical Features

Presenting Symptoms

The most common symptom of cervical cancer is abnormal vaginal bleeding or discharge. Abnormal bleeding may take the form of postcoital spotting, intermenstrual bleeding, menorrhagia, or postmenopausal spotting. If bleeding has been chronic, a patient may complain of fatigue or other symptoms related to anemia. Serosanguineous or yellowish vaginal discharge, frequently associated with a foul odor, may accompany an advanced or necrotic carcinoma. Pelvic pain may result from locally advanced disease or tumor necrosis. Tumor extension to the pelvic side wall may cause sciatic pain or back pain associated with hydronephrosis. Metastatic tumor to the iliac and paraaortic lymph nodes can extend into the lumbosacral nerve roots and present as lumbosacral back pain. Urinary or rectal symptoms (i.e., hematuria, hematochezia) can be associated with bladder or rectal invasion by advanced-stage cervical carcinoma.

Physical Findings

Invasive carcinoma of the cervix displays a wide range of gross appearances. Early lesions may be focally indurated or ulcerated, or present as a slightly elevated and granular area that bleeds readily on contact (Fig. 15). More advanced tumors have two major types of gross appearance: exophytic and endophytic. Exophytic tumors characteristically have a polypoid or papillary appearance. Endophytic tumors are usually ulcerated or nodular. They tend to develop within the endocervical canal and frequently invade deep into the cervical stroma to produce an enlarged, hard, barrel-shaped cervix.

Spread of Disease

Paracervical and Parametrial Extension

Tumor cells commonly spread through parametrial lymphatic vessels, expanding and replacing parametrial lymph nodes (Fig. 16). These individual tumor masses enlarge and become

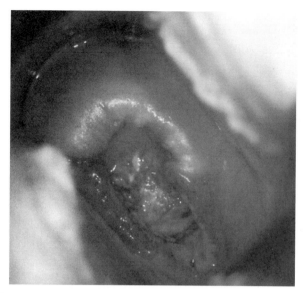

FIG. 15. Gross appearance of squamous cell carcinoma of the cervix. This is an ulcerative type of lesion.

confluent, eventually replacing the normal parametrial tissue. Less commonly, the central tumor mass reaches the pelvic side wall by direct contiguous extension through the cardinal (Mackenrodt's) ligament. Significant involvement of the medial portion of this ligament may result in ureteral obstruction.

Vaginal Extension

When the primary tumor has extended beyond the confines of the cervix, the upper vagina is frequently involved (50% of cases). Anterior extension through the vesicovaginal septum is most common, often obliterating the dissection plane between the bladder and underlying cervical tumor, making surgical therapy difficult or impossible. Posteriorly, a deep peritoneal cul-de-sac (pouch of Douglas) can represent an anatomic barrier to direct tumor spread from the cervix and vagina to the rectum.

Bladder and Rectal Involvement

In the absence of lateral parametrial disease, anterior and posterior spread of cervical cancer to the bladder and rectum is uncommon. Only 20% of patients with tumor extending to the pelvic side wall have biopsy-proven bladder invasion.

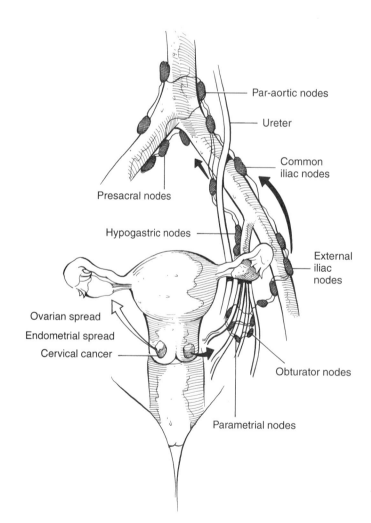

FIG. 16. Anatomic pathways of spread in invasive cervical carcinoma.

Endometrial Involvement

The endometrium is involved in 2% to 10% of cervical cancer cases treated with surgery, although the overall incidence (including nonsurgical cases) is unknown. Endometrial extension is associated with decreased survival and a higher incidence of distant metastases.

Ovarian Metastasis

Ovarian involvement with cervical cancer is rare but, when present, most likely occurs through the lymphatic connections between the uterus and adnexal structures. In patients undergoing surgical treatment, ovarian metastasis are present in fewer than 1% of squamous cell carcinomas and slightly more than 1% of adenocarcinomas.

Lymph Node Involvement

Lymphatic spread of cervical carcinoma follows an orderly and reasonably predictable pattern. The lymph node groups most commonly involved are the obturator, external iliac, and hypogastric. The inferior gluteal and presacral lymph nodes are less frequently involved. Secondary nodal involvement (i.e., common iliac, paraaortic) rarely occurs in the absence of primary nodal disease (i.e., pelvic). The percentage of involved lymph nodes increases directly with primary tumor volume. Rarely, retrograde lymphatic embolization may occur to the inguinal lymph nodes. In patients with clinically advanced or recurrent disease, metastatic spread may be detected in the scalene nodes.

Hematogenous Spread

The most common areas for hematogenous spread are the lung, liver, and bone. Metastasis to the bowel, adrenal gland, spleen, and brain are less frequent.

Diagnosis and Staging

Diagnosis

An international convention of staging permits comparison of results between institutions and definition of codes of treatment within an institution. The International Federation of Gynecology and Obstetrics (FIGO) staging system for the diagnosis and evaluation of cervical carcinoma is based on clinical evaluation (inspection, palpation, colposcopy), radiographic examination of the chest, kidneys, and skeleton, and ECC and biopsies. Lymphangiograms, arteriograms, computed tomographic (CT) scans, magnetic resonance imaging, and laparoscopy or laparotomy should not be used for clinical staging. Staging procedures allowed by FIGO convention are shown in Table 5.

In 1995, FIGO revised the clinical staging system of cervical carcinoma (Table 6). Stage I neoplasms are those that are clinically confined to the cervix. In the current staging classi-

TABLE 5. *Staging procedures for cervical carcinoma*

Physical examination	Examination under anesthesia recommended
Radiologic studies	Chest x-ray
	Intravenous pyelogram
	Barium enema
	Skeletal x-ray
Procedures	Colposcopy
	Cervical biopsy
	Conization
	Endocervical curettage
	Cystoscopy
	Proctoscopy
Optional studies[a]	Computed tomography
	Lymphangiography
	Ultrasonography
	Magnetic resonance imaging
	Radionucleotide scanning
	Laparoscopy/laparotomy

[a]Not allowed for staging purposes by the International Federation of Gynecology and Obstetrics (FIGO).

fication, stage IA1 (microinvasive carcinoma) is defined as a tumor with stromal invasion no greater than 3 mm in depth beneath the basement membrane and no wider than 7 mm. This definition reflects data indicating that patients with less than 3 mm of invasion are at very low risk of metastatic disease and may be treated more conservatively. The 1995 staging system also subclassifies stage IB lesions into stage IB1 (no greater than 4 cm in maximal diameter) and stage IB2 (greater than 4 cm in maximal diameter), reflecting the importance of tumor volume for macroscopic lesions limited to the cervix. The distribution of patients by clinical stage is stage I 38%, stage II 32%, stage III 26%, and stage IV 4%.

Evaluation of Disease Extent

Determination of clinical stage depends on careful inspection and palpation of the cervix, vagina, and pelvis. It is important to palpate the entire vagina to determine whether disease is limited to the cervix (IB), extends to the upper two-thirds of the vagina (IIA), or also involves the lower third of the vagina (IIIA) (Fig. 17). Tumor extension into the parametrial tissue (IIB) or to the pelvic side wall (IIIB) is best appreciated on rectovaginal examination. It is impossible at clinical examination to decide whether a smooth and indurated parametrium is truly cancerous or only inflammatory, and the case should be considered stage III only if the parametrium is nodular on the pelvic wall or if the growth itself extends to the pelvic wall.

When there is doubt concerning which stage a tumor should be assigned, the earlier stage is mandatory. Once a clinical stage has been determined and treatment initiated, subsequent findings on either extended clinical staging (CT, etc.) or surgical exploration should not alter the assigned stage. Assignment of a more advanced stage during treatment will result in an apparent but deceptive improvement in the results of treatment for earlier-stage disease.

TABLE 6. *FIGO staging of cervical carcinoma*

Stage	Features
0	Carcinoma *in situ*, intraepithelial carcinoma
I	Carcinoma is strictly confined to the cervix
IA	Invasive cancer identified only microscopically. All gross lesions even with superficial invasion are stage IB cancers. Invasion is limited to measured stromal invasion ≤ of 5 mm deep and < 7 mm wide
IA1	Measured invasion of stroma ≤ 3 mm deep and < 7 mm wide
IA2	Measured invasion of stroma > 3 mm but ≤ 5 mm deep and < 7 mm wide
IB	Clinical lesions confined to the cervix or preclinical lesions greater than stage IA
IB1	Clinical lesions ≤ 4 cm in size
IB2	Clinical lesions > 4 cm in size
II	Carcinoma extends beyond the cervix but has not extended to the pelvic wall. Carcinoma involves the vagina but not as far as the lower third
IIA	No obvious parametrial involvement
IIB	Obvious parametrial involvement
III	Carcinoma has extended to the pelvic wall. On rectal examination, there is no cancer-free space between the tumor and the pelvic wall. The tumor involves the lower third of the vagina. All cases of hydronephrosis or non-functioning kidney are included, unless known to be due to another cause
IIIA	No extension to the pelvic wall
IIIB	Extension to the pelvic wall, hydronephrosis, or nonfunctioning kidney
IV	Carcinoma has extended beyond the true pelvis or has clinically involved the mucosa of the bladder or rectum. Bullous edema does permit a case to be allocated to stage IV
IVA	Spread of growth to adjacent organs
IVB	Spread to distant organs

FIGO, International Federation of Gynecology and Obstetrics.

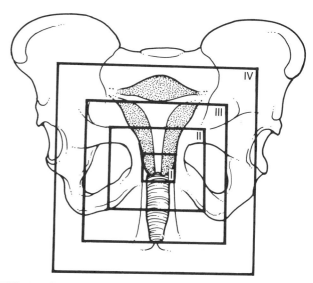

FIG. 17. Clinical stages of carcinoma of the cervix. In stage I, only the cervix is involved. In stage II, the parametrium or upper two-thirds of the vagina is involved. In stage III, the malignancy extends to the pelvic side wall or involves the lower third of the vagina.

Surgical Staging

The current FIGO staging classification for cervical cancer is based on pretreatment clinical findings. Only the subclassification of stage I (IA1, IA2) requires pathologic assessment. Discrepancies between clinical staging and surgicopathologic findings range from 17.3% to 38.5% in patients with clinical stage I disease, to 42.9% to 89.5% in patients with stage III disease. This has lead some to emphasize surgical staging of cervical carcinoma to identify occult tumor spread and determine the presence of extrapelvic disease, so that adjunctive or extended-field radiation therapy may be offered. Transperitoneal surgical staging procedures, when followed by abdominopelvic irradiation, are associated with appreciable complications, particularly enteric morbidity. The extraperitoneal surgical approach can be performed through a paraumbilical or paramedian incision and allows accurate assessment of disease status. It is associated with few compli-

cations and does not delay institution of radiation therapy. The role of laparoscopic surgical staging for cervical cancer has yet to be determined.

Prognostic Variables

Tumor Characteristics

Prognostic variables directly related to surgicopathologic tumor characteristics and their effect on survival were compiled by the NCI's Surveillance, Epidemiology, and End Results (SEER) program for the period 1973 through 1987. This study included 17,119 cases of invasive cervical cancer and found that FIGO stage, tumor histology, histologic grade, and lymph node status are all independent prognostic variables relating to survival (Kosary, 1994). In addition, tumor volume and depth of invasion have also been shown to have an impact on survival.

Stage

Clinical stage of disease at the time of presentation is the most important determinant of subsequent survival, regardless of treatment modality. Five-year survival declines as FIGO stage at diagnosis increases from stage IA (97%) to stage IV (12.4%). Significantly lower survival is seen for every stage compared to stage IA.

Histology

Squamous carcinomas accounted for 74.9% of cases in the SEER data, while 15.1% of cases were adenocarcinomas. No differences in overall survival were observed between these two histologic subtypes; however, adenosquamous histology was associated with decreased survival.

Histologic Grade

Overall survival is correlated with the degree of tumor differentiation. Five-year survival for patients with well differentiated tumors is 74.5%; for those with moderately differentiated tumors it is 63.7%, and falls to 51.4% for those patients with poorly differentiated carcinomas.

Lymph Node Invovement

Among surgically treated patients, survival is directly related to the number and location of lymph node metastasis. The frequency of positive lymph nodes increases with the stage of disease (Table 7). For all stages of disease, when both pelvic and paraaortic lymph nodes are negative, the 5-year survival rate is 75.2%. Survival decreases to 45.6% with positive pelvic nodes, and the risk of recurrence is related to the number of nodes involved. The recurrence rate is 35% with one positive pelvic lymph node, 59% with two or three positive nodes, and 69% with metastases to more than three pelvic lymph nodes. When paraaortic nodes are involved, the 5-year survival rate drops to 15.4%.

Tumor Volume

The revised FIGO staging system for cervical cancer reflects the fact that lesion size is an important predictor of survival. However, Finan et al., (1996) showed that the division of stage IB patients into subclasses IB1 and IB2 does not necessarily have an independent impact on survival. Rather, in stage IB patients, lesion size acts through nodal status in its impact on survial. Larger tumor volume is associated with higher rates of parametrial involvement and decreased survival. For stages IB through IIB, the 5-year survival rates decrease from 84.9% to 69.6% when the parametria are involved with tumor.

Depth of Invasion

Survival is strongly correlated with depth of tumor invasion into the stroma, with 3-year survival rates of 86% to 94% for

invasion of less than 10 mm, 71% to 75% for 11 to 20 mm, and 60% for greater than 21 mm of invasion.

Host Factors

Age

Whether or not younger women have a lower survival rate compared to older women with the same stage of disease remains controversial. Some investigators have observed decreased survival in women younger than 35 to 40 years, who have a greater frequency of poorly differentiated tumors. Others have found no significant difference in survival between younger and older patients.

Hematologic Factors

The incidence of pretreatment anemia (hemoglogin of 12 g/dl or less) increases with advancing stage of disease, occuring in 25%, 33%, and 45% of patients with stages I, II, and III disease, respectively. Anemia is associated with a higher incidence of pelvic recurrences and decreased survival, primarily due to more frequent radiation therapy failures. Tumor hypoxia is the proposed mechanism of radioresistance in the presence of anemia. Another prognostic hematologic parameter is thrombocytosis (greater than $400,000/mm^3$), which has been associated with decreased survival after controlling for cell type, stage, and age.

Coexistent Medical Conditions

Diabetes and hypertension are frequently associated with significant vascular disease and potentially contribute to both tumor hypoxia and decreased blood supply to normal pelvic tissues. Patients with these conditions are subject to a higher incidence of treatment complications and pelvic tumor recurrence, as well as decreased survival.

Pathology

Squamous cell carcinoma (SCC) constitutes 75% to 90% of cervical cancers and can be arbitrarily classified into three different histologic grades.

Grade 1 SCC

Grade 1 is a well differentiated tumor composed of sheets and cords of cells with abundant acidophillic cytoplasm, clearly visible intercellular bridges, and often production of variable amounts of keratin. Formation of an epidermoid pearl is characteristic of these well differentiated tumors, and relatively few mitoses are found. Grade 1 tumors constitute about 5% of cervical SCCs.

Grade 2 SCC

Grade 2 is the most common variety, with 85% of SCCs falling in this category (Fig. 18). It is characterized by masses

TABLE 7. *Incidence of pelvic and paraaortic lymph node metastasis by FIGO stage of cervical carcinoma*

Stage	n	Positive pelvic nodes (%)	Positive paraaortic nodes (%)
IA1	179	0.5	0
IA2	178	6.2	<1
IB	1926	15.9	2.2
IIA	110	24.5	11
IIB	324	31.4	19
III	125	44.8	30
IVA	23	55	40

FIGO, International Federation of Gynecology and Obstetrics.

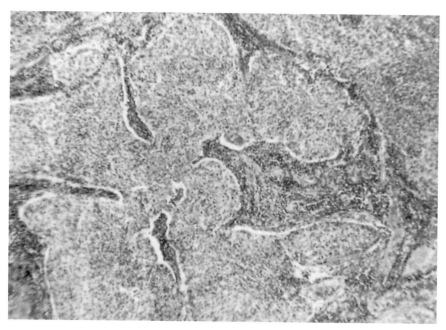

FIG. 18. Moderately differentiated squamous cell carcinoma of the cervix.

and cords of spindle-shaped squamous cells with elongated nuclei and scant cytoplasm. There may be a few areas in which the cells have become enlarged and well differentiated to form pearls, but in general there are no intercellular bridges and little keratin formation. The number of mitoses is higher than in well differentiated tumors.

Grade 3 SCC

Grade 3, or undifferentiated, tumors have a rapid growth rate, with numerous mitoses and cells with closely crowded nuclei and scant cytoplasm. These tumors are difficult to recognize as having originated in squamous cells and constitute approximately 10% of cervical SCCs.

Treatment

General Management by Stage

Surgery and radiation therapy are the two therapeutic modalities most commonly used to treat invasive cervical carcinoma. In general, primary surgical management is limited to stages I and IIA. There are several advantages to surgical therapy over radiation. Surgery provides the opportunity to perform a thorough pelvic and abdominal exploration, which can identify patients with a disparity between the clinical and surgicopathologic stages. Such patients can then be offered an individualized treatment plan based on their precise disease status. In younger patients, surgery permits conservation of the ovaries, which may be transposed out of subsequent radiation fields. Radical hysterectomy results in vaginal shortening; however, with sexual activity gradual lengthening will occur. Urinary and bowel fistula formation and incisional complications related to surgical treatment tend to occur early in the postoperative period and are usually amenable to sur-

gical repair. Other reasons for the selection of radical surgery over radiation include concomitant inflammatory bowel disease, previous radiation for other disease, and the presence of a simultaneous adnexal neoplasm.

Radiation therapy can be used for all stages of disease and for most patients regardless of age, body habitus, or coexistent medical conditions. Sexual function may be compromised, as pelvic irradiation produces persistent vaginal fibrosis and atrophy with loss of both vaginal length and caliber. Ovarian function is lost in virtually all patients undergoing radiation therapy to the pelvis. In contrast to surgical therapy, fistulous complications associated with radiation therapy tend to occur late and are more difficult to repair secondary to poorly vascularized tissues from radiation fibrosis and vasculitis.

Stage IA1

The 5-year survival rate of these patients approaches 100% with primary surgical therapy. Extrafascial hysterectomy is adequate treatment for this group of patients. Conization may be used selectively if preservation of fertility is desired, provided the surgical margins are free of disease. In the absence of lymph-vascular invasion, the incidence of pelvic lymph node metastasis is 0.3%, and lymphadenectomy is not indicated. In the presence of lymph-vascular involvement, the risk of pelvic node metastasis increases to 2.6%. Pelvic lymphadenectomy and extrafascial hysterectomy should be performed in these cases. In medically inoperable patients, stage IA1 carcinoma can be effectively treated with intracavitary radiation.

Stage IA2

Microinvasive carcinoma with stromal invasion of 3.1 to 5.0 mm is associated with positive pelvic lymph nodes in 6.2% of patients. The preferred treatment for these lesions is modified radical (type II) hysterectomy with pelvic lymphadenectomy.

Stages IB1, IB2, IIA

Both radical surgery and radiation therapy are equally effective in treating stages IB and IIA carcinoma of the cervix. Numerous uncontrolled studies support the merits of each modality, with no significant differences in pelvic tumor control or overall survival. Zander et al. reported on 1092 patients with stages IB and II cervical cancer treated with radical (type III) hysterectomy and pelvic lymphadenectomy. Five-year survival rates were 84.5% for stage IB and 71.1% for stage II disease. Similar survival rates are obtained with primary radiation therapy. In one series, Perez et al. (1986) reported 5-year survival rates of 85% for 312 patients with stage IB disease and 70% for 98 patients with stage IIA disease treated with primary radiation therapy.

Treatment should be individualized for patients with bulky stage I (IB2) tumors. Tumor expansion of the upper endocervix and lower uterine segment can distort cervical anatomy and lead to suboptimal placement of intracavitary radiation sources. Consequently, the central failure rate has been reported as high as 17.5% in patients with cervical lesions greater than 6 cm treated with radiation alone. In such situations, a "completion" extrafascial hysterectomy is usually performed following radiation therapy. While many clinicians limit the use of radical hysterectomy to patients with small stage IB (less than 3 to 4 cm) or stage IIA lesions, there

is evidence that acceptable survival rates can be obtained with primary surgical treatment in patients with bulky disease confined to the cervix. Five-year survival rates range from 73.6% to 82% after radical hysterectomy and pelvic lymphadenectomy for cervical lesions greater than 4 cm. Survival decreases to 66% at 5 years for lesions greater than 6 cm.

Stages IIB, III, IVA, and IVB

Radiation therapy is the treatment of choice for patients with stage IIB and more advanced disease. Radiation therapy for invasive cervical cancer is given as a combination of external and intracavitary treatments (see Chapter 53). Long-term survival rates are approximately 60% for stage II, 45% for stage III, and 18% for stage IV disease. Patients with stage IVB disease are usually treated with chemotherapy alone or chemotherapy in combination with local irradiation. These patients have a uniformly poor prognosis regardless of treatment modality.

Surgical Therapy

Types of Hysterectomy

There are five distinct variations or types of hysterectomy used in the treatment of cervical cancer.

Type I. A type I hysterectomy refers to the standard extrafascial total abdominal hysterectomy. This procedure ensures complete removal of the cervix with minimal disruption

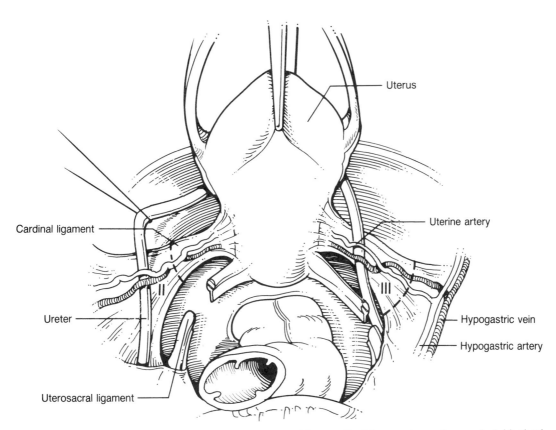

FIG. 19. Anatomic dissection of radical hysterectomy. The cardinal ligaments are transected *(dashed line)* at the level of the ureter (type II) or at the pelvic side wall (type III).

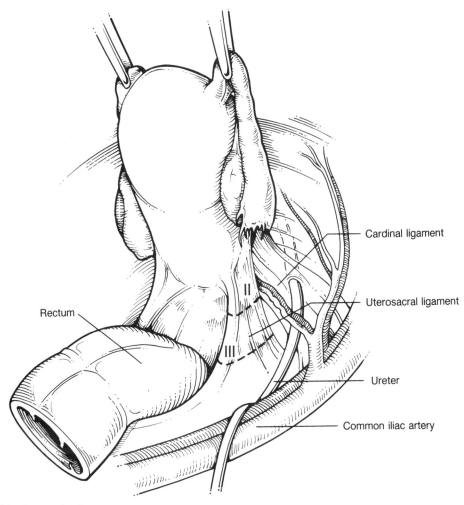

FIG. 20. Anatomic dissection of radical hysterectomy. The uterosacral ligaments are divided at the sacrum (type III) or midway between the sacrum and the uterus (type II).

to surrounding structures and is appropriate treatment for stage IA1 disease.

Type II. A type II hysterectomy is also referred to as a modified radical or Wertheim hysterectomy (Figs. 19 to 21). This procedure involves dissection of the ureters from the parametrial and paracervical tissues down to the ureterovesical junction. This permits removal of all parametrial tissue medial to the ureters, as well as the medial half of the uterosacral ligament and proximal 1 to 2 cm of vagina. This operation may be performed with pelvic lymphadenectomy.

Type III. In a type III or radical abdominal (Meigs) hysterectomy, the ureters are completely dissected from within the paracervical tunnel, and the bladder and rectum are extensively mobilized (Figs. 19 to 21). Establishing the paravesical and pararectal spaces facilitates removal of all the parametrial tissue out to the pelvic side wall, complete resection of the uterosacral ligaments, and excision of the upper one-third to one-half of the vagina. Bilateral pelvic lymphadenectomy is performed with this procedure.

Type IV/Type V. A type IV or extended radical hysterectomy includes removal of the superior vesical artery, peri-

ureteral tissue, and up to three-fourths of the vagina. In a type V or partial exenteration operation, the distal ureters and a portion of the bladder are resected. Type IV and type V procedures are rarely performed today because most patients with disease extensive enough to require these operations can be more adequately treated with primary radiation therapy.

Complications of Radical Abdominal Hysterectomy

Modern surgical techniques and anesthesia have reduced the operative mortality associated with radical hysterectomy to 0.6%. Potentially lethal pulmonary embolism occurs in 1% to 2% of patients. Ureterovaginal and vesicovaginal fistulas occur in 2% and 0.9% of patients, respectively. The most commonly observed complication after radical hysterectomy is urinary dysfunction resulting from partial denervation of the detrusor muscle during excision of the paracervical and paravaginal tissue. Pelvic lymphocyst formation occurs in 2% to 6.7% of patients following radical hysterectomy and pelvic lymphadenectomy. The incidence is somewhat lower when the retroperitoneal spaces are left open. Most lymphocysts

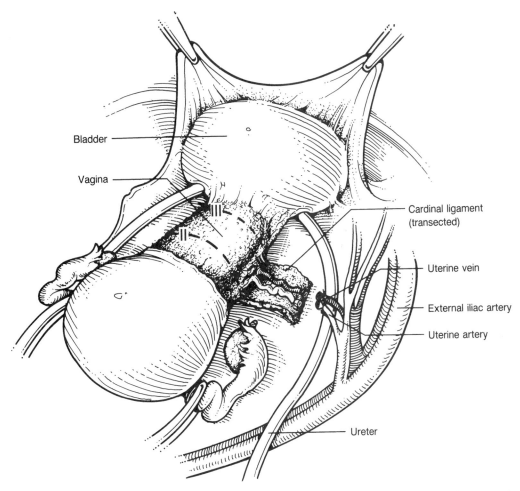

Bladder

Vagina

Cardinal ligament
(transected)

Uterine vein

External iliac artery

Uterine artery

Ureter

FIG. 21. Anatomic dissection of radical hysterectomy. In a type II radical hysterectomy, the upper 1 to 2 cm of vagina are excised. In type III radical hysterectomy, the proximal one-third to one-half of the vagina is removed.

are asymptomatic and do not require intervention. However, lymphocysts may occassionally produce pelvic pain, ureteral obstruction, or partial venous obstruction with thrombosis.

Adjuvant Therapy Following Surgery

Data are limited concerning the efficacy of postoperative pelvic irradiation in patients at high risk of recurrence after radical hysterectomy and pelvic lymphadenectomy. High-risk prognostic factors include microscopic parametrial invasion, pelvic lymph node metastases, deep cervical invasion, and positive or close surgical margins. The survival benefit of receiving postoperative radiation therapy for patients with one or two positive lymph nodes is yet to be conclusively shown. Although there are no controlled studies, retrospective data suggest that postoperative irradiation after radical hysterectomy may provide a modest gain in survival in patients with three or more positive pelvic lymph nodes. Combined surgical and radiation therapy results in increased morbidity, however, as lower-extremity lymphedema has been reported in up to 23.4% of patients receiving combined therapy.

The administration of chemotherapeutic agents before radical hysterectomy has been termed neoadjuvant chemotherapy. Cisplatin (Platinol), bleomycin sulfate (Blenoxane), and vinblastine sulfate (Velban) have been the most extensively used combination. When chemotherapy is administered prior to surgery, complete clincal response rates range from 17% to 44%, with overall response rates of 80% to 90%. In addition to increasing surgical resectability, preoperative chemotherapy also decreases the number of positive pelvic lymph nodes and, in some studies, has seemingly improved 2- and 3-year survival rates.

Radiation Therapy

External-beam irradiation is usually delivered to the pelvis from a linear accelerator. The purpose of external therapy is to decrease tumor volume and reduce the anatomic distortion produced by larger tumor masses, allowing optimization of subsequent intracavitary therapy. Following external therapy, brachytherapy is delivered using a variety of intracavitary techniques, including intrauterine tandem and vaginal colpostats, vaginal cylinders, or interstitial needle implants.

Radiation therapy is associated with both acute and chronic complications. Perforation of the uterus may occur at the time of intracavitary insertion and, if unrecognized, may result in significant blood loss, radiation damage, and peritonitis. Appropriate management consists of removal of the implant and broad-spectrum antibiotic coverage if signs of infection are present. Proctosigmoiditis occurs in up to 8% of patients undergoing radiation therapy for cervical cancer. Symptoms include abdominal pain, diarrhea, and nausea. An antispasmodic agent, a low-gluten and low-lactose diet, and steroid enemas may be useful; however, severe cases may require hyperalimentation and a diverting colostomy. Hemorrhagic cystitis is seen in approximately 3% of patients undergoing radiation therapy for cervical cancer.

Vaginal stenosis is the most common chronic complication of radiation therapy for cervical cancer and is seen in up to 70% of cases. Rectovaginal and vesicovaginal fistulas each occur in approximately 1% of cervical cancer patients treated with irradiation. In such cases, biopsy specimens should be obtained from the edge of the fistula to rule out recurrent cancer. Diversion of the fecal (colostomy) or urinary (percutaneous nephrostomy) stream is usually required to allow adequate healing (3 to 6 months) prior to surgical repair. Two percent of patients experience small bowel obstruction as a consequence of radiation therapy, more commonly in those patients with vascular disease or a history of previous abdominal surgery. The most common site of small bowel obstruction is the terminal ileum, which is relatively fixed within the radiation field by the cecum. Complete small bowel obstruction or cases recalcitrant to conservative management require surgical intervention.

Chemotherapy

Chemotherapy is indicated for patients with extrapelvic metastases or those with recurrent disease who are not candidates for radiation therapy or exenterative surgery. Cisplatin has been the most extensively studied agent and has demonstrated the most consistent clinical response rates. Complete clinical responses have been observed in 24% of patients, with an additional 16% demonstrating a partial response. Unfortunately, in most series, responses to cisplatin are short-lived (3 to 6 months). Other agents demonstrating at least partial activity against cervical cancer include carboplatin (Paraplatin), ifosfamide (IFEX), doxorubicin hydrochloride (Adriamycin), vinblastine, vincristine sulfate (Oncovin), 5-fluorouracil, methotrexate, and altretamine (Hexalen). There is little objective evidence to suggest that combination chemotherapy is superior to single-agent cisplatin treatment in improving the overall survival of patients with advanced or recurrent cervical cancer.

Posttreatment Surveillance

Among patients with recurrent cervical cancer, recurrence is detected within 1 year in 50% of patients and within 2 years

in more than 80%. Pelvic examination and lymph node evaluation, including supraclavicular nodes, should be performed every 3 months for 2 years and then every 6 months for an additional 3 years. Over 70% of patients with recurrent cervical cancer in the pelvis will have abnormal cervical or vaginal cytology; therefore, appropriate cytologic smears should be obtained at the time of each routine examination. Any palpable pelvic mass should be evaluated by CT with fine-needle aspiration cytology if indicated. A chest x-ray should be obtained annually to detect pulmonary metastases.

Treatment of Recurrent Cervical Cancer

Cervical cancer detected within the first 6 months after primary therapy is often termed *persistent* cancer, while that diagnosed later is referred to as recurrent disease. Appropriate treatment of recurrent cervical cancer is dictated by both the site of recurrence and the modality of primary therapy. In general, patients in whom recurrent disease develops following primary surgery should be considered for radiation therapy. Conversely, surgical treatment should be considered for those patients with recurrent disease who initially received irradiation. Distantly metastatic recurrent tumor is not amenable to either modality alone and is an indication for palliative chemotherapy and possibly radiation therapy for local control.

Surgical Treatment of Recurrent Cervical Cancer

Only patients with recurrent tumor confined to the central pelvis are candidates for surgical intervention. Total hysterectomy is inadequate treatment for centrally recurrent cervical cancer. Additionally, when radical hysterectomy is performed following maximum-dose radiation therapy, 20% to 50% of patients will experience ureteral strictures, urinary fistulas, or other serious complications. Therefore, pelvic exenteration is usually the procedure of choice for centrally recurrent cervical cancer.

Prior to exenterative surgery, a thorough investigation should be undertaken to rule out extrapelvic metastases. The clinical triad of unilateral leg edema, sciatic pain, and ureteral obstruction heralds tumor extension to the pelvic side wall and is a contraindication to surgery. In most series, approximately 25% of patients with recurrent cervical cancer are deemed satisfactory candidates for exenterative surgery.

Anterior exenteration is indicated for treatment of recurrent cervical cancer limited to the cervix, anterior vagina, and/or bladder. The procedure combines radical cystectomy with radical hysterectomy and vaginectomy. *Posterior exenteration* combines abdominal perineal resection of the rectum with radical hysterectomy and vaginectomy and is indicated for lesions confined to the posterior fornix and rectovaginal septum. *Total pelvic exenteration* is most often required for recurrent cervical cancer. The procedure involves the *en bloc* excision of the bladder, uterus, rectum, and vagina (Fig. 22).

Using current surgical stapling devices, low-rectal reanastomosis can be performed in approximately 70% of cases. Reconstruction of the urinary system is accomplished using

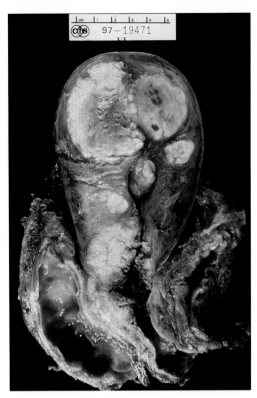

PLATE 24. Total pelvic exenteration performed for recurrent cervical cancer involves *en bloc* resection of the bladder, vagina, uterus, and rectum. In this specimen, recurrent cervical cancer has replaced the cervix (uterine leiomyomata occupy the uterine fundus). (This plate is printed in black and white as Figure 49-22.)

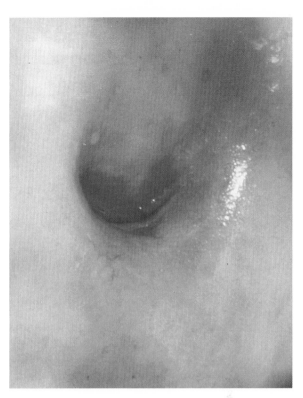

PLATE 25. In the original squamous epithelium, the superficial spider-like network of capillaries is barely visible (original magnification 316). (This plate is printed in black and white as Figure 49-24.)

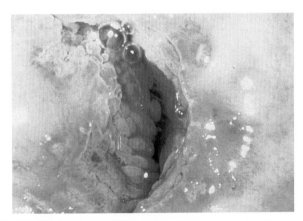

PLATE 26. In the normal transformation zone, islands of squamous metaplasia and tongues of columnar epithelium (i.e., grape-like structures) are visible on the patient's right external cervical os. (This plate is printed in black and white as Figure 49-25.)

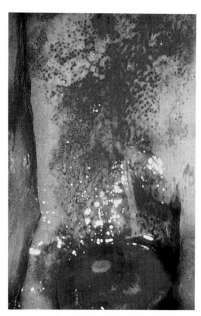

PLATE 27. Punctation on the anterior lip of the cervix is mixed with some white epithelium. A biopsy specimen from the area showed severe dysplasia. (This plate is printed in black and white as Figure 49-26A.)

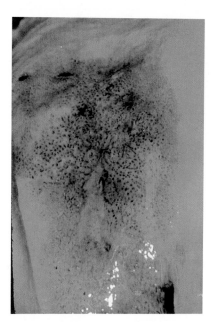

PLATE 28. Use of a green filter on the colposcope enhances the appearance of punctation. (This plate is printed in black and white as Figure 49-26B.)

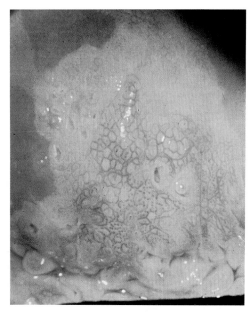

PLATE 29. A mosaic pattern is seen within the white epithelium. A biopsy from the area showed carcinoma *in situ.* (This plate is printed in black and white as Figure 49-27.)

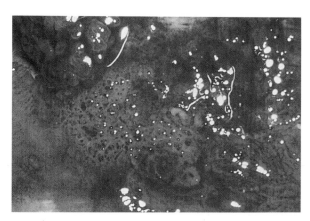

PLATE 30. Atypical vessels. The terminal vessels are irregular in size, shape, and arrangement. Biopsy specimens revealed invasive carcinoma. (This plate is printed in black and white as Figure 49-28.)

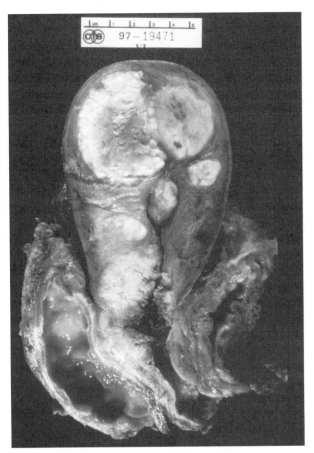

FIG. 22. Total pelvic exenteration performed for recurrent cervical cancer involves *en bloc* resection of the bladder, vagina, uterus, and rectum. In this specimen, recurrent cervical cancer has replaced the cervix (uterine leiomyomata occupy the uterine fundus). (This figure is printed in color as Plate 24.)

either an intestinal urinary conduit or one of the many techniques of continent urinary diversion (Miami pouch, Indiana pouch). A neovagina can be created by a variety of techniques using myocutaneous flaps (e.g., bulbocavernosus, gracilis, transverse rectus abdominus).

With modern surgical techniques and intensive care unit support, perioperative mortality does not exceed 7% in recent series. With proper patient selection and sound surgical judgment, 5-year survival rates after pelvic exenteration range from 45% to 61%.

◊ ADENOCARCINOMA

Adenocarcinoma of the cervix accounts for approximately 10% to 15% of all invasive cervical neoplasms. As with to SCC, tumor size, depth of invasion, and histologic tumor grade have been identified as predictors of pelvic lymph node metastasis and overall survival. Although cervical adenocarcinoma has been reported to have a worse prognosis than similar stage SCC, this difference is due, at least in part, to the tendency of adenocarcinoma to grow endophytically and establish a large tumor volume prior to clinical detection. When cervical adenocarcinoma and SCC are comparatively

matched by patient age, clinical stage, tumor volume, and treatment method, survival outcomes are not significantly different.

◊ SMALL CELL CARCINOMA

Small cell carcinoma of the uterine cervix is similar to small cell "neuroendocrine" tumor of the lung and other anatomic locations. These tumors are clinically aggressive, demonstrating a marked propensity to metastasize to local and distant sites. At the time of presentation, disease is often widely disseminated, with bone, brain, and liver being the most common sites. Because of the high metastatic potential of small cell carcinoma, local therapy alone (surgery and/or radiation) rarely results in long-term survival. Multiagent chemotherapy, in combination with external-beam and intracavitary radiation therapy, is a therapeutic approach currently under study. The two most commonly used chemotherapeutic regimens are vincristine, doxorubicin (Adriamycin), and cyclophosphamide (VAC) and etoposide and cisplatin (EP).

◊ CARCINOMA OF THE CERVICAL STUMP

The natural history and patterns of spread of carcinoma of the cervical stump are similar to those of carcinoma of the intact uterus. The diagnostic evaluation, clinical staging, and principles of staging are also unchanged. In appropriate surgical candidates, early stage disease can be treated with simple or radical trachelectomy with or without lymphadenectomy, depending on the volume of disease. Advanced-stage disease is treated with radiation therapy. However, the lack of a uterine cavity can make placement of intracavitary radiation sources difficult or impossible. In this case, vaginal ovoids alone or an interstital needle implant technique can be used with external-beam therapy.

◊ INCIDENTAL CERVICAL CANCER FOUND AT SIMPLE HYSTERECTOMY

Invasive cervical cancer may be incidentally discovered in the surgical specimen after hysterectomy has been performed. For disease more advanced than stage IA1 (without lymph-vascular involvement), simple hysterectomy is inadequate treatment, as the parametria, vaginal cuff, and pelvic lymph nodes may harbor residual tumor. Additional treatment is dictated by the volume of disease and the status of the surgical margins of resection.

Radical surgery following simple hysterectomy for invasive cervical cancer generally includes radical parametrectomy, resection of the cardinal ligaments, excision of the vaginal stump, and pelvic lymphadenectomy. Although it may be technically difficult to perform an adequate radical resection, reoperation should be considered in selected clinical situations, particularly for young patients in whom ovarian preservation is desired. Use of postoperative adjuvant radiation therapy is dictated by surgical and pathologic findings.

Cervical carcinoma at the margins of resection after simple hysterectomy or the presence of gross residual tumor are absolute indications for radiation therapy. Patients with such findings have a much less favorable prognosis than those without residual tumor and those with comparable disease who have been appropriately staged and treated with radiation alone. Radiation therapy is also well suited for older patients or those who are poor surgical candidates. Five-year survival is 95% to 100% for patients with microscopic disease, while 82% to 84% of those with macroscopic disease and negative surgical margins survive 5 years. If the surgical margins of resection are microscopically involved with carcinoma, 5-year survival ranges from 38% to 87%; survival drops to 20% to 47% for patients with gross residual tumor.

◊ COLPOSCOPY

Colposcopy was developed by Hinselmann in 1925, and although it was used extensively in German-speaking countries and in South America, it made relatively little impression in the English-speaking world, except in Australia. The delay in adopting of colposcopy in Great Britain and the United States was mainly because of Hinselmann's highly technical and difficult terminology, most of which originated from visual impressions not necessarily related to the underlying histopathologic processes. The development of diagnostic exfoliative cytology also delayed the introduction of colposcopy in English-speaking countries. Learning how to take an adequate cervical smear is much easier than learning how to use the colposcope. Training in colposcopy is time-consuming, but without adequate training, good results are impossible.

Colposcopy and cytology were long considered competitive methods of early cancer detection. However, each method has its particular limitations and strengths in cancer detection, and the two methods complement one another. Cytology is a laboratory method of detection; colposcopy is a clinical method. Each deals with a different aspect of neoplasia. Cytology evaluates the morphologic changes in the exfoliated cells; colposcopy evaluates the changes in the terminal vascular network of the cervix that reflect the biochemical and metabolic changes in the tissue.

Technique

The colposcope is basically a stereoscopic microscope by which the cervix can be seen, magnified 6- to 40-fold, in bright light (Fig. 23). The examination technique is rapid, requiring little more time than inspection of the cervix with an unaided eye. After a specimen for cell study has been obtained, the mucus is carefully removed from the cervix by means of a swab. The colposcope is then focused on the cervix. In routine colposcopic examination, a magnification of ×16 is used. The cervix is then soaked with acetic acid 3% to 5% to accentuate the appearance of abnormal areas. Metaplastic, dysplastic, or CIS epithelium is delineated by its white appearance. Optimal contrast of the vessels is achieved

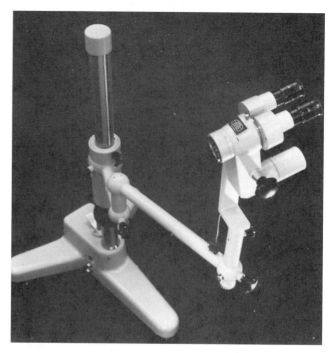

FIG. 23. Zeiss colposcope.

by insertion of a green filter. The effect of the acetic acid lasts for only a few minutes, but the cervix may again be soaked with acetic acid if further examination is desirable.

Colposcopic Findings

Terminology and Classification of Lesions

In 1978, during the Third World Congress for Cervical Pathology and Colposcopy in Orlando, Florida, a new colposcopic terminology was adopted. Colposcopic findings are divided into four groups: normal, abnormal, unsatisfactory, and other.

Normal Colposcopic Findings

Original squamous epithelium is the smooth, pink, featureless epithelium originally established on the cervix and vagina. No remnants of columnar epithelium, such as mucus-secreting epithelium, cleft openings, or nabothian cysts, are identified (Fig. 24).

Columnar epithelium is a single layer of tall, mucus-producing epithelium that extends into the endocervix from the original squamous epithelium or the metaplastic epithelium. The area covered with columnar epithelium has an irregular surface, with long stromal papillae and deep clefts. After application of acetic acid, this epithelium reveals a typical grape-like structure. Columnar epithelium may be present on the portio or may extend into the vagina.

The transformation zone is the area between the original squamous epithelium and the columnar epithelium in which metaplastic epithelium of various degrees of maturity is identified. Components of a normal transformation zone include

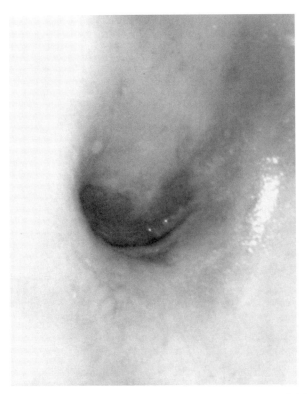

FIG. 24. In the original squamous epithelium, the superficial spider-like network of capillaries is barely visible (original magnification ×16). (This figure is printed in color as Plate 25.)

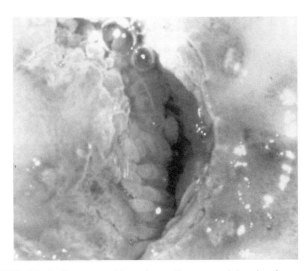

FIG. 25. In the normal transformation zone, islands of squamous metaplasia and tongues of columnar epithelium (i.e., grape-like structures) are visible on the patient's right external cervical os. (This figure is printed in color as Plate 26.)

islands of columnar epithelium surrounded by metaplastic epithelium, gland openings, and nabothian cysts. In a normal transformation zone, there are no colposcopic findings suggestive of cervical neoplasia (Fig. 25).

Abnormal Colposcopic Findings

An atypical transformation zone contains one or more findings that suggest cervical neoplasia: acetowhite epithelium, punctuation, mosaic vascular pattern, hyperkeratosis, and abnormal blood vessels.

◊ *Aceteowhite epithelium* is a focal, abnormal colposcopic lesion seen after application of acetic acid. This transient phenomenon is seen in the area of increased nuclear density.
◊ *Punctuation* is a focal abnormal colposcopic lesion with a stippled vascular pattern caused by capillary loops in stromal papillae seen on end. The vascular changes are sharply demarcated against normal epithelium (Fig. 26).
◊ In a focal abnormal colposcopic lesion with a *mosaic pattern,* the fields of mosaic are separated by reddish borders caused by capillary loops seen transversing the epithelium (Fig. 27).
◊ *Hyperkeratosis* is a focal colposcopic pattern in which hyperkeratosis or parakeratosis appears as an elevated whitened plaque. This whitened plaque is identified before the application of acetic acid. Some cases of

hyperkeratosis may be identified outside the transformation zone.
◊ *Abnormal blood vessels* constitute a focal abnormal colposcopic pattern in which the blood vessels appear not as punctuation, mosaic, or delicately branching vessels, but as irregular vessels with abrupt courses appearing as commas, corkscrew capillaries, or spaghetti-like forms running parallel to the surface (Fig. 28).

Another type of abnormal finding is colposcopically obvious invasive cancer that is not evident on clinical examination (Fig. 29).

Unsatisfactory Colposcopic Findings

The designation of unsatisfactory colposcopy is applied when the squamocolumnar junction cannot be delineated or the endocervical extent of an observed lesion cannot be visualized.

Other Colposcopic Findings

There are several other colposcopic findings. In vaginocervicitis, there is a diffuse colposcopic pattern of hyperemia, in which the blood vessels appear in a stippled pattern similar to the vascular pattern in punctuation (Fig. 30). In true erosion, the colposcopic examination reveals an area denuded of epithelium. The condition is usually caused by trauma. Atrophic epithelium is an estrogen-deprived squamous epithelium in which the vascular pattern is more readily identified because of the relative thinness of the overlying squamous epithelium. Condyloma and papilloma are exophytic lesions that may be inside or outside the transformation zone.

Correlation of Colposcopic and Histologic Findings

Table 8 correlates the colposcopic terminology with the colposcopic appearance and the expected histologic changes.

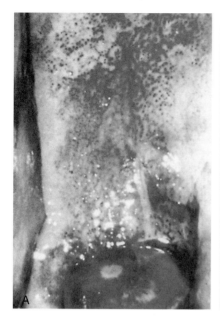
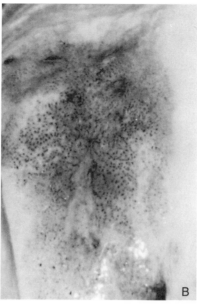

FIG. 26. A: Punctation on the anterior lip of the cervix is mixed with some white epithelium. A biopsy specimen from the area showed severe dysplasia. B: Use of a green filter on the colposcope enhances the appearance of punctation. (These figures are printed in color as Plates 27 and 28.)

Normal colposcopic findings are original cervical epithelium (i.e., squamous or columnar) or metaplastic squamous epithelium. In patients with normal colposcopic findings in whom the squamocolumnar junction is fully visible, cervical neoplasia should not exist in the tissue.

The most common abnormal colposcopic findings are acetowhite epithelium, punctuation, and a mosaic pattern. Because the pathogenesis of these patterns is similar, combinations of these findings are common. The histologic counterparts of these patterns range from minimal dysplastic changes to CIS. For prediction of histopathologic changes in a directed biopsy, it is not important whether the lesion viewed colposcopically appears as white epithelium, punctuation, or a mosaic pattern. These histopathologic changes can be predicted by reference to easily observable colposcopic features: vascular pattern, intercapillary distance, surface pattern, color tone, and clarity of demarcation.

The vascular pattern is one of the most important diagnostic features. Changes in the vascular pattern closely correspond to the degree of histologic changes. During the first stage of carcinogenesis, the morphology of the tissue is unaltered, but the blood vessels react to these changes in tissue metabolism and cell biochemistry, and the vascular alterations constitute the first morphologic abnormality in the development of cervical neoplasia. For a detailed description of the different patterns of vessels and their diagnostic significance, the reader is referred to the colposcopic literature.

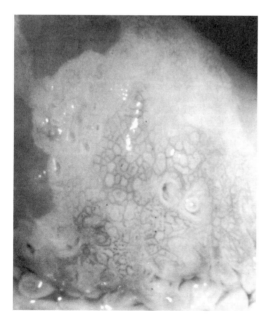

FIG. 27. A mosaic pattern is seen within the white epithelium. A biopsy from the area showed carcinoma *in situ*. (This figure is printed in color as Plate 29.)

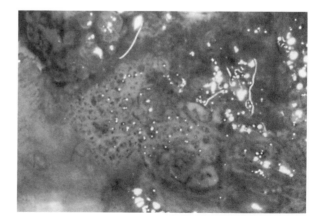

FIG. 28. Atypical vessels. The terminal vessels are irregular in size, shape, and arrangement. Biopsy specimens revealed invasive carcinoma. (This figure is printed in color as Plate 30.)

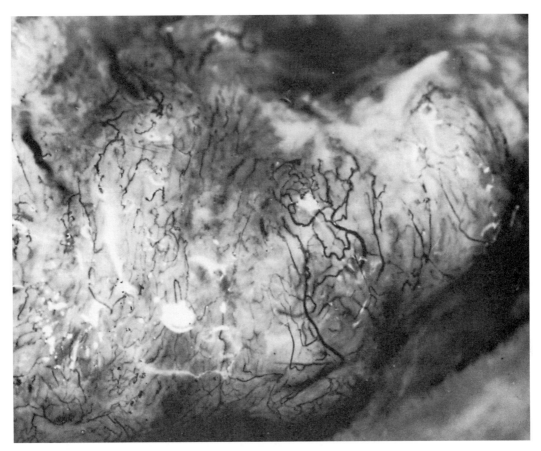

FIG. 29. Suspected frank invasive cancer. Atypical branching and network vessels are compatible with frank invasive cancer. A biopsy confirmed the diagnosis (original magnification ×16). (From Kolstad P, Stafl A. *Atlas of colposcopy.* Oslo, Norway: Universitetsforlaget, 1972; with permission.)

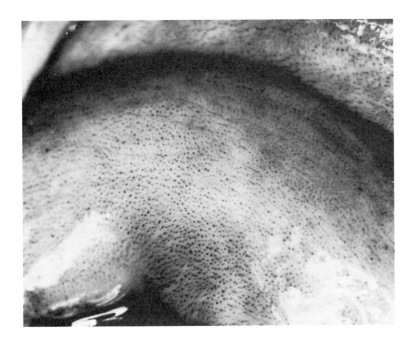

FIG. 30. Original squamous epithelium with inflammatory changes. The terminal vessels in trichomonal infection may give a colposcopic picture resembling punctation; however, capillaries are diffusely distributed over the ectocervix and vaginal wall (original magnification ×16). (From Kolstad P, Stafl A. *Atlas of colposcopy.* Oslo, Norway: Universitetsforlaget, 1972; with permission.)

TABLE 8. *Correlation of colposcopic and histologic findings*

Colposcopic term	Colposcopic appearance	Histologic correlate
Original squamous epithelium	Smooth, pink Indefinitely outlined vessels No change after application of acetic acid	Squamous epithelium
Columnar epithelium	Grape-like structures after application of acetic acid	Columnar epithelium
Transformation zone	Tongues of squamous metaplasia Gland openings Nabothian cysts	Metaplastic squamous epithelium
White epithelium	White, sharp-bordered lesion visible only after application of acetic acid No vessels visible	Minimal dysplasia to carcinoma *in situ*
Punctation	Sharp-bordered lesion Red stippling Epithelium whiter after application of acetic acid	Minimal dysplasia to carcinoma *in situ*
Mosaic	Sharp-bordered lesion Mosaic pattern Epithelium whiter after application of acetic acid	Minimal dysplasia to carcinoma *in situ*
Hyperkeratosis	White patch Rough surface Visible before application of acetic acid	Usually hyperkeratosis or parakeratosis; seldom carcinoma *in situ* or invasive carcinoma
Atypical vessels	Horizontal vessels running parallel to surface Constriction or dilatation of vessels Atypical branching, winding course	Carcinoma *in situ* to invasive carcinoma

The intercapillary distance refers to the amount of cervical tissue that separates blood vessels. During a colposcopic examination, the intercapillary distance in a colposcopically abnormal lesion can be estimated by comparison with that of the capillaries in the adjacent normal epithelium. In cervical neoplasia, the intercapillary distance increases as the stage of the disease advances.

The colposcope provides a stereoscopic magnification that greatly facilitates the study of the surface contour, which can be described as smooth, uneven, granulated, papillomatous, or nodular. Normal squamous epithelium or minimal dysplasia has a smooth surface; CIS and early-stage invasive cancer have an uneven, slightly elevated surface.

Colposcopic lesions have different color tones, varying from white to deep red. The difference between the surface color of the cervix before and after the application of acetic acid is diagnostically significant. When there is a marked change from deep red to white after application of acetic acid, a severe histologic lesion may be expected. It is important to examine the cervix colposcopically before and after application of acetic acid.

An important feature of a colposcopically abnormal lesion is the clarity of demarcation between the lesion and the adjacent normal tissue. The borderline between normal squamous epithelium and inflammatory changes or minimal dysplasia is diffuse and irregular. Severe dysplasia or CIS usually produces a lesion with sharp borders that distinctly demarcate it from the adjacent normal epithelium.

The main value of colposcopy is in the evaluation of patients whose cytologic studies are abnormal and who are at high risk for significant cervical neoplasia. Colposcopy makes it possible to localize the lesions, evaluate their extent, and obtain a directed biopsy from which the histopathologic diagnosis can be established. Colposcopy is accurate in differentiating invasive from noninvasive lesions and inflammatory atypia from neoplasia. In patients with abnormal cells on cytology, colposcopy can immediately differentiate between inflammatory and neoplastic changes. The limitation of colposcopy is its inability to detect a lesion deep in the endocervical canal; the results of the colposcopy evaluation may be unsatisfactory because the squamocolumnar junction is not visible. Further diagnostic steps are required. The frequency of unsatisfactory colposcopic findings in premenopausal women is 12% to 15%. After menopause, the frequency of unsatisfactory colposcopy rises significantly, so that the value of colposcopy in the evaluation of the cervix of postmenopausal women is somewhat more limited. However, in patients whose squamocolumnar junction is fully visible, the false-negative rate of colposcopy is low.

Like every diagnostic method, colposcopy has limitations that must be fully recognized. The importance of adequate training and experience cannot be overemphasized. Inexperience can lead to serious mistakes in the diagnosis and management of cervical cancer that may significantly discredit colposcopy. The limitation of colposcopy in the diagnosis of lesions in the endocervical canal should be fully appreciated, and when the squamocolumnar junction is not fully visible, other methods of evaluation (e.g., ECC, conization) must be used. When used intelligently with a thorough understanding of all the morphologic details, colposcopy is an important diagnostic tool for clinical practice and research.

◊ RECOMMENDED READINGS

Ahern JK, Allen HM. Cervical hemangioma. *J Reprod Med* 1978;21:228.

American College of Obstetrics and Gynecology. Committee opinion: recommendations on frequency of Pap test screening. *Int J Gynaecol Obstet* 1995;49: 210.

Anderson GH, Boyes DA, Benedet JL, et al. Organization and results of the cervical cytology screening programme in British Columbia, 1955–85. *BMJ* 1988;296:975.

Arena B, Valentine BH. Evaluation of cytology and colposcopy in the follow-up of laser ablation for cervical intra-epithelial neoplasia. *J Obstet Gynecol* 1991;11:290.

Brunaham RC, Paavonen J, Stevens CE, et al., Mucopurulent cervicitis—the ignored counterpart in women of urethritis in men. *N Engl J Med* 1984; 311:1.

Centers for Disease Control and Prevention. Morbitity and mortality weekly report. *MMWR* 1993;42:51.

Conti M. Prevalence and risk of progression of genital intraepithelial neoplasia in women with human immunodeficiency virus infection. *Adv Gynecol Obstet Res* 1991;3:283.

Delgado G, Bundy BN, Fowler WC, et al. A prospective surgical pathological study of stage I squamous carcinoma of the cervix: a Gynecologic Oncology Group Study. *Gynecol Oncol* 1989;35:314.

Eddy GL. Screening for cervical cancer. *Ann Intern Med* 1990;113:214.

Evan AS, Monaghan JM, Beattie AB. Carbon dioxide laser treatment of cervical warty atypias. *Gynecol Oncol* 1984;17:296.

Finan MA, DeCesare S, Fiorca JV, et al. Radical hysterectomy for stage IB1 vs. IB2 carcinoma of the cervix: does the new staging system predict morbidity and survival? *Gynecol Oncol* 1996;62:139.

Fluhmann CF. *The cervix uteri and its diseases.* Philadelphia: WB Saunders, 1961.

Hatch KD, Shingleton HM, Orr JW, et al. Role of endocervical curettage in colposcopy. *Obstet Gynecol* 1985;65:403.

Herbst AL, Bern HA, eds. *Developmental effects of diethylstilbestrol (DES) in pregnancy.* New York: Thieme-Stratton, 1981.

Kaufman RH, Noller KL, Adam E, et al. Genital tract abnormalities and pregnancy outcome in diethylstilbesterol-exposed progeny. *Am J Obstet Gynecol* 1984;148:973.

Kosary CL. FIGO stage, histology, histologic grade, age and race as prognostic factors in determining survival for cancers of the female gynecologic system: an analysis of 1973–87 SEER cases of cancers of the endometrium, cervix, ovary, vulva, and vagina. *Semin Surg Oncol* 1994;10:31.

Krebs HG. Treatment of vaginal condylomata acuminata by weekly topical application of 5-fluorouracil. *Obstet Gynecol* 1988;70:68.

Maiman M, Fruchter RG, Guy L, Cuthill S, Levine P, Serur E. Human immunodeficiency virus infection and invasive cervical carcinoma. *Cancer* 1993;71:402.

Meisels A, Morin C, Casas-Cordoro C. Human papillomavirus infection of the uterine cervix. *Int J Gynecol Pathol* 1982;1:75.

Moberg PJ, Einhorn N, Silfversward C, Soderberg G. Adenocarcinoma of the uterine cervix. *Cancer* 1986;57:407.

National Institutes of Health. *Cervical cancer. NIH consensus statement.* 1996;14:1.

Oster AG. Natural history of cervical intraepithelial neoplasia: a critical review. *Int J Gynecol Pathol* 1993;12:186.

Perez CA, Camel HM, Kuske RR, et al. Radiation therapy alone in the treatment of carcinoma of the uterine cervix: a 20-year experience. *Gynecol Oncol* 1986;23:127.

Peterson F. *Annual report on the results of treatment of gynecologic cancer.* Radiumhemmet, Stockholm, Sweden: International Federation of Gynecology and Obstetrics, 1994:132.

Poyner EA, Barakat RR, Hoskins WJ. Management and follow-up of patients with adenocarcinoma *in situ* of the uterine cervix. *Gynecol Oncol* 1995;57:158.

Ranade V, Palermino DA, Tronik B. Cervical pregnancy. *Obstet Gynecol* 1978;51:502.

Raskin MM. Diagnosis of cervical pregnancy by ultrasound: a case report. *Am J Obstet Gynecol* 1978;130:234.

Richart RM, Barron BA. A follow-up study of patients with cervical dysplasia. *Am J Obstet Gynecol* 1969;105:386.

Robboy SJ, Noller KL, O'Brien P, et al. Increased incidence of cervical and vaginal dysplasia in 3,980 diethylstilbesterol (DES)-exposed young women: experience of the National Collaborative DES-Adenosis (DESAD) Project. *JAMA* 1984;252:2979.

Schink JC, Lurain JR. Microinvasive cervix cancer. *Int J Gynaecol Obstet* 1991;36:5.

Szarewski A, Cuzick J, Edwards R, et al. The use of cervicography in a primary screening service. *Br J Obstet Gynaecol* 1991;98:313.

Wright TC, Ferenczy A. Benign diseases of the cervix. In: Kurman RJ, ed. *Blaustein's pathology of the female genital tract,* 4th ed. New York: Springer-Verlag, 1994:203.

Zander J, Baltzer J, Lohe KJ, Ober KG, Kaufman C. Carcinoma of the cervix: an attempt to individualize treatment. Results of a 20-year cooperative study. *Am J Obstet Gynecol* 1981;139:752–759.

Zuna RE. Association of condylomas with intraepithelial and microinvasive cervical neoplasia: histopathology of conization and hysterectomy specimens. *Int J Gynecol Pathol* 1984;2:364.

Zweizig S, Noller K, Reale F, Collis S, Resseguie L. Neoplasia associated with atypical glandular cells of undetermined significance on cervical cytology. *Gynecol Oncol* 1997;65:314.

CHAPTER 50

Diseases of the Uterus

—— ◇ ——

Patricia S. Braly

The uterus is a hollow, muscular organ lying in the true pelvis between the bladder and the rectum and composed of three discreet layers: serosa or outer peritoneal covering, myometrium, and endometrium. Because of its position and its physiologic responses to many factors, such as hormone levels and infection, the uterus may develop many organ-related disorders and symptoms, both benign and malignant, which will be discussed in this chapter.

◇ UTERINE ANOMALIES

Congenital Anomalies: Uterine Effects of Diethylstilbestrol Exposure

The observation that intrauterine exposure to diethylstilbestrol (DES) is associated with upper genital tract abnormalities was first reported by Kaufman et al. in 1977.[15] They described a T-shaped appearance to the uterus, constricting bands in the uterine cavity, a hypoplastic uterus and, less frequently, intrauterine polypoid defects and synechiae (Figs. 1 and 2). In their original article, they speculated that these defects might adversely affect subsequent pregnancies. Over the next 10 years, Kaufman and other investigators evaluated pregnancy outcomes in relation to upper genital tract abnormalities documented on hysterosalpingography.[14,16] From these studies, several interesting findings were noted, including the fact that the frequency of uterine abnormalities varied according to whether subjects were identified from record review or from self-referral of interested patients (Table 1). Another finding was the clear association between cervical and vaginal epithelial changes (e.g., adenosis) and upper genital tract abnormalities. The third conclusion was that women documented to have upper genital tract abnormalities were more likely to have poor pregnancy outcomes, with the most consistent being preterm delivery and ectopic pregnancies, compared to DES-exposed women with normal hysterosalpingograms (Table 2). Animal studies have suggested that the anatomic basis of these uterine abnormalities is related to stunted growth of the upper müllerian ducts with

failure of the inner and outer stromal layers of the uterine walls to segregate normally when these animals were exposed *in utero* to DES. Although several studies addressed the question of fertility in DES-exposed women, there is no clear consensus on the impact of *in utero* DES exposure and the frequency of infertility. Although there is no clear evidence that infertility is increased in women with an abnormal hysterosalpingogram per se, there appear to be subsets of abnormalities, such as the finding of a T-shaped uterus along with constriction of the upper cavity, that are are associated statistically with the inability to conceive.

The clinical management options for patients with upper genital tract abnormalities and poor pregnancy outcomes have unfortunately been quite limited.[4] Since very little can be done to improve outcome prior to conception, the knowledge of either uterine abnormalities as documented by hysterosalpingography or even the findings of cervical structural or vaginal epithelial changes should alert the clinician to the increased likelihood of either an ectopic pregnancy or a preterm delivery. Early in pregnancy these patients should be evaluated with transvaginal sonography to document an intrauterine gestational sac, and then as the pregnancy develops, consideration should be given to serial ultrasound and/or digital examinations to evaluate the cervix for premature effacement and dilation. If these changes are documented, patients should be considered for cervical cerclage. Interestingly, as opposed to other, non-DES-related congenital upper genital tract abnormalities, there seems to be no increase in urinary tract abnormalities in women with DES-related uterine abnormalities examined with intravenous pyelography.

Acquired Anomalies: Asherman Syndrome

Asherman syndrome represents an obliteration of all or most of the endometrial cavity, almost always as a result of a dilation and curettage (D&C) performed for postpartum bleeding 1 or more days after delivery, multiple D&Cs performed for persistent uterine bleeding, or a D&C performed for an

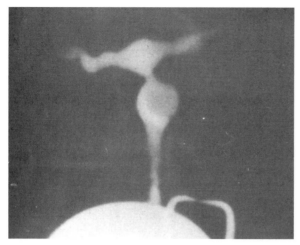

FIG. 1. T-shaped uterus with constriction. Lower half of uterine cavity has a bulbous appearance, and expected area of cervical canal has a funnel shape. (From Kaufman, RH, Adam E, Binder GL, Gerthoffer E. Upper genital tract changes and pregnancy outcome in offspring exposed in utero to diethylstilbestrol. *Am J Obstet Gynecol* 1980;137: 301–302; with permission.)

infected abortion. In the absence of sufficient endometrium and particularly when an inflammatory process is present, the residual endometrial tissue is replaced by collagen, causing the development of intrauterine adhesions or synechiae. Although the usual presenting complaint is amenorrhea or hypomenorrhea, Asherman syndrome may result in infertility or recurrent spontaneous abortion with or without amenorrhea. Once this history is obtained, further workup includes a hysterosalpingogram, which often demonstrates no endometrial cavity or severe deformity and obliteration of parts of the cavity. Prior to this procedure, the presence or absence of functioning endometrium can be demonstrated with an

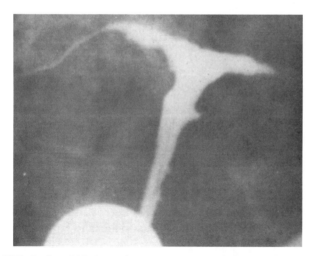

FIG. 2. Small T-shaped uterus with dye extending out from cavity into myometrium. (From Kaufman, RH, Adam E, Binder GL, Gerthoffer E. Upper genital tract changes and pregnancy outcome in offspring exposed in utero to diethylstilbestrol. *Am J Obstet Gynecol* 1980;137:301–302; with permission.)

TABLE 1. *Hysterosalpingographic findings in 676 women: cavity shape*

Cavity shape	Record reviews (%)	Walk-ins, referrals, others (%)
Normal	58.4[a]	39.0[a]
T-shape	29.9	46.5[a]
Constriction	30.2	59.2[a]
Wide Clover segment	12.7	19.5
Arcuate	11.6	6.0[a]
Hypoplastic	6.5	20.0[a]
Bicornuate	1.4	1.6
Unicornuate	0.3	0.8
Other	2.4	2.1
Women examined (*n*)	291	385

[a]Significance of difference between the cohorts: $p < 0.01$.

estrogen–progestin challenge test, since the only requirement for withdrawal bleeding after estrogen and progestin stimulation is functioning endometrium. For this evaluation, the patient is treated with conjugated estrogens daily for 21 days, and for the last 10 days of this cycle, a progestin is added to the estrogen. Withdrawal bleeding should occur approximately 5 to 7 days after completion of the hormonal therapy. Of course, pregnancy should be ruled out prior to the administration of these hormones.

The optimal treatment for Asherman syndrome involves hysteroscopic lysis of the intrauterine synechiae. After the operative procedure, an intrauterine device is often placed into the uterine cavity in an attempt to maintain its patency and keep the endometrial surfaces apart. Cyclic high-dose estrogen and progestin therapy is administered in an attempt to induce endometrial proliferation. In most patients, this treatment is sufficient, but on occasion the intrauterine synechiae reform.

◊ BENIGN DISORDERS OF THE UTERUS

Pyometra and Hematometra

An enlarged, fluid-filled endometrial cavity usually represents a hematometra or pyometra. Both conditions are associated with either congenital or acquired cervical stenosis or other outflow obstruction, such as an imperforate hymen or transverse vaginal septum. In young patients, common presenting signs and symptoms include primary amenorrhea, dysmenorrhea, endometriosis, and infertility. On occasion, if the uterine fluid collection represents purulent material (pyometrium), pressure can cause this fluid to escape through the fallopian tubes into the peritoneal cavity, thus causing peritonitis and sepsis. When a lower genital tract anomaly has been ruled out, the presumption is that the patient has acquired cervical stenosis, which most commonly is iatrogenic in nature. Frequent causes of iatrogenic cervical stenosis include conization, cryocautery, and hot cautery of the cervix for premalignant lesions. Patients at highest risk for cervical stenosis following ablative or excisional therapy are women who have been exposed to DES *in utero*, presumably because

TABLE 2. *Relationship of first pregnancy outcome to cavity shape*

Cohort (%)	Cavity shape	Women (n)	Outcome of pregnancy												Any unfavorable outcome
			Term live birth		Preterm live birth		Spontaneous abortion		Ectopic pregnancy		Stillbirth					
			n	%	n	%	n	%	n	%	n	%				n
Record reviews																
25[a]	Normal	99	74	75	8	8	15	15	1	1	1	1				25
49[a]	Abnormal	70	36	51[a]	11	16[b]	15	21	7	10[b]	1	1				34
Walk-ins, referrals, others																
56	Normal	63	28	44	15	24	14	22	6	9	0	0				35
65	Abnormal	95	32	34	26	27	19	20	14	15	4	4				63
All																
37	Normal	162	102	63	23	14	29	18	7	4	1	1				60
59[a]	Abnormal	165	68	41[a]	37	22	34	21	21	13[a]	5	3				97

[a]Significance of difference between abnormal and normal hysterosalpingography groups: $p < 0.01$.
[b]Significance of difference between abnormal and normal hysterosalpingography groups: $p < 0.05$.
(From ref. 16; with permission.)

of defective cervical stroma. Other causes of cervical stenosis include malignancy involving either the endo- or exocervix or lower uterine segment, cervicitis, senile atrophy, or trauma from childbirth. Treatment of acquired cervical stenosis obviously depends on patient symptoms and desire for future fertility. Often, attempts to dilate the cervix will be associated with recurrent stenosis. Currently, the most effective treatment appears to be laser ablation of the fibrotic cervical tissue surrounding the endocervical canal.

The diagnosis of hematometra or pyometra should be suspected when a patient complains of amenorrhea and cramping lower abdominal pain, and pelvic examination documents an enlarged, globular uterus. The diagnosis can be confirmed by sonogram, and treatment includes D&C, as well as correction of the obstruction if possible. When a diagnosis of pyometra is made, in addition to drainage of the fluid collection, patients should also be given antibiotics to treat common organisms such as bacteroides, anaerobic staphylococci, streptococci, and aerobic coliforms. Placement of a large mushroom catheter has been attempted with variable success, but often repeated cervical dilation every few days is more effective in draining the pyometra.

Endometritis

Endometritis is an inflammatory reaction of the endometrium occurring in acute and chronic forms, depending on the type of inflammatory infiltrate. Chronic endometritis can often be subdivided by the identification of various etiologic agents. Acute endometritis is diagnosed by the finding of focal collections of polymorphonuclear leukocytes (PML) that form microabscesses or fill gland lumina. This is in contrast to the findings of a PML infiltrate in the stroma with necrosis and hemorrhage during the normal menstrual phase of the cycle.

Most episodes of acute endometritis appear to arise from infections ascending through the disrupted cervical barrier. The usually effective cervical barrier is compromised during menses, instrumentation, abortion, and parturition. When this barrier is disrupted, various organisms can gain access to the endometrial cavity but usually do not produce an infection. The most common clinically important cases of acute endometritis are associated with pregnancy or abortion and are usually caused by *Streptococcus, Staphylococcus, Neisseria*, or *Clostridium* organisms. Culture of the endometrial tissue either by swab or at the time of curettage is important for identifying the causative agent and helping select the appropriate antibiotic.

Chronic endometritis is diagnosed by the identification of plasma cells as a component of the inflammatory infiltrate, along with lymphocytes and macrophages. Often, the endometrium lacks the typical features that make dating it possible. Additional histologic findings include the characteristic spindle-cell alteration of the stromal cells. Squamous metaplasia may also be seen with chronic endometritis. The clinical presentation of chronic endometritis is quite variable, ranging from asymptomatic, to irregular bleeding, to salpin-

gitis. Patients may present with menometrorrhagia, uterine tenderness, and a mucopurulent vaginal discharge. The histologic findings of chronic endometritis can be found in up to 10% of endometrial biopsy specimens performed for irregular bleeding. Chronic endometritis has been identified with abortion in 41% of cases, with salpingitis in 25%, with an intrauterine device in 14%, and with a recent pregnancy in 12%.[17] Chronic endometritis also occurs with the presence of necrotic endometrial tissue, such as an infarcted polyp or carcinoma, or in association with cervical stenosis related to previous radiation or cervical malignancy.[17] In patients diagnosed with chronic endometritis not associated with an obvious etiology, an endocervical culture for *Neisseria* and *Chlamydia* should be performed because cervical cultures will often be positive for one of these organisms, even though the endometrial culture will be negative.

Chronic endometritis may also be associated with specific organisms such as *Mycoplasma, Mycobacterium tuberculosis*, fungi, viruses, and parasites. In tubercular infection, endometrial involvement is thought to occur by spread of organisms from the fallopian tubes following either hematogenous or lymphatic spread from a primary focus in the lung or gastrointestinal tract. Genital tuberculosis is thought to occur in 3% to 8% of women with pulmonary disease and is often an incidental finding at laparotomy for either pelvic inflammatory disease or infertility. Every attempt to identify the causative organism should be made so that appropriate therapy can be instituted.

Adenomyosis

Adenomyosis is a benign disease of the uterus characterized by areas of ectopic endometrial glands and stroma situated within the myometrium (Fig. 3). Adenomyosis arises spontaneously from glands of the basalis layer of the endometrium, and therefore these glands do not usually undergo the cyclic proliferative and secretory changes seen in the more superficial layers of the endometrium. It is unusual to identify any continuity between the basilar layer of the endometrium and foci of adenomyosis, with most cases having at least one low-power field (2.5 mm) of normal myometrium between the two. The documented frequency of adenomyosis is quite variable, depending on the thoroughness of the histologic evaluation. With multiple serial sections of the uterine wall, the incidence may exceed 60% in women undergoing hysterectomy between 40 and 50 years of age. With routine histologic evaluation, adenomyosis is reported in 5% to 10% of postmenopausal women and 15% of women under the age of 40. Adenomyosis is associated with uterine leiomyomata 50% of the time and with endometriosis less than 20% of the time.

Histogenesis and Pathology

The numerous theories of histogenesis of adenomyosis are largely unproven, with the most widely accepted being an actual invasion of the myometrium by the basal endometrium.

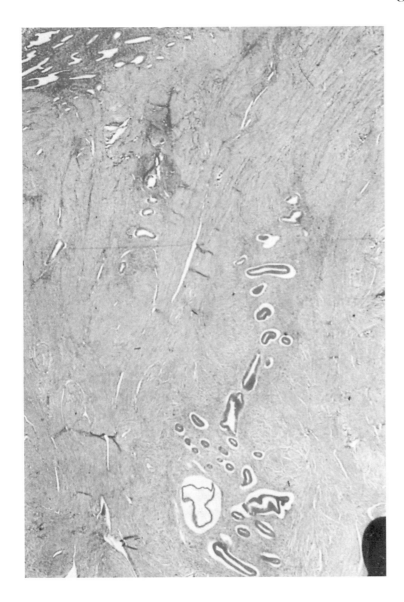

FIG. 3. Microscopic section of uterus with adenomyosis. Foci of endometrium are present deep to endometrium within myometrium.

Because adenomyosis is most often found in parous women, one hypothesis is that chronic postpartum endometritis may be associated with a disruption of the barrier between the endometrium and the myometrium. It is thought that first the stroma and then the glands begin to invade the myometrium along lymphatic and vascular channels.

Grossly, adenomyosis presents in two different ways: diffuse and focal involvement of the myometrium. Most commonly, the uterus is grossly enlarged and somewhat globular, with diffuse involvement of both anterior and posterior walls but usually greater involvement of the posterior wall. On sectioning, the myometrium is thickened with an irregular cut surface. There may be tiny foci of translucent tissue protruding from the cut surface, and on microscopic examination areas of endometrial glands and stroma are found to be scattered throughout the myometrium. The second type of presentation occurs as focal areas known as adenomyomas, which may result in an asymmetric uterus. These focal areas may be difficult to distinguish grossly from a myoma. The

cut surface reveals the nodule to be poorly demarcated from the surrounding myometrium, and it typically does not bulge above the myometrium as a myoma usually does.

Clinical Presentation

Most women with adenomyosis are asymptomatic or report minor symptoms such as slight menorrhagia or dysmenorrhea. The vast majority of symptomatic cases are documented in women between the ages of 35 and 50 years. The classic symptoms of adenomyosis include secondary dysmenorrhea (15% to 30%) and menorrhagia (40% to 50%), with increasingly severe dysmenorrhea as the disease progresses. With advanced disease, deep, midline dyspareunia may become a problem. On pelvic examination, the uterus tends to be diffusely enlarged and is often tender, especially in the premenstrual phase of the cycle. Because of the variable presentation of this disorder, adenomyosis is correctly diagnosed preoperatively in only 25% of cases. Both transvaginal ultrasound and magnetic resonance (MR) imaging may be helpful in delineating adenomyosis from uterine myomata, which may be important when conservative surgery such as myomectomy is being considered.

Therapy of Adenomyosis

There is no long-term successful medical treatment for adenomyosis. In selected patients, cyclic oral contraceptives may be tried, but success is variable, and anecdotal reports exist of worsening symptomatology when the oral contraceptives are discontinued. Prostaglandin synthetase inhibitors may relieve pain and decrease bleeding, but again success is unpredictable and often short-lived. While gonadotropin-releasing hormome (Gn-RH) agonists may be effective in suppressing adenomyosis, any benefit lasts only as long as these compounds are administered, with recurrence of symptoms and growth occurring promptly after drug therapy is stopped. Since there is no conservative surgical therapy that exists for adenomyosis, preoperative therapy with Gn-RH agonists is not appropriate. In patients who are symptomatic and do not desire future fertility, hysterectomy is the definitive therapy. Depending on associated gynecologic and medical factors, a hysterectomy for adenomyosis may be performed either abdominally or vaginally.

Endometrial Disorders

Functional Disorders

Irregular shedding of the endometrium is characterized by prolonged, heavy bleeding at the time of menses, with bleeding often lasting longer than 2 weeks. The diagnosis is substantiated by curettage of the uterus after the the fifth or sixth day of menstrual flow. Microscopic examination of these endometrial curettings shows areas of typical postovulatory menstrual endometrium, as well as areas of early proliferative endometrium. This abnormality appears to be caused by persistent function of the corpus luteum, with excessive production of progesterone, and is often associated with a corpus luteum cyst. Both the clinical symptoms and the resulting endometrial pathology can be reproduced by administration of progesterone during the premenstrual phase of the cycle. This condition is typically seen in women ages 24 to 50 years and may occur repeatedly or be limited to a single cycle. Time and curettage of the uterus that was required for diagnosis are often therapeutic.

Polyps

Endometrial polyps are pedunculated areas of overgrowth of endometrial glands and stroma that project above the endometrial surface and occasionally prolapse through the endocervical canal. They develop as solitary or multiple polyps, frequently composed of hyperplastic endometrium. The size of endometrial polyps varies from millimeters to several centimeters in diameter, being either sessile (broad based) or pe-

dunculated. Most polyps are asymptomatic and those that are symptomatic present with varied bleeding patterns. Since endometrial polyps are often associated with uterine leiomyomata and endometrial hyperplasia, it is difficult to determine which symptoms are actually caused by the polyps. Endometrial polyps are often an incidental finding at the time of D&C or hysterectomy. When symptoms do exist, the clinical picture is one of nonspecific abnormal uterine bleeding, including postmenopausal bleeding. Although the peak incidence of endometrial polyps is between 40 and 50 years of age, they have been documented in patients from 12 years to over 80 years of age.

Grossly, endometrial polyps are tan to red-brown in color with a vascular core. Histologically, a polyp consists of glands, stroma, and vasculature, with approximately two-thirds having immature endometrium that will have a cystic hyperplastic appearance regardless of the cycle phase (Fig. 4). The other one-third of polyps will consist of functional endometrium that will undergo cyclic histologic change. Low-grade malignant transformation occurs in 0.5% of polyps, and coexisting endometrial cancer occurs in approximately 10% of postmenopausal women with polyps.

The diagnosis of endometrial polyps is usually established at the time of curettage or hysterectomy, although with the increasing use of transvaginal sonography and sonohysteroscopy these structures are being identified preoperatively with increasing frequency. Occasionally, an endometrial polyp may protrude through the cervical os and be mistaken for a cervical polyp (Fig. 5).

Polyps are often missed at curettage unless a grasping instrument is also used to carefully explore the endometrial cavity. Therefore, a polyp forceps is recommended for routine use at the time of D&C. Hysteroscopy provides visual guidance to ensure that all polyps have been identified and removed, and without use of this technique up to 25% of endometrial polyps will be missed.

Other Benign Uterine Tumors

Other benign disorders of the uterus include adenomyoma, teratoma, and lymphangioma, as well as the presence of heterologous tissue (i.e., tissue not native to the endometrium). Most of these tumors are quite rare with few reported cases and no specific clinical syndromes associated with them. They are often diagnosed as incidental findings at the time of hysterectomy and, if noted prior to surgery, are usually mistaken for leiomyomata.

Atypical polypoid adenomas grossly resemble endometrial polyps and often arise from the lower uterine segment. They are typically seen in women in the reproductive and perimenopausal age groups and are often associated with irregular uterine bleeding. Microscopically, the lesion is composed of irregularly shaped hyperplastic glands within smooth muscle and on a curettage specimen may be difficult to distinguish from endometrial hyperplasia, invasive adenocarcinoma, and mixed müllerian tumors. Despite the cytologic atypia of this

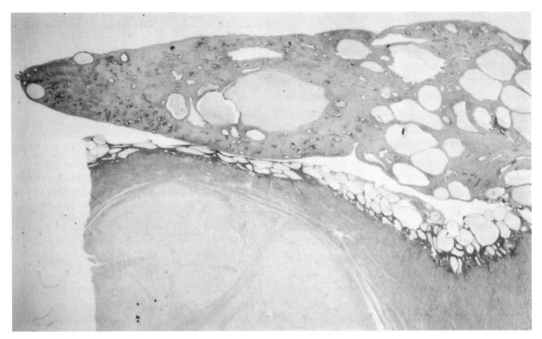

FIG. 4. Subcutaneous myoma, cystic atrophy of the endometrium, and an endometrial polyp with cystic hyperplasia and slight congestion of the tip were unexpected findings in a uterus removed from a postmenopausal patient.

lesion, its clinical course is benign, and simple curettage may be curative in women who wish to maintain fertility.[17]

Uterine teratoma is an extremely rare lesion that microscopically resembles ovarian teratoma. Typically, this neoplasm is lined by squamous epithelium and contains respiratory epithelium, adipose tissue, and sebaceous glands.[17]

Lymphangiomas are usually small, circumscribed nodules composed of a maze of lymphatic channels with a background of fibrous connective tissue.

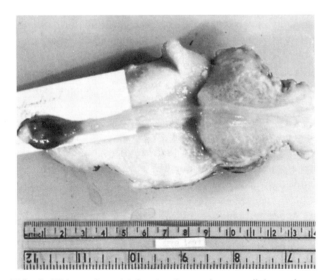

FIG. 5. This endometrial polyp has a long pedicle and protruded through the cervical os; as a result, the tip of the polyp is hemorrhagic and necrotic.

Hemangiopericytoma is a rare tumor composed of non-neoplastic capillaries surrounded by collars of neoplastic pericytes. It is usually found incidentally and is sometimes confused with stromal adenomyosis.

Lipoma is a lobulated, encapsulated yellow growth composed of adult adipose tissue. It is usually possible to distinguish a lipoma from a myoma with fatty degeneration by the remaining areas of smooth muscle in the latter tumor.

Cysts or small adenomatous growths in the lateral wall of the uterus are rare. These lesions presumably arise from remnants of the mesonephric duct or tubules. Even more rarely, such lesions may give rise to malignant neoplasms. The presence of heterologous tissue within the uterus, including bone, cartilage, smooth muscle, and glial tissue, has been reported. If these tissues are malignant, they represent a malignant mixed müllerian tumor. One possible explanation for the finding of benign heterologous tissue within the uterus is that this represents implantation of fetal tissue after abortion and instrumentation.

Endometrial Hyperplasia

Endometrial hyperplasia, which represents an overgrowth of endometrial glands and stroma, usually develops within a background of proliferative endometrium in response to prolonged unopposed estrogen stimulation. For many years, it has been suggested that endometrial hyperplasia reflects the histologic representation of the continuum between normal proliferating endometrium and adenocarcinoma *in situ.* This theory was based on prospective studies first reported by Gusberg and Kaplan in 1963.[12] In that study, the authors reported that 20% of patients who had a hysterectomy were found to have a coexisting adenocarcinoma and that endometrial cancer developed in almost 12% of the remaining patients with an average follow-up of 5.3 years. They concluded that the risk of cancer was significantly higher in women with endometrial hyperplasia than those without this diagnosis and that at 10 years the cumulative risk for cancer was approximately 30%.

During the ensuing years, several different classification schemes were developed, with resulting confusion regarding both diagnostic criteria and prognosis of the various subtypes of hyperplasia. Recently, the International Society of Gynecological Pathologists endorsed a classification schema that utilizes both architectural features (the degree of glandular crowding and complexity) and cytologic features, especially cellular atypia.[10] Simple hyperplasia is defined as abnormally thickened endometrium with histologic evidence of an increased ratio of glands to stroma; the glands are cystically dilated and somewhat irregular with some infolding and budding. Complex hyperplasia represents glandular crowding with even less intervening stroma, and the glands show significant infolding and budding. Atypical hyperplasia refers to either simple or complex architectural patterns in which the cells lining the glands show loss of polarity, nuclear enlargement with increased nucleus-to-cytoplasm ratio and prominent nucleoli, and irregularly condensed chromatin.

Since the study by Gusberg and Kaplan, additional studies have clarified some of the questions regarding this disorder. In an important paper, Kurman et al.[18] reported that the risk of progression of endometrial hyperplasia to cancer varied according to the subtype. In 170 patients with untreated endometrial hyperplasia, 74% regressed spontaneously and 18% remained stable for more than 10 years. The risk of progression to cancer was 1% for patients with simple hyperplasia, 3% for those with complex hyperplasia, 8% for those with atypical simple hyperplasia, and 29% for patients with atypical adenomatous hyperplasia. In addition to differences in overall prognosis, the various subtypes of endometrial hyperplasia also show differences in the ability of progestin therapy to reverse them. Ferenczy and Gelfand[9] reported on the results of progestin therapy in 85 postmenopausal women with endometrial hyperplasia. In patients who had hyperplasia without atypia, complete reversal of the abnormality was seen following treatment with medroxyprogesterone acetate, 10 to 20 mg daily, with only 50% responding to the same treatment if cellular atypia was present. In patients with atypical hyperplasia, there was also an increased risk of recurrent hyperplasia or cancer after completion of the progestin therapy (50% vs. 6%).

Clinical Management

Therapy for endometrial hyperplasia must be individualized and depends on histologic criteria, predisposing factors, patient age, and desire to maintain fertility (Fig. 6). Premenopausal women can be treated with oral contraceptives for 3 months if they have no significant contraindications to their use. Most studies suggest that cancer will eventually develop in about 20% to 30% of patients with atypical adenomatous hyperplasia, but some studies have suggested a risk as high as 82% for untreated atypical hyperplasia. The risk of progression appears to be higher for postmenopausal than premenopausal women. The mean duration of progression from endometrial hyperplasia to carcinoma is about 10 years for lesions without atypia and 4 years for atypical lesions. In patients with atypical hyperplasia diagnosed in an endometrial biopsy specimen, a formal D&C should be performed to rule out a coexisting adenocarcinoma. It has been suggested that if gland epithelium is found within the stroma (i.e., stromal invasion) of the curettage specimen, even if the diagnosis is hyperplasia, there is a significant chance that the uterus still contains an endometrial cancer. If a diagnosis of carcinoma *in situ* is made on endometrial biopsy or D&C, in almost all circumstances a hysterectomy should be performed, because this is not a clearly reproducible diagnosis and may actually represent early invasive cancer or sampling error.

In patients with endometrial hyperplasia without atypia, progestin therapy is very effective in reversing this abnormality. For these patients, either cyclic or continuous therapy is appropriate, using medroxyprogesterone acetate, 10 to 20 mg per day, or megestrol acetate (Megace), 20 to 40 mg per day, for either 14 days each month or daily. Therapy should be continued for 3 months, and then the endometrium should again be sampled to document response. The hyperplasia will revert to normal in 75% to 90% of patients treated with progestins. In patients who desire pregnancy, ovulation induction can be considered using either clomiphene or menotropins (Pergonal). If a patient does not desire pregnancy, oral contraceptive therapy should be considered. In those patients with persistent hyperplasia, definitive surgery should be strongly considered.

Patients with atypical hyperplasia will often opt for a hysterectomy and bilateral salpingo-oophorectomy, when made aware of the risk of coexisting adenocarcinoma (approximately 20%) and the premalignant potential of these lesions. A truly postmenopausal woman (last menses 2 or more years ago) should be strongly encouraged to undergo hysterectomy, with progestin therapy reserved for patients with severe medical problems that would make them very poor surgical candidates. If the decision is made to treat a patient medically, daily progestin therapy for 3 months is recommended, followed by repeat endometrial sampling. If hyperplasia persists in these patients, a D&C should be performed to rule out a coexisting malignancy, or a hysterectomy should be performed. At the time of hysterectomy, the uterus should be opened intraoperatively, with frozen section if indicated to document the presence and extent of any malignancy so that surgical staging can be performed at the same setting if appropriate.

An interesting but still experimental approach is insertion of an intrauterine contraceptive progesterone system (ICPS) that releases continuous therapeutic doses of progesterone or

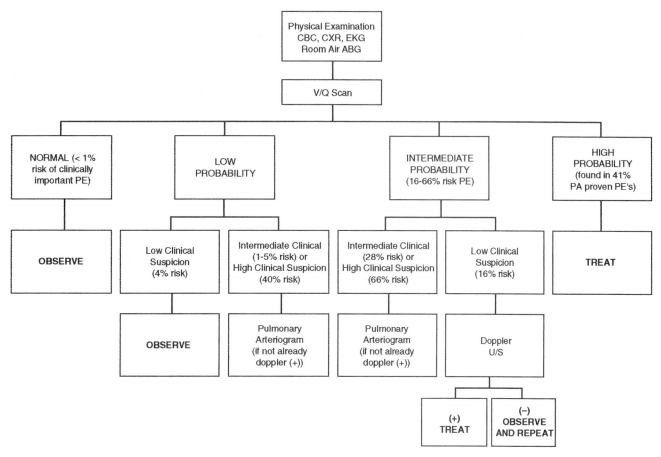

FIG. 6. Workup for abnormal bleeding.

levonorgestrel. Until more experience is gained with the ICPS, it should not be employed outside a research setting. Two preliminary studies reported on the use of danazol (Danocrine) to treat women with adenomatous hyperplasia, and in both studies all women treated were noted to have reversal of the hyperplasia on repeat endometrial sampling. In all premenopausal women, menses resumed within 1 to 2 months following therapy. In the first study, atrophic changes were noted on repeat endometrial sampling even though the patients had normal serum estradiol levels, suggesting a direct effect on the endometrium.[26]

A relatively recently described risk factor for the development of endometrial hyperplasia and carcinoma is the use of tamoxifen citrate (Nolvadex) as an adjuvant treatment for breast cancer. Tamoxifen has been associated with a two- to threefold increased risk of endometrial cancer and an increased risk of endometrial hyperplasia, polyps, and growth of fibroids. Currently, the best method for monitoring women taking tamoxifen is unknown. Obviously, patients should have an annual pelvic examination and Pap smear. Endometrial sampling should be performed in all patients with abnormal uterine bleeding. Since tamoxifen acts as a weak estrogen, it is not unreasonable to consider annual endometrial biopsy or sonographic evaluation of endometrial stripe thickness. This recommendation, however, is not based on prospective studies, but rather on an intuitive approach. According to a study by Uziely et al.,[27] women who have been on tamoxifen for more than 12 months have a high risk for development of a thickened endometrium, which is associated with abnormal findings on biopsy. Based on the published studies to date, sonography is only useful for ruling out significant pathology if the endometrial stripe is less than 5 mm in thickness.

In summary, the management of endometrial hyperplasia should be individualized depending on the histologic findings and the patient's age and reproductive desires. Treatment options include hormonal therapy and surgery. Due to the increasing use of tamoxifen, gynecologists should expect to see more women on this medication and should be aware of the risk of both benign and malignant changes of the endometrium.

◊ UTERINE MALIGNANCIES

Endometrial Cancer

Endometrial carcinoma is the most common female genital tract malignancy, accounting for approximately 7% of all cancers in women, with an estimated 31,600 new cases and 6300 deaths in 1998.[19] In the United States, endometrial cancer will develop in about 1 in every 45 women during their lifetime. The great majority of these tumors are adenocarcinomas arising from the endometrium. Approximately 5%

of uterine malignancies are sarcomas, and an even smaller number represent mixed tumors with both carcinomatous and sarcomatous elements (mixed müllerian tumors).

The incidence of endometrial carcinoma has increased over the last 50 years, most likely because of the aging population, the increased frequency of certain predisposing conditions such as obesity, and the availability of improved methods of diagnosis. Adenocarcinoma of the endometrium is mainly a malignancy of postmenopausal women and is increasingly virulent with advancing age. Peak age at diagnosis of this malignancy is between 50 and 65 years, with approximately 25% of all cases of endometrial carcinoma being diagnosed in premenopausal women and 5% in women younger than 40 years. Usually, but not always, these young women are either obese, chronically anovulatory, or both.

It appears that there may be two different types of endometrial cancer, one estrogen-dependent and the other estrogen-independent.[1] The first type of malignancy typically occurs in younger, perimenopausal women with a history of exposure to unopposed estrogen. These tumors tend to arise in areas of hyperplasia and to be well differentiated and associated with a more favorable prognosis. The latter type of cancer occurs in older women without estrogen stimulation of the endometrium, is not often associated with endometrial hyperplasia, and tends to be poorly differentiated with a poor prognosis.

Risk Factors

The main risk factor predisposing to the development of endometrial adenocarcinoma is chronic unopposed estrogen exposure of either endogenous or exogenous origin. Obesity, nulliparity, and late menopause appear to be associated with high endogenous levels of unopposed estrogen. In obese women, there is an increased peripheral conversion of androstenedione to estrone by fat cells. Nulliparity seems to be associated with the development of endometrial cancer because ovarian dysfunction (chronic anovulatory cycles and polycystic ovaries) contributes both to the nulliparity and unopposed estrogen levels. Estrogen-secreting tumors such as granulosa cell tumors are associated with endometrial cancer up to 25% of the time. Other risk factors include a history of pelvic radiation, a history of breast or ovarian cancer, and use of tamoxifen.

Diagnosis

Currently, there are no accepted screening methods for detecting endometrial hyperplasia or cancer in asymptomatic women. Clinical studies have evaluated routine endometrial biopsy, transvaginal ultrasound, and Pap smears, but none of these techniques is sensitive or specific enough to be applied to the general population. Even though a routine Pap smear cannot be relied on to screen for endometrial cancer, this malignancy should be suspected in any nonpregnant woman with atypical endometrial cells or in any postmenopausal woman with normal endometrial cells on a Pap smear.[22]

Abnormal uterine bleeding is the most common presenting symptom of endometrial cancer. Any bleeding in a postmenopausal woman must be promptly evaluated, although overall only about 20% of these patients are found to have a genital malignancy. The likelihood that postmenopausal bleeding is indicative of a uterine cancer clearly increases with increasing age. Perimenopausal women with abnormal bleeding must also undergo thorough investigation, with the most suspicious patterns being increased menstrual flow, a decreased menstrual interval, and intermenstrual bleeding. Whenever possible, the diagnostic procedure for evaluating the endometrium should be an office endometrial biopsy, which under optimal conditions approaches the accuracy of a formal D&C (approximately 90%). An endocervical curettage (ECC) should always be performed in the evaluation of postmenopausal bleeding to rule out an endocervical carcinoma as the etiology. If the endometrial biopsy and ECC are satisfactory (with adequate tissue for a diagnosis) and demonstrate no significant abnormality, no further evaluation is necessary. If postmenopausal bleeding is persistent or recurrent or other high-risk factors exist, a fractional D&C should be considered. High-risk factors include the diagnosis of atypical hyperplasia or endometrial polyps. Hysteroscopy should be considered if bleeding is recurrent or if either polyps or submucous fibroids are suspected. Many clinical studies now support the usefulness of transvaginal ultrasound for evaluating the thickness of the endometrium in patients with postmenopausal bleeding. Various studies have suggested that when the endometrial stripe is less than 5 mm, the cause of bleeding is usually related to atrophy, but there have been occasional reports of biopsy-proven malignancy even in patients with thin endometrial stripes.

If endometrial adenocarcinoma is diagnosed, further evaluation of is necessary prior to deciding on the therapeutic approach. A careful physical examination should be performed, with particular attention to supraclavicular and inguinal lymph nodes, thorough abdominal palpation, and a bimanual rectovaginal examination to evaluate the size and mobility of the uterus, the size and consistency of the cervix, the adnexal structures and parametrium, and the entire vagina, vulva, and rectum, checking for nodules, masses, induration, and plaque-like lesions that might signify metastatic disease. Any suspicious genital lesions should be biopsied, and the stool should be tested for occult blood. The histologic subtype and grade of tumor can be determined from the endometrial biopsy or D&C specimen, but it is important to remember that approximately one-third of the time the final grade of tumor as determined on the hysterectomy specimen will differ from the original. Additional studies that should be obtained include a two-view chest x-ray and routine laboratory studies. Based on other risk factors and symptoms, consideration should be given to performing a barium enema examination or colonoscopy and preoperative computed tomography or MR imaging to evaluate the uterus for depth of invasion and document occult metastatic disease. An additional test that has been reported to successfully predict either deep myometrial invasion or distant disease is the serum tumor marker CA 125. Several studies have documented that 53% to 87% of patients with clinical stage I disease later found to have extrauterine disease at the time of surgery had elevated CA 125, compared to only 2% to 12% of patients with surgical stage I disease. These studies may not be routinely necessary if the decision for full surgical staging can be made intraoperatively (i.e., if the necessary surgical expertise is available to perform pelvic and periaortic lymphadenectomy).

Since endometrial cancer is now staged surgically as opposed to the old clinical schema, several practical considerations should be noted. In the past, preoperative radiation was used in many patients, especially those with grade 2 or 3 lesions, a positive ECC, or a large uterus. Depending on where the patient was treated, preoperative radiation could consist of intracavitary radium or cesium for approximately 72 hours or external-beam irradiation of 4000 to 4500 cGy to the pelvis. Using these types of treatment plans, many patients would receive either unnecessary radiation or radiation that did not encompass all of their disease (e.g., paraaortic node metastases). A second consideration is that all patients should at least be evaluated for full surgical staging, including selective pelvic and paraaortic node dissection. With the adoption of the new surgical staging scheme (see below), most patients should undergo primary surgical therapy, including a hysterectomy, bilateral salpingo-oophorectomy, peritoneal cytology, and selective pelvic and paraaortic node dissection, as indicated. Since endometrial cancer can spread via both the lymphatics and the blood stream, as well as transmurally or transtubally into the peritoneal cavity (Fig. 7), a thorough exploration of the entire abdominal cavity is necessary to document any extrauterine sites of metastases. Only patients with technically inoperable tumors or medical conditions that make them poor operative candidates should be considered for primary radiation therapy. In these cases, patients should be staged using the older clinical staging schema.

Prognostic Factors

Several well recognized factors can be used to predict the prognosis of patients with adenocarcinoma of the endometrium.

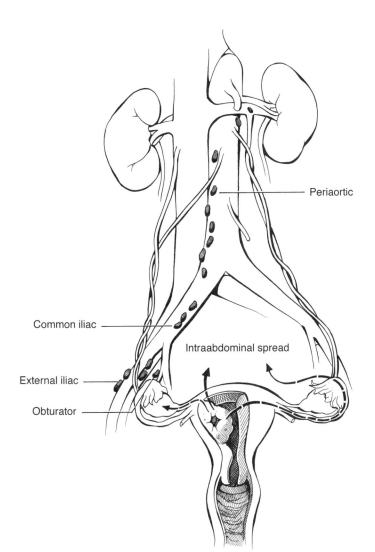

FIG. 7. Spread pattern of endometrial cancer with particular emphasis on potential lymph node spread. Pelvic and periaortic nodes are at risk, even in stage I disease.

These factors are also important in selecting appropriate therapy for patients.

Staging

Until the late 1980s, endometrial cancer was clinically staged using clinical information obtained from examination of the patient and the fractional D&C. This staging system, however, failed to recognize important prognostic factors, such as deep myometrial invasion and clinically occult extrauterine disease, and often underestimated the extent of disease.[23] Because of these inadequacies, the International Federation of Gynecologists and Obstetricians (FIGO) modified this staging schema in 1988 to reflect the information obtained from surgical exploration and pathologic evaluation of removed tissue. Endometrial cancer is now staged according to the FIGO staging system (Table 3). The current recommendation is for all medically operable patients with clinical stage I disease, regardless of tumor grade, to undergo an extrafascial total abdominal hysterectomy and bilateral salpingo-oophorectomy for both staging and therapeutic purposes.[5,8] The abdominal wall incision should be adequate to perform both pelvic and periaortic lymph node sampling, if indicated by tumor grade and depth of invasion into the myometrium. Immediately after entering the peritoneal cavity, fluid (either ascites or a washing) is obtained for cytologic analysis.

Despite the fact that the FIGO surgical staging schema has been in effect for 10 years, there is still considerable controversy as to which patients should undergo the pelvic and periaortic lymph node sampling as required by this schema. It is also unclear how to select these patients and which preoperative and intraoperative findings can be used to define the patient population that is most likely to benefit from this procedure. Many institutions send the uterus for frozen-section analysis intraoperatively and use the pathologic determination of tumor grade and depth of invasion to determine the need for full surgical staging. Others use preoperative information obtained from the endometrial biopsy specimen and radiographic information, especially where patients need to be triaged to another referral center for surgical staging.

In a large study by the Gynecologic Oncology Group (GOG) of 621 women with clinical stage I disease, 22% of patients were found to have disease outside the uterus.[7] The sites of distant disease were evenly divided between periaortic and pelvic lymph nodes and positive peritoneal cytology. Adnexal involvement was less likely than nodal involvement or positive peritoneal cytology. Equally important, an additional study documented that only 24% of patients with clinical stage II disease actually had pathologic confirmation of cervical involvement at the time of hysterectomy. On occasion, patients are found to have simultaneous endometrial and ovarian cancers, with a reported incidence rate of 1.4% to 3.8%.[25] Although the difference between metastatic and synchronous primaries can usually be determined by routine pathologic examination, this determination occasionally cannot be made with any degree of certainty.

TABLE 3. *FIGO staging for carcinoma of the corpus uteri*

Stage IA G123	Tumor limited to endometrium
Stage IB G123	Invasion to less than one-half the myometrium
Stage IC G123	Invasion to more than one-half the myometrium
Stage IIA G123	Endocervical glandular involvement only
Stage IIB G123	Cervical stromal invasion
Stage IIIA G123	Tumor invades serosa and/or adnexa, and/or positive peritoneal cytology
Stage IIIB G123	Vaginal metastases
Stage IIIC G123	Metastases to pelvic and/or paraaortic lymph nodes
Stage IVA G123	Tumor invasion of bladder and/or bowel mucosa
Stage IVB	Distant metastases including intra-abdominal and/or inguinal lymph nodes

Histopathology—degree of differentiation:
Cases of carcinoma of the corpus should be classified (or graded) according to the degree of histologic differentiation, as follows:

G1 = 5% or less of a nonsquamous or nonmorular solid growth pattern
G2 = 6%–50% of a nonsquamous or nonmorular solid growth pattern
G3 = more than 50% of a nonsquamous or nonmorular solid growth pattern

Notes on pathological grading:
1. Notable nuclear atypia, inappropriate for the architectural grade, raises the grade of a grade 1 or grade 2 tumor by 1
2. In serous adenocarcinoma, clear-cell adenocarcinoma, and squamous cell carcinoma, nuclear grading takes precedence
3. Adenocarcinoma with squamous differentiation is graded according to the nuclear grade of the glandular component

Rules related to staging:
1. Because corpus cancer is now staged surgically, procedures previously used for determination of stages are no longer applicable, such as the findings from fractional dilation and curettage to differentiate between stage I and stage II
2. It is appreciated that there may be a small number of patients with corpus cancer who will be treated primarily with radiation therapy. If that is the case, the clinical staging adopted by FIGO in 1971 would still apply, but designation of that staging system would be noted
3. Ideally, width of the myometrium should be measured along with the width of tumor invasion

(From International Federation of Gynecology and Obstetrics. Annual report on the results of treatment in gynecologic cancer. *Int J Gynaecol Obstet* 1989;28:189–190; with permission.)

Tumor Grade

Grading provides a measure of tumor aggressiveness, and it is now an essential part of the FIGO staging for endometrial cancer. Tumor grade is one of the most important prognostic factors in predicting overall survival. Assignment of tumor grade is based on both architectural patterns such as gland formation and nuclear atypia and is significantly affected by interobserver reproducibility. It is also not unusual for the tumor grade from the endometrial biopsy to vary from the final tumor grade from the hysterectomy specimen. The higher the grade is, the more likely the patient will have deep myometrial invasion, as well as lymph node and other metastases.

Histologic Subtype

The histologic subtype of adenocarcinoma may independently impact on patient outcome. Approximately 80% of endometrial cancers are endometrioid, with 15% to 25% of these tumors demonstrating squamous differentiation. The significance of squamous differentiation is unclear, and its impact has been debated for many years. In the past, the terms "adenoacanthoma" and "adenosquamous carcinoma" were used to identify adenocarcinomas with either benign or malignant squamous differentiation. More recently, Zaino et al.[28] recommended that these terms be replaced with the more descriptive term *adenocarcinoma with squamous differentiation*. Papillary serous and clear cell cancers of the endometrium are both quite rare (approximately 5% each) but have a significantly worse prognosis, compared to endometrioid adenocarcinoma. Both of these histologies are more common in older women and tend to present with distant disease, even when clinically stage I.

Age

Although it is clearly recognized that advancing patient age at diagnosis is associated with a poorer outcome, there is no agreement as to why this is true. In a study by Lurain et al.,[21] increasing patient age was an independent prognostic factor associated with recurrent disease. No patient under age 50 years developed recurrent cancer, compared with 12% of women between 50 and 75 years and 33% of women older than 75 years. For every 1-year increase in age over 50 years, there was a 7% increase in the rate of recurrence. Younger patients tend to have early, well differentiated lesions with no or minimal myometrial invasion, compared to older patients. Younger patients also tend to be in better general health, thereby allowing more aggressive definitive surgery. It has also been suggested that older women are more likely to ignore signs of vaginal bleeding, thereby delaying diagnosis until the stage is more advanced. Interestingly, however, the length of time between onset of bleeding and presentation to a clinician does not correlate with tumor stage, and patients with advanced-stage disease have not necessarily delayed seeking medical care.

Race

Even with correction for age and tumor stage, black women with endometrial cancer have a much poorer prognosis than white women. For all stages of endometrial cancer, white women have an 86% 5-year survival compared to a 55% 5-year survival for black women, and within each stage the relative survival is worse for blacks.

Depth of Myometrial Invasion

Depth of myometrial invasion is another important prognostic factor that directly correlates with the likelihood of extrauterine disease. In the new surgical staging criteria, maximum depth of myometrial invasion determines the subcategories within stage I disease. It is believed that increasing depth of invasion is associated with a higher likelihood of access to the lymphatic system, thereby increasing the incidence of both pelvic and periaortic lymph node metastases. In a study by Boronow et al.,[2] only 1% of patients without myometrial invasion had pelvic lymph node involvement, compared to 25% having positive pelvic lymph nodes with outer-third involvement. Survival was also shown to be affected by depth of invasion, with a 80% to 90% 5-year survival with minimal invasion compared with 60% survival with deep invasion.

Peritoneal Cytology

The significance of malignant peritoneal cytology obtained during surgical staging for endometrial cancer is controversial. In essentially all studies in the literature, a positive peritoneal cytology result is associated with other high-risk features such as deep myometrial invasion, adnexal spread, positive lymph node metastases, and cervical involvement. Several studies showed a two- to threefold increase in the risk of recurrent disease in patients with positive peritoneal cytology, but often these patients have one or more other high-risk factors and many times the recurrent disease is outside the peritoneal cavity. In patients found to have positive cytology, it is unclear whether any currently available therapy would have any impact on eventual outcome.

Lymph Node Metastases

For patients with clinical stage I endometrial cancer, the presence of lymph node involvement is the most important independent prognostic factor, being associated with a sixfold increase in the risk of recurrent disease. In these patients with clinical stage I cancer, approximately 10% will have positive pelvic lymph nodes, and 6% will have positive periaortic lymph nodes, with periaortic node involvement being the most important predictor of survival. The incidence of lymph node involvement correlates with stage and grade of tumor, depth of myometrial involvement, and location of the cancer in the uterus (i.e., fundal versus lower uterine segment). In patients with stage II disease, lymph node metastases occur in approximately 35%.

Adnexal and Intraperitoneal Involvement

Clinically occult adnexal metastases occur in approximately 10% of patients with stage I disease, with most patients having other high-risk factors such as deep myometrial invasion or lymph node involvement. In patients with adnexal metastases as their only high-risk factor, overall survival seems to be minimally affected. Other extrauterine intraperitoneal disease is associated with a significant decrease in survival.

Other Factors

Many other factors have been shown to affect prognosis, including hormone receptor status of the tumor, DNA content or ploidy, proliferative index, and oncogene expression. Both estrogen receptor and progesterone receptor levels have been shown to be prognostic factors independent of tumor grade, with the progesterone receptor level being the more important for predicting overall survival. Progesterone receptor levels can also be used to predict which patients with advanced or recurrent disease are more likely to respond to hormonal therapy.

Treatment

The primary treatment for endometrial cancer is surgery, consisting of removal of the uterus, cervix, and adnexal structures. Surgical staging procedures including careful exploration of the abdomen and pelvis and lymphadenectomy are often done at the same time, as described above. As soon as the uterus has been removed, it should be sent to the pathology laboratory for frozen section to determine tumor grade and depth of invasion, as well as to obtain tissue for estrogen and progesterone receptor levels and other studies as indicated. For patients in whom lymph node sampling is indicated (Table 4), representative samples of lymph node–bearing tissue from the lower aorta and vena cava are removed. Pelvic lymph node sampling should remove nodes from common and external iliac and obturator regions. An omental biopsy may be performed and is indicated for patients with papillary serous and clear cell cancers. In patients who are very poor

candidates for exploratory laparotomy (e.g., morbidly obese), consideration of vaginal hysterectomy or laparoscopically assisted vaginal hysterectomy should be made. Every effort should be made to remove the adnexal structures, and therefore laparoscopically assisted vaginal hysterectomy may be preferable. If appropriate surgical expertise is available, the full surgical staging including pelvic and periaortic lymphadenectomy can be performed through the laparoscope. Until additional information is obtained, vaginal hysterectomy should be limited to very select patients who otherwise might be given radiation therapy only. In patients with clinically apparent cervical involvement, radical hysterectomy with bilateral salpingo-oophorectomy and lymph node dissection may be considered.

Following surgery and review of the final pathology report, patients may be divided into risk groups based on the many prognostic factors discussed above. This classification can then be used to individualize the recommended postoperative therapy, if needed. A suggested protocol for the treatment of surgically staged adenocarcinoma of the endometrium is shown in Figure 8. Since formal surgical staging has been widely utilized for less than 10 years, most of the information on recommendations for postoperative radiation therapy are based on clinically staged patients. The risk of pelvic recurrence in patients with high-risk factors but negative surgical staging is largely unknown. The GOG study based on surgicopathologic correlation found that even when sampled lymph nodes were negative, patients with deep myometrial invasion and poorly differentiated cancers were still at a higher risk of recurrence. Even though the surgical staging procedures failed to document extrauterine pelvic disease, postoperative pelvic radiation was associated with a decreased risk of local recurrence. It is not yet clear whether surgical staging can define a subgroup of stage I patients, other than the already identified low-risk patients, who can be treated without adjuvant radiation treatment.

Treatment for patients with stage II disease remains somewhat controversial. Most studies suggest that patients with cervical involvement are at a higher risk for vaginal vault recurrence, and often recommend adjuvant vaginal cuff radiation. Whether or not those patients with otherwise negative surgical staging also need pelvic radiation remains to be confirmed. With clinically apparent cervical involvement, treatment recommendations include either radical hysterectomy or preoperative radiation followed by extrafascial hysterectomy.

Treatment for patients with documented extrauterine disease (stages III and IV) should be individualized to encompass the true extent of the disease. Therapeutic options include pelvic radiation, extended-field radiation to cover the periaortic lymph nodes, whole-abdomen radiation, and systemic hormonal therapy or chemotherapy. In most cases, treatment of distant metastases with either high-dose progestins or chemotherapy is palliative only, with little expectation for long-term control of disease. The most widely used chemotherapy agents include doxorubicin hydrochloride (Adriamycin) and cisplatin (Platinol) or carboplatin (Paraplatin).[24]

TABLE 4. *Surgical therapy of endometrial cancer*

Risk group (incidence)	Positive pelvic nodes (%)	Surgery
Low risk (30%)		
Stage 1A, 1B	3	TAH-BSO
Grade 1		Peritoneal cytology
Moderate risk (50%)		
Stage 1B	9	TAH-BSO, LND
Grade 2,3		Peritoneal cytology
High risk (20%)		
Stage 1C	18	TAH-BSO, LND
Grade 1, 2, 3		Peritoneal cytology

LND; TAH-BSO
(Modified from ref. 5.)

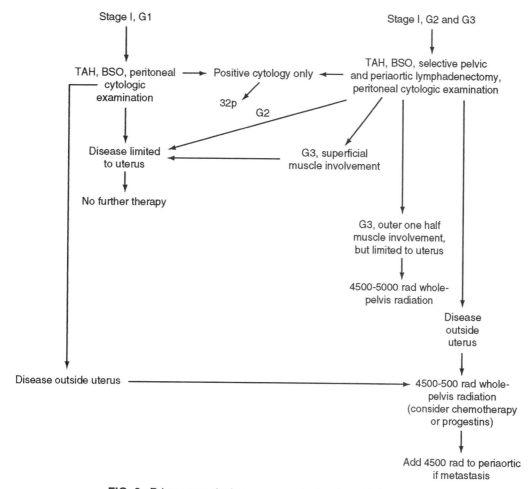

FIG. 8. Primary surgical management of endometrial cancer.

Progestins have been used for many years in the treatment of recurrent endometrial carcinoma, with approximately one-third of patients having a favorable response. Patients with well differentiated tumors have a higher response rate than those with moderately or poorly differentiated cancers. Although the role of estrogen and progesterone receptors in endometrial cancer therapy has not yet been widely accepted, it does appear that the responsiveness of recurrent tumor to progestin therapy is related to the content of both estrogen and progesterone receptors. If both receptors are present, the likelihood of a favorable response is good regardless of tumor grade or other high-risk factors. If the concentration of receptors is low, it is unlikely that the recurrent tumor will respond to progestins, and chemotherapy should be considered.

Approximately 10% to 15% of patients with endometrial cancer are inoperable, usually because of morbid obesity or severe intercurrent disease. In these patients, primary radiation therapy should be considered. In most cases, a combination of external-beam and intracavitary radiation should be used, and with definitive therapy approximately 85% to 90% of patients with early-stage disease will have control of uterine disease by this technique. The overall risk of recurrence in these patients with stage I disease correlates with tumor

grade, with a 5-year survival of 94% for grade I, 92% for grade II, and 78% for grade III tumors.[11]

Posttreatment Surveillance

Many studies have confirmed that the majority of recurrences after treatment of endometrial cancer will occur within 3 years. Approximately one-half of these recurrences will be asymptomatic, and thus the traditional recommendation has been to follow patients with examination and vaginal cytology every 3 to 4 months for the first 2 to 3 years and then at 6-month intervals for at least 5 years. Serial serum CA 125 measurements have also been suggested for posttreatment surveillance of patients treated for endometrial cancer, although the level may be normal in patients with early recurrent disease. Since treated endometrial cancer will not recur in the great majority of patients, however, several studies have addressed the cost effectiveness of this traditional recommendation.[13] In a study from the M.D. Anderson Cancer Center, 59% of recurrences were asymptomatic, with over one-half being picked up on examination, 26% by an elevated CA 125, and only 4% by vaginal cytology. Because of these findings, these authors recommended that physical examination, serum

CA 125 assay, and vaginal cytology be performed only every 6 to 12 months on asymptomatic patients. A Canadian study reported that only one recurrence was documented during more than 200 routine follow-up visits after treatment for endometrial cancer, using a schedule of examinations of every 3 months for the first year, every 4 months for the second year, and every 6 months thereafter. There was no difference in the salvage rates of recurrent disease picked up during routine surveillance compared to recurrent disease documented in symptomatic patients. In this study, no recurrence was picked up by vaginal cytology alone. In a third study from Duke University, an analysis of various follow-up techniques demonstrated that routine vaginal cytology and chest x-ray were not cost-effective. The recommendation of these investigators is to follow patients every 6 months with examination alone, using additional testing to evaluate any symptoms.

Estrogen Replacement Therapy after Treatment

For many years, it has been thought that a history of endometrial cancer, even successfully treated, was an absolute contraindication to estrogen replacement therapy (ERT) because adenocarcinoma of the endometrium is considered an estrogen-dependent neoplasm. Because no scientific data support the contention that ERT is dangerous for patients who have had a hysterectomy for endometrial cancer and because the body of evidence is increasing in supporting the value of ERT in decreasing morbidity and mortality from heart disease, strokes, and osteoporosis, many physicians and patients are questioning the earlier proscription. In the last decade, there have been several small retrospective studies of patients given ERT following treatment for early-stage endometrial cancer (Table 5). In 1986, Creasman et al.[6] reported on 221 patients with stage I endometrial cancer, of whom 47 (21%) were given postoperative estrogen replacement for a median of 26 months. Statistical analysis revealed no increased risk of recurrence or death between those who received ERT and those who did not when adjustments were made for tumor grade, myometrial invasion, nodal metastases, peritoneal cytology, and age. In fact, the risk of recurrence was significantly higher in the nontreated group (15% vs. 2%), as was the risk of dying of intercurrent disease. Similar study design and conclusions were reported 3 years later by Lee et al.[20] In both of these studies, selection bias may have contributed to the results, but it does appear that a low-risk

group of patients can be selected who can safely take estrogen replacement. Chapman et al.[3] retrospectively reviewed information on 123 patients with stages I and II endometrial cancer, of whom 62 received ERT, and again documented no increase in recurrences or deaths from this malignancy. In a Committee Opinion in August 1993, the American College of Obstetricians and Gynecologists concluded that there are no definitive data to support specific recommendations regarding the use of ERT in women previously treated for endometrial cancer. The opinion states that estrogens could be used for the same indications as for any other woman, except that the selection of appropriate candidates should be based on prognostic indicators and the risk that a patient is willing to assume. The need for progestational agents in addition to estrogens could not be evaluated by the gynecologic practice committee due to the paucity of data.

Other Uterine Malignancies

Sarcomas of the uterus are rare, constituting only 3% to 5% of all uterine malignancies. These lesions arise primarily from two tissues: endometrial sarcomas from endometrial glands and stoma, and leiomyosarcomas from the myometrium itself. Other sarcomas, such as angiosarcoma and fibrosarcoma, arise in supporting tissues. In general, uterine sarcomas are the most malignant type of uterine tumor and tend to differ significantly from endometrial adenocarcinomas with regard to patterns of spread and prognosis.

Numerous classification schemes for uterine sarcomas have been proposed, depending on both cell type and site of origin. Pure tumors are composed of only one cell type, whereas mixed tumors have more than one cell type. Homologous tumors contain tissue elements that are indigenous to the uterus, whereas heterologous tumors are defined as those that contain tissue elements foreign to the uterus, such as rhabdomyosarcoma and chondrosarcoma (Table 6). Since the great majority of uterine sarcomas fall into one of four categories, the GOG has accepted a more simplified classification:

◊ Leiomyosarcoma,
◊ Endometrial stromal sarcoma,
◊ Mixed homologous müllerian sarcoma (carcinosarcoma),
◊ Mixed heterologous müllerian sarcoma (mixed mesodermal sarcoma).

TABLE 5. *Effect of estrogen replacement therapy (ERT) on endometrial cancer recurrence*

| Investigator | Subjects (n) | Stage | | | Interval to treatment postsurgery (mo) | Duration follow-up on ERT (mo) | Recurrence |
		IA	IB	II			
Baker	31	—	—	—	0–120	—	0
Bryant (letter)	20	19	—	1	18–24	42–168	0
Creasman et al. (1986)[6]	47	30	17	0	0–81	25–150	0
Lee et al. (1990)[21]	44	24	20	0	1–≥60	24–84	1
Chapman et al. (1996)[3]	62	—	60	2	0–108	57	2
Gitsch et al.	8	—	—	—	—	12–78	0

TABLE 6. *Classifications of uterine sarcomas*

Homologous	Heterologous
Ober classification	
Pure	
Stromal sarcoma (endolymphatic stromal myosis)	Rhabdomyosarcoma
Leiomyosarcoma	Chondrosarcoma
Angiosarcoma	Osteosarcoma
Fibrosarcoma	Liposarcoma
Mixed	
Carcinosarcoma	Mixed müllerian tumors (mixed mesodermal tumor)
Gynecologic Oncology Group classification	
Leiomyosarcomas	
Endometrial stromal sarcomas	
Mixed homologous müllerian sarcomas (carcinosarcoma)	
Mixed heterologous müllerian sarcomas (mixed mesodermal sarcoma)	
Other uterine sarcomas	

The relative incidence of the various subtypes of uterine sarcomas differs significantly in the literature, with mixed mesodermal sarcomas being the most common in recent studies. The staging criteria for uterine sarcomas are based on the FIGO classification for endometrial cancers (see Table 3).

Patients diagnosed with uterine sarcomas are usually postmenopausal. Leiomyosarcoma is most common in women in their 40s and 50s, whereas mixed mesodermal sarcoma and endometrial stromal sarcoma occur most commonly in women who are 10 years older (Fig. 9). The most common presenting symptoms in women with a uterine sarcoma are an abdominal mass and pain. A rapidly enlarging uterus is common, but in postmenopausal women this should not be attributed to uterine leiomyomata; instead a sarcoma must be ruled out. Abnormal vaginal bleeding is also a frequent complaint, and on examination a friable polypoid mass may be seen extending through the dilated cervix. When these symptoms and signs are present, histologic evaluation of the uterus is mandatory. If a tumor is found to be protruding through the cervix, tissue is readily accessible, but if the diagnosis is a leiomyosarcoma, the lesion is usually high in the uterus and accessible only with a D&C. Approximately 50% of all patients with uterine sarcomas present with clinical stage I disease, but as many as one-third of these patients will have more advanced disease documented at the time of surgery.

Leiomyosarcoma

The older literature suggests that leiomyosarcoma is the most common uterine sarcoma, but more recent data indicate that it represents less 25% of these tumors. As noted previously, this malignancy is found in younger women with a median age at diagnosis between 43 and 53 years. Leiomyosarcoma

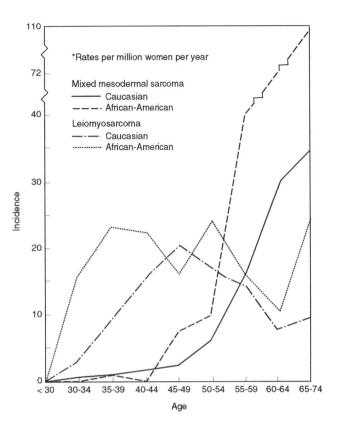

FIG. 9. Incidence of uterine sarcomas among women by age, race, and histology: SEER areas, 1973 to 1981. (Adapted from Harlow BL, Weiss NS, and Lofton S. The epidemiology of sarcomas of the uterus. *J Natl Cancer Inst* 1986;76: 399–402.)

is more common in black women and is associated with a poorer prognosis in these patients. The patterns of spread for leiomyosarcoma appear to be via both lymphatics and the vasculature, since distant metastases will develop in many patients even if lymph node biopsies are negative at the time of surgery.

Although there is some disagreement about the exact histologic criteria required for a diagnosis of leiomyosarcoma, the most important factor appears to be the mitotic count of the tumor. Cellular myomas and bizarre leiomyomas may appear to be malignant, but if there are fewer than five mitoses per 10 high-power fields (HPFs), the lesion is considered to be benign. Tumors with more than 10 mitoses per 10 HPFs are malignant, and those with 5 to 10 mitoses per 10 HPFs are thought to have an uncertain potential for malignancy. Many investigators agree that 5-year survival is related to the number of mitoses per 10 HPF, with a 95–98% survival with fewer than 5 MF/10 HPF, approximately 40% survival with 5–10 MF/10 HPF and very poor survival (15–20%) with more than 10 MF/10 HPF.

Endometrial Stromal Tumor

Endometrial stromal tumors are usually divided into two groups: endolymphatic stromal myosis and endometrial stromal sarcoma. The former usually follows an indolent course and is considered a low-grade stromal sarcoma. On gross inspection of the surgical specimen, it often has an infiltrative growth pattern and can project from the cut surface in a worm-like manner that may also extend into blood vessels in the broad ligament. Microscopically, there are little cellular atypia and few, if any, mitoses. The clinical course is slowly progressive and treatment is by surgery alone.

Endometrial stromal sarcoma, on the other hand, has a much more aggressive course, with frequent and widespread metastases and a very poor prognosis. As with leiomyosarcoma, the differentiation between these two entities depends on the number of mitoses per 10 HPFs, with 10 mitoses being the cutoff to categorize the tumor as an endometrial stromal sarcoma. These tumors exhibit high concentrations of both estrogen and progesterone receptors, and occasional responses have been seen when high-dose progesterone therapy is administered.

Mixed Müllerian Tumor

This tumor is the most common uterine sarcoma, accounting for more than 50% of all cases in recent series. Histologically, it is composed of both sarcoma and carcinoma, with the sarcomatous element being divided into homologous types (tissue normally found in the uterus) and heterologous types (tissue such as cartilage or bone). This malignancy is more common in blacks and is associated with prior pelvic radiation in up to one-third of patients. The main presenting symptom is vaginal bleeding and on examination, most patients are found to have an enlarged uterus, often with a polypoid mass protruding through the cervix. This tumor tend to be aggressive, with early metastases to pelvic and periaortic lymph nodes and adjacent tissue. Hematogenous spread, especially to the liver and lungs, is common.

Treatment of Uterine Sarcomas

The first step in the treatment of early uterine sarcoma should be surgical, with an exploratory laparotomy, total abdominal hysterectomy, and bilateral salpingo-oophorectomy. Because of the propensity of these lesions to metastasize to the pelvic and periaortic lymph nodes, some authors have suggested selective sampling in these areas. Even with clinical stage I disease, approximately one-half of patients will already have disease outside the uterus; in such cases, the prognosis is extremely poor. Based on the surgicopathologic findings, additional therapy with either pelvic radiation or chemotherapy can be tried. On rare occasion, surgical excision of a solitary pulmonary metastasis can be curative. Patients with recurrent disease do very poorly and should be considered for clinical trials in an attempt to identify active chemotherapy agents.

◊ REFERENCES

1. Bokhman JV. Two pathogenetic types of endometrial carcinoma. *Gynecol Oncol* 1983;15:10–17.
2. Boronow RC, Morrow CP, Creasman WT, et al. Surgical staging in endometrial cancer: clinical-pathologic findings of a prospective study. *Obstet Gynecol* 1984;63:825–832.
3. Chapman JA, Di Saia PJ, Osann K, Roth PD, Gillotte DL, Berman ML. Estrogen replacement in surgical stage I and II endometrial cancer survivors. *Am J Obstet Gynecol* 1996;175:1195–1200.
4. Copeland LJ, ed. *Textbook of gynecology.* Philadelphia: WB Saunders, 1993.
5. Creasman WT. Limited disease: role of surgery. *Semin Oncol* 1994; 21:79–83.
6. Creasman WT, Henderson D, Hinshaw W, Clarke-Pearson DL. Estrogen replacement therapy in the patient treated for endometrial cancer. *Obstet Gynecol* 1986;67:326–330.
7. Creasman WT, Morrow CP, Bundy BN, Homesley HD, Graham JE, Heller PB. Surgical pathological spread patterns of endometrial cancer: a Gynecologic Oncology Group study. *Cancer* 1987;60:2035–2041.
8. DiSaia PJ, Creasman WT. *Clinical gynecologic oncology,* 5th ed. St. Louis, MO: Mosby–Year Book, 1997.
9. Ferenczy A, Gelfand M. The biologic significance of cytologic atypia in progestin-treated endometrial hyperplasia. *Am J Obstet Gynecol* 1989;160:126–131.
10. Gordon MD, Ireland K. Pathology of hyperplasia and carcinoma of the endometrium. *Semin Oncol* 1994;21:64–70.
11. Grigsby P, Kuske R, Perez C, et al. Medically inoperable stage I adenocarcinoma of the endometrium treated with radiotherapy alone. *Int J Radiat Oncol Biol Phys* 1987;13:483–488.
12. Gusberg SB, Kaplan AL. Precursors of corpus cancer. IV. Adenomatous hyperplasia as stage 0 carcinoma of the endometrium. *Am J Obstet Gynecol* 1963;87:662–678.
13. Karasek K, Faul C. Changing concepts in the management of endometrial cancer. *Oncology* 1996;10:1099–1110.
14. Kaufman RH, Adam E, Binder GL, Gerthoffer E. Upper genital tract changes and pregnancy outcome in offspring exposed *in utero* to diethylstilbestrol. *Am J Obstet Gynecol* 1980;137:299–308.

15. Kaufman RH, Binder GL, Gray PM, Adam E. Upper genital tract changes associated with exposure *in utero* to diethylstilbestrol. *Am J Obstet Gynecol* 1977;128:51–59.

16. Kaufman RH, Noller K, Adam E, et al. Upper genital tract abnormalities and pregnancy outcome in diethylstilbestrol-exposed progeny. *Am J Obstet Gynecol* 1984;148:973–984.

17. Kurman RJ, ed. *Blaustein's pathology of the female genital tract*, 4th ed. New York: Springer-Verlag, 1994.

18. Kurman RJ, Kaminski PF, Norris HJ. The behavior of endometrial hyperplasia: a long-term study of untreated hyperplasia in 170 patients. *Cancer* 1985;56:403–412.

19. Landis SH, Murray T, Bolden S, Wingo PA. Cancer statistics, 1988. *CA Cancer J Clin* 1998;48:6–30.

20. Lee RB, Burke TW, Park RC. Estrogen replacement therapy following treatment for stage I endometrial cancer. *Gynecol Oncol* 1990;36:189–191.

21. Lurain JR, Rice BL, Rademaker AW, Poggensee LE, Schink JC, Miller DS. Prognostic factors associated with recurrence in clinical stage I adenocarcinoma of the endometrium. *Obstet Gynecol* 1991;78:63–69.

22. Mencaglia L, Valle RF, Perino A, Keith LG. Early detection of endometrial carcinoma and its precursors. *Curr Probl Obstet Gynecol Fertil* 1988;11:173–202.

23. Morrow CP, Bundy BN, Kurman RJ, et al. Relationship between surgical-pathological risk factors and outcome in clinical stages I and II carcinoma of the endometrium: a Gynecologic Oncology Group study. *Gynecol Oncol* 1991;40:55–65.

24. Muss HB. Chemotherapy of metastatic endometrial cancer. *Semin Oncol* 1994;21:107–113.

25. Prat J, Matias-Guiu X, Barreto J. Simultaneous carcinoma involving the endometrium and the ovary. *Cancer* 1991;68:2455–2459.

26. Terakawa N, Inoue M, Shimizu I, et al. Preliminary report on the use of danazol in the treatment of endometrial hyperplasia. *Cancer* 1988;62:2618–2621.

27. Uziely B, Lewin A, Brufman G, et al. The effect of tamoxifen on the endometrium. *Breast Cancer Res Treat* 1993;26:101–105.

28. Zaino RJ, Kurman R, Herbold D, et al. The significance of squamous differentiation in endometrial carcinoma. *Cancer* 1991;68:2293–2302.

CHAPTER 51

Uterine Leiomyoma

——— ◊ ———

William N. Spellacy

Uterine leiomyomas, sometimes referred to as myomas or fibromas, are very frequently found benign tumors of the uterus. In one careful study, approximately 75% of women had myomas diagnosable by serial histologic sections of the uterus. Only about 20% to 30% of women will have uterine myomas clinically, and most myomas are asymptomatic. Nevertheless, myomas represent the most common reason for gynecologic surgery and are, therefore, a very important gynecologic problem. This chapter will discuss the epidemiology, tumor biology, pathology, symptoms, unusual complications, diagnosis, and management of uterine myomas.

◊ EPIDEMIOLOGY

Myomas are more common in black women than in any other race. This increased frequency is approximately three times higher than that found in Caucasians. For all races, the frequency of myomas increases as a woman moves through her reproductive years. They are rare before menarche. The highest frequency of symptomatic myomas occurs in the perimenopausal time period. Myoma growth is rare in menopausal women, and indeed, they usually shrink in size after menopause. Myomas are also more common in obese women. Smoking has been found to decrease the frequency of uterine myomas. This is most probably because smoking interferes with the conversion of androgens to estrogen via the aromatase enzyme pathway, and thus, women who smoke have lower circulating estrogen levels. High levels of exogenous estrogen and progestins can increase myoma growth, but the currently used low-dose oral contraceptives have no effect on myoma growth. This is in contradistinction to the data reported in the 1960s to 1980s from the use of high-dose oral contraceptives, where myoma growth was accelerated by those compounds. The long-term use of Depo-Provera reduces the size of myomas because this drug suppresses LH and FSH and therefore ovarian steroids. It thus becomes clear that the women at greatest risk for myoma growth are those who are black, obese, perimenopausal, and nonsmokers (Table 1).

◊ TUMOR BIOLOGY

Biochemical studies have shown that myomas begin from a single muscle cell. The best evidence for this relates to the fact that normal uterine myometrial cells produce one of two isoenzymes of glucose-6-phosphate dehydrogenase. Thus, if one takes a portion of the uterus with many myometrial cells and chromatographically studies G-6-PD, both types A and B will be found. However, when tissue from a myoma is similarly studied, only type A or type B isoenzyme is detected. Other biochemical testing supports these studies, showing that a myoma originates from a single muscle cell and that all cells in this tumor are of the same genetic type.

A number of studies have been performed to look for chromosome abnormalities in these tumors to learn more about their biology. Approximately 20% of studied myomas show an abnormal karyotype. Abnormalities frequently found are rearrangements 6p, deletions 7q, and transformations (12:14). This is interesting in that other benign tumors such as lipomas commonly have abnormalities like these (6p). When multiple myomas in the same uterus are studied, there is often karyotype discordance, again supporting the concept that each myoma begins from a single muscle cell.

Because epidemiologic studies show that myomas generally grow and become symptomatic during the reproductive years of a woman, it has been postulated for years that their growth is regulated by ovarian steroids. Studies from the same uterus of myoma and myometrial tissue show that the myoma contains a higher concentration of progesterone receptors than does the adjacent myometrium. The content of progesterone receptors is determined by estrogen levels. Studies of uterine cell turnover rates and mitotic index frequency show that the highest rates occur during the secretory phase of the menstrual cycle. These data show that estrogen is necessary in order to develop progesterone receptors in

TABLE 1. *Risk factors for uterine myomas*

Black race
Obese
Perimenopausal
Nonsmoker
High estrogen - progesterone levels

uterine myometrium and myoma cells and that progesterone binding to the nuclear receptors is the stimulating steroid to cause growth and turnover. Progesterone seems to work by increasing the production of several growth factors. Studies have shown that myoma tissue contains an increased concentration of growth stimulators, such as insulin-like growth factor-1 and epidermal growth factor. There is also evidence that inhibitory growth factors, such as transforming growth factor-β, are reduced in myoma tissue. Finally there is evidence that progesterone increases the production of Bal-2 gene protein in myoma cells, and this protein prevents cell death, thus resulting in tumor growth. In summary, myoma development depends on growth of a single muscle cell into a benign tumor. Some of these cells have an abnormal karyotype, but most do not. A high concentration of estrogen causes these cells to produce progesterone receptors. Progesterone then binds to the cells' nuclear receptors and produces cell growth by altering intracellular growth factors and by preventing cell death (Table 2).

◊ PATHOLOGY

It is rare that only a single myoma develops in a uterus, and usually many exist. This is seen in the examples in Fig. 1. As the abnormal myoma cell replicates and expands, its gross appearance becomes that of a white swirling compact cellular tumor that creates a pseudocapsule by its expansion within the myometrium. The gross appearance of a cut myoma is seen in Fig. 2. This pseudocapsule can easily be demonstrated at the time of surgery, and it allows for the easy shelling out of myomas from their uterine bed. Myomas may occupy any position within the uterus or Müllerian ductal system, and their development will distort the uterine shape accordingly. Clinically, they present as firm irregular enlarged pelvic masses on physical examination. The myomas may be just under the serosa of the uterus (subserosal) and be palpated as round masses on the surface. Some develop on a stalk (pedunculated). On occasion a torsion of the pedicle may occur, resulting in ischemic necrosis of the surface peritoneum with

TABLE 2. *Development of myomas*

Begin from a single muscle cell
Cell karyotype abnormality in about 20%: chromosome
   6, 7, 12, or 14 most common
Estrogen increases nuclear progesterone receptors
Progesterone increases tissue growth factors
Growth factors cause myoma to grow

acute pain. Myomas may also develop within the central wall of the uterus (intramural), and these myomas are generally less symptomatic and produce a more symmetric pelvis mass. Finally, myomas may develop under endometrium (submucous), and these myomas distort the endometrial lining, usually producing abnormal uterine bleeding. The submucous myoma may also develop a stalk and prolapse through the cervix and into the vagina.

Histologically myomas demonstrate uniform spindle-shaped smooth muscle cells, and few mitoses are usually present (Fig. 3). A number of degenerative changes may be seen, including cystic degeneration, calcifications, hyaline degeneration, fatty degeneration, and necrosis.

On rare occasions the myoma may become a sarcoma. The overall frequency of sarcoma formation in myomas is approximately 0.7%, but this frequency increases with age, and in the menopausal woman the frequency doubles. The risk of sarcoma development does not justify hysterectomy for all myomas. However, a rapidly expanding myoma in a menopausal woman is a concern and usually warrants surgery. The diagnosis of sarcoma should be suspected on gross examination. The sarcoma tends to be hemorrhagic and soft, presenting what has been described as a "raw pork" appearance (Fig. 4). In addition, on gross exam, the pseudocapsule will be invaded by the tumor so that the myoma cannot be easily shelled out of its bed. On microscopic examination mitoses are frequent, and usually one sees more than 10 mitoses in 10 high-power fields. The tumor cells are pleomorphic with enlarged hyperchromatic nuclei and numerous mitoses (Fig. 5). The large number of mitoses seen in these tumors is, therefore, the diagnostic criterion of a sarcoma.

◊ SYMPTOMS

The three major presenting symptoms of patients with myomas are abnormal uterine bleeding, a pelvic mass, and sensations of pressure in the pelvis. Myomas rarely cause pain. Abnormal bleeding is a frequent symptom and results from submucous myomas that distort the endometrial cavity. The endometrium covering a submucous myoma has glands that grow parallel to the surface of the myoma rather than perpendicular to the base, as is seen in the rest of the uterus. Thus, with a menstrual period, the shedding of the endometrium across the submucous myoma leaves a large raw surface that must be reepithelialized from the periphery of the tumor rather than from nearby adjacent glands. The uterine cavity may also be enlarged in surface area and thus have more blood loss with menstruation. As a result, the bleeding pattern is usually one of prolonged heavy menses.

An expanding myoma can also be first noticed by the woman or examining physician as a pelvic mass. On examination, this mass is firm, nontender, irregular, attached to the uterus, and generally in the midline. The expanding pelvic mass may produce symptoms not dissimilar to those of early pregnancy, where the uterus is also enlarging. These pressure symptoms could include frequent urination as the bladder is

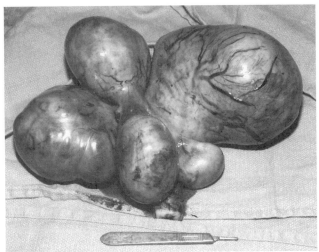

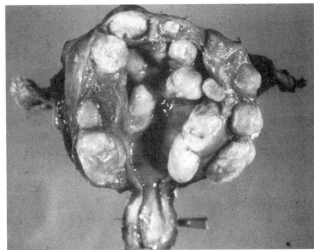

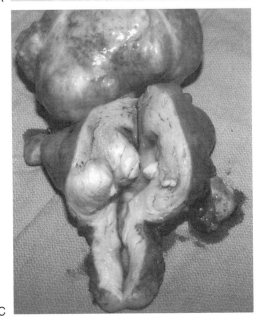

FIG. 1A–C: Uterus with multiple leiomyomas demonstrating subserosal, intramural, pedunculated, and submucous types.

compressed or pressure on other pelvic structures creating such problems as ureteral obstruction and hydronephrosis or colon pressure and gastrointestinal symptoms.

If a subserous pedunculated myoma twists and interrupts its blood supply, acute necrosis will occur, producing acute pelvic pain with tenderness localized to the myoma. If a submucous myoma develops a long stalk and is delivered by uterine contractions through the cervix, the patient will experience cramps, vaginal discharge, and perhaps find a mass exiting the introitus.

Most uterine myomas, however, are asymptomatic and require no treatment. An asymptomatic myoma should be followed at regular intervals by physical examination to document the rate of growth. These exams are usually done every 6 months. The growth is most easily determined in abdominally palpable myomas by measuring the uterine size with a tape measure from the symphysis to the top of the mass. This measurement, which is similar to that performed on the preg-

nant uterus during prenatal care, allows a quantified description of myoma growth. Asymptomatic myomas that are less than 12 weeks of pregnancy size (or 280 g) rarely need treatment (Table 3).

◊ UNUSUAL COMPLICATIONS

Polycythemia

The literature contains many reports describing polycythemia in women with myomas. When the myoma is surgically removed, the polycythemia abates. Recent biochemical studies have shown that the myometrium has the ability to produce erythropoietin, and in those patients with polycythemia, excess erythropoietin has been measured. Presumably the myoma is producing an excessive amount of this erythrocyte-stimulating factor, resulting in the increased red blood cell mass. If the patient has excessively heavy menses, the re-

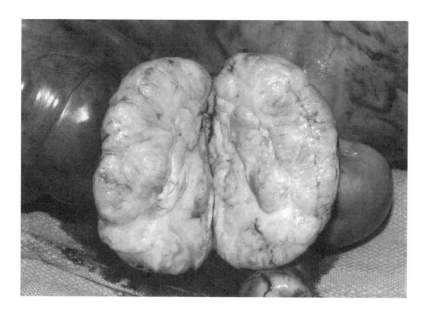

FIG. 2. Gross appearance of a cut myoma.

sulting anemia and iron loss may mask the polycythemia. These tumors tend to be large and are more frequent in menopausal women.

Pregnancy

Pregnancy in a uterus with myomas is a frequent ocurrence because myomas are so common. Several complications can result from this combination. Occasionally a subserous myoma will go through acute hemorrhagic carious degeneration during pregnancy. This will result in uterine cramps as well as extreme pain localized over the myoma as a result of the irritation of the serosal nerves covering this necrotic tumor. In general, these will not initiate preterm labor, and in a short time the pain will subside, and the myoma will then generally decrease in size. Surgery is contraindicated, and the patient should be managed with appropriate analgesics to control the pain until resolution has occurred.

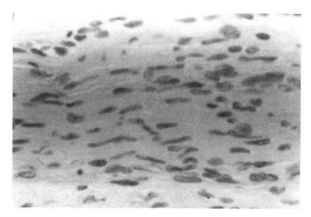

FIG. 3. Histologic appearance of a myoma with uniform, spindle-shaped smooth muscle cells. A few mitoses are present.

Occasionally tocolytic drugs will be needed to stop uterine contractions.

A more serious problem is placental abruption. If a portion of the placenta is implanted over a submucous myoma, there is defective implantation, and the risk of abruption increases significantly. Early pregnancy loss as spontaneous abortion can also result. The frequency of late pregnancy abruption depends on the size of the myoma and on how much of the placenta is implanted at that site. A submucous myoma more than 5 cm in diameter with the placenta covering this area produces an approximately 50% abruption rate. The potential problem can be anticipated by antepartum ultrasound exams, and if large myomas are found near or under the placenta, then early elective delivery seems reasonable.

Myomas developing in the lower uterine segment and cervix can also create a problem with malpresentation of the fetus and labor. A large myoma in the lower uterine segment may prevent a vertex presentation and result in a breech or transverse lie. If the myoma involves the lower segment and/or cervix, it may prevent cervical dilation during labor. These two complications will often result in a significantly increased chance for cesarean section delivery.

Serial studies of myomas during pregnancy show that about 20% enlarge, 20% decrease in size, and 60% remain unchanged. Although cramps and uterine contractions are common in these pregnancies, preterm delivery rates are usually not increased (Table 4).

◊ DIAGNOSIS

The clinician can usually easily diagnose myomas by abdominal and pelvic examination. Although the abdominal examination may fail to reveal small myomas, the pelvic exam will show an irregular, firm, usually mobile and nontender midline pelvic mass. Myomas may extend into the parametrial area, but it is unusual to find this without a distortion of

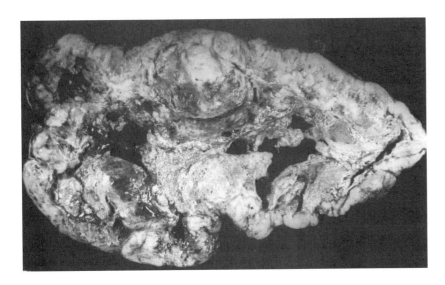

FIG. 4. Soft, yielding, hemorrhagic sarcoma with a "raw pork" appearance.

the uterus as well. An occasional patient may not present until late in her myoma growth phase and have a large abdominal mass sometimes extending into the upper abdomen.

All imaging techniques have been used with myomas. On x-ray examination, calcifications can frequently be seen in myomas and appear as discrete, calcified, round masses in the abdomen (Fig. 6). If a hysterosalpingogram is performed on a patient with submucous myomas, there will be distinct areas lacking contrast in the endometrial cavity outline (Fig. 7). Ultrasound studies of the myoma show a "snow-storm" image not dissimilar from that seen with a hydatidiform mole. The pseudocapsule can often be delineated. By measuring the dimensions of a myoma and using formulas for calculating the volume of a sphere, one can estimate the myoma volume, and therefore, its rate of growth can be followed with serial examinations. Myomas can also be easily imaged with nuclear magnetic resonance studies. Thus, the

diagnosis of a myoma is easily accomplished. If the myoma is large, additional imaging of adjacent structures such as intravenous pylograms or barium enemas may be needed to determine if mechanical compression damage is occurring.

◊ MANAGEMENT

Two forms of management are available for women with symptomatic myomas, and the choice depends in part on their desire to have more children. If future childbearing is important to the patient, then a conservative management program should be attempted. This could be medical treatment or conservative surgery.

Medical Treatment

The most commonly used medical treatment is to administer gonadotropin-releasing hormone (GnRH) agonists. The GnRH agonists are at higher concentrations than those normally secreted by the arcuate nucleus of the hypothalmus, and as a result, they down-regulate the anterior pituitary gonadotropin cell receptors, which results in a suppression of both LH and FSH blood levels. The ovary then fails to develop a follicle, and there is a concomitant decrease of estradiol and progesterone. Thus, this form of medical therapy results in a temporary reversable castration and moves the woman to a menopause-like condition. Because myomas are dependent on estrogen and progesterone for their maintanence and

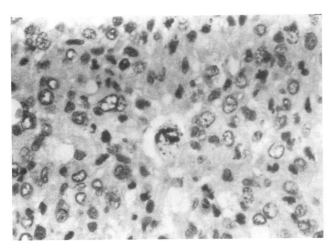

FIG. 5. Pleomorphic tumor cells with enlarged hyperchromatic nuclei and numerous mitoses. A large number of mitoses in a myoma is one diagnostic criterion of a sarcoma.

TABLE 3. *Common symptoms from myomas*

Abnormal bleeding
Pelvic mass
Pressure symptoms on other organs
Acute pain from torsion
Asymptomatic

TABLE 4. *Pregnancy complications with myoma*

Carious degeneration and pain
Abruption/abortion
Malpresentation
Failure of cervix to dilate
Preterm contractions
Increased cesarean section rates

growth, the result will be a shrinkage of the myoma. Many studies have now shown that the myoma size will decrease by about 50% after 3 months of treatment. When the treatment is discontinued, the reproductive cycles will recur, and the myoma will regrow to its pretreatment size in 2 to 3 months.

For the young woman being treated with GnRH who is medically transformed to a menopausal-like state, there are significant side effects, including vasomotor instability and hot flushes, pelvic tissue atrophy with dysuria and dyspareunia, memory loss, osteoporosis and an adverse effect on lipids potentially damaging the arterial vascular system. These side effects, plus the high cost of the medication, limit the duration of its use to no more than 6 months. In order to minimize some of the side effects, treated women have been also given low doses of hormone replacement therapy with estrogen and progestins as an add-back regimen. Because myoma cell turnover is related directly to progesterone, a progestin add-back regimen should not be used with myoma GnRH treat-

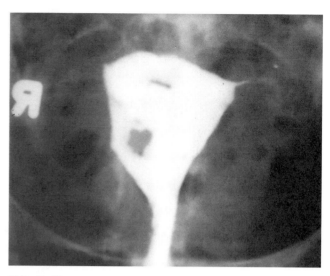

FIG. 7. Hysterosalpingogram performed on a patient with submucous myomas. Note that there are distinct areas lacking contrast in the endometrial cavity outline.

ment, as it will prevent tumor regression. Only estrogen add-back should be used until tumor reduction has occured.

The use of GnRH in myoma treatment offers five potential advantages. First, if the patient's problem is bleeding, GnRH treatment will decrease the bleeding and allow time for the patient to rebuild her red blood cell mass and thus reduce the need for blood transfusions at the time of surgery. Second, by decreasing the size of the myoma mass by 50%, it may allow a different surgical procedure to be done, such as vaginal as opposed to abdominal hysterectomy. Vaginal hysterectomy has a lower morbidity for the patient and therefore would be an advantage. Third, if the myomas are reduced in size, an abdominal hysterectomy may be performed with a transverse (Pfannenstiel) incision rather than a midline incision. The transverse incision is stronger, has less morbidity, and is cosmetically preferred by many women. Fourth, by decreasing the size of the myomatous mass, it may make the surgical procedure less difficult at the time of hysterectomy, with less bleeding during surgery. Finally, if the patient is perimenopausal, the medical therapy may be continued until the time when the patient is in menopause, when discontinuing the medical treatment will not result in the regrowth of the myomas (Table 5).

Another type of medical treatment that is being utilized is with antiprogestins. Studies using compounds like RU-486

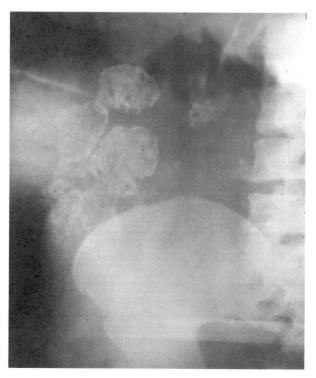

FIG. 6. Radiograph of myoma calcifications, which appear as discrete, calcified, round masses in the abdomen.

TABLE 5. *Possible advantages of GnRH treatment for myoma*

Stops bleeding so anemia can be corrected without blood transfusion
Allow vaginal rather than abdominal hysterectomy
Allow transverse abdominal incision rather than midline
Make surgery simpler with less blood loss
Carry patient until time of natural menopause

have shown that the decrease in myoma size achieved with this treatment is almost identical to that seen with GnRH treatment. Thus, it can be expected that there will be a 50% decrease in size by approximately the third month of treatment. Studies have shown that as little as 25 mg per day of this compound achieves those results. There are fewer side effects with the antiprogestins, and therefore, they can be used for extended periods of time. These new antiprogestin compounds may offer a significant improvement in medical therapy for prevention as well as treatment of uterine myomas. They are not yet approved for this use in the United States, but there is a broad experience published from other centers in the world.

Other medical therapies have been utilized with varying success including Depo-Provera an GnRH antagonists and weak androgens such as danazol. Depo-Provera treatments suppress LH and FSH and result in ovarian shutdown. Therefore, even if a progestin is given, the lack of estrogen decreases progesterone receptors in the myoma, so the cells will decrease in size. Their use, however, seems to have been displaced by the GnRH agonists and antiprogestins, as described above.

Conservative Surgery

Conservative surgery removing myomas while attempting to leave the intact uterus can be offered to some women desiring future fertility. This procedure is called myomectomy. At the time of myomectomy, several myomas frequently are present that need excision. The surgeon needs to carefully inspect the uterus and to attempt to make the uterine incision at a site where most if not all of the myomas can be removed with one uterine incision. Before incising the uterus, the surgeon should make an attempt to limit blood flow to the uterus during the surgical procedure. This can usually be achieved with either a clamp or a rubber tourniquet placed around the lower uterine segment to impede blood flow through the uterine arteries during the surgical procedure. Other techniques involve injections of vasoconstrictors such as vasopressin. If possible, the incision should be placed on the anterior side of the uterus. These incisions are associated with much less postoperative adhesion formation compared to posterior incisions and will, therefore, have less impairment of future fertility because of scarring. If necessary, incisions can be put in the posterior wall of the uterus, but they are much less desirable.

After the uterine incision is made over the myoma, the myoma is shelled out of its pseudocapsule. The uterine defect left by the myoma needs to be closed with multiple layers of suture, achieving hemostasis. A risk of the procedure is postoperative bleeding, which may require a hysterectomy to control. Following conservative myomectomy, the pregnancy rate is approximately 60%. Placing adhesion-preventing bioresorbable membranes over the uterine incision seems to improve pregnancy rates. These patients have a weakened uterine wall independent of whether the initial incision went into the endometrial cavity or not, and therefore, at the time

of term pregnancy, they may need an elective cesarean section for delivery, depending on the depth of the myometrial incision. This is usually performed at approximately 38 weeks of gestation.

Hysterectomy

The definitive surgical procedure for the symptomatic myomatous uterus is hysterectomy. For women under the age of 50 in whom no adnexal disease is present, the tubes and ovaries are usually left in place. Removing one ovary significantly decreases estrogen production, and therefore, it is best to leave both ovaries if they are normal. At times the uterine myomatous mass is so large it is technically difficult to do a hysterectomy. Several myomectomies can be performed first, which will make the hysterectomy technically easier. If the patient had abnormal bleeding, then endometrial sampling must be done before the hysterectomy to be certain endometrial cancer is not present. If there is no symptomatology other than a pelvic mass, the recommendation by the American College of Obstetricians and Gynecologists is that the uterus should not be surgically removed unless it has reached the size of a 12-week pregnancy, which is equivalent to 280 g in weight.

The patient with the asymptomatic myomatous uterus who is being followed conservatively will experience a shrinkage of her myomas when she reaches menopause. In the postmenopausal woman with asymptomatic myomas, it is important to recommend hormone replacement treatment with low doses of estrogen and progestin to prevent cardiovascular disease, osteoporosis, vasomotor instability and hot flashes, and pelvic tissue atrophy. The asymptomatic myomatous uterus is not a contraindication to hormone replacement therapy in the menopausal woman. It has been found, however, that women who develop irregular bleeding during hormone replacement treatment frequently have a submucous myoma that is the site of the bleeding. Some of these small submucous myomas can be resected through the cervix using a hysteroscope, which will eliminate the bleeding problem.

◊ CONCLUSION

Uterine myomas are the most common gynecologic pelvic tumors. They are usually multiple, each developing from a single myometrial cell, and are stimulated in growth by growth factors under the control of progesterone, which is attached to nuclear receptors regulated by estrogen. Only approximately 25% of women with myomas have symptoms like bleeding, a large pelvic mass, or pelvic pressure. Sarcomatous degeneration is a rare problem, occurring in less that 1% of uteri. Myomas may complicate pregnancy by leading to such problems as abruption, pain, and malpresentation requiring cesarean section. Most myomas can be observed and require no treatment. Conservative management includes medical therapy with GnRH agonists or antiprogestins or conservative surgical management with myomectomy. Some women need aggressive surgical management with hysterectomy when their myomatous uterus is symptomatic. Myomas represent the most frequent reason for performing hysterectomy. Menopausal women with asymptomatic myomas should be offered hormone replacement therapy.

◊ RECOMMENDED READINGS

American College of Obstetricians and Gynecologists. *Technical bulletin no. 192: Uterine leiomyomata.* 1994.

Benagiano G, Kivenen ST, Fadini R, Cronje H, Klintorp S, Spuy ZM. Zoladex (goserelin acetate) and the anemic patient: Results of a multicenter fibroid study. *Fertil Steril* 1996;66:223.

Brosens I, Deprest J, Dal Cin P, Van den Berghe H. Clinical significance of cytogenetic abnormalities in uterine myomas. *Fertil Steril* 1998; 69:232.

Cramer SF, Patel A. The frequency of uterine leiomyomas. *Am J Clin Pathol* 1990;94:435.

Deligdisch L, Hirschmann S, Altchek A. Pathologic changes in gonadotropin releasing hormone agonist analogue treated uterine leiomyomata. *Fertil Steril* 1997;67:837.

Fayed YM, Tsibris JCM, Langenberg PW, Robertson AL Jr. Human uterine leiomyoma cells: Binding and growth responses to epidermal growth factor, platelet-derived growth factor and insulin. *Lab Invest* 1989; 60:30.

Friedman AJ, Barbieri RL, Doubilet PM, Fine C, Schiff I. A randomized double-blind trial of a gonadotropin releasing hormone agonist (leuprolide) with or without medroxyprogesterone acetate in the treatment of leiomyomata uteri. *Fertil Steril* 1988;49:404.

Friedman AJ, Hoffman DI, Comite F, Browneller RW, Miller JD. Treatment of leiomyomata uteri with leuprolide acetate depot: A double-blind placebo-controlled, multicenter study. *Obstet Gynecol* 1991;77:720.

Kawaguchi K, Fujii S, Konishi I, Nanbu Y, Nonogaki H, Mori T. Mitotic activity in uterine leiomyomas during the menstrual cycle. *Am J Obstet Gynecol* 1989;160:637.

Koutsieris M. Pathophysiology of uterine leiomyomas. *Biochem Cell Biol* 1992;70:273.

Leibsohn S, d'Ablaing G, Mishell DR Jr, Schlaerth JB. Leiomyosarcoma in a series of hysterectomies performed for presumed uterine leiomyomas. *Am J Obstet Gynecol* 1990;162:968.

Levgur M. The enlarged uterus—relation of uterine size to symptoms and histopathologic findings. *J Reprod Med* 1996;41:166.

Linder D, Gartler SM. Glucose-6-phosphate dehydrogenase mosaicism: Utilization as a cell marker in the study of leiomyomas. *Science* 1965; 150:67.

Matsuo H, Maruo T, Samoto T. Increased expression of Bcl-2 protein in human uterine leiomyoma and its up-regulation by progesterone. *J Clin Endocrinol Metab* 1997;82:293.

Mizutani T, Sugihara A, Nakamuro K, Terada N. Suppression of cell proliferation and induction of apoptosis in uterine leiomyoma by gonadotropin-releasing hormone agonist (leuprolide acetate). *J Clin Endocrinol Metab* 1998;83:1253.

Murphy AA, Morales AJ, Kettel LM, Yen SSC. Regression of uterine leiomyomata to the antiprogesterone RU-486: Dose-response effect. *Fertil Steril* 1995;64:187.

Nilbert M, Heim S. Uterine leiomyoma cytogenetics. *Genes Chromosomes Cancer* 1990;2:3.

Parazzini F, Negri E, LaVecchia C, Rabaiotti M, Luchini L, Villa A, Fedele L. Uterine myomas and smoking—results from an Italian study. *J Reprod Med* 1996;41:316.

Parker WH, Fu YS, Berek JS. Uterine sarcoma in patients operated on for presumed leiomyoma and rapidly growing leiomyoma. *Obstet Gynecol* 1994;83:414.

Phelan JP. Myomas and pregnancy. *Obstet Gynecol Clin North Am* 1995;22:801.

Porter KB, Tsibris JCM, Nicosia SV, Murphy JM, O'Brien WF, Rao PS, Spellacy WN. Estrogen-induced guinea pig model for uterine leiomyomas: do the ovaries protect? *Biol Reprod* 1995;52:824.

Raj R, Lake Y. Polycythemia associated with leiomyoma of the uterus. *Br J Obstet Gynaecol* 1992;99:923.

Rein MS, Barbieri RL, Friedman AJ. Progesterone: A critical role in the pathogenesis of uterine myomas. *Am J Obstet Gynecol* 1995;172:14.

Spellacy WN, LeMaire WJ, Buhi WC, Birk SA, Bradley BA. Plasma growth hormone and estradiol levels in women with uterine myomas. *Obstet Gynecol* 1972;40:829.

Tulandi T, Murray C, Guralnick M. Adhesion formation and reproductive outcome after myomectomy and second-look laparoscopy. *Obstet Gynecol* 1993;82:213.

Vollenhoven BJ, Lawrence AS, Healy DL. Uterine fibroids: A clinical review. *Br J Obstet Gynecol* 1990;97:285–298.

West CP, Lumsden MA, Lawson S, Williamson J, Baird DT. Shrinkage of uterine fibroids during therapy with goserelin (Zoladex): A luteinizing hormone-releasing hormone agonist administered as a monthly subcutaneous depot. *Fertil Steril* 1987;48:45.

CHAPTER 52

Diseases of the Ovary and Fallopian Tubes

———— ◊ ————

Dennis Yi-Shin Kuo
Joan G. Jones
Carolyn D. Runowicz

Abnormalities of the ovary or fallopian tubes may result from physiologic changes, infectious processes, or benign or malignant neoplasms. Patients may present with a pelvic mass with or without other signs or symptoms. Diseases of the ovary or fallopian tube may occur at any age from childhood to senescence. Depending on patient age, the physiologic and pathologic processes will differ. For example, for patients presenting with a pelvic mass, the incidence of ovarian cancer increases with age, with an overall risk of malignancy of 13% in premenopausal women and 45% in elderly post-menopausal women. Therefore, the differential diagnosis and workup may vary, depending on a patient's age (Fig. 1).

◊ AGE LESS THAN 20 YEARS

Benign Fallopian Tube Diseases

Pelvic inflammatory disease and *ectopic pregnancy* are common findings in young women presenting with adnexal masses (see Chapters 34 and 11, respectively). Each has distinct clinical findings and must be high on the differential diagnostic list. Other benign fallopian tube pathologies in this age group are rare and often incidentally detected during surgical procedures for other indications.

Inclusion Cyst and Walthard Nest

Inclusion cysts are formed by invagination of the tubal serosa, resulting in one or multiple, small (1 to 2 mm) unilocular cysts. The cells lining these inclusion cysts can be transformed by a process of metaplasia to polygonal epithelial cells forming a Walthard nest. Less commonly, the inner layer of epithelial cells may also undergo columnar metaplasia. These cysts are benign and are usually incidentally detected.

Broad Ligament Cyst

Similar to inclusion cysts, broad ligament cysts are often incidental findings. They are of mesonephric or paramesonephric origin. *Hydatid cysts of Morgagni* are pedunculated broad ligament cysts that are usually small and translucent, measuring 1 cm or less in diameter. They are often bilateral and have a slender stalk attached to the fimbria. *Intraligamentous cysts,* on the other hand, can range from 1 cm to greater than 15 cm in diameter. They are usually unilocular and, like hydatid cysts of Morgagni, are thin-walled. They are often referred as para-ovarian cysts. Although malignant transformation is rare, large intraligamentous cysts (greater than 5 cm) should be removed.

Benign Ovarian Diseases

Functional Cysts

Corpus Luteum Cyst

Corpus luteum cysts occur during the reproductive period. They are thin-walled and unilocular, measuring from 3 to 11 cm in diameter. They are often filled with serous or serosanguineous fluid or blood clots (Figs. 2 and 3). During pregnancy, they may grow and may rarely become palpable. In the absence of pregnancy, corpus luteum cysts may enlarge as a result of unusual growth or hemorrhage into the lumen. Microscopically, they are composed of luteinized granulosa cells and theca interna cells.

Corpus luteum cysts are usually an incidental finding. Even if they are noted on routine examination, most often

Differential diagnosis

A. **Benign fallopian tube disease**
    1. **Infection**
        a. Acute or chronic salpingitis
        b. Tubo-ovarian abscess
    2. **Ectopic pregnancy**
    3. **Benign lesions**
        a. Inclusion cysts and walthard nests
        b. Broad ligament cysts
           i. Hydatid cyst of Morgagni
B. **Benign ovarian disease**
    1. **Functional cysts**
        a. corpus lutein cysts
        b. theca lutein cysts
        c. follicular cysts
    2. **Germ cell tumors**
        a. Mature teratomas
           i. Struma ovarii
    3. **Sex cord-Stromal tumors**
           i. Fibromas(see age 20-40)
C. **Malignant ovarian disease**
    1. **Germ cell tumors**
        a. **Dysgerminomas**
        b. **Endodermal sinus tumors(yolk sac tumor)**
        c. **Immature teratomas**
        d. **Embryonal carcinomas**
        e. **Polyembryomas**
        f. **Choriocarcinomas**
        g. **Mixed germ cell tumors**
        h. **Mixed form - Gonadoblastomas**

    2. **Sex cord-stromal tumors:**
        a. **Juvenile granulosa-cell tumors**
        b. **Sertoli-Leydig cells(see age 20-40)**
    3. **Malignant epithelial tumors (see age >40)**

FIG. 1. Differential diagnosis for patients less than 20 years of age.

they will spontaneously regress within 1 to 2 months in menstruating patients. Occasionally, patients may present with symptoms of hemorrhage, rupture, or torsion. Conservative management of these patients is usually attempted. Oral contraceptives are often used for 2 to 3 menstrual cycles in an attempt to hasten resolution of the cysts. However, recent data

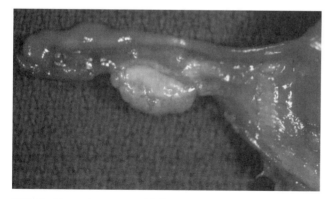

FIG. 2. Normal ovary and fallopian tube. This is the normal gross appearance of a postmenopausal ovary and fallopian tube.

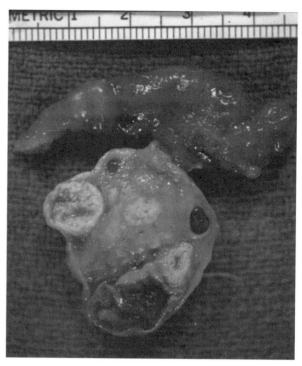

FIG. 3. Corpus luteum and follicle cysts. On section, the lower aspect of this ovary contains a cystically dilated corpus luteum. It is grossly recognizable by its convoluted yellow rim. Also present in this ovary are corpora albicancea and follicle cysts.

challenge the effectiveness of this therapy. If surgical intervention is indicated, an ovarian cystectomy with preservation of ovarian tissue is the treatment of choice.

Follicle Cyst

Follicle cysts are a common occurrence in the neonatal, childhood, and reproductive periods (Fig. 4). They are the most commonly seen cystic enlargements of the ovary, as they can attain a size of 8 to 9 cm in diameter. Microscopically, follicle cysts are lined by an inner layer of granulosa cells and an outer layer of theca interna cells, which may or may not be luteinized.

In menstruating women, persistent follicular cysts are the result of ovulatory failure, most likely related to abnormalities in the release of anterior pituitary gonadotropins with continued growth of the follicles. Hyperstimulation of the ovary from the use of fertility drugs may also result in significant enlargement of multiple follicle cysts. They may be multiple, recurrent, bilateral, or associated with pregnancy.

The management of enlarged follicle cysts is similar to that of corpus luteum cysts. Persistently enlarged cysts require further investigation, such as laparoscopy and/or laparotomy. Ovarian cystectomy with conservation of the ovarian tissue is the treatment of choice, if surgery is indicated. Treatment for hyperstimulated ovaries from fertility drugs is usually supportive only.

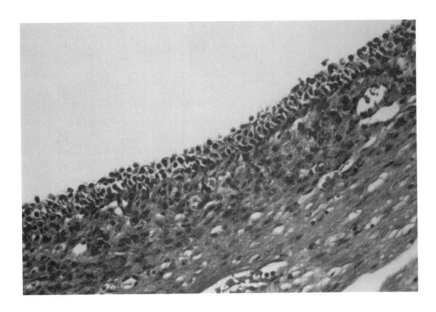

FIG. 4. Follicle cyst. The lining is composed of an inner layer of granulosa cells and an outer layer of theca interna cells.

Theca-lutein Cyst

Theca-lutein cysts are the least common type of functional cyst (Fig. 5). They result from bilateral follicular cyst enlargement and are often seen with hydatidiform mole, choriocarcinoma, or multiple pregnancies. Cyst enlargement is most likely due to elevated human chorionic gonadotropin (hCG) associated with these clinical entities. These cysts may grow to as large as 15 cm in diameter. Microscopically, the cysts are lined by theca cells that may or may not be luteinized. Granulosa cells may or may not be present.

After evacuation of the uterus for a hydatidiform mole or at the end of a pregnancy, theca-lutein cysts usually regress, as the ovary return to its normal size. Surgery is reserved for cases with complications, such as torsion or hemorrhage.

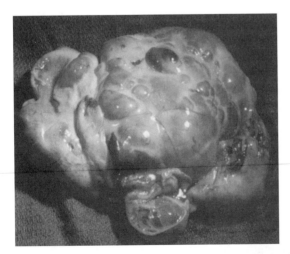

FIG. 5. Theca-lutein cysts. Ovarian enlargement due to the presence of multiple luteinized follicle cysts secondary to human chorionic gonadotropin stimulation is also called hyperreactio luteinalis.

Germ Cell Tumor

The most common ovarian tumor in children and young women is germ cell tumor, accounting for 90% of prepubertal tumors and 60% of tumors in women younger than 20 years. These tumors arise from the germ cells originating in the embryonic yolk sac. Patients usually present with complaints of abdominal pain and have an associated pelvic or abdominal mass. Others might present with acute abdominal pain as a result of ovarian rupture, hemorrhage, or torsion. A misdiagnosis of acute appendicitis has been made in these circumstances.

Mature Cystic Teratoma

Mature cystic teratomas, also known as dermoid cysts, are the most common benign ovarian neoplasm, with a peak incidence from ages 20 to 40 years. However, they can also be seen in infancy as well as menopausal woman. Mature cystic teratomas originate from primordial germ cells and are composed of well differentiated derivatives of any combination of the three germ layers: ectoderm, mesoderm, endoderm. Ectodermal elements usually predominate. Although they are in general benign, on rare occasion they may undergo malignant transformation in one of the elements, usually a squamous cell carcinoma.

Grossly, the tumors are round or oval with a smooth, glistening, gray-white surface. The majority of tumors measure 5 to 10 cm in diameter, with 8% to 15% of cases being bilateral. The tumors are usually unilocular but occasionally multilocular, and are filled with fatty material similar to sebum and with hair. A solid portion located at one pole of the cyst and projecting into the cavity is known as a *Rokitansky protuberance, embryonic node, dermoid nipple,* or *dermoid protuberance,* where hair, teeth, bone, or any other tissue may be found (Fig. 6).[15] Microscopically, ovarian stroma is noted on the outside wall, with the cyst being lined by mostly squamous

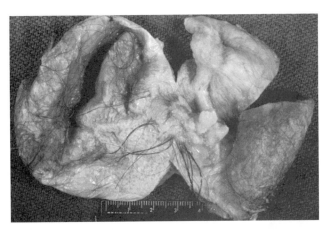

FIG. 6. Mature cystic teratoma. This mature cystic teratoma contains hair and teeth.

cell epithelium with underlying sebaceous and sweat glands. Other tissues can also be found at the protuberance, such as glia, neurons, bone, cartilage, retina, smooth muscle, fibrous and fatty tissue, gastrointestinal and bronchial mucosa, and thyroid and salivary gland tissue (Fig. 7).[15]

In the past, a diagnosis of benign cystic teratoma was usually made on an abdominal x-ray, which easily visualizes teeth. Sonography, however, has become the diagnostic test of choice in most centers. Torsion is a frequent complication in children and pregnant patients. Cyst rupture may result in a chemical peritonitis due to the spillage of the tumor contents, causing formation of dense adhesions. Because benign cystic teratomas are more prevalent in young women, treatment is usually ovarian cystectomy with preservation of ovarian tissue.

Struma Ovarii

Struma ovarii is a subset of mature cystic teratomas in which the tumor is composed entirely or predominantly of thyroid tissue. Grossly, the cut surface shows gelatinous red to green-brown colloid, and microscopically mature thyroid tissue is seen (Figs. 8 and 9). Struma ovarii accounts for less than 3% of mature teratomas, with similar age distribution and similar clinical findings. However, occasionally thyroid gland enlargement is seen, and about 5% of patients with the struma ovarii will experience signs and symptoms of thyrotoxicosis. Malignant changes in a struma ovarii are rare but can occur, and 30% of reported cases of malignant struma ovarii are associated with metastasis.

The surgical management of a benign ovarian neoplasm is summarized in Figure 10.

Malignant Ovarian Disease

Germ Cell Tumor

Malignant ovarian germ cell tumors account for less than 5% of all ovarian cancers. Table 1 provides a listing of the World Health Organization classification of germ cell tumors of the ovary. Their male counterpart, testicular cancer, is approximately 10 times more common than ovarian germ cell tumors. Many of the recent advances in the management of malignant ovarian germ cell tumors are a result of clinical trials in patients with testicular cancer.

Dysgerminoma

Dysgerminoma is the most common malignant germ cell tumor of the ovary, accounting for 2% of all ovarian malignancies. Approximately 50% of the patients with this tumor are younger than 20 years and 80% are younger than 30 years. Children with dysgerminoma may present with precocious puberty or primary amenorrhea. The serum lactate dehydrogenase level is almost always elevated and serves as a tumor marker during treatment and follow-up. Occasionally, serum

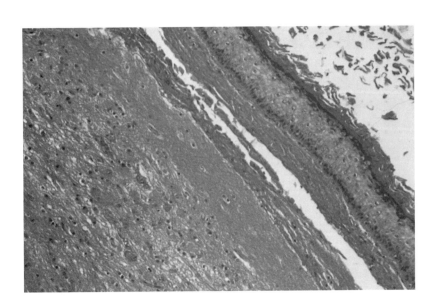

FIG. 7. Mature cystic teratoma. Microscopically, there is keratinizing squamous epithelium on the right and mature glial tissue on the left.

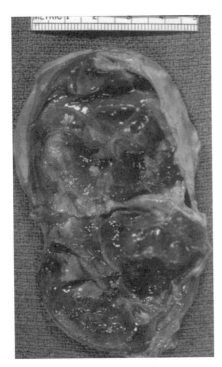

FIG. 8. Struma ovarii. The color of the glistening colloid in struma ovarii can be the expected red-brown or may have a green tinge.

β-hCG may also be elevated. Table 2 outlines the serum tumor markers typically associated with germ cell tumors.

Although dysgerminoma tends to be unilateral, approximately 10% to 15% of tumors are bilateral. It is usually gray-white, smooth, and fleshy in appearance, and on cut surface it is usually solid (Fig. 11). Hemorrhage and necrosis may be seen. Cystic areas suggest the presence of mixed germ cell elements that would require further careful sampling of the specimen. The microscopic appearance of an ovarian dysgerminoma is similar in histology to its male counterpart, testicular seminoma, with aggregates of tumor cells surrounded by connective tissue stroma containing lymphocytes and foreign-body giant cells (Fig. 12).[15] The tumor cells are usually large, with clear or lightly granular cytoplasm containing abundant glycogen. Nuclei are vesicular and large, occupying half the cells and containing one or more nucleoli. Mitotic activity is almost always present. In fewer than 10% of patients, syncytiotrophoblastic giant cells may be detected, producing hCG that may be demonstrated in tissue section by immunohistochemical techniques and in the serum by an elevated hCG level. Syncytiotrophoblastic cells in a dysgerminoma do not have prognostic significance. Serum β-hCG levels can be used to monitor patients' response to treatment and in follow-up.

Treatment is determined by patient age. The management of dysgerminoma is illustrated in Figure 13. Since most patients with dysgerminoma are of reproductive age, unilateral salpingo-oophorectomy and a full staging procedure with preservation of the contralateral ovary and the uterus are recommended, as long as there is no evidence of disease in the other ovary. Table 3 is a listing of procedures required when a full staging procedure is performed. Table 4 illustrates the widely used International Federation of Gynecology and Obstetrics (FIGO) staging system for all ovarian cancers. Observational studies have revealed identical remission rates for conservative treatment (e.g., unilateral salpingo-oophorectomy) and aggressive therapy (e.g., bilateral salpingo-oophorectomy with or without a hysterectomy) in early-stage disease.[12] Routine biopsy of the contralateral ovary should be avoided in normal-appearing contralateral ovaries. If gross tumor is noted in both ovaries, a unilateral salpingo-oophorectomy of the larger ovary, a unilateral cystectomy, and a full staging procedure followed by chemotherapy may be appropriate in those patients who desire fertility, after appropriate counseling and consultation with a gynecologic oncologist. Patients with advanced disease may require complete removal of the reproductive organs, which should be performed in consultation with a gynecologic oncologist.

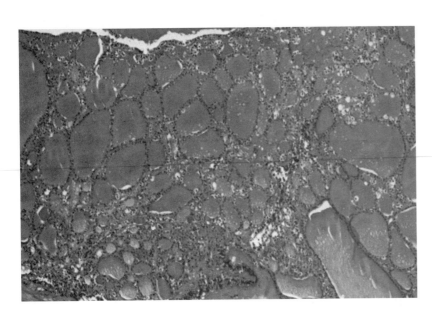

FIG. 9. Struma ovarii. Microscopically, the tumor is composed of normal thyroid tissue.

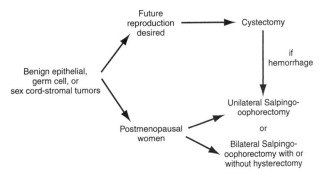

FIG. 10. Management of a benign ovarian neoplasm.

Dysgerminoma is very sensitive to radiation and chemotherapy. Since it is a disease of young women, chemotherapy is the most appropriate postoperative treatment in these patients and should be offered to those with disease more advanced than stage Ia. Although combination therapy with vincristine sulfate (Oncovin), dactinomycin (Cosmegen), and cyclophosphamide (VAC) or vinblastine sulfate (Velban), bleomycin sulfate (Blenoxane), and cisplatin (Platinol) (VBP) has been used with excellent results, especially in stage I patients, the combination of bleomycin, etoposide, and cisplatin (BEP) has been found to be even more effective in treating all stages of disease, with a sustained remission in essentially 100% of patients. The M.D. Anderson Cancer Center group and the Gynecologic Oncology Group (GOG) have used BEP in their treatment of dysgerminoma in all stages of disease and have reported prolonged disease-free interval with three to six cycles of therapy, depending on disease status, residual disease, and tumor markers.[12,13] Based on these descriptive studies (type III evidence), BEP should be used as first-line therapy. In patients with pure dysgerminoma seemingly confined to the ovary who were inadequately staged, administration of three cycles of adjuvant BEP is recommended due to a recurrence rate of 20%. However, the scientific merit of this treatment plan requires further investigation. Another option is to offer a repeat surgery to fully stage the disease.

There have been several reports of secondary neoplasm, especially hematologic malignancies, after the use of BEP and other etoposide-based regimens.[23] Although these are rare occurrences, careful long-term follow-up and evaluation of risk–benefit ratio may be warranted to assess the efficacy of this regimen with and without etoposide.

TABLE 1. *World Health Organization classification of germ cell tumors*

Dysgerminoma
Endodermal sinus tumor
Teratomas
   Immature
   Mature (dermoid cyst)
   Monodermal (struma ovarii, carcinoid)
Embryonal carcinoma
Polyembryoma
Choriocarcinoma
Mixed forms
Gonadoblastoma: mixed germ cells and sex cord–stromal
   derivatives

(From Serov SF, Scully RE, Robin IH. *Histological typing of ovarian tumors: international histological classification of tumors, no. 9.* Geneva: World Health Organization, 1973; with permission.)

Endodermal Sinus Tumor (Yolk Sac Tumor)

Endodermal sinus tumor is the second most common germ cell tumor, representing 1% of all ovarian malignancies. It may be pure or part of a malignant mixed germ cell tumor. The reported age distribution ranges from 16 months to 46 years, but most patients are younger than 30 years. The serum alpha-fetoprotein (AFP) level is frequently elevated in these tumors (see Table 2), making it a useful diagnostic test in the initial workup, in the assessment of response to therapy, and in follow-up for recurrence. Symptoms are typical of those observed with other germ cell tumors. Several cases have presented in pregnancy. No endocrine manifestations have been seen with the pure form of endodermal sinus tumor. More than 70% of endodermal sinus tumors present in stage I, although they are biologically virulent.

Grossly, tumors are usually gray-yellow, large, and solid, ranging from 3 to 30 cm in diameter. Bilateral involvement has been noted only in patients with metastatic spread to other organs. Foci of hemorrhage, necrosis, and gelatinous changes are present. Microscopically, endodermal sinus tumors display a wide range of histologic patterns. The microcystic pattern is characterized by a loose network of channels and spaces forming a honeycomb lined by flat pleomorphic mesothelial-like cells with large hyperchromatic or vesicular nuclei. Hyaline globules or droplets, which are positive with periodic acid–Schiff stain, are commonly found. The endo-

TABLE 2. *Tumor markers associated with germ cell neoplasms: likelihood of elevation*

Neoplasm	AFP (normal, <10 ng/ml)	CA 125 (normal, <35 U/ml)	CEA (normal, <5 ng/ml)	hCG (normal, <5 mIU/ml)	LDH (normal, ≤240 IU/L)
Endodermal sinus tumor	Always	Usually	May be	May be	Usually
Immature teratoma	May be	May be	May be	May be	May be
Dysgerminoma	Not elevated	Rarely	Not elevated	Rarely	Usually
Choriocarcinoma	Not elevated	Not elevated	Not elevated	Always	Not elevated

AFP, alpha-fetoprotein; CEA, carcinoembryonic antigen; hCG, human chorionic gonadotropin; LDH, lactate dehydrogenase.

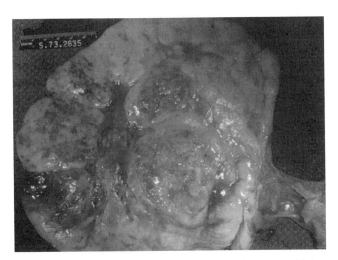

FIG. 11. Dysgerminoma. Cut surface is soft, tan, and lobulated, with areas of hemorrhage and necrosis.

dermal sinus pattern is characterized by perivascular formations called Schiller-Duval bodies (Fig. 14). Other patterns include the alveolar-glandular pattern, composed of alveolar, gland-like, or cystic spaces lined by flat or cuboidal epithelium; the polyvesicular vitelline pattern, in which numerous small vesicles are surrounded by connective tissue; and the solid pattern, consisting of aggregates of small pleomorphic undifferentiated cells.[15] These histologic patterns do not have prognostic significance.

In the past, patients with endodermal sinus tumors, even those with early-stage tumors, did poorly in spite of aggressive surgical and radiation treatments. With adjuvant chemotherapy after conservative pelvic surgery and staging laparotomy (see Table 3), there has been a marked improvement in the prognosis of patients with this malignancy. Adjuvant chemotherapeutic regimens for all nondysgerminomatous germ cell tumors (including endodermal sinus tumors, immature cystic teratoma, embryonal cell tumors, and others) are similar, as

they are grouped together in treatment protocols in several major studies.[12,13] The VAC regimen, first introduced in the 1970s, resulted in a successful cure rate of greater than 80% in stage I disease but less than 50% in patients with more advanced stage, as reported by a GOG study and the M.D. Anderson experience. The VBP regimen has shown superior results, compared to VAC, but toxicity is increased. However, no randomized clinical trials have been performed to compare the two regimens due to the rarity of these malignancies. More recently, the BEP regimen has shown an excellent response rate of over 95% in patients with local or advanced disease, and has become the primary therapeutic regimen.[12] Further studies, however, are needed to explore alternative regimens to reduce the rate of toxicity while maintaining the same efficacy. Second-look laparotomy should not be a part of posttherapy surveillance for this tumor or any other germ cell tumors. Salvage therapies, such as surgery followed by chemotherapy, in patients who have failed primary chemotherapy have shown some success; however, they are anecdotal at best due to the limited number of cases.

Immature Cystic Teratoma

Like mature cystic teratoma, immature cystic teratoma is composed of tissues derived from all three germinal layers, except that they also contain embryonic tissue. This group of tumors is the third most common malignant germ cell tumor, representing about 25% of all such tumors in patients younger than 20 years. Unlike mature cystic teratoma, which occurs in all ages but more frequently in the reproductive years, immature cystic teratoma is essentially found in the first two decades of life. It usually grows rapidly through its capsule, forming adhesions to the surrounding structures and implants in the peritoneal cavity.

Tumors are usually smooth and unilateral, ranging from 9 to 28 cm. A mature cystic teratoma may be present in the other ovary. Tumors are predominantly solid with some cystic

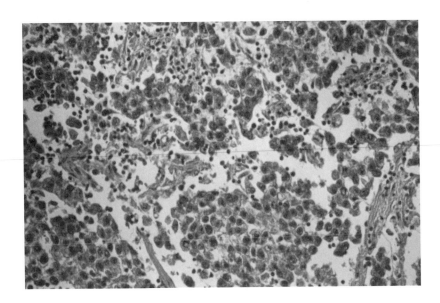

FIG. 12. Dysgerminoma. Loose aggregates of tumor cells are separated by connective tissue containing abundant lymphocytes.

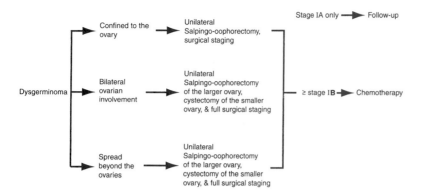

FIG. 13. Management of dysgerminoma.

areas filled with serous or mucinous fluid or fatty material (Fig. 15). The cut surface is soft and usually gray to pink to brown. Foci of cartilage or bone, hair, and calcified areas may be noted. Microscopically, the most common immature tissue present is neural, derived from the ectoderm (Fig. 16). A histologic grading system was therefore proposed based on the relative amount of mature and immature neuroepithelial tissues, mitotic activity, and degree of differentiation:[15]

Grade 0   Mature tissue only
Grade 1   Limited immature neuroepithelial tissue and mitotic activity
Grade 2   Moderate amount of immature tissue and mitotic activity.
Grade 3   Large quantities of immature tissue and mitotic activity

Prognosis correlates with histologic grade of tumors, as the presence of immature elements worsens the prognosis. In patients with stage Ia/grade 1 disease, surgery alone, consisting of an exploratory laparotomy, unilateral salpingo-oophorectomy, and a complete staging procedure (see Table 3), is sufficient. For more advanced disease, adjuvant chemotherapy after surgery is

TABLE 3. *Complete staging procedure for ovarian malignancy*

Removal of ascites for cytologic evaluation
If there is no ascites, do peritoneal washing with 50–100 ml of normal saline in the pelvis, the paracolic spaces, and infradiaphragmatic area
Cytoreductive surgery, reducing tumor size, including lymph nodes, to ≤1 cm residual size whenever possible

If tumor appears to be confined to the pelvis, the following procedures should be carried out:
  Right diaphragmatic scraping or biopsy
  Thorough examination of the peritoneal surface, intestine, and other viscera
  Routine biopsies from the cul-de-sac, right and left pelvic side walls and the right and left paracolic spaces
  Infracolic omentectomy
  Biopsy of all suspicious areas or adhesions
  Evaluation and sampling of paraaortic and pelvic lymph nodes

TABLE 4. *FIGO staging for ovarian cancer*

Stage I	Growth limited to the ovaries
Stage Ia	Growth limited to one ovary; no ascites; no tumor on the external surface; capsule intact
Stage Ib	Growth limited to both ovaries; no ascites; no tumor on the external surfaces; capsules intact
Stage Ic	Tumor either stage Ia or Ib but with tumor on the surface of one or both ovaries
Stage II	Growth involving one or both ovaries with pelvic extension
Stage IIa	Extension and/or metastases to the uterus and/or tubes
Stage IIb	Extension to other pelvic tissues
Stage IIc	Tumor either stage IIa or IIb but with tumor on the surface of one or both ovaries; or with capsules(s) ruptured; or with ascites present containing malignant cells or with positive peritoneal washings
Stage III	Tumor involving one or both ovaries with peritoneal implants outside the pelvis and/or positive retroperitoneal or inguinal nodes. Superficial liver metastasis equals stage III. Tumor is limited to the true pelvis but with histologically verified malignant extension to small bowel or omentum
Stage IIIa	Tumor grossly limited to the true pelvis with negative nodes but with histologically confirmed microscopic seeding of abdominal peritoneal surfaces
Stage IIIb	Tumor of one or both ovaries with histologically confirmed implants of abdominal peritoneal surfaces ≤2 cm in diameter. Nodes negative
Stage IIIc	Abdominal implants >2 cm in diameter and/or positive retroperitoneal or inguinal nodes
Stage IV	Growth involving one or both ovaries with distant metastasis. If pleural effusion is present, there must be positive cytologic test results to allot a case to stage IV. Parenchymal liver metastasis equals stage IV

(From International Federation of Gynecology and Obstetrics (FIGO). *Annual report on the results of treatment in gynecological cancer,* vol 21. Stockholm: FIGO, 1991; with permission.)

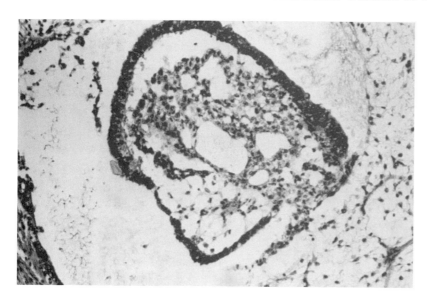

FIG. 14. Yolk sac tumor. A characteristic finding in the endodermal sinus pattern is the Schiller-Duval body.

necessary. Depending on disease extent, preservation of the contralateral ovary and the uterus is usually feasible. Serum AFP levels may be elevated (see Table 2). Chemotherapy is discussed in detail in the section of endodermal sinus tumor (see above).

Embryonal Carcinoma

Embryonal carcinoma is rare, accounting for less than 5% of all germ cell tumors. It usually occurs in children, with a median age of 15 years. Like its testicular counterpart, embryonal carcinoma is a highly malignant neoplasm. Because it is often seen as part of mixed germ cell tumors, serum AFP and hCG levels are often elevated (Fig. 17). Clinically, it may be associated with precocious puberty, as well as abnormal vaginal bleeding in adults.

The gross pathologic picture is variable, but the tumor is usually large and soft, with a cut surface that is solid and

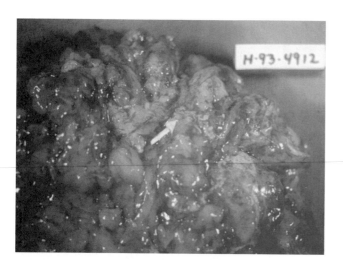

FIG. 15. Immature teratoma. This bulky neoplasm, removed from a 20-year-old woman, weighed 1800 g. The neuroectodermal elements appeared opaque and friable (*arrow*).

gray-white with areas of hemorrhage and necrosis. Microscopically, embryonal carcinoma consists of primitive, undifferentiated sheets of variably sized epithelial cells (Fig. 18). Nuclei are vesicular, and mitoses are frequent. Syncytiotrophoblastic giant cells are frequently seen in the stroma or directly adjacent to clusters of embryonal carcinoma cells.

Polyembryoma

Polyembryoma is a rare germ cell tumor, characterized by numerous embryoid bodies that morphologically resemble normal presomite embryos. It is usually part of a mixed germ cell neoplasm and has similar symptoms. The median age of patients with polyembryoma is 15 years. The tumor is usually unilateral, ranging from 10 cm to a mass that fills the entire abdominal cavity; cut section reveals mostly solid areas with hemorrhage and necrosis. Microscopically, embryonic bodies including an embryonic disk, amniotic cavity, yolk sac, and extraembryonic mesenchyme of varying degrees of differentiation are noted (Fig. 19). Syncytiotrophoblastic cells have also been detected. AFP, hCG, and sometimes human placental lactogen can be demonstrated in the serum and in cells by immunohistochemical staining.

Choriocarcinoma

Choriocarcinoma is a rare germ cell tumor that may be present in either pure or mixed form. Pure choriocarcinoma is usually found in prepubertal children. Isosexual precocious puberty is a common clinical finding in premenarcheal patients. In postmenarcheal patients, the presence of other germ cell components is helpful in distinguishing ovarian germ cell tumors from a gestation choriocarcinoma. A diagnosis of ectopic pregnancy is often entertained in postmenarcheal patients due to the shared signs and symptoms.

The gross appearance of choriocarcinoma depends on the composition of the germ cell elements. The tumor is usually

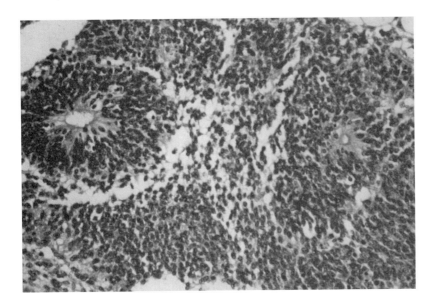

FIG. 16. Immature teratoma. These tumors are graded based on the presence and extent of neuroepithelial elements. Note the rosettes.

large, unilateral, and solid with areas of necrosis and hemorrhage. Microscopically, both cytotrophoblasts and syncytiotrophoblasts are present (Fig. 20). Treatment is as described previously for the other germ cell tumors.

Gonadoblastoma

Gonadoblastoma almost always arises in a congenitally abnormal gonad with associated sexual maldevelopment.[26] Patients with gonadoblastoma most often have pure or mixed gonadal dysgenesis or are male pseudohermaphrodites. Predominantly, karyotypes 46,XY, 45X/46,XY mosaicism, and, rarely, 46,XX or 45,X have been associated with this tumor. Gonadoblastoma is much more common in phenotypic females than in phenotypic males, with a ratio of 4 : 1. It is frequently associated with dysgerminoma and occasionally with

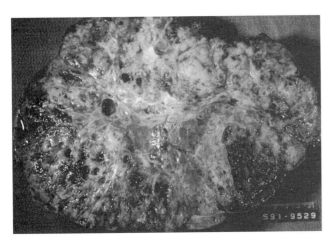

FIG. 17. Mixed germ cell tumor. Embryonal carcinoma frequently is found as part of a mixed germ cell tumor. This example is firm, solid, and cystic with extensive hemorrhage and necrosis.

other germ cell neoplasms, including yolk sac tumor, embryonal carcinoma, and choriocarcinoma.

Patients with gonadoblastoma usually complain of primary amenorrhea, virilization, or developmental abnormalities of the genitalia. It is during the workup of these conditions that gonadoblastoma is usually diagnosed. It is most frequently detected in the second decade. Hot flushes and other menopausal symptoms have been noted after tumor excision, suggesting the presence of estrogen-secreting cells in these tumors. However, the exact source of the androgen or estrogen production is unknown, as the steroid production was noted in the absence of Leydig or lutein cells.

Gonadoblastoma is more common in the right gonad than in the left, and is bilateral in 38% of patients. The tumor can range from a microscopic lesion to a mass, measuring up to 8 cm in diameter, that is soft and fleshy to firm and hard, depending on the degree of calcification. When mixed with other malignant germ cell elements, it can grow to even larger sizes. Microscopically, gonadoblastoma is composed of cellular nests containing a mixture of germ cells and immature sex cord–stromal cells, such as Sertoli and granulosa cells (Fig. 21).[14] Hyaline bodies and calcification are often present in the nests. In 50% of patients, a supervening dysgerminoma displaces most of the gonadoblastoma, pushing the cell nests to the periphery.

Treatment for patients with gonadal dysgenesis is a bilateral gonadectomy, as they have an increased risk for a germ cell tumor, especially gonadoblastoma. If the gonads are not removed and tumors develop, the prognosis of patients with pure gonadoblastoma is excellent, as long as the tumor and the other ovary are both removed. The prognosis in patients with gonadoblastoma associated with dysgerminomatous elements remains very good, even with metastases. If the gonadoblastoma is associated with other germ cell tumors, such as endodermal sinus tumor, embryonal carcinoma, or choriocarcinoma, the prognosis is poor, if untreated. However,

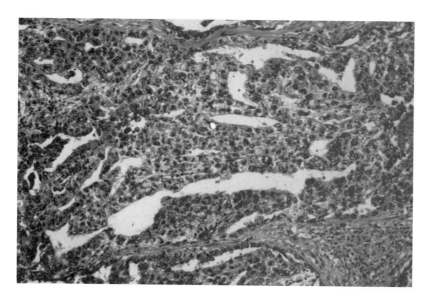

FIG. 18. Embryonal carcinoma. Tumor cells form syncytial aggregates and surround cleft-like spaces.

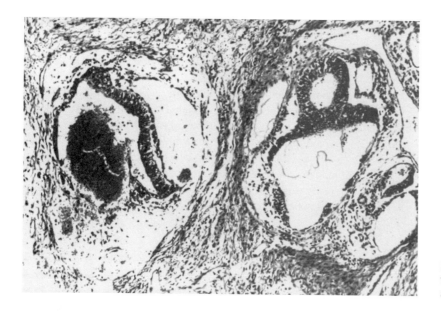

FIG. 19. Polyembryoma. In less differentiated forms, embryoid bodies may have a bizarre appearance.

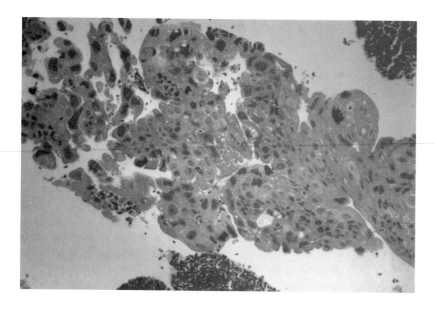

FIG. 20. Choriocarcinoma. There is a dimorphic population of malignant cytotrophoblasts and syncytiotrophoblasts. Associated hemorrhage is a common finding.

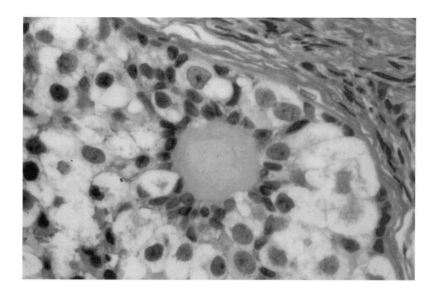

FIG. 21. Gonadoblastoma. Large germ cells are admixed with smaller sex cord derivatives that surround rounded hyaline material resembling a Call-Exner body.

combination chemotherapy (BEP) results in significant improvement, as described previously.

Sex Cord–Stromal Tumor

Sex cord–stromal tumor accounts for approximately 8% of all ovarian tumors. The origin of tumor cells may be the coelomic and mesonephric epithelium or the mesenchymal stroma of the genital ridge. This category includes an array of tumors derived from the sex cords (granulosa and Sertoli cells) and from the gonadal stroma (theca and Leydig cells). The most common types of sex cord–stromal tumor are granulosa cell tumors and fibrothecomas, whose peak age incidence is approximately 50 years. These tumors have the potential for steroid-hormone secretion, with estrogen being the predominant hormone. They are usually not seen in women younger than 20 years, except for juvenile granulosa cell tumors. (The classification of sex cord–stromal cell tumors is outlined in Table 5.)

Juvenile Granulosa Cell Tumor

Approximately 44% of all juvenile granulosa cell tumors occur in the first decade of life, and 97% in the first three decades. Isosexual pseudoprecocious puberty is commonly associated with this tumor, along with Ollier disease (enchondromatosis), Maffucci syndrome (enchondromatosis and hemangiomatosis), and abnormal karyotypes with ambiguous genitalia. Symptoms usually include abdominal pain, increasing abdominal girth, and hemoperitoneum due to rupture. Occasionally, it may be associated with pregnancy.

The gross appearance of juvenile granulosa cell tumor is commonly a large yellow-to-gray, solid and cystic mass, similar to the adult form. A mixture of granulosa and theca cells may be present. Microscopic features that distinguish juvenile granulosa cell tumor from the adult form are hyperchromatism of the tumor cells, which generally lack grooves, and the frequent luteinization of both the granulosa and theca cells.[14] The follicles are usually immature (Fig. 22). Call-Exner bod-

ies, which are pathognomonic of adult granulosa cell tumor, are rarely present in the juvenile form.

Treatment in young women usually consists of a unilateral salpingo-oophorectomy with a complete staging (see Table 3), especially if preservation of reproductive function is desired and the tumor appears to be grossly confined to one ovary. While the survival rate for stage I disease is greater than 90%, juvenile granulosa cell tumor appears to behave more aggressively in advanced disease, with a survival rate of less than 50%.[23] Isolated reports of successful treatment with various combination chemotherapies have been recorded. Due to the rarity of these tumors, a standard chemotherapeutic regimen has not emerged.

◊ AGE 20 TO 40 YEARS

Many of the tumors, both benign and malignant, that occur in the under-20-years age group are also prevalent in the 20- to 40-year age group (Fig. 23). Benign and low-malignant-potential epithelial ovarian tumors are more common in women aged 20 to 40 years. Although invasive ovarian malignancies occur in patients younger than 40 years, few are of epithelial origin. When an invasive epithelial ovarian carcinoma does occur in this age group, it may represent an inherited genetic predisposition. However, fewer than 5% of all epithelial ovarian carcinomas occur in this age group. (For discussion of malignant germ cell tumors, see the preceding section, "Age Less Than 20 Years.")

Benign Ovarian Disease

Functional Ovarian Cysts

Functional cysts may be found in postmenarcheal women who are younger than 20 years, as well as in the 20- to 40-year age group. Many of these benign ovarian cysts are associated with abnormal hormone production and are prevalent in patients of

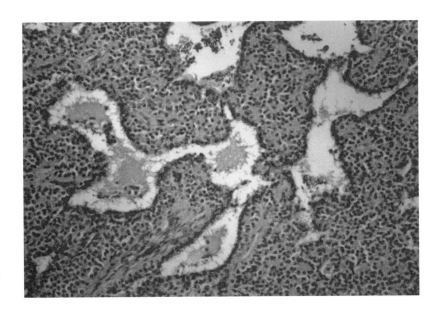

FIG. 22. Juvenile granulosa cell tumor. Tumor cells form follicles of varying sizes and shapes that contain weakly basophilic secretions.

Differential diagnosis

A.   **Benign fallopian tube disease**
    1.   **Infection(See chapter 37 on PID)**
        a.   **Acute or chronic salpingitis**
        b.   **Tuboovarian abscess**
    2.   **Ectopic pregnancy(See chapter 11 on ectopic pregnancy)**
    3.   **Benign lesions**
        a.   **Inclusion cysts and Walthard nests**
        b.   **Broad ligament cysts**
            i. **Hydatid of Morgagni**

B.   **Benign ovarian disease**
    1.   **Functional ovarian cysts(Described in preceding section)**
    2.   **Endometrioma(See chapter 42 on endometriosis)**
    3.   **Infectious process: tuboovarian abscess(See chapter 37 on PID)**
    4.   **Hyperplastic conditions**
        a.   **Polycystic ovary syndrome**
        b.   **Pregnancy luteoma**
    5.   **Germ cell tumors**
        a.   **Mature cystic teratomas(Described in previous section)**
    6.   **Benign epithelial neoplasms**
        a.   **Serous cystadenomas**
        b.   **Mucinous cystadenomas**
        c.   **Cystadenofibromas**
        d.   **Brenner tumors**
    7.   **Sex cord-stromal tumors**
        a.   **Granulosa-stromal cell tumors**
            i. **thecomas**
            ii. **fibromas**
        b.   **Androblastomas; Sertoli-Leydig cell tumors**
            i. **Leydig cell tumors: Hilus cell tumors**

C.   **Tumors of low malignant potential or atypical proliferating tumors**

E.   **Malignant ovarian disease**
    1.   **Sex cord-stromal tumors**
        a.   **Androblastomas; Sertoli-Leydig cell tumors**
            i. **Sertoli-cell tumors**
            ii. **Sertoli-Leydig cell tumors**
           iii. **Steroid-cell tumors, not otherwise specified (NOS)**

FIG. 23. Differential diagnosis for patients aged 20 to 40 years.

reproductive age. Recognizing their physiologic characteristics permits conservative therapy in the majority of patients.

Hyperplastic Conditions

Polycystic Ovarian Syndrome

Polycystic ovarian syndrome (PCO), also known as Stein-Leventhal syndrome, typically affects patients in the third decade, although it may rarely be seen in adolescent girls. It is estimated that 3.5% to 7% of the female population have this syndrome. Patients may present with multiple symptoms, including endocrine abnormalities related to anovulation, premenarcheal obesity, secondary amenorrhea or oligomenorrhea, infertility, and hirsutism. Ovarian enlargement may not always be detected on physical examination or pelvic ultrasound. PCO most likely represents a spectrum of disorders from a centralized hypothalamic–pituitary abnormality to a localized ovarian dysfunction that leads to the common clinical findings described above. A familial tendency has been postulated with an autosomal-dominant or X-linked inheritance.

Other important clinical findings due to unopposed estrogen are endometrial hyperplasia or endometrial carcinoma. These patients are usually premenopausal and obese. The pathology is usually a noninvasive well differentiated adenocarcinoma, reflecting unopposed estrogen stimulation due to chronic anovulation.

PCO characteristically involves both ovaries, which are typically round to oval and two to five times normal size. Cut surface usually reveals a thickened, white, superficial cortex and numerous follicle cysts (Fig. 24). Microscopically, the cysts lie beneath the superficially fibrotic cortex, lined by an inner layer of nonluteinized granulosa cells and an outer thicker layer of luteinized theca interna cells. Both maturing and atretic follicles may be present, but there is no evidence of ovulation. Ovarian hyperthecosis or any other hormone-producing ovarian lesion should be distinguished from PCO. Treatment may include oral contraceptives, danazol (Danocrine), or a gonadotropin-releasing hormone agonist; in those who desire pregnancy, ovary-stimulating drugs may be used.

Luteoma of Pregnancy

Pregnancy luteoma is a nonneoplastic, hyperplastic condition that may affect both ovaries and usually occurs in the third or fourth decades. In some women, the condition is noted as an incidental finding during cesarean section or postpartum tubal ligation. In others, it may result in late-pregnancy hirsutism or virilization or, if very large, obstruction of the birth canal. Virilization of a female infant may occasionally be seen, characterized by clitoromegaly and labial fusion. Spontaneous regression of these lesions usually occurs after termination of the pregnancy.

The ovary appears as a large, solid, fleshy, red-gray nodular mass measuring up to 20 cm in diameter. Microscopically, there is nodular hyperplasia of the luteinized granulosa and theca cells of adjacent follicles (Fig. 25). These cells usually contain abundant eosinophilic cytoplasm and little or no lipid. Production of hCG probably plays an important role in the pathogenesis of this condition. Surgical treatment is not usually needed, unless the diagnosis is unclear.

Benign Epithelial Neoplasms

Serous Cystadenoma

Serous and mucinous cystadenomas are the most common benign epithelial ovarian neoplasms. Serous tumors account for approximately 25% of all benign ovarian neoplasms, with an age range of 20 to 50 years; they are bilateral in 12% to 20% of patients. Symptoms are variable. For many patients, the diagnosis is made during routine pelvic examination.

Grossly, serous cystadenoma is a cystic, usually unilocular lesion, ranging from 5 to 15 cm in diameter. The inner

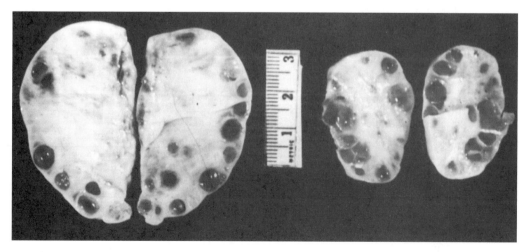

FIG. 24. Gross appearance of the cut surfaces of bilateral polycystic ovaries.

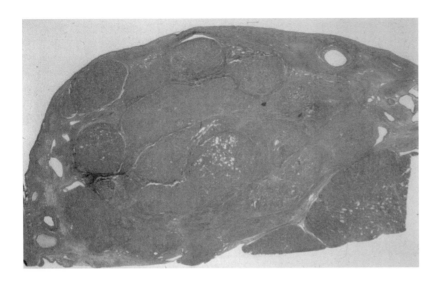

FIG. 25. Pregnancy luteoma. The ovary is replaced by nodular proliferations of luteinized cells.

lining of the cyst wall may be flat or partially covered by papillary projections (Fig. 26). Microscopically, the epithelial lining can range from simple cuboidal cells, resembling the ovarian surface epithelium, to tall columnar cells, resembling the fallopian tube (Fig. 27).[15] Ciliated and secretory cells may be present. Mitoses are rare, and nuclear atypia is absent. Psammoma bodies, which are concentric calcifications, are seen in 15% of tumors. Multiple, large, calcified deposits may be visible on radiologic examination of the abdomen. The stroma may vary from fibrous to cellular to hyalinized with marked stromal edema. The papillary processes are fibrous and lined by a single layer of epithelial cells.

The preoperative workup depends on patient age and the degree of suspicion of malignancy. A unilateral salpingo-oophorectomy is usually performed in patients who have completed childbearing. In those desiring future reproduction, a ovarian cystectomy is usually performed. A bilateral salpingo-oophorectomy may be performed in selected individuals, particularly in those with bilateral tumors. In such cases, discussion of a hysterectomy is reasonable but not necessary.

Mucinous Cystadenoma

Mucinous cystadenoma accounts for approximately 25% of all benign ovarian neoplasms, with an age range of 20 to 50; in 2% to 3% of patients it is bilateral. The tumor arises from the surface epithelium of the ovary, resembling müllerian-type epithelium of the endocervix, intestinal-type epithelium, or both these types. Because of the large size that this tumor attains, patients usually present with a palpable pelvic/abdominal mass and may have associated pain.

Gross evaluation of a mucinous cystadenoma reveals that it is usually multilocular and larger than its serous counterpart, ranging up to 50 cm or more in diameter. The external surface is usually smooth, pinkish gray, and sometimes lobulated. Inside, locules tend to be small and contain thick, sticky, tenacious mucinous material (Fig. 28). Microscopically, the epithelium consists of a single layer of uniform tall columnar cells that resemble a picket fence in the endocervical type (Fig. 29). The cytoplasm is clear, and nuclei are small and basally oriented. Goblet, argentaffin, and Paneth cells may be seen, depending on tumor type. Tumor stroma is fibrocollagenous and variably cellular.

Treatment is similar to that for serous cystadenoma. The appendix should be carefully inspected for an associated mucocele, which would require removal.

Cystadenofibroma

As the name suggests, cystadenofibroma is a variant of serous cystadenoma, containing both cystic and solid components. This benign tumor is usually unilateral and has a similar age distribution to that of serous cystadenoma. It is variably papillary to solid (Fig. 30). Papillae are broad, firm, and nonfriable.

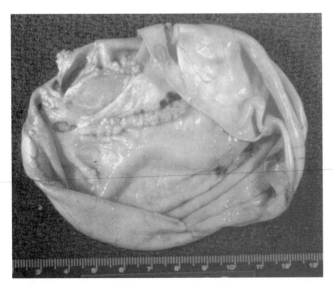

FIG. 26. Serous cystadenoma. Coarse papillations cover part of the inner lining.

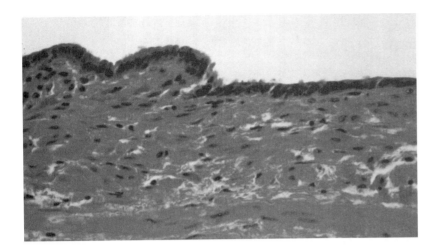

FIG. 27. Serous cystadenoma. The lining epithelium commonly appears tubal.

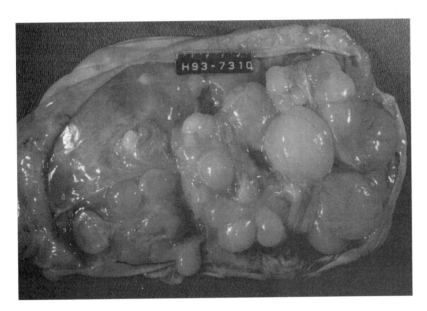

FIG. 28. Mucinous cystadenoma. The tumor is multilocular.

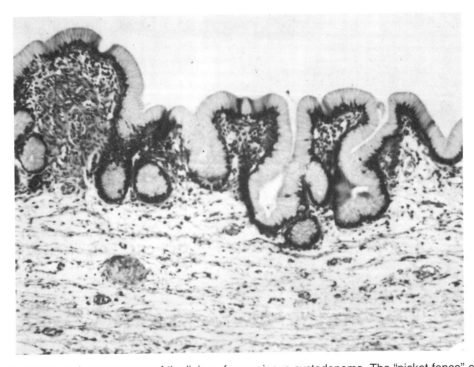

FIG. 29. Microscopic appearance of the lining of a mucinous cystadenoma. The "picket fence" epithelium is characteristic of this tumor.

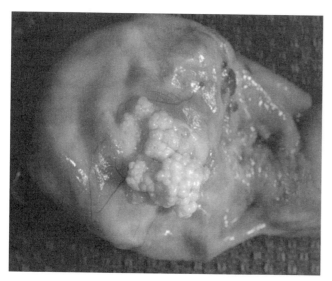

FIG. 30. Cystadenofibroma. Blunt, coarse papillations are seen in this example.

Microscopically, solid areas are found to contain small cystic structures that are histologically identical to serous cysts. As with other benign epithelial ovarian tumors, treatment is individualized based on patient age and reproductive desire.

Brenner Tumor

Also known as transitional cell tumor, Brenner tumor constitutes 2% of all primary ovarian tumors. Patients with this tumor range in age from 30 to 70 years, with a mean age of 50 years. Brenner tumor is thought to be derived from ovarian surface epithelium that undergoes a metaplastic transformation to cells resembling urothelium. It may occur synchronously with mucinous cystadenoma. Most transitional cell tumors are benign, but transformation to a malignant form

has been observed. Presentation may be variable, as the tumor may be asymptomatic or may present with a palpable mass or pain. Occasionally, patients may present with vaginal bleeding, probably due to hormonal activity in the stroma.

Grossly, the tumor is solid—less commonly cystic—and usually unilateral, although 6% to 7% of tumors are bilateral (Fig. 31). Ranging in size from microscopic to as large as 30 cm in diameter, it is usually gray, white, or yellow, with a faintly lobulated cut surface. Microscopic review depicts a characteristic pattern of circumscribed epithelial nests of cells embedded in an abundant fibromatous stroma (Fig. 32).[15] Epithelial cells may be round to polygonal, with eosinophilic or clear cytoplasm. When longitudinal grooves of the nuclei are present, the cells are described as having a "coffee bean" appearance. Often, these nests of epithelial cells undergo benign cystic changes lined by either transitional cells or mucinous cells. Treatment is usually resection of the tumor, and this may involve a cystectomy or salpingo-oophorectomy with or without a hysterectomy, depending on patient age and reproductive desires.

Sex Cord–Stromal Tumors

Although benign sex cord–stromal tumors are seen in any age group, they are more common in the over-40-years age group.

Thecoma

Thecoma is a benign tumor affecting all ages, with a predominance in the postmenopausal group; it is rare in patients younger than 35 years. It accounts for 2% of all ovarian tumors. Many women with a thecoma present with abnormal or postmenopausal uterine bleeding; some present with an endometrial adenocarcinoma as a result of unopposed estrogen production by the tumor. Thecoma is composed of lipid-laden

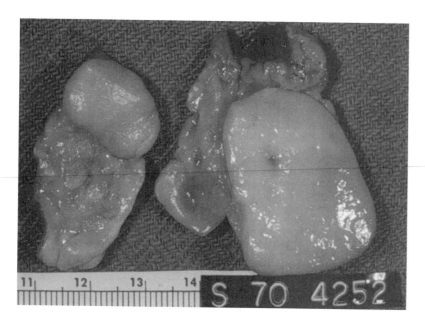

FIG. 31. Brenner tumor. The tumor is solid and circumscribed.

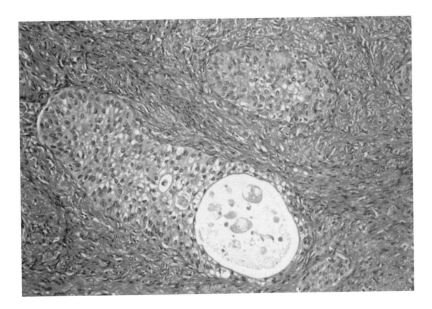

FIG. 32. Brenner tumor. Epithelial nests embedded in a fibromatous stroma may show cystic change. Longitudinal grooves in the cells can impart a "coffee bean" appearance.

stromal cells resembling theca cells. Rather than arising as a *de novo* neoplasm, it may represent changes occurring in background cortical stromal hyperplasia.

Tumor size ranges from a nonpalpable incidental finding to a large solid mass with a diameter of 15 to 20 cm. It is usually unilateral and almost never malignant. Its outer surface is smooth, and its cut surface is typically solid, lobulated, and yellow (Fig. 33). Cystic change may be seen. Microscopic evaluation reveals masses of oval or round cells with abundant, pale, lipid-containing cytoplasm. Hyaline plaques are often noted. A luteinized thecoma sometimes occurs, usually in younger women.

Treatment for thecoma is tailored to patient age and ranges from a total abdominal hysterectomy and bilateral salpingo-oophorectomy for menopausal or postmenopausal women to a salpingo-oophorectomy or ovarian cystectomy, if possible, in patients who desire future fertility.

Fibroma

Like thecoma, fibroma is also a benign tumor affecting all ages, although most occur in women aged 40 to 60 years; fewer than 10% of patients are 30 years of age or younger. Fibroma is not associated with hormone production. In some cases, hydrothorax and ascites are found in association with a pelvic mass—a constellation of findings known as Meigs syndrome. In other cases, fibroma is seen in patients with a hereditary basal cell nevus syndrome, characterized by early-appearing basal cell carcinomas, keratocysts of the jaw, calcification of the dura, and mesenteric cysts.

Fibroma, like thecoma, ranges in size from a nonpalpable incidental finding to larger than 20 cm; it is usually unilateral but multinodular. Cut surface is firm and hard and has a whorled appearance (Fig. 34). Microscopically, fibroma is composed of bundles of collagen-producing spindle cells arranged in a stori-

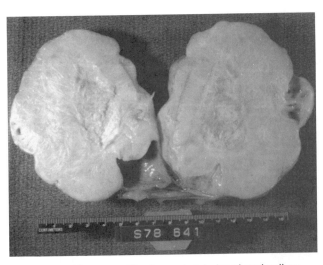

FIG. 33. Thecoma. The tumor is lobulated and yellow.

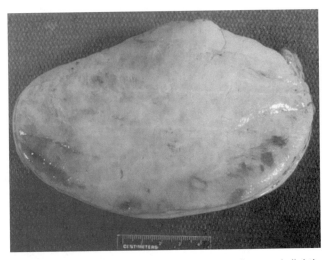

FIG. 34. Fibroma. Cut surface is solid, white, firm, and slightly edematous.

form pattern (Fig. 35). Hyalinization and intercellular edema are characteristic. The cytoplasm of tumor cells may contain small quantities of lipid, making distinction from thecoma difficult.

Treatment is similar to that for thecoma. In patients with Meigs syndrome, the hydrothorax and ascites usually resolve after resection of the pelvic tumor.

Androblastoma and Sertoli-Leydig Cell Tumor

Leydig Cell Tumor: Hilus Cell Tumor is a subtype of Leydig cell tumor, originating from the ovarian hilus. The other subtype, which is very rare, is a nonhilar-type Leydig cell tumor, derived from ovarian stromal cells and having similar clinical and pathologic features. The average age of patients with a hilus cell tumor is 58 years, and many present with symptoms of abnormal menstruation, hirsutism, and virilization. Some may present with estrogenic manifestations. Hilus cell tumor is are almost always benign.

Grossly, this tumor is circumscribed, lobulated, solid, soft, and red to yellow. Tumor enlargement is usually minimal, and the tumor is often physically undetectable. Sometimes, it is incidentally discovered when the ovaries are pathologically sectioned for another purpose. Microscopic evaluation reveals circumscribed masses of steroid cells with abundant eosinophilic cytoplasm. Lipochrome pigment may also be present.[15] The diagnostic elongate eosinophilic crystalloids of Reinke must be found for the tumor to be definitively classified as a Leydig cell neoplasm. Treatment of this benign tumor is unilateral salpingo-oophorectomy or ovarian cystectomy if future fertility is desired.

Tumors of Low Malignant Potential (Atypical Proliferating Tumors)

Epidemiology

Ovarian tumors of low malignant potential (LMP), also known as atypical proliferating tumors, comprise a group of tumors showing greater epithelial proliferation than that seen in benign serous cystadenoma, although they are by definition noninvasive.[3,18] Recognized by FIGO in 1971, LMP ovarian tumors account for approximately 15% of all epithelial ovarian cancers; mean age of occurrence is 40 years. A metaanalysis performed by the Collaborative Ovarian Cancer Group found that, as with malignant epithelial ovarian cancer, parity, multiple births, history of breast-feeding, and oral contraceptive use are protective against LMP tumors. A history of infertility and use of infertility drugs increase the risk of developing an LMP tumor, although the data are weak and controversial. Prospective trials are needed to resolve the controversy surrounding the use of infertility drugs and these tumors.

Clinical Features

Patients usually present with a pelvic mass and complaints of abdominal and pelvic pain, increasing abdominal girth, or abnormal bleeding. Ultrasound or computed tomography (CT) scan may be helpful in making the diagnosis of an ovarian mass. Serum CA 125 levels are not always elevated. When they are, the tumor is usually of serous histology, and CA 125 levels are not as high as when a malignancy is present. LMP tumors usually have an indolent course. Many biomarkers, such as DNA ploidy, tumor markers, oncogenes, and defects in tumor suppressor genes, have been studied in an attempt to define a high-risk group or predict aggressive tumor behavior, and thus indicate which patients might benefit from adjuvant treatment. To date, no such marker has been identified.

Pathology

LMP ovarian tumors have been described for all epithelial ovarian subtypes; the most common types are serous and mucinous tumors. The absence of stromal invasion is an absolute criterion for making the diagnosis. Careful examination of the tissue blocks is necessary to minimize the potential for omitting

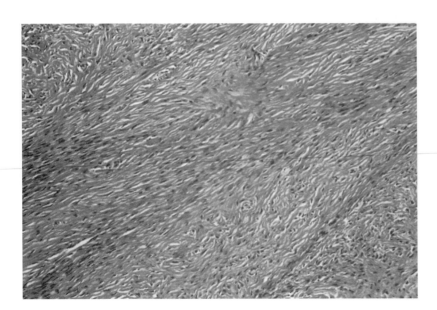

FIG. 35. Fibroma. The tumor is composed of intersecting bundles of spindled cells.

an area of invasive carcinoma in LMP tumors. Approximately 20% to 30% of ovarian tumors diagnosed as borderline at frozen section prove to be carcinomas on review of the permanent section.[34] The mean diameter of serous LMP tumors is 12 cm, and bilateral tumors are reported in 33% to 75% of patients. These tumors are usually cystic with mural clusters of papillary projections (Figs. 36 and 37).

Mucinous LMP tumors are larger than their serous counterparts, with an average diameter of 17 to 20 cm; they are infrequently bilateral. They are characterized by multiloculated cystic masses, with smooth outer surfaces and areas of papillations and solid thickening on the inner surface (Fig. 38). Microscopically, the epithelial lining of the cysts consists of tall, columnar, mucin-secreting cells, resembling the epithelium of the endocervix or intestine. Stratified epithelial cells may be atypical with hyperchromatic nuclei and mitotic figures, but without stromal invasion (Fig. 39). More than 80% of women with advanced-staged disease present with a syndrome of pseudomyxoma peritonei, which is now thought to develop secondary to a mucinous tumor of the appendix.[36] Thus, in the setting of pseudomyxoma peritonei, an appendectomy should be performed, regardless of the gross appearance of the appendix.

Recognizing that some (5% to 10%) advanced LMP tumors (stage II or higher) recur and behave aggressively as an ovarian carcinoma, while others are very indolent like a benign ovarian tumor, Seidman and Kurman[31] recently examined this classification of ovarian tumors, especially serous and mucinous borderline tumors. Distinct histologic features were identified in the serous borderline tumors that are believed to be predictors of prognostic outcome. These investigators believe that LMP tumors are actually a heterogeneous group of tumors, both histologically and clinically, that can be divided into three groups:

◊ Micropapillary serous carcinoma,
◊ Serous borderline tumor with noninvasive implants,
◊ Serous borderline tumor with invasive implants.

Stage for stage, the 5-year survival rate for patients with LMP epithelial ovarian tumors is far better than that for patients with malignant epithelial ovarian cancer. A review of the literature by several investigators revealed a survival rate of greater than 95% in patients with stage I LMP ovarian tumors. Furthermore, Kurman and Trimble found that a majority of patients with LMP tumors actually died with the disease, not from it, as invasive carcinoma developed in only 8 (0.8%) of 953 patients with a mean follow-up of 7 years.[16] The other patients died from radiation- or chemotherapy-associated complications. Using the new classification for LMP tumors, patients with micropapillary serous carcinoma were found to have 5- and 10-year survival rates of 81% and 71%, respectively. Patients with a serous borderline tumor without invasive implants (atypical proliferative serous tumor) had 5- and 10-year survival rates of greater than 98%. However, in serous borderline tumor with invasive implants, survival rates drop to 33% at 5 and 10 years. Thus, atypical proliferative serous tumor and serous borderline tumor without invasive implants follow in a very benign clinical course. Micropapillary serous carcinoma has a tendency for late recurrence. Finally, serous borderline tumor with invasive implants has a clinical behavior and survival rate similar to those of an invasive primary epithelial ovarian carcinoma.

Micropapillary serous carcinoma is characterized by thin, elongated micropapillae with minimal or no fibrovascular support arising directly from thick, more centrally located papillary structures (Fig. 40). Cells are uniform and round with minimal nuclear atypia and scanty cytoplasm. Mitotic activity may be seen in some of the cases, ranging from one to three figures per 10 high-power fields. Peritoneal implants associated with micropapillary serous carcinoma are invasive in most cases. The distinction between serous borderline tumors with or without invasive implants may be difficult. Noninvasive implants usually have a scant epithelial component surrounded by reactive spindle cells with imperceptibly meshed epithelial and stromal cells (Fig. 41). On the other hand, invasive implants usually have a more cellular epithelial component, with complex epithelial proliferation composed of multiple micropapillae and small round nests that display a destructive infiltrative growth (Fig. 42). Sometimes, a tumor with invasive implants may not show any evidence of invasion in the primary tumor. It should be considered a borderline tumor with concomitant extraovarian (peritoneal) serous carcinoma and should be treated accordingly.

Treatment

The primary surgical treatment for patients with LMP tumors who have completed childbearing is identical to the recom-

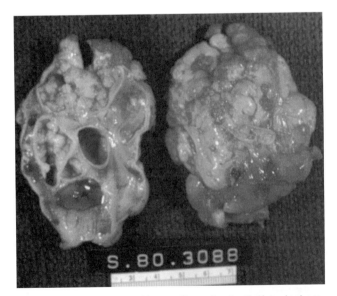

FIG. 36. Serous tumor of low malignant potential/atypical proliferating tumor. On the right is the external surface of the ovary; on the left the cut surface. The tumor is multicystic, and within some cysts are complex papillary projections.

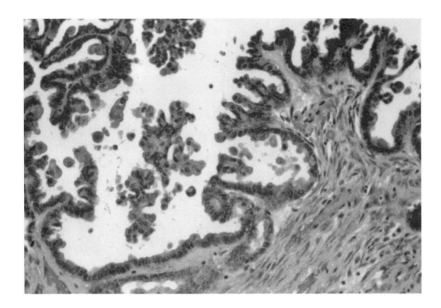

FIG. 37. Serous tumor of low malignant potential/atypical proliferating tumor. Ramifying papillae are lined by a relatively bland serous epithelium that forms tufts and seemingly free-floating clusters.

mendation for invasive ovarian disease, including a total abdominal hysterectomy, bilateral salpingo-oophorectomy, tumor debulking, and full staging (see Table 3). An appendectomy should be performed in patients with a mucinous LMP tumor because of the association with a synchronous primary appendiceal tumor.

In younger patients with early-stage diagnosis and a desire for future childbearing, conservative surgery with preservation of the uterus, the contralateral ovary, and in some cases the ipsilateral ovary (i.e., cystectomy) may be the appropriate treatment. Consultation with a gynecologic oncologist and pathologist can identify those patients who are candidate for conservative management. Several studies, both cohort and observational, have reported excellent outcome with conservative management of such patients (*n*=147). Fewer than 10% (10/147) of reported cases had recurrent disease.[18] The feasibility of doing a cystectomy for an LMP ovarian tumor and conserving the rest of the ovarian tissue in early-stage disease has been reported; however, the data are mostly observational (4/35 with recurrence).[3,18]

LMP ovarian tumors have also been diagnosed during pregnancy. Conservative surgery is usually performed, and pregnancy does not appear to be deleterious in regard to the prognosis for these patients. Most patients went on to deliver at full term without any complications.

Postoperative Therapy

Presently, there is no evidence to suggest that adjuvant chemotherapy in early-stage disease or in patients with optimal cytoreduction of advanced disease improves survival in patients with LMP tumors. In fact, patients may be more likely to die from the side effects of adjuvant therapy than from the disease itself. Therefore, adjuvant therapy is not recommended after surgery. Although recurrence of the disease has been reported during long-term follow-up, there is meager evidence to suggest the use of chemotherapy in these patients. An ongoing prospective Gynecologic Oncology Group trial will address these issues. Second-look laparotomy should not be a part of the standard therapy in treating these patients. Patients with pseudomyxoma peritonei should be treated similarly to patients with primary appendiceal cancer with widespread metastasis.

Malignant Ovarian Disease

Malignant ovarian disease occurring in the 20- to 40-years age group is commonly a sex cord–stromal cell tumor. Epithelial ovarian carcinoma does occur but is rare. Genetic predisposition may be a factor associated with epithelial ovarian carcinomas in this age group. The management of these patients

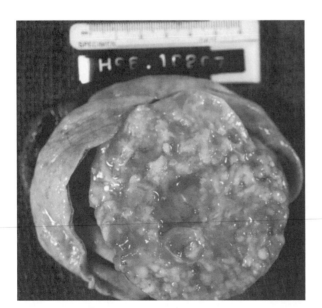

FIG. 38. Mucinous tumor of low malignant potential/atypical proliferating tumor. The tumor is multilocular and cystic, but the cysts are smaller and more compact than in mucinous cystadenoma.

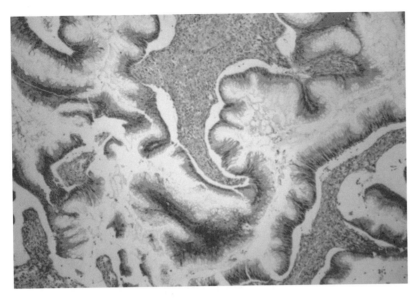

FIG. 39. Mucinous tumor of low malignant potential/atypical proliferating tumor. Epithelial proliferation results in pseudostratification and tufting. Mild cytologic atypia is present.

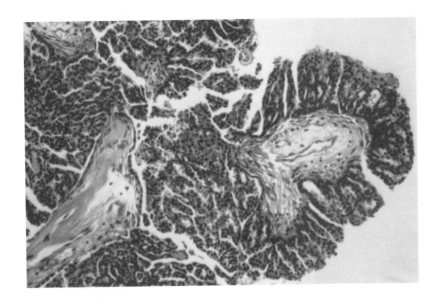

FIG. 40. Micropapillary serous carcinoma. In this fully malignant serous carcinoma, strands of neoplastic cells stream from thick, fibrous cores, stimulating a Medusa-head.

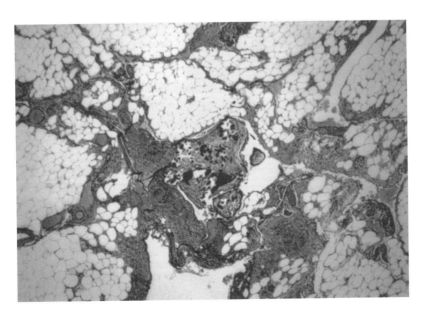

FIG. 41. Noninvasive implant in a serous borderline tumor. A circumscribed focus of tumor is surround by fibroadipose tissue that shows no stromal reaction. Cell nests are heavily calcified.

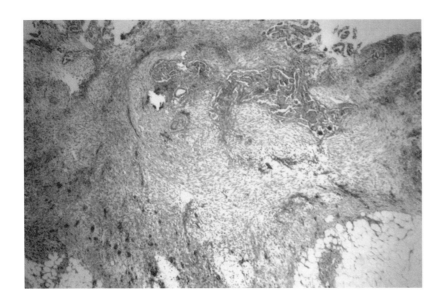

FIG. 42. Invasive implant in a serous border-line tumor. The tumor here is more cellular. The invasive implant extends below the peritoneal surface and is associated with reactive desmoplasia.

(discussed in the next section) presents an interesting challenge to the gynecologist.

Sex Cord–Stromal Tumors: Sertoli-Leydig Cell Tumors

Sertoli-Leydig cell tumors are also termed Sertoli–stromal cell tumors and can be further divided into several subtypes (Table 5). Stage and tumor differentiation seem to be important prognostic factors. Despite the name of these tumors, hormone production is not always associated with them. Tumors that produce hormones may result in masculine or feminine phenotypes, as few of the tumors actually produce estrogen or progesterone.

Sertoli Cell Tumor

Sertoli cell tumor is very rare. Patients, ranging in age from 7 to 79 years (median, 33 years), usually present with a pelvic and/or abdominal mass. If the mass is functional, patients may present with some form of estrogenic effect, such as endometrial hyperplasia or isosexual precocious pseudopuberty. Androgenic and progestogenic effects may also occur. Most tumors are stage I unilateral masses that are well circumscribed, averaging about 9 cm in diameter. Cut surface reveals solid, yellow-to-brown, lobulated masses. Microscopic evaluation discloses closely packed hollow or solid tubules lined by Sertoli cells that can also contain abundant cytoplasmic lipid.[15] An association between Sertoli cell tumors and Peutz-Jeghers syndrome has been reported in the literature.

Most Sertoli cell tumors are benign or early-stage malignant neoplasms that are cured with surgery. Conservative surgery with a unilateral salpingo-oophorectomy is indicated in many of these patients who are young and desire preservation of ovarian function. Only rarely are these tumors poorly differentiated and aggressive. Experience with chemotherapy in these tumors is limited due to their rarity.

Sertoli-Leydig Cell Tumor

Sertoli-Leydig cell tumor accounts for less than 0.5% of all ovarian tumors. It is most often seen in young women, with a mean age of occurrence of 25 years. Fewer than 10% of these tumors occur in women older than age 50 years, and fewer than 5% occur in prepubertal girls. Sertoli-Leydig cell tumor is often associated with androgen production; however, virilization develops in only 50% patients. This may be due to a lack of hormone production or insufficient androgen production. Typically, patients complain of oligomenorrhea followed by amenorrhea, breast atrophy, acne, hirsutism, temporal balding, deepening of the voice, and enlargement of the clitoris. The latter two symptoms may not resolve after tumor removal. Patients without endocrine manifestations may present with complaints of abdominal swelling or pain. Occasionally, symptoms of estrogen production, due to the Sertoli cell component of the tumor or peripheral androgenic

TABLE 5. *World Health Organization classification of sex cord–stromal tumors*

Granulosa stromal cell
  Granulosa cell
  Thecoma-fibroma
Androblastoma: Sertoli-Leydig cell tumors
  1. Well differentiated
    Sertoli cell tumor
    Sertoli-Leydig cell tumor
    Leydig cell tumor; hilus cell tumor
    Steroid cell tumors
  2. Intermediate differentiation
  3. Poorly differentiated (sarcomatoid)
  4. With heterologous elements
Gynandroblastoma
Unclassified

(From Serov SF, Scully RE, Robin IH. *Histological typing of ovarian tumors: international histological classification of tumors, no. 9.* Geneva: World Health Organization, 1973; with permission.)

conversion, may be seen such as menorrhagia or menometror-rhagia. Sertoli-Leydig cell tumor must be distinguished from other virilizing tumors, such as adrenal tumors, which are often associated with an elevated urinary level of 17-ketosteroids; the urinary level of 17-ketosteroids in Sertoli-Leydig cell tumor is usually normal or only slightly elevated. Serum AFP level may be increased and may be useful as a tumor marker.

The gross appearance of Sertoli-Leydig cell tumor is highly variable. Overall, it has an average diameter of 12 to 15 cm, and its cut surface is usually tan or yellow and may be cystic (Fig. 43). Hemorrhage and necrosis are frequently seen in the poorly differentiated tumors. On microscopic examination, the tumor is composed of a mixture of Sertoli, Leydig, and undifferentiated gonadal stromal cells, with or without heterologous components, in varying proportions and degrees of differentiation.[15] In well differentiated lesions, Sertoli cells from tubules and Leydig cells are found in the intervening stroma (Fig. 44). Sertoli cells are cytologically bland, and mitotic figures are rare. Leydig cells may contain abundant lipochrome pigment or crystalloids of Reinke. Intermediate and poorly differentiated tumors are characterized by more immature components of the Sertoli and Leydig cells. Cartilage, mucinous epithelium, skeletal muscle, and other heterologous elements are found in 20% to 25% of these tumors, most of which are of intermediate differentiation. In those instances in which heterologous elements have been found in poorly differentiated neoplasms, the tumors are clinically malignant. Sertoli-Leydig cell tumor with a reti-form pattern may be seen with prominent hyalinized cores and papillae lined by stratified epithelial cells.

The treatment for Sertoli-Leydig cell tumor usually depends on patient age and tumor stage, degree of differentiation, and presence of heterologous elements in the tumor. The most important prognostic factor is stage. In young women with a stage Ia well differentiated tumor who desire future pregnancy, a unilateral salpingo-oophorectomy and a staging procedure are adequate treatment (see Table 3). However, more aggressive cytoreductive surgery, including

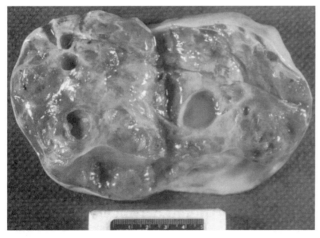

FIG. 43. Sertoli-Leydig cell tumor. Cut surface is yellow-brown, soft, and partially cystic.

a hysterectomy and bilateral salpingo-oophorectomy, tumor resection and staging procedure may be indicated in post-menopausal patients or those with more advanced disease.

Adjuvant therapy is recommended for patients who have stage Ia lesions with poorly differentiated elements or heter-ologous components or for those who have heterologous elements or metastatic disease. However, due to the limited number of cases, no standard adjuvant therapy has been accepted for these patients. Most of the information available comes from small series and case reports. Treatment of advanced sex cord–stromal cell tumors, unlike germ cell tumors, has not met with much success. Platinum-based therapies have yielded the best results with an overall survival of approximately 50%.[12] These include the PAC, VBP, and BEP regimens. Similar to chemotherapy, radiotherapy has been used successfully in limited cases.

Steroid Cell Tumors Not Otherwise Specified

Termed lipid cell or lipoid tumors in the past, these are tumors composed entirely of cells resembling typical steroid hormone–secreting cells (e.g., lutein cells, Leydig cells, and adrenal cortical cells), except that specific features such as location of origin in the hilus or crystalloids of Reinke are not identified. Steroid cell tumors not otherwise specified (NOS) account for approximately 0.1% of all ovarian tumors, with a mean age of occurrence of 43 to 60 years. Androgenic changes, occurring in 75% to 90% of patients, may be of many years' duration. Estrogenic and progestogenic changes are occasionally noted. Although the estrogenic manifestations may be a result of estrogen production by the tumors, the aromatization of androgen to estradiol in adipose tissue may be more plausible. Cushing syndrome may also be found in some patients, accompanied by elevated serum cortisol levels. Diagnosis is often dependent on the clinical manifestation of virilization or the rare occasion of isosexual pseudoprecocity. Tumor removal results in rapid resolution of most of the hormonal effects, except for deepening of the voice and clitoromegaly.

Grossly, steroid cell tumors NOS are solid, well circum-scribed, and yellow to orange-tan, measuring 5 to 8 cm in diameter. Hemorrhage, necrosis, and cystic degeneration are occasionally observed. Cut surface of the tumor is soft and lobulated. Microscopically, tumor cells may resemble Leydig or hilar cells (Fig. 45). In other instances, cells have abundant pale cytoplasm, resembling adrenocortical cells.[15] These cells are polygonal to round and larger than Leydig cells, with central nuclei and lipid-rich cytoplasm. The striking resemblance of many of these tumors to adrenocortical tumors has led some to speculate that they may arise from the adreno-cortical rests. The association with manifestations of Cushing syndrome would seem to support this theory, and detailed examination has revealed the presence of these rests in the broad ligament and the ovarian hilus. Alternatively, given the fact that steroid cell tumors NOS are often confined to the ovary may simply mean that adrenocortical hormones are being produced by cells of ovarian origin rather than by

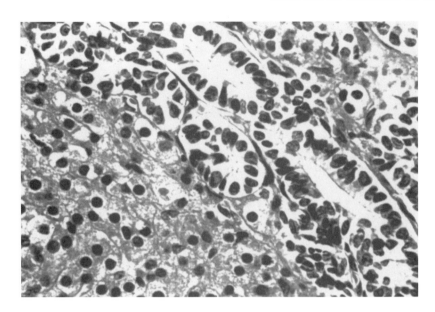

FIG. 44. Sertoli-Leydig cell tumor. This well differentiated tumor is composed of hollow tubules lined by Sertoli cells and adjacent sheets of Leydig cells.

an ectopic adrenal tumor. Steroid cell tumors NOS are rarely malignant; approximately 10% to 15% of them recur or metastasize.

A unilateral salpingo-oophorectomy is adequate for stage Ia disease in young, reproductive-age women. An abdominal hysterectomy and bilateral salpingo-oophorectomy with staging and resection of all extraovarian disease are indicated in women with advanced disease or in those beyond reproductive age.

◊ AGE 40 YEARS AND BEYOND

The most common ovarian malignancy in women aged 40 years and older is epithelial ovarian carcinoma, with the incidence increasing after age 55 years. Many patients present with signs and symptoms of metastatic disease. Others may present with an adnexal mass, for which a spectrum of differential diagnostic possibilities must be considered (Fig. 46). Careful preoperative evaluation of patients should provide the clinician with sufficient information to accurately predict whether a mass is benign or malignant. The most appropriate surgical team can then be assembled.

Fallopian Tube Carcinoma

Primary Fallopian Tube Epithelial Carcinoma

More than 96% of all fallopian tube tumors are invasive epithelial tumors, yet fallopian tube carcinoma is still one of the rarest gynecologic malignancies, with an average annual incidence of 3.6 per 1 million women. The youngest reported age of occurrence is 14 years, with the rate rising sharply, peaking at ages 60 to 64 years. Recent epidemiologic observational data suggest that age and nulliparity are factors associated with fallopian tube carcinoma, similar to endometrial and ovarian carcinoma.[25] In the past, others have reported the frequent occurrence of salpingitis in patients with fallopian tube carcinoma

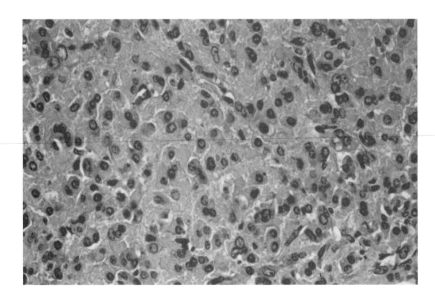

FIG. 45. Steroid cell tumor not otherwise specified. If crystalloids of Reinke were identified in these cells, the tumor would be classified as a Leydig cell tumor or possibly a hilus cell tumor, depending on the tumor's location. The granular appearance of the cytoplasm in these polygonal-to-rounded tumor cells suggests that they contain little lipid.

Differential diagnosis

A.   **Benign fallopian tube disease**
B.   **Fallopian tube cancers**
       1.   **Epithelial tumors**
       2.   **Sarcomas**
       3.   **Choriocarcinomas**
       4.   **Metastatic tumors**
C.   **Benign ovarian disease**
       1.   **Functional cysts**
       2.   **Endometriomas(see chapter 42 on endometriosis)**
       3.   **Infectious process: tuboovarian abscess(see chapter 37 on PID)**
       4.   **Benign epithelial neoplasms**
            a.   **Serous cystadenomas**
            b.   **Mucinous cystadenomas**
            c.   **Cystadenofibromas**
            d.   **Brenner tumors**
       5.   **Sex cord-stromal tumors**
            a.   **thecomas**
            b.   **fibromas**
            c.   **Hilus cell tumors**
D.   **Tumor of low malignant potential**
E.   **Malignant epithelial tumors**
       1.   **Serous tumors**
       2.   **Mucinous tumors**
       3.   **Endometrioid tumors**
       4.   **Clear cell tumors**
       5.   **Undifferentiated carcinomas**
       6.   **Brenner tumors**
       7.   **Müllerian mesenchymal and Mixed tumors**
            a.   **Adenosarcoma**
            b.   **Malignant mixed mesodermal tumor**
F.   **Sex-cord stromal tumors**
       1   **Granulosa cell tumors**
       2.   **Androblastomas; Sertoli-stromal cell tumors**
            a.   **Sertoli-leydig cell tumors**
            b.   **Steroid cell tumors**

FIG. 46. Differential diagnosis for patients aged 40 years and older.

and have indicated that tubal infection may play an important role in the pathogenesis of the disease. However, the prevalence of pelvic inflammatory disease and the rarity of fallopian tube carcinoma make the argument suspect.

Patients may present with symptoms of pelvic pain, a pelvic mass, and serosanguineous vaginal discharge. Hydrops tubae profluens is characterized by colicky lower abdominal pain relieved by a profuse, serous, watery, yellow intermittent vaginal discharge.[25] Although not present in all cases, it is thought to be the classic finding in fallopian tube carcinoma. Other symptoms include abnormal vaginal bleeding, abdominal distention, urinary urgency, altered bowel function, lower back pain, and an acute abdomen from torsion or intraperitoneal bleeding. The most common physical sign is a pelvic or abdominal mass. This mass is often thought to be an ovarian mass, with the correct diagnosis made at surgery. Occasionally, a Pap smear revealing abnormal glandular cells with negative cervical or endometrial findings may lead the clinician to the correct location of the neoplasm. Serum CA 125 levels are often elevated in advanced disease, as is noted in 80% of ovarian carcinoma patients. Unlike those with ovarian cancer, many patients with fallopian tube cancer present with early-stage disease. In a review of several series, two-thirds of patients with fallopian tube carcinoma presented with stage I (33%) or stage II (34%) disease.[25] A staging classification for fallopian tube cancer, established by FIGO in 1991, is listed in Table 6.

Fallopian tube carcinoma is usually characterized by swollen tubes secondary to intraluminal growth. An infectious etiology is ruled out only after opening the specimen. Cut section reveals a lumen filled and dilated by papillary or solid tumor (Fig. 47). Focal areas of hemorrhage and necrosis may be present. The tumor is bilateral in 10% to 26% of patients; however, the nature of the bilaterality has not been well characterized, with some favoring metastatic spread and others multifocality. The majority of fallopian tube adenocarcinomas are serous, histologically identical to ovarian serous carcinoma. Other types of epithelial fallopian tube carcinoma have been reported but are very rare; these include mucinous, endometrioid, clear cell, and squamous cell. Well differentiated serous adenocarcinoma is composed of fine, branching papillae. Poorly differentiated tumor usually contains solid sheets of cells, with areas of necrosis (Fig. 48).

Several diagnostic criteria have been established and must be met to differentiate fallopian tube malignancy from ovar-

TABLE 6. *FIGO staging for fallopian tube cancer*

Stage 0	Carcinoma *in situ* (limited to tubal mucosa)
Stage I	Growth limited to the fallopian tubes
Stage Ia	Growth is limited to one tube with extension into the submucosa and/or muscularis but not penetrating the serosal surface; no ascites
Stage Ib	Growth is limited to both tubes with extension into the submucosa and/or muscularis but not penetrating the serosal surface; no ascites
Stage Ic	Tumor either stage Ia or Ib with tumor extension through or onto the tubal serosa; or with ascites present containing malignant cells or with positive peritoneal washings
Stage II	Growth involving one or both fallopian tubes with pelvic extension
Stage IIa	Extension and/or metastasis to the uterus and/or ovaries
Stage IIb	Extension to other pelvic tissues
Stage IIc	Tumor either stage IIa or IIb and with ascites present containing malignant cells or with positive peritoneal washings
Stage III	Tumor involves one or both fallopian tubes with peritoneal implants outside of the pelvis and or positive retroperitoneal or inguinal nodes. Superficial liver metastases equals stage III. Tumor seems limited to the true pelvis but with histologically proven malignant extension to the small bowel or omentum
Stage IIIa	Tumor is grossly limited to the true pelvis with negative nodes but with histologically confirmed microscopic seeding of abdominal peritoneal surfaces
Stage IIIb	Tumor involving one or both tubes with histologically confirmed implants of abdominal peritoneal surfaces ≤2 cm in diameter. Lymph nodes are negative
Stage IIIc	Abdominal implants >2 cm in diameter and/or positive retroperitoneal or inguinal nodes
Stage IV	Growth invading one or both fallopian tubes with distant metastases. If pleural effusion is present, there must be positive cytology to be stage IV. Parenchymal liver metastases equal stage IV

Note: Staging for fallopian tube is by the surgical pathological system. Operative findings designating stage are determined prior to tumor debulking.

(From International Federation of Gynecology and Obstetrics (FIGO). *Annual report on the results of treatment in gynecological cancer,* vol 21. Stockholm: FIGO, 1991; with permission.)

ian and other primary tumors. Microscopically, the tumor must arise from the endosalpinx, with a histologic pattern consistent with tubal mucosal epithelium. The transition from benign to malignant epithelium is desirable. The ovaries and endometrium are either normal or have tumor smaller than that in the tube. As in epithelial ovarian carcinoma, fallopian tube epithelial tumors may spread by direct extension, lymphatic channels, or the hematogenous route. Distant metastases are infrequent.

Treatment of primary fallopian tube epithelial tumors is based on the standard management for ovarian carcinoma, due to the lack of any large-scale studies for this rare tumor. Surgery remains the principal treatment, including a total abdominal hysterectomy, bilateral salpingo-oophorectomy, tumor debulking, and a full staging, as with ovarian cancer (see Table 3). Platinum-based therapies are recommended following surgery, based on several series showing a 5-year survival of greater than 50% in advanced-stage (stages III and IV) patients.[25] Due to the rarity of fallopian tube cancer, paclitaxel (Taxol) has not yet been widely used in this disease. However, based on data from patients with ovarian cancer, it could be an active agent in fallopian tube cancer. Medroxprogesterone acetate and megestrol acetate (Megace) have been used in treating fallopian tube carcinomas. Early indications suggest that these progestational agents do not appear to be beneficial. Other agents, such as tamoxifen citrate (Nolvadex), may have some activity in these tumors.

As in ovarian carcinoma, the prognosis is dependent on the extent of disease and the amount of residual tumor at the end of surgery. Second-look surgery may be helpful in determining treatment efficacy and persistent disease, but, as in ovarian carcinoma, it should not be considered standard therapy at this time.

Fallopian Tube Sarcoma

Sarcomas of the fallopian tubes may be classified as pure or mixed. They are exceedingly rare—fewer than 50 cases have been reported—and are usually found in postmenopausal women. Abdominal pain and watery or bloody vaginal discharge with signs of peritoneal spread are common findings. An ovarian origin must be ruled out by clearly identifying residual normal ovarian structure. The life expectancy of patients with these sarcomas is usually measured in months. As described in case reports, radiation and chemotherapy have not been effective.

Fallopian Tube Choriocarcinoma

Compared to fallopian tube sarcoma, choriocarcinoma of the fallopian tube is even rarer. It may arise from gestational trophoblastic disease within an ectopic pregnancy or from a remnant of an extraovarian germ cell tumor. Its histology is similar to that of uterine choriocarcinoma. Treatment is also patterned after that of uterine choriocarcinoma. Currently, there is no standard recommended therapy for this disease, as the reported results are based on case reports only.

Metastatic Disease

Metastatic fallopian tube disease is actually more common than primary tumors of the fallopian tubes. It commonly originates

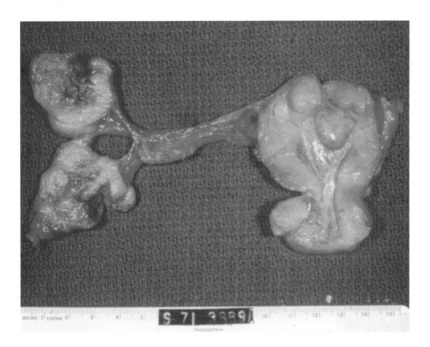

FIG. 47. Fallopian tube carcinoma. The fallopian tube lumen and its wall have been replaced by tumor.

from a primary tumor of the ovary or endometrium and rarely from a primary of the breast, gastrointestinal tract, or uterine cervix. Lymphatic involvement and an intact tubal epithelium distinguish a metastatic tumor from a primary fallopian tube tumor. The diagnostic criteria for differentiating between primary versus metastatic fallopian tube tumors were discussed earlier.

Benign Ovarian Disease

Many of the benign ovarian diseases seen in over-40-years age group are also seen in patients 20 to 40 years old. These include endometrioma, tuboovarian abscess, functional cysts, tumors of low malignant potential, and benign epithelial and sex cord–stromal tumors. These topics have been discussed earlier or are dealt with in other chapters.

Malignant Epithelial Tumors

Epidemiology[37]

Epithelial ovarian carcinomas account for 80% to 90% of all ovarian malignancies. Incidence rates in the United States are about 12 to 15 per 100,000 for white women, compared to about 8 to 10 per 100,000 for the United States residents of non-European heritage. The incidence rate continues to increase to about 40 cases per 100,000 women by age 50 years, and then continues to slowly increase to about 50 cases per 100,000 by age 65. Although the incidence rates in Asian na-

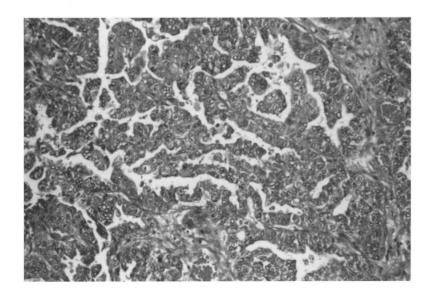

FIG. 48. Fallopian tube carcinoma. Serous carcinoma of the fallopian tube has the same microscopic appearance as an ovarian primary. In this example, cells are arranged in strands, nests, and delicate papillae.

tions are lower, studies have indicated increasing incidence rates in these countries. Other than race, epidemiologic studies have identified risk factors for ovarian cancer, including age over 60 years, early menarche, late menopause, nulliparity, infertility, personal history of breast or colon cancer, and family history of ovarian, breast, or colon cancer. In some inherited cases, the increased risk of ovarian cancer may be more than 50%, depending on the type and number of family members afflicted and age of onset. Other factors that have been implicated but lack adequate epidemiologic evidence include high-fat diets, talcum powder, and use of infertility drugs. Use of an oral contraceptive, bilateral tubal ligation, and hysterectomy are protective. Data from the United States Collaborative Analysis support the suppression of ovarian activity as a means of preventing ovarian cancer.[37]

Epithelial tumors are derived from the ovarian surface epithelium, which is the site of ovulation. Many of these risk factors are associated with incessant ovulation. A recent study suggests that a high number of ovulatory cycles may be associated with increased amounts of proliferation-associated DNA damage and increased risk of development in p53-positive but not p53-negative epithelial ovarian cancer.[29]

Clinical Presentation

Many patients with epithelial ovarian cancer present with advanced-stage disease with symptoms of abdominal fullness, pain, distention, early satiety, and weight loss. Other gastrointestinal symptoms include nausea, dyspepsia, constipation, or diarrhea. Abdominal distention can be due to ascites or a large abdominopelvic mass. Abdominal pain may result from rupture, torsion, or hemorrhage of the mass. Abnormal vaginal bleeding is seen in 30% of the cases. The most common physical signs are ascites, manifested by a fluid wave and the absence of shifting dullness, and the presence of a pelvic mass. The mass is frequently firm, hard, and fixed with multiple nodularities. Small tumors may not be easily palpated in the presence of ascites. Possible sites of spread within the abdomen are multiple (Fig. 49).

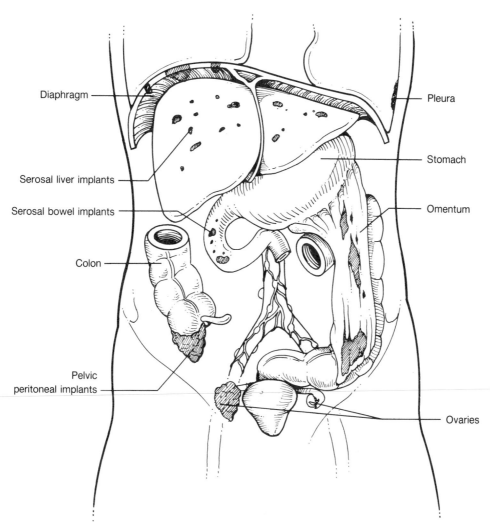

Diaphragm

Serosal liver implants

Serosal bowel implants

Colon

Pelvic peritoneal implants

Pleura

Stomach

Omentum

Ovaries

FIG. 49. Possible sites of spread of epithelial ovarian cancer.

Preoperative Evaluation[6]

All patients should have a complete blood cell count and serum chemistries including liver function tests performed. These tests, though routinely done preoperatively, will select out patients who may be at higher anesthetic risk. For example, any liver or kidney dysfunction may require further investigation, or the presence of anemia may justify a workup and transfusion prior to surgery. Serum tumor markers should be assayed. Although CA 125, a commonly used marker, can be observed in a variety of benign conditions and other nongynecologic malignancies, it is elevated in 80% of epithelial ovarian cancers. As a diagnostic aid, it appears to have a higher sensitivity in postmenopausal than in premenopausal women. CA 19-9, which is elevated in 87.5% of mucinous ovarian carcinomas, and carcinoembryonic antigen, which may be elevated in 7% to 37% of patients with ovarian cancer, are other less frequently used tumor markers. Preoperatively, tumor markers may be useful in helping predict the potential for malignancy. If elevated, they can be used to follow response to therapy and detect an early recurrence.

Chest x-rays are routinely performed to look for malignant pleural effusions, which occur in 10% of patients, and metastatic pulmonary disease, which is very rare. Barium enema examination is not routinely performed but may be helpful in patients with a left lower quadrant mass, blood in the stool, obstipation, or anemia, or in patients with carcinomatosis in whom a primary gastrointestinal tract malignancy must be ruled out. Barium enema examination is not very useful in predicting the need for colon resection. Mammography is necessary to rule out a possible metastatic or synchronous breast carcinoma. Although frequently ordered, CT scan is not a superior test, compared to pelvic sonography, in the evaluation of ovarian masses. It is an excellent for characterizing the liver, lymphatic spread, the omentum, and the mesentery. CT scan may be helpful in distinguishing a gynecologic malignancy from a metastatic pancreatic neoplasm for which surgery may not be warranted. If retroperitoneal or diffuse abdominal disease is noted, CT scan can be helpful in identifying those patients who require the surgical expertise of a gynecologic oncologist. Magnetic resonance imaging in patients with an ovarian mass has not been shown to have any clear advantage, except for the evaluation of pregnant patients whose ultrasound examination was inconclusive and CT scan would result in undesirable ionizing irradiation.

Sonography is the most useful diagnostic examination in the evaluation of a pelvic mass. It is an easily accessible and inexpensive imaging modality that provides an accurate description of ovarian pathology. Some characteristics easily detected by sonography include irregular borders, solid versus cystic elements, papillary projections, bilateral involvement, ascites, and liver parenchymal involvement. Some of these characteristics are even better delineated by transvaginal sonography. With strict criteria, some investigators have suggested a morphology index in identifying ovarian cancer;

the structural components included in the index are ovarian volume, wall structure, and septal structure.[10] Color Doppler imaging that evaluates blood flow to an ovarian mass has shown some promise but lacks the ability to distinguish absolutely between benign and malignant masses. Therefore, even though it is used frequently in practice, color Doppler imaging has a role that has not been clearly defined.

Other studies such as bone and liver scintigraphy do not add any useful information. Intravenous pyelograms or renal scans may be helpful in patients with abnormal renal function or abnormal findings on ultrasound, but they are rarely used. Immunoscintigraphy using CYT-103 or OC125 that detects occult extraabdominal or miliary metastasis is experimental but may be helpful in patients prior to second-look laparotomy or with recurrent disease. Positron emission tomography (PET) is a form of computer-assisted imaging that uses radiopharmaceuticals labeled with positron-emitting isotopes. PET has been examined in several preliminary studies involving the preoperative evaluation for suspected recurrent or metastatic ovarian tumors. Although the results are promising, PET's role in the preoperative evaluation of such patients awaits further study.

The nutritional status of patients with epithelial ovarian carcinoma must also be evaluated. Malnourished surgical patients are at greater risk for postoperative complications, which translates to longer hospital stays and higher health care costs. One way of correcting this would be the use of preoperative total parenteral nutrition (TPN). A large randomized, prospective study published by the Veterans Administration Cooperative Study Group found that preoperative TPN was associated with higher rates of pneumonia, wound infection, and septic complications during long-term use (more than 7 days). In addition, mortality in the TPN group was not decreased. The study group concluded that TPN may benefit fewer than 5% of patients, and careful screening is required to select those patients who are severely malnourished.

Staging

Staging is a very important step in the treatment of ovarian cancer, especially epithelial ovarian carcinoma. It is done at the time of surgical exploration in accordance with the FIGO system revised in 1987 (see Table 4). Proper staging is absolutely necessary, as it impacts on both prognosis and subsequent treatment method (see Table 3). Observational studies have shown that 30% of patients who were thought to have stage I or stage II disease at initial surgery had more advanced disease at restaging laparotomy.

A midline vertical incision is recommended, and it should be extended to above the umbilicus, if necessary, to allow proper exposure of the upper abdominal cavity. If an ovarian malignancy is discovered unexpectedly through a low transverse incision, the rectus muscle can be either severed or detached from the pubic symphysis. A J-shaped-extension incision should be avoided, unless it is absolutely necessary.

Pathology[14]

Serous Tumor

Serous tumor is the most common epithelial ovarian carcinoma, accounting for 40% to 50% of all such tumors. In the majority (50% to 60%) of patients, serous tumor is bilateral and is disseminated at the time of diagnosis. Grossly, tumors vary from microscopic size to 20 cm in diameter. They are soft, friable, mostly cystic, and multilocular tumors, containing turbid or bloody fluid and having extensive papillary projections. Papillary excrescences may also be seen on the external surface or attached to adjacent structures (Fig. 50).

Microscopic evaluation in well differentiated serous carcinoma reveals well formed papillary structures that grow into cystic spaces or on the peritoneal surface of the tumor. Psammoma bodies are present in the majority of cases (Fig. 51). With less differentiated tumors, the papillary pattern becomes less visible, the mitotic activity more brisk, and tumors become solid sheets of uniform, dark cells that are often slightly spindled and have a high nucleus-to-cytoplasm ratio. Furthermore, bizarre mononuclear or syncytial-like giant cells may be seen in many poorly differentiated carcinomas.

Mucinous Tumor

Mucinous carcinoma represents 5% to 10% of all epithelial ovarian malignancies. Bilaterality is present in 15% to 20% of cases. Disseminated spread is seen much less frequently than in patients with serous carcinoma. Mucinous carcinoma is usually larger than its serous counterpart, measuring approximately 15 to 30 cm in diameter. The tumor is multiloculated, solid and cystic, and filled with thick, viscous mucin.

Microscopically, invasive well differentiated mucinous carcinoma is typically composed of intestinal-type cells (Fig. 52). It may show only subtle irregularities in gland contour and irregular budding, with no other stromal signs of invasion. Mucin production is prominent. In moderately differentiated carcinoma, the glands are more back-to-back, with obvious stromal invasion, cellular stratification, and

nuclear atypia. In poorly differentiated mucinous carcinoma, cells are disorganized, embedded in a dense reactive ovarian stroma. Signet-ring cells may be present, as in a Krukenberg tumor. Mucinous tumor often contains a wide range of histologic differentiation; therefore, extensive sampling must be performed to obtain the correct diagnosis.

Endometrioid Tumor

Endometrioid carcinoma accounts for 20% of all epithelial ovarian malignancies. It is the second most common type of epithelial ovarian carcinoma and is bilateral in 30% of cases. In up to 30% of patients, endometriosis has been noted in the same ovary or elsewhere in the pelvis. In addition, a synchronous endometrial adenocarcinoma has been seen in 20% of patients; these tumors are usually small and superficial and are associated with endometrial hyperplasia.

Grossly, endometrioid tumor smooth and ranges from 12 to 20 cm in diameter. On cut surface, both cystic and solid components may be seen with mucin and polypoid projections (Fig. 53). Similar to endometrial adenocarcinoma, well differentiated ovarian endometrioid adenocarcinoma is characterized by well developed glands lined by tall, columnar, pseudostratified or multilayered epithelium (Fig. 54). Squamous differentiation may be seen in about 30% of tumors and is usually benign. As tumors become less differentiated, the glandular pattern becomes less organized, and a solid growth pattern becomes predominant. Mitoses are more frequent, and nuclei are more high-grade.

Clear Cell Tumor

Clear cell carcinoma constitutes 5% to 10% of malignant epithelial ovarian tumors. It is bilateral in 15% to 20% of patients and confined to the ovary in 60%. This is somewhat deceiving because clear cell carcinoma is a biologically virulent tumor, even stage I. It is frequently associated with endometriosis, with 25% of tumors arising from the lining of the endometriotic cysts. A mixed form of epithelial ovarian carcinoma with

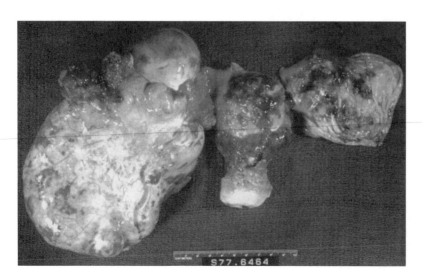

FIG. 50. Serous carcinoma. The tumor forms large, bilateral, solid and cystic masses that have grown through the capsule. Tumor also involves the uterine serosa.

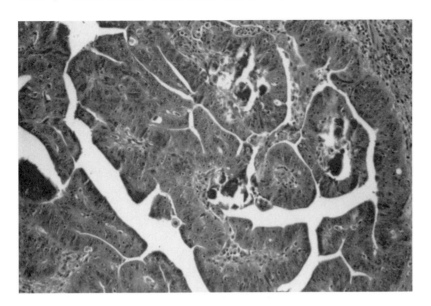

FIG. 51. Serous carcinoma. In this tumor, papillae are lined by high-grade tumor cells with prominent nucleoli. Psammoma bodies are present.

clear cell tumor and endometrioid or serous carcinoma can occur, suggesting a similar histogenesis.

Grossly, clear cell tumor can measure up to 30 cm in diameter, with an average of 15 cm, and is usually cystic. Although adhesions are frequently seen, they are inflammatory rather than neoplastic. Cut surface reveals papillary projections, polyps, or fleshy yellow nodules that invade the thick cyst wall. Microscopically, clear cell tumor may be characterized by sheets of polyhedral clear cells divided by fine connective tissue septa. Cells usually have abundant glycogen in the cytoplasm that is responsible for the clear appearance of the cells. The other characteristic feature is the tubulopapillary pattern formed by the columnar secretory cells with nuclei that bulge into the lumina of the glands, giving a hobnail appearance (Fig. 55). Eosinophilic cells instead of secretory columnar cells may surround tubules or papillae, or a mixture of these cells may be present.

Undifferentiated Tumor

Accounting for 5% to 10% of all ovarian malignancies, undifferentiated tumor exhibits such poor differentiation that it can not be classified into any of the above described categories. There is a variable histologic pattern, ranging from sheets of large anaplastic cells, to undifferentiated small cells, to large pleomorphic giant cells with eosinophilic cytoplasm. The prognosis is usually very poor because patients often present in advanced stage with large tumor burdens.

Brenner Tumor

Malignant Brenner tumor is very rare (see also "Brenner Tumor" above). It ranges from 10 to 30 cm in diameter and is usually unilateral. Cut surface reveals cystic and solid components consisting of friable polypoid mural nodules. Micro-

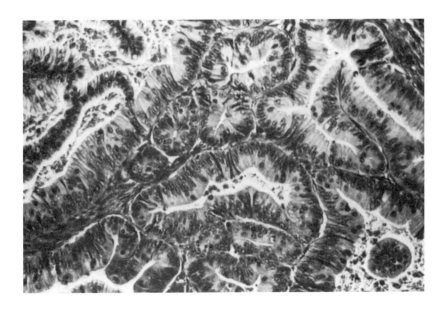

FIG. 52. Mucinous carcinoma. Infiltrating, crowded glands are lined by tall columnar cells with pale cytoplasm. Note the atypical, stratified nuclei (original magnification ×160).

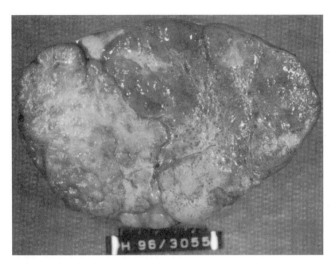

FIG. 53. Endometrioid carcinoma. The tumor is tan to brown in the softer more friable areas.

scopically, malignant Brenner tumor exhibits solid sheets of heterogeneous epithelial cells with minimal stroma. Nuclear grade and mitotic activity are high. Histologically, these cells resemble transitional cells, like those in the urologic tract. Differentiation from a carcinoma of urinary origin is based on clinical presentation and surgical findings. Origin in the ovary is supported by finding a transition from a benign or proliferating Brenner tumor.

Müllerian Mesenchymal and Mixed Tumors[17]

These rare ovarian tumors are divided into subtypes, including adenosarcoma and malignant mixed mesodermal tumor; they are associated with a poor prognosis. Histologically, they resemble their uterine counterparts. Adenosarcoma usually measures 10 cm in diameter and contains a benign epithelial component and a sarcomatous mesenchymal component. Malignant mixed mesodermal tumor has both malignant epithelial and malignant mesenchymal components (i.e., carcinosarcoma).

Similar to epithelial ovarian tumors, these tumors are usually surgically staged. However, optimal cytoreduction and adjuvant chemotherapies for these patients may not be as effective as they are for patients with the other types of epithelial tumors. The chemotherapeutic regimens are also different, but studies are limited by the rarity of these tumors. Agents that have been tried include doxorubicin (Adriamycin), cisplatin, and ifosfamide (IFEX).

Treatment

Surgery

Surgery is the most important aspect in the initial care of patients with epithelial ovarian cancer.[14] Surgery alone is curative for patients with stage Ia, grades 1 to 2 ovarian carcinoma. For more advanced disease, surgery establishes the diagnosis and allows appropriate staging and cytoreduction, optimally to less than 1 cm residual disease. A unilateral salpingo-oophorectomy with a full staging procedure is recommended only for young women with stage Ia, grades 1 to 2 disease who desire future fertility. The contralateral ovary should be carefully evaluated, as there is a 5% chance of occult metastasis or a separate primary carcinoma. Biopsy of the contralateral ovary is no longer recommended, unless there are grossly apparent abnormalities. Such patients must also have strict subsequent follow-up. Although a hysterectomy and removal of remaining adnexae is recommended for women who have completed childbearing, this recommendation is not based on randomized clinical trials.

Primary cytoreduction of ovarian carcinoma has been recommended for more than two decades. The theory is that removal of large hypoxic tumors allows better penetration of chemotherapeutic agents to residual tumor nodules. Optimal cytoreduction is defined as residual disease less than 1 cm. Several reports over the last 20 years have shown that the

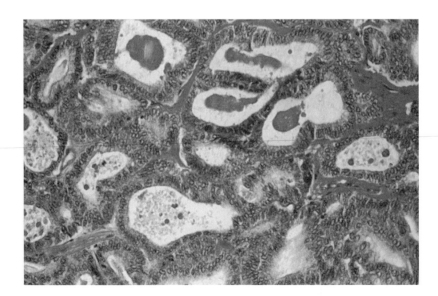

FIG. 54. Endometrioid carcinoma. In a well differentiated endometrioid carcinoma, the glands are smoothly rounded, closely packed, and lined by an endometrioid type of columnar epithelium.

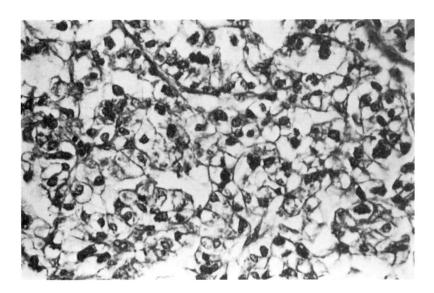

FIG. 55. In clear cell carcinoma, tumor cells are polygonal, with central nuclei and abundant clear cytoplasm (original magnification ×250).

diameter of the largest residual disease correlates with response rate, progression-free interval, and overall survival. The Gynecologic Oncology Group (GOG) evaluated survival by maximum diameter of residual disease (combined protocol 52 and 97) and found that the survival rate for patients with residual disease of 2 cm or greater is about 20% at 4 years, as compared with a 60% survival rate at 4 years in those with only microscopic residual disease.[14] For patients with residual disease less than 2 cm, the survival rate was 40% at 4 years (Fig. 56). Another GOG study (protocol 52) compared survival in stage III patients who were found to have intraabdominal disease of 1 cm or less at the time of initial surgery to those who were surgically cytoreduced to disease of 1 cm or less.[14] The patients with 1-cm-or-less disease preoperatively had better survival rates than those who were cytoreduced to 1 cm or less (Fig. 57). Patient age, tumor grade, and number of tumor nodules also affected outcome, suggesting that factors influencing the "biology of the tumor" are also important in determining survival rates and that operability may be determined by tumor biology rather than the aggressiveness of surgeons.

At the end of chemotherapy, patients who are clinically in complete remission may be offered second-look laparotomy to determine the success of therapy, as measured by the presence of any residual tumor.[11] The purpose of a second-look laparotomy is to determine disease presence, thus allowing continued therapy in an attempt to improve survival. A laparoscopic approach may reduce the length of hospital stay, but it is limited to surgeons with adequate expertise and to patients whose entire abdomen and retroperitoneal spaces are to be thoroughly evaluated. A diagnostic laparoscopy, however, may obviate the need for a laparotomy if gross disease is detected. Older studies have shown that survival rates for those who underwent second-look surgery as compared to those who did not were essentially the same, suggesting no benefit for the procedure. However, these studies have not evaluated the effect of newer chemotherapy and more effective salvage therapies. Thus, second-look surgery should be

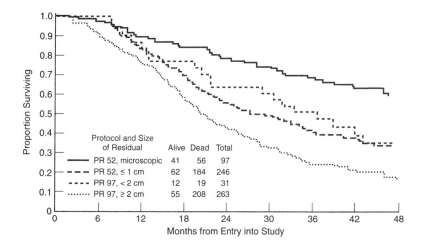

FIG. 56. Survival by residual disease: Gynecologic Oncology Group, protocols 52 and 97. (From Hoskins WJ, McGuire WP, Brady MF, et al. The effect of diameter of largest residual disease on survival after primary cytoreductive surgery in patients with suboptimal residual epithelial ovarian carcinoma. *Am J Obstet Gynecol* 1994;170:974–980; with permission.)

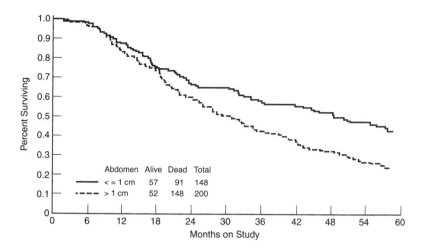

FIG. 57. Survival time by initial maximum abdominal tumor diameter (including omentum). (From Hoskins WJ, Bundy BN, Thigpen JT, Omura GA. The influence of cytoreductive surgery on recurrence-free interval and survival in small volume stage III epithelial ovarian cancer: a Gynecologic Oncology Group study. *Gynecol Oncol* 1992;47:159–166; with permission.)

performed in patients enrolled in clinical trials to evaluate the efficacy of newer first-line therapies and the efficacy of better salvage therapies in improving survival.

Secondary cytoreduction at the time of second-look laparotomy has also been examined in several studies that revealed a benefit in a select group of patients with gross disease that is successfully cytoreduced to microscopic disease.[5,38] However, gross disease sometimes cannot be detected until the time of surgery, subjecting many patients to an unnecessary procedure. Therefore, until more accurate diagnostic tests can be identified to determine macroscopic residual disease after standard treatment, secondary cytoreduction should not have a large role in the treatment of epithelial ovarian carcinoma, except as a part of a research protocol.

Interval debulking surgery is performed after induction of neoadjuvant chemotherapy in patients with advanced ovarian cancer. Although it remains a controversial subject, the Gynecological Cancer Cooperative Group of the European Organization for Research and Treatment of Cancer recently conducted a large randomized study ($n=278$).[35] All patients received three cycles of cyclophosphamide and cisplatin followed by randomization to debulking versus no debulking surgery, and then three more cycles of chemotherapy. The study revealed that interval debulking surgery showed a statistical significance in improving both the progression-free and overall survival in advanced epithelial ovarian cancer, with a 6-month improvement in median overall survival (Fig. 58). Although the difference is small and requires confirmation with further studies, interval debulking surgery may be considered in patients who, based on the clinician's judgment, could not be optimally cytoreduced at initial surgery. This study, however, did not compare patients with optimal primary cytoreductive surgery to those with interval cytoreductive surgery.

Secondary cytoreductive surgery in patients with recurrent epithelial ovarian carcinoma has also been evaluated in several studies.[5,11] The majority of these reports show a statistically significant survival benefit for patients who were optimally cytoreduced at surgery for recurrent ovarian cancer. Patients who benefit the most are those who had 1 year or more of

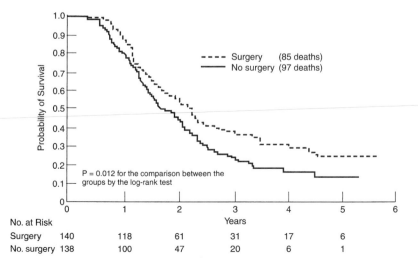

FIG. 58. Survival of patients with advanced epithelial ovarian cancer according to whether or not they underwent debulking surgery. (From ref. 35; with permission.)

disease-free interval, suggesting again the importance of the biologic properties of these tumors in determining outcome.

Chemotherapy

Following surgery, most patients will require chemotherapy. In patients with stage Ia, grade 1 tumor, no further therapy is required. It is not clear that all patients with stage Ia or stage Ib grades 2 or 3 tumors need additional therapy. The GOG and the Gruppo Italiano Collaborativo in Oncologia Ginecologica (GICOG) studies showed no difference in survival rate (greater than 80%) whether patients received chemotherapy (melphalan [Alkeran] or cisplatin) or intraperitoneal phosphorus 32.[9] Another GICOG randomized study compared no further treatment to six cycles of cisplatin (*n*=186) and found a statistically significant difference in 5-year disease-free survival (cisplatin 83% vs. observation only 64%); however, there was no difference in overall survival.[9] While the debate continues regarding the need for treatment in these patients, as well as the choice of treatment, there is no argument for treating patients with disease higher than stage Ic.

Various chemotherapeutic agents have been found to be active against ovarian cancer. Single-agent cisplatin or cisplatin-based combination therapy is the most effective regimen. Other active agents include paclitaxel, topotecan hydrochloride (Hycamtin), doxorubicin, cyclophosphamide, ifosfamide, etoposide, and altretamine (Hexalen). Although a higher complete response is achieved with multiagent therapy (greater than 50%), there is insufficient evidence to suggest a longer overall survival rate in these patients, compared to those treated with single-agent cisplatin.

Recently, paclitaxel, a microtubule stabilizer, was found to have significant activity in many cancers, including epithelial ovarian carcinoma. In 1996, the GOG published a study comparing the efficacy of paclitaxel and cisplatin with cyclophosphamide and cisplatin as first-line adjuvant therapy in patients with suboptimally debulked epithelial ovarian carcinoma (stages III or IV).[20] Disease-free survival and overall survival for the paclitaxel/cisplatin group was statistically higher than for the cyclophosphamide/cisplatin group (median survival, 38 to 24 months) but more toxic (Fig. 59). If this regimen is more effective for patients with gross residual disease, intuitively, it should be as effective for patients with advanced cancer optimally cytoreduced. Further ongoing studies by the GOG will evaluate the efficacy of substituting carboplatin (Paraplatin) for cisplatin in this combination regimen and of using a 3-hour infusion schedule, a more economically favorable practice in this cost-conscious health care system.

GOG study 132 compared single-agent paclitaxel (24-hour) with single-agent cisplatin and the combination of 24-hour paclitaxel and cisplatin as adjuvant therapy in the treatment of patients with suboptimally debulked advanced-stage ovarian cancer.[21] Patients who received paclitaxel only had a lower progression-free interval, compared to patients in the other groups, but the overall survival rate among the patients was the same, which was attributed to crossover treatment. This study suggests that paclitaxel alone may not be as good as cisplatin or a combination of paclitaxel and cisplatin.

Since paclitaxel, many new drugs have been approved by the U.S. Food and Drug Administration as second-line regimens in ovarian cancer; these include topotecan, gemcitabine hydrochloride (Gemzar), vinorelbine tartrate (Navelbine), and doxorubicin hydrochloride liposome injection (Doxil).[28] Topotecan, a topoisomerase inhibitor, has been shown in small series to be slightly more effective than paclitaxel in the treatment of patients with recurrent or persistent ovarian cancer. A large-scale randomized study is needed to evaluate topotecan and cisplatin as a first-line therapy, compared to paclitaxel and cisplatin.

Neoadjuvant chemotherapy to reduce the tumor load before performing a laparotomy is being investigated.[30] Based on available noninvasive testing, it is difficult to accurately predict which patients will not be candidates for a successful cytoreduction. Furthermore, neoadjuvant therapy has only been employed in small retrospective observational series.

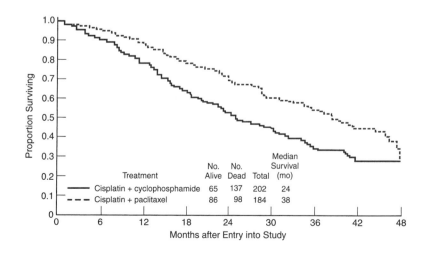

FIG. 59. Survival of 546 eligible patients with stage III ovarian cancer who were randomly assigned to treatment with intravenous or intraperitoneal cisplatin. (From ref. 20; with permission.)

Although neoadjuvant chemotherapy has permitted subsequent optimal cytoreductive surgery, this has not translated into higher survival rates in the limited number of patients studied.

Intraperitoneal therapy may be advantageous in a select group of patients.[2,19] It allows direct exposure of a tumor to a drug concentration that may be 10- to 1000-fold higher than that achieved with systemic therapy. The ideal drugs must have minimal local peritoneal toxicity, a steep dose–response curve, low peritoneal permeability, rapid clearance from the plasma, and immediate activity without the need for conversion to an active form. At the same time, patients should have limited peritoneal adhesions to ensure adequate drug distribution, and small-volume disease, preferably microscopic or 5 mm or less in diameter. The clinical situations in which intraperitoneal therapy may be considered include salvage therapy of patients with disease of 5 mm or less, consolidation therapy of patients with surgically documented complete chemotherapeutic response, initial therapy of patients with high-grade early-stage tumors, or combination adjuvant therapy with systemic infusion. Drugs that have been used via the intraperitoneal route include cisplatin, carboplatin, mitoxantrone hydrochloride (Novantrone), doxorubicin, and mitomycin (Mutamycin). Paclitaxel has recently been evaluated in several studies and has shown some potential. In preclinical studies, AD-32 (N-trifluoroacetyladriamycin-14-valerate), an analog of doxorubicin, was found to be superior to doxorubicin in many areas, including toxicity and antitumor efficacy. A phase I trial was performed using AD-32 as an intraperitoneal agent in patients with gynecologic malignancies confined to the abdomen in whom standard therapy had failed. The drug appears to be well tolerated and can be safely administered. Further studies are ongoing to evaluate its efficacy in selected patients.

A randomized trial of intraperitoneal cisplatin with intravenous cyclophosphamide versus intravenous cisplatin and cyclophosphamide for optimally debulked stage III ovarian cancer (less than 2 cm residual tumor nodules) was recently published.[2] It showed significant improvement in survival and less toxicity in patients who received intraperitoneal cisplatin, with a median survival of 49 versus 41 months (Fig. 60). This study suggests that combination intraperitoneal cisplatin with an intravenous agent as primary therapy may be advantageous. However, optimal intraperitoneal regimens remain to be defined and will require randomized trials comparing intraperitoneal infusion with other approaches. The GOG is currently conducting a phase III study comparing the use of intraperitoneal or intravenous cisplatin combined with intravenous paclitaxel after optimal cytoreductive surgery.

Radiation Therapy

Abdominopelvic radiation therapy has been used postoperatively in selected patients who have microscopic or small-volume residual disease. Except for phosphorus 32, radiation therapy is an infrequently used adjuvant therapy in ovarian cancer in the United States. One of the largest series, compiled by the Toronto group in treating stage II and III patients with abdominopelvic radiation, showed a 10-year disease-free survival of 38% (n=91) for patients with residual less than 2 cm and 6% (n=91) for patients with residual greater than 2 cm.[33] The details of radiation therapy are discussed in Chapter 53.

Prognosis

Despite of the addition of several innovative therapeutic regimens that have enhanced the length of survival of patients with epithelial ovarian cancer, significant strides have not been made in treating patients with advanced ovarian cancer. The overall 5-year survival may have improved, but it still lingers around 42%. Efforts in both basic and clinical research must continue so that an understanding of the etiopathogenesis can help in the development of prevention strategies, screening for early detection, and better therapies.

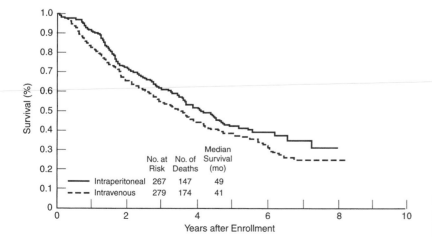

FIG. 60. Survival with intravenous versus intraperitoneal cisplatin therapy. (From ref. 2; with permission.)

Sex Cord–Stromal Tumors

Granulosa Cell Tumor

The adult form of granulosa cell tumor accounts for 1% to 2% of all ovarian tumors and 95% of all granulosa cell tumors. Although these tumors average 10 to 12 cm in diameter, a pelvic mass is not always detectable. Peak age of occurrence is 50 to 55 years, and most granulosa cell tumors produce estrogen, which in premenopausal women is manifested by menstrual irregularities such as menorrhagia, amenorrhea due to anovulation, or metrorrhagia. In postmenopausal women, vaginal bleeding results from endometrial stimulation. Endometrial hyperplasia or carcinoma is a common occurrence, approximately twice that seen in premenopausal women. The best estimate for the frequency of associated endometrial carcinoma is 5%.

Grossly, the tumors are solid and gray-white or yellow, with cystic areas and hemorrhage (Fig. 61). Microscopically, they are composed of granulosa cells and theca cells or fibroblasts, or both.[15] Theca cells and fibroblasts are most likely a response of the ovarian stroma to granulosa cell proliferation, as only granulosa cells are found in metastatic sites. Granulosa cells may be round, polygonal, or spindle-shaped, with scant cytoplasm and round or ovoid nuclei. Many different histologic patterns may be seen separately or together; these include the microfollicular pattern with its distinctive Call-Exner bodies (Fig. 62), macrofollicular, insular, trabecular, solid-tubular, and, rarely, hollow-tubular patterns. Less differentiated forms include the watered-silk or diffuse pattern. Rarely, a granulosa cell tumor undergoes sarcomatous transformation, producing the most aggressive form of the disease.

Although most granulosa cell tumors have a very low potential for malignant behavior, with 90% of tumors being stage Ia, they do have a propensity for late recurrence up to 10 to 20 years or more after initial diagnosis. In addition to full surgical staging (see Table 3), surgery should include a total abdominal hysterectomy and bilateral salpingo-oophorectomy in postmenopausal patients. Conservative surgery is indicated in younger patients who wish to maintain fertility, if the tumor is confined to one ovary. Stage appears to be the most important prognostic factor. Although other prognostic factors include capsular rupture, tumor size, nuclear atypia, mitotic activity, and histologic pattern, studies of these factors have not been conclusive. It is difficult to evaluate the efficacy of chemotherapy in this group of tumors. Most retrospective series have been limited by their small sample size and short follow-up. Platinum-based therapy including the PAC, VBP, and BEP regimens have been reported to be the most successful, with a 5-year survival of 50%.[12,13] Radiotherapy has also been used with varying success in studies limited by small numbers. In recurrent disease, surgery may offer the best mode of therapy. Chemotherapy and radiation therapy have been used in this setting.

Management of an Adnexal Mass: Surgery Versus Conservative Management, Laparoscopy Versus Laparotomy

The risk of a malignant ovarian neoplasm in premenopausal women is 13%. It becomes an important issue for the clinician to assess patients with an adnexal mass in a complete and thorough fashion prior to surgery to determine whether the mass is most likely benign or malignant. The clinician must determine whether an adnexal mass can be managed conservatively in the hope of a spontaneous resolution without surgical intervention. If an adnexal mass needs to be removed, the clinician must determine whether laparoscopy or laparotomy is the ideal surgical approach. For details on the laparoscopic management of adnexal mass, please see Chapter 46.

◊ HEREDITARY OVARIAN CANCER

Hereditary Forms Ovarian Cancer[4]

Approximately 5% to 10% of patients with ovarian cancer are thought to have an inherited genetic predisposition. Al-

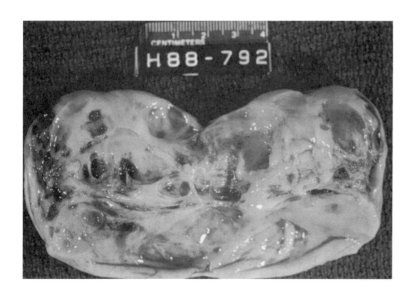

FIG. 61. Granulosa cell tumor. Cut surface is soft, yellow, solid and cystic, with the cysts containing clotted blood.

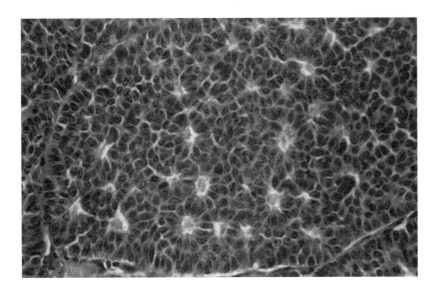

FIG. 62. Granulosa cell tumor. The microfollicular pattern is characterized by granulosa cells with angulated nuclei surrounding small cavities that simulate the Call-Exner bodies of the developing follicle.

though this represents a small percentage of patients with ovarian cancer, great emphasis has been placed on these genetic mutations, given their clinical, social, and ethical implications.

To date three distinct types of hereditary ovarian cancer syndrome have been described:

◊ Breast–ovarian cancer syndrome, which is frequently linked with the susceptible *BRCA1* gene;
◊ Hereditary nonpolyposis colon cancer (HNPCC) syndrome, which is also known as cancer family syndrome and lynch syndrome II;
◊ Site-specific ovarian cancer family syndrome, which is now linked to the *BRCA1* gene and thought to be a variant of the breast–ovarian cancer syndrome.

Families with site-specific ovarian family syndrome simply do not manifest early-onset breast cancer. A detailed family history must be obtained to determine the genetic susceptibility for the members of each family. Average age at diagnosis for this group of patients is usually 10 years younger than for the general population. Most tumors are of the serous type, and mucinous tumors and LMP tumors are rarely linked to *BRCA1*.

The breast–ovarian cancer syndrome accounts for up to 85% of all hereditary ovarian cancer cases. A pedigree of the family with the breast–ovarian cancer syndrome should show at least five first- or second-degree relatives with breast or ovarian cancers or three cases of early-onset (before age 60 years) breast or ovarian cancers. A sample pedigree of a breast–ovarian cancer syndrome family is illustrated in Fig 63. Almost all of the cancers are linked to the *BRCA1* gene, located on chromosome 17q12-21. Those not linked to *BRCA1* are most likely linked to the *BRCA2* gene, located on chromosome 13q12-13. This is especially true in the cases of male breast cancer. However, the incidence of ovarian cancer is much lower in *BRCA2*-linked families, at a cumulative risk of approximately less than 10% by age 70 years.[6]

The HNPCC syndrome accounts for approximately 15% of all hereditary ovarian cancer cases. It is an autosomal-dominant genetic syndrome characterized by three or more first-degree relatives with colon cancer (over 70% in the proximal colon) or endometrial cancer, where two of them must be diagnosed with cancer before age 50 years.[8] In addition, the HNPCC syndrome family members are also at risk for cancer

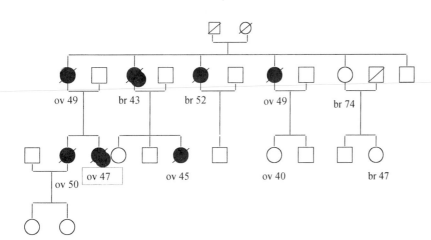

FIG. 63. Sample family pedigree.

of other gastrointestinal sites, urologic tract, and the ovary. Limited studies have reported a 3.5-fold increase in the risk of ovarian cancer in members of these families.[8] Recently, four gene foci—all part of the DNA mismatch repair (MMR) pathway—have been identified as being responsible for the HNPCC phenotype. Genetic heterogeneity for this syndrome is suggested by the fact that a defect of any one of these genes may result in the manifestation of the HNPCC syndrome.

Molecular Genetics of Hereditary Ovarian Cancer[4]

BRCA1

The existence of the *BRCA1* gene was confirmed by linkage analysis in several studies in the early 1990s. The candidate gene for *BRCA1* was then described in 1994. It consists of 22 coding exons spanning over 100 kilobases of genomic DNA on chromosome 17q21 with 5.7-kilobase coding regions, expressed in abundance in the testis and thymus and at lower levels in the breast and ovary. The exact function of the *BRCA1* gene remains unclear, but studies support its role as a tumor suppressor.

Many mutations have been described, located throughout the entire gene, with nonsense mutations or frameshift mutations being predominant. Nonsense mutations occur when a single nucleotide substitution results in a stop codon, and frameshift mutation occurs when one or more nucleotides are deleted to produce a downstream stop codon. In addition, the loss of alleles at or around the *BRCA1* region, documented by loss of heterozygosity, can also affect the phenotype of this gene.

BRCA2

The *BRCA2* gene was also recently cloned in a similar fashion to the *BRCA1* gene. It is even larger than the *BRCA1* gene, as it is composed of 26 coding exons that span over 70 kilobases of genomic DNA with 10.2 kilobases of coding regions, located on chromosome 13q12-13. It is also found in abundance in testis and thymus and at lower levels in breast and ovary. The two genes share many structural and functional similarities. Mutations are also scattered throughout the entire gene, with frameshift mutation being the most common. The *BRCA2* gene is also believed to function as a tumor suppressor.

Mismatch Repair Genes

The HNPCC syndrome is due to an inherited mutation in any one of four genes: *hMSH2* (chromosome 2p), *hMLH1* (chromosome 3p), *hPMS1* (chromosome 2q), or *hPMS2* (chromosome 7p). The products of these genes are involved in the same DNA-MMR pathway. The majority of affected patients are found to have defects in either *hMSH2* or *hMLH1*, which also are thought to function as tumor suppressor genes. In addition, there are multiple simple repeat sequences located throughout all of the genomes. Alteration of the length of

these repeating sequences may disrupt the basic DNA structure or the replicating efficiency of the genes in question, which in this case are the MMR genes. This is a phenomenon called microsatellite instability. The exact mechanism of tumorigenesis due to microsatellite instability is unknown, but this in combination with the gene defect may contribute to HNPCC-associated cancer and other sporadic cases.

Clinical Implications

Genetic Testing

The first major concerns in genetic testing are those dealing with scientific and technical issues; these include the reliability of tests, their predictive value, their interpretation, and ultimately their ability to prevent cancer in patients who test-positive with them. With the numbers of mutations that have already been discovered and with more such discoveries likely to come, testing for these genes may be technically difficult, and the results may not be easily interpreted. The second major concern relates to the ethical, legal, and social implications of gene testing because of the potential misuse of the information, including insurance and employment discrimination, testing of minors, and the prenatal diagnosis of *BRCA1* and other mutations. The estimated risk of ovarian cancer in patients with *BRCA1* mutations ranges from 26% to 85% by age 70 years,[7] with much lower rates for the *BRCA2* and HNPCC MMR genes.[7,8] For breast cancer, the estimated risk ranges from 50% to 85% for *BRCA1* and *BRCA2* gene. Tables 7 and 8 list the risk of cancer associated with these susceptibility genes. The proper selection of patients for testing is very important. Genetic counseling is imperative. As testing for these genes becomes more available to the public in both commercial and academic settings, clinicians and patients must work together to ensure that the results are used in a fashion that will carefully consider the ethical, legal, and psychosocial issues that may arise from genetic testing. Multidisciplinary services that include pre- and posttest counseling, screening, treatment, and psychosocial sessions should be established in the major referral centers and done in a research setting to further enhance the impact of genetic testing.

TABLE 7. *Risk of cancer associated with* BRCA1 *and* BRCA2 *genes*

Type of cancer	Proposed gene	Estimated risk[a] by age 70 yr
Breast cancer, women	BRCA1	85%
	BRCA2	Similar to BRCA1
Ovarian cancer	BRCA1	26%–85%
	BRCA2	<10%
Colon cancer, men and women	BRCA1	6%
Prostate cancer, men	BRCA2	8%

[a]Risk estimates are derived from high-risk families enrolled in research protocols.
(From ref. 7; with permission.)

TABLE 8. *Risk of cancer associated with the HNPCC genes*

Type of cancer	Proposed HNPCC gene	Associated risk
Ovarian cancer	*hMLH1, hMSH2, hPMS1, hPMS2*	Relative risk, 3.5
Colon cancer in men and women	*hMLH1, hMSH2, hPMS1, hPMS2*	68%–75% by age 65 yr
Endometrial cancer	*hMLH1, hMSH2, hPMS1, hPMS2*	30%–39% by age 70 yr

HNPCC, hereditary nonpolyposis colon cancer.
(From ref. 8; with permission.)

Risk Analysis

Family history remains the most reliable predictor of ovarian cancer risk. While many women will have relatives with ovarian cancer, the majority will not be identified with hereditary ovarian cancer syndromes. As noted earlier, the estimated risk of ovarian cancer in patients with a defective *BRCA1* allele is 26% to 85% by age 70 years. The higher estimates reflect initial studies on families with multiple affected members. In addition, the penetrance for ovarian cancer may be variable, depending on the specific *BRCA1* mutation. Other factors affecting the estimated risks may include environmental, reproductive circumstances, or other epidemiologic factors. First- or second-degree relatives of an affected individual from a breast–ovarian cancer syndrome family carrying the *BRCA1* gene are considered at high risk for ovarian cancer. In the general population, the risk for women with a single affected first-degree relative is increased to 5%, and with two affected first-degree relatives, it is increased to 7%. Compared to the general risk of 1 in 70 (1.4%), the risk is increased three- to fivefold. Patients who are carriers of *BRCA2* or the HNPCC genes and whose risks for ovarian cancer are 10%, or increased approximately sevenfold, are definitely not at the same level of risk as *BRCA1* carriers, whose risks may be as high as 85%, although probably lower based on population-based studies.

Follow-up and Management

Screening[7,8]

Follow-up and management of patients with an inherited genetic predisposition is complex due to the variable estimated risk attributed to different genetic alterations and their predisposition to other cancers (i.e, breast cancer for *BRCA1* and *BRCA2* genes and colon cancer for HNPCC MMR gene). A multidisciplinary approach based on the most current information may be necessary to meet the needs of each individual or family. Several studies have examined the screening technology available for ovarian cancer in both the general population and patients at risk. Transvaginal ultrasound with color Doppler flow and morphologic indices and serial serum CA 125 levels are the two modalities that have shown potential usefulness in surveying these patients. Transvaginal ultrasound is very sensitive in detecting early-stage ovarian cancer; however, it is limited by its ability to distinctively differentiated between malignant and benign masses, resulting in a high false-positive rate and perhaps unnecessary surgery, especially in premenopausal women. CA 125 levels may be elevated in other benign diseases and may not be elevated in early-stage I ovarian cancer; thus, it lacks sufficient sensitivity. Consequently, screening of the general population does not appear to be warranted with the currently available technology.

Although the utility of screening in the general population may be limited by the relatively low prevalence of the disease and currently available technology, the National Institute of Health *Consensus Statement on Ovarian Cancer*[24] and the Cancer Genetic Studies Consortium (CGSC)[7] recommend screening starting at ages 25 to 35 years as part of the annual or semiannual routine examination for women carrying the *BRCA1* mutation. The benefit, however is not absolutely proven, as the evidence is based on expert opinion only. The CGSC also recommended screening tests for other organs in this group of patients. Patients with the *BRCA2* mutation are at much lower risk for ovarian cancer, such that the benefits of this testing may be significantly reduced. Table 9 lists the provisional recommendations for cancer surveillance for the carriers of *BRCA1* and *BRCA2* mutations. Screening and prophylactic surgery for patients with HNPCC-associated mutations is also based on expert opinion, although colonoscopy and stool occult blood testing have been shown in randomized clinical trials to reduce the incidence of and mortality from colon cancer. The provisional recommendations for surveillance and treatment of these patients are listed in Table 10.

Prophylactic Oophorectomy[22]

In hereditary forms of ovarian cancer, onset usually occurs between ages 35 and 45 years. Prophylactic oophorectomy is therefore an option that could be offered to carefully selected patients at unequivocally high genetic risk for ovarian cancer who have completed their childbearing or are at least age 35 years. However, the evidence for performing prophylactic oophorectomy in these patients is inconclusive, and the optimum age has not been established. Several other issues remain unresolved:

◊ Physiologic adjustments to premature surgical menopause, especially vasomotor symptoms;
◊ Psychosocial adjustments to premature menopause;
◊ Prevention of cardiovascular disease and osteoporosis;
◊ Hormone replacement therapy (HRT), especially in those at high risk for breast cancer.

Data also suggest that there is poor compliance with long-term hormonal therapy.

TABLE 9. *Options for surveillance for carriers of BRCA1 and BRCA2 mutations*

Intervention	Provisional recommendation	Quality of evidence[a]	Cautionary issues
Breast cancer			
Breast self-examination	Education regarding monthly self-examination	III (expert opinion only)	Benefit not proven
Clinician breast examination	Annually or semi-annually, beginning at age 25–35 yr	III (expert opinion only)	Benefit not proven
Mammography	Annually beginning at age 25–35 yr	III (expert opinion only) I (randomized trial, average-risk women aged 50–69 yr)	Risks and benefits not established for women under age 50 yr
Ovarian cancer			
Transvaginal ultrasound with color Doppler and CA-125 level	Annually or semiannually beginning at age 25–35 yr	III (expert opinion only)	Benefit not proven; level of ovarian cancer risk estimated to be lower in *BRCA2* mutation carriers
Prostate cancer			
Prostate cancer surveillance (*BRCA1*-mutation carriers only)	Inform regarding options for screening involving rectal examination and prostate-specific antigen level, annually beginning at age 50 yr	III (expert opinion only)	Benefit not proven; many agencies do not recommend screening due to uncertainty of benefit from early detection
Colon cancer			
Colon cancer surveillance	Follow recommendations for general population: fecal occult blood test annually and flexible sigmoidoscopy every 3–5 yr beginning at age 50 yr	Evidence from average-risk populations: I (randomized trials fecal occult blood test) II-2 (case–control study; sigmoidoscopy)	Relevance of population-based data uncertain

[a]Quality of evidence based on criteria of the U.S. Preventive Service Task Force: I, highest quality (randomized, controlled trial); II, intermediate quality (nonrandomized trials and observational studies); (II-3, multiple time series with and without intervention); III, lowest quality (expert opinion and case reports).
(From ref. 8; with permission.)

If a patient at risk for ovarian cancer is having abdomino-pelvic surgery, a prophylactic oophorectomy should be performed. It has been reported that elective routine removal of the ovaries after age 40 years would eliminate approximately 12% to 14% of all ovarian cancer. The added surgical morbidity of oophorectomy at the time of laparotomy/laparoscopy for other indications is minimal. The physiologic and psychosocial issues associated with premature menopause and HRT need to be addressed.

Patients considered for prophylactic surgery should have completed their desired childbearing. They should receive genetic counseling and must understand that the surgery will

TABLE 10. *Options for surveillance and prophylactic surgery for carriers of HNPCC-associated mutations*

Intervention or surgery	Provisional recommendation	Quality of evidence[a]	Cautionary issues
Transvaginal ultrasound or endometrial aspiration	Annually, beginning at age 25–35 yr	II-3 (expert opinion only)	Benefit not proven, limited sensitivity
Hysterectomy and oophorectomy	Insufficient data to recommend for or against the intervention	III (expert opinion only)	Efficacy uncertain risk not fully eliminated

[a]Quality of evidence based on criteria of the U.S. Preventive Service Task Force: I, highest quality (randomized, controlled trial); II, intermediate quality (nonrandomized trials and observational studies); II-3, multiple time series with and without intervention; III, lowest quality (expert opinion and case reports).
(From ref. 8; with permission.)

produce a premature menopause and irreversible infertility when combined with a total hysterectomy. They must be informed about HRT, and the issue of noncompliance with long-term medication should be addressed. The risk of osteoporosis and heart disease need to be considered in presurgical counseling.

The efficacy of prophylactic oophorectomy in hereditary breast–ovarian cancer syndrome has been evaluated in several observational studies. Failure does occurs in the form of primary peritoneal carcinoma that is similar in histology to the primary ovarian carcinoma. These cancers have been reported in several patients 1 to 27 years after prophylactic oophorectomy: 3 (11%) of 28 women in one study and 6 (2%) of 324 women in another.[6] These observational studies suggest that there is some protective effect in a significant number of these high-risk patients, given that their lifetime risk of ovarian cancer may be high as 85%. Although the number of patients was small, a prospective cohort study did not achieve statistical significance in the incidence of "ovarian cancer" between oophorectomized and nonoophorectomized high-risk patients.[32]

Recommendations from other agencies or groups are as follows:

◊ American College of Obstetricians and Gynecologists (1992).[1] Women with familial ovarian or hereditary breast–ovarian cancer syndromes who do not wish to maintain their reproductive capacity may be offered prophylactic bilateral salpingo-oophorectomy. Such women should have a documented familial syndrome, preferably established via a full pedigree analysis by a geneticist. These women should be informed that removal of the tubes and ovaries does not provide 100% protection; primary peritoneal carcinoma has been reported after bilateral salpingo-oophorectomy in some cases.

◊ National Institutes of Health *Consensus Statement on Ovarian Cancer* (1994).[24] The probability of a hereditary ovarian cancer syndrome in a family pedigree increases with the number of affected relatives, with the number of affected generations, and with young age of onset of disease. Therefore, prophylactic oophorectomy should be considered in these settings, with careful weighing of the risks and potential benefits. The risk of ovarian cancer in women from families with hereditary ovarian cancer syndrome is sufficiently high to recommend prophylactic oophorectomy at age 35 years or after completion of childbearing.

◊ The CGSC. There is insufficient evidence to recommend for or against prophylactic oophorectomy as a measure for reducing ovarian cancer risk. Women with *BRCA1* mutations should be counseled that this is an option available to them. Those considering prophylactic oophorectomy should be counseled that cancer has been documented to occur after the procedure. Observational data have so far failed to demonstrate statistically significant evidence for risk reduction.

Prevention

Clearly established protective factors, as mentioned earlier, include greater than one full-term pregnancy, oral contraceptive use, breast-feeding, tubal ligation, and hysterectomy. However, the role of these protective factors in the management of women with known genetic risks for ovarian cancer has not been thoroughly examined. Therefore, further epidemiologic studies are required to determine their efficacy as preventive means in the care of these high-risk patients before they can be accepted as effective strategies in this subgroup of patients.

SUMMARY POINTS

◊ The differential diagnosis of a patient presented with an adnexal mass depends on patient age.

◊ Germ cell tumors are the most common gynecologic malignancy in young women. The cure rate is now approaching 100% due to the significant advancement of chemotherapeutic regimens. The most commonly used regimen is BEP. The risk of secondary malignancy, especially hematologic, with the use of etoposide must always be considered when this regimen is administered.

◊ Although significant strides have been made in the treatment of epithelial ovarian cancer, the 5-year survival rate remains less than 50%. Continual efforts are needed to understand the etiology, which will ultimately result in the development of prevention strategies, early detection, and innovative therapies.

◊ Identification of the *BRCA1* gene and other genes that are responsible for several familial cancer syndromes has opened up new areas of investigation and provided with valuable information for understanding the development of both hereditary and sporadic ovarian carcinoma.

◊ Although there is no level I evidence to support the use of screening and prophylactic surgery in patients who are at high risk for ovarian cancer, they remain the only modalities currently available to these patients to reduce the chance of disease development.

◊ REFERENCES

1. American College of Obstetrics and Gynecology Committee opinion. *Genetic risk and screening techniques for epithelial ovarian cancer* 1992:117.

2. Alberts DS, Liu PY, Hannigan EV, et al. Intraperitoneal cisplatin plus intravenous cyclophosphamide versus intravenous cisplatin plus intravenous cyclophosphamide for stage III ovarian cancer. *N Engl J Med* 1996;335:1950–1955.

3. Barakat R. Borderline tumors of the ovary. *Obstet Gynecol Clin North Am* 1994;21:93–105.

4. Boyd J, Rubin SC. Hereditary ovarian cancer: molecular genetics and clinical implications. *Gynecol Oncol* 1997;64:196–206.

5. Bristow RE, Lagasse LD, Karlan BY. Secondary surgical cytoreduction for advanced epithelial ovarian cancer: patient selection and review of the literature. *Cancer* 1996;78:2049–2062.

6. Brooks S. Preoperative evaluation of patients with suspected ovarian cancer. *Gynecol Oncol* 1994;55:S80–S90.

7. Burke W, Daly M, Garber J, et al., for the Cancer Genetic Studies Consortium. Recommendations for follow-up care of individuals with an inherited predisposition to cancer II: BRCA1 and BRCA2. *JAMA* 1997; 227:997–1003.

8. Burke W, Petersen G, Lynch P, et al. Recommendations for follow-up care of individuals with an inherited predisposition to cancer I: hereditary nonpolyposis colon cancer. *JAMA* 1997;277:915–919.

9. Colombo N, Chiari S, Maggioni A, Bocciolone L, Torri V, Mangioni C. Controversial issues in the management of early epithelial ovarian cancer: conservative surgery and role of adjuvant therapy. *Gynecol Oncol* 1994;55:S47–S51.

10. DePriest PD, Varner E, Powell J, et al. The efficacy of a sonographic morphology index in identifying ovarian cancer: a multi-institutional investigation. *Gynecol Oncol* 1994;55:174–178.

11. Creasman WT. Second-look laparotomy in ovarian cancer. *Gynecol Oncol* 1994;55:S122–S127.

12. Gershenson DM. Chemotherapy of ovarian germ cell tumors and sex cord-stromal tumors. *Semin Surg Oncol* 1994;10:290–298.

13. Gershenson DM. Management of early ovarian cancer: germ cell and sex cord-stromal tumors. *Gynecol Oncol* 1994;55:S62–S72.

14. Hoskins WJ. Epithelial ovarian carcinoma: principles of primary surgery. *Gynecol Oncol* 1994;55:S91–S96.

15. Kurman RJ. *Blaustein's pathology of the female genital tract*, 4th ed. New York: Springer-Verlag, 1994.

16. Kurman RJ, Trimble CL. The behaviour of serous tumors of low malignant potential: are they ever malignant? *Int J Gynecol Path* 1993; 12:120–127.

17. Le T, Krepart GV, Lotocki RJ, Heywood MS. Malignant mixed mesodermal ovarian tumor treatment and prognosis: a 20-year experience. *Gynecol Oncol* 1997;65:237–240.

18. Liu Trimble C, Trimble EL. Management of epithelial ovarian tumors of low malignant potential. *Gynecol Oncol* 1994;55:S52–S61.

19. Markman M. Salvage therapy in ovarian cancer: is there a role for intraperitoneal drug delivery? *Gynecol Oncol* 1993;51:86–89.

20. McGuire WP, Hoskins WJ, Brady MF, et al. Cyclophosphamide and cisplatin compared with paclitaxel and cisplatin in patients with stage III and stage IV ovarian cancer. *N Engl J Med* 1996;334:1–6.

21. Muggia FM, Braly PS, Brady MF, et al. Phase III of cisplatin (P) or paclitaxel (T), versus their combination in suboptimal Stage III and IV epithelial ovarian cancer (EOC): Gynecologic Oncology Group (GOG) #132. Abstract 1257. Program/Proceedings. American Society of Clinical Oncology, thirty-third annual meeting, May 17–20, 1997.

22. Nguyen HN, Averette HE, Janicek M. Ovarian carcinoma: a review of the significance of familial risk factors and the role of prophylactic oophorectomy in cancer prevention. *Cancer* 1994;74:545–555.

23. Nichols CR, Breeden ES, Lowrer PJ, Williams SD, Einhorn LH. Secondary leukemia associated with a conventional dose of etoposide: review of serial germ cell tumor protocols. *J Natl Cancer Inst* 1993; 85:36–40.

24. NIH Consencus Conference. Ovarian cancer screening, treatment and follow-up. *JAMA* 1995;273:491–497.

25. Nordin AJ. Primary carcinoma of the fallopian tube: a 20-year literature review. *Obstet Gynecol Surv* 1994;49:349–361.

26. Obata NH, Nakashima N, Kawai M, Kikkawa F, Mamba S, Tomoda Y. Gonadoblastoma with dysgerminoma in one ovary and gonadoblastoma with dysgerminoma and yolk sac tumor in the contralateral ovary in a girl with 46XX karyotype. *Gynecol Oncol* 1995;58:124–128.

27. Powell JL, Johnson NA, Bailey CL, Otis CN. Management of advanced juvenile granulosa cell tumor of the ovary. *Gynecol Oncol* 1993; 48: 119–123.

28. Runowicz CD, Fields AL, Goldberg GL. Promising new therapies in the treatment of advanced ovarian cancer. *Cancer* 1995;76:2028–2033.

29. Schildkraut JM, Bastos E, Berchuck A. Relationship between lifetime ovulatory cycles and overexpression of mutant p53 in epithelial ovarian cancer. *J Natl Cancer Inst* 1997;89:932–938.

30. Schwartz PE, Chambers JT, Makuch R. Neoadjuvant chemotherapy for advanced ovarian cancer. *Gynecol Oncol* 1994;53:33–37.

31. Seidman JD, Kurman RJ. Subclassification of serous borderline tumors of the ovary into benign and malignant types. *Am J Surg Pathol* 1996; 20:1331–1345.

32. Struewing JP, Watson P, Easton DF, Ponder BAJ, Lynch HT, Tucker MA. Prophylactic oophorectomy in inherited breast/ovarian cancer families. *Monogr Natl Cancer Inst* 1995;17:33–35.

33. Thomas GM, Dembo AJ. Integrating radiation therapy into the management of ovarian cancer. *Cancer* 1993;71:1710–1718.

34. Twoalfhoven FCM, Peters AAW, Trimbos JB. The accuracy of frozen section diagnosis of ovarian tumors. *Gynecol Oncol* 1991;41:189–192.

35. van der Burg MEL, van Lent M, Buyse M, et al. The effect of debulking surgery after induction chemotherapy on the prognosis in advanced epithelial ovarian cancer. *N Engl J Med* 1995;332:629–634.

36. Young RH, Gilks CB, Sculy RE. Mucinous tumors of the appendix associated with mucinous tumors of the ovary and pseudomyxoma peritonei: a clinicopathologic analysis of 22 cases supporting an origin in the appendix. *Am J Surg Pathol* 1991;15:415–429.

37. Westhoff C. Ovarian cancer. *Annu Rev Public Health* 1996;17:85–96.

38. Williams L, Bruetto VL, Yordan E, Di Saia PJ, Creasman WT. Secondary cytoreductive surgery at second-look laparotomy in advanced ovarian cancer: a Gynecologic Oncology Group study. *Gynecol Oncol* 1997;66: 171–178.

CHAPTER 53

Radiation Therapy in Gynecology

◇

Philip J. Di Saia

All life has evolved in a milieu in which the major source of energy essential for most biological processes is in the form of radiant energy. Sunlight provides heat, light, and energy for plant photosynthesis, and radio waves provide a means of communication. These radiations benefit life processes and are not harmful in ordinary quantities. Certain types of high-energy or ionizing radiations are not so harmless, but they provide useful tools in gynecology for diagnostic and therapeutic purposes. These high-energy radiations can be traumatic to biological material, and they are used in oncology because of their ability to inflict an injury from which normal tissue recovers more effectively than malignant tissue. They produce deleterious effects on all forms of life, from the relatively simple unicellular plants and animals to the complex higher organisms.

The change produced by ionizing radiations may be grossly apparent and visible soon after exposure of the living organism, but more often, the radiation does not appear on cursory examination to have affected the organism. The radiation may produce small changes that can be detected only by careful chemical or microscopic study, and the effects may not become apparent for many years or may manifest themselves only in the offspring of the irradiated organism. Radiation exposure from diagnostic tests, therapeutic irradiation, and radiation acquired incidentally from the environment may all be detrimental, and although the chance of injury often is slight, the possibility of damage from a known exposure must always be weighed against the importance of the information to be gained or the effect desired. Incidental exposure must be avoided through control of environmental hazards whenever possible.

◇ NATURE AND EFFECTS OF IONIZING RADIATION

The electromagnetic spectrum encompasses a broad range of photon energies, which extends from long radio waves to short γ-rays (Fig. 1).

The radiation emitted by radioactive isotopes (e.g., radium, cesium, iridium) is used to treat many malignancies. During the past 40 years, machines capable of producing radiant energy of high intensity (e.g., supervoltage, megavoltage) have become available and are used extensively in the treatment of malignancies. Machines that emit energies greater than 1 million electron volts (1 MeV) are most commonly used and include cobalt generators, betatrons, and linear accelerators (Table 1).

Physical and Chemical Nature

The physical forces of concern are called ionizing radiations because of their characteristic ability to transfer their energy to matter by separating orbital electrons from their atoms, forming physical ion pairs. The term is an inclusive one, because the phenomenon may be caused by particulate radiations or electromagnetic waves. This discussion is limited to electromagnetic radiations with wavelengths in the range of 10^{-7} to 10^{-10} cm (1 to 0.001 nm).

Radiations that originate from decay of an atomic nucleus are called γ-rays; those that originate outside the atomic nucleus are x-rays and are produced when high-energy charged particles (i.e., electrons) bombard a suitable target, such as tungsten. When these fast-moving electrons approach the fields around the nuclei of the atoms of the target material, they are deflected from their path, and energy is emitted in the form of electromagnetic radiation. The emitted x-rays may have any energy from zero to a maximum determined by the kinetic energy of the impinging electrons. Machines such as the betatron are capable of generating electrons at high accelerations, and the x-rays generated by these machines have high energies. A continuous spectrum of x-ray energy can be produced if a large number of impinging electrons are involved in the process.

Some x-rays are produced when a high-speed electron impinging on the target material knocks out an orbital electron (i.e., ionization) from a target atom. When this electron is from

909

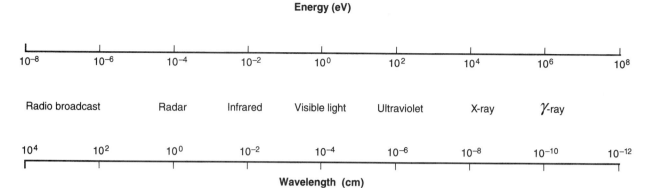

FIG. 1. The electromagnetic spectrum. There are no sharp boundaries between most regions. Only the band of visible light is well defined.

an inner shell, its place is immediately taken by an electron from an outer shell; during this transition, an x-ray is given off. The photon energy of that x-ray represents the difference in energies of the inner and outer orbital electron levels.

The γ-rays and x-rays can be collectively called photons. It is the energy of the photon, not its source, that is important in terms of its biological effects. The interaction of photons with matter takes place primarily through three mechanisms: the photoelectric effect, Compton scattering, and pair production. All of these processes result in ionization of molecules within the target or free radical formation. Free hydrogen atoms and free hydroxyl radicals commonly result from the bombardment of water by high-energy photons (Fig. 2).

Approximately one-half of the hydrogen (H) atoms encounter hydroxy (OH) radicals and form peroxide (H_2O_2). In the irradiation of water by electrons or photons, few of the H atoms or OH radicals are formed close enough to one another to react quickly before they diffuse. The addition of oxygen (O_2) causes the H atoms to react to form the radical HO_2. This molecule is less reactive than the OH radical and permits the decomposition of water to H_2O_2 to proceed. These excited and ionized molecules are unstable, and they react with proteins and other key substances within the cell. Many other events may occur with photon bombardment: long-chain molecules may be split and regrouped, aggregates may be pro-

duced, and ring forms may be disrupted indiscriminately. Certain chemical bonds may be vulnerable to inactivation by oxidation, resulting in loss of functional capacity. All of these chemical changes may ultimately be translated into biological injury at the cellular level.

Biological Effects

The mechanism of cell injury from radiation varies, and the effects may become manifest at different intervals after the primary event, depending on the type of intracellular target affected and the time in which certain chemical constituents are called on to perform. After some injury by ionization, a mature cell in a state of low metabolic activity may be grossly unaffected, but an actively growing cell may be destroyed. Cells that are in the act of dividing are more vulnerable than those resting between mitoses. Low oxygen tension, dehydration, freezing, and the presence of chemical reducing agents may significantly protect cells from radiation injury.

Radiation injury manifests itself as swelling of the cell, vacuolization of the cytoplasm, giant cell formation, and fragmentation or partial separation of the chromosomes at the time of division (Fig. 3). After a latent period, there is evidence of cell death, with loss of nuclear and cytoplasmic structures. The response is the typical inflammatory reaction: edema, capillary dilation and proliferation, infiltration of round cells, and fibroblastic growth. This immediate reaction is followed gradually by fibrosis, avascularity, and walling off of the injured area. Very late changes are scarification and contracture, with occasional inelastic, dilated blood vessels pinched off by essentially avascular stroma.

The selective destruction of tissues forms the basis of therapeutic radiology. Neoplastic cells are always more easily killed by radiation than are the parent cells of the surrounding normal tissues. The magnitude of the difference in radiovulnerability between normal and cancerous tissues largely determines whether the particular portion of the disease considered for radiation can be eradicated. This relative differ-

TABLE 1. *Modalities of external radiation*

Modality	Voltage	Source
Low voltage (superficial)	85–150 kV	X-ray
Medium voltage (orthovoltage)	180–400 kV	X-ray
Supervoltage	500 kV–8 MV	X-ray, ^{60}Co, ^{137}Cs, ^{226}Ra
Megavoltage	Above super-voltage energy	Betatron, Synchrotron, Linear accelerator

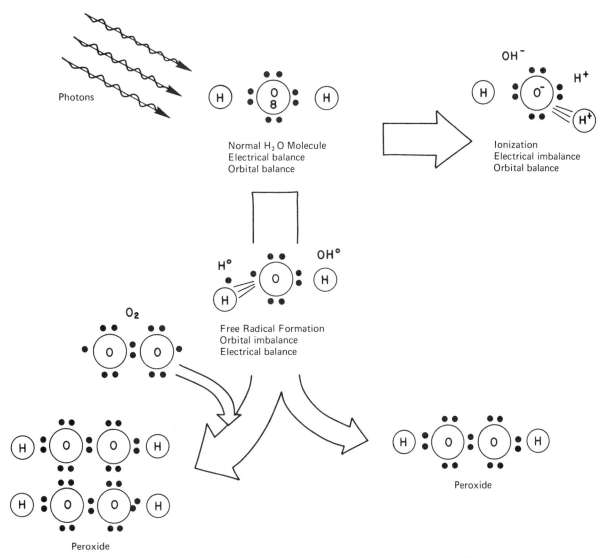

FIG. 2. Effects of radiation on water. Ionizing radiation produces water ions and may initiate free radical formation, yielding peroxide. The latter process is enhanced by addition of pure oxygen. (From Nolan JF. Basic radiation physics. *Clin Obstet Gynecol* 1961;4:504.)

ence in local radiovulnerability is referred to as a difference in radiosensitivity. Radiosensitivity and radiocurability are not identical. Relatively radioresistant tumors accessible to high-dose local radiotherapy are curable, but radiosensitive tumors that at the start of therapy or shortly thereafter are widely metastasized can only be controlled locally. An excellent example of a curable relatively radioresistant tumor is squamous cell carcinoma of the cervix. This malignancy remains one of the most curable tumors because of its accessibility to high-dose radiation and the relatively radioresistant nature of the hosting normal tissues of the cervix and vagina. The ability to place in juxtaposition to the malignancy a dose of radium that is tolerated by the surrounding normal tissue contributes to the success.

As a result of the chemical changes in response to irradiation, the very large molecules common in biological systems undergo a variety of structural changes that may alter their

function. Large molecules are degraded or broken into smaller units by irradiation. Cross-linking is another common structural change. A long molecule that is somewhat flexible in structure can undergo intramolecular cross-linking if a chemically active locus is produced on it and if the spot comes in contact with another reactive area. If the cross-linking is extensive, the molecules become incapable of normal function, and they may no longer be soluble in the system. Many macromolecules are held in a rigid configuration by intramolecular cross-linking bonds (i.e., specific chemical groups are linked together), frequently by hydrogen atoms, to form a three-dimensional structure. The hydrogen bonds are among the weakest in the molecule and are the first to be broken by irradiation. Such structural changes can lead to severe alterations in the biochemical properties of the molecule.

The radiation effects on molecules such as proteins, enzymes, nucleic acids, and certain lipids can profoundly affect

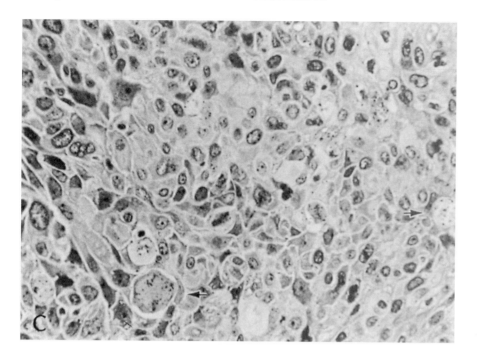

FIG. 3. Epidermoid carcinoma of cervix immediately after removal of the intracavitary radiation source. The most dramatic morphologic change occurs in the cells undergoing mitosis. Notice the swelling and disruption of the mitotic spindles *(arrow)*. The cytoplasm and nuclei of the interphase cells are vacuolated; the cytoplasm appeared swollen compared with the tumor pattern before irradiation. (Original magnification ×255; from Kraus KT. Irradiation changes in the uterus. In: Norris HJ, Hertig AT, Abell MR, eds. *The Uterus.* Baltimore: Williams & Wilkins, 1973.)

the cells and alter the organ and organism. The initial chemical change occurs in a fraction of a second and is seldom detected directly. Some of these chemical changes are repaired almost immediately; others that occur within less important structures may result in alterations that are seldom recognizable. In most cases, the transition between a chemical change in a system and the biological manifestation of this change is complicated and often obscure. The absorption and use of energy by a cell constitutes a complex chain of events in which many proteins are involved; radiation damage to these vital proteins can result in loss of cell membrane integrity and cell death.

In calculating tissue injury, the quantity of radiation is expressed in roentgens (R) or centigrays (cGy). The roentgen is the unit of exposure, and the centigray is the unit of absorbed dose. In the case of x- or γ-rays, exposure to 1 R results in an absorbed dose in soft tissue that is equivalent to 1 cGy. For many years, the rad was used as a measure of absorbed radiation dose, especially when physicians referred to external irradiation. One rad represents 100 ergs per gram of energy absorbed in a tissue. The gray (1 Gy = 100 rad = 100 cGy) was later adopted and is now used throughout the world in professional and scientific publications.

Although a variety of morphologic and functional changes have been described in irradiated cells, the bulk of direct and inferential evidence suggests that the cell nucleus is the major site of radiation damage leading to cell death. It has been calculated that 1×10^6 cGy are required to damage a cell membrane, but chromosomal aberrations and mutations can be produced by low radiation doses. Because only a few hundred centigrays are needed to kill most proliferating cells in tissue culture, it seems logical that the nuclear changes produced by the low doses are responsible for cell death.

Cell Cycle Effects

Mammalian cells growing exponentially are distributed randomly throughout the four compartments of the cell cycle. These compartments are known as G_1, S, G_2, and M, which represent the presynthetic phase, DNA synthesis, the postsynthetic phase, and mitosis, respectively. Compartmental analysis of the cell cycle depends on the observation of certain morphologic events. The first is the process of mitosis. In an appropriately stained population of exponentially growing mammalian cells, the proportion of mitoses can be calculated, and the mitotic index (i.e., ratio of cells undergoing mitosis to the total cell population observed) can be calculated. In most mammalian cell populations, the mitotic index is in the range of 2% to 7%. The second period of interest is that of DNA synthesis. To estimate the proportion of cells in DNA synthesis, exponentially growing cells are exposed to a precursor of DNA that has been labeled with an appropriate isotope. During a brief exposure to the labeled precursor, only cells replicating DNA are labeled, and these cells can be identified. The labeling index gives the portion of *growing* cells in DNA synthesis, which is usually between 50% and 60%.

It is important to understand several principles of cell growth. In exponentially growing populations, the portion of cells in each of the four compartments remains constant. The proportion of cells in each compartment is roughly proportional to the time required for completion of that particular cell activity. Important macromolecular events occur between each division, and accurate estimates of cell cycle distributions can be obtained rapidly with modern technology.

Radiobiological studies have determined several important features of the radiosensitivity of cell populations. When cells are in the process of DNA synthesis, they are most resistant to radiation. When cells are in G_2 or mitosis, they are most sensitive to radiation. Cells in G_1 may be sensitive if time in the compartment is short, or they may exhibit a period of increased resistance if G_1 occupies a more significant portion of total cell cycle time.

Radiation must be considered a classic cell-cycle-specific agent. It follows that the radiation response of certain human tumors may be related to the cell cycle distributions of tumor cells. The normal tissue bed response may depend on similar kinetic considerations.

Oxygen Effect

Molecular oxygen influences the radiation exposure of normal and neoplastic tissues, and the oxygen effect is one of the most important in radiation biology. Oxygen functions as a radiosensitizer, making cells more vulnerable to lethal damage. Conversely, hypoxic cells may be radioresistant. The issue of hypoxic cells in human neoplastic tissue may be important in radiation therapy of at least two types of tumors of the female reproductive tract. In advanced carcinoma of the cervix, the probability of local control of pelvic disease with external beam irradiation is low, a result that may reflect the presence of large numbers of hypoxic tumor cells. Women with carcinoma of the ovary who present with ascites are more effectively treated with chemotherapeutic agents and whole-abdomen irradiation after paracentesis and surgical debulking. Whether the improved efficiency of these modalities is cause by the reduction of tumor burden or removal of populations of hypoxic cells has not been determined, but radiation and chemotherapeutic agents are more effective when tumor cells are well oxygenated and the tumor cell burden is low.

Oxygen is an important modifier of radiation sensitivity, and mammalian cells are 2.5 to 3.5 times more resistant when irradiation is conducted in the absence of oxygen (Fig. 4). This difference is called the oxygen enhancement ratio. Whether this effect influences the probability of local control of *large* human tumors is a subject of continuing study, as is the role of oxygen in determining radiotherapeutic results.

Genetic Effects

It is not possible to assign a specific mutation rate to a specific radiation dose. Gene loci differ markedly in their mutability, and the rather random damage exerted by radiation on any particular chromosome makes predictability exceedingly difficult. Mitotic stage, cell type, sex, species, and dose rate all influence the rate of mutation production in lower animals and bacteria. Data accumulated in lower animals are difficult to extrapolate to humans, and predictions about mutation rates cannot be expected on the basis of the evidence accumulated from various types of radiation exposure; direct evidence of radiation-induced mutation in humans is lacking. The largest group of humans available for study are descendants of those exposed to radiation in Hiroshima and Nagasaki, and although there has been no detectable effect on the frequency

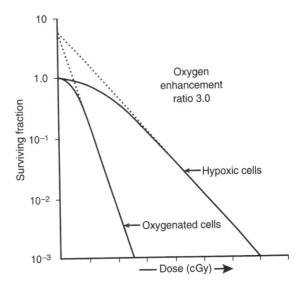

FIG. 4. Survival curves for mammalian cells exposed to x-rays in oxygenated and hypoxic environments. The difference in radiation sensitivity is threefold.

of prenatal or neonatal deaths or on the frequency of malformations in the offspring of these people, this does not mean that no hereditary effects have been produced by the radiation. The number of exposed parents was small, and doses were so low that it would be surprising if an increase in mutation had been detected. Several generations are needed to reveal recessive damage.

It is logical to expect that radiation exposure can increase the mutation rate in humans. This expectation is based largely on experiments on mice. It is estimated that the dose that doubles the spontaneous mutation rate for humans lies between 10 and 100 cGy. For an acute exposure to radiation, the probable value is between 15 and 30 cGy; for chronic irradiation, it is probably around 100 cGy. The Committee of Genetics of the Atomic Energy Commission has recommended that no person from conception to the years be subjected to more than 10 cGy. With appropriate shielding to prevent scatter, improved x-ray film, and image intensifiers, it is possible to attain satisfactory roentgenographic visualization of internal structures with reduced exposure. The average radiation doses to a developing fetus and to the maternal gonads inflicted by some common diagnostic techniques are shown in Table 2.

Effects on the Fetus

The classic effects of radiation on the mammalian embryo are intrauterine and extrauterine growth retardation; embryonic, fetal, or neonatal death; and gross congenital malformations. The structure most readily and consistently affected by radiation is the central nervous system. If the *in utero* absorbed dose is below 25 cGy, these classic effects of radiation are never observed together in laboratory animals or, in all likelihood, in humans. The absorbed dose, the stage of gestation,

TABLE 2. *Average radiation dose to the fetus and maternal gonads from diagnostic examinations*

Examination	Dose to fetus and maternal gonads (1×10^{-5} Gy)
Lower extremity roentgenography	1
Cervical spine roentgenography	2
Skull roentgenography	4
Chest roentgenography	8
Pelvimetry	750
Chest fluoroscopy	70
Cholecystography	300
Lumbar spinal roentgenography	275
Abdominal roentgenography	185/film
Hip roentgenography	100
Intravenous or retrograde pyelography	585
Upper gastrointestinal roentgenography	330
Lower gastrointestinal roentgenography	465

and the dose rate are important in determining the effect of radiation on a mammalian embryo. Embryonic damage can be reduced significantly by decreasing the dose rate to allow recovery processes to function.

Gross malformations occur most often when the fetus is irradiated during the early organogenic period, although cell, tissue, and organ hypoplasia can be produced by radiation throughout organogenic, fetal, and neonatal periods if the dose is high enough. There is no stage of gestation during which exposure to 50 cGy is not associated with significant probability of observable embryonic defect: death during the preimplantation period, malformations during the early organogenic stage, and cell deletions and tissue hypoplasia during the fetal stages. Animal experiments indicate that all embryos exposed to 100 cGy or more after implantation exhibit some degree of growth retardation. Finding and recognizing radiation-induced deleterious effects in offspring irradiated *in utero* become increasingly difficult with decreasing doses (<10 cGy) because such small doses are unlikely to produce such defects and because the natural incidence of defects is high. Clinically, an absorbed dose of 10 cGy to the fetus at any time during gestation can be considered a practical threshold for the induction of congenital defects, below which the probability of producing adverse effects becomes exceedingly small. Diagnostic x-ray procedures (Table 2) should be avoided in managing the pregnant woman unless there is overwhelming urgency. In women of childbearing age, possible damage to an early conceptus may be prevented by performing such tests immediately after the commencement of a normal menstrual period.

◊ CLASSIFICATION OF IONIZING RADIATIONS USED IN THERAPY

The radiations of main interest in radiotherapy are described as ionizing radiations. These can be subdivided according to their nature: electromagnetic radiations and particle radia-

tions. These groups may be further subdivided according to their origin and method of production. The terms x-rays and γ-rays are used for the ionizing electromagnetic radiations. Although these radiations are of an identical nature, the difference in terminology has evolved because x-rays can be produced by suitable generators, but γ-rays are radiations emitted spontaneously by radioactive materials undergoing nuclear transitions (Fig. 5). The use of the term x-ray or γ-ray depends on the origin of irradiation, not the energy of the photons. The field of particle irradiation has become complex, and among the particles in this classification are protons, helium, pions, neutrons, and heavy ions.

X-rays are produced when fast-moving electrons strike matter. Any apparatus designed to produce x-rays must provide a source of electrons, a method of accelerating the electrons (e.g., application of high voltage, acceleration by a linear accelerator), and a target that the electrons strike, producing the x-radiation.

The atoms of a radioactive material are unstable and spontaneously undergo radioactive decay, as a result of which they give out radiation as electromagnetic radiation (i.e., photons), particles, or both. An example of the medical use of the electromagnetic emission of a radioactive isotope is seen in the use of cobalt 60 (^{60}Co) as a source for teletherapy machines. An example of a source of particle emission used in medical therapy is radioactive phosphorus (^{32}P), which emits β particles, which are identical with electrons.

◊ PRINCIPLES OF RADIATION THERAPY

The technical modalities used in modern radiation therapy can be classified as external irradiation and local irradiation. External irradiation refers to radiant energy from sources at a distance from the body (e.g., ^{60}Co, linear accelerator, betatron, standard orthovoltage x-ray machines). Local irradia-

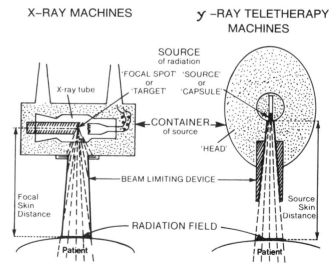

FIG. 5. Comparison of two devices used to produce ionizing electromagnetic radiation.

tion refers to radiant energy from sources in direct proximity to the tumor. Examples are intracavitary irradiation by means of applicators loaded with radioactive material such as radium or cesium (e.g., vaginal ovoids, vaginal cylinder); interstitial irradiation usually delivered in the form of removable needles containing radium, cesium, or iridium; and direct therapy (e.g., transvaginal irradiation), usually delivered by means of cones from an orthovoltage machine.

External Irradiation

The energy and penetrating power of ionizing radiation increase as the photon wavelength decreases. Differences in the physical characteristics of the radiation used are of great importance in therapeutic radiology (Table 3). The clinically important changes occur with radiation generated in the range of 400 to 800 kV (Table 1). Above this energy, the advantages are reduced absorption of radiation by bone, less damage to the skin at the portal of entry, better tolerance by the vasculoconnective tissue, greater radiation at the depth relative to the surface dose, and reduced lateral scatter of radiation in the tissues.

Supervoltage radiation has a reduced skin effect compared with orthovoltage radiation. With the higher-energy supervoltage radiation, forward scattering (i.e., in the direction of the primary beam) of radiation in the absorber is greater, and lateral scattering is diminished. With supervoltage radiation, the maximal ionization occurs below the level of the epidermis. For example, with ^{60}Co teletherapy, maximal ionization

TABLE 3. *The electromagnetic spectrum*

Type of wave	Wave energy[a]	Wavelength
Radio	10^{-10}–10^{-4} eV	3×10^5–1 cm
Infrared	0.01–1 eV	0.01–10^{-4} cm
Visible	2–3 eV	700–400 nm
Ultraviolet	3–124 eV	400–10 nm
X-ray	124 eV–124 MeV	10–0.00001 nm

[a] An electron volt (eV) is the energy of motion acquired by an electron accelerated through a potential difference of 1 V; 1 kiloelectron volt (keV) = 1000 eV; 1 megaelectron volt (MeV) = 1,000,000 eV.

occurs about 5 mm below the surface, and the surface dose may be only 40% of this maximum (Fig. 6).

An isodose curve is a line that connects points in the tissue that receive equivalent dosages of irradiation. Figure 53-6 contrasts the isodose curves for 250 kV, ^{60}Co, and 22-MeV machines. For the ^{60}Co machine, the maximal dose is near the surface (i.e., 0.5 cm below the skin), with a more rapid falloff in deeper tissues compared to the 22-MeV machine, which has its maximal dose well beneath the surface (i.e., 4 cm), with a more gradual falloff in the tissue. At a given depth, the higher dose of radiation can be achieved with a 22-MeV machine, sparing the effects of the radiation on the skin and subcutaneous tissue. These high-energy machines are particularly useful for treating deep tumors and for treating obese patients.

As the energy of radiation increases, it becomes more penetrating. As photons and resultant electrons become more energetic, they travel a greater distance into absorbing mate-

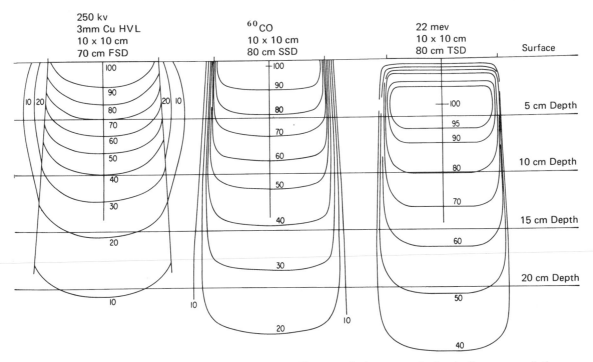

FIG. 6. Three isodose curves showing kilovoltage differences in tissue penetration by the same radiation dose generated by orthovoltage (250 kV), supervoltage (^{60}Co), and megavoltage (22 MeV). Cu HVL, copper half-value layer; FSD, focal–skin distance; SSD, source–skin distance; TSD, tumor–source distance.

rial. The percentage of radiation at any specific depth, compared with the surface dose, increases as the energy increases. This advantage of supervoltage and megavoltage is of clinical importance in the treatment of tumors located deep within the organism (e.g., carcinomas of the bladder and cervix), where the introduction of a sufficiently high dose with orthovoltage radiation is difficult or impossible.

Figure 6 demonstrates the isodose curves from various machines given a single portal of entry (i.e., one field). However, in the practice of gynecologic radiotherapy, two- or four-field techniques are commonly used. A two-field technique or parallel and opposed treatment of the pelvis has the great advantage of simplicity, and because adequate lateral margins are given, small variations in day-to-day setup do not introduce appreciable differences in a dose delivered to a target volume. The isodose curves for this two-field parallel and opposed treatment of the pelvis is seen in Figure 7, using a 22-MeV machine. Notice the reduced exposure of normal tissue anteriorly and posteriorly with a substantial dose at the target, which is the central pelvis.

Four fields, also called a box technique, can be used to reduce the subcutaneous doses and the total normal tissue volume subjected to a high dose. For a patient with an anteroposterior separation of 24 cm, a volume of approximately 6000 cc is irradiated to approximately the prescribed dose (e.g., 5000 cGy) with parallel and opposed fields, but with a four-field plan, the volume is reduced to about 3500 cc. Although the total volume of normal tissue irradiated with some dose is increased with the four-field technique, spreading the dose will reduce the normal tissue reactions. The need for treating all fields each day has been documented many times in the literature. Figure 8 illustrates the isodose curves for a four-field technique using the same 22-MeV machine.

In the supervoltage range, absorption of radiation by bone approximates that by water or soft tissue per unit density, but with orthovoltage, absorption of radiation is considerably greater by bone than soft tissue. The vasculoconnective tissue immediately adjacent to the bone around the haversian canals receives a higher dose because of static irradiation. This higher dose increases the risk of bone necrosis by destruction of the osteoblastic elements and damage to the vascular system. As radiation energy increases, similar tumor effects can be produced with less damage to important adjacent normal structures. The incidence of mucosal and skin reactions is reduced, and there is less damage to the vasculoconnective tissue. This greater tolerance of vasculoconnective tissue to a higher dose of properly protracted supervoltage radiation therapy is one of the factors that permits the planned combination of preoperative radiation and surgery without appreciably increasing the surgical risks beyond those associated with surgery alone.

Local Irradiation

Local application of radiation permits delivery of very high doses to restricted tissue volumes. Some of the high cure rates possible in gynecologic cancer result from the accessibility of vaginal and uterine cancer to local irradiation. This accessibility allows relatively high doses of radiation to be delivered to the neoplasm with safe amounts of normal tissue exposure.

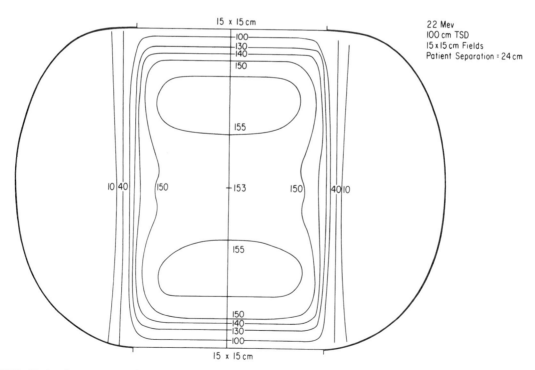

FIG. 7. Isodose curves from a two-field treatment plan on a 22-MeV linear accelerator. TSD, tumor–source distance.

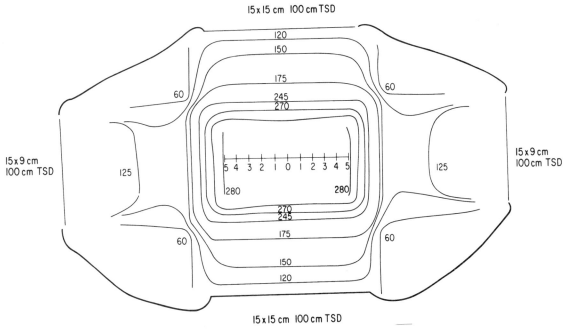

FIG. 8. Isodose curves from a four-field treatment plan on a 22-MeV machine (e.g., betatron). TSD, tumor–source distance.

Regardless of the source of electromagnetic or photon radiation, the transmitted energy from the source diverges as the distance from the source increases. This divergence causes a decrease in energy, and the relation is described by the inverse square law, which indicates that the energy dose of radiation per unit area decreases proportionately to the square of the distance from the site and the source. For example, the dose of radiation 2 cm from a point source is only one-fourth of the value of the dose at 1 cm. The depth dose (relative to the surface dose) increases with the use of larger vaginal ovoids associated with brachytherapy of cervical cancer (Fig. 9). In this situation, the principle that the intensity of irradiation rapidly decreases with distance from the radiation source (i.e., inverse square law) is used to advantage.

Local irradiation is suitable for a small tumor with well-defined limits and a clinical situation in which it is desirable to restrict the volume of tissue irradiated. A larger volume of tissue is best treated with external irradiation. In the past, radium was the isotope most frequently used, in tubes and in needles, for local application to the genital tract. With the other materials (Table 4) currently available for local application, the major disadvantage is an appreciably shorter half-life. Several can be incorporated into a solid material, such as ceramic or various metals, and need not be used as a powder or gas, as is the case with radium. Radium tubes and needles contain radium powder, and many of its decay products are in gas form within the same container. For these reasons, cesium has replaced radium in most institutions. In the past, gold 198 ([198]Au) was used as a permanent tumor implant. It was difficult to prepare and had a rather rapid radioactive decay, and a homogeneous dose was dif-

ficult to obtain. Iodine 125 (^{125}I) has replaced [198]Au in permanent implants.

If the radiation intensity decreases rapidly with increasing depth in tissue, as is the case with local irradiation, the tissue adjacent to the radiation source theoretically may be treated adequately without damage to the underlying structures. The effectiveness of this distribution of radiation depends on care-

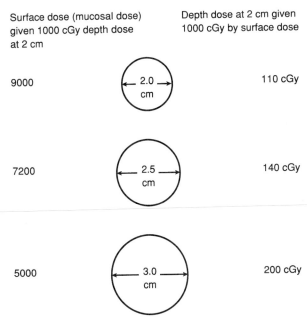

FIG. 9. Brachytherapy with vaginal ovoids, comparing the increased depth dose with the size of the ovoids used.

TABLE 4. *Isotopes commonly used in radiation therapy*

Isotope[a]	Energy (MeV)	Half-life
^{137}Cs	0.662	30 years
^{60}Co	1.173, 1.332	5.3 years
^{125}I	0.027–0.035	60 days
^{192}Ir	0.47	74 days
^{226}Ra	0.8	1620 years
^{222}Rn	0.8	3.83 days
^{182}Ta	1.18	115 days

^{a} ^{226}Ra, ^{137}Cs, ^{192}Ir, and ^{182}Ta are suitable for temporary implants; ^{222}Rn is suitable for permanent implants that remain in the patient; ^{60}Co has some uses in intracavitary therapy.

ful application of the source. Interstitial application of a radioactive source is much more difficult than intracavitary application. A system of multiple, discrete sources often results in a less homogeneous isodose pattern than irradiation from an external source or from a well-placed intracavitary source. On the other hand, higher doses can be attained within the tissue at risk.

Interstitial therapy consists of the use of cesium or iridium needle implants to the tumor tissue. Because of the high concentration of dose around the source, many sources are usually necessary to produce a uniform dose covering a large volume. Isodose curves can be calculated or measured for such implants. Needle implants are often used to deliver a high, localized dose to vaginal lesions. The use of perineal templates has expanded the use of radioactive needle implants to parametrial areas for cervical and vaginal lesions (Fig. 10).

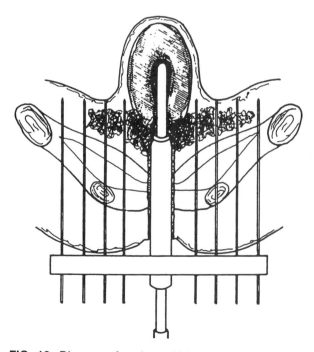

FIG. 10. Diagram of an interstitial implant used to treat a stage IIIB cervical cancer with a Syed-Noblett applicator.

◊ IONIZING RADIATION IN GYNECOLOGIC THERAPY

For practical purposes, the modern use of ionizing radiation in gynecology is limited to the treatment of malignant diseases. In the recent past, radiation was used for sterilization, in the treatment of dysfunctional or climacteric bleeding, to produce ovulation in cases of infertility, and in the treatment of eczematoid and other benign diseases of the vulva. A single dose of 400 to 500 cGy to the ovaries is often sufficient to permanently arrest menses in a premenopausal woman. However, a dose of 1200 to 2000 cGy in 10 days to 2 weeks is often required to produce complete arrest of ovarian steroidogenesis in younger patients. This technique for producing cessation of menses still has applicability in some women with severe menorrhagia who are not good surgical candidates, such as a premenopausal, acutely leukemic woman with thrombocytopenia and menorrhagia. However, with this possible exception, all of the benign conditions listed above are now managed by other means.

Tolerance of Pelvic Organs

The tolerance to radiation of the pelvic organs varies slightly from patient to patient and is subject to the factors previously described, such as volume, fractionation, and energy of radiation received. The administration of isotopes by different techniques may also result in different dose distributions and considerable differences in tolerance. The more advanced the lesion, the greater is the dose necessary for its eradication, and the greater is the likelihood of morbidity. With advanced disease, higher risks of injury are justified. In advanced cervical, vaginal, or corpus cancer, the integrity of the bladder and rectum may be already compromised, and serious sequelae may follow irradiation of such lesions.

The cervix and corpus of the uterus can tolerate very high doses of radiation. They withstand higher doses than any other comparable volume of tissues in the body; doses of 20,000 to 30,000 cGy in about 2 weeks are routinely tolerated. This remarkable tolerance level permits a large dose and enables a high rate of control of cervical cancer. The unusual tolerance of the uterus and the vagina to radiation accounts for the success of radium and cesium in the treatment of cervical lesions. In addition to the tissue tolerance, the epithelium of the uterus and vagina appears to have a remarkable ability to recover from radiation injury.

The sigmoid, rectosigmoid, and rectum are more susceptible to radiation injury than other pelvic organs (small bowel excluded). The frequency of injury to the large bowel often depends on its proximity to the treating isotope and on the total dose administered by external beam plus intracavitary sources. When an external beam is used alone, the large bowel is the most sensitive of pelvic structures to radiation. An acute early reaction is heralded by diarrhea and tenesmus. A later manifestation of injury, usually occurring 6 to 12 months after treatment, is chronic pelvic pain associated with constriction of the bowel lumen and partial bowel obstruction. The maximal dose that the rectum can tolerate depends on many factors, including the time–dose relationship of the external beam and local isotope source. Kottmeier calculated that the dose to the bladder and rectum from the Stockholm technique of intracavitary application of radium is about 4000 cGy per 3 cm^2 of rectum and bladder.

The bladder tolerates slightly more radiation than the rectum, according to most calculations. A convenient rule of thumb proposed by Fletcher gives upper limits of radiation dose and indirectly estimates the tolerance of the bladder and rectum: the sum of the central dose delivered by the external beam plus the number of milligram hours (mgh) of radium or cesium administered by intracavitary techniques should never exceed 10,000. This rule of thumb may not be valid unless the Fletcher-Suit intercavitary system is used. If a heavy dose of intracavitary radium or cesium is applied centrally for a small lesion, the amount of external-beam irradiation applied centrally must be kept to a minimum. Conversely, if the lesion is large and the vaginal geometry poor, a minimal intracavitary dose can be given, and the dose administered centrally by external beam may be quite high (6000 to 7000 cGy).

Because irradiation for carcinoma of the cervix is primarily directed to the pelvic contents, only limited portions of small bowel are included. The small bowel is normally in constant motion, and this tends to prevent any one segment from receiving an excessive dose. If loops of small bowel are immobilized as a result of adhesions from previous pelvic surgery, they may be held directly in the path of the radiation beam and be injured. The resultant injury usually becomes symptomatic 1 year or more after the completion of radiation and is manifested as a narrowed lumen with or without associated mucosal ulceration.

Injury to normal tissue may be permanent. When any area of the body is subjected to tumoricidal doses of radiation, the normal tissues of that area suffer an injury that is only partially repaired, even if the person survives for several decades after treatment. Radiobiologists estimate that, in the case of injury to normal tissues, only 5% to 20% of the damage is repaired. The normal tissues in the irradiated area can retain a considerable handicap. If a second malignant neoplasm arises in that same area many years later, additional tumoricidal radiation would result in a normal tissue injury level that could be unacceptable. In general, the same area must not be subjected to tumoricidal radiation on more than one occasion; the result is inevitably massive loss of normal tissue.

Treatment Planning

A prescription for radiation therapy should be based on many factors. The physician should have performed an evaluation of the full extent of the lesion by whatever means available, including palpation, imaging studies, and surgical observations. Knowledge of the pathologic characteristics of the disease including potential areas of metastases that may influence the treatment plan also need to be considered. An

example of the latter is a rationale for elective irradiation of the regional lymphatics in the pelvis.

The therapist must then decide on the goal of therapy, either cure or palliation. A selection for the appropriate treatment from several modalities should include the possibility of combining radiation with surgery or chemotherapy. Such a choice may have significant impact on the volume treated and the total dose of radiation delivered. The determination of the optimal dose of radiation and the volume to be treated is influenced greatly by the anatomic location, histologic type, stage, and other characteristics of the lesion as well as the normal tissue bed in the radiation field.

The radiation oncologist should work closely with the gynecologist to integrate the various modalities. The physicist will help with the treatment planning and the dosimetry to ensure the greatest possible accuracy. Periodic evaluation of the patient's general condition, tumor response, and normal tissue status is essential during and after therapy. The ultimate responsibility for treatment decisions and the technical execution of the radiation therapy rests with the radiation oncologist.

Radiocurability

Radiocurability is often confused with radiosensitivity. Radiocurability implies eradication of the tumor at the primary and regional sites as a direct result of the irradiation. Radiosensitivity is an expression of the response of the tumor to the radiation and may not be associated with cure. The sensitivity of a particular malignant lesion depends on many factors including the degree of hypoxia, the proportion of cells in cycle during radiation, the inherent radiosensitivity of the tumor cells in cycle, and the efficiency of the repair mechanism for radiation damage in the tumor cells. Most unresponsive tumors have a high hypoxic fraction and fail to reoxygenate during fractionated irradiation. This concept of hypoxia underlying radioresistance has been validated in experimental models, but clinical trials designed to reverse the hypoxia have had limited success in improving outcome. Repair of sublethal damage is found in most cell tumor lines. Potentially lethal damage varies greatly from one cell line to another and tends to correlate with the clinical radiocurability, with less curable tumors showing the greatest degree of sublethal recovery. There is no consistent correlation between the responsiveness of a tumor to irradiation and curability, and relatively radioresistant and still curable lesions are found in most tumor types.

Cancer of the Cervix

External pelvic irradiation is justified in cervical cancer for several reasons. Because intracavitary radium or cesium obeys the inverse square law of all radiation that emanates from radioactive isotopes (Fig. 11), it cannot safely deliver a cancericidal dose beyond 3 cm from the external cervical os. Moreover, structures other than the uterus, the upper part

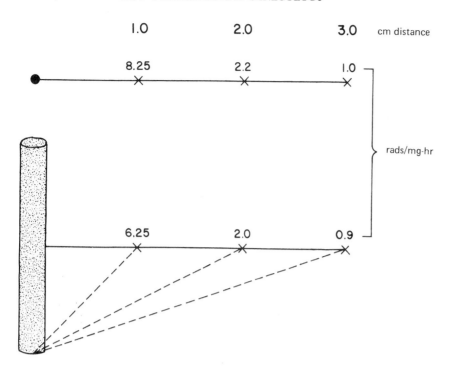

FIG. 11. Radiation effects at various distances from a 1-mg point source of radium and a 1-mg, 2-cm-long tubular source of radium.

of the vagina, and medial portions of the broad ligament, such as the lateral portions of the broad ligament, uterosacral ligaments, uterovesical ligaments, and pelvic lymph nodes, also must be considered within the spread pattern of uterine cancer and within the field to be treated. The amount of intracavitary radium that can be safely applied is limited by the sensitivity of neighboring structures, such as the bowel and bladder. Although the normal tissue of the uterus and vagina is extremely radioresistant, certain limits to the quantity of intracavitary radium must be set, and external pelvic irradiation remains the only method capable of delivering an effective dose homogeneously throughout the large volume of tissue at risk.

In the treatment of cervical cancer, the careful combination of external irradiation and intracavitary application of radium or cesium is crucial. For stage IB lesions, in which regional metastases are unlikely, intracavitary radium may be used alone, delivering a total of 10,000 mgh in two applications by the Fletcher technique. For stage III lesions, especially those with poor vaginal geometry for radium use, external-beam irradiation may be the major component of the treatment plan, and whole-pelvis irradiation can be 6000 to 7000 cGy. The distribution of disease must be carefully assessed by palpation and diagnostic techniques, and intracavitary application of radium and external-beam irradiation must be done judiciously to direct the greatest dose to the tumor that is compatible with acceptable morbidity.

The objectives of treatment are to sterilize the central lesion and to destroy neoplastic cells in the paracervical tissues and regional lymph nodes. External irradiation commonly is used first to destroy metastases to the lateral lymph nodes and to reduce the size of the central lesion. Reduction in the size of the central lesion is desirable because the lateral effect of an iso-

tope source diminishes according to the square of the distance. The smaller the cervix, the greater is the isotope effect lateral to the cervix. The use of external irradiation before local therapy also allows resolution of badly infected cervical lesions and shrinkage of fungating exophytic lesions that interfere with the accurate placement of intracavitary devices.

To quantify the amount of radiation reaching certain areas in the pelvis, concomitant with the development of the Manchester system (see Intracavitary Radiation Techniques), British workers suggested specific landmarks designated as point A and point B. They defined a point 2 cm above the mucosa at the lateral vaginal fornix and 2 cm lateral to the uterine canal as point A and another point 5 cm lateral using the same landmarks as point B. This enables calculation of the dose of radium and x-rays delivered and of the dose absorbed in the paracervical triangle (i.e., point A) and in the region of the pelvic nodes (i.e., point B). It was suggested that a tumor dose of 7000 to 8000 cGy was necessary to control squamous cell carcinoma of the cervix, and most followers of the Manchester system attempted to administer a minimum of 7000 cGy to point A. This precipitated concern about positioning of the radium or cesium, because it was desirable to keep the rectal dose at 6000 cGy to point A. Careful placement of radium makes this possible.

Intracavitary Radiation Techniques

Stockholm Technique

The Stockholm technique (Fig. 12A) usually employs two intracavitary applications of radium or cesium 3 weeks apart. Each application is approximately 25 to 28 hours in duration, and the intrauterine applicator contains between 50 and 75 mg

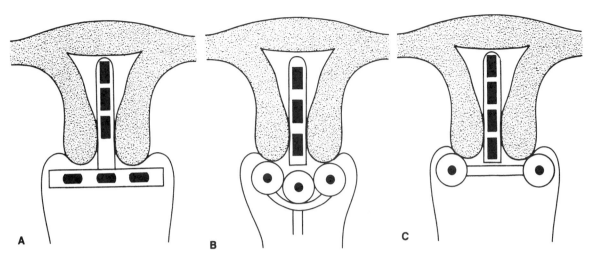

FIG. 12. Application of radium in the treatment of cervical cancer. **(A)** Stockholm technique. **(B)** Paris technique. **(C)** Manchester technique.

of isotope. In an attempt to reduce the chance of overdose to the cervix and adjacent midline structures, the lower 2 cm of the uterine tandem contains no radium; the uterine applicator is otherwise evenly distributed with sources. The vaginal applicator consists of boxes or cylinders in series. In this manner, two to four rows of sources can be used to cover the cervical lesion; a total of 60 to 80 mg of radium is commonly used. This technique uses a hot loading of radium over a relatively brief period. In the Stockholm technique, the dose at point A averages slightly less than 6000 cGy; the dose at point B is usually about 1900 cGy.

Paris Technique

The Paris technique (Fig. 12B) was initiated by the Curie Foundation. It uses a uterine tandem and vaginal sources. The tandem extends the length of the uterine cavity, and in a typical case, it contains 6.6 mg of radium in the cervical canal and two sources of 13.3 mg cephalad for a total of three sources within the tandem. A 10- or 15-mg source can be substituted for the 13.3-mg source. In the typical case, two cork cylinders containing 13.3 or 15 mg of radium are pushed into the lateral vaginal fornices by a connecting spring. A third cork containing 6.6 mg is placed directly against the external os. With the Paris technique, the dose at point A is similar to that delivered by the Manchester technique. When equivalent milligram hours are used, this dose is about 5700 cGy in 6 days. One treatment period of 96 to 200 hours is the rule for the Paris technique.

Manchester Technique

The Manchester technique (Fig. 12C), a convenient and popular modification of the Paris system, differs from the Paris technique in that the source placed in the area of the cervical canal is considered as unit strength. The remaining sources in the corpus and vagina are applied as multiples of this unit,

and they are selected and arranged to produce the equivalent isodose curves in each case and an optimal dose to preselected points A and B in the pelvis (Fig. 13). The Manchester system is designed to yield constant isodose patterns regardless of the size of the uterus and vagina (Fig. 14).

A modification that has gained wide popularity because of its ability to accommodate to afterloading is the Fletcher-Suit radium system (Fig. 15). Many institutions have discontinued the use of radium for the less expensive isotope cesium at equivalent doses and use cesium in all applicators.

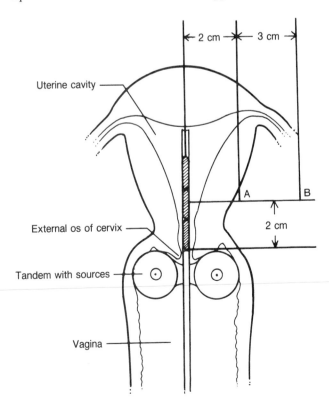

FIG. 13. Diagram of a tandem and ovoid placement for cervical cancer with points A and B identified.

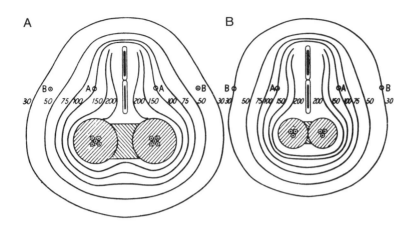

FIG. 14. Isodose curves show the dose delivered by the Manchester technique to different depths in two cases in which different amounts of radium could be used. In each, the dose is calculated as 100% at point A or *x* centigrays (cGy). Other numbers show the percentage of this dose delivered at other depths. **(A)** Standard applicators for a large vagina. **(B)** Standard applicators for a small vagina. The dose at points A and B is considerably improved by using larger vaginal ovoids. With the larger ovoids, the same maximal normal tissue tolerance of the bladder, rectum, and vaginal mucosa is arrived at, with more radiation being delivered to the parametria as represented by point A and point B. (From Paterson R. *The treatment of malignant disease by radiotherapy.* London: Arnold, 1963; with permission.)

External Pelvic Irradiation

Whole-pelvis irradiation is usually administered through an anterior and posterior field approximately 15 to 18 cm² (Fig. 16). When the lesion is central and small, it may be judicious to conserve the tolerance of the bladder and rectum for radium and use a 4-cm lead block in the midline of the field. This technique, called parametrial irradiation (Fig. 17), allows the parametrium and pelvic wall to be irradiated homogeneously and conserves the tolerance of the midline structures for future intracavitary techniques. Supervoltage or megavoltage radiation has the advantages mentioned earlier and, whenever possible, should be used for whole-pelvis or parametrial irradiation.

Individualized therapy with judicious use of external-beam and intracavitary irradiation can result in gratifying survival rates (Tables 5 and 6). Other considerations affecting the treatment of cancer of the cervix are discussed in Chapter 49.

Cancer of the Vagina and Vulva

Squamous cell carcinoma of the vagina usually occurs in elderly women who are not good candidates for surgery. Most lesions are treated by whole-pelvis irradiation, which effectively treats the pelvic lymph nodes and markedly reduces the size of the central lesion. The central lesion is additionally treated by local irradiation delivered by a transvaginal cone or by interstitial implantation of radium, cesium, or iridium within the lesion. Overall cure rates of 40% to 50% with radiation therapy have been reported from some institutions. Approximately 80% of stage I lesions are effectively eradicated.

Although some large squamous cell cancers of the vulva have responded dramatically to radiation therapy, ionizing radiation is not considered the treatment of choice for this lesion. The normal tissues of the cervix and vagina can tolerate large doses of radiation, but the vulva is exquisitely sensitive to ionizing radiation. Some radiobiologists think this area contains a disproportionately large number of end arteries, in which damage by radiation results in vasculitis and radiation necrosis. Radiation to the vulva is inevitably associated with severe vulvitis that almost invariably requires interruption of therapy. Surgical excision of the vulvar lesion by means of vulvectomy remains the treatment of choice. The rationale for a combination of wide local surgery followed by radiation to the regional nodes has some merit, especially for patients who are unable to undergo surgical removal of these regional nodes.

Carcinoma of the Endometrium

The most common malignant lesion of the uterus is endometrial carcinoma. This lesion often invades deeply into the myometrium. Treatment primarily with radiation therapy has been attempted in the past. However, placing isotope sources in proximity to the disease to deliver optimal radiation to all the central lesion is usually not possible. Removal of the uterus and both adnexa has proved essential for optimal results (see Chapter 50). When large series of patients are analyzed, it is apparent that the addition of hysterectomy to the treatment plan for endometrial cancer improves survival by at least 20%, even when the data are corrected for death caused by intercurrent disease. Unlike cervical cancer, the treatment of endometrial cancer by irradiation alone is not advisable.

The staging of endometrial lesions is now surgical in nature, essentially eliminating the prior practice of preoperative intracavitary and external radiation therapy. Initial surgical staging allows radiation therapy to be tailored to the high-risk pathologic findings, such as deep myometrium invasion, involvement of the endocervix, or adnexal metastases.

Some institutions assume that radiation alone constitutes adequate treatment of stage II endometrial cancer that has extended to involve the endocervical canal. However, this remains controversial. Most clinicians prefer to treat suspected stage II patients with surgery first and to tailor radiation therapy to the operative findings. Some patients with a large amount of tumor in the cervix may need a radical hysterectomy.

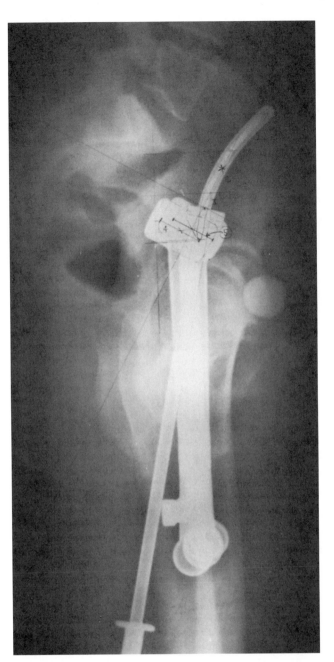

FIG. 15. Fletcher-Suit afterloading radium system. All radium is placed into a hollow tandem and ovoids after the placement films (similar to that seen here) are inspected and approved. The metal seed in the posterior lip of the cervix can be seen above the ovoids, marking the cervical tissue on the film.

Postoperative External Irradiation

Most institutions have discontinued the use of preoperative radiation therapy for endometrial carcinoma and substituted postoperative external and intracavitary (i.e., vaginal vault) irradiation in selected cases. Much of the data collected in the literature in the last decade suggest that cervical or isthmic involvement, deep myometrial invasion, and anaplastic histology significantly increase the possibility of pelvic recurrence and mandate the need for whole-pelvis irradiation. The cus-

tomary dose is between 4000 and 5000 cGy in fractionated doses administered over 5 to 6 weeks. Unequivocal proof that this improves survival is nonexistent, but the control of pelvic recurrences, especially vaginal cuff recurrence, appears to be well documented.

Postoperative Radioisotopes

The intraperitoneal instillation of colloidal ^{32}P is recommended by some authorities for stage I patients in whom positive peritoneal washings are the only evidence of extrauterine disease. The technique is discussed further in the section on carcinoma of the ovary.

Postoperative Application of an Isotope to the Vaginal Vault

Several studies have strongly suggested that postoperative adjunctive radiation therapy for endometrial carcinoma is as effective as preoperative radiation in the prevention of vaginal cuff recurrence. Some institutions advocate primary hysterectomy with bilateral salpingo-oophorectomy if there is no indication of cervical involvement or anaplastic histology. The specimens are then carefully reviewed by the pathologist, and if an occult area of undifferentiated disease, occult involvement of the cervix or isthmus, deep myometrial invasion, or adnexal metastases is found, postoperative whole-pelvis irradiation is applied. If none of these indicators of nodal involvement is found, the postoperative radiation therapy may be avoided or take the form of cuff irradiation delivered by a variety of vaginal applicators as early as 1 week after hysterectomy. The cuff irradiation, which may also be delivered by transvaginal cone, is relatively simple and usually can be accomplished without an additional anesthetic. No prospective randomized study has been conducted to ascertain the true value of cuff irradiation alone or after external irradiation in patients with high-risk factors who have undergone a hysterectomy for endometrial carcinoma. The application of cuff irradiation to these patients is intuitive and not based on demonstrated improved outcome.

Radiation Treatment of Recurrent Cancer

The development of a pelvic mass in a patient previously treated for endometrial carcinoma may indicate a pelvic side wall recurrence. Laparotomy should be performed, if possible, to confirm the diagnosis and delineate the extent of the disease. Patients with an unresectable localized recurrence are candidates for a permanent implant with ^{125}I seeds or a removable transperineal implant with iridium sources.

If whole-pelvis irradiation has not already been used, consideration should be given to outlining the recurrence with metal clips and delivering external irradiation to the affected area after the operation. If the recurrence is at the apex of the vaginal vault, treatment depends on the size of the lesion. External irradiation should be considered if normal tissue toler-

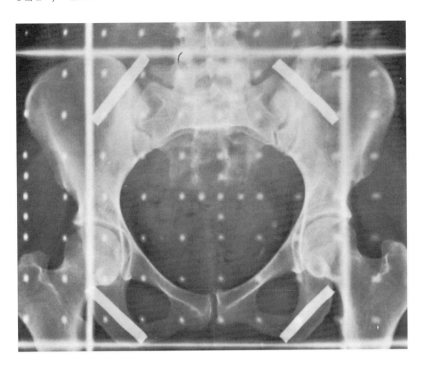

FIG. 16. Whole-pelvis irradiation for cervical cancer extending into the upper part of the vagina. The lower margin of the 18-cm by 18-cm field is well below the pubic symphysis. Lead tapes (white strips) are used for excluding the corners of a square field, reducing the irradiated volume by roughly 10%.

ance has not been approached by previous radiation therapy. For vaginal recurrence, external irradiation is usually supplemented by an interstitial implant or the use of a transvaginal cone. Di Saia et al. reported on a technique of open implant at laparotomy for such recurrences occurring after previous hys-

terectomy (Fig. 18). Unfortunately, these pelvic recurrences are often in a field of fibrosis and avascularity secondary to previous radiation therapy, and the response of pelvic recurrence to systemic progestin therapy or chemotherapy is much less favorable than that of distant recurrences.

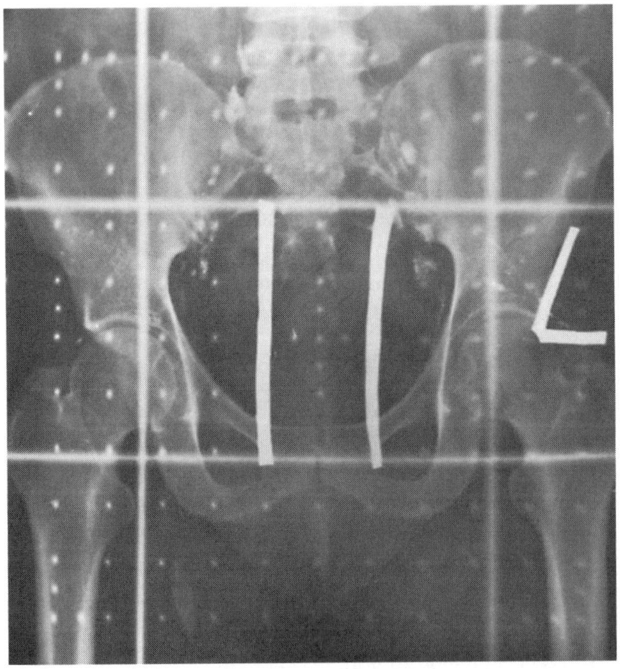

Carcinoma of the Ovary

Approximately 80% of primary ovarian carcinomas arise from germinal epithelium, and this histogenesis is associated with limited radiosensitivity. Except for dysgerminomas, the typical bulky ovarian carcinomas are not easily treated with irradiation. Although adenocarcinomas have limited radiosensitivity, other ovarian tumors, such as malignant teratoma or embryonal carcinoma, are notoriously poor in their response to irradiation. In addition to the limited radiovulnerability of most ovarian lesions, radiation therapy is severely handicapped by the fact that the disease is usually widely distributed within the peritoneal cavity.

Complete surgical extirpation of all grossly visible tumor considerably enhances the response to radiation therapy.

FIG. 17. Parametrial irradiation for cervical cancer. A 4-cm lead block is placed between strips of lead tape, sparing the midline. The height of the field is considerably reduced compared with that in Fig. 16. Only a 10-cm height needs to be blocked in the midline, and in a larger field, the top center portion should not be spared because this represents the node-bearing areas.

TABLE 5. Epidermoid carcinoma of the uterine cervix: 5-year disease-free survival rates with irradiation treatment only[a]

Stage	No. of cases	%
IA	29	100
IB	302	87.7
IIA	249	70.9
IIB	249	66.3
III	226	36.7

[a]From Grisby PW, Perez CA, Kuske RR, et al. Adenocarcinoma of the uterine cervix. Radiother Oncol 1988:12:289; with permission.

TABLE 6. *Adenocarcinoma of the cervix: 5-year disease-free survival rates*

Stage	No. of cases	%
IB		
<3 cm	91	88
3–4 cm	65	65
4.1–5.9 cm	37	62
>6 cm	22	45
IIA	22	38
IIB	38	28
III	46	31

[a]From Eifel PJ, Morris M, Oswald MJ, et al. Adenocarcinoma of the uterine cervix; prognosis and patterns of failure in 367 cases treated at the MD Anderson Cancer Center between 1965–1985. *Cancer* 1990;65:2057; with permission.

Dembo reported excellent survival results for a series of patients with minimal residual disease after surgery who were treated with irradiation therapy to the abdomen and pelvis with and without chemotherapy. Confirmatory studies are needed.

Although bulky ovarian cancer within the pelvis may respond satisfactorily to standard pelvic irradiation, large residual areas of disease in the upper abdomen present a difficult problem for the radiotherapist. The difficulty arises whenever the entire abdomen is at risk because the tolerance for whole-abdomen irradiation is low and the dose that can be safely delivered is well below a tumoricidal dose. The abdomen does not tolerate a dose higher than 2500 cGy. Fletcher proposed that the peritoneal cavity be irradiated by moving-strip technique, in which small segments of the abdomen are systematically irradiated at high intensity. This technique theoretically keeps the morbidity at an acceptable level and permits radiobiologically greater effective doses to be delivered. Many institutions have been unable to adopt this technique successfully, and its value remains uncertain (Fig. 19).

There is interest in a treatment technique for stage I and stage II ovarian cancer that includes the postoperative intraperitoneal instillation of colloidal ^{32}P. This technique has considerable theoretical merit if all gross disease is removed after hysterectomy and bilateral salpingo-oophorectomy, with only microscopic implants or cellular spill remaining for postoperative therapy. ^{32}P emits β-rays, which penetrate only to a depth of 1 to 4 mm. The colloidal substances adhere to or are phagocytized by peritoneal surfaces and can discharge their ionizing radiation to malignant cells *in situ*. No prospective randomized studies have been published showing superiority to chemotherapy.

◊ IMPROVED THERAPEUTIC STRATEGIES

By the combined use of hyperthermia in radiation therapy, it is possible to double the complete response rates obtained with the radiation alone in certain malignant disease states. Although hyperthermia is not of practical value in the therapy of most forms of clinical cancer, there is reason to hope that this treatment modality will become valuable during the next century because of the continuing increase in our understanding

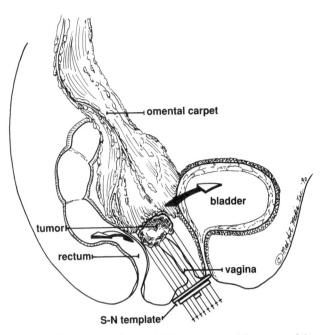

FIG. 18. Placement of omental tissue around the apex of the vagina containing neoplasm after reflecting the bladder and the rectum. (From Di Saia PJ, Creasman WT. *Clinical gynecologic oncology, 5th ed.* St Louis: CV Mosby, 1997.)

of the mechanisms of cytotoxicity of elevated temperatures, the growing technical power and precision of machines that heat tissues and monitor the degree of heating, and the introduction of the concept of the multimodality therapy in which hyperthermia, radiation therapy, and chemotherapy are combined in bimodality or trimodality regimens.

It is unlikely that hyperthermia itself will be capable of producing major tumor regression with sufficient predictability to make it a practical treatment modality, but under optimal conditions, hyperthermia can enhance the effectiveness of radiation therapy, as demonstrated by several preclinical models and by work with superficial cancers that can be adequately heated. A strongly positive cytotoxic interaction exists between hyperthermia and a variety of drugs that injure cellular DNA or interfere with cellular energy metabolism. The initial observations on the trimodality interactions of irradiation, hyperthermia, and chemotherapy are highly encouraging.

Radiation therapy is an integral part of curative cancer therapy, but the tolerance of normal tissues traversed by radiation and the resistance that tumor cell populations can develop have limited the curability of certain tumors, especially those in higher clinical stages. Research in radiobiology and radiation physics may provide methods to increase cure while decreasing morbidity. Computer-controlled dynamic treatment, radioprotector drugs, hyperbaric oxygen, particle irradiation, and hypoxic cell-sensitizing drugs are undergoing clinical evaluation, with some preliminary encouraging results.

Among the various strategies for improving on conventional radiotherapy clinical results in cancer, the use of

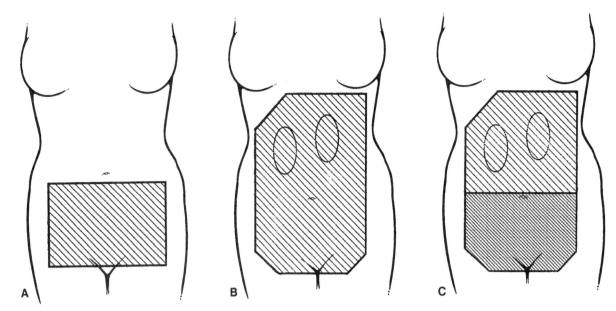

FIG. 19. Three radiation fields are commonly used. **(A)** A pelvic field is used for whole-pelvis irradiation. **(B)** A whole-abdomen field is used for early-stage ovarian cancer and endometrial cancer with positive peritoneal cytologic results. **(C)** A whole-abdomen field with a pelvic boost is used for ovarian cancer postoperative therapy after removal of most gross disease.

charged or uncharged particle radiotherapy is particularly attractive. Depending on the particle beam in question, such radiation offers a biological advantage, a dose distribution advantage, or both over photon or electron radiation. Fast neutrons, which are uncharged particles, have radiobiological properties that may be superior to those of x-rays or γ-rays.

Among the charged particles, protons and helium ions exhibit superior dose distribution properties. Pions and heavy ions such as carbon 12, neon 20, silicon 28, and argon 40 have dose distribution and potential biological advantages. The theoretical ranking of particle beams suggests that heavy ions and pions may be better than the other for therapy. Although much of the theory may be true, clinical correlations are far from being demonstrated. Most clinical investigations of particle irradiation in the United States have involved neutrons, protons, or helium ions. The choices are largely determined by considerations of cost. Heavy ions and pions are theoretically better than neutrons, protons, and helium ions, but they are much more expensive to produce. Despite the difficulty in production and other problems, particle radiation therapy has been impressively effective against several cancers in small trials, but additional studies are necessary for confirmation.

◊ RECOMMENDED READINGS

Dembo AJ. Radio therapeutic management of ovarian cancer. *Semin Oncol* 1984;11:238.

Dische S. Chemical sensitizers for hypoxic cells: a decade of experience in clinical radiotherapy. *Radiother Oncol* 1985;3:97.

Di Saia PJ, Creasman WT. Clinical gynecologic oncology. Appendix B. In: *Basic principles in gynecologic radiotherapy, 5th ed.* St Louis: CV Mosby, 1997.

Di Saia PJ, Syed AMN, Puthawala AA. Malignant neoplasia of the upper vagina endocrurrie, hypertherm. *Oncology* 1990;6:251.

Dusenbery KE, Carson L, Potish RA. Perioperative morbidity and mortality of gynecologic brachytherapy. *Cancer* 1991;67:2786.

Elkind MM. DNA damage and cell killing: cause and effect. *Cancer* 1985;45:2123.

Fajardo LJ. *Pathology of radiation injury.* New York: Mason Publishing, 1982.

Fletcher GH. *Textbook of radiotherapy, 3rd ed.* Philadelphia: Lea & Febiger, 1980.

Hall EJ. Radiation biology. *Cancer* 1985;55:2051.

Hall EJ. *Radiobiology for the radiologist, 4th ed.* Philadelphia: JB Lippincott, 1994.

Hand JW, James JR, eds. *Physical techniques in clinical hyperthermia.* New York: John Wiley & Sons, 1986.

Hilaris BS, Nori D, Anderson LL. *An atlas of brachytherapy.* New York: Macmillan, 1988.

Khan FM. *The physics of radiation therapy, 2nd ed.* Baltimore: Williams & Wilkins, 1994.

National Council on Radiation Protection and Measurements. *Report no. 116, Limitation of exposure to ionizing radiation.* Bethesda, MD: NCRP, 1993.

Nori D, Hilaris B. *Radiation therapy of gynecological cancer.* New York: Alan R Liss, 1987.

Overgaard J. The current and potential role of hyperthermia in radiotherapy. *Int J Radiat Oncol Biol Phys* 1989;16:535.

Perez CA, Garcia DM, Gigsby PW, Williamson J. Clinical applications of brachytherapy. In: Perez CA, Brady LW, eds. *Principles and practice of radiation oncology, 2nd ed.* Philadelphia: JB Lippincott, 1992.

Perez CA, Purdy JA. Biologic and physical aspects of radiation oncology. In: Hoskins W, Young R, Perez C, eds. *Principles and practice of gynecologic oncology.* Philadelphia: JB Lippincott, 1992:217.

Perez CA, Camel HM, Galakatos AE, et al. Definitive irradiation in carcinoma of the vagina: long term evaluation of results. *Int J Radiat Oncol Biol Phys* 1988;15:1283.

Phillips TL, Wasserman TH. Promise of radiosensitizers and radioprotectors in the treatment of human cancer. *Cancer Treat Rep* 1984;68:291.

Pistenmaa DA. Particle beam radiation therapy. In: Devita VT Jr, Hellman S, Rosenberg SA, eds. *Cancer: principles and practice of oncology, 2nd ed.* Philadelphia: JB Lippincott, 1985:2280.

Suit H, Urie M, Efrid JT. Proton beams in clinical radiation therapy. *PPO Updates* 1992;6:1.

Swartz HM. Hazards of radiation exposure for pregnant women. *JAMA* 1978;239:1907.

CHAPTER 54

Gestational Trophoblastic Neoplasms

——— ◇ ———

Charles B. Hammond

Gestational trophoblastic neoplasia (GTN) is an unusual spectrum of benign and malignant tumors derived from the trophoblast of the human placenta. Although rare in incidence, they have the potential to be rapidly fatal diseases that afflict young women in their peak reproductive years.

Traditionally, GTN have been divided histologically into three categories: hydatidiform mole, invasive mole (chorioadenoma destruens), and choriocarcinoma. Partial hydatidiform moles and placental site tumors (PST) are now recognized as being histologically and clinically separate entities under the broad classification of GTN.

Despite the apparent diversity of these entities, they are all derived from the human placenta, trophoblast, and the paternal genome, with an occasional maternal contribution. Human chorionic gonadotropin (hCG) is secreted by these neoplasms and serves as a sensitive tumor marker that correlates well with the clinical course for all but the PST.

In 1956, metastatic gestational choriocarcinoma, the most malignant form of these diseases, was shown to be curable by chemotherapy.[14] Now, many studies show the extreme curability of most of these patients, although individualization of therapy is an important fundamental.

This chapter is an attempt to review this unusual group of human neoplasms and to provide a review of the important concepts reading diagnosis, therapy, and follow-up for patients with GTN.

◇ PATHOLOGY

Patients may be treated for malignant GTN on the basis of clinical, radiographic, and hCG level determinations without an exact histologic diagnosis. For this reason, the generic term of GTN is useful, especially when treating patients with metastatic disease that is not readily accessible for histologic analysis. Except for PST, the initial histologic features of any lesion identified as a GTN are less important than the clinical data and hCG level, which indicate how a particular patient and her GTN interact.

Hydatidiform Mole

All hydatidiform moles were once categorized together, but two distinct types of molar gestations have now been described: partial and complete hydatidiform moles, which have distinct cytogenetic origin, pathologic features, and clinical behavior. It is not as clear whether partial hydatidiform mole represents a form of GTN or an extreme form of hydropic degeneration of the placenta in a chromosomally abnormal pregnancy. Until larger numbers of patients with partial molar pregnancies are studied, they should be considered as being a variant of the complete hydatidiform mole and having the risk (albeit less) of malignant sequelae. Most patients with primary molar gestations do not require chemotherapy and can be safely monitored after evacuation with serial hCG level determinations until either spontaneous regression occurs or the patient develops criteria for beginning chemotherapy for malignant sequelae.

Partial Hydatidiform Mole

Approximately 1% of pregnancies have a triploid karyotype and resolve in spontaneous abortion. A portion of these have some histologic features in common with hydatidiform mole; these have been described as partial hydatidiform moles. A comparison of karyotypic, pathologic, and clinical features of partial and complete hydatidiform moles is given in Table 1.[8] Partial moles are often associated with an identifiable fetus or with amniotic membranes. Grossly, the placenta has a mixture of normal and hydropic villi. Microscopic features include an intermingling of normal and hydropic chorionic villi with focal mild hyperplasia of trophoblastic elements. Scalloping of the hydropic villi is common, with trophoblastic inclusions in the stroma. Fetal vessels are frequently observed with nucleated fetal erythrocytes within the vessels. Normal amniotic membranes are often identified, even if a fetus is not found.[11]

Partial moles are almost always associated with one haploid maternal and two haploid paternal sets of chromosomes. Pre-

TABLE 1. *Complete and partial hydatidiform moles*

Feature	Partial hydatidiform mole	Complete hydatidiform mole
Karyotype	Triploid paternal and maternal origin	Most 46,XX paternal origin
Pathology		
Fetus or amnion, fetal vessels	Present	Absent
Hydropic villi	Variable, often focal	Pronounced, generalized
Trophoblastic proliferation	Focal	Variable, often marked
Clinical		
Mole clinical diagnosis	Rare	Common
Uterus large for dates	Rare	30–50%
Malignant sequelae	<5%	6–36%

sumably, this results from dispermic fertilization of a haploid ovum or fertilization of a haploid ovum with a diploid sperm.

Women with partial hydatidiform mole usually have a clinical diagnosis of spontaneous abortion or missed abortion. Often, hydropic villi are not identified on ultrasound, and the diagnosis is not suspected until after evacuation of the pregnancy. Initial hCG levels are lower than those seen in patients with complete hydatidiform mole, and a prompt postevacuation regression of hCG level usually occurs. Unlike patients with complete moles, who have a 10% to 30% incidence of malignant sequelae, fewer than 5% of the patients with partial moles require chemotherapy for malignant GTN.

Although patients with partial hydatidiform mole appear to have a low incidence of malignant sequelae, it is recommended that all undergo hCG level surveillance after evacuation, similar to that recommended for patients with complete hydatidiform mole. If there is any doubt that the products of a conception are molar, hCG monitoring should be done.

Complete Hydatidiform Mole

Complete hydatidiform mole is identified macroscopically by edema and swelling of virtually all chorionic villi with a lack of fetus or amniotic membranes. Hydropic villi are usually 1 to 3 cm in diameter, giving the gross appearance of a mass of grape-like vesicles. Microscopically, the chorionic villi are hydropic with marked interstitial edema. Fetal vessels are absent in the stroma of the villi. Proliferation of cytotrophoblast and syncytiotrophoblast is observed. Regardless of the degree of trophoblastic proliferation, all patients should be followed in similar fashion. All hydatidiform moles secrete hCG, and this marker is used to monitor regression after evacuation.

Complete moles are almost uniformly diploid with paternal chromosomal markers. Most are 46,XX, although a few have a 46,XY karyotype. The most common origin of complete hydatidiform mole is fertilization of an empty egg by a haploid sperm, which reduplicates, although a few may result from dispermic fertilization of an empty egg.

Unlike patients with partial hydatidiform moles, approximately one-third to one-half of these patients have uterine enlargement greater than expected for gestational dates. A few will be smaller. Fetal heart tones are absent. Patients often present with vaginal bleeding and spontaneous abortion of the atypical hydropic vesicles. Theca lutein cysts are detected clinically in approximately 20% of patients with complete moles. Pulmonary decompensation, pregnancy-induced hypertension, and hyperthyroidism are occasionally observed. The clinical diagnosis of molar gestation is supported by a characteristic mixed echogenic image filling the uterus on an ultrasound scan.

Invasive Mole

The diagnosis of invasive mole (chorioadenoma destruens) rests on the demonstration of a complete hydatidiform mole invading into the myometrium without intervening endometrial stroma. Otherwise, histologic features are identical to a complete mole. Invasive moles usually are diagnosed within 6 months of molar evacuation. Untreated invasive moles tend to invade the uterine wall locally, which can result in uterine perforation and hemorrhage. Direct vascular invasion and metastasis can also occur. Rarely, biopsies of distant metastases have the hydropic villi of invasive mole rather than the expected solid sheets of anaplastic cells seen in choriocarcinoma.

The identification of an invasive mole from uterine curettings can be difficult unless there is sufficient myometrium to document direct myometrial invasion.

Choriocarcinoma

Choriocarcinoma is a highly anaplastic malignancy derived from trophoblastic elements. No chorionic villi are identified. Grossly, the tumor has a red, granular appearance on cut section with focal, often extensive central necrosis and hemorrhage. Histologically, the lesion consists of intermingled syncytioblastic and cytotrophoblastic elements with many abnormal mitoses, multinucleated giant cells, and extensive areas of necrosis and hemorrhage. Choriocarcinoma rapidly invades the myometrium and uterine vessels, and systemic metastasis results from hematogenous embolization. The lung and vagina are the most common metastatic sites, with secondary dissemination to the central nervous system (CNS), kidney, liver, gastrointestinal tract, and other distant sites.

Choriocarcinoma can follow any type of pregnancy. Approximately one-half of choriocarcinomas are preceded by hydatidiform mole, and the remaining one-half are equally distributed between a normal antecedent term gestation and abortion or ectopic pregnancy. Gestational choriocarcinoma has been observed several years after the last known pregnancy. Spontaneous regression of the primary uterine site has been well documented from autopsy series of patients before the development of effective chemotherapy.

Placental Site Tumor

Placental site tumors are locally invasive neoplasms derived from intermediate cells of the placenta. These rare neoplasms are composed of a monomorphic population of intermediate cytotrophoblast cells that secrete placental lactogen and relatively small amounts of hCG. They produce local myometrial invasion with rare systemic metastasis. Placental site tumors are much more resistant to standard chemotherapy than other forms of GTN. Hysterectomy is the initial therapy of choice, although some patients have been apparently cured by curettage alone.

◊ INCIDENCE AND EPIDEMIOLOGY

Hydatidiform mole is identified in approximately one of 1500 to 2000 pregnancies in the United States. There appears to be marked variation in the incidence of hydatidiform mole, with the incidence 5- to 15-fold higher in the Far East and Southeast Asia than in the Western industrialized nations. Some of this variation may be accounted for by the methodology of studies reporting the incidence of molar gestation, because many studies were reported from the experience at referral centers and may overestimate the true incidence of molar pregnancies in the general population.

Racial differences may account for some of the geographic variations, as suggested by observations that Japanese immigrants to Hawaii have an incidence of molar gestation intermediate between that of native Hawaiians and native Japanese. The risk of developing a subsequent molar gestation is four to five times higher than the risk of the first. Maternal age appears to influence the risk of hydatidiform mole. Several studies have suggested that the risk increases with increasing maternal age, and other studies have suggested an increased risk for younger women or adolescents. The impact of paternal age on the incidence of hydatidiform mole is difficult to separate from the effect of maternal age.

Nutritional factors may also be important in the development of hydatidiform mole, including deficiencies of protein or animal fat and fat-soluble carotene. These nutritional causes may partially explain the observed geographic differences in hydatidiform mole.

The incidence of partial hydatidiform mole is unknown. Presumably, many are undiagnosed because of insufficient histologic analysis of tissue from spontaneous and induced abortions. Some pathologists are not familiar with the diagnosis of partial hydatidiform mole, and karyotyping is seldom performed on material obtained from spontaneous abortions. Szulman and colleagues reclassified approximately 10% of all moles in their studies as partial hydatidiform moles on the basis of histologic analysis.

Invasive mole follows approximately 10% to 15% of complete hydatidiform moles. In the United States, approximately one of 40 moles, one of 5000 ectopic pregnancies, one of 15,000 abortions, and one of 150,000 normal pregnancies result in choriocarcinoma. Approximately 3000 cases of hydatidiform mole and 500 to 750 cases of malignant GTN are diagnosed in the United States each year.

◊ MANAGEMENT OF HYDATIDIFORM MOLE

The basic principles for managing the patient with hydatidiform mole include establishing the diagnosis, evacuating the molar gestation, and providing adequate hCG level monitoring after evacuation to aid in the detection of malignant GTN. Patients with complete hydatidiform moles frequently present with spontaneous abortion of hydropic villi, which are pathognomonic for molar pregnancy. Absent fetal heart tones, uterine enlargement different from that expected for the gestational age, and a markedly elevated hCG level are all useful clues to the diagnosis of hydatidiform mole. Ultrasound is now the diagnostic method of choice for evaluating patients with suspected hydatidiform mole. Ultrasound gives a characteristic image of multiple echogenic regions within the uterus corresponding to hydropic villi and focal intrauterine hemorrhage (Fig. 1).

Evaluation of the patient before evacuation of the hydatidiform mole is directed toward preparing the patient for evacuation, obtaining baseline hCG level information, screening for occult metastatic disease, and screening for associated hyperthyroidism. The following studies are recommended:

◊ Complete physical and pelvic examinations,
◊ Complete blood count,
◊ Blood chemistries, including renal, hepatic, and thyroid function tests,
◊ Baseline serum hCG level,
◊ Chest radiograph,
◊ Pelvic ultrasound.

Suction curettage (D&C) offers a safe, rapid, and effective method of evacuation of hydatidiform mole in most patients. Some patients who do not desire preservation of reproductive function may benefit from primary hysterectomy for evacuation of hydatidiform mole and concurrent sterilization. However, these patients must be closely followed after hysterectomy because malignant sequelae develop in a few women, even after hysterectomy for hydatidiform mole. Hysterotomy or induction of labor for molar evacuation are no longer recommended.

Suction D&C for evacuation of hydatidiform mole has a low complication rate among patients with uterine sizes corresponding to less than 16 weeks of gestation. Oxytocic agents are given after cervical dilation and partial evacuation to aid in postoperative hemostasis. Patients with excessive uterine enlargement have a high risk of pulmonary complications associated with D&C, which may be related to trophoblastic deportation, preeclampsia, fluid overload, anemia, and hyperthyroidism. For patients with hydatidiform mole complicated by uterine enlargement greater than that of 16 weeks of gestation, baseline arterial blood gases should be obtained preoperatively with an electrocardiogram, radionucleotide-gated heart pool scan for ejection fraction, and a valvular function

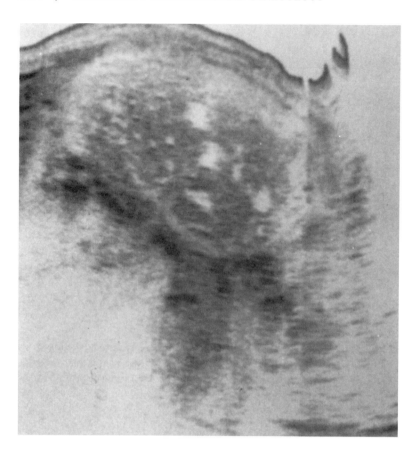

FIG. 1. A longitudinal ultrasound reveals a hydatidiform mole. The mixed echoic pattern is caused by hydropic villi and focal intrauterine hemorrhage.

assessment by cardiac ultrasound. Evacuation should be performed with a laparotomy set and facilities for central hemodynamic monitoring on hand.

Primary hysterectomy is a reasonable alternative for termination of molar gestation in patients with hydatidiform mole who have completed childbearing and desire sterilization. Hysterectomy reduces the incidence of malignant sequelae after evacuation of hydatidiform mole from approximately 20% after suction D&C to less than 5% after hysterectomy. However, this does not eliminate the need for careful follow-up or complete hCG surveillance after termination of hydatidiform mole, because malignant GTN may develop even after hysterectomy.[6] We would base decision regarding regarding extirpation of the adnexa on similar grounds as any other benign process.

Theca lutein cysts are clinically detected in approximately 20% of patients with molar gestations. These cysts are thin-walled and highly vascular. Theca lutein cysts develop as a response to ovarian hyperstimulation from the high hCG levels produced by hydatidiform moles. They usually regress spontaneously over several weeks after molar evacuation. It is preferable to avoid operation or ovarian manipulation in patients with uncomplicated theca lutein cysts. Rarely, because of abdominal distension and respiratory compromise, they may require aspiration by ultrasonic guidance. These cysts may become enlarged and undergo torsion, infarction, or rupture, and in these circumstances, oophorectomy may be life saving.

Prophylactic short courses of methotrexate or dactinomycin chemotherapy have been used at the time of molar evacuation, and they appear to decrease the incidence of malignant sequelae in patients with high-risk features. Such chemotherapy does not eliminate the chance of subsequent malignancy and does not eliminate the need for hCG surveillance. We do not recommend prophylactic chemotherapy at the time of molar evacuation for patients with uncomplicated hydatidiform mole if reliable hCG surveillance is available.

Surveillance After Molar Evacuation

Since sensitive hCG assays became readily available, histologic grading of molar tissue after evacuation of hydatidiform mole has assumed less importance in predicting the potential for malignant postmolar sequelae. Several sensitive hCG assays are available, measuring the β-subunit of hCG by radioimmunoassay or by radioimmunometric assay. These assays are able to detect hCG levels elevated above the baseline variations of pituitary gonadotropins. These sensitive hCG assays should be used to monitor patients with GTN after evacuation of hydatidiform mole and during therapy of patients with malignant GTN. Urinary or serum pregnancy screening tests should not be used to follow patients with GTN, because the assays do not have sufficient sensitivity to permit detection of minimal elevations of hCG levels.

The recommendations for postmolar follow-up include baseline physical examination, pelvic examination, and chest radiographs; determination of serum β-hCG levels every 1 to 2 weeks after evacuation until hCG level is normal; determination of the hCG level 2 to 4 weeks after first normal level to confirm spontaneous hCG regression; and hCG surveillance every 1 to 2 months for 6 months after the first normal hCG level.

Most women with molar pregnancies undergo hCG level regression after evacuation to normal limits and require no further therapy. We recommend strict contraception during hCG surveillance to avoid an intercurrent pregnancy that would interfere with monitoring. The hCG elevation of an early normal pregnancy could mask the hCG rise associated with postmolar malignant GTN.

Although an early report implicated oral contraceptives as increasing the risk for the development of postmolar malignant GTN, subsequent investigators found no significant increase in the risk of malignant GTN associated with the use of oral contraceptives after molar evacuation. Because oral contraceptives are the most reliable form of contraception in young patients, my colleagues and I routinely use these after evacuation of hydatidiform mole. After completion of 6 months of hCG level surveillance with normal results, patients are allowed to achieve pregnancy if desired. Because patients are at a fourfold to fivefold increased risk of recurrent molar pregnancy, they should undergo early screening of future pregnancies with ultrasound to exclude recurrent molar gestations. Figure 2 illustrates our algorithm for diagnosis and follow-up of patients with hydatidiform mole.

◊ MALIGNANT GESTATIONAL TROPHOBLASTIC NEOPLASMS

Malignant Sequelae After Molar Evacuation

The spectrum of malignant sequelae after evacuation of hydatidiform mole includes intrauterine molar proliferation without invasion (i.e., retained mole), invasive mole, choriocarcinoma, and the clinical identification of metastatic GTN without a histologic diagnosis. The purpose of hCG level surveillance is early detection of trophoblastic neoplasia before the development of complications related to local proliferation, uterine invasion, or distant metastases.

Before the development of effective chemotherapy against GTN, Delfs reported that approximately 9% of women required hysterectomy for malignant sequelae after evacuation of hydatidiform mole. Many series of patients have been reported since the development of chemotherapy, with a wide range in the rate (9% to 36%) of patients requiring therapy after evacuation of hydatidiform mole. These observed differences in the frequency of malignant GTN probably reflect inclusion of partial moles in some studies, a different incidence of metastatic disease in patient populations, or different hCG level regression criteria used to define malignant GTN and assign therapy in the various studies.

Histologic and clinical features can be used to define high- and low-risk groups of patients after molar evacuation but are of little value in determining the need for therapy in individual patients. Trophoblastic proliferation, uterine enlargement, theca lutein cysts, respiratory distress syndrome after molar evacuation, and postevacuation uterine hemorrhage are all associated with a higher frequency of postmolar malignant GTN. Prompt uterine involution and regression of theca lutein cysts are favorable prognostic signs. However, the definitive method for predicting development of postmolar malignant GTN is observation of the pattern of hCG regression.

Serial hCG levels are obtained at 1-week intervals with chest radiographs every 2 to 4 weeks as long as the hCG levels are elevated. Patients are treated with chemotherapy according to several criteria: hCG level rise; hCG level plateau for 3 or more consecutive weekly levels (x, $x + 7$ days, $x + 14$ days); appearance of metastases; or histologic evidence of invasive mole or choriocarcinoma. On the basis of these criteria, the incidence for therapy of postmolar malignant GTN at our center is approximately 20%.

Diagnosis

The diagnosis of malignant GTN is made when a woman has a rising or plateauing hCG level or develops metastases after

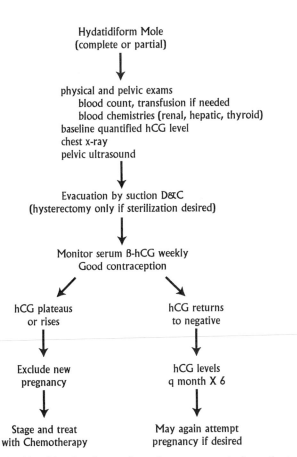

Hydatidiform Mole
(complete or partial)

↓

physical and pelvic exams
    blood count, transfusion if needed
    blood chemistries (renal, hepatic, thyroid)
baseline quantified hCG level
chest x-ray
pelvic ultrasound

↓

Evacuation by suction D&C
(hysterectomy only if sterilization desired)

↓

Monitor serum β-hCG weekly
Good contraception

↙   ↘

hCG plateaus   hCG returns
or rises   to negative

↓   ↓

Exclude new   hCG levels
pregnancy   q month X 6

↓   ↓

Stage and treat   May again attempt
with Chemotherapy   pregnancy if desired

FIG. 2. Algorithm for diagnosis and management of a patient with hydatidiform mole.

evacuation of a hydatidiform mole. Histologic diagnosis of invasive mole or choriocarcinoma is the criterion for malignant GTN. Patients who developed malignant GTN after non-molar gestations often present with atypical symptoms referable to distant metastases. Gastrointestinal or urologic hemorrhage, hemoptysis, or cerebral hemorrhage may be the initial symptoms. Irregular uterine bleeding or amenorrhea may be observed. Rarely, patients present with clinical hyperthyroidism. Under these circumstances, the diagnosis of malignant GTN is facilitated with an alert examiner, serum hCG testing, and the exclusion of normal pregnancy. The possibility of metastatic GTN should be considered for any woman of the reproductive age group presenting with metastatic disease involving the lungs or distant sites from an unknown primary site of malignancy.

After the diagnosis has been made, the following clinical, laboratory, and radiographic evaluations are recommended for a patient with malignant GTN:

◊ Physical and pelvic examinations,
◊ Baseline hCG level,
◊ Complete blood count and baseline chemistries,
◊ Chest radiograph,
◊ Pelvic ultrasound,
◊ Computed tomography (CT) of brain, chest, and abdomen–pelvis.

Before a woman is treated for malignant GTN with chemotherapy, it is essential to rule out an intrauterine pregnancy with a pelvic ultrasound scan. Approximately 50% of patients with malignant GTN have pulmonary metastases detected by routine chest radiographs. The clinical significance of small pulmonary metastases detected only by whole-lung CT scans is unknown. Because CNS and hepatic metastases occasionally have been encountered without clinical or radiographic evidence of pulmonary or vaginal metastases, the remainder of the radiologic studies are strongly recommended regardless of whether abnormalities are detected by physical examination or chest radiograph. The role of magnetic resonance imaging studies in the evaluation of women with GTN is not yet defined.

Occult CNS metastases may be detected using lumbar puncture with simultaneous serum and cerebrospinal fluid (CSF) hCG determinations. The plasma–CSF hCG level ratio is normally greater than 60:1 in the absence of CNS metastases and is usually less than 60:1 in patients with CNS metastases.[1] Some investigators have reported falsely lowered plasma–CSF hCG ratios for patients without GTN undergoing first-trimester abortions and for patients with nonmetastatic GTN. My colleagues and I have used CSF hCG determinations most frequently to evaluate patients who have developed resistance to chemotherapy and who have residual disease documented by elevated serum hCG levels, although the site of disease has remained obscure.

Surgery may be useful for patients with malignant GTN, but it is rarely indicated for staging or diagnosis alone. Histologic evaluation of tissue obtained by D&C may yield prognostic information related to the response to first-line chemotherapy, but the procedure runs the risk of uterine perforation and hemorrhage. Laparoscopy, craniotomy, and thoracotomy are rarely justified to establish the primary diagnosis of malignant GTN because this diagnosis can be made on the basis of an elevated hCG levels with radiographic evidence of metastases after excluding pregnancy.

All patients with malignant GTN must be thoroughly evaluated for metastatic disease. Selection of the initial therapy and subsequent survival largely depend on identification of poor prognostic factors in patients with metastatic disease. See Fig. 3 for our algorithm of management of malignant GTN.

Staging and Classification

Because there is considerable overlap in the clinical course of the histologic entities that comprise malignant GTN, and because a complete histologic evaluation of an individual patient with GTN is rarely possible, a variety of classification and staging systems have been used to assess risk and assign initial therapy and prognosis for these patients. Several clinical findings are important in categorizing patients for treatment, and any classification system must take these factors into consideration to be clinically useful.

A simple clinical classification system has been used at our institution since 1968 to assign initial therapy for patients with malignant GTN.[9] This system takes into account factors that

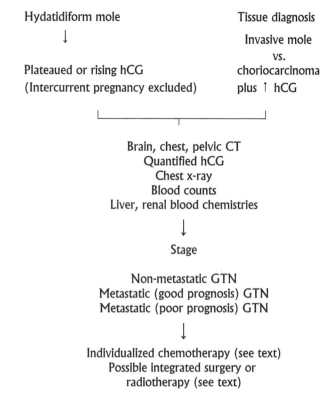

FIG. 3. Algorithm for management of a patient with malignant gestational trophoblastic disease.

TABLE 2. *Clinical classification of malignant gestational trophoblastic neoplasia*

I. Nonmetastatic GTN[a]
  A. Not defined in terms of good versus poor prognosis
II. Metastatic GTN
  A. Good prognosis (i.e., absence of high-risk factors)
    1. Pretreatment hCG level <40,000 mIU/ml serum β-hCG
    2. <4-Month duration of symptoms attributable to disease
    3. No evidence of brain or liver metastasis
    4. No significant prior chemotherapy
    5. No antecedent term pregnancy
  B. Poor prognosis (i.e., any single high-risk factor)
    1. Pretreatment hCG level >40,000 IU/ml serum β-hCG
    2. >4-Month duration of symptoms attributable to disease
    3. Brain and/or liver metastasis
    4. Failed prior chemotherapy
    5. Antecedent term pregnancy

[a]GTN, gestational trophoblastic neoplasms; hCG, human chorionic gonadotropin.

predict failure of the initial single-agent chemotherapy and allows identification of patients who would benefit from initial aggressive multidrug chemotherapy (Table 2). After the radiographic studies have been completed, the patient is considered to have nonmetastatic GTN if there is no evidence of extrauterine metastases. This category is not subdivided into good-prognosis and poor-prognosis categories because these patients can achieve approximately 100% remission rates using current chemotherapeutic regimens. The histologic diagnosis of choriocarcinoma, although mandating treatment, does not change the initial choice of therapy. If there is any clinical or radiographic evidence of extrauterine metastases, the patient is classified as having metastatic GTN. These patients are further divided into good-prognosis and poor-prognosis categories on the basis of factors that predict the failure of primary single-agent chemotherapy with methotrexate or dactinomycin.

The International Federation of Gynecologists and Obstetricians (FIGO) developed a staging system for GTN that is based on the anatomic site of disease, conforming to the FIGO staging systems for other gynecologic malignancies:

Stage I: Disease confined to the uterine corpus
Stage II: Metastases to the vagina or pelvis
Stage III: Metastases to the lung
Stage IV: Other extrapelvic metastases

Although essentially all patients with stage IV disease are at high risk, this system does not recognize the prognostic importance of other factors, such as the initial hCG level, other direct and indirect measurements of tumor burden, or duration of disease. The World Health Organization (WHO) devised a prognostic index scoring system (Table 3) based on Bagshawe's analysis of the prognostic factors of his patient population. In addition to using a weighted scale for risk factors analyzed by the clinical classification, such as hCG level and duration of disease, the system identifies a graded range of additional risk factors. Ectopic pregnancies and abortions are considered to have an intermediate risk between molar and term pregnancies. Blood types and age contribute to the score. The size of the largest tumor, the number of metastatic sites, and site of metastases are considered as indirect approximations of tumor burden. After computation of each risk factor, the patient is considered to be at low risk if the score is 4 or less, at intermediate risk with a score of 5 to 7, and at high risk with a score of 8 or more.

The WHO prognostic index scoring system has been found to correlate well with survival after conventional approaches to chemotherapy. However, not all of the factors have been critically evaluated to determine whether the graded scoring system is valid. Figure 3 illustrates our plan of evaluation and therapy for patients with malignant GTN.

Therapy

Before the development of effective chemotherapy against malignant GTN, surgical therapy was unsatisfactory for most

TABLE 3. *World Health Organization prognostic scoring system for gestational trophoblastic neoplasia*

Prognostic factor	Score[a]			
	0	1	2	4
Age	≥39	>39		
Antecedent pregnancy	Hydatidiform	Abortion; ectopic	Term pregnancy	
Interval (months)[b]	<4	4–6	7–12	>12
hCG level (IU/liter)	<10^3	10^3–10^4	10^4–10^5	>10^5
ABO blood groups (female/male)		O/A A/O	B AB	
Largest tumor (cm)	<3	3–5	>5	
Site of mestastasis		Spleen, kidney	Gastrointestinal tract, liver	Brain
Number of metastases		1–3	4–8	>8
Prior chemotherapy			Single drug	Multiple drugs

[a]Low risk, ≤4; intermediate risk, 5–7; high risk, ≥8.
[b]Interval: time between antecedent pregnancy and start of chemotherapy.

patients, even for women with nonmetastatic disease confined to the uterus. Since the introduction of methotrexate in the 1950s, malignant GTN has become the most curable of human solid tumors.[14,15,25] Therapy should be conducted by physicians who have considerable experience in the management of these diseases, and a reliable hCG assay should be available so that therapeutic changes can be instituted when necessary. Brewer and associates originally observed a worse prognosis for patients with metastatic GTN who received primary therapy outside of a trophoblastic center many years ago, and we continue to have patients referred for therapy after failure of inappropriate regimens for malignant GTN. Although chemotherapy has largely replaced surgery and radiation therapy as the first-line management of malignant GTN, these modalities continue to play an important part in the management of patients with malignant GTN.

Chemotherapy

The initial chemotherapy for malignant GTN should be selected on the basis of one of the systems of classification of malignant GTN (Table 4). We use the clinical classification system. Patients with nonmetastatic GTN are initially treated with single-agent chemotherapy regimens using less vigorous therapy with methotrexate, as are patients with good-prognosis metastatic GTN. Patients are treated with 5-day courses of methotrexate or actinomycin D, and those with poor-prognosis metastatic GTN require initial chemotherapy using combinations of active agents. The most frequently used combination now is the EMA-CO regimen.

Chemotherapy for Nonmetastatic Disease

The most widely used initial chemotherapy regimens for patients with nonmetastatic GTN include cyclical courses or alternating doses of methotrexate at a dose of 1 mg/kg (maximum 50 mg) on days 1, 3, 5, and 7 with folinic acid rescue administered intramuscularly at a dose of 0.1 mg/kg on days 2, 4, 6, and 8.[3,4,17,21] A variety of other agents and schedules have been used to treat nonmetastatic GTN with essentially equivalent remission rates. Recent reports indicate that weekly courses of methotrexate administered intravenously as a single dose of 30 mg/m^2 have an advantage over other schedules of methotrexate in reducing cost and toxicity and seem equally effective.[13] Hematologic and liver chemistry monitoring must be done. Multiple studies show remission rates in this stage of disease to be 98% to 100% when patients are appropriately treated.

The major goals of therapy for patients with nonmetastatic GTN include administration of active, relatively nontoxic regimens of chemotherapy with close hCG level monitoring. For most of these patients, chemotherapy alone is adequate treatment, and surgery is unnecessary. However, primary hysterectomy may be used for patients who desire sterilization because this reduces the amount of chemotherapy necessary to achieve remission.

Chemotherapy for Good-Prognosis Metastatic Disease

Initial therapy with repetitive cycles of 5-day courses of single-agent methotrexate or dactinomycin is preferred for patients with good-prognosis metastatic GTN.[20] For such patients without high-risk factors, the ultimate sustained remission rate approaches 100%. Patients are initially treated with repetitive 5-day cycles of methotrexate administered intravenously at a dose of 0.4 mg/kg per day or dactinomycin administered intravenously daily at a dose of 500 µg. Chemotherapy is recycled every 14 days or as soon as permitted by the toxic effects. Again, hematologic and liver chemistry monitoring must be done. Remission rates with either agent are approximately 60%, and most drug-resistant patients are salvaged with the alternative single agent. Occasionally, patients may require hysterectomy or other surgical procedures to extirpate loci of disease or a change in therapy to multidrug chemotherapy.[2,7,12]

Chemotherapy for Poor-Prognosis Disease

Multidrug chemotherapy is selected as the initial therapy for patients with poor-prognosis metastatic GTN.[5,16,19,25] Survival is poor for this group if the initial therapy is with only a single agent, and it is important to diagnose poor-prognosis, high-risk features in these patients so that appropriate initial therapy may be selected.

The most successful and least toxic multiagent regimen now seems to be EMA-CO (etoposide, methotrexate with folic acid rescue, dactinomycin alternating with vincristine [Oncovin], and cyclophosphamide). Other salvage regimens include MAC (methotrexate, actinomycin D, and cytoxan), and the modified Bagshawe regimen of hydroxyurea, methotrexate, vincristine, cyclophosphamide, dactinomycin and adriamycin (doxorubicin).[23,24] Because VP-16, cisplatin, 5-FU, vinca alkaloids, and bleomycin all have some activity

TABLE 4. *Chemotherapy for malignant gestational trophoblastic neoplasms*

Type of disease	Initial treatment[a]	Salvage treatment
Nonmetastatic GTN[a]	MTX/FA or weekly MTX	Single agent, dactinomycin Combination chemotherapy
Good-prognosis metastatic GTN	Single agent, methotrexate in 5-day courses	Single agent, dactinomycin Combination chemotherapy
Poor-prognosis metastatic GTN	EMA-CO	Other combination chemotherapy

[a]GTN, gestational trophoblastic neoplasms; MTX/FA, methotrexate–folinic acid; EMA-CO (see text).

against GTN, other salvage regimens are based on combinations employing some of these agents. Regardless of regimen, another cycle of chemotherapy is administered as soon as toxicity from the previous cycle has cleared. Although toxicity may be marked with these combinations, aggressive initial multiagent chemotherapy is usually necessary to ensure optimal survival for patients in this category. Patients with poor-prognosis metastatic GTN should be treated at centers that specialize in the therapy of patients with GTN, as physician experience with the therapy of this disease appears to improve the outcome for these patients.

Patients with poor-prognosis metastatic GTN who have failed standard chemotherapy regimens are extremely challenging in terms of designing appropriate coordinations of chemotherapy and other therapeutic modalities to produce salvage. Frequently, patients must be treated without regard for toxicity and must be supported through episodes of profound marrow suppression, sepsis, and nutritional deprivation to have a chance at salvage.

Surgical and Radiation Therapy

Hysterectomy

Brewer and associates documented poor survival among women, even those with nonmetastatic GTN, who were treated with hysterectomy alone. Because of improvements in chemotherapy, hysterectomy is rarely indicated as the initial therapy for women with malignant GTN. However, for patients with nonmetastatic or good-prognosis metastatic GTN with uterine disease, hysterectomy appears to decrease the duration of hospital stay and number of courses of chemotherapy required to achieve remission. Delayed or secondary hysterectomy is required for approximately 10% of patients as salvage therapy in these categories, but chemotherapy alone is successful in curing approximately 85% of patients with nonmetastatic and good-prognosis metastatic GTN. Among women with poor-prognosis metastatic GTN, preservation of childbearing capacity must be of secondary importance, but primary or delayed hysterectomy does not appear to offer as many benefits as in the therapy of patients with low-risk disease.[22]

Surgical procedures for the purpose of removing sites of GTN are performed during a cycle of chemotherapy. Theoretically, this prevents dissemination of disease caused by embolization of GTN during the surgical manipulation of tissues. The complications of surgery and wound healing do not appear to be increased using this approach.

Thoracotomy

Thoracotomy with pulmonary segmental resection has been the most frequently performed procedure other than hysterectomy to remove drug-resistant disease. The radiographic regression of pulmonary nodules may lag far behind the response measured by hCG levels, and the persistence of a lung nodule after hCG normalization should not necessarily be interpreted as indicating persistent disease.

There have been reports of success with resection of solitary pulmonary nodules in highly selected women with drug-resistant disease. Before considering pulmonary resection, it is important to exclude the possibility of disease elsewhere. If the patient has not had a hysterectomy, occult pelvic GTN should be evaluated with arteriography or other imaging techniques, such as magnetic resonance imaging. Prompt hCG remission after pulmonary resection predicts a favorable outcome.

Brain and Liver Metastases

Whole-brain and whole-liver irradiation are often used as adjuncts to chemotherapy in the treatment of patients with metastases to these sites. Whole-brain irradiation of approximately 3000 cGy over 10 days is begun immediately in conjunction with chemotherapy after brain metastases are diagnosed. The rationale for this treatment is to prevent hemorrhage from these highly vascular metastases. With this approach, survival rates of approximately 85% are achieved for patients receiving primary therapy for brain metastases; survival rates of approximately 50% are achieved for all patients with brain metastases, including those developing metastases during chemotherapy or at the time of recurrence. An alternate approach includes the combined use of high-dose systemic methotrexate with intermittent intrathecal methotrexate.[1]

Craniotomy is not often required for the primary therapy or diagnosis of brain metastases from GTN and usually is not successful when used alone. However, neurosurgical consultation should be obtained early in the course of therapy in the event that hemorrhage into brain lesions occurs and craniotomy is required for stabilization of the patient.

Whole-organ irradiation of approximately 2000 cGy delivered over 10 days may be used to treat liver metastases and prevent hepatic hemorrhage. Some investigators have not used hepatic irradiation to avoid exacerbation of the toxic hepatic effects of chemotherapy. Others have advocated selective occlusion of the hepatic artery by means of ligation or embolization when bleeding has occurred. Patients with hepatic metastases have a dismal prognosis and require aggressive chemotherapy with careful monitoring during therapy to maximize the chances for survival. Whole-organ irradiation does not appear to compromise tolerance of aggressive chemotherapy.

Placental Site Tumors

A PST is a rare placental neoplasm that is histologically and clinically distinct from other forms of GTN. Because PST lack significant numbers of syncytiotrophoblast elements and do not secrete high levels of hCG, serum hCG levels are not as reliable a tumor marker as seen in other forms of GTN. The PST usually are locally aggressive, invading into the myometrium. They are not usually sensitive to traditional chemotherapeutic agents. Most women with PST require hysterectomy, although a few have apparently been cured by D&C alone. Rarely, PST pursue a more aggressive course, marked by distant metastases and rapidly progressive disease.[10]

Monitoring Therapy

Laboratory Evaluations

During chemotherapy, hematologic, renal, and hepatic indices should be monitored carefully. Toxicity from methotrexate- and dactinomycin-based chemotherapy is relatively predictable. Unless a patient is receiving salvage chemotherapy for drug-resistant or recurrent GTN, new cycles of therapy should be withheld unless the total leukocyte count is greater than 3000 cells/mm³, the platelet count is greater than 100,000/mm³, and the renal and hepatic indices are normal. Radiographic studies of metastatic lesions and pelvic examination should be repeated frequently to monitor response to therapy.

More important than radiographic surveillance is closely following the hCG level response during therapy. Sensitive assays of the hCG levels should be performed at 1-week intervals during therapy. Chemotherapy should be changed if the hCG titer has not dropped at least 25% after a treatment cycle or if toxicity does not permit adequate dosage or frequency of administration.

Human Chorionic Gonadotropin Level Remission and Surveillance

Complete remission is defined as three consecutive weekly hCG levels in the normal range. After remission has been achieved, hCG levels should be followed every 1 to 2 weeks for the first 3 months after completion of therapy, every 2 to 4 weeks for the next 3 months, and every 1 to 2 months for the completion of the first year of surveillance. Recurrent episodes of GTN usually develop within a few months after completion of therapy, but late recurrences develop in a few cases. The assay of hCG levels should be repeated indefinitely at 6-month intervals. Patients are counseled to avoid pregnancy through the first year of hCG surveillance; most are treated with oral contraceptives for efficiency and to avoid low-level interference with the hCG assays caused by luteinizing hormone.

Prevention of Recurrent Disease

Despite the accuracy of hCG assays, a tumor burden of 10⁴ cells may exist despite normal serum hCG levels. Recurrence rates after therapy for GTN have been 3% to 26%, depending on the patient population being studied. Patients with poor-prognosis metastatic GTN usually have a much higher recurrence rate than patients with low-risk disease. Most investigators agree that maintenance chemotherapy beyond the first normal hCG level should be administered. I administer one cycle of chemotherapy beyond the first normal hCG level for patients with nonmetastatic disease, two cycles of maintenance chemotherapy for patients with good-prognosis metastatic GTN, and three to four cycles of maintenance chemotherapy for patients with poor-prognosis metastatic GTN. Toxicity must be considered in continuing therapy for these patients.

Reproduction After Therapy

Most women treated for GTN are successfully cured by chemotherapy without resorting to hysterectomy.[9,18] Several reports have documented that there is little or no increased risk of congenital malformation of infants from subsequent pregnancies. There may be a slight increase in the incidence of spontaneous abortions in this population, but this increase may be an artifact of increased hCG level surveillance and identification of preclinical pregnancies in women who have previously received treatment for GTN. There is also an increased incidence of repeat molar gestation in patients who have had a prior hydatidiform mole. Patients who have received intensive therapy for poor-prognosis metastatic GTN often undergo hysterectomy during therapy or may develop ovarian failure as a result of prolonged multidrug chemotherapy. Only a few patients in this category with uterine conservation are able to conceive or desire to attempt pregnancy after therapy.

Although the risk of congenital anomalies is not significantly increased after chemotherapy for malignant GTN, obstetric complications may be increased. Major obstetric complications can be observed in as many as 9% of these pregnancies. The incidence of placenta accreta in particular appears to be increased.

Women who have been treated successfully for GTN should be advised that pregnancy should be deferred for at least 1 year of hCG level surveillance after therapy. They should be reassured about the incidence of congenital malformations and recurrent GTN in subsequent pregnancies. An ultrasound scan should be performed early in pregnancy to exclude the possibility of recurrent molar gestation. A chest radiograph and serum hCG level should be obtained 6 to 8 weeks after delivery to screen for the rare case of recurrent choriocarcinoma developing after a subsequent normal pregnancy.

SUMMARY POINTS

◊ Gestational trophoblastic neoplasms are a spectrum of human neoplasia, spanning the range from benign with potential malignant sequelae to highly malignant.

◊ Primary hydatidiform mole (complete) usually presents as a pregnancy with threatened first trimester vaginal bleeding. Other frequent findings include discordant uterine size, ovarian cystic enlargement, and hyperemesis but may also include hyperthyroidism and preeclampsia.

(continues)

(*summary points continued*)

◊ Evacuation of hydatidiform mole is best done by suction D&C with caution used regarding trophoblastic deportation and pulmonary embolization.

◊ Individualization of therapy is critical for successful treatment of patients with GTN. Although chemotherapy is the primary modality for therapy, surgery and radiotherapy may also have a role.

◊ Human chorionic gonadotropin (hCG) is a sensitive and reliable marker for GTN and can be effectively used to aid in diagnosis, monitor therapy, and maintain follow-up evaluation.

◊ REFERENCES

1. Athenassion A, Begent RH, Newlands ES, et al. Central nervous system metastases of choriocarcinoma: 23 years' experience at Charing Cross Hospital. *Cancer* 1983;52:1728.

2. Berkowitz RS, Goldstein DP, eds. Advances in gestational trophoblastic disease, a symposium. *J Reprod Med* 1991;36:1.

3. Berkowitz RS, Goldstein DP, Bernstein MR. Management of nonmetastatic trophoblastic tumors. *J Reprod Med* 1981;26:219.

4. Berkowitz RS, Goldstein DP, Bernstein MR. Ten years' experience with methotrexate and folinic acid as primary treatment for gestational trophoblastic disease. *Gynecol Oncol* 1986;23:111.

5. Curry SL, Blessing JA, DiSaia PJ, et al. A prospective randomized comparison of MAC versus CHAMOCA chemotherapy in poor prognosis metastatic gestational trophoblastic disease, a GOG study. *Obstet Gynecol* 1989;73:357.

6. Curry SL, Hammond CB, Tyrey L, et al. Hydatidiform mole:diagnosis, management and long-term follow-up in 347 patients. *Obstet Gynecol* 1975;45:1.

7. DuBeshter B, Berkowitz RS, Goldstein DP, et al. Metastatic gestational trophoblastic disease: experience at the New England Trophoblastic Disease Center, 1965 to 1985. *Obstet Gynecol* 1987;69:390.

8. Elston CW. The histopathology of trophoblastic tumors. *J Clin Pathol* 1977;29(Suppl 10):111.

9. Hammond CB, Borchert LG, Tyrey L, et al. Treatment of metastatic trophoblastic disease: good and poor prognosis. *Am J Obstet Gynecol* 1973;115:4.

10. Hancock BW, Newlands ES, Berkowitz RS, eds. *Gestational trophoblastic disease*. London: Chapman and Hall, 1997.

11. Hertig AT, Sheldon WM. Hydatidiform mole: a pathologico-clinical correlation of 200 cases. *Am J Obstet Gynecol* 1947;53:1.

12. Hertz R, Lewis JL Jr, Lipsett MG. Five years' experience with the chemotherapy of metastatic choriocarcinoma and related trophoblastic tumors in women. *Am J Obstet Gynecol* 1961;82:631.

13. Holmesly HD, Blessing JA, Rettenmeier M, et al. Weekly methotrexate for nonmetastatic gestational trophoblastic disease. *Obstet Gynecol* 1988;72:413.

14. Li MC, Hertz R, Spencer DB. Effects of methotrexate upon choriocarcinoma and chorioadenoma. *Proc Soc Exp Biol Med* 1956;93:361.

15. Lurain JR, Brewer JI, Torok EE, et al. Gestational trophoblastic disease: treatment results at the Brewer Trophoblastic Disease Center. *Obstet Gynecol* 1982;60:354.

16. Lurain JR, Brewer JI. Treatment of high-risk gestational trophoblastic disease with methotrexate actinomycin-D, and cyclophosphamide chemotherapy. *Obstet Gynecol* 1985;65:830.

17. Lurain JR, Elfstrand EP. Single agent methotrexate for treatment of nonmetastatic gestational trophoblastic tumors. *Am J Obstet Gynecol* 1995; 172:574.

18. Matsui H, et al. Reproductive status in patients with gestational trophoblastic disease treated with etoposide. *J Reprod Med* 1997;42(2):104.

19. Newlands ES, Bagshawe KD. The role of VP16-23 (etoposide: NCD-141540) in gestational choriocarcinoma. *Cancer Chemother Pharmacol* 1982;7:211.

20. Ross GT, Goldstein DP, Hertz R, et al. Sequential use of methotrexate and actinomycin-D in the treatment of metastatic choriocarcinoma and related trophoblastic tumors in women. *Am J Obstet Gynecol* 1965; 93:223.

21. Smith EB, Weed JC Jr, Tyrey L, et al. Treatment of nonmetastatic gestational trophoblastic disease: results of methotrexate alone versus methotrexate-folinic acid. *Am J Obstet Gynecol* 1982;144:88.

22. Soper JT, Hammond CB. Role of surgical therapy and radiotherapy in gestational trophoblastic disease. *J Reprod Med* 1987;32:663.

23. Soper JT, Evans AC, Rodriguez GC, et al. Etoposide-platinum combination chemotherapy for chemorefractory gestational trophoblastic neoplasms. *Gynecol Oncol* 1995;56:421.

24. Soto-Wright D, et al. Management of gestational trophoblastic tumors with etoposide, methotrexate and actinomycin-D. *Gynecol Oncol* 1997; 64(1):156.

25. Surwit EA, Hammond CB. Treatment of metastatic trophoblastic disease with poor prognosis. *Obstet Gynecol* 1980;55:565.

CHAPTER 55

Ethical and Legal Issues

——— ◊ ———

Frank A. Chervenak
Laurence B. McCullough

Physicians in obstetric and gynecologic practice confront ethical concerns and issues that arise when the physician's judgment about what is in the patient's interest differs from the patient's judgment about what is in her or her fetus's interest.[1-6] One way to manage such differences is to assert the primacy of the physician's judgment. This strategy is discredited because it leads to paternalism in the care of patients.[7] Paternalism can occur when medical judgments fail to take account of the patient's values and beliefs regarding her own health and medical care.[8] To avoid paternalism, one might opt for the alternative of the primacy of the patient's judgment.[9] The problem with this approach is that it reduces the physician to the status of a mere technician and may require the physician to act in ways that contradict reasonable medical judgment.

In this chapter we apply the methods of ethics to the problem of differences between the obstetrician-gynecologist and the patient about what is in the patient's interest in a way that avoids these two extremes. We develop a framework for clinical judgment and decision making about the ethical dimensions of the obstetrician-gynecologist–patient relationship. To achieve this goal, we first define ethics, medical ethics, and the fundamental ethical principles of medical ethics, beneficence, and respect for autonomy. Second, we show how these two principles should interact in gynecologic clinical judgment and practice. Third, we show how these two principles should interact in obstetric judgment and practice, emphasizing the example of cesarean delivery. Fourth, we examine ethical issues in managed care, emphasizing the virtues of the physician as a professional. We emphasize a preventive ethics approach that appreciates the protocol for ethical conflict and adopts ethically justified strategies to prevent those conflicts from occurring.[5,10] Preventive ethics helps to build and sustain a strong physician–patient relationship.

◊ ETHICS, MEDICAL ETHICS, AND ETHICAL PRINCIPLES

Ethics is the disciplined study of morality and draws on the disciplines of the humanities, especially philosophy. Medical ethics is the disciplined study of morality in medicine and concerns the obligations of physicians and institutions to patients as well as the obligations of patients. It is important not to confuse ethics with the many sources of morality in a pluralistic society.[11] These include, but are not limited to, law, our political heritage as a free people, the world's religions (most of which now exist in our country), ethnic and cultural traditions, families, the traditions and practices of medicine (including medical education and training), and personal experience. These sources of morality are useful reference points for ethical inquiry.

The traditions and practices of medicine, including education and training, constitute an obvious source of morality for physicians. They provide an important reference point for ethics in medicine because they are based on the obligation to protect and promote the interests of the patient.[5,12] This obligation tells physicians what morality in medicine ought to be, but in very general, abstract terms. Providing a more concrete, clinically applicable account of that obligation is the central task of medical ethics.

To make concrete the general obligation of protecting and promoting the interests of the patient, medical ethics focuses on the question of "How *ought* the physician conduct himself or herself with patients?" Among relevant tools of ethics for answering this question are ethical principles because they help the physician to interpret and implement his or her general moral obligation to protect and promote the interests of the patient, which has been the traditional moral foundation of the physician–patient relationship.[5,12]

The Principle of Beneficence

The principle of beneficence requires one to act in a way that is expected reliably to produce the greater balance of goods over harms in the lives of others.[5,8,12] To put this principle into clinical practice requires a reliable account of the goods and harms relevant to the care of the patient and of how those goods and harms should be reasonably balanced against each other when not all of them can be achieved in a particular situation. In medicine, the principle of beneficence requires the physician to act in a way that is reliably expected to produce the greater balance of clinical goods over harms for the patient.

Beneficence-based clinical judgment has an ancient pedigree, with its first expression found in the Hippocratic Oath and accompanying texts.[5,8] It makes an important claim: to interpret reliably the interests of the patient from medicine's perspective.[5] This perspective is provided by accumulated scientific research, clinical experience, and reasoned responses to uncertainty. It is thus not the function of the individual clinical perspective of a particular physician and therefore should not be based merely on the clinical impression or intuition of an individual physician.

On the basis of this rigorous, clinical perspective, beneficence-based clinical judgment identifies the goods that can be achieved for the patient in clinical practice based on the competencies of medicine. The goods that medicine is competent to seek for patients are the prevention and management of disease, injury, handicap, and unnecessary pain and suffering and the prevention of premature or unnecessary death.[5] Pain and suffering become unnecessary when they do not result in achieving the other goods of medical care.

It is important to note that there is an inherent risk of paternalism in beneficence-based clinical judgment. By this we mean that beneficence-based clinical judgment, if it is, *mistakenly* considered to be the sole source of moral responsibility and therefore moral authority in medical care, invites the unwary physician to conclude that beneficence-based judgments can be imposed on the patient in violation of her autonomy.[5,8,12] Paternalism is a dehumanizing response to the patient and, therefore, should be avoided in the practice of obstetrics and gynecology.

The preventive ethics response to this inherent paternalism is for the physician to explain the diagnostic, therapeutic, and prognostic reasoning that leads to his or her clinical judgment about what is in the interest of the patient so that the patient can assess that judgment for herself. This general rule can be put into clinical practice in the following way. The physician should disclose and explain to the patient the major factors of this reasoning process, including matters of uncertainty. (Note that this does not require that the patient be provided with a complete medical education.) The physician should then explain how and why other clinicians might reasonably differ from his or her clinical judgment. The physician should then present a well-reasoned response to this critique. The outcome of this process is that beneficence-based clinical judgments take on a rigor that they sometimes lack, and the process of their formulation includes explaining them to the patient. It should be apparent that beneficence-based clinical judgment will frequently result in the identification of a continuum of clinical strategies that protect and promote the patient's interests, such as the choice of a particular method of contraception. Awareness of this feature of beneficence-based clinical judgment provides an important preventive ethics antidote to paternalism by increasing the likelihood that one or more of these alternatives will be acceptable to the patient. This feature of beneficence-based clinical judgment also provides a preventive ethics antidote to "gag" rules that restrict physician discussions with the managed care patient. All beneficence-based alternatives must be identified and explained to all patients, regardless of how the physician is paid.

The very process of explaining beneficence-based clinical judgment enhances the patient's ability to understand and deal effectively with the technical aspects of medical care, an important consideration in obstetric-gynecologic practice, for example, prophylactic oophorectomy at the time of hysterectomy or the nature and limits of obstetric ultrasound. Recent data suggest the need for such enhancement. The Louis Harris survey prepared for the recent President's Commission on Ethics in Medicine presents an important finding: "The vast majority of physicians report that they address most aspects of the condition and treatment with their patients as a matter of course. This is substantiated by the large majority of the public, who report that their physicians usually discuss these matters with them."[13] This survey also reports a "large and reliable difference of approximately 15 to 25 percentage points" between the proportion of physicians who report themselves as discussing some aspects of medical care and the proportion of the public who report that their physicians discuss such matters as diagnosis and prognosis, nature and purpose of treatment, pros and cons of the treatment, and side effects.[13] The process of disclosure described above, if adopted as a standard of care, could well close these significant gaps in the care of female and pregnant patients, especially in the managed care setting.

One advantage for the physician in carrying out this approach to communicating with the patient would be, we believe, to increase the likelihood of compliance. This is an especially pertinent consideration in gynecologic practice, where the patient often must monitor herself for clinical changes (e.g., a woman at risk for ectopic pregnancy) and take an active role in preventive medicine (e.g., breast self-examination) as well as in obstetric practice (e.g., self-observation for unusual weight gain or bleeding). Another advantage would be to provide the patient with a better-informed opportunity to make a decision about whether to seek a second opinion. The approach outlined above should make such a decision less threatening to her physician, who has already shared with the patient the limitations on clinical judgment. A final advantage may be a reduction in the percentage (20%) of physicians who reportedly dismiss patients who disagree with them and in the high percentage (36%) of patients who report that they have changed physicians who disagree with them.[13]

The Principle of Respect for Autonomy

In addition to the principle of beneficence, there has been increasing—even dominant—emphasis in the literature of ethics in medicine on the principle of respect for autonomy.[8,11] This principle requires one always to acknowledge and carry out the value-based preferences of others, irrespective of what one might think the consequences of their doing so might be.

The female or pregnant patient increasingly brings to her medical care her own perspective on what is in her interest. The principle of respect for autonomy translates this fact into autonomy-based clinical judgment, a creature of the 20th century that finds its roots in the law of malpractice, dating from the second decade of our century, and then in ethics, dating from three decades ago.[5,14] Because each patient's perspective on her interests is a function of her values and beliefs, it is impossible to specify the goods and harms of autonomy-based clinical judgment in advance. Indeed, it would be inappropriate to do so, because the definition of her goods and harms and their balancing are the prerogative of the patient. Not surprisingly, autonomy-based clinical judgment is strongly antipaternalistic in nature.

To understand the moral demands of this principle, we need an operationalized concept of autonomy to make it relevant to clinical practice. To do this, we identify three sequential autonomy-related behaviors on the part of the patient: (1) absorbing and retaining information about her condition and alternative diagnostic and therapeutic responses to it, (2) understanding that information (i.e., evaluating and rank-ordering those responses), and (3) expressing a value-based preference for a particular response. The physician has a role to play in each of these. They are, respectively, (1) to recognize the capacity of each patient to deal with medical information (and not to underestimate that capacity), provide information (i.e., disclose and explain all alternatives supported in beneficence-based clinical judgment), and recognize the validity of the values and beliefs of the patient, (2) not to interfere with but, when necessary, to assist the patient in her evaluation and ranking of diagnostic and therapeutic alternative responses to her condition, and (3) to elicit and implement the patient's value-based preference.[11]

The legal obligations of the physician regarding informed consent were established in a series of cases during the twentieth century.[14] *Schloendorff v. The Society of The New York Hospital* established the concept of simple consent, i.e., whether the patient says "yes" or "no" to medical intervention. "Every human being of adult years and sound mind has the right to determine what shall be done with his body, and a surgeon who performs an operation without his patient's consent commits an assault for which he is liable in damages."[14] The legal requirement of consent further evolved to include disclosure of information sufficient to enable patients to make informed decisions about whether to say "yes" or "no" to medical intervention. There are two legal standards for such disclosure. The professional community standard defines adequate disclosure in the context of what the relevantly trained and experienced physician tells patients. The reasonable person standard goes further and requires the physician to disclose "material" information, what the lay person of average sophistication should not be expected to know. This second standard has emerged as the ethical standard,[14] and we therefore urge obstetrician-gynecologists to adopt it. On this standard the physician should disclose to the patient her or the fetus's diagnosis (including differential diagnosis when that is all that is known), the medically reasonable alternatives to diagnose and manage the patient's condition, and the short-term and long-term benefits and harms of each alternative.

A particularly important dimension of informed consent in practice involves what have come to be known as "advance directives." Spurred by the famous case of Karen Quinlan in New Jersey in 1976, all but two legislatures have enacted "living will" legislation, and, in as many states, there is legislative or common law authority for durable power of attorney for health care.[5]

The basic idea of an advance directive is that a patient, when autonomous, can make decisions regarding her medical management in advance of a time during which she becomes incapable of making health care decisions. The ethical dimensions of autonomy that are relevant here are the following:

1. A patient may exercise her autonomy now in the form of a refusal of life-prolonging interventions.
2. Autonomy-based refusal, expressed in the past and left unchanged, remains in effect for any future time during which the patient becomes nonautonomous.
3. That past autonomy-based refusal should therefore translate into physician obligations at the time the patient becomes unable to participate in the informed consent process.
4. In particular, refusal of life-prolonging medical intervention should translate into the withholding or withdrawal of such interventions.

The living will is an instrument that permits the patient to make a direct decision to refuse life-prolonging medical intervention in the future. The living will becomes effective when the patient is a "qualified patient," usually terminally or irreversibly ill, and is also not able to participate in the informed consent process. Obviously, terminally or irreversibly ill patients who are able to participate in the informed consent process retain their autonomy to make their own decisions. Some states prescribe the wording of the living will, and others do not. The physician should become familiar with the legal requirements in the his or her own jurisdiction. A living will, to be useful and effective, should be as explicit as possible. The legal basis for the living will is the legal right of self-determination, the right of any competent adult to determine what shall be done to her body. A number of state courts have made it clear that this right extends to the refusal of both hydration and nutrition. The recent U.S.

Supreme Court ruling in the famous *Cruzan* case is ambiguous about whether there is such a right based in the U.S. Constitution.[5] As a consequence, hospitals and other health care institutions have begun to reconsider the refusal of hydration and nutrition based on a living will. The reader should become familiar with those institutional policies that affect such patients.

The concept of a durable power of attorney is that any autonomous adult, in the event that that person later becomes unable to participate in the informed consent process, can assign decision-making authority to another person. The advantage of the durable power of attorney for health care is that it applies only when the patient becomes nonautonomous. It does *not*, as does the living will, also require that the patient also be terminally or irreversibly ill. However, unlike the living will, the durable power of attorney does not necessarily provide explicit direction, only the explicit assignment of decision-making authority to an identified individual or "agent." Obviously, any patient who assigns durable power of attorney for health care to someone else has an interest in communicating her values, beliefs, and preferences to that person. The physician can play a facilitating role in this process. Indeed, in order to protect the patient's autonomy, the physician should play an active role in encouraging this communication process so that there will be minimal doubt about whether the person holding durable power of attorney is faithfully representing the wishes of the patient.

The main clinical advantages of these two forms of advance directives are that they encourage patients to think carefully in advance about the refusal of medical intervention and that these directives, therefore, help to prevent ethical conflicts and crises in the management of nonautonomous patients and nonautonomous terminally or irreversibly ill patients. Unfortunately, the use of advance directives is not as widespread as it should be. The reader is encouraged to think of advance directives as powerful, practical strategies for preventive ethics and to encourage patients to consider them carefully, especially patients with gynecologic disease—particularly gynecologic cancers—that could become or are life threatening.

◊ THE INTERACTION OF BENEFICENCE AND RESPECT FOR AUTONOMY IN GYNECOLOGIC JUDGMENT AND PRACTICE

Beneficence-based and autonomy-based clinical judgments in gynecologic practice are usually in harmony (Fig. 1). A woman may present with an adnexal mass of 10 cm. The gynecologist would explain this diagnostic finding and the potential for malignancy and torsion of the mass as well as the unlikelihood of spontaneous resolution. In beneficence-based clinical judgment, surgical management provides a clear-cut greater balance of medical goods over harms for the

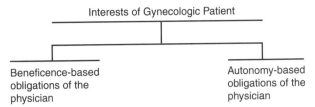

FIG. 1. Moral obligations in gynecologic care.

patient, whereas nonsurgical management provides a clear-cut greater balance of medical harms over goods for the patient. Beneficence-based clinical judgment requires a careful explanation of these matters to the patient, with no restriction from managed care "gag" rules, and supports a definitive recommendation for surgical management. Respect for the patient's autonomy also requires explanation of these matters but goes further and obligates the physician to elicit the patient's value-based priorities for the management of the newly diagnosed condition, which almost always coincide with beneficence-based clinical judgment. Synergy between beneficence and respect for autonomy occurs when the physician's management plan is carried out in conjunction with the patient's informed consent.[14]

Sometimes, beneficence-based and autonomy-based clinical judgments are in conflict. In situations of conflict, neither beneficence nor respect for autonomy in and of itself should be viewed as a "trump," to borrow a term from the game of bridge. That is, beneficence does not always override respect for autonomy, nor vice versa. Instead, both principles should be understood as theoretically equally weighted. Thus, their differences must be negotiated in clinical judgment and practice. The competing demands of both principles must be balanced and negotiated to determine which management strategies protect and promote the patient's interests. In the technical language of ethics, we are treating these principles as *prima facie* or potentially overriding in nature.[5,8,12]

The process of negotiating conflict between the two principles is a function of several factors involved in gynecologic clinical judgment: subject matter; probability of net medical benefit; availability of reasonable alternatives; and the ability of the patient to participate in the informed consent process (Fig. 2).

When the subject matter is primarily technical in nature, such as the selection of an effective antibiotic regimen or intraoperative surgical technique, clinical judgment is justifiably beneficence-based. This is because technical matters largely concern the calculus of medical goods and harms for aggregates of patients with a particular diagnosis and treatment plan. Such decisions are justifiably within the gynecologist's purview. The individual values and beliefs of a particular patient cannot readily be taken into account in this process. By contrast, when the patient's basic values and beliefs are at stake, e.g., the treatment of infertility or elective

	Factors that increase the weight of beneficence-based obligations relative to autonomy-based obligations	Factors that increase the weight of autonomy-based obligations relative to beneficence-based obligations
Subject matter	Technical matters (e.g., selection of effective antibiotic regimen, intra-operative surgical technique)	Basic values or beliefs of the patient (e.g., treatment of infertility, elective abortion)
Probability of net medical benefit for the patient of diagnostic or therapeutic indication	High (chemotherapy for treatment for gestational trophoblastic disease, surgical correction of prolapsed uterus)	Low (experimental therapy for advanced ovarian malignancy, prophylactic oöphorectomy at time of hysterectomy at 40–45 years of age)
Availability of reasonable alternative management options	No (removal of ruptured ectopic pregnancy, screening for cervical cancer by Pap smear)	Yes (surgery versus radiotherapy for management of stage 1A cancer of the cervix, method of contraception or tubal ligation)
Ability of patient to participate in informed consent process	Low (e.g., severe or profound mental retardation, life threatening emergency with no time for consent)	Not low (e.g., speaker of a foreign language, existence of advanced directives)

FIG. 2. Factors that influence the relative weight of beneficence-based and autonomy-based obligations to the gynecologic patient.

abortion, clinical judgment is justifiably autonomy-based. This is because particular diagnostic or treatment interventions can directly and adversely affect the basic values and beliefs of a particular patient, a matter that only each individual patient can decide.[5] Such decisions are justifiably within the patient's purview.

When the probability of net medical benefit for the patient of diagnostic or therapeutic medical intervention is high, e.g., chemotherapy for some forms of gestational trophoblastic disease, or surgical correction of a prolapsed uterus, beneficence-based clinical judgment is dominant. This is because, in such circumstances, the net benefit is clear-cut. The gynecologist is therefore justified in recommending interventions that have a high probability of net medical benefit. By contrast, when that probability is low, e.g., experimental therapy for advanced ovarian malignancy or prophylactic oophorectomy at 40–45 years of age, clinical judgment is justifiably autonomy-based. This is because, when there is no clear-cut benefit and significant risks of intervention exist, the patient is in the best position to determine which trade-off makes the most sense. The gynecologist is therefore justified in offering these alternatives but not in recommending one as indisputably the best.

When there is no reasonable alternative to manage the patient's condition (e.g., removal of a ruptured ectopic pregnancy or screening for cervical cancer by Pap smears), clinical judgment is appropriately beneficence-based because there is no other alternative that to any degree protects and promotes the interests of the patient.[15] The gynecologist is

therefore justified in strongly recommending the intervention in question. By contrast, when there are reasonable alternatives, such as surgery versus radiotherapy for stage 1A cervical cancer or a method of contraception versus tubal ligation, clinical judgment is appropriately autonomy-based. This is because reasonable alternatives all promote the patient's interests to a significant degree, and no one alternative can exclude any other as unreasonable. The gynecologist is justified only in presenting the reasonable alternatives.

When the ability to implement the informed consent process is low, as for a patient with severe or profound mental retardation or in a life-threatening emergency without time for consent, clinical judgment is justifiably beneficence-based. This is because it is impossible to determine the patient's relevant values and beliefs because of either significant irreversible cognitive impairment or urgent lack of time. The gynecologist is therefore justified in basing clinical decision making primarily on beneficence. By contrast, when the ability of the patient to participate in the informed consent process is not low, as in a speaker of a foreign language or the existence of a legally valid advance directive, then clinical judgment is justifiably autonomy-based. This is because the ability of the patient to participate in the informed consent process is presumed in the absence of compelling reasons to the contrary.[14]

As a rule, the result of the informed consent process should be implemented. When the patient refuses to accept any of the alternatives supported in beneficence-based clinical judgment, the physician is ethically and legally obligated to engage in what is known as "informed refusal." This legal and ethical obligation arises from the case of *Truman v. Thomas*.[16] Dr. Thomas had delivered several of Mrs. Truman's babies and, on the delivery of her last child, had recommended that she have a Pap smear. She refused to have this test until she could pay for it and did not accept Dr. Thomas's offer to perform it without charge. Mrs. Truman next presented to Dr. Thomas with advanced cervical cancer, from which she died. In the malpractice action brought by her survivors, Dr. Thomas stated that, although they were of clinical concern to him in the management of Mrs. Truman, he did not tell Mrs. Truman of the risks of having presymptomatic changes in her cervix indicative of cervical cancer or that he was concerned that she could die from such disease. The California Supreme Court ruled that, because risks were of clinical salience to Dr. Thomas—they were the motivation for his offering the Pap smear—he should have informed Mrs. Thomas about these risks so that her refusal would be informed. This case changed practice and introduced the concept of informed refusal into medical law and ethics.

The ethical and legal obligation of the physician in the matter of informed refusal is very clear and not difficult to fulfill. The patient should be informed in straightforward, but not harsh or hostile, terms the medical risks that she is taking in her refusal of a diagnostic or therapeutic intervention supported in beneficence-based clinical judgment. The risks to be disclosed are those that are salient in clinical judgment: if they are important to the physician, that is, motivating the offering or recommending of the diagnostic test or therapy, they are salient and should be disclosed. This is all that the law requires. Good ethical practice suggests strongly that this disclosure should be followed by a recommendation that the patient reconsider her refusal. As a matter of good ethical practice, the physician should respond, in the end, to adamant refusal by offering a trial of respect for the patient's refusal, asking her to return for an office visit and to reconsider her refusal once she has had some experience with it. This preventive ethics approach avoids the need to abandon the patient, keeps lines of communication open, and sends a powerful signal of concern by the physician to the patient about the medical folly of her refusal.

Patients' demands for inappropriate management are the reverse side of this coin. We suggest the following preventive ethics strategy in response:[17]

1. Is the intervention reliably expected to have its intended, usual anatomic or physiological effect? If in reliable beneficence-based clinical judgment it is not expected to do so, then the physician should not offer it. There is no obligation to offer or to perform medical interventions that are futile in this strict sense, such as providing a feeding tube for a patient with cancer cachexia.

2. Is the intervention reliably expected to have some minimal clinical benefit, defined as maintaining some minimal level of ability to interact with the environment and thus grow and develop as a human being? Is the patient in a permanent vegetative state? If, in reliable beneficence-based clinical judgment, it is not expected to do so, then the physician should offer the intervention and then recommend against it. We suggest this approach to respect a patient's or surrogate decision makers who are vitalists, i.e., who value the preservation of life at any cost. The physician should explain that this is *not* a value in medical ethics and never has been. Moreover, the intervention in question, whether it is initiated or continued, will just sustain a false hope of recovery.

3. If the patient or the patient's surrogate persists in the demand, then the physician should consult with colleagues and then the Ethics Committee, which should have a clear policy on response to demands by patients or their surrogates for futile intervention.[18,19]

◊ THE INTERACTION OF BENEFICENCE AND RESPECT FOR AUTONOMY IN OBSTETRIC CLINICAL JUDGMENT AND PRACTICE

The ethical principles of beneficence and respect for autonomy play a more complex role in obstetric clinical judgment and practice (Fig. 3). There are obviously beneficence-based and autonomy-based obligations to the pregnant patient:[5] the physician's perspective on the pregnant woman's interests provides the basis for the physician's beneficence-based obligations to her, whereas her own perspective on those interests provides the basis for the physician's autonomy-based obligations to her. Because of an insufficiently developed central nervous system, the fetus cannot meaningfully be said to possess values and beliefs. Thus, there is no basis for saying that a fetus has a perspective on its interests. There can therefore be no autonomy-based obligations to any fetus.[5] Hence, the language of fetal rights has no meaning and there-

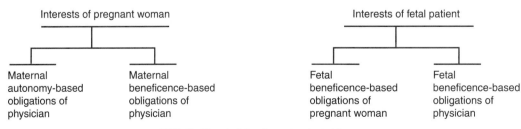

FIG. 3. Moral obligations in obstetric care.

fore no application to the fetus in obstetric clinical judgment and practice despite its popularity in public and political discourse in the United States and other countries. Obviously, the physician has a perspective on the fetus's health-related interests, and the physician can have beneficence-based obligations to the fetus, *but only when the fetus is a patient.* Because of its importance for obstetric clinical judgment and practice, the topic of the fetus as a patient requires detailed consideration.

Two Senses of the Concept of the Fetus as a Patient

The concept of the fetus as a patient is essential to obstetric clinical judgment and practice. Developments in fetal diagnosis and management strategies to optimize fetal outcome[20–23] have become widely accepted,[24–31] encouraging the development of this concept. This concept has considerable clinical significance because, when the fetus is a patient, directive counseling, that is, recommending a form of management, for fetal benefit is appropriate, and when the fetus is not a patient, nondirective counseling, that is, offering but not recommending a form of management for fetal benefit, is appropriate. However, these apparently straightforward roles for directive and nondirective counseling are often difficult to apply in actual perinatal practice because of uncertainty about when the fetus is a patient. One approach to resolving this uncertainty would be to argue that the fetus is or is not a patient in virtue of personhood,[6,11,32–37] or some other form of independent moral status.[38–41] We now show that this approach fails to resolve the uncertainty, and we therefore defend an alternative approach that does resolve the uncertainty.[5]

The Independent Moral Status of the Fetus

One prominent approach for establishing whether or not the fetus is a patient has involved attempts to show whether or not the fetus has independent moral status. This is the first sense of the concept of the fetus as a patient. Independent moral status for the fetus means that one or more characteristics that the fetus possesses in and of itself and, therefore, independently of the pregnant woman or any other factor, generate and therefore ground obligations to the fetus on the part of the pregnant woman and her physician.

A striking variety of characteristics have been nominated for this role, e.g., moment of conception, implantation, central nervous system development, quickening, and the moment of birth.[42–44] It should come as no surprise that, given the variability of proposed characteristics, there is considerable variation among ethical arguments about when the fetus acquires independent moral status. Some take the view that the fetus has independent moral status from the moment of conception or implantation.[45–47] Others believe that independent moral status is acquired in degrees, thus resulting in "graded" moral status.[6,38,40] Still others hold, at least by implication, that the fetus never has independent moral status so long as it is *in utero.*[39]

Despite an ever-expanding theological and philosophical literature on this subject, there has been no closure on a single authoritative account of the independent moral status of the fetus.[48,49] This is an unsurprising outcome because, given the absence of a single method that would be authoritative for all of the markedly diverse theological and philosophical schools of thought involved in this endless debate, closure is impossible. For closure ever to be possible, debates about such a final authority within and between theological and philosophical traditions would have to be resolved in a way satisfactory to all, an inconceivable intellectual and cultural event. We therefore propose to abandon these futile attempts to understand the fetus as a patient in terms of independent moral status of the fetus and turn to an alternative approach that makes it possible to identify ethically distinct senses of the fetus as a patient and their clinical implications for directive and nondirective counseling.[5] In its first sense, that of the independent moral status of the fetus, the fetus as a patient has no stable or clinically applicable meaning. We therefore consider a second sense of the concept of the fetus as a patient.

The Dependent Moral Status of the Fetus

Our analysis of this second sense of the concept of the fetus as a patient begins with the recognition that being a patient does not require that one possess independent moral status.[41] Rather, being a patient means that one can benefit from the applications of the clinical skills of the physician. Put more precisely, a human being without independent moral status is properly regarded as a patient when two conditions are met: that a human being (1) is presented to the physician, and (2) there exist clinical interventions that are reliably expected to be efficacious, in that they are reliably expected to result in a greater balance of goods over harms for the human being in question.[50] This is the second sense of the concept of the fetus as a patient, what we call the dependent moral status of the fetus.

The authors have argued elsewhere that beneficence-based obligations to the fetus exist when the fetus is reliably expected *later* to achieve independent moral status (sometime during the second year postpartum.[5] That is, the fetus is a patient when the fetus is presented for medical interventions, whether diagnostic or therapeutic, that reasonably can be expected to result in a greater balance of goods over harms for the child or person the fetus can *later* become during early childhood. The ethical significance of the concept of the fetus as a patient, therefore, depends on links that can be established between the fetus and its later achieving independent moral status.

The Viable Fetal Patient

One such link is viability. Viability is not, however, an intrinsic property of the fetus because viability must be understood in terms of both biological and technological factors.[49,51,52] It is only by virtue of both factors that a viable fetus can exist *ex utero* and thus achieve independent moral status. Moreover, these two factors do not exist as a function of the autonomy of the pregnant woman. When a fetus is viable, that is, when it is of sufficient maturity so that it can survive into the neonatal period and achieve independent moral status given the availability of the requisite technological support, and when it is presented to the physician, the fetus is a patient.

Viability exists as a function of biomedical and technological capacities, which are different in different parts of the world. As a consequence, there is, at the present time, no worldwide, uniform gestational age to define viability. In the United States, we believe, viability presently occurs at approximately 24 weeks of gestational age.[53,54]

When the fetus is a patient, directive counseling for fetal benefit is ethically justified. In clinical practice, directive counseling for fetal benefit involves one or more of the following: recommending against termination of pregnancy; recommending against nonaggressive management; or recommending aggressive management. Aggressive obstetric management includes interventions such as fetal surveillance, tocolysis, cesarean delivery, or delivery in a tertiary care center when indicated. Nonaggressive obstetric management excludes such interventions. Directive counseling for fetal benefit, however, must take account of the presence and severity of fetal anomalies, extreme prematurity, and obligations to the pregnant woman.

It is very important to appreciate in obstetric clinical judgment and practice that the strength of directive counseling for fetal benefit varies according to the presence and severity of anomalies. As a rule, the more severe the fetal anomaly, the less directive counseling should be for fetal benefit.[5,55,56] In particular, when there is "(1) a very high probability of a correct diagnosis and (2) either (a) a very high probability of death as an outcome of the anomaly diagnosed or (b) a very high probability of severe irreversible deficit of cognitive developmental capacity as a result of the anomaly diagnosed,"[57] counseling should be nondirective in recommending between aggressive and nonaggressive management. By contrast, when lethal anomalies can be diagnosed with certainty, there are no beneficence-based obligations to provide aggressive management.[15,55,58] Such fetuses are not patients; they are appropriately regarded as dying fetuses, and the counseling should be nondirective in recommending between nonaggressive management and termination of pregnancy but directive in recommending against aggressive management for the sake of maternal benefit.[55]

The strength of directive counseling for fetal benefit in cases of extreme prematurity of viable fetuses does not vary. In particular, this is the case for what we term just-viable fetuses,[5] those with a gestational age of 24 to 26 weeks, for which there are significant rates of survival but high rates of mortality and morbidity.[53,54] These rates of morbidity and mortality can be increased by nonaggressive obstetric management, whereas aggressive obstetric management may favorably influence outcome. Thus, it appears that there are sub-stantial beneficence-based obligations to just-viable fetuses to provide aggressive obstetric management. This is all the more the case in pregnancies beyond 26 weeks of gestational age.[53,54] Therefore, directive counseling for fetal benefit is justified in all cases of extreme prematurity of viable fetuses, considered by itself. Of course, such directive counseling is appropriate only when it is based on documented efficacy of aggressive obstetric management for each fetal indication. For example, such efficacy has not been demonstrated for routine cesarean delivery to manage extreme prematurity.[53]

Any directive counseling for fetal benefit must occur in the context of balancing beneficence-based obligations to the fetus against beneficence-based and autonomy-based obligations to the pregnant woman (Fig. 3).[5,59] Any such balancing must recognize that a pregnant woman is obligated only to take reasonable risks of medical interventions that are reliably expected to benefit the viable fetus or child later. A unique feature of obstetric ethics is that the pregnant woman's autonomy influences whether, in a particular case, the viable fetus ought to be regarded as presented to the physician.

Obviously, any strategy for directive counseling for fetal benefit that takes account of obligations to the pregnant woman must be open to the possibility of conflict between the physician's recommendation and a pregnant woman's autonomous decision to the contrary. Such conflict is best managed preventively through informed consent as an ongoing dialogue throughout the pregnancy, augmented as necessary by negotiation and respectful persuasion.[5,10]

The Previable Fetal Patient

The only possible link between the previable fetus and the child it can become is the pregnant woman's autonomy. This is because technological factors cannot result in the previable fetus becoming a child. The link, therefore, between a fetus and the child it can become when the fetus is previable can be established only by the pregnant woman's decision to confer the status of being a patient on her previable fetus. The previable fetus, therefore, has no claim to the status of being a patient independently of the pregnant woman's autonomy. The pregnant woman is free to withhold, confer, or, having once conferred, withdraw the status of being a patient on or from her previable fetus according to her own values and beliefs. The previable fetus is presented to the physician solely as a function of the pregnant woman's autonomy.

Counseling the pregnant woman regarding the management of her pregnancy when the fetus is previable should be nondirective in terms of continuing the pregnancy or having an abortion if she refuses to confer the status of being a patient on her fetus. If she does confer such status in a settled way, at that point beneficence-based obligations to her fetus come into existence, and directive counseling for fetal benefit becomes appropriate for these previable fetuses. Just as for viable fetuses, such counseling must take account of the presence and severity of fetal anomalies, extreme prematurity, and obligations owed to the pregnant woman.

For pregnancies in which the woman is uncertain about whether to confer such status, the authors propose that the fetus be *provisionally* regarded as a patient.[5] This justifies directive counseling against behavior that can harm a fetus in significant and irreversible ways, e.g., substance abuse, until the woman settles on whether to confer the status of being a patient on the fetus.

In particular, nondirective counseling is appropriate in cases of what we term near-viable fetuses,[5] that is, those that are 22 to 23 weeks of gestational age, for which there are anecdotal reports of survival.[5] In our view, aggressive obstetric and neonatal management should be regarded as clinical investigation (i.e., a form of medical experimentation), not a standard of care.[60] There is no obligation on the part of a pregnant woman to confer the status of being a patient on a near-viable fetus because the efficacy of aggressive obstetric and neonatal management has yet to be proven.

The *In Vitro* Embryo Patient

A subset of previable fetuses as patients concerns the *in vitro* embryo. It might seem that the *in vitro* embryo is a patient because such an embryo is presented to the physician. However, for beneficence-based obligations to a human being to exist, medical interventions must be reliably expected to be efficacious.

Recall that, in terms of beneficence, whether the fetus is a patient depends on links that can be established between the fetus and its eventual independent moral status. Therefore, the reasonableness of medical interventions on the *in vitro* embryo depends on whether that embryo later becomes viable. Otherwise, no benefit of such intervention can meaningfully be said to result. An *in vitro* embryo, therefore, becomes viable only when it survives *in vitro* cell division, transfer, implantation, and subsequent gestation to such a time that it becomes viable. The process of achieving viability occurs only *in vivo* and is therefore entirely dependent on the woman's decision regarding the status of the fetus(es) as a patient, should assisted conception successfully result in the gestation of the previable fetus(es). Whether an *in vitro* embryo will become a viable fetus, and whether medical intervention on such an embryo will benefit the fetus, are both functions of the pregnant woman's autonomous decision to withhold, confer, or, having once conferred, withdraw the moral status of being a patient on the previable fetus(es) that might result from assisted conception.

It therefore is appropriate to regard the *in vitro* embryo as a previable fetus rather than as a viable fetus. As a consequence, any *in vitro* embryo(s) should be regarded as a patient only when the woman into whose reproductive tract the embryo(s) will be transferred confers that status. Thus, counseling about how many *in vitro* embryos should be transferred and about preimplantation diagnosis should be nondirective.[5,61] As to the first, information should be presented about prognosis for a successful pregnancy and the possibility of confronting a decision about selective reduction, de-

pending on the number of embryos transferred. However, no definitive recommendation should be made about these matters, because directive counseling for fetal benefit is not appropriate until the woman confers the status of being a patient on the *in vitro* embryo. In short, the woman should have the final say about how many embryos are to be transferred. Preimplantation diagnostic counseling should be nondirective because the woman may elect not to implant abnormal embryos. These embryos are not patients, and so there is no basis for directive counseling.

When to Offer, Recommend, and Perform Cesarean Section

When to offer, recommend, and perform cesarean delivery is a common clinical ethical challenge in day-to-day obstetric practice, a challenge that will only increase with the growing influence of managed care. In this section we provide an ethically justified and clinically comprehensive algorithm for offering, recommending, and performing cesarean delivery, with particular reference to managed care, based on the ethical principles of beneficence and respect for autonomy and the concept of a fiduciary (Fig. 4).

Our algorithm begins by asking, "Is cesarean delivery substantively supported and vaginal delivery not supported in beneficence-based clinical judgment?" For example, when there is a previous classical incision on the uterus, cesarean is clearly preferable to vaginal delivery because cesarean prevents the fetal and maternal risk of a ruptured classical incision in the uterus in up to 12% of cases.[62] Vaginal delivery in these circumstances would result in a substantial increase in maternal–fetal morbidity and mortality. Because vaginal delivery involves unnecessary and preventable harms that are both quantitatively and qualitatively important, and cesarean prevents these harms, no well-founded beneficence-based clinical judgment could support offering vaginal delivery to women with a previous classical uterine incision. Only cesarean delivery should be offered and recommended to such patients. With the patient's consent, it should then be performed.

In some clinical circumstances, such as frank breech presentation, there is scientific controversy as to whether cesarean delivery is the better alternative. Competing well-founded beneficence-based clinical judgments regarding how to balance the fetal benefit of preventing harm against the maternal risk of cesarean delivery generate these controversies.[63] Whenever multiple management strategies are substantively supported in beneficence-based clinical judgment, all should be offered to the pregnant woman so that she can exercise her autonomy meaningfully. Such disclosure empowers the woman to emphasize her own perspective in balancing maternal and fetal risks. Not offering all management options substantively supported in beneficence-based clinical judgment is an unjustified form of paternalism. It is ethically appropriate to offer and perform either cesarean or vaginal delivery. A physician who is unable to perform vagi-

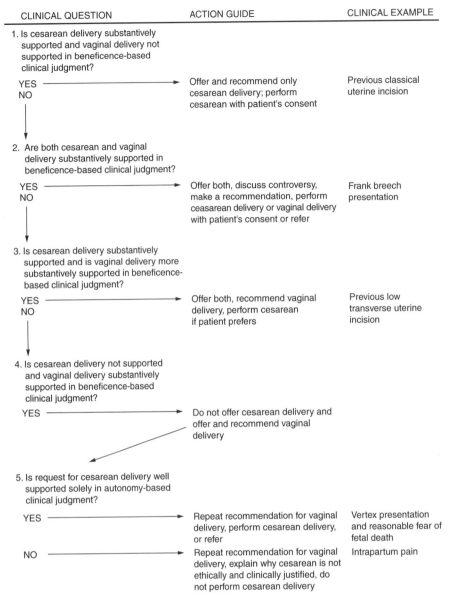

CLINICAL QUESTION	ACTION GUIDE	CLINICAL EXAMPLE

1. Is cesarean delivery substantively supported and vaginal delivery not supported in beneficence-based clinical judgment?

YES → Offer and recommend only cesarean delivery; perform cesarean with patient's consent — Previous classical uterine incision

NO ↓

2. Are both cesarean and vaginal delivery substantively supported in beneficence-based clinical judgment?

YES → Offer both, discuss controversy, make a recommendation, perform ceasarean delivery or vaginal delivery with patient's consent or refer — Frank breech presentation

NO ↓

3. Is cesarean delivery substantively supported and is vaginal delivery more substantively supported in beneficence-based clinical judgment?

YES → Offer both, recommend vaginal delivery, perform cesarean if patient prefers — Previous low transverse uterine incision

NO ↓

4. Is cesarean delivery not supported and vaginal delivery substantively supported in beneficence-based clinical judgment?

YES → Do not offer cesarean delivery and offer and recommend vaginal delivery

5. Is request for cesarean delivery well supported solely in autonomy-based clinical judgment?

YES → Repeat recommendation for vaginal delivery, perform cesarean delivery, or refer — Vertex presentation and reasonable fear of fetal death

NO → Repeat recommendation for vaginal delivery, explain why cesarean is not ethically and clinically justified, do not perform cesarean delivery — Intrapartum pain

FIG. 4. An ethically justified, clinically comprehensive algorithm for offering, recommending, and performing cesarean delivery. (From ref. 68.)

nal delivery for breech presentation is required to offer to refer the patient to a colleague who will be able to carry out the patient's preference.

In clinical circumstances when cesarean delivery is substantively supported in beneficence-based clinical judgment but vaginal delivery is more substantively supported, vaginal delivery is the better alternative, but not the only one. It is widely accepted that vaginal delivery after a previous low transverse cesarean involves low risk of harm to both the mother and fetus and prevention of the higher risk of harm of elective repeat cesarean to the mother. Nevertheless, uterine rupture occurs in fewer than 1% of women during labor,[62] a nontrivial qualitative risk. Thus, although cesarean is substantively supported in beneficence-based clinical judgment,

trial of labor is more substantively supported. To avoid unjustified paternalism, both cesarean and vaginal delivery should be offered. Because trial of vaginal delivery is the better option, it should be recommended. Because cesarean is also substantively supported in beneficence-based clinical judgment, it is justified to perform a cesarean if that is the patient's preference.

All remaining cases (i.e., most obstetric practice) should not be offered cesarean delivery when beneficence-based clinical judgment concludes that vaginal delivery is the only reasonable alternative. Cesarean delivery involves a quantitative increase of risks of unnecessary and preventable maternal morbidity and mortality, risks that are avoided by vaginal delivery. The qualitative nature of the unnecessary and preventable risks of cesarean delivery loom large in this beneficence-based calculus. As a consequence, it is not ethically justified to offer cesarean delivery, and only vaginal delivery should be offered and recommended.

In rare cases, patients request cesarean delivery not indicated on beneficence-based grounds, raising the challenging concept that autonomy-based indications in limited and rare circumstances can be well supported.[15] For example, one of us (F.A.C.) approved a cesarean delivery for a patient who expressed a legitimate fear of spontaneous fetal death and for whom there were no maternal contraindications for cesarean. She understood and accepted the maternal morbidity and mortality associated with cesarean delivery. An effort was made to dissuade the patient, but she considered and rejected it. A patient's preference that is based on deeply held values that are reaffirmed after a serious attempt to change her decision meet the test for being well supported in autonomy-based clinical judgment.

We can now answer a question that Feldman and Freiman[64] asked 10 years ago: "If an informed patient opts for prophylactic cesarean section at term, can it be denied?" If such a request is well supported in autonomy-based clinical judgment, which will be rare, it should be carried out by the physician, or an appropriate referral should be made. Feldman and Freiman also suggested that patients should be informed of the "very real risks associated with the passive anticipation of vaginal delivery after fetal maturity has been reached."[64] However, we conclude that this obligation does not exist because an affirmative answer makes the incorrect assumption that cesarean delivery is supported in beneficence-based clinical judgment.

Well-supported requests for cesarean delivery contrast with those that are not well supported in autonomy-based clinical judgment (i.e., when the goals expressed in the patient's preference for cesarean can be achieved without delivering by cesarean). For example, a woman who is in pain during labor may request cesarean delivery for relief of the pain. However, this goal can be achieved by administration of analgesia, whereas cesarean delivery for pain relief will result in more pain and unnecessary risk of morbidity and mortality. The preference is internally inconsistent and therefore not well supported in autonomy-based clinical judgment.

On the basis of our algorithm, there are four ethical indications for cesarean delivery: (1) when it is the only reasonable alternative in beneficence-based clinical judgment; (2) when it is the more substantively supported beneficence-based clinical judgment; (3) when it is substantively supported and the patient prefers it; and (4) when it is well supported in autonomy-based clinical judgment, a purely autonomy-based indication.

This algorithm underscores the importance of the professional integrity of the physician's role in the informed-consent process. In some clinical situations, such as a previous low transverse uterine incision, there are advantages of elective repeat cesarean delivery for the physician, including time saved, convenience, and possibly increased remuneration. It is a clear and unacceptable violation of the professional integrity of the physician's role in the informed consent process for the physician to distort this process in pursuit of such advantages.[5,65]

One business strategy of managed care models is to impose shared economic risk on the physician and sometimes on the patient, with a view toward influencing both to use resources with economic efficiency.[66] Strategies such as capitation for covered lives will put the economic interests of obstetricians and other physicians at risk every time they use a costly surgical intervention such as cesarean delivery. On the basis of our algorithm, the response of the physician always should be to offer a cesarean delivery when it is substantively supported in beneficence-based clinical judgment (i.e., when question 1, 2, or 3 in our algorithm of Fig. 4 is answered in the affirmative). "Gag" rules, in contrast, are inconsistent with good ethical practice.

We believe the doctor and the patient should be insulated from shared economic risk when the first clinical question is answered in the affirmative because vaginal delivery would fall below standard of care, and managed care providers, like physicians, are fiduciaries of patients.[5] As such, physicians are ethically obligated not to practice below standard of care, which is established by beneficence-based clinical judgment. Physicians who recommend cesarean delivery in response to clinical question 2 should negotiate payment plans that insulate them from risk when no one else is available to deliver breech-presenting infants vaginally. This is because economic attempts to resolve genuine clinical controversies in any specialty are scientifically arbitrary and therefore inconsistent with the integrity of medicine as a profession.

Payment for cesarean delivery in response to question 3 is ethically complex. Managed care organizations want the lowest possible rate of cesareans, yet an ethically more important consideration is that physicians have fiduciary obligations to be advocates for their patients.[66] For example, some women are justifiably averse to a trial of vaginal delivery after low transverse cesarean delivery and cannot be persuaded to change their decision.[67] Such factors justifiably influence the definition of the lowest acceptable rate of cesarean delivery. The imposition of shared economic risk is an ethically acceptable strategy only when physicians take the leading role in defining acceptable rates of use or an acceptable cesarean delivery rate for this clinical circumstance. To do otherwise violates the integrity of medicine as a profession.

For cesarean delivery and other procedures that are performed in the clinical circumstances of question 5 (Fig. 4), physicians should negotiate payment arrangements that require the patient to bear all the economic risk because the indication for the procedure is solely autonomy based. Managed care plans and other payers have an ethical obligation as fiduciaries, or under a principle of justice, to provide care that is consistent with well-formed beneficence-based clinical judgment. Claims on resources that are based solely on autonomy and not on beneficence are, in principle, limited. It follows that patients have, at best, disputable justice-based claims on such resources when the indication for their use is purely autonomy-based. In general, when the only justification for a procedure or other use of resources is autonomy-based, physicians are justified in negotiating payment arrangements that shift some degree of economic risk to the patient.

Shared economic risk should have no effect on offering and recommending procedures that are substantively supported in beneficence-based clinical judgment. This aspect of the informed consent process should be kept immune from shared economic risk by managed care companies. The physician's role as the fiduciary of the patient in advocating ethically defensible degrees of shared economic risk cannot be overemphasized. In our view, the degree of shared economic risk should be nonexistent for clinical questions 1 through 4 and imposed entirely on patients who want cesarean delivery for question 5 (Fig. 4).[68]

◊ MANAGED CARE AND THE VIRTUES OF THE OBSTETRICIAN-GYNECOLOGIST

In the previous sections we have made reference to managed care. In this section we provide a more detailed analysis of the ethics of managed care, with particular reference to the virtues of the obstetrician-gynecologist. The practice of obstetrics and gynecology is coming under managed care, which involves a set of strategies used by both private and public payers to control the cost of medical care. Two main business tools are used to achieve this goal: (1) creating conflicts of interests in how physicians are paid, diplomatically called "sharing economic risk"; and (2) strict control of clinical judgment and practice through such means as practice guidelines, critical pathways, physician report cards, and retrospective chart review. These business tools generate ethical challenges to obstetrician-gynecologists that seriously threaten the virtues that define the fiduciary character of medicine as a profession.[69]

In medicine, the physician-fiduciary, as a primary consideration, is expected as a matter of routine and habit to fulfill obligations to protect and promote patients' interests rather than pursue his or her own interests. Virtues are those traits and habits of character that routinely focus the concern and behavior of an individual on the interests of others and thereby habitually blunt the motivation to act on self-interest as the physician's primary consideration. We believe that four virtues constitute the physician–patient relationship based on the physician as fiduciary.

The first virtue is *self-effacement.* This requires the physician not to act on the basis of potential differences between the patient and the physician such as race, religion, national origin, education, gender, manners, socioeconomic status, hygiene, or proficiency in speaking English. Self-effacement prevents biases and prejudices arising from these differences that could adversely impact on the plan of care for the patient.

The second virtue is *self-sacrifice.* This requires physicians to accept reasonable risks to themselves. As one example, physicians manifest this virtue in their willingness to care for patients with infectious diseases such as tuberculosis, hepatitis, and HIV infection, all of which are a potential threat to the physician's health. In both fee-for-service and managed care, this virtue of self-sacrifice obligates the physician to turn away from economic self-interest and focus on the patient's need for relief when the two are in conflict.

The third virtue, *compassion,* motivates the physician to recognize and seek to alleviate the stress, discomfort, pain, and suffering associated with the patient's disease and illness. Self-effacement, self-sacrifice, and compassion provide the basis for a powerful ethical response to the business tool of conflicts of interest by the physician.

This response is strengthened by the fourth virtue, *integrity.* This virtue imposes an intellectual discipline on the physician's clinical judgments about the patient's problems and how to address them. Integrity prescribes rigor in the formation of clinical judgment. Clinical judgment is rigorous when it is based on the best available scientific information or, when such information is lacking, consensus clinical judgment and on careful thought processes of an individual physician that can withstand peer review. In settings that lack such quality control mechanisms, physicians confront a powerful incentive to make the pursuit of remuneration via fee-for-service the primary consideration. Integrity is thus an antidote to the pitfalls of bias, subjective clinical impressions, and unexamined clinical "common sense." Integrity provides the basis for the physician's ethical response to the business tool of control of clinical judgment and practice.

None of these four virtues is absolute in its ethical demands. The task of medical ethics is to identify both the application and the limits of these four virtues. The concept of legitimate self-interest provides the basis for these limits.[5] Legitimate self-interest includes protecting the conditions for practicing medicine well, fulfilling obligations to persons in the physician's life other than the patient, and protecting activities outside the practice of medicine that the physician finds deeply fulfilling.

Managed Care and the Physician as Fiduciary

Fee for service unconstrained by fiduciary obligations could and did lead to harm to patients from nonindicated overutilization of resources. It is a violation of the standard of care to subject patients to unnecessary active intervention in order to achieve personal economic gain.

Managed care unconstrained by fiduciary obligations puts patients at risk of harm by denying access to the standard of care. This will occur if patients are subjected to unnecessary risk from withholding appropriate care and intervention in order to achieve economic efficiency.[70] A primary goal of managed care is to achieve this economic efficiency through price competitiveness in order to retain and grow market share.

Financial incentives to the physician and supervision of clinician decision making with strict controls of utilization of services are the business tools managed care uses. Forms of payment by managed care plans, such as capitation and with-hold, deliberately impose an economic conflict of interest on the physician. Every time the physician uses a resource, e.g., consultation, diagnostic testing, or surgical procedures, the physician pays an economic penalty. The ethical challenge occurs when the patient's interests are subordinated to the pursuit of financial rewards and thereby harmed by this underutilization. This conflict of interest becomes actual when a physician signs such a payment contract.

The physician's decision in signing contracts is subject to considerations of legitimate self-interest. For example, failure to sign a contract with a plan that has captured 20% of one's present patients will result in a very significant loss of income that the physician may not be able to replace through other contracts. Because there is usually an excess of physician supply in large markets, physicians as suppliers who fail to sign contracts in a buyer's market do so at their economic peril. Therefore, rational calculation of one's legitimate concern to protect income from very significant reduction may strongly incline a physician to sign virtually every contract presented as a matter of prudent protection of legitimate self-interest.

However, the virtue of self-sacrifice prohibits the physician from making the avoidance of such financial risk the *primary* consideration. Avoiding financial risk as one's *primary* consideration involves an ethically pathologic process that leads naturally and quickly to the abandonment of self-effacement (economically driven managed care for some patients but not for others), compassion (patients' health-related concerns do not matter but are only a means to maximize revenues), and integrity (the standard of care is sacrificed to maximize revenues). Importantly, physicians are not sanctioned by society to engage in the destruction of medicine as a fiduciary profession.

Adhering to the demands of the virtues provides the antidote to this unacceptable sequence of ethical failure. Physicians should negotiate changes in payment contracts to make economic conflicts of interest as manageable as possible. It is not realistic to call for elimination of conflict of interest, as some have done.[71] It is important to recall that fee-for-service involves conflicts of interest that also cannot be eliminated.

Physicians should not assume that managed care organizations (MCOs) are unwilling to negotiate contracts to reduce the severity of economic conflicts of interest. Physicians should therefore make a good faith effort to negotiate these matters. If the MCO refuses to negotiate and the economic risk of not signing the contract is very significant, then the physician should voluntarily accept the ethical responsibility to be alert to and manage these conflicts of interest well. First, integrity requires that the physician avoid the self-deception of underestimating any potential influence on clinical judgment and practice by the conflict of interest. Second, once these contracts are signed, the virtues add an important di-

mension to total quality management: diligent monitoring of conflicts of interest to prevent them from resulting in substandard care should be among the physician's "accountabilities." Third, the realities of managed care mean that, for the near term at least, increasing financial sacrifice may be required to protect the integrity of medicine as a fiduciary profession. Fourth, in group practice, there should be a fair sharing of economic self-sacrifice. In particular, individual efforts to tune the system to one's economic advantage in a group, for example, avoiding the care of high-risk pregnancies, and to the disadvantage of colleagues should be avoided.

The second business tool of managed care, strict control of clinical judgment and practice, is a heterogeneous phenomenon. Some managed care plans are poorly capitalized and poorly managed. They compete by price, with little or no attention given to the quality of their services. A "bottom line" mentality dominates, with economic savings and net revenue maximization the overriding values. These poorly managed companies have little or no understanding of or interest in the fiduciary nature of medicine, and so their controls of clinical judgment and practice are driven almost entirely by economic considerations.

Physicians subject to management controls by such companies face the very difficult challenge of trying to get such companies to constrain their economic interests by their fiduciary obligations, a daunting task[72] but not, we believe, an impossible task. The concerns of ethics, especially to protect the integrity of the fiduciary enterprise, may frequently be swept aside when they are not ignored altogether. Nonetheless, physicians in such managed care organizations are the ultimate bulwark on which patients and society must be able to rely at the present time to protect patients from management's unbridled pursuit of economic self-interest. Physicians, therefore, should strenuously resist and seek to change management controls driven solely by economic considerations. If physicians refused to cooperate with such poorly managed companies, systematic dissociation would result in a loss of market share or, more optimistically, better management.

Antitrust legislation needs to be changed to permit group responses to this kind of managed care organization. We realize that this may not be a politically realistic proposal at the present time. Antitrust legislation may presently legally prevent physicians from banding together to deal with this problem. Thus, regulatory relief through state and federal governments becomes an ethically justified strategy to stop the abuse of these plans.

There is a contrast that provides a cause for optimism. Well-managed and well-capitalized plans can be as much concerned with quality as with economic efficiency. The trend of some large, Fortune 500 employers to require National Committee on Quality Assurance certification[73] will reinforce the importance of quality. The virtues, as we have shown above, have an important role to play in the definition of quality. The concept of quality should be expanded beyond the usual measures of morbidity, mortality, and customer satisfaction to include monitoring for and managing threats to the fiduciary character of medicine.

One approach to doing so concerns the development and use of practice guidelines. It appears that well-managed plans will rely increasingly on this as their primary business tool rather than the strategy of creating conflicts of interest with its disruptive and demoralizing effects. Nonetheless, practice guidelines pose a number of ethical concerns.

First, guidelines have the potential to impede economic efficiency, an important value of all managed care organizations. Economically inefficient plans are threatened with significant loss of market share or even extinction through local market competition by managed care organizations competing solely by price.

Second, every step of a guideline absorbs monetary resources that would otherwise be available for, among other purposes, physician remuneration, or return to investors in the case of for-profit plans. An interest in job security and maximizing income could therefore subtly enter into physicians' judgments about the value of deleting, adding, or altering diagnostic and therapeutic steps to a guideline. As a consequence, uncertainty about whether a particular step of a guideline adds clinical value may lead to the elimination of that step if doing so increases economic efficiency. This subtle form of conflict of interest should be monitored closely so that the virtues of integrity and self-sacrifice are not unduly threatened.

Third, curtailment of steps in a guideline also might result in physicians concentrating only on the clinical care for which they have direct and immediate answers. The failure to pursue unanswered questions may result in less complete care and failure to develop new clinical competencies, a long-term negative effect on the standard of care.

The integrity of medicine as a fiduciary enterprise justifies, indeed requires, practice guidelines that acknowledge the heterogeneity of patients' conditions and the natural history of diseases and their management, to avoid inadvertent and preventable harm to patients' interests. In defense of such guidelines, which must be as scientifically rigorous as possible—integrity requires this, too, physicians will be obligated by the virtue of integrity to take the unpopular and at times antibusiness position of defending economic inefficiency as the necessary price of protecting medicine as a fiduciary profession. Failure to do so amounts to willful failure of the physician's fiduciary responsibilities.

Legislative proposals currently being considered in Congress will permit provider groups to start managed care organizations without the levels of capitalization required of insurance companies. The goal of this proposed legislation is for physicians to recapture control of capital and revenue and thus retake control of patient care. Inevitably, these new entities, in order to survive and grow, will have to use the business tools of conflict of interest and control of clinical judgment and practice. Being physician-controlled provides no immunization against the ethical challenges of the business tools of managed care. These new physician-owned provider entities will not provide a solution in and of themselves to the

ethical threats of conflict of interest and control of clinical judgment and practice. The virtue-based arguments we made will apply to these new entities without exception.

There is no conclusive evidence that preserving medicine as a fiduciary profession is impossible, even given the enormous economic power of managed care organizations. Ethics teaches us that business and economic power are not absolute and should always be called to account for their consequences. Society has not given MCOs the moral authority or permission to destroy the fiduciary character of medicine as a consequence of the pursuit of economic interest and power. Nor has society given physicians moral authority or permission to cooperate willfully with this destruction. Quite the opposite, society counts on physicians because ultimately society can count on no one else to preserve and advocate for the fiduciary character of the medical profession.

◇ CONCLUSION

In this chapter we have provided a general ethical framework for both gynecologic and obstetric clinical judgment and practice. Implementing this framework on a daily basis is essential to creating and sustaining the physician–patient relationship in obstetrics and gynecology. This framework emphasizes preventive ethics, i.e., an appreciation that the potential for ethical conflict is built into clinical practice and the use of such clinical tools as informed consent and negotiation to prevent such conflict from occurring. We have provided guidelines for preventing conflict about futile management in gynecologic practice and about cesarean delivery in obstetric practice. We have also shown how the virtues provide a basis for a powerful and effective preventive ethics response to the business tools of managed practice.

◇ REFERENCES

1. Cain J, Stacy L, Jusenius K, Figge D. The quality of dying: Financial, psychological, and ethical dilemmas. *Obstet Gynecol* 1990;76:149–152.
2. Park RC. Old bedfellows: Ethics and obstetrics and gynecology. *Obstet Gynecol* 1989;73:1–3.
3. Jennings JC. Ethics in obstetrics and gynecology: A practitioner's review and opinion. *Obstet Gynecol Surv* 1989;44:656–661.
4. Skrzydelwski WB. Gynaecology and ethics. *Eur J Obstet Gynaecol Reprod Biol* 1990;36:274–282.
5. McCullough LB, Chervenak FA. *Ethics in obstetrics and gynecology*. New York: Oxford University Press, 1994.
6. Strong C. *Ethics in reproductive medicine: A new framework*. New Haven: Yale University Press, 1997.
7. Veath R. *A theory of medical ethics*. New York: Basic Books, 1981.
8. Beauchamp TL, Childress JF. *Principles of biomedical ethics, 4th ed.* New York: Oxford University Press, 1994.
9. Annas GJ. Protecting the liberty of pregnant patient. *N Engl J Med* 1988;316:1213–1214.
10. Chervenak FA, McCullough LB. Clinical guides to preventing ethical conflicts between pregnant women and their physicians. *Am J Obstet Gynecol* 1990;162:303–307.
11. Engelhardt HT Jr. *The foundations of bioethics, 2nd ed.* New York: Oxford University Press, 1996.
12. Beauchamp TL, McCullough LB. *Medical ethics: The moral responsibilities of physicians.* Englewood Cliffs, NJ: Prentice-Hall, 1984.
13. Louis Harris and Associates. Views on informed consent and decision making: Parallel surveys of physicians and the public. In: *President's*

Commission for the Study of Ethical Problems in Medicine and Biomedical and Behavior Research, Making health care decisions, vol 2, Appendices: Empirical studies of informed consent. Washington, DC: US Government Printing Office, 1982.

14. Faden RR, Beauchamp TL. A history and theory of informed consent. New York: Oxford University Press, 1986.

15. Brett A, McCullough LB. When patients request specific interventions: Refining the limits of the physician's obligations. N Engl J Med 1986;315:1347–1351.

16. Truman v Thomas. 27 Cal. 3d 285, 165 Cal. rptr, 308,611 p. 2d 902.

17. Rabenech L, McCullough LB, Wray NP. Ethically justified, clinically comprehensive guidelines for percutaneous endoscopic gastrotomy tube placement. Lancet 1997;349:496–498.

18. Brody BA, Halevy A. A multi-institutional collaborative policy in medical fertility. JAMA 1996;276:571–574.

19. Chervenak FA, McCullough LB. Identifying and managing ethical conflict in the gynecolgist–patient relationship. J Reprod Med 1993;38:553–557.

20. American College of Obstetricians and Gynecologists, Committee on Ethics. Patient choice: Maternal–fetal conflict. Washington, DC: American College of Obstetricians and Gynecologists, 1987.

21. American College of Obstetricians and Gynecologists. Technical bulletin. Ethical decision-making in obstetrics and gynecology. Washington, DC: American College of Obstetricians and Gynecologists, 1989.

22. Harrison MR, Golbus MS, Filly RA. The unborn patient. New York: Grune & Stratton, 1984.

23. Liley AW. The foetus as a personality. Aust NZ J Psychiatry 1972;6:99–105.

24. Fletcher JC. The fetus as patient; ethical issues. JAMA 1981;246:772–773.

25. Mahoney MJ. Fetal–maternal relationship. In: Reich WT, ed. Encyclopedia of bioethics. New York: Macmillan. 1978:485–489.

26. Mahoney MJ. The fetus as patient. West J Med 1989;150:517–540.

27. Murray TH. Moral obligations to the not-yet born: The fetus as patient. Clin Perinatol 1987;14:313–328.

28. Newton ER. The fetus as patient. Med Clin North Am 1989;73:517–540.

29. Pritchard JA, MacDonald PC, Gant NF. Williams obstetrics, 17th ed. Norwalk, CT: Appleton-Century-Crofts, 1985:xi.

30. Shinn RL. The fetus as patient: A philosophical and ethical perspective. In: Milunsky A, Annas GJ, eds. Genetics and the law III. New York: Plenum Press, 1985:317–324.

31. Walters L. Ethical issues in intrauterine diagnosis and therapy. Fetal Ther 1986;1:32–37.

32. Anderson G, Strong C. The premature breech: Cesarean section or trial of labor? J Med Ethics 1988;14:18–24.

33. Engelhardt HT, Jr. The foundations of bioethics. New York: Oxford University Press, 1986.

34. Fleming L. The moral status of the fetus: A reappraisal. Bioethics 1987;1:15–34.

35. Ford NM. When did I begin? Conception of the human individual in history, philosophy and science. Cambridge: Cambridge University Press, 1988.

36. Strong C. Ethical conflicts between mother and fetus in obstetrics. Clin Perinatol 1987;14:313–328.

37. Strong C, Anderson G. The moral status of the near-term fetus. J Med Ethics 1989;15:25–27.

38. Dunstan GR. The moral status of the human embryo. A tradition recalled. J Med Ethics 1984;10:38–44.

39. Elias S, Annas GJ. Reproductive genetics and the law. Chicago: Year Book Medical Publishers, 1987.

40. Evans MI, Fletcher JC, Zador IE, et al. Selective first-trimester termination in octuplet and quadruplet pregnancies: Clinical and ethical issues. Obstet Gynecol 1988;71:289–296.

41. Ruddick W, Wilcox W. Operating on the fetus. Hastings Cent Rep 1982;12:10–14.

42. Macklin R. Abortion: Contemporary ethical and legal aspects. In Reich WT, ed. Encyclopedia of bioethics, 2nd ed. New York: Macmillan, 1995:6–16.

43. Hellegers AE. Fetal development. Theol Stud 1970;31:3–9.

44. Noonan JT, ed. The morality of abortion. Cambridge: Harvard University Press, 1970.

45. Bopp J, ed. Restoring the right to life: The human life amendment. Provo, UT: Brigham Young University, 1984.

46. Bopp J, ed. Human life and health care ethics. Frederick, MD: University Publications of America, 1985.

47. Noonan JT. A private choice. Abortion in America in the seventies. New York: The Free Press, 1979.

48. Callahan S, Callahan D, eds. Abortion: Understanding differences. New York: Plenum Press, 1984.

49. Roe v Wade, 410 US 113 (1973).

50. Chervenak FA, McCullough LB. What is obstetric ethics? J Perinat Med 1996;23:331–341.

51. Fost N, Chudwin D, Wikker D. The limited moral significance of fetal viability. Hastings Cent Rep 1980;10:10–13.

52. Mahowald M. Beyond abortion: Refusal of cesarean section. Bioethics 1989;3:106–121.

53. Hack M, Fanaroff AA. Outcomes of extremely-low-birth-weight infants between 1982 and 1988. N Engl J Med 1989;321:1642–1647.

54. Whyte HE, Fitzhardinge PM, Shennan AT, Lennox K, Smith L, Lacy J. External immaturity: outline of 568 pregnancies of 23–26 weeks' gestation. Obstet Gynecol 1993;82:1–7.

55. Chervenak FA, McCullough LB. An ethically justified, clinically comprehensive management strategy for third-trimester pregnancies complicated by fetal anomalies. Obstet Gynecol 1990;75: 311–316.

56. Chervenak FA, McCullough LB. Does obstetric ethics have any role in the obstetrician's response to the abortion controversy? Am J Obstet Gynecol 1990;163:1425–1429.

57. Chervenak FA, McCullough LB. Nonaggressive obstetric management: An option for some fetal anomalies during the third trimester. JAMA 1989;261:3439–3430.

58. Chervenak FA, Farley MA, Walters L, et al. When is termination of pregnancy during the third trimester morally justifiable? N Engl J Med 1984;310:501–504.

59. Chervenak FA, McCullough LB. Perinatal ethics: A practical method of analysis of obligations to mother and fetus. Obstet Gynecol 1985;66:442–446.

60. Chervenak FA, McCullough LB. The limits of viability. J Perinat Med. 1997;25:418–420.

61. Grifo JA, Boyle A, Tang XY, Ward DC. Preimplantation genetic diagnosis. Arch Pathol Lab Med 1992;116:393–397.

62. American College of Obstetricians and Gynecologists, Committee on Obstetric Practice. Vaginal delivery after a previous cesarean birth. ACOG committee opinion no. 143. Washington, DC: American College of Obstetricians and Gynecologists, 1994.

63. American College of Obstetricians and Gynecologists. Management of the breech presentation. ACOG technical bulletin no. 95. Washington, DC: American College of Obstetricians and Gynecologists, 1986.

64. Feldman GB, Freiman JA. Prophylactic cesarean section at term? N Engl J Med 1985;312:1264–1267.

65. Rodwin MA. Conflicts in managed care. N Engl J Med 1995;322:604–607.

66. American Medical Association Council on Ethical and Judicial Affairs. Ethical issues in managed care. JAMA 1995;273:330–335.

67. Abitbol MM, Castillo I, Taylor UB, Rochelson BL, Shmoys S, Monheit AG. Vaginal birth after cesarean section: the patient's point of view. Am Fam Physician 1993;47:129–134.

68. Chervenak FA, McCullough LB. An ethically justified algorithm for offering, recommending, and performing cesarean delivery and its application in managed care practice. Obstet Gynecol 1996;87: 302–305.

69. Chervenak FA, McCullough LB. Responding to the ethical challenges posed by the business tools of managed care in the practice of obstetrics and gynecology. Am J Obstet Gynecol 1996;175:524–527.

70. Council on Ethical and Judicial Affairs of the American Medical Association. Ethical issues in managed care. JAMA 1995;273:330–335.

71. Emanuel EJ, Dobler NN. Preserving the physician–patient relationship in the era of managed care. JAMA 1995;273:323–329.

72. Woodhandler S, Himmelstein DS. Extreme risk—the new corporate proposition for physicians. N Engl J Med 1996;333:1706–1708.

73. National Committee for Quality Assurance. Standards for the accreditation of managed care organizations. Washington, DC: National Committee for Quality Assurance, 1995.

Subject Index

Page numbers followed by f *refer to figures; page numbers followed by* t *refer to tables.*